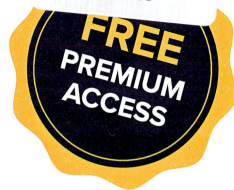
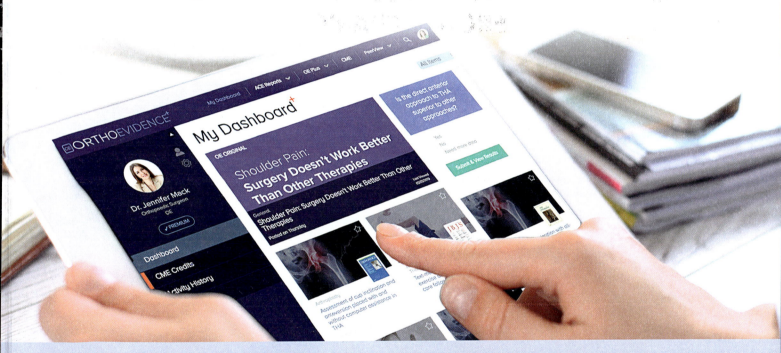

VuMedi Partnership

ELSEVIER

The Editors and Publisher have partnered with VuMedi, the Healthcare Video Education Network, to provide direct links to sections of videos that complement the content in this book.

VuMedi aims to help clinicians make optimal patient care decisions through comprehensive video education from a variety of trustworthy institutions and practitioners. Through VuMedi, clinicians can gain access to information on thousands of topics covering new advances, alternative approaches, challenging treatments, diagnostics, rare pathologies, complications, and more.

To view the videos, you will need to register for VuMedi and log into your account.

Please note the Editors and Publisher did not create these videos. The Editors and Publisher do not own nor endorse these videos and are not responsible for the content on VuMedi.

To view this video content, please visit the links below:

Pediatrics
Pediatric Trauma - https://www.vumedi.com/term/pediatricpediatric-trauma

GREEN'S SKELETAL TRAUMA
IN CHILDREN

6th EDITION

GREEN'S SKELETAL TRAUMA IN CHILDREN

Gregory A. Mencio, MD
Neil E. Green Professor and Vice Chairman
Department of Orthopaedics
Vanderbilt University Medical Center
Chief, Pediatric Orthopaedics
Monroe Carell, Jr. Children's Hospital at Vanderbilt
Nashville, Tennessee

Steven L. Frick, MD
Professor and Vice Chairman
Orthopaedic Surgery
Stanford University School of Medicine,
Stanford, California
Chief, Pediatric Orthopaedics
Orthopaedic Surgery
Lucile Packard Children's Hospital Stanford,
Stanford, California

ELSEVIER

Elsevier
1600 John F. Kennedy Blvd.
Ste 1800
Philadelphia, PA 19103-2899

GREEN'S SKELETAL TRAUMA IN CHILDREN, SIXTH EDITION   ISBN: 978-0-323-61336-1
Copyright © 2020 by Elsevier, Inc. All rights reserved.

Notice

Previous editions copyrighted 2015, 2009, 2003, 1998, and 1992.

Library of Congress Control Number: 2019949250

Senior Content Strategist: Belinda Kuhn
Senior Content Development Specialist: Kathryn DeFrancesco
Publishing Services Manager: Shereen Jameel
Project Manager: Rukmani Krishnan
Design Direction: Ryan Cook

Printed in the United States of America

Last digit is the print number: 9 8 7 6 5 4 3 2 1

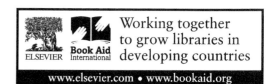

Madelyn Anne Mencio
Alyson Mencio Stevens
Marissa Mencio Lichliter

Lisa Kahn Frick
Eric Altman Frick
Rachel Ivy Frick

We dedicate this book to our teachers, colleagues,
and students.
We single out the memory of our departed colleagues,
Neil Green, MD, and Kathy Cramer, MD.
This book is created to improve the care of the injured
child; Neil and Kathy dedicated their lives
to this goal. Both are fondly remembered and deeply
missed.

Contributors

Alexandre Arkader, MD
Associate Professor of Orthopaedic Surgery
Perelman School of Medicine at University of Pediatrics
    Pediatric Orthopedic and Orthopedic Oncology Surgeon
Children's Hospital of Philadelphia (CHOP)
Philadelphia, Pennsylvania

Richard E. Bowen, MD
Clinical Professor
Orthopaedic Surgery
David Geffen School of Medicine at UCLA
Los Angeles, California
Orthopaedic Institute for Children
Los Angeles, California

Andrea C. Bracikowski, MD
Associate Professor
Orthopedics and Rehabilitation
Vanderbilt University School of Medicine
Nashville, Tennessee
Associate Professor
Pediatrics
Vanderbilt Children's Hospital
Nashville, Tennessee
Associate Professor
Emergency Medicine
Vanderbilt University School of Medicine
Nashville, Tennessee

Kevin M. Dale, MD
Assistant Professor of Orthopaedics and Rehabilitation
Department of Orthopaedic Surgery
Vanderbilt University School of Medicine
Nashville, Tennessee

Jaime R. Denning, MD, MS
Assistant Professor
Orthopaedic Surgery
Cincinnati Children's Hospital Medical Center
University of Cincinnati School of Medicine
Cincinnati, Ohio

Aleksei B. Dingel, BS
Research Coordinator
Department of Orthopaedic Surgery
Stanford University School of Medicine
Stanford, California

Eric W. Edmonds, MD, FAOA
Professor of Orthopedic Surgery
University of California San Diego
Director of Orthopedic Research and Sports Medicine
Division of Orthopedic Surgery
Rady Children's Hospital San Diego
San Diego, California

John B. Erickson, DO
Assistant Professor
Pediatric Orthopedic Surgery
Medical College of Wisconsin
Milwaukee, Wisconsin

Steven L. Frick, MD
Professor and Vice Chairman
Orthopaedic Surgery
Stanford University School of Medicine
Stanford, California
Chief, Pediatric Orthopaedics
Orthopaedic Surgery
Lucile Packard Children's Hospital Stanford
Stanford, California

Christopher Greeley, MD, MS
Professor
Pediatrics
Baylor College of Medicine
Houston, Texas
Chief
Section of Public Health Pediatrics
Texas Children's Hospital
Houston, Texas

Nathan L. Grimm, MD
Orthopaedic Surgery Pediatric & Adult
    Sports Medicine Fellow
UConn Health Center
Department of Orthopaedic Surgery
Farmington, Connecticut

Christina K. Hardesty, MD
Assistant Professor of Orthopaedic Surgery
Pediatric Orthopaedic Surgery
Rainbow Babies and Children's Hospitals at Case Western
    Reserve University
Cleveland, Ohio

Ginger E. Holt, MD
Professor and Vice Chair, Orthopaedic Surgery
Vanderbilt University Medical Center
Nashville, Tennessee

Elizabeth W. Hubbard, MD
Assistant Professor of Orthopaedic Surgery
Duke University School of Medicine
Durham, North Carolina

Megan E. Johnson, MD
Assistant Professor
Orthopaedics
Vanderbilt University Medical Center
Nashville, Tennessee

Sheila M. Jones, MD
Medical Director, Pediatric Emergency Department
Centennial Women's & Children's Hospital
Nashville, Tennessee
Adjunct Assistant Professor of Pediatrics
Vanderbilt Children's Hospital
Nashville, Tennessee

Kevin E. Klingele, MD
Chief
Orthopedic Surgery
Nationwide Children's Hospital
Columbus, Ohio

Scott H. Kozin, MD
Clinical Professor
Orthopedics Surgery
Lewis Katz School of Medicine
Temple University
Philadelphia, Pennsylvania
Clinical Professor
Orthopaedic Surgery
Sidney Kimmel Medical College
Thomas Jefferson University
Philadelphia, Pennsylvania
Chief of Staff
Shriners Hospital for Children
Philadelphia, Pennsylvania

Ying Li, MD
Associate Professor
Department of Orthopaedic Surgery
C.S. Mott Children's Hospital
Ann Arbor, Michigan

Kristin Livingston, MD
Assistant Professor of Orthopaedic Surgery
University of California, San Francisco
San Francisco, California

Raymond W. Liu, MD
Associate Professor and Victor M. Goldberg Endowed
    Chair in Orthopaedics
Pediatric Orthopaedic Surgery
Rainbow Babies and Children's Hospitals at Case Western
    Reserve University
Cleveland, Ohio

Steven Lovejoy, BS, MD
Assistant Professor
Pediatric Orthopedic Surgery
Vanderbilt Children's Hospital
Nashville, Tennessee

Jeffrey E. Martus, MD, MS
Associate Professor
Pediatric Orthopaedic Surgery
Vanderbilt University Medical Center
Nashville, Tennessee

Gregory A. Mencio, MD
Neil E. Green Professor and Vice Chairman
Department of Orthopaedics
Vanderbilt University Medical Center
Chief, Pediatric Orthopaedics
Monroe Carell, Jr. Children's Hospital at Vanderbilt
Nashville, Tennessee

Amirhossein Misaghi, MD
Orthopedic Surgeon
CHOC (Children's Hospital of Orange County)
Orange, California

James F. Mooney III, MD
Chief of Staff
Medical Affairs
Shriners Hospital for Children-Springfield
Springfield, Massachusetts

Robert F. Murphy, MD
Assistant Professor
Department of Orthopaedics
Medical University of South Carolina
Charleston, South Carolina

Unni G. Narayanan, MBBS, MSc, FRCS(C)
Professor
Department of Surgery & Rehabilitation Sciences
    Institute
University of Toronto
Divisions of Orthopaedic Surgery and Child Health
    Evaluative Sciences
The Hospital for Sick Children
Toronto, Ontario
Canada

James P. Norris IV, MD
Clinical Instructor
Orthopaedic Surgery
Vanderbilt University Medical Center
Nashville, Tennessee

Shital N. Parikh, MD
Professor
Orthopaedic Surgery
Cincinnati Children's Hospital Medical Center
University of Cincinnati School of Medicine
Cincinnati, Ohio

Anthony I. Riccio, MD
Associate Professor of Orthopaedic Surgery
University of Texas Southwestern Medical Center
Dallas, Texas

Sanjeev Sabharwal, MD, MPH
Professor
Orthopedics
University of California
San Francisco
Oakland, California

Walter Samora, MD
Assistant Professor
Orthopedic Surgery
Nationwide Children's Hospital
Columbus, Ohio

Brian Scannell, MD
Associate Professor
Department of Orthopaedic Surgery
Atrium Health
Charlotte, North Carolina
Physician
OrthoCarolina
Charlotte, North Carolina

Jonathan G. Schoenecker, MD, PhD
Associate Professor and Mast Chair of Pediatric Trauma
    and Hip Surgery
Vanderbilt University Medical Center
Monroe Carell, Jr. Children's Hospital at Vanderbilt
Nashville, Tennessee

Herbert S. Schwartz, MD
Professor and Chair Emeritus
Orthopaedic Surgery
Vanderbilt University Medical Center
Nashville, Tennessee

Kevin G. Shea, MD
Orthopedic Surgeon
Sports Medicine
Stanford University
Stanford, California
Professor
Orthopaedics
Stanford University
Stanford, California

Jeffrey Shilt, MD
Chief of Community Surgery
The Woodlands
Texas Children's Hospital
The Woodlands, Texas
Associate Professor
Department of Orthopaedics & Scoliosis Surgery
Baylor School of Medicine
Houston, Texas
Medical Director of Motion Analysis & Human
    Performance
Texas Children's Hospital
Houston, Texas

Eric D. Shirley, MD
Pediatric Orthopaedic Surgeon
Pediatric Orthopaedic Associates
Woodstock, Georgia

Mauricio Silva, MD
Medical Director
Orthopaedic Institute for Children
Los Angeles, California
Clinical Professor
UCLA-Orthopaedic Hospital Department of Orthopaedic
    Surgery
David Geffen School of Medicine
University of California Los Angeles
Los Angeles, California

Louise Z. Spierre, MD
Director Pediatric Rehabilitation
Wolfson Children's Hospital
Assistant Professor
Department of Pediatrics
University of Florida Health Science Center
Jacksonville, Florida

Chris Stutz, MD
Assistant Professor
Orthopedic, Hand, and Microvascular Surgery
Texas Scottish Rite Hospital for Children
Dallas, Texas

George H. Thompson, MD
Director
Division of Pediatric Orthopaedic Surgery
Rainbow Babies and Children's Hospital
Cleveland, Ohio
Professor, Orthopaedic Surgery and Pediatrics
Case Western Reserve University
Cleveland, Ohio

Rachel M. Thompson, MD
Assistant Professor-in-Residence
Orthopaedic Surgery
UCLA/OIC
Los Angeles, California

Dan A. Zlotolow, MD
Adjunct Clinical Associate Professor of Orthopaedics
The Hospital for Special Surgery
New York, New York
Attending Physician
Shriners Hospital for Children
Philadelphia, Pennsylvania

Preface

The second edition of *Skeletal Trauma in Children* provided the reader with advanced analysis and recommendation for the full spectrum of musculoskeletal injuries in children. We added more advanced forms of fracture care than were available in the first edition and provided expanded reference lists and treatment recommendations based on greater analysis of outcome.

The recognition that children's diaphyseal fractures are not always best treated by nonoperative means was clearly explained in the chapters of the second edition. Additional treatment options for diaphyseal fractures involving minimal surgical incisions were spelled out in detail. For example, the morbidity coming from traditional traction and cast treatment of femur fractures was clearly described. The risk of complications from operative management of long bone fractures, such as overgrowth, infection, and nonunion, were detailed. The second edition added new chapters on the assessment of outcome of musculoskeletal injury, which has proved to be a widely used reference in the pediatric musculoskeletal injury community. In fact, evidence obtained by this relatively new field has provided much of the rationale for more invasive treatment of skeletal injuries in children.

In the third edition, we added two new chapters. The chapter on Anesthesia and Analgesia for the Ambulatory Management of Children's Fractures stems from our long-standing academic interest in the best ways to manage pain in children while achieving safe and accurate reduction. As is the tradition of this book with management of individual injuries, we provided descriptors for the full spectrum of options with recommended treatment. Second, we added a chapter on Rehabilitation of the Child with Multiple Injuries. This chapter has proved to be a useful reference in defining the role of rehabilitation services in obtaining optimum outcomes for children with multiple injuries, especially those with a concomitant head injury.

In the fourth edition, we expanded the detail in the Rehabilitation chapter and Anesthesia chapter and added material on new methods of internal fixation, both indications and results. In addition, a new chapter on Sports Injuries was added.

In the fifth edition, we added chapters on Casting Techniques and Nerve Injury and Repair. We felt that the former was a useful addition because the vast majority of fractures in children are still best treated by casting, splinting, and/or immobilization, and we wanted this edition to be a more comprehensive tool for individuals treating injured children. The Nerve Injury and Repair in Children chapter was also thought to add to the scope of the book because nerve repair is more often appropriately indicated in injured children than it is in adults with corresponding better functional outcomes. Finally, we added levels of evidence to the reference list to help readers easily identify the research design of the cited references and note those that, because of a higher-quality research design, should impact practice decisions the most.

The sixth edition adds updated chapters with a focus on innovative, evolving techniques for pediatric fracture care, such as expanded use of minimally invasive bridge plating and elastic nailing, while providing methods and tips for modern application of tried-and-true principles of closed treatment for children's fractures. Newly developed surgical approaches, such as surgical hip dislocation approaches for pediatric hip injuries and arthroscopically assisted techniques for pediatric intraarticular injuries, are reviewed.

As in the first five editions, we did not spend much time reviewing treatment of historical interest only. We updated the treatment of all musculoskeletal injuries in this volume to continue to enable the reader to find quickly and review the details about what is considered to be the current best method of treatment for individual pediatric musculoskeletal injuries. Our contributors again labored many hundreds of hours individually and in teams to provide you, the reader, with this current compendium. Most important, organizing the material in a way that is useful to working surgeons should provide the orthopedic surgeon with more confidence and result in better outcomes for children with musculoskeletal injuries.

Gregory A. Mencio, MD
Steven L. Frick, MD

Levels of Evidence for Primary Research Question[1]

	Therapeutic Studies—Investigating the Results of Treatment	Prognostic Studies—Investigating the Effect of A Patient Characteristic on the Outcome of Disease	Diagnostic Studies—Investigating A Diagnostic Test	Economic and Decision Analyses—Developing An Economic or Decision Model
Level I	• High-quality randomized controlled trial with statistically significant difference or no statistically significant difference but narrow confidence intervals • Systematic review[2] of Level I randomized controlled trials (and study results were homogeneous[3])	• High-quality prospective study[4] (all patients were enrolled at the same point in their disease with ≥80% follow-up of enrolled patients) • Systematic review[2] of Level I studies	• Testing of previously developed diagnostic criteria in series of consecutive patients (with universally applied reference "gold" standard) • Systematic review[2] of Level I studies	• Sensible costs and alternatives; values obtained from many studies; multiway sensitivity analyses • Systematic review[2] of Level I studies
Level II	• Lesser-quality randomized controlled trial (e.g., <80% follow-up, no blinding, or improper randomization) • Prospective[4] comparative study[5] • Systematic review[2] of Level II studies or Level I studies with inconsistent results	• Retrospective[6] study • Untreated controls from a randomized controlled trial • Lesser-quality prospective study (e.g., patients enrolled at different points in their disease or <80% follow-up) • Systematic review[2] of Level II studies	• Development of diagnostic criteria on basis of consecutive patients (with universally applied reference "gold" standard) • Systematic review[2] of Level II studies	• Sensible costs and alternatives; values obtained from limited studies; multiway sensitivity analyses • Systematic review[2] of Level II studies
Level III	• Case-control study[7] • Retrospective[6] comparative study[5] • Systematic review[2] of Level III studies	• Case-control study[7]	• Study of nonconsecutive patients (without consistently applied reference "gold" standard) • Systematic review[2] of Level III studies	• Analyses based on limited alternatives and costs; poor estimates • Systematic review[2] of Level III studies
Level IV	• Case series[8]	• Case series	• Case-control study • Poor reference standard	• No sensitivity analyses
Level V	• Expert opinion	• Expert opinion	• Expert opinion	• Expert opinion

[1]A complete assessment of the quality of individual studies requires critical appraisal of all aspects of the study design.

[2]A combination of results from two or more prior studies.

[3]Studies provided consistent results.

[4]Study was started before the first patient enrolled.

[5]Patients treated one way (e.g., with cemented hip arthroplasty) compared with patients treated another way (e.g., with cement-less hip arthroplasty) at the same institution.

[6]Study was started after the first patient enrolled.

[7]Patients identified for the study on the basis of their outcome (e.g., failed total hip arthroplasty), called "cases," are compared with those who did not have the outcome (e.g., had a successful total hip arthroplasty), called "controls."

[8]Patients treated one way with no comparison group of patients treated another way.

From the *Journal of Bone and Joint Surgery* (jbjs.org). Originally adapted from material published by the Centre for Evidence-Based Medicine, Oxford, UK. For more information, please see www.cebm.net.

Acknowledgments

Many individuals at Elsevier provided an important role in the development, writing, and editing of this text. We would like to particularly thank Katie DeFrancesco for her efforts to oversee preparation of the sixth edition. We would be remiss not to acknowledge the significant contributions by Dr Mark Swiontkowski as co-editor of the previous 5 editions of Skeletal Trauma in Children and whose shared vision along with Dr Green was foundational in the development of this text.

I, Gregory Mencio, acknowledge that my editorial contribution to this text is based on the knowledge and experience that I have gained from my practice at Vanderbilt University Medical Center since 1991. In particular, I want to thank Dr. Neil Green, with whom I had the pleasure of working for more than 25 years at Vanderbilt. Dr. Green was a great surgeon, tremendous partner, outstanding role model, and loyal friend. He was an educator par excellence and a superb surgeon who has had a major influence on the evolution of pediatric orthopedic trauma care. I am grateful to Mark Swiontkowski for his friendship over the years and guidance in coediting the fifth edition of *Skeletal Trauma in Children* and to Steve Frick for his support and collaboration as coeditor on this edition of the book. I would also like to recognize the many other mentors who have had meaningful impact on my career, including Drs. Frank Bassett, J. Leonard Goldner, James Urbaniak, and Robert Fitch at Duke University Medical Center and Dan Spengler at Vanderbilt. Finally, I would like to thank Drs. Steven Lovejoy, Jeffrey Martus, Jonathan Schoenecker, Christopher Stutz, Megan Johnson, Kevin Dale, and David Ebenezer, current and former partners at Monroc Carell Jr. Children's Hospital at Vanderbilt for the expertise, enthusiasm, and skill they display daily in managing all aspects of pediatric orthopedic trauma. Their commitment to excellence in patient care, orthopedic education, and scholarly exchange continues to make coming to work a fulfilling experience.

I, Steve Frick, want to acknowledge the mentorship provided me by many orthopedic surgeons during my career, including Drs. Green and Swiontkowski, and Dr. Mencio for the opportunity to assist with this edition. Learning from Drs. Edward Hanley Jr., Jeffrey Kneisl, James Kellam, Michael Bosse, Stephen Sims, Scott Mubarak, Dennis Wenger, Peter Newton, Henry Chambers, and Douglas Wallace prepared me for a career taking care of injured patients. Thanks to my professional colleagues at Carolinas Medical Center, Nemours Children's Hospital, and Stanford University and the dedicated members of the Pediatric Orthopaedic Society of North America for providing ongoing dialogue and research to improve our care for injured children.

Contents

Video Contents

Skeletal Growth, Development, and Healing as Related to Pediatric Trauma

1

Brian Scannell | Steven L. Frick

INTRODUCTION

Consideration of growth potential is the major difference in treating injuries in children as compared with adults. Pediatric skeletal trauma can result in enhanced or diminished growth. Future growth is usually helpful because some angular and length deformities can correct themselves as the child grows. Loss of growth potential can be one of the more difficult problems to treat. Adult bone is dynamic; it is constantly involved in bone turnover and remodeling in response to aging and changes in stress on the skeleton. The pediatric skeleton not only remodels in response to alterations in stress but also grows in length and width and changes shape, alignment, and rotation as it matures. Understanding growth potential and the changing forces after skeletal trauma in children are important in determining the appropriate treatment for injured bones.

The following are the most common clinical questions in caring for children with fractures: (1) is the physis injured with an accompanying risk of growth disturbance, and (2) is the length and alignment of the fracture acceptable or unacceptable (i.e., will it improve with growth enough that function and cosmesis will not be adversely affected)? If the answer is no, a reduction is indicated. The response to these two questions requires knowledge of normal growth mechanisms and studies of fractures in children (the science), whereas applying this knowledge to an individual patient and making decisions about how to care for the fracture require an assessment of multiple factors related to the child and the fracture (the art).

Principles of fracture treatment are the same for all ages—the goal is to achieve restoration of normal length, alignment, rotation, and the anatomic reduction of articular surfaces. In children, attempting to preserve normal growth potential is also critical; thus, assessment of the integrity and alignment of the physis is important. Although some angulation is acceptable when treating fractures in children, it is best to keep the amount of angulation as small as possible by closed fracture treatment methods, regardless of the patient's age. On the other hand, multiple attempts at anatomic reduction in a child, particularly in fractures involving the physis, may cause harm and should be avoided. The small amount of angulation associated with torus or so-called buckle fractures in children is almost always acceptable. Marked bowing that causes clinical deformity, which can be seen in plastic deformation and "greenstick" fractures in the forearm, should usually be corrected.[1,2]

Bone healing in children is generally rapid, primarily because of the thickened, extremely osteogenic periosteum. The age of the patient directly affects the rate of healing of any fracture: the younger the child, the more rapidly the fracture heals. The periosteum thins as the child grows older and has less osteogenic capability. Injuries to the growth plate heal more rapidly than shaft fractures do. Physeal injuries, in almost all parts of the body, heal in approximately 3 weeks.[3]

Treatment of trauma to the pediatric skeleton is generally straightforward. Dislocations and ligamentous injuries are uncommon in children in comparison with adults because the physis and bones in children are usually weaker mechanical links in the system and thus more susceptible to injury. Ligamentous injuries may occur, especially in older children, as physiologic physeodeses begin to occur, resulting in more secure attachments of the epiphyseal and metaphyseal regions.[4,5] Most injuries, though, are simple fracture patterns caused by low-velocity trauma such as falls. In most cases, closed reduction followed by a short period of immobilization restores normal function to a pediatric extremity. However, a number of pitfalls can make treatment of pediatric fractures, particularly fractures of the growth plate, difficult and demanding.

HISTORY, DIAGNOSIS, AND INJURY MECHANISMS

In infants, skeletal trauma may be related to the birthing process or may be the only sign of child abuse because young children are at higher risk for abuse.[6] The presenting sign may be deformity, swelling, or lack of movement in an extremity. Caregivers should be questioned about the circumstances of the injury, and a lack of a plausible mechanism of injury should prompt an evaluation for nonaccidental trauma. Radiographs of an infant can be difficult to obtain and interpret, especially those of bones in the elbow and hip region, which may require comparison views. Anteroposterior and lateral views, including the joints above and below the injured area, constitute a minimal radiographic evaluation. Usually, routine radiographs coupled with a good physical examination can establish the diagnosis. Arthrograms, ultrasonography, or magnetic resonance imaging (MRI) can be useful as a diagnostic aid when radiographs are confusing.[3,7] Additionally, a skeletal survey can be used in the young patient because unsuspected fractures may be present up to 20% of the time.[8]

Children with multiple trauma or head injuries or both can have occult axial fractures and physeal injuries that may not be suspected or may be difficult to diagnose, even with a good physical examination. This is more commonly seen in patients with a lower Glasgow Coma Scale and higher Injury Severity Score.[9] In these children, historically, a bone scan assisted in diagnosing fractures unidentified by routine screening radiographs[10]; however, they can be difficult to obtain in multiply injured children. More recently, radiographic skeletal surveys and multiplanar imaging with computed tomography or MRI are favored for identifying occult injuries.[11]

Fractures through the growth plate in children can be difficult to interpret if the fracture is not displaced. A thorough physical examination can usually identify this type of injury; the sign is swelling and maximal tenderness occurring over the injured physis, which occurs most commonly at the distal end of the radius or fibula. Palpation at or distal to the tip of the lateral malleolus usually identifies a ligamentous injury; swelling and tenderness at the growth plate may suggest a fracture undetected by radiographs. However, studies evaluating children with lateral ankle pain after injury but normal radiographs were not found to frequently have a physeal fracture by ultrasound[5] or MRI.[12] Another recent MRI study challenges the perception that distal fibular physeal injuries are common after twisting ankle injuries in skeletally immature patients.[4] Often, a small metaphyseal fragment on the radiograph suggests physeal injury. Repeated radiographs in 1 to 2 weeks can confirm the physeal injury because the healing physis appears wider, and periosteal reaction may be seen.

Each age group has typical injury mechanisms and common fractures. Most infants and newborns (≤12 months of age) sustain fractures by having someone else injure them. When children are older, walking and running, accidental injuries are more common. Children most commonly fracture the forearm, usually the distal end of the radius.[13–15] Clavicle fractures are common in infancy and in the preschool age group, but their incidence decreases with increasing age. Elbow hyperextension in early and midchildhood predisposes children in these age groups to supracondylar humerus fractures. Forearm fractures, although common in young children, show a progressive increase into the teenage years.

Most injuries occur when the child falls. Severe, high-energy injuries are less common in children and are frequently caused by automobiles, lawn mowers, or motorcycles/all-terrain vehicles. As a child approaches the midteens, injuries are much like those of an adult. The age at which the growth plates close varies greatly and depends on hereditary factors and hormonal variation. Skeletal age is an important factor in the consideration of injuries in children, in that the closer the child is to the end of growth, the less prominent the role of the growth plate in treatment of the injury and the less the remodeling potential. Healing capacity is inversely related to age.

Finally, child abuse must be considered in all children's injuries, and, as noted earlier, it should especially be considered when treating very young children with fractures.[6,16] Care must be taken to ensure that the child is checked for signs of abuse on the initial assessment and for possible subsequent injuries during follow-up. Repeating a skeletal survey at 2 to 3 weeks is strongly recommended in young patients to increase diagnostic yield in patients with suspected abuse injuries.[17] Parents or guardians of children who are not brought back for follow-up appointments for fractures should be contacted and asked to schedule a return visit.

FORMATION OF BONE

Embryonic bone forms through either membranous or endochondral ossification. In the former, mesenchymal cells proliferate to form membranes primarily in the region in which flat bones are fabricated.[18,19] Endochondral ossification is bony replacement of a cartilage model and is the mode of formation of long bones.

MEMBRANOUS BONE FORMATION

Membranous bone formation increases the diameter of long bones and is responsible for the creation of flat bones such as the scapula, skull, and, in part, the clavicle and pelvis. Flat bones are formed as mesenchymal cells condense into sheets that eventually differentiate into osteoblasts. Surface cells become the periosteum. Primary bone is remodeled and transformed into cancellous bone, to which the periosteum adds a compact cortical bone cover. This type of growth is independent of a cartilage model.

As endochondral ossification lengthens bones, proliferation of bone occurs beneath the periosteum through membranous bone formation, thus enlarging the diameter of the diaphysis in long bones. This type of bone formation is also apparent in subperiosteal infection and after bone injury when periosteal bone forms around a fracture hematoma (Fig. 1.1). The osteogenic periosteum of children contributes to rapid healing because the callus and periosteal new bone increase the diameter of the bone and provide early biomechanical strength.

ENDOCHONDRAL OSSIFICATION

Endochondral ossification requires the presence of a cartilage anlage. Early in gestation, mesenchymal cells aggregate to form models of the future long bones. A cartilage model develops, and the peripheral cells organize into a perichondrium.[18,19] Cartilage cells enlarge and degenerate, and the matrix surrounding them calcifies. This calcification begins in the center of the diaphysis and becomes the primary ossification center. Vascular buds enter the ossification center and transport new mesenchymal cells capable of differentiating into osteoblasts, chondroclasts, and osteoclasts. These cells align themselves on the calcified cartilage and deposit bone. Primary cancellous bone is thus formed, and ossification expands toward the metaphyseal regions.

Long bone growth continues as the terminal ends of the cartilage model keep growing in length by cartilage cell proliferation, hypertrophy, and production of extracellular matrix. This growth continues in this manner until after birth, when secondary ossification centers (epiphyses) develop.

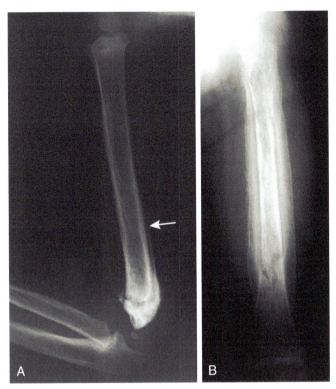

Fig. 1.1 (A) Radiograph of a healing supracondylar fracture illustrating the periosteum stripped (*arrow*) to nearly the midshaft of the humerus. The bridging periosteal bone stabilizes this fracture in about 3 weeks. (B) The large periosteal involucrum surrounds the former bone (sequestrum) in a femur with osteomyelitis. The periosteum can be stimulated to remanufacture an entire cortex around this area, such that when the sequestered bone is removed, the periosteal bone will form a new (larger-diameter) femoral diaphysis.

The mass of cartilage found between the epiphyseal and diaphyseal bones in later postnatal development thins to become the epiphyseal plate, which continues as the principal contributor to the growth (in length) of long bones until maturation is reached. The girth of the long bone is provided by the cambium layer of the periosteum.[13,18] Successive surfaces of compact bone are added to the exterior while remodeling by resorption of the interior (endosteal) surface takes place.

Once the physis is established between the epiphysis and metaphysis, the periosteal ring becomes relatively firmly attached at the level of the zone of hypertrophied cells. This periphyseal periosteal collar is referred to as the fibrous ring of LaCroix.[3,13,18] The zone of Ranvier, the cellular segment responsible for growth in diameter of the physis,[13] is located in the same area. The periosteum is firmly attached at this level. Even when the periosteum is torn over the metaphysis or diaphysis, it usually remains attached at the physis.

REGULATION OF GROWTH AND DEVELOPMENT

Factors affecting skeletal growth vary and are incompletely understood. Although commonly used growth curve charts suggest that growth is smoothly continuous throughout childhood, a saltation and stasis model of human growth is now recognized,[20,21] with bursts of growth in length (growth spurts) occurring after prolonged periods of stasis. Growth in length occurs only at the physis and can occur through three mechanisms: an increase in the number of cells, an increase in the size of cells, or an increase in the amount of extracellular matrix. The physis responds to various growth-regulating hormones (e.g., growth hormone, thyroxine, estrogen, and testosterone), parathyroid hormone, and corticosteroids, as well as the peptide-signaling proteins—transforming growth factor β (TGF-β), platelet-derived growth factor (PDGF), and bone morphogenetic proteins (BMPs)—and immunoregulatory cytokines (interleukin-1 [IL-1] and IL-6).[22–26] Further research is still needed to better understand these growth pathways. However, recently it was suggested that differential expression of gene pathways specifically for BMP-2 and BMP-6 may contribute to further physeal growth.[27]

Local paracrine regulators have recently been identified as critical in controlling bone development and remodeling. An important feedback loop controlling chondrocyte development involves Indian hedgehog protein (Ihh) and parathyroid hormone-related peptide. These paracrine factors control the decision for chondrocytes to leave the proliferative pool and undergo hypertrophic differentiation.[28,29] Fibroblast growth factor (FGF) signaling also appears crucial in regulating chondrocyte proliferation and differentiation in the physis and appears to have an opposite effect from the BMPs, decreasing chondrocyte proliferation, increasing production of Ihh, and accelerating differentiation of hypertrophic chondrocytes.[29] An example of abnormal growth related to FGF signaling is in achondroplasia. A gene mutation affecting FGF receptor 3 suppresses proliferation and maturation of growth plate chondrocytes, causing decreased growth plate size and decreased bone elongation.[30] Thyroxine is also involved in the cellular and molecular events of terminal chondrocyte differentiation and morphogenesis of columnar cartilage.[31]

Diurnal variation in the growth of bone has been shown to reflect the levels of the different hormones, and animal studies suggest mechanical factors may also be critical because 90% of growth occurred during periods of recumbency in a study of growth in sheep.[21] Physeal growth is slowed by excessive compression and accelerated by distraction, recognized in the American literature as the Hueter-Volkmann law,[32] but noted earlier by Delpech in 1829.[33] This theory affects growth but also fracture healing, which is one of many differences between pediatric and adult fracture healing.

Growth in length ceases at skeletal maturity with fusion of the physes and occurs at different times in individual bones; it also varies based on gender, hereditary factors, and hormone levels. Physiologic physiodesis is the normal, gradual replacement of the growth plate by bone during adolescence, and physeal closure is induced at skeletal maturity by estrogen levels in both males and females.[28]

BIOLOGY OF FRACTURE HEALING

Fracture healing is usually divided into three stages: (1) inflammatory, (2) reparative, and (3) remodeling. Fracture healing involves both membranous and endochondral ossification. Injuries to the pediatric skeleton always involve a variable amount of surrounding soft tissue injury. Unlike the soft tissues, which heal by replacement of the injured tissue with collagen scar tissue, bone heals by replacing the area that is injured with normal bony tissue.

The blood supply to the bone is an important part of fracture healing, and significant soft tissue injury delays healing because the blood supply to bone enters at sites of soft tissue attachment. The normal process of fracture healing in any part of the bone follows a set chronologic order. Any of these phases may be disrupted or delayed by excessive adjacent soft tissue injury.

INFLAMMATORY PHASE

The inflammatory phase of fracture healing "sets the stage" for cartilage and bone formation by supplying the building blocks necessary for repair and remodeling. When bone is injured, the bone, periosteum, and soft tissue (mostly muscle) around the fracture begin to bleed. Hematomas form at the fracture site, both inside and outside the bone. The hematoma may dissect along the periosteum, which is easily elevated or was elevated at the time that the fracture was maximally displaced. The more severe the soft tissue injury, the more displaced the fracture; in addition, the more the periosteum is torn, the larger the area that fills with the hematoma. The role of a hematoma is to serve as a source of signaling agents capable of initiating cellular events critical to fracture healing. This also explains why some minimally displaced or greenstick fractures (minimal to no hematoma) may be slow to heal.

Research has focused on factors controlling fracture healing in two groups: peptide-signaling proteins (TGF-β, FGF, PDGF, and BMPs) and immunoregulatory cytokines (IL-1 and IL-6).[25] The peptide-signaling proteins are derived from platelets and extracellular bone matrix and are critical for regulation of cell proliferation and mesenchymal stem cell differentiation. TGF-β is a multifunctional growth factor that controls tissue differentiation in fracture repair. FGFs increase the proliferation of osteoblasts and chondrocytes and may stimulate the formation of new blood vessels. PDGF acts on mesenchymal cell precursors to stimulate osteoblast differentiation. BMPs are a class of proteins produced in the early stages of fracture repair and strongly stimulate endochondral ossification. The sole criterion for BMP classification is the induction of bone formation in a standard in vivo rodent assay, and at least 14 BMPs, grouped in the TGF superfamily of growth and differentiation factors, have been identified. BMPs are present in bone matrix in a form that allows for presentation to marrow stromal cells to induce differentiation into osteoblasts. Furthermore, osteoblasts have been shown to synthesize and secrete BMPs. Cells that synthesize new bone during fractures also have been shown to be targets of BMPs and to possess BMP receptors. BMPs (BMP 2, 3, 4, 5, and 8) and BMP receptors are upregulated in the periosteum as early as 3 days after fracture.[34]

Studies utilizing microarray analysis of the genetic response to a fracture demonstrate that the genomic response to a fracture is complex and involves thousands of genes, including the BMPs and other growth factors noted earlier, as well as immunoregulatory cytokines.[10,34–36] The immunoregulatory cytokines are released from inflammatory cells present in the hematoma and serve to regulate the early events in fracture healing.

Pediatric bone is more vascular than that of an adult and is able to generate a greater hyperemic and inflammatory response. The more mature (less porous) the cortex, the slower the vascular response to injury. Vasodilatation and the cellular inflammatory response begin shortly after a fracture, and the injured area is filled with inflammatory cells such as polymorphonuclear leukocytes and macrophages. The hematoma and inflammatory response also incite the release of molecules such as growth factors and cytokines from the platelets.[37] In the initial phase of fracture healing, after the hematoma has formed, a scaffolding of fibrovascular tissue replaces the clot with collagen fibers. These fibers eventually become the collagen of the woven bone of the primary callus that forms around the fracture.

The primary callus is later ossified as the microvascular supply returns to the area. However, the bone, for at least a millimeter or two directly adjacent to the fracture site, loses its blood supply early in the inflammatory stage. After initial reabsorption of the dead bone along the fracture line, the fracture line in children usually becomes more visible radiographically 2 or 3 weeks after injury. The dead bone at the fracture surface is revascularized in a process that occurs faster in more vascular areas such as the metaphysis (as compared with the diaphysis).

The vascular response aids in initiating the cellular response to the fracture. A number of TGF-β subtypes help mediate cellular and tissue responses to inflammation and tissue repair.[37] During the inflammatory phase of fracture healing, TGF-β from the extracellular matrix of bone and also from platelets controls the mesenchymal precursor cells that may form osteoblasts and osteoclasts. The maximal cellular response is ongoing within 24 hours of injury and occurs first in the subperiosteal region of the fracture.[38,39]

Osteogenic induction is stimulation by growth factors to convert the multipotential cells into osteoprogenitor cells. The osteoprogenitor cells on the undersurface of the periosteum help form periosteal bone. The osteogenic cells that originate from the periosteum help manufacture the external callus. Endochondral bone formation from the endosteal areas combines with subperiosteal bone formation to bridge the fracture.

The subperiosteal callus in children initially stabilizes the area so that the external callus may clinically heal the fracture by the end of the reparative phase. During remodeling, this callus decreases and is replaced with the endochondral ossified bone that has formed at the fracture surface.

REPARATIVE PHASE

The reparative phase of fracture healing is highlighted by the development of new blood vessels and the onset of cartilage formation. The surrounding soft tissue provides vascular ingrowth initially to the periosteal area and subsequently to the endosteal area. Before the fracture, the cortical blood supply was primarily from endosteal bone and branched out radially from inside the medullary canal. During the reparative phase, most of the blood supply to the cortex arises from outside the bone rather than inside.

Rat models of fracture healing reveal that intramembranous and endochondral bone formation is initiated during the first 10 days. Inflammatory mediators in the fracture hematoma recruit chondrocytes capable of producing fracture

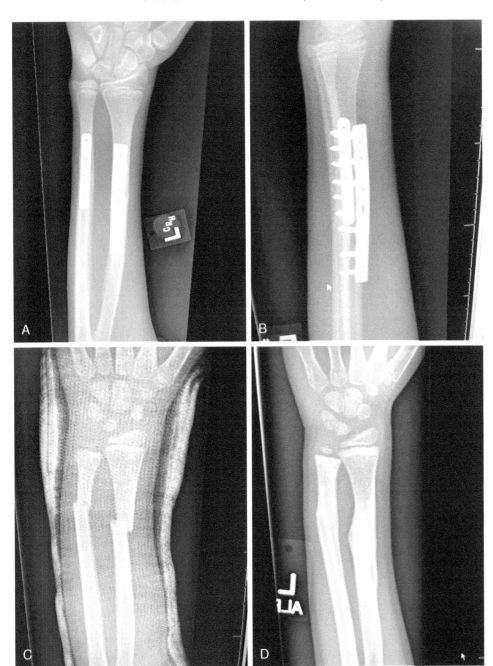

Fig. 1.2 Anteroposterior (A) and lateral (B) radiographs of a forearm in a 15-year-old male who underwent open reduction and internal fixation with plates/screws. The fracture healing demonstrates primary bone healing with rigid fixation. An anteroposterior radiograph of a forearm in a 5-year-old at the time of original cast immobilization (C) and at 10 weeks (D) with complete fracture union demonstrates secondary bone healing. The motion that occurs with secondary bone healing results in abundant callus formation.

callus. The hematoma is eventually replaced by the ingrowth of fibrovascular tissue. This developing construct provides structural support to stabilize the bone ends. This primitive tissue is eventually replaced through endochondral and intramembranous bone formation.

Tissue differentiation during the reparative phase is strongly influenced by local mechanical factors. Fracture stability has a critical effect on bone healing. Fracture healing is classically divided into primary and secondary healing. Primary healing results from rigid stabilization (i.e., plate immobilization) and involves a direct attempt by the cortex to bridge the fracture gap. Bridging occurs through direct haversian remodeling by intramembranous bone formation (Fig. 1.2A, B).

Secondary healing results from treatment of fractures with less rigid methods (i.e., fracture bracing, casts). In secondary healing, more motion at the fracture site leads to lower

oxygen tension, and more cartilage is formed. Motion at the fracture site, the presence of a fracture gap, and an intact soft tissue envelope all encourage the formation of abundant callus (Fig. 1.2C, D). The increased diameter of the callus enhances biomechanical stability because the rigidity of the bone is proportional to its radius. The callus formed subsequently undergoes endochondral ossification. Ideal fracture treatment involves enough rigidity to ensure adequate vessel ingrowth, followed by progressive loading and motion to stimulate ample callus formation.[36,40]

As the periosteum produces bone beneath it, the periosteum is pushed away from the bone and makes a collar of bone around the area of injury. Initially, this tissue is more cartilaginous and fibrous and is not very well ossified. It may not show up well on a radiograph until the blood supply is adequate enough to allow mineralization and conversion to bone.

An important process that occurs between the reparative and remodeling phases is clinical union of the fracture, which takes place when the bony callus surrounds the fracture fragments and joins the callus coming from the other side. At this point, the bone may be stable clinically, and although some plastic deformation is still possible with force, the bone is usually strong enough that the patient can begin to use the extremity in a more normal way.

Although there are many ways suggested in the literature to determine union, clinical examination with radiographic evidence of healing is the most important in assessing union.[41] Clinical union has occurred when the fracture site is no longer tender and does not move during examination and when physiologic loading does not cause pain. Radiographic union occurs later when radiographs demonstrate bone bridging across the fracture. This point demarcates the end of the reparative phase and the beginning of the remodeling phase.

REMODELING PHASE

Remodeling is the final phase of bone healing. It may last for a short time in a young child, or continue throughout growth or even beyond the end of growth in an older child. Once the bone is clinically stabilized, the ongoing stresses and strains on the bone that normally cause modeling are responsible for remodeling this early soft woven bone. After fractures in children, the bone usually returns to normal radiographically and clinically.

One complete skeletal turnover occurs during a child's first year of life. This turnover declines to about 10% per year in late childhood and continues at about this rate or a little slower for life.[24] Remodeling does not result from the activity of a single type of cell, such as osteoclasts or osteoblasts, but rather results from coordinated absorption and formation of bone over large regions around the fracture. The control mechanisms for the remodeling phase of bone are believed to be the bioelectric behavior that is responsible for modeling bone, according to Wolff's law. As bone is subjected to the stresses of use during normal activities, the bone remodels appropriately for those stresses. Because a child's bone is normally modeling anyway (actively changing in response to growth and stress), a child's bone remodels significantly faster than an adult's. This remodeling typically involves addition of bone to the concavity of angular deformities (compression side) and subtraction of bone from the convexity (tension side), resulting in a "rounding off" of the angle.

Systemic factors can affect the rate of bone healing. In addition to the age of the patient, hormonal factors that may help promote bone healing are growth hormone, thyroid hormone, calcitonin, insulin, anabolic steroids, and vitamins A and B.[19]

Factors that have been shown to discourage bone healing are diabetes, corticosteroids, exposure to cigarette smoke, and certain endocrinopathies. Denervation, irradiation, and high doses of hyperbaric oxygen may also slow the healing of fractures.

Historically, nonsteroidal antiinflammatory medications in children were avoided because of concern for fracture healing. However, more recent basic science and clinical studies suggest that it is unlikely to affect healing of fractures in children.[42–44]

PHYSEAL FRACTURE HEALING

Cartilage does not heal in the same phases as bone. When the physis is injured, it does not heal by the formation of callus within the physis. Inflammatory and reparative phases occur in cartilage healing, but cartilage healing has no remodeling phase.[19,23] In 1958, Dale and Harris used a rhesus monkey model of physeal fractures and described the process of physeal fracture healing: initially the gap in the physis is filled with fibrin, and new bone formation ceases. The calcified cartilage cells on the metaphyseal side of the fracture line persist unaltered, while the cells on the epiphyseal side of the fracture continue to grow. These two processes lead to a temporary but pronounced increase in the thickness of the physeal plate in healing physeal fractures, which creates widening at the physis radiographically. Finally, callus grows from the metaphysis and periosteum of the shaft across the physeal fracture gap and reunites the epiphysis to the metaphysis and shaft. Once this occurs, the vascular supply is restored and normal endochondral ossification resumes; the physeal thickness rapidly returns to normal as the dead and dying chondrocytes on the metaphyseal side of the physis are calcified, and the calcified cartilage is then replaced with bone.[45]

Most physeal fractures heal uneventfully, and normal growth resumes. Occasionally, however, physeal bars form after fractures through the physis, and shortening or angular deformity develops. There are a few theories for physeal bar etiology: (1) axial compression causes injury to germinal chondrocytes;[33,46] (2) anastomoses between epiphyseal and metaphyseal blood supplies lead to bone formation between the two;[16] and (3) fractures extending to the physeal-epiphyseal border may disrupt the vascular supply to the physis.[47] The axial compression theory seems less likely because chondrocytes are better able to withstand compressive loads than immature bone, and metaphyseal bone would likely fail first. Occasionally, fractures occur that result in metaphyseal bone contacting epiphyseal bone; in addition, some authors have suggested that repeated attempts at closed reduction may result in "grinding away" the physis[14] or predisposing to growth arrest.[48] The vascular theories differentiate physeal fracture prognosis based on the plane of the fracture within the physis. Previously, it was believed that physeal fractures almost always occurred within the zone of hypertrophy of the physis,[46] but now the variability of the fracture plane has been noted.[19,47]

Basic science studies of physeal bar formation demonstrate that bars form by primary ossification[47,49] along vertical septa created when fractures extend to or through the physeal-epiphyseal border.[47] Some clinical research suggests that periosteum interposed in physeal fractures may contribute to bar development,[50] although basic science work shows only minor shortening without an increase in bar formation.[51] Physeal arrest appears to be less likely to occur when it involves only the hypertrophic zone but more likely to occur when involving the basement plate of the physis.[52]

Anatomic reduction of displaced physeal fractures seems to decrease the rate of premature physeal closure, especially for fractures that involve the epiphyseal-articular surface (Salter-Harris types III and IV),[16,53] and perhaps for some physeal-metaphyseal fractures (Salter-Harris type II).[50] This is controversial because surgical reduction of distal tibial fractures was not shown to reduce the incidence of premature physeal closure, which still remained high at 43%.[54] Physeal fracture healing in clinical and basic science studies is rapid; almost all fractures heal within 3 weeks.

DIFFERENCES BETWEEN PEDIATRIC AND ADULT FRACTURE HEALING

One of the primary differences between pediatric and adult bone is that the periosteum in children is very thick. The periosteum around the fracture site walls off the hematoma and is stripped from the bone as bleeding occurs—a primary factor in the amount of new bone formed around a fracture. The area of bone necrosis on either side of the fracture surface must be replaced by viable bone through the process of bone resorption and deposition. This process leads to an initial radiographic appearance of sclerosis at the fracture site because new bone is being formed on the existing necrotic bone. The area around the necrotic bone elicits an inflammatory response. Because pediatric bone is more vascular than adult bone, the inflammatory (hyperemic) response is more rapid and significant. Temperatures as high as 40°C may be noted after major long bone fractures. This hyperemic inflammatory reaction may also be responsible for growth stimulation, which may result in overgrowth of the bone. The early stage of fracture healing is shorter in a child than in an adult.[14,19]

The major reason for the increased speed of healing of children's fractures is the periosteum, which contributes the largest part of new bone formation around a fracture. Children have significantly greater osteoblastic activity in this area because bone is already being formed beneath the periosteum as part of normal growth. This already active process is readily accelerated after a fracture. Periosteal callus bridges fractures in children long before the underlying hematoma forms a cartilage anlage that goes on to ossify. Once cellular organization from the hematoma has passed through the inflammatory process, repair of the bone begins in the area of the fracture. In most children, by 10 days to 2 weeks after the fracture, a rubberlike bone forms around the fracture and makes it difficult to manipulate. The fracture site is still tender, however, and not yet ready for mobilization of the adjacent joints.

As part of the reparative phase, cartilage formed as the hematoma organizes is eventually replaced by bone through the process of endochondral bone formation. Fracture healing is a recapitulation of bone development that, as noted previously, involves a complex interaction of multiple cell types and cellular processes.[55]

The remodeling phase of fracture healing may continue for some time, particularly in more displaced fractures. The motion of the adjacent joints and the use of the extremity accelerate remodeling. The stresses and strains of regular use of the bone directly promote remodeling of the fractured bone into a bone that closely resembles the original structure.

Children also vary from adults as bone overgrowth has been seen in pediatric fracture healing. Fractures distant from the physis can also result in changes in growth patterns. This is particularly evident in overgrowth after femoral shaft fractures; some investigators have hypothesized that disruption of the periosteal sleeve or increasing vascularity of the bone after a fracture increases longitudinal growth.[19,23] This phenomenon most frequently compensates for fractures that heal with shortening but occasionally results in the injured limb being longer. The same cells and processes that govern normal growth are involved in fracture healing.[55] Studying growth mechanisms with microarray technology demonstrates the complexity of the genetic response to a fracture. In a study of femoral overgrowth mechanisms in a rat model, more than 5000 genes in the proximal femoral physis were noted to respond significantly to fractures. Genes related to vascular development and growth were downregulated, which casts doubt on the widely held assertion that femoral overgrowth is a consequence of increased vascularity in the limb after a fracture.[35] It has been postulated that mechanical factors, such as tension within the surrounding periosteum, may have some control over the growth rate.[18,19] This is clinically best exemplified by posttraumatic tibia valgus after proximal tibial metaphyseal fractures in children (the Cozen phenomenon).[56–58] Recent basic science data by Halanski et al[59] confirmed that disruption of the periosteum would accelerate growth. This pattern of overgrowth is not observed in adult fracture healing, and thus, fracture shortening at union will be permanent.

GROWTH ARREST LINES OR GROWTH SLOWDOWN LINES

In radiographs of bones that were fractured several weeks to months previously, transverse lines may be seen in the metaphyseal region. These lines are usually referred to as Harris growth arrest lines, or the transverse lines of Park,[60] and are unique to children's bones after a fracture or injury. These transversely oriented trabeculae occur in bones that are normally growing rapidly (e.g., femur or tibia) and in those in which the trabeculae are predominantly longitudinally oriented (Fig. 1.3). When growth deceleration occurs, as happens immediately after a fracture of an extremity, the bone is, in effect, standing still and making transversely oriented trabeculae. The calcified cartilage and bone formed has increased density and is evident radiographically after further growth. Arrest lines should parallel the physeal contour if the physis is growing normally. After a fracture, these lines are typically visible 6 to 12 weeks after injury and can provide the orthopedist with the ability to assess and predict abnormal growth.[60] A specific effort should be made to look for these arrest lines during radiographic evaluation of childhood fractures, especially those involving the physes, because lines that do not parallel the physis indicate an area of physeal damage or an osseous bridge.[60,61] Arrest lines that do not parallel the physis point to an area of abnormal physeal growth.

The physes that grow more rapidly (e.g., the distal end of the femur or the proximal end of the tibia) have arrest lines farthest from the physis. In the metaphyseal areas of bones, where the slowest growth occurs, transverse trabeculae may be difficult to see radiographically or may not form at all.

Transversely oriented Harris lines may also result from any type of stress on the bone that causes a temporary slowdown in the formation of longitudinally oriented bone. Such stresses include systemic illness, fever, and starvation,

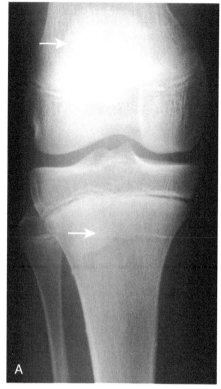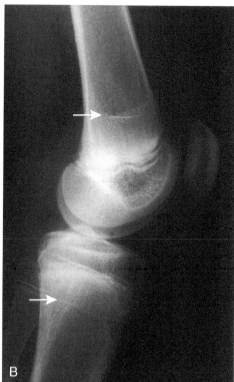

Fig. 1.3 Anteroposterior (A) and lateral (B) radiographs of the knee of a 12-year-old child 6 months after a femoral shaft fracture. Arrest lines parallel to the physis can be seen in the metaphyseal area of the distal end of the femur and proximal tibia (arrows). The temporary depression of growth at the time of injury results in more horizontal trabeculae being laid down, thereby increasing the density of bone at that level.

as well as skeletal trauma.[62] Similar lines can be seen in skeletally immature patients being treated with bisphosphonates, and are called zebra lines in osteogenesis imperfecta patients.[63,64]

REMODELING AFTER A FRACTURE IN CHILDHOOD

The remodeling ability of bone in children may make reduction accuracy less important than it is in adults. *Remodeling* is a commonly used term in pediatric fracture care, implying that the child has the ability to straighten and correct residual deformity with growth. This capability depends not only on the mechanisms of bone remodeling described earlier during the remodeling phase of fracture healing (Wolff's law) but also on reorientation of the physis by asymmetric growth after a fracture (Hueter-Volkmann law or Delpech's law). Younger children have greater remodeling potential. The amount depends on the age of the child, location of the injury in the bone (proximity to the physis), degree of deformity, and whether the deformity is in the plane of motion of the adjacent joint.[3,65,66] Clinical judgment and experience are required to guide decision-making regarding defining "acceptable" reductions, but obtaining the best reduction possible during initial treatment is advisable because it will lessen reliance on remodeling. Remodeling does not occur in displaced intraarticular fractures; thus reduction, usually by open methods, is needed. In children, remodeling is often relied on for the treatment of proximal humeral and distal radial injuries because these physes contribute greatly to the length of the respective segment, and the joints have wide ranges of motion. Remarkable remodeling has been documented in cases of these fractures (Fig. 1.4).

The effect of growth on fracture healing usually aids in fracture treatment because some angulation and deformity remodels with growth. Remodeling of angular deformities of immature long bones occurs at the growth plate and along the shaft.[67] Accelerated growth of the injured bone (as well as surrounding bones) can occur, leading to limb length discrepancy (usually the femur or humerus).[68] Growth, however, can produce deformity if the growth plate is injured or if trauma has altered muscle forces on an extremity, as may occur after a spinal cord injury or traumatic brain injury.

Remodeling may occur readily in the plane of a joint (Fig. 1.5), but it occurs far less readily, if at all, in children with rotational deformity or angular deformity not in the plane of the joint.[14,65,66,69] Abraham[67] studied the remodeling potential of immature monkeys and found that remodeling occurred at the growth plate and along the concavity of the shaft deformity, with minimal resorption on the convexity of the shaft. Diaphyseal remodeling and physeal reorientation with growth contributed similar amounts to the degree of remodeling. In femoral shaft fractures in children, 75% of the remodeling of angular deformities takes place in the physis, and 25% comes from appositional remodeling of the diaphysis.[70] The physis adjacent to a fracture realigns itself with asymmetric growth to become perpendicular to the forces acting through the bone, and most authors believe this is the primary mechanism for remodeling.[66]

Significant angulation in the midportion of long bones is not usually acceptable and does not remodel very well, depending on the age of the child. In children younger than 8 years, residual angulation is more acceptable. If the angulation is less than 30 degrees and is within the plane of the joint, remodeling toward normal alignment can be expected.[2,19] The potential for remodeling to an acceptable functional and cosmetic outcome depends on many factors, including which bone is fractured, how close the fracture is to a joint, the orientation to the joint axis, and the amount of growth remaining for the child.[66] Side-to-side (bayonet or

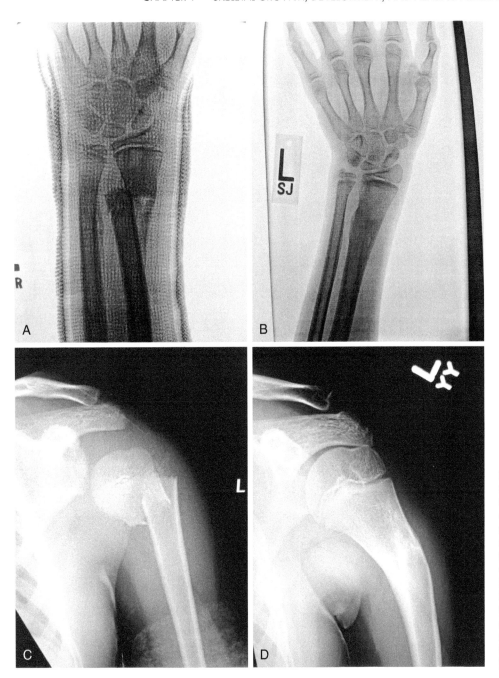

Fig. 1.4 Anteroposterior of a 9-year-old with a distal radius fracture that was pinned in poor position (A), now 4 weeks out from pinning (x-ray after pin removal). Anteroposterior of the same distal radius fracture (B) at 12 months from the injury with complete remodeling. Anteroposterior of a proximal humerus fracture in an 11-year-old at the time of injury (C) and at 6 months (D). Similar to the distal radius, these anatomic locations have tremendous remodeling potential secondary to the large contribution of growth from adjacent physes.

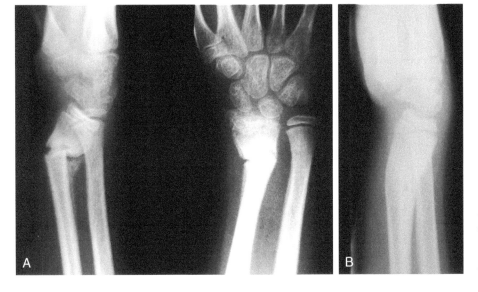

Fig. 1.5 (A) Radiograph of the distal portion of the radius in an 11-year-old girl at the time of cast removal 6 weeks after injury. (B) A lateral radiograph taken 3 months later shows considerable remodeling of the fracture in the plane of the joint.

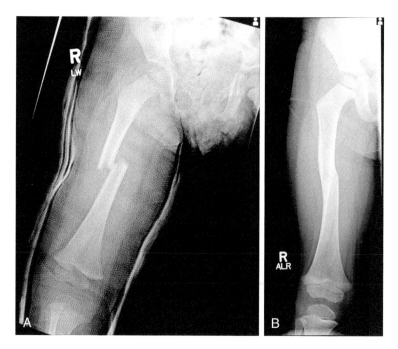

Fig. 1.6 Radiograph of a femoral shaft fracture in a 2-year-old boy in a spica cast at the time of injury (A) and at 12 months postinjury (B). The fracture demonstrates bayonet apposition with otherwise good alignment. The bayonet apposition remodeled within 12 months in this young child.

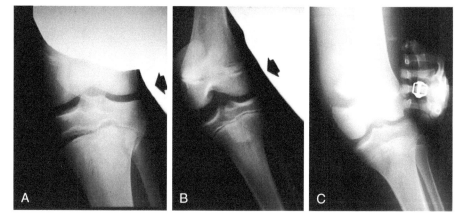

Fig. 1.7 Stress films illustrating injuries to the proximal tibial physis (A), the medial collateral ligament (B), and the distal femoral physis (C) in skeletally immature children. Stress films are no longer recommended. The diagnosis of a nondisplaced Salter I physeal fracture is made based on local tenderness and swelling over the physis.

overriding) apposition of bone is acceptable as long as alignment is accurate (Fig. 1.6). This position leads to prompt, strong union with solid periosteal bone bridging.[57]

COMPLICATIONS OF FRACTURES IN CHILDREN OTHER THAN PHYSEAL ARREST

Delayed union and nonunion rarely occur in healthy children. In a series of more than 2000 fractures in children, not a single case of nonunion was seen.[71] Lateral condyle fractures of the distal humerus are one of the few childhood injuries with a predilection for nonunion, but displaced fractures treated with accurate reduction and fixation rarely fail to heal.[72] Exceptions to uneventful fracture healing occur in older children with open injuries that have severe soft tissue injury or that become infected. Refracture is uncommon, although in malaligned forearm fractures, refracture may occur after mobilization.[73] Myositis ossificans and stiffness in joints secondary to fractures are rare. Physical therapy to regain motion is seldom necessary in children because return of motion and function is typical as the child resumes normal activities and play.

ANATOMIC DIFFERENCES OF PEDIATRIC BONES

As the skeleton of a child grows, it develops from a relatively elastic and rubbery type of biomechanical material to the more rigid structure of an adult skeleton. Because of the amount of radiolucent cartilaginous material in pediatric bone, comparison films are sometimes necessary to determine whether a radiograph is abnormal, and this lack of clarity in the radiograph can make diagnosis of fractures difficult. The types of injuries may also be different in children; for example, ligamentous injuries and dislocations are rare. Injuries around the knee frequently lead to ligamentous and meniscal injuries in adults. In children, the distal femoral or proximal tibial physis is more likely to be injured because it is the weak link (Fig. 1.7). Previously, stress radiographs were recommended, but these are usually unnecessary because the diagnosis can be made by a complete history and physical examination and confirmed at follow-up when radiographs demonstrate a widened physis consistent with a healing growth plate injury. Ligamentous injuries in skeletally immature children are uncommon, but they do occur and become more frequent in adolescence as

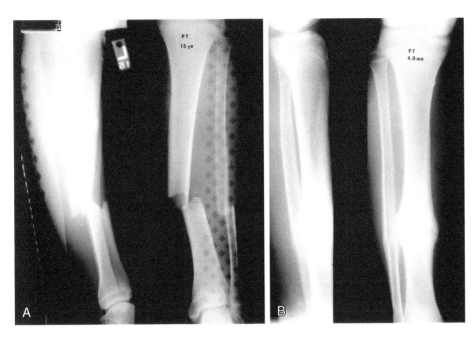

Fig. 1.8 (A) Anteroposterior and lateral radiographs of a 15-year-old boy who sustained a displaced transverse fracture of the diaphysis of his tibia. (B) Follow-up at 4 months shows abundant periosteal healing, although a portion of the fracture line is still evident. It is characteristic for pediatric long bone fractures to heal early with periosteal callus; secondarily, the diaphyseal cortex heals and remodels.

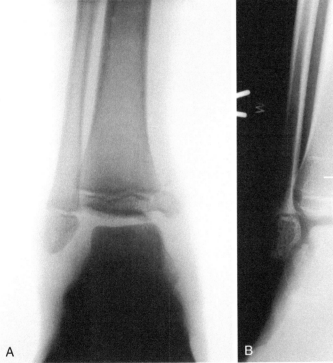
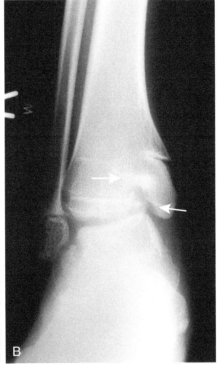

Fig. 1.9 (A) Radiograph of a 7-year-old boy who sustained a fracture of the medial malleolus, as shown in this mortise view. The fracture was treated with closed reduction and application of a long leg cast. (B) Mortise view of the ankle of the same patient 4 years after his injury. The medial malleolus portion of the epiphysis has healed to the metaphyseal area of this Salter-Harris type IV injury. He has not only an incongruous growth plate but also an incongruous ankle joint *(arrows)*. Intraarticular fractures such as this one should be treated with open reduction and internal fixation to anatomically restore both the joint surface and the growth plate.

the transition to skeletal maturity occurs.[5] As noted earlier, traditional teaching that twisting ankle injuries cause distal fibular physeal injuries more commonly than ligamentous injuries in children has been challenged by studies using advanced imaging techniques.[4,5]

Pediatric bony injuries are more often treated by closed reduction than by open reduction because of the short time to union and the ease of obtaining and maintaining near-anatomic reductions, as well as the potential for remodeling (Fig. 1.8). The quality of anesthesia/analgesia provided to the child is strongly correlated with the quality of the reduction.[22]

The most obvious anatomic differences in the pediatric skeleton are the presence of growth plates and the thick periosteum. Growth plate injuries and epiphyseal injuries can lead to growth disturbance that may be significant (Fig. 1.9). Treatment of injury to the growth plate and epiphysis parallels adult intraarticular injuries in that pediatric articular injuries require anatomic reduction to preserve joint function and growth potential. As noted earlier, the periosteum in children is much thicker, more active, less readily torn, and more easily stripped from the bone than in adults. The periosteum helps both in reduction (where intact periosteum on the concavity of the deformity serves as a hinge) and in maintenance of reduction and contributes immensely to rapid fracture healing. The intact periosteum helps reduce the amount of displacement and is the primary reason for more stable fractures in children.

EPIPHYSIS

At birth, most epiphyses are completely cartilaginous structures. The length of time for formation of the secondary ossification center within the epiphysis varies, with the distal portion of the femur being formed first.[65] A global type of growth plate is present in the epiphysis, as evidenced by columns of chondrocytes and growth potential at the physis occurring between the epiphysis and metaphysis and also just beneath the articular surface. When the epiphysis is entirely cartilaginous, it is almost completely protected from injury; traumatic forces tend to fracture the diaphysis or metaphysis, or infrequently, they may disrupt the physis, as is seen in distal humeral physeal separations in infants. Once bone has formed within the epiphysis, it is more likely to be broken, but epiphyseal fractures are much less common than fractures of the diaphysis and metaphysis. When the epiphysis is nearly all bone, it is subject to injury, much like the remainder of the bones.

PHYSIS

The growth plate remains cartilaginous throughout development. As the child grows older, the physis becomes thinner, and it is easier to disrupt the growth plate by injury. The most common location of injury in Salter-Harris type I injuries is classically described as through the lower hypertrophic zone of the physis, but variation in the plane of physeal fractures has been noted.[47] Physeal anatomy changes markedly with growth. Infants and newborns have fewer mammillary processes that stabilize the epiphysis on the metaphysis. However, with further growth, particularly in the distal femoral region, prominent mammillary processes help the physis secure the epiphysis to the metaphysis, which is likely a response to physiologic demand and the need to resist torsional forces. The proximal femoral physis changes considerably with growth and eventually forms two separate physeal areas: the capital femoral epiphysis and, below it, the trochanteric physis.

METAPHYSIS

The metaphysis is the trumpet-shaped end of long bones. It has a thinner cortical area and increased trabecular bone and is wider than the corresponding diaphyseal part of the bone. Porosity in the metaphyseal area is greater than in the diaphyseal area, and the periosteum is more firmly attached in the metaphyseal area as it gets closer to the physis.

Much bone remodeling occurs in the metaphyseal region of a bone after a fracture. Periosteal bone forms in the area joining the diaphysis to the epiphysis. This area progressively transforms back into a trumpet-shaped metaphyseal cortex with longitudinal growth.

The remodeling of the metaphyseal region to create the trumpet shape can be an issue after plates and screws are placed in the metaphysis for fractures. Physeal growth results in the physis "growing away" from the plate, and the "cut-back" remodeling can result in long screws that are prominent medially (Fig. 1.10).[74] In addition to this problem, lateral plates placed on the distal femur adjacent to the

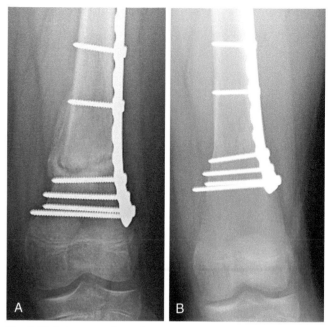

Fig. 1.10 Anteroposterior radiographs of 12-year old male who underwent open reduction and internal fixation of a supracondylar femur fracture at 1 month (A) and 18 months (B) postoperative. The significant growth of the distal femur resulted in physis "growing away" from the screws and the screws becoming prominent on the medial side.

physis that are left in growing patients can result in substantial valgus deformity.[75,76]

DIAPHYSIS

The diaphysis is the principal portion of the long bone and is extremely vascular in the newborn. With further growth it becomes less vascular, and the cortical bone thickens. The diaphysis grows in diameter by periosteum-mediated membranous bone formation.

BIOMECHANICAL DIFFERENCES AND CHANGES WITH GROWTH

Pediatric bone is less dense, more porous, and is penetrated by more vascular channels than adult bone.[62] It has a comparatively lower modulus of elasticity, lower bending strength, and lower mineral content.[77] Immature bone has greater porosity on cross section, and immature cortical bone has a greater number of osteon systems traversing the cortex than mature bone. The increased porosity of pediatric bone helps prevent propagation of fracture lines, explaining the infrequency of comminuted fractures in children. A comparison of load deformation curves of fractures in pediatric and adult bone shows a long plastic phase in children.[77] The porosity and rough mechanical fracture surface prolong the time and energy absorption before bone is broken. Adult bone almost always fails in tension, whereas bone in children can fail either in tension or in compression (buckle or torus fractures).[62]

When bones are bent, stress on the tension side is about the same as on the compression side. Because bone has a lower yield stress in tension than in compression, bone yields first on the tension side. As the bending continues, a crack travels across the bone from the tension side toward the

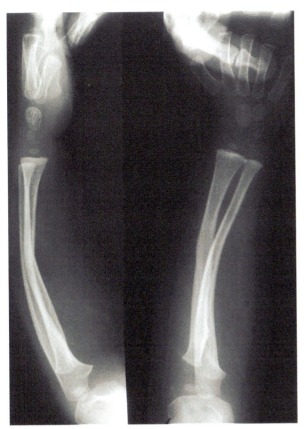

Fig. 1.11 Plastic deformation in the radius and ulna of a 2-year-old patient after a fall. The bones are plastically deformed at the midshaft, with volar compression and dorsal tension failure, but without fracture propagation.

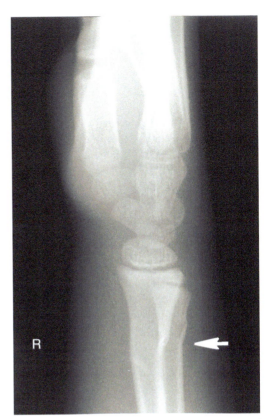

Fig. 1.12 Torus fractures usually occur at the junction (arrow) of metaphyseal and diaphyseal bone. The more porous metaphyseal bone fails in compression.

compression side. Depending on the amount of energy to be absorbed, the large pores in growing bone may stop propagation of the fracture line, which may leave a portion of the cortex intact on the compression side and result in a greenstick fracture.[1]

Bone is said to be elastic if it returns to its original shape after the load is removed. If bone does not return to its original shape and residual deformity remains after the load is released, bone has undergone plastic deformation. Incomplete failure in tension in which the fracture line does not propagate through bone results in plastic deformity of bone (Fig. 1.11). If enough plastic deformity is present in the remaining cortex, it may be necessary to complete the fracture as part of treatment. Completing the fracture is usually done by reversing the deformity so that the remaining cortex is placed under tension until it fails.[1]

CLASSIFICATION OF CHILDREN'S FRACTURES

The anatomic and biomechanical differences in the pediatric skeleton necessitate different classification systems to describe children's fractures. Pediatric fractures can be classified into five types: (1) plastic deformation, (2) buckle fractures (near the metaphysis), (3) greenstick fractures, (4) complete fractures, and (5) physeal fractures.

PLASTIC DEFORMATION

Plastic deformation of bone is essentially unique to children. It is most commonly seen in the ulna and, occasionally, the fibula. If no hematoma is formed, periosteal elevation and significant callus formation may not occur to promote remodeling, and the bone may be permanently deformed. If the deformity occurs in a child younger than 4 years or if the deformation is less than 20 degrees, the angulation usually corrects with growth.[1] Plastic deformation that produces clinically evident deformity should usually be reduced because remodeling can be unreliable.

BUCKLE FRACTURES

A buckle fracture, also an injury primarily of childhood, is a compression failure of bone that usually occurs at the junction of the metaphysis and diaphysis. In the metaphysis, where porosity is greatest, bone in compression may be buckled by the denser bone of the diaphysis (Fig. 1.12). The more cortical diaphyseal bone may be pushed into the more porous metaphyseal bone and may create a torus fracture, so named because of its similarity to the raised band around the base of a classical Greek column.[62]

GREENSTICK FRACTURES

Greenstick fractures occur when a bone is bent, and the tension side of the bone fails. The bone begins to fracture, but the fracture line does not propagate entirely through the bone. Incomplete failure on the compression side of the bone allows plastic deformity to occur. In children, if bone undergoes plastic deformation, it does not recoil to an anatomic position and usually must be completely broken to restore normal alignment. Bone is viscoelastic, meaning that its response to loading depends on the rate at which the load is applied. Remembering this when correcting plastic deformation and greenstick fractures can be helpful because slow application of steadily increasing amounts of force over a fulcrum can result in gradual return of more normal alignment.

COMPLETE FRACTURES

Fractures that propagate completely through a bone may be described in several ways, based on the pattern of the fracture.

SPIRAL FRACTURES

Spiral fractures are usually created by a rotational force on the bone. They are typically low-velocity injuries. An intact periosteal hinge enables reduction of the fracture by reversing the rotational injury.

OBLIQUE FRACTURES

Oblique fractures occur diagonally across diaphyseal bone, usually at about 30 degrees to the axis of the bone. Analogous to complete fractures in an adult, these injuries usually cause more significant disruption of the soft tissues, including the periosteum. Because these fractures are unstable and may be difficult to hold in anatomic reduction, alignment is important. Fracture reduction is attempted by immobilizing the extremity while applying traction.

TRANSVERSE FRACTURES

Transverse fractures through pediatric bone usually occur from three-point bending and are readily reduced by use of the periosteum on the concave side of the fracture force. The periosteum on the side opposite the force is typically torn. The three-point mold type of immobilization usually maintains this diaphyseal fracture in a reduced position (Fig. 1.13).

Butterfly fragments are not common in pediatric injuries but result from a mechanism similar to that causing a transverse fracture; the butterfly fragment remains on the side of the apical force of the three-point bend. This injury occurs in the highly cortical area of the diaphysis—usually in the midshaft of the femur, tibia, or ulna (Fig. 1.14).

PHYSEAL FRACTURES

Injuries to the epiphysis of a bone almost always involve the growth plate, but most physeal fractures do not involve the epiphysis (or therefore the articular surface). Problems after injury to the growth plate are not common, but any time the physis is injured, the potential for growth disturbance exists. The distal radial physis is often cited as the most frequently injured physis.[15] Usually, the growth plate repairs well and rapidly, and most physeal injuries heal within 3 weeks. The rapid healing provides a limited window for reduction of deformity because late reduction (later than 1 week) after early physeal healing has occurred may cause physeal damage.[48,78] Damage to the plate can occur by crushing, vascular

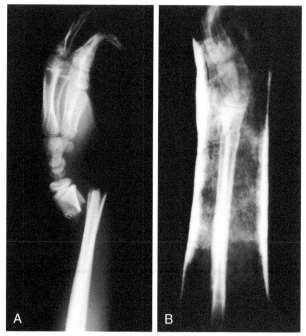

Fig. 1.13 (A and B) Lateral radiographs of a dorsally displaced transverse distal radial and ulnar fracture, which is easily reduced by use of the intact dorsal periosteum to aid in locking the distal fragments in place.

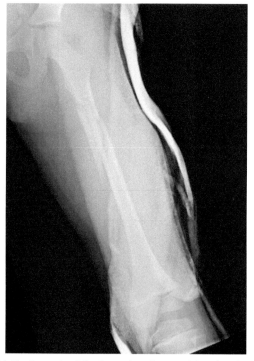

Fig. 1.14 Radiograph of the femur in a 7-year-old patient involved in a motor vehicle collision. The butterfly fragment typically lies on the side of the apical force of the three-point bend.

compromise of the physis, or bone growth bridging from the metaphysis to the bony portion of the epiphysis. The damage can result in progressive angular deformity, limb length discrepancy, or joint incongruity.

Injury to the physis has been studied extensively.[3,14,45,78] These studies show an age-dependent change in the stability

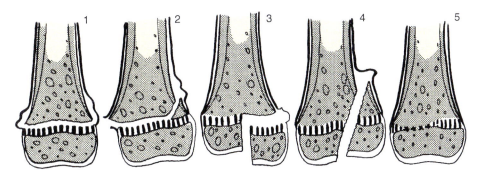

Fig. 1.15 Illustration of the Salter-Harris classification of epiphyseal injuries (see text). (From Salter RB, Harris WR. Injuries involving the epiphyseal plate. *J Bone Joint Surg Am.* 1963;45:587.)

of the epiphysis on the metaphysis. The physis and epiphyses are firmly connected externally by periosteum and internally by the mammillary processes. The physis is a hard, rubbery material that is more susceptible to injury by rotation than by angulation or traction.

Injuries involving the growth plate usually occur at the junction of calcifying cartilage cells or those that are uncalcified, although recent studies demonstrate the variability of the fracture plane within the physis.[46,47] With epiphyseal injury, the growth plate is generally attached to the epiphyseal side of the fracture, and anatomic reduction of the joint surface usually results in anatomic reduction of the growth plate. The fracture plane does not always propagate directly through the hypertrophic zone but may at some places undulate into the germinal zone of the physis or into the epiphysis or metaphysis. Changes in physeal contour are caused by the mammillary processes extending into the metaphysis and play a role in determining the fracture plane. The distal femoral growth plate is shaped such that fragments of the metaphysis are often broken off when the growth plate is injured, and its propensity for physeal bar formation may be related to its large number of mammillary processes.

Physeal injuries are usually classified by the Salter-Harris classification system,[46] which is based on the radiographic appearance of the fracture (Fig. 1.15). Injury may occur to the epiphysis, growth plate, metaphysis, or perichondrial ring.

In a type I fracture, the epiphysis separates completely from the metaphysis without any radiographically evident fracture through ossified bone. The periosteum usually remains attached to the growth plate, thereby preventing significant displacement of the epiphysis from the metaphysis. In patients with very little periosteal disruption, a slight widening of the physis may be the only radiographic sign of an injury through the physis. Although type I injuries are not usually associated with vascular change, complete separation of the capital femoral epiphysis can result in avascular necrosis and growth arrest of the proximal end of the femur. The larger the ossification center, the greater the tendency of the injury to produce a metaphyseal fragment on the compression side of the injury.

In a type II fracture, the most common Salter-Harris fracture pattern,[79] the injury passes through the growth plate and out through a portion of the metaphysis. The periosteum is usually damaged on the tension side, but the fracture leaves the periosteum intact in the region of the metaphyseal fragment. As in a type I injury, the line of fracture separation usually occurs along the hypertrophic and calcified zones of the physis. However, propagation along this junction is more variable in a type II injury. As the fracture line courses toward the compression side of the injury, it propagates through the metaphyseal area. The periosteal attachment along the metaphyseal fragment can be used to aid in reduction of the injury.

Growth disruption secondary to type I and type II injuries is infrequent, although it can occur, particularly if the circulation to the epiphysis is disrupted. Anatomic reduction is not generally required with type I and type II injuries, although one study in distal tibia fractures describes persistent gaps (>3 mm) after reduction as correlated with an increased incidence of premature physeal closure,[50] but a later study by the same group did not confirm this finding.[54] These injuries are adjacent to the joint, and the entire epiphysis is intact.

A type III fracture is intraarticular and passes through the epiphysis until it reaches the growth plate. The fracture line then courses through the growth plate to the periosteal surface. This type of fracture usually occurs when the growth plate is beginning to undergo closure. As such, problems pertaining to growth arrest may not be major. With anatomic reduction of the articular surface, the physis is usually anatomically reduced as well, and growth arrest after anatomic reduction usually does not occur.

A type IV injury is also intra-articular and involves the epiphysis as well as the metaphysis. The fracture line crosses through the growth plate. The injury is similar to a type III fracture in that the articular surface must be anatomically reduced. A more vertical split of all zones of the physis occurs, and the physis must be anatomically reduced to restore the architecture of the growth plate and minimize the risk of osseous bridge formation.

Considerable debate exists concerning type V injuries. The original type V injury as described by Salter was a crush injury to the growth plate.[14] A type V fracture cannot be recognized on initial radiographs because it appears to be a type I injury. These injuries are very uncommon, but any injury accompanied by clinical swelling and tenderness around the growth plate and associated with considerable axial load could possibly become a type V fracture, as evidenced by early closure of the physis after injury.

The Salter-Harris classification is useful as a rapid means of describing a physeal injury based on radiographic interpretation. A more complex and inclusive classification scheme was proposed by Ogden.[19,80] It includes nine types of fractures that are further divided into subtypes A through D. Peterson also developed a physeal injury classification.[19,79–82] The Ogden and Peterson classifications have not been used as often.

Other injuries to the epiphysis are avulsion injuries, commonly of the tibial spines or distal tibia (Tillaux fractures). Apophyseal injuries occur with traction injuries to tendon and muscle attachments, commonly seen in the pelvis, tibial tubercle, and medial epicondyle of the elbow. Osteochondral fractures of the articular surface of the femur, patella, and talus are among other epiphyseal injuries that do not involve the growth plate.

SUMMARY

Injury to the growing skeleton is common both as an isolated event and in a multiply injured child. Skeletal injuries in children should be treated as early as possible because they heal more rapidly than adult injuries do. Growth usually aids in the care of a traumatized extremity in that it speeds fracture healing; the mechanisms responsible for normal growth are also those that repair bone and are thus ongoing. The thick osteogenic periosteum aids in reduction of the fracture and rapidly provides a bridge over the broken bone as it ossifies.

Porous growing bone affords fracture patterns that are biomechanically different from those of adult bone but that are, in general, easier to treat. Nearly all fractures in children suitable for nonoperative treatment can be treated with a cast without worry about stiff joints or the need for physical therapy to mobilize injured joints.

Although growing bone is well equipped to deal with trauma, some injuries may damage the growth mechanisms so severely that they cannot recover. Others have that potential if the orthopedist is not wary and ready to act rapidly to restore normal anatomy for preservation of growth as well as function.

ACKNOWLEDGMENT

We would like to acknowledge and thank Dr. Eric T. Jones for his contributions to the previous versions of this chapter.

REFERENCES

The level of evidence (LOE) is determined according to the criteria provided in the Preface.

1. Mabrey JD, Fitch RD. Plastic deformation in pediatric fractures: mechanism and treatment. *J Pediatr Orthop.* 1989;9(3):310–314. **(LOE IV)**
2. Noonan KJ, Price CT. Forearm and distal radius fractures in children. *J Am Acad Orthop Surg.* 1998;6(3):146–156. **(LOE V)**.
3. Wenger DR, Pring ME, Pennock AT, Upasani VV. *Rang's Children's Fractures.* 4th ed. Philadelphia: J.B. Lippincott; 2017. **(LOE N/A)**.
4. Boutis K, Narayanan UG, Dong FF, et al. Magnetic resonance imaging of clinically suspected Salter-Harris I fracture of the distal fibula. *Injury.* 2010;41(8):852–856. **(LOE II)**.
5. Farley FA, Kuhns L, Jacobson JA, DiPietro M. Ultrasound examination of ankle injuries in children. *J Pediatr Orthop.* 2001;21(5):604–607. **(LOE II)**.
6. Wu SS, Ma CX, Carter RL, et al. Risk factors for infant maltreatment: a population-based study. *Child Abuse Negl.* 2004;28(12):1253–1264. **(LOE II)**.
7. Davidson RS, Markowitz RI, Dormans J, Drummond DS. Ultrasonographic evaluation of the elbow in infants and young children after suspected trauma. *J Bone Joint Surg Am.* 1994;76(12):1804–1813. **(LOE II)**.
8. Barber I, Perez-Rossello JM, Wilson CR, Kleinman PK. The yield of high-detail radiographic skeletal surveys in suspected infant abuse. *Pediatr Radiol.* 2015;45(1):69–80. **(LOE IV)**.
9. Podolnick JD, Donovan DS, Atanda AW Jr. Incidence of delayed diagnosis of orthopaedic injury in pediatric trauma patients. *J Orthop Trauma.* 2017;31(9):e281–e287. **(LOE IV)**.
10. Heinrich SD, Gallagher D, Harris M, Nadell JM. Undiagnosed fractures in severely injured children and young adults. Identification with technetium imaging. *J Bone Joint Surg Am.* 1994;76(4):561–572. **(LOE II)**.
11. Nguyen A, Hart R. Imaging of non-accidental injury; what is clinical best practice? *J Med Radiat Sci.* 2018;65(2):123–130. **(LOE V)**.
12. Boutis K, Plint A, Stimec J, et al. Radiograph-negative lateral ankle injuries in children: occult growth plate fracture or sprain? *JAMA Pediatr.* 2016;170(1):e154114. **(LOE II)**.
13. Neer CS 2nd, Horwitz BS. Fractures of the proximal humeral epiphysial plate. *Clin Orthop Relat Res.* 1965;41:24–31. **(LOE IV)**.
14. Ogden JA. Injury to the growth mechanisms of the immature skeleton. *Skeletal Radiol.* 1981;6(4):237–253. **(LOE IV)**.
15. Randsborg PH, Gulbrandsen P, Saltyte Benth J, et al. Fractures in children: epidemiology and activity-specific fracture rates. *J Bone Joint Surg Am.* 2013;95(7):e42. **(LOE II)**.
16. King J, Diefendorf D, Apthorp J, Negrete VF, Carlson M. Analysis of 429 fractures in 189 battered children. *J Pediatr Orthop.* 1988;8(5):585–589. **(LOE IV)**.
17. Kleinman PK, Nimkin K, Spevak MR, et al. Follow-up skeletal surveys in suspected child abuse. *AJR Am J Roentgenol.* 1996;167(4):893–896. **(LOE IV)**.
18. Alman BA. The immature skeleton. In: Flynn JM, Skaggs DL, Waters PM, eds. *Rockwood and Wilkins' Fractures in Children.* 8th ed. Philadelphia: J.B. Lippincott; 2014:1–86. **(LOE N/A)**.
19. Ogden JA. Anatomy and physiology of skeletal development. *Skeletal Injury in the Child.* 3rd ed. New York: Springer; 2000:1–37. **(LOE N/A)**.
20. Lampl M, Veldhuis JD, Johnson ML. Saltation and stasis: a model of human growth. *Science.* 1992;258(5083):801–803. **(LOE II)**.
21. Noonan KJ, Farnum CE, Leiferman EM, Lampl M, Markel MD, Wilsman NJ. Growing pains: are they due to increased growth during recumbency as documented in a lamb model? *J Pediatr Orthop.* 2004;24(6):726–731. **(LOE N/A)**.
22. Grauer JN, ed. *Orthopaedic Knowledge Update.* Vol. 12. Rosemont, IL: American Academy of Orthopaedic Surgeons; 2017. **(LOE N/A)**.
23. Brighton CT. The growth plate and its dysfunctions. *Instr Course Lect.* (36):3–25. **(LOE N/A)**.
24. Buckwalter JA, Glimcher MJ, Cooper RR, Recker R. Bone biology. I: Structure, blood supply, cells, matrix, and mineralization. *Instr Course Lect.* 1996;45:371–386. **(LOE N/A)**.
25. O'Keefe RJ, Jacobs JJ, Chu CR, Einhorn TA, eds. *Orthopaedic Basic Science: Foundation of Clinical Practice.* 4th ed. Rosemont, IL: American Academy of Orthopaedic Surgeons; 2018. **(LOE N/A)**.
26. Karsenty G. The complexities of skeletal biology. *Nature.* 2003;423(6937):316–318. **(LOE N/A)**.
27. Teunissen M, Riemers FM, van Leenen D, et al. Growth plate expression profiling: large and small breed dogs provide new insights in endochondral bone formation. *J Orthop Res.* 2018;36(1):138–148. **(LOE N/A)**.
28. Ballock RT, O'Keefe RJ. The biology of the growth plate. *J Bone Joint Surg Am.* 2003;85-A(4):715–726. **(LOE N/A)**.
29. Kronenberg HM. Developmental regulation of the growth plate. *Nature.* 2003;423(6937):332–336. **(LOE N/A)**.
30. Ornitz DM, Legeai-Mallet L. Achondroplasia: development, pathogenesis, and therapy. *Dev Dyn.* 2017;246(4):291–309. **(LOE N/A)**.
31. Ballock RT, Reddi AH. Thyroxine is the serum factor that regulates morphogenesis of columnar cartilage from isolated chondrocytes in chemically defined medium. *J Cell Biol.* 1994;126(5):1311–1318. **(LOE N/A)**.
32. Mehlman CT, Araghi A, Roy DR. Hyphenated history: the Hueter-Volkmann law. *Am J Orthop (Belle Mead NJ).* 1997;26(11):798–800. **(LOE N/A)**.
33. Arkin AM, Katz JF. The effects of pressure on epiphyseal growth; the mechanism of plasticity of growing bone. *J Bone Joint Surg Am.* 1956;38-A(5):1056–1076. **(LOE V)**.
34. Yu YY, Lieu S, Lu C, Miclau T, Marcucio RS, Colnot C. Immunolocalization of BMPs, BMP antagonists, receptors, and effectors during fracture repair. *Bone.* 2010;46(3):841–851. **(LOE N/A)**.

35. Ashraf N, Meyer MH, Frick S, Meyer RA Jr. Evidence for overgrowth after midfemoral fracture via increased RNA for mitosis. *Clin Orthop Relat Res.* 2007;454:214–222. **(LOE N/A).**

36. Heiner DE, Meyer MH, Frick SL, Kellam JF, Fiechtl J, Meyer RA Jr. Gene expression during fracture healing in rats comparing intramedullary fixation to plate fixation by DNA microarray. *J Orthop Trauma.* 2006;20(1):27–38. **(LOE N/A).**

37. Einhorn TA. Enhancement of fracture-healing. *J Bone Joint Surg Am.* 1995;77(6):940–956. **(LOE N/A).**

38. Tonna EA, Cronkite EP. Use of tritiated thymidine for the study of the origin of the osteoclast. *Nature.* 1961;190:459–460. **(LOE N/A).**

39. Tonna EA, Cronkite EP. Autoradiographic studies of cell proliferation in the periosteum of intact and fractured femora of mice utilizing DNA labeling with H3-thymidine. *Proc Soc Exp Biol Med.* 1961;107:719–721. **(LOE N/A).**

40. Perren SM. Evolution of the internal fixation of long bone fractures. The scientific basis of biological internal fixation: choosing a new balance between stability and biology. *J Bone Joint Surg Br.* 2002;84(8):1093–1110. **(LOE N/A).**

41. Axelrad TW, Einhorn TA. Use of clinical assessment tools in the evaluation of fracture healing. *Injury.* 2011;42(3):301–305. **(LOE N/A).**

42. Cappello T, Nuelle JA, Katsantonis N, et al. Ketorolac administration does not delay early fracture healing in a juvenile rat model: a pilot study. *J Pediatr Orthop.* 2013;33(4):415–421. **(LOE N/A).**

43. DePeter KC, Blumberg SM, Dienstag Becker S, Meltzer JA. Does the use of ibuprofen in children with extremity fractures increase their risk for bone healing complications? *J Emerg Med.* 2017;52(4):426–432. **(LOE IV).**

44. Kay RM, Directo MP, Leathers M, Myung K, Skaggs DL. Complications of ketorolac use in children undergoing operative fracture care. *J Pediatr Orthop.* 2010;30(7):655–658. **(LOE IV).**

45. Dale GG, Harris WR. Prognosis of epiphysial separation: an experimental study. *J Bone Joint Surg Br.* 1958;40-B(1):116–122. **(LOE IV).**

46. Salter RB. Injuries of the epiphyseal plate. *Instr Course Lect.* 1992;41:351–359. **(LOE N/A).**

47. Wattenbarger JM, Gruber HE, Phieffer LS. Physeal fractures, part I: histologic features of bone, cartilage, and bar formation in a small animal model. *J Pediatr Orthop.* 2002;22(6):703–709. **(LOE N/A).**

48. Aitkin A. Further observation on the fractured radial epiphysis. *J Bone Joint Surg Am.*;17:922–927. **(LOE IV).**

49. Lee MA, Nissen TP, Otsuka NY. Utilization of a murine model to investigate the molecular process of transphyseal bone formation. *J Pediatr Orthop.* 2000;20(6):802–806. **(LOE N/A).**

50. Barmada A, Gaynor T, Mubarak SJ. Premature physeal closure following distal tibia physeal fractures: a new radiographic predictor. *J Pediatr Orthop.* 2003;23(6):733–739. **(LOE IV).**

51. Gruber HE, Phieffer LS, Wattenbarger JM. Physeal fractures, part II: fate of interposed periosteum in a physeal fracture. *J Pediatr Orthop.* 2002;22(6):710–716. **(LOE N/A).**

52. Wattenbarger JM, Marshall A, Cox MD, Gruber H. The role of the basement plate in physeal bar formation. *J Pediatr Orthop.* 2018;38(10):e634–e639. **(LOE N/A).**

53. Crawford SN, Lee LS, Izuka BH. Closed treatment of overriding distal radial fractures without reduction in children. *J Bone Joint Surg Am.* 2012;94(3):246–252. **(LOE II).**

54. Russo F, Moor MA, Mubarak SJ, Pennock AT. Salter-Harris II fractures of the distal tibia: does surgical management reduce the risk of premature physeal closure? *J Pediatr Orthop.* 2013;33(5):524–529. **(LOE IV).**

55. Gerstenfeld LC, Cullinane DM, Barnes GL, Graves DT, Einhorn TA. Fracture healing as a post-natal developmental process: molecular, spatial, and temporal aspects of its regulation. *J Cell Biochem.* 2003;88(5):873–884. **(LOE N/A).**

56. Cozen L. Knock-knee deformity after fracture of the proximal tibia in children. *Orthopedics.* 1959;1:230–234. **(LOE IV).**

57. Green NE. Tibia valga caused by asymmetrical overgrowth following a nondisplaced fracture of the proximal tibial metaphysis. *J Pediatr Orthop.* 1983;3(2):235–237. **(LOE IV).**

58. Ogden JA, Ogden DA, Pugh L, Raney EM, Guidera KJ. Tibia valga after proximal metaphyseal fractures in childhood: a normal biologic response. *J Pediatr Orthop.* 1995;15(4):489–494. **(LOE IV).**

59. Halanski MA, Yildirim T, Chaudhary R, Chin MS, Leiferman E. Periosteal fiber transection during periosteal procedures is crucial to accelerate growth in the rabbit model. *Clin Orthop Relat Res.* 2016;474(4):1028–1037. **(LOE N/A).**

60. Lee TM, Mehlman CT. Hyphenated history: Park-Harris growth arrest lines. *Am J Orthop (Belle Mead NJ).* 2003;32(8):408–411. **(LOE N/A).**

61. Ogden JA. Growth slowdown and arrest lines. *J Pediatr Orthop.* 1984;4(4):409–415. **(LOE N/A).**

62. Light TR, Ogden DA, Ogden JA. The anatomy of metaphyseal torus fractures. *Clin Orthop Relat Res.* 1984;188:103–111. **(LOE N/A).**

63. Loizidou A, Andronikou S, Burren CP. Pamidronate "zebra lines": a treatment timeline. *Radiol Case Rep.* 2017;12(4):850–853. **(LOE N/A).**

64. Sarraf KM. Images in clinical medicine. Radiographic zebra lines from cyclical pamidronate therapy. *N Engl J Med.* 2011;365(3):e5. **(LOE IV).**

65. Blount W. *Fractures in Children.* Baltimore: Williams & Wilkins. **(LOE N/A).**

66. Wilkins KE. Principles of fracture remodeling in children. *Injury.* 2005;36(suppl 1):A3–A11. **(LOE N/A).**

67. Abraham E. Remodeling potential of long bones following angular osteotomies. *J Pediatr Orthop.* 1989;9(1):37–43. **(LOE N/A).**

68. Edvardsen P, Syversen SM. Overgrowth of the femur after fracture of the shaft in childhood. *J Bone Joint Surg Br.* 1976;58(3):339–342. **(LOE IV).**

69. Davids JR. Rotational deformity and remodeling after fracture of the femur in children. *Clin Orthop Relat Res.* 1994;(302):27–35. **(LOE IV).**

70. Wallace ME, Hoffman EB. Remodelling of angular deformity after femoral shaft fractures in children. *J Bone Joint Surg Br.* 1992;74(5):765–769. **(LOE IV).**

71. Beckman F, Sullivan J. Some observations of fractures of long bones in children. *Am J Surg.* 1941;51:722–741. **(LOE V).**

72. Thomas DP, Howard AW, Cole WG, Hedden DM. Three weeks of Kirschner wire fixation for displaced lateral condylar fractures of the humerus in children. *J Pediatr Orthop.* 2001;21(5):565–569. **(LOE IV).**

73. Tisosky AJ, Werger MM, McPartland TG, Bowe JA. The factors influencing the refracture of pediatric forearms. *J Pediatr Orthop.* 2015;35(7):677–681. **(LOE IV).**

74. Gamble JG, Zino C, Imrie MN, Young JL. Trans-metaphyseal screws placed in children: an argument for monitoring and potentially removing the implants. *J Pediatr Orthop.* 2019;39(1):e28–e31. **(LOE IV).**

75. Ezzat A, Iobst C. Extreme femoral valgus and patella dislocation following lateral plate fixation of a pediatric femur fracture. *J Pediatr Orthop B.* 2016;25(4):381–384. **(LOE V).**

76. Kelly B, Heyworth B, Yen YM, Hedequist D. Adverse sequelae due to plate retention following submuscular plating for pediatric femur fractures. *J Orthop Trauma.* 2013;27(12):726–729. **(LOE IV).**

77. Currey JD, Butler G. The mechanical properties of bone tissue in children. *J Bone Joint Surg Am.* 1975;57(6):810–814. **(LOE N/A).**

78. Egol KA, Karunakar M, Phieffer L, Meyer R, Wattenbarger JM. Early versus late reduction of a physeal fracture in an animal model. *J Pediatr Orthop.* 2002;22(2):208–211. **(LOE N/A).**

79. Peterson HA, Madhok R, Benson JT, Ilstrup DM, Melton LJ 3rd. Physeal fractures: Part 1. Epidemiology in Olmsted County, Minnesota, 1979-1988. *J Pediatr Orthop.* 1994;14(4):423–430. **(LOE IV).**

80. Ogden JA. Injury to the growth mechanisms. *Skeletal Injury in the Child.* 3rd ed. New York: Springer; 2000:147–208. **(LOE N/A).**

81. Peterson HA. Physeal fractures: Part 3. Classification. *J Pediatr Orthop.* 1994;14(4):439–448. **(LOE IV).**

82. Peterson HA. Physeal fractures: Part 2. Two previously unclassified types. *J Pediatr Orthop.* 1994;14(4):431–438. **(LOE V).**

2 Physeal Injuries

Amirhossein Misaghi | Jonathan G. Schoenecker | Alexandre Arkader

INTRODUCTION

Preservation of the structure and function of the growth plate, or physis, is essential for normal growth. Physes are composed of cartilage. They may be weaker than surrounding bone and ligaments and therefore are prone to injuries in tension or shear. Different physes respond differently to injury, and each must be approached as a distinct entity; careful attention should be paid to the child's age, the growth potential of the affected area, the location, and the type of injury. Long-term complications of physeal injuries include growth arrest and progressive angular deformities, and these are often best managed with early recognition.

RELEVANT BASIC SCIENCE

The physis is the primary center for skeletal growth of long bones and should be distinguished from the epiphysis, or secondary ossification center. Physes have been described as either pressure (compression) or traction (tensile) responsive; the latter are also referred to as apophyses. Primary physes are initially discoid areas of rapidly maturing cartilage, but with increasing biomechanical stress, especially shear stress, they undergo changes in contour known as undulations.[1] Planar physes contribute primarily to longitudinal growth, and spherical physes contribute almost exclusively to circumferential expansion of bone. The physes also differ in morphology according to their skeletal location. The rapidly growing distal femoral physis, for example, has elongated cell columns, in contrast to the shortened cell column formation in the slowly growing phalangeal physis.

Cartilage cells grow continually toward the side of the physis facing the epiphysis of a long bone, whereas on the metaphyseal side, cartilage is continually replaced by bone. When growth is complete, the physes are resorbed and replaced by primary spongiosa (bone) that fuses the epiphysis permanently to the metaphysis. In males, most physes are closed at about 18 years of age, although the medial clavicle physis may not close until age 25 years; in females, growth in the length of the bones ceases about 2 years earlier.

The physis can be divided into zones according to its function (Fig. 2.1).[2] In the resting and proliferative layers, the cells are relatively small and surrounded by a mechanically strong, thick layer of matrix. It is in the resting layer that germinal cells of stem cell origin are found. They exist in an area of low oxygen tension and respond to circulating hormones. As the cells proliferate, they appear as thin disks and palisades. In the extracellular matrix, longitudinal orientation of the collagen fibers occurs. This is an area of high oxygen tension. With hypertrophy of the chondrocytes (to 5–10 times their original size), there is physically less space for the extracellular matrix and its strengthening effect. The hypertrophic zone is therefore the weakest layer of the physis under tension, shear, and bending stress,[3] and it is the most common area for fractures. In the zone of provisional calcification, metaphyseal vascular invasion allows mineralization of the matrix to occur, and programmed cell death of the chondrocytes is initiated. With the vascular invasion come osteoblasts and osteoclasts, allowing the formation of the primary spongiosa and its subsequent remodeling to more mature secondary spongiosa that no longer contains remnants of the cartilaginous precursor.

The physis is connected to the epiphysis and metaphysis peripherally via the zone of Ranvier and the perichondral ring of LaCroix. The zone of Ranvier is a circumferential notch containing cells (i.e., osteoblasts, chondrocytes, and fibroblasts), fibers, and a bony lamina located at the periphery of the physis. It also contributes to latitudinal or

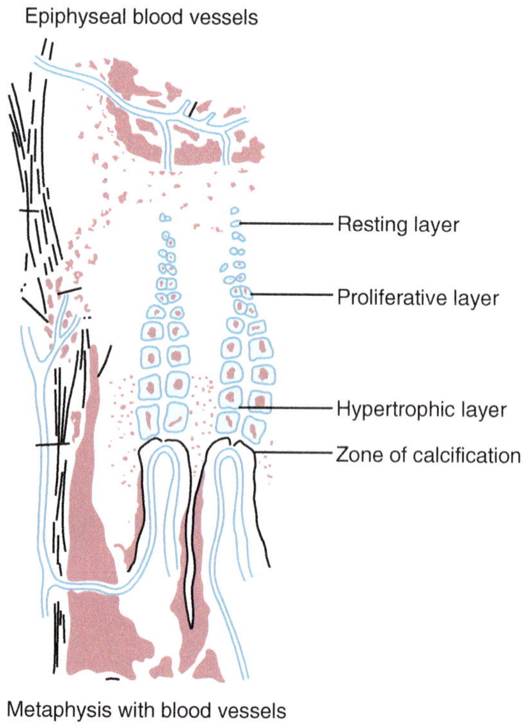

Fig. 2.1 Diagrammatic representation of the zones of the physis. (From Ramachandran M: *Basic orthopaedic sciences: the Stanmore guide,* New York, 2007, Oxford University Press.)

appositional growth. The periosteal sleeve is firmly attached to each end of a bone at the zone of Ranvier and the perichondrium of the epiphysis, and is thought to be an anatomic restraint to rapid, uncontrolled longitudinal growth.[4,5] The perichondral ring of LaCroix is a strong, fibrous structure that secures the epiphysis to the metaphysis.

There are three sources of blood supply to the physis: the epiphyseal, metaphyseal, and perichondral circulations. The epiphyseal vessels (arteries, veins, and capillary network) disperse throughout the chondroepiphysis, except for the avascular articular cartilage region, within cartilage channels, occasionally communicating with the metaphyseal circulation. The pattern of this vascular network may be of two types.[6] In type A epiphyses, which are covered almost entirely by articular cartilage, the blood supply enters from the metaphyseal side of the physis and is therefore prone to injury during epiphyseal separation. The proximal femur and proximal radius are the only two type A epiphyses. In type B epiphyses, which are only partially covered by articular cartilage, the blood supply enters from the epiphyseal side of the physis and is therefore protected from injury during epiphyseal separation.

The metaphysis contributes to the strength of the physis by way of its trabeculae, although these are susceptible to compressive forces. When the epiphysis is mainly cartilaginous, it acts as a shock absorber. As the epiphysis ossifies, its shock-absorbing ability diminishes.

EPIDEMIOLOGY

Physeal injuries have been reported to occur in approximately 30% of children's long bone fractures.[7] They are twice as common in boys as in girls, possibly because the physes are open for a longer period of time in boys, and boys participate in more risk-taking behavior and athletics. Most physeal injuries occur between the ages of 12 and 16 in boys and between the ages of 10 and 12 in girls. The most common physeal fractures involve the phalanges of the fingers, distal radius, and distal tibia. Distal physes tend to be injured more frequently than proximal physes. Injuries occur approximately equally on right and left limbs, and upper limbs tend to be more commonly injured than lower limbs.

MECHANISM OF INJURY

The mechanism depends on the age of the child. The physis is relatively thick in infancy and childhood and is therefore more prone to injury secondary to shear or tensile forces. In older children and adolescents, a fracture–separation of the physis is more common and occurs as the result of a combination of shear and compressive forces. Intraarticular fractures may also be caused by transient or near dislocation of a joint secondary to a tensile or shear force. Compressive forces may be transmitted to the physis secondary to severe abduction or adduction, angular forces applied to a joint that normally only flexes and extends.

Repetitive microtrauma can also injure the physis, as seen in examples such as Little League elbow and gymnast wrist. Other mechanisms of injury include iatrogenic causes (e.g., insertion of hardware, medications, or irradiation),

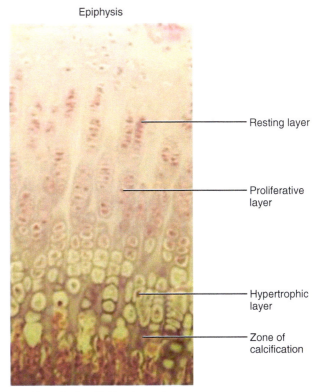

Epiphysis

Resting layer

Proliferative layer

Hypertrophic layer

Zone of calcification

Metaphysis with blood vessels

Fig. 2.2 Zones of the physis as seen on histologic examination.

diseases including infections and neoplasms, vascular insults, and thermal injuries such as those caused by frostbite or lightning.

CONSEQUENCES OF INJURY

The most characteristic consequence of a physeal injury is the disruption or cessation of longitudinal bone growth. Complete growth arrest can result in significant limb length inequality with functional impairment. Partial growth arrest can lead to angular deformities. Other consequences of physeal injuries include nonunion (e.g., after a lateral humeral condylar fracture), malunion, and avascular necrosis.

The prognosis for future growth is dependent on the type and mechanism of injury and on the location of the injury within the physis (Fig. 2.2). If the fracture is limited to the hypertrophic layer, healing is usually uncomplicated. If the fracture line involves the resting zone or affects multiple zones of the physis, growth disturbance is far more likely.[8] Although the exact mechanism that leads to physeal bar formation is unclear, Gruber et al hypothesize that injury to the basement plate of the physis results in an inability of the physis to heal itself and thus to subsequent physeal bar formation.[9] Also, physeal bar formation may occur when the layers of the physis are not realigned properly, leading to bony bar formation between the bone of the metaphysis and that of the epiphysis.

ASSOCIATED INJURIES

Neurovascular and ligamentous structures adjacent to the physis may be injured as a result of physeal fractures.

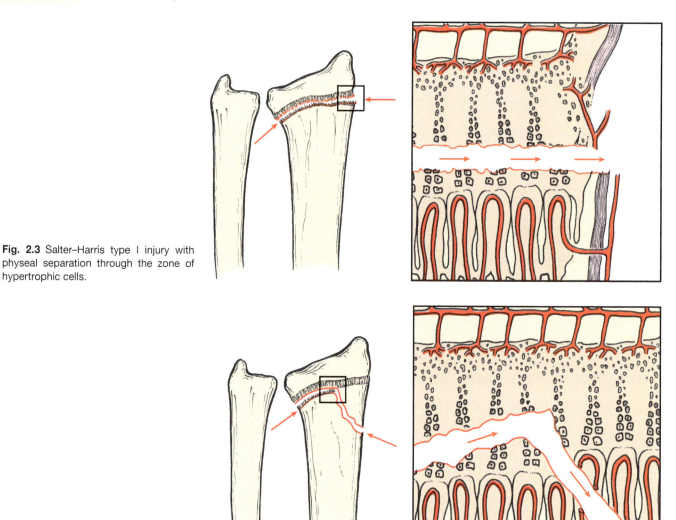

Fig. 2.3 Salter–Harris type I injury with physeal separation through the zone of hypertrophic cells.

Fig. 2.4 Salter–Harris type II injury, similar to type I but with a metaphyseal spike (known as the Thurston–Holland sign).

Ligamentous injuries that result in physeal avulsion occur most often at the tibial spine, at the ulnar styloid, and in the phalanges. Combinations of physeal injury and ligamentous disruption are most common in the knee, such as tibial spine avulsion associated with anterior cruciate ligament avulsion.

Compartment syndrome is not commonly associated with physeal fractures but has been reported with proximal and distal tibial fractures. A displaced distal radius physeal injury can lead to acute carpal tunnel syndrome. Joint dislocation or an ipsilateral shaft fracture is seen most frequently with medial epicondylar fractures about the elbow, approximately half of which are associated with partial or complete elbow dislocation.

CLASSIFICATION

A number of classification systems have been described for physeal fractures, including those by Aitken, Li et al, Ogden, and Poland.[10–13] The most widely used classification, however, is the Salter–Harris (SH) system described in 1963.[8] It is based on the relationship of the fracture line to the layers of the physis, and it has prognostic value with respect

to subsequent growth disturbance. Five types of fractures are described in the classification. The first four types are, in fact, combinations of those injuries described by Poland[13] (types I to III) and Aitken[10] (types I to III), and the last type was added by Salter and Harris.

An SH type I (SH I) fracture occurs entirely through the zone of hypertrophic cells, but the surrounding bone is not fractured. This may result in complete separation of the epiphysis from the metaphysis (Fig. 2.3). Because the resting layer remains with the epiphysis, growth is usually undisturbed unless there is damage to the epiphyseal blood supply (e.g., proximal femoral epiphyseal traumatic separation).

SH II injuries are similar to type I, except that the fracture line exits through the metaphysis on the compression side of the fracture (Thurston–Holland fragment) (Fig. 2.4). The periosteum remains intact on the metaphyseal side of the fragment and provides stability once the fracture has been reduced. Again, growth disturbance is unusual because the resting layer is intact. This pattern is the most common type.

SH III fractures are intraarticular injuries with a fracture line running through the epiphysis and exiting through the physis (Fig. 2.5). There is a high risk of growth arrest, and any displacement needs to be corrected.

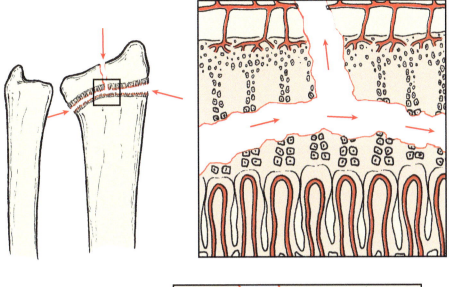

Fig. 2.5 Salter–Harris type III injury with physeal separation and extension across the epiphysis into the joint.

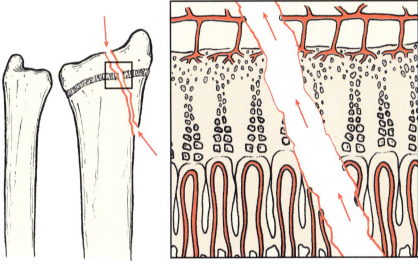

Fig. 2.6 Salter–Harris type IV injury with a metaphyseal spike; the physis and epiphysis are both involved.

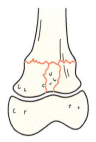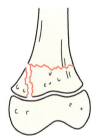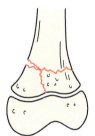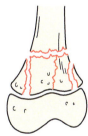

Fig. 2.7 Peterson type I injuries of the metaphysis, with various patterns of extension to the physis.

SH IV injuries involve a fracture through the metaphysis, physis, and epiphysis (Fig. 2.6). Because the fracture line crosses the resting layer and enters the joint, anatomic reduction is necessary to prevent articular incongruity and osseous bridging across the physis. The risk of growth arrest is high.

SH V fractures involve a compression or crushing injury to the physis. They are rare and cannot be immediately diagnosed because of the lack of radiographic signs. These fractures are recognized once a growth disturbance occurs.

Certain physeal injuries do not fit into the SH classification scheme. Rang[14] described an injury to the perichondral ring of LaCroix, naming it a type VI physeal injury.

This is most often seen in injuries about the medial malleolus caused by lawnmowers or after an individual has been dragged along the street by a motor vehicle. Peterson introduced a novel classification in 1994 based on a review of 951 fractures.[15] Although there are similarities to the SH scheme, two previously undescribed injury types were added. In a Peterson type I fracture, seen commonly in the distal radius, a transverse fracture of the metaphysis occurs with longitudinal extension into the physis (Fig. 2.7). In a Peterson type VI fracture, an open injury occurs, associated with loss of a portion of the physis. Peterson recommended emergent treatment in the form of débridement, often with wound packing, and secondary closure, occasionally with a skin graft or flap closure for this type of fracture. This fracture type may also require later reconstructive surgery as a result of premature physeal closure and bar formation on the exposed bone surface (Fig. 2.8).

DIAGNOSIS

Most children with physeal injuries can recall a specific traumatic event and can localize their symptoms to a specific anatomic region. The most common symptoms are pain and localized tenderness; swelling and effusion are variable signs depending on the severity of the injury. Nontraumatic physeal injuries, such as infection, neoplasia, or congenital conditions, are usually evident from the history.

Orthogonal radiographs, most often anteroposterior and lateral, are usually sufficient to diagnose the physeal injury and plan treatment. Some physeal injuries may not be visible on standard views because of the irregular contour and chondro-osseous nature of the physis. Slight physeal widening may be the only sign of minimal displacement of an epiphyseal fragment. The Thurston–Holland metaphyseal fragment may sometimes be difficult to appreciate. Comparison radiographs of the contralateral extremity may be helpful for diagnosis, particularly for nondisplaced or minimally displaced SH type I and II fractures. Occasionally, stress views can help to demonstrate gapping between the epiphysis and metaphysis, particularly in injuries about uniplanar joints such as the knee, ankle, and elbow. However, alternatives such as magnetic resonance imaging (MRI) (Fig. 2.9) or repeated radiographs 10 days after immobilization and protection can allow the diagnosis to be made without causing the patient discomfort.

Imaging modalities that can be used for diagnosis include arthrography, MRI, ultrasound, and computed tomography (CT). Arthrography can be helpful in diagnosing fractures in areas where there is a large volume of cartilage, such as the distal humerus, although MRI and ultrasound are increasingly being used to evaluate such injuries. MRI is particularly useful in diagnosing occult fractures about the physis when plain radiography is negative. In a prospective study evaluating injuries to the elbow, distal femur, and distal tibia in children age 3 to 15 years with negative plain radiographs, MRI was able to detect a fracture in 34.8% of patients.[16] Ultrasound may also be used to document soft tissue injury without fracture and has also been shown to be a safe and effective tool for evaluating SH I fractures with subperiosteal hematoma as well as other pathologies involving periosteal reaction, including infection and tumor.[17] CT is helpful in complex fracture patterns, such as triplane ankle fractures. Furthermore, MRI and CT are particularly helpful in assessing the size and location of bony bars after growth arrest.

Nonaccidental injury may be suspected from the history and examination and, occasionally, on radiographs. The pathognomonic sign of a "corner fracture" of the metaphysis (also known as a bucket-handle fracture when seen "en face") indicates the application of torsional or shear forces (such as severe twisting or wrenching) to a limb (Fig. 2.10). Note that although this finding may indicate nonaccidental trauma, it may also be a normal finding in some. Nonaccidental trauma is discussed in more detail in Chapter 20.

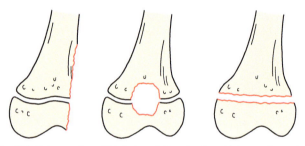

Fig. 2.8 Peterson type VI injuries of the physis, which are characterized by a portion of the physis being missing.

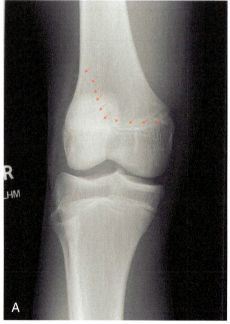
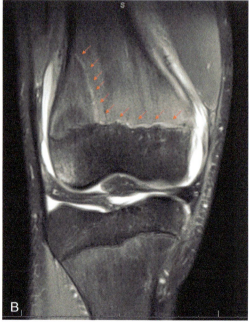

Fig. 2.9 Plain radiograph demonstrating minimally displaced Salter–Harris type II fracture of the distal femur that was initially missed (A) and then clearly identified on magnetic resonance imaging (B). Images courtesy of the Children's Hospital of Philadelphia.

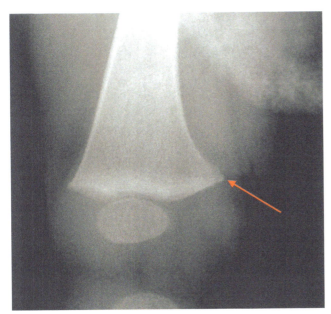

Fig. 2.10 Corner fracture of the distal femoral metaphysis, indicative of a nonaccidental injury.

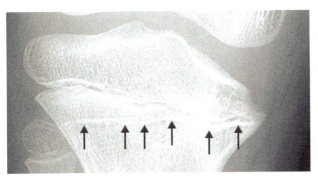

Fig. 2.11 Partial growth arrest confirmed by a Harris growth arrest line *(arrows)* lying oblique to the proximal tibial physis. (From Skaggs DL, Flynn JM: *Staying out of trouble in pediatric orthopaedics,* ed 1, Philadelphia, 2006, Lippincott Williams & Wilkins, p 320.)

Previous injury to the physis may be evident by the presence of Harris growth arrest lines, which are transverse striations in the metaphysis thought to represent a period of slowing or cessation of growth.[18] These lines may be present in either a single long bone after an isolated traumatic injury, or all long bones after a significant systemic illness. If the Harris growth arrest lines run parallel to the physis and continue to move away from the physis with time, the physis can be assumed to be growing normally after the injury. If they are asymmetric or oblique moving toward the physis, partial growth arrest is likely to have occurred (Fig. 2.11). No growth arrest lines are seen after complete physeal arrest.

TREATMENT

As with all patients with fractures, a child must be fully assessed with use of the basic ABCs (airway, breathing, and circulation) of trauma management, and all life- and limb-threatening injuries should be identified and treated. The goal of treating any physeal fracture is to obtain and maintain an acceptable reduction by closed or open means

without causing any further injury to the resting cell layer of the physis. The specific treatment of physeal injuries is dictated by several factors, such as the severity of the injury, the anatomic location, the degree of residual deformity, the amount of time elapsed from the injury, and the age of the child.

Neurovascular and open injuries can coexist with physeal fractures and must be managed first on an emergent basis before attention is turned to the physeal injury. With respect to anatomic location, the capacity for remodeling is dependent on the location of the injury within a respective long bone. For example, the proximal humeral physis contributes 80% of the longitudinal growth of the humerus and therefore has great remodeling potential.

There is no exact degree of deformity that can be defined as acceptable in children's fractures. In general, more valgus deformity can be tolerated than varus deformity, and more flexion deformity can be tolerated than extension deformity. In the lower extremity, more deformity can be tolerated proximally than distally. Angular deformities correct to the greatest extent when they are in the plane of motion of a nearby hinge joint, whereas angulation in other directions may persist to some extent. Rotational deformities do not tend to remodel.

The following numbers are approximate but worth remembering as a general guide when treating skeletal injuries in children. Most children's fractures heal twice as fast as adult fractures, and most epiphyseal separations heal in half the time of a child's long bone fracture. For example, in the tibia, an adult fracture may need 12 to 18 weeks to heal, a child's fracture may only need 6 to 9 weeks, and a pure epiphyseal separation (SH I injury) heals in only 3 to 5 weeks.

The delay between injury and treatment is an important factor. Ideally, all reductions should be performed as soon after the injury as possible. If there is a delay, the decision to perform a reduction is dependent on the age of the child and the plane and severity of the deformity. The younger the patient, the more likely the correction will be through remodeling, particularly if the angulation is in the plane of motion of the adjacent joint. If the delay is more than 7 to 10 days in an SH I or II fracture, it is safer to perform an osteotomy later on to correct the deformity than to risk damaging the physis through a traumatic reduction of a healing physeal fracture. In intraarticular SH III and IV injuries with significant intraarticular displacement, anatomic reduction must be performed regardless of the amount of time elapsed from the injury.

With respect to age, the same injury that may lead to disabling sequelae in a young child, in whom injury to the physis has a longer time to negatively impact normal growth, may result in little disability in an adolescent nearing skeletal maturity. On the other hand, if a child has several years of growth remaining and the physis has not been damaged, the majority of deformities in the plane of motion of the joint will remodel.

GENERAL PRINCIPLES

Treatment of specific physeal injuries is discussed in the relevant chapters by anatomic location, but several general principles are worth considering. If displacement is minimal or

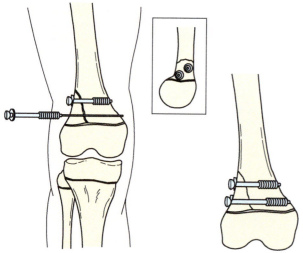

Fig. 2.12 Drawing of a Salter–Harris type II fracture of the distal femur showing screw fixation parallel to the physis through a large metaphyseal (Thurston–Holland) fragment. Depending upon fracture characteristics, fixation with threaded implants should preferably be parallel to the physis in the epiphysis and/or the metaphysis.

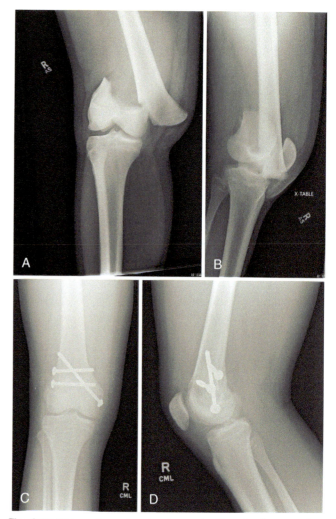

Fig. 2.13 Plain radiographs showing a significantly displaced Salter–Harris type II fracture in a near skeletally mature 130-kg male (A and B) that was treated by closed reduction and fixed percutaneously with two metaphyseal screws placed parallel to the physis plus a third transphyseal fixation for added stability to valgus stress (C and D). (Images courtesy of the Children's Hospital of Philadelphia.)

absent, or if the diagnosis is in doubt, the extremity should be immobilized and the injury reexamined in 1 or 2 weeks for a periosteal reaction indicating an SH I fracture. When a physeal fracture is reduced, traction rather than forceful manipulation is preferred, and care should be taken not to "grate" the physis on metaphyseal or epiphyseal fragments. The rule of thumb of 90% traction and 10% translation is useful. Multiple attempts at reduction may cause further physeal damage. If the fracture cannot be reduced after a few attempts with the patient under local or regional anesthesia, closed reduction under general anesthesia is the next step. If significant deformity persists after closed reduction, especially in SH III and IV fractures, open reduction and internal fixation is indicated.

Some of the anatomic landmarks surrounding the physis should be taken into consideration. The periosteum in particular is of interest. It has been shown that the periosteum around the epiphysis may be resected or reflected for more accurate exposure and reduction, but care should be taken to ensure that the fragment is not completely denuded of its soft tissue attachments, through which it receives its blood supply. Bright[19] recommended careful resection of about 1 cm of periosteum on either side of the physis to prevent bony bridge formation between the epiphysis and metaphysis; however, there is no definitive evidence to support this concept. The role of interposed periosteum in bony bridge formation is controversial. Although histologic studies in a rat model showed that in the presence of interposed periosteum the physis was able to repair itself,[20,21] clinical studies have shown that interposition of periosteum may be associated with an increased incidence of growth arrest for fractures around the ankle.[22]

When a growth plate warrants fixation for adequate stability, ideally, the fixation should be inserted parallel to the physis in the epiphysis and metaphysis (Fig. 2.12). However, at times, the need for stability will warrant transphyseal fixation (Fig. 2.13). If the patient has growth remaining, transphyseal fixation should be performed with the use of smooth rather than threaded pins (Fig. 2.14). Every physeal

fracture should be closely monitored to ensure that there is no loss of reduction. SH I and II fractures do not tend to redisplace after the second week; however, SH III and IV fractures are unstable and may redisplace up to 3 weeks after the injury.

For every growth plate injury, adequate counseling is essential. The family should be informed of the possibility of complications, which can be as high as 40% after physeal fractures of the distal femur, with 85% to 100% of SH IV and V fractures experiencing complications.[23] Follow-up should occur for at least 6 to 12 months after the injury to evaluate for growth arrest. During follow-up, Harris growth arrest lines should be examined closely to ensure that they remain parallel to the physis.

SALTER–HARRIS FRACTURES

SH I fractures are generally treated by closed reduction and immobilization without internal fixation. Healing usually occurs within 3 to 4 weeks, and complications are rare. The same is generally true of SH II injuries. The intact hinge of periosteum in SH II injuries usually aids reduction. Often, the reduction is stable because of the presence of the metaphyseal fragment and its associated intact periosteum. If reduction is unstable, the orthopedist may use pins or screws to fix the metaphyseal fragment to the metaphysis, avoiding the physis. When closed reduction is performed in the operating room, fixation is generally used to prevent loss of reduction. In distal femoral physeal fractures, fixation should always be used for any fracture requiring reduction. Thomson et al[24] demonstrated that 43% of distal femoral physeal fractures treated without internal fixation displaced, whereas no fractures with internal fixation displaced. If the metaphyseal fragment is too small, smooth pins can be used across the physis. Growth arrest is more likely in SH II fractures with larger physeal fragments, with larger degrees of displacement, in irregular undulating physes such as the distal femur and proximal tibia, and after repeated attempts at reduction.

Anatomic reduction is essential for SH III injuries, and it is most often achieved by open reduction so that the articular surfaces can be visualized. Fixation may be achieved by fixing the epiphyseal fragment across the fracture site parallel to the physis within the epiphysis (Fig. 2.15). There needs to be a high index of suspicion for an intraarticular injury in adolescents with an injury mechanism and pain because plain radiographs may show a large effusion, but the SH III fracture may be difficult to diagnose, with as many as 39% of these injuries being missed on initial plain imaging and the amount of displacement being greater than 3 versus 6 mm on further advanced imaging.[25] In SH IV injuries, open reduction and internal fixation are again usually required for alignment of the physis and articular surface if there is any displacement. Fixation is best achieved from epiphysis to epiphysis or metaphysis to metaphysis, and long-term follow-up is needed because the growth arrest rate is very high. SH V injuries are rarely diagnosed immediately, and treatment is usually delayed until growth arrest is evident.

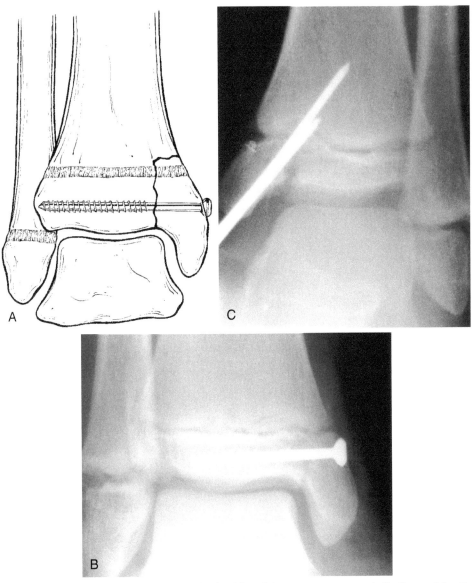

Fig. 2.14 Smooth oblique pins may be used to fix across the physis, although transverse screw or pin fixation avoiding the physis is preferred. (A) A cancellous screw should be placed in the epiphysis only, parallel to the physis. (B) Radiograph showing screw in place. (C) Smooth pins may cross the physis, as in this Salter–Harris type III fracture, even though parallel transverse pins are preferred when possible.

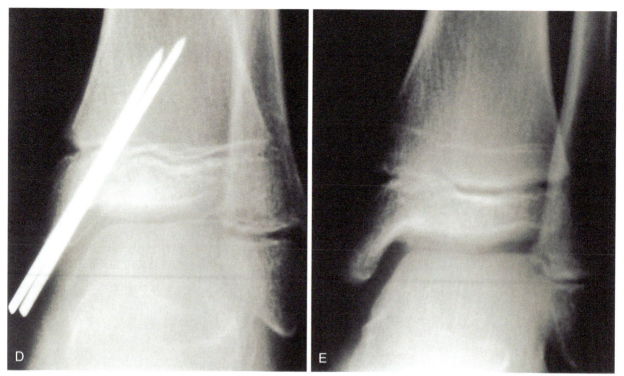

Fig. 2.14, cont'd (D) At the time of union and pin removal. (E) At 2 years, symmetric growth (note the parallel "injury line" proximally) and no bony bridge formation. (B–E, From Canale ST, Beaty JH, editors: *Operative pediatric orthopaedics,* St. Louis, 1991, Mosby-Year Book.)

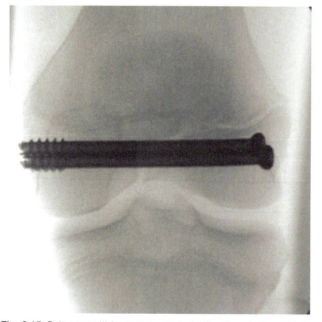

Fig. 2.15 Salter type III fracture treated with fixation wholly within the epiphysis. Ideally, washers could have been used to prevent migration of the screw heads into the soft epiphyseal bone.

ISSUES BASED ON SPECIFIC ANATOMIC LOCATION

PROXIMAL HUMERUS

The most common injuries here are SH II fractures, which often occur in younger children, rarely require fixation, and

remodel satisfactorily as long as sufficient growth remains. Rarely, if soft tissue, such as deltoid muscle, biceps tendon, or periosteum, becomes trapped at the fracture site, open reduction and/or percutaneous pin fixation may be necessary (Fig. 2.16).

DISTAL HUMERUS

Care should be taken not to confuse fracture–separations of the distal humerus with elbow dislocations or fractures of the lateral condyle (Fig. 2.17). Normal secondary ossification centers of the olecranon should not be confused with physeal fractures. The growth potential of the distal humerus is relatively small, which means it has very little remodeling potential; thus, these fractures often require reduction and fixation.

DISTAL RADIUS AND ULNA

Distal radius fractures are extremely common pediatric injuries, and most SH I and II injuries here can be treated by closed means with the use of the intact periosteal hinge to effect a closed reduction. Rarely, a periosteal flap may become interposed at the fracture site and prevent reduction, which would necessitate open reduction and internal fixation. Reduction may also be challenging to achieve in completely displaced simultaneous fractures of both the distal radius and ulna. Although growth arrest of the distal radius is rare, with rates between 1% and 7% reported, these injuries should still be followed 3 to 6 months postreduction to evaluate for premature physeal closure and possible ulnar overgrowth. Factors that may lead to physeal injury include severity of the fracture as well as attempts at reduction made greater than 7 to 10 days

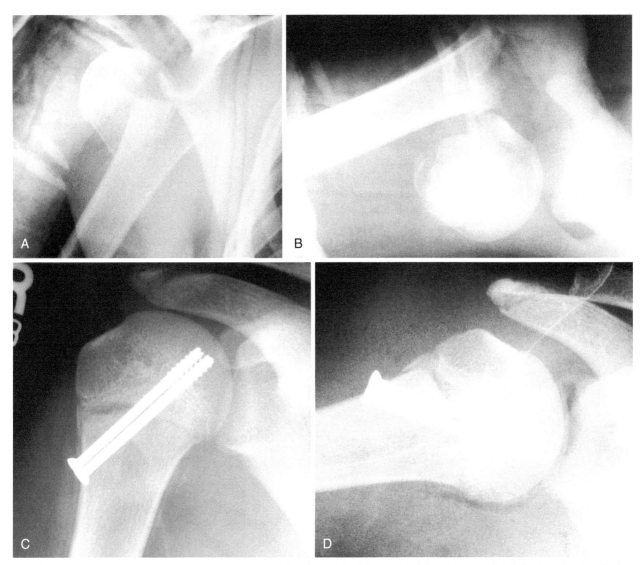

Fig. 2.16 Series of radiographs showing the remodeling potential of a proximal humeral epiphyseal separation following closed reduction and percutaneous pinning. (A and B) Anteroposterior and lateral views of the displaced proximal humeral fracture in an unacceptable position. (C and D) After limited open reduction and internal fixation.

postinjury.[26] Physeal injuries of the distal ulna may be difficult to diagnose because of the late ossification of the distal ulnar physis. In injuries to the distal radius, it is important to exclude concomitant ulnar physeal injuries, especially when an ulnar styloid or metaphyseal fracture is not readily obvious. The sequelae of ulnar physeal injuries include premature physeal closure, ulnar shortening, radial bowing, ulnar angulation of the distal radius, and ulnar translocation of the carpus.[27]

PROXIMAL FEMUR

The avascular necrosis rate is high after epiphyseal separations of the proximal femur, regardless of displacement of the fragment (Fig. 2.18). In children nearing skeletal maturity, closed reduction and pinning can be performed, and although premature physeal closure occurs, there is little functional limb length discrepancy. Urgent capsular release may be associated with a lower rate of avascular necrosis and is becoming common in many centers, although conclusive data are lacking for this approach. The treatment for this injury is unique in that rigid fixation may be placed across an open growth plate, sacrificing growth for stability and fracture healing, if needed.

DISTAL FEMUR

All SH fractures have the potential for instability. Types III and IV injuries have a high incidence of growth arrest, 50% to 85%, which should be shared with the family at presentation. The level of energy and amount of displacement are important factors in the development of growth arrest.[23]

PROXIMAL TIBIA

SH III injuries, if unrecognized, can cause premature physeal closure, with resulting varus or valgus deformity.[28] Hyperextension deformity can occur as a result of anterior physeal closure. SH I or II injuries with posterior displacement can compromise the popliteal vessels and cause compartment syndrome, even in fractures showing minimal displacement on radiographs.

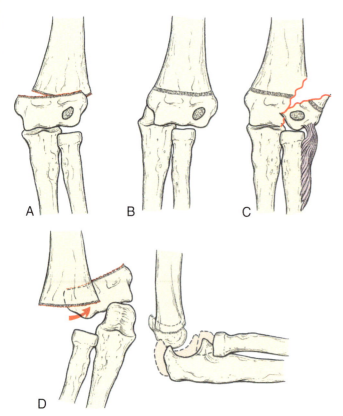

Fig. 2.17 Elbow injuries that may be confused clinically include (A), separation of the distal humeral epiphysis, (B) dislocation of the elbow, (C) fracture of the lateral condyle, and (D) fracture–separation of the distal humeral epiphysis with posteromedial displacement (note that the radial head and proximal part of the ulna are displaced as a unit in relation to the distal end of the humerus. (A–C, Modified from Mizuno K, Hirohata K, Kashiwagi D: Fracture-separation of the distal humeral epiphysis in young children. *J Bone Joint Surg Am* 61:570–573, 1979. D, Modified from Barrett WP, Almquist EA, Staheli LTJ: Fracture separation of the distal humeral physis in the newborn. *J Paediatr Orthop* 4:618, 1984.)

DISTAL TIBIA

Type I and II injuries are most often treated by closed means, but this approach has been recently questioned by one study, in which the rate of premature physeal closure was found to be 3.5 times higher (60% premature closure) in Salter I and II fractures if there was residual fracture displacement of greater than 3 mm in postreduction films.[22] The authors attributed this to interposed periosteum. These fractures often occur in older children in which a premature physeal closure may not have clinical relevance.

In type III injuries of the medial malleolus, growth disturbance has been reported in up to 38% of patients treated nonoperatively; thus, only a very low threshold is required before proceeding to an anatomic reduction via operative means, which decreases the rate of growth disturbance.[29] In type IV injuries with significant growth remaining, fixation should not cross the physis but should be from epiphysis to epiphysis and from metaphysis to metaphysis (Fig. 2.19).

OTHER MECHANISMS OF PHYSEAL INJURY

Although less common, several mechanisms of injury other than trauma can lead to partial or complete growth arrest.

It is not uncommon for radiographic results to be normal at the time of the insult but to have physeal arrest diagnosed weeks, months, or years later.

IATROGENIC INJURIES

Inadvertent surgical insult to the physis during the treatment of fractures, deformities, infection, or tumors can lead to premature growth arrest. Subperiosteal dissection adjacent or extending to the perichondral ring may injure the peripheral part of the physis, an area that is more prone to arrest than the center. At times, pathology involving the physis, such as trauma, infection, or a tumor, may have to be treated by violating part or all of the physis with resection or fixation. Steinmann pins or Kirschner wires are more likely to cause arrest if they are multiple, threaded, not perpendicular to the center of the physis, larger in diameter, or are left in for a long period of time. Screws are more likely to cause growth arrest than smooth pins. Intentional iatrogenic growth arrest may be part of the treatment for certain pediatric orthopedic conditions, such as a slipped capital femoral epiphysis.

Growth modulation utilizing staples or bridging plates and screws may lead to permanent growth arrest if devices are left in for a long period of time, if there is an iatrogenic injury to the perichondral ring at the time of insertion, or if a peripheral bone bridge forms after removal.

Although drilling across the physis can lead to growth arrest, anterior cruciate ligament reconstruction surgery can be safely done in the immature skeleton, as long as soft tissue (e.g., tendon) material is interposed in the bone tunnel[30] and screw fixation across the physis is avoided.[31] However, even procedures adjacent to the physis may lead to premature growth arrest if unrecognized iatrogenic injury occurs in the process of tunnel preparation or graft fixation because of close working relationships and proximity to the physis (Fig. 2.20).

INFECTIONS

Both osteomyelitis and septic arthritis can lead to growth arrest, and this may not be evident until late after the infection is controlled; therefore, long-term follow-up is recommended. Partial arrest is more common and may result in angular deformity and limb length discrepancy. Although the infection is brought under control when arrest is clinically noted, reactivation may occur if further surgery, such as bar excision, is needed. Systemic infections, such as meningococcal septicemia, may also lead to multicenter physeal arrest through a generalized vascular insult.[32]

NEOPLASMS

Growth arrest may occur either by direct tumor invasion of the growth plate or as a result of the treatment of tumors. The latter may be as a result of the proximity of the tumor to the physis or as a result of local (e.g., surgery or radiation therapy) or systemic treatment of a neoplastic process (e.g., chemotherapy).

Radiation therapy has a growth-inhibiting effect on the physis, primarily by alteration of chondroblastic activity. The extent of injury to the physis is determined by the age of the patient, the amount of radiation delivered, the field size, the site, and its growth potential.[33]

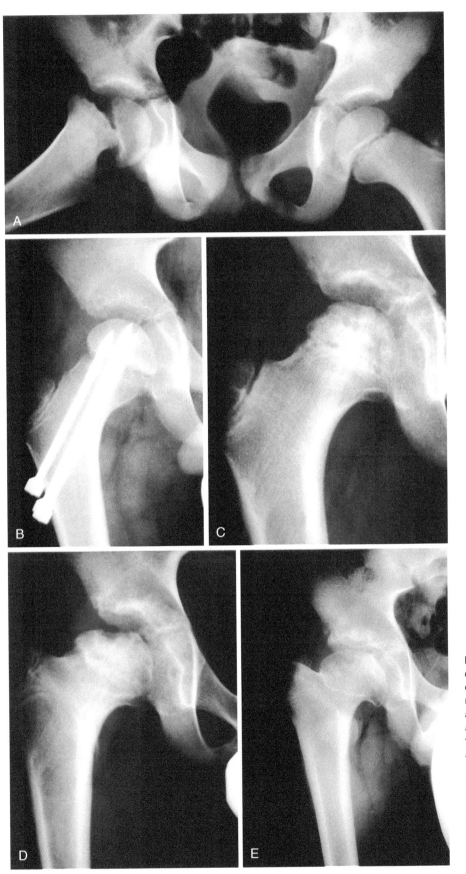

Fig. 2.18 Transepiphyseal fracture–separation of the proximal femur treated with closed reduction and pinning that resulted in avascular necrosis. (A) Type I transepiphyseal fracture in a 6-year-old child. (B) After closed reduction and fixation with smooth pins. (C) One year after the fracture, the pins have been removed, and avascular necrosis has developed. (D) During the course of abduction treatment. (E) Four years after treatment of avascular necrosis, the femoral neck is short because of premature physeal closure; however, the head is reasonably well shaped, and the result is acceptable. (A–E, From Canale ST, Beaty JH, editors: *Operative pediatric orthopaedics,* St. Louis, 1991, Mosby-Year Book.)

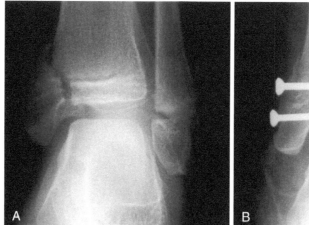
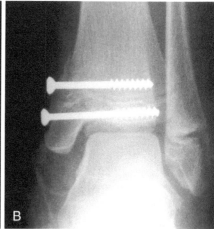

Fig. 2.19 (A) Salter–Harris type IV fracture of the distal tibia treated by open reduction, and (B) internal fixation with cancellous screws inserted parallel to the physis.

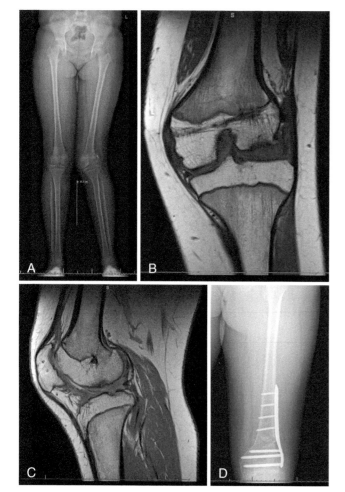

Fig. 2.20 Significant valgus deformity of the left knee (A) following anterior cruciate ligament reconstruction in a skeletally immature patient. Despite using an "all epiphyseal" technique, the magnetic resonance (MR) image shows proximity of the femoral tunnel within millimeters of the physis on coronal and sagittal MR images (B) and (C), presumably causing iatrogenic injury to the physis. (D) The resulting deformity was later corrected by opening wedge osteotomy to address valgus angulation and length deficiency. (Images courtesy of the Children's Hospital of Philadelphia.)

THERMAL INJURIES

Cold injuries such as frostbite are more often seen in the fingers and toes and may result in various skeletal changes as a result of premature closure of the physes.[34] Features include involvement of the index and little fingers, shorter and smaller phalanges than normal, and complete disappearance or a V-shaped appearance of the involved physes on radiographs. Surgical treatment is rarely needed emergently, but late sequelae such as deformities and degenerative joint disease may need intervention, such as osteotomy, arthrodesis, or resection arthroplasty. Excessive heat injuries include burns, electric shock, and those caused by laser treatment; the injuries most often damage the perichondral ring of LaCroix.

METABOLIC ABNORMALITIES

Both vitamin deficiency (e.g., vitamin C) and excess (e.g., vitamin A) can predispose to premature physeal closure.[35,36] In the case of vitamin C deficiency (scurvy), dietary replacement can spontaneously correct the condition.[35] Chronic illnesses in childhood, such as chronic renal failure, can lead to growth retardation because of impairment of growth plate chondrogenesis. This occurs as a result of a combination of inflammation, protein/calorie deprivation, uremic/metabolic acidosis, glucocorticoids, and impaired growth hormone/insulin growth factor-I axis.[37]

REPETITIVE STRESS INJURIES

Repetitive shearing or compression stresses to the physis can cause irregularity and sclerosis of the metaphysis and widening of the physis without separation, and can lead to premature physeal closure if long-standing. These changes have been described in adolescent athletes as a result of repetitive compression or distraction. Compression injuries have been reported in gymnasts, most commonly at the distal radius and ulna physes (gymnast wrist) (Fig. 2.21).[38,39] Little League shoulder is an example of a tension injury of the proximal humerus in which pain is localized to the physis during the

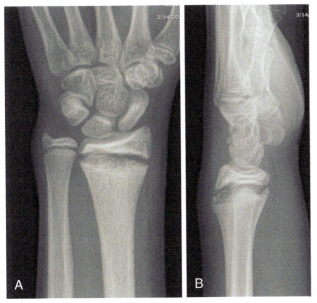

Fig. 2.21 (A) Anterior–posterior and (B) lateral radiographs of a high-level, competitive 11-year-old female gymnast complaining of chronic wrist pain of several months' duration. Note the irregularity and widening of the physis consistent with chronic/stress physeal fracture. (Images reproduced with permission from Children's Orthopaedic Center, Children's Hospital Los Angeles, Los Angeles, CA.)

follow-through phase of throwing. Also, MRI studies in elbows of Little League baseball players have shown that as many as 35% of players have signal abnormalities in their medial elbow preseason.[40] Symptoms and signs include pain and tenderness localized to the involved physis that increases with the sporting activity and is relieved by rest and painful limitation of motion at the adjacent joint. Treatment is symptomatic and involves temporary reduction or cessation of physical activity.

COMPLICATIONS

Physeal injuries may be complicated by growth disturbances, nonunion, malunion, infection, and avascular necrosis. Of these complications, only growth disturbances are unique to physeal fractures and will be further considered. Specific treatment of other complications is discussed under the individual injuries in the relevant chapters.

Growth acceleration is rare and may be caused by the injury itself or by transitory changes in the bone vascular supply, or associated with the implants used to fix the injury. It rarely leads to a significant limb length discrepancy. The types of growth arrest and their management are discussed here.

GROWTH ARREST

Growth arrest develops when there is bridging or union between the epiphysis and metaphysis. There are several factors that increase the chances of growth arrest. The greater the severity of the injury, such as from high-energy mechanism with resultant comminution, the more likely the chance of growth arrest. Injuries that cross the resting layer of the physis, such as SH III and IV, are more likely to lead to growth disturbance. Growth arrest may be partial (more common) or complete, such as seen with SH V (Fig. 2.22).[41]

EPIDEMIOLOGY

Growth arrest is twice as common in boys as in girls. The most common cause is trauma or fractures. The vast majority of cases of growth arrest are partial, and 60% are peripheral. The most frequently affected physes are the distal femur, the distal and proximal tibia, and the distal radius. Although the distal femur and proximal tibia account for only 2% of all physeal injuries, these physes are responsible for two-thirds of the lower extremity growth, and together, they are responsible for 50% of the bony bars requiring treatment.

Bone bridges may be detected within weeks to months after an injury, but it may take years until they become clinically evident. Thus, long-term follow-up is recommended for children at risk of physeal bar formation.[42] Early detection of growth arrest makes management easier because treatment can be aimed at the growth arrest rather than at its sequelae, such as angular deformity or limb length discrepancy.

PARTIAL GROWTH ARREST

This is caused by the formation of a bone bridge or bar across the physis from the metaphysis to the epiphysis. Partial growth arrest can be classified into peripheral, central, or combined.[19,42] Peripheral (type I) bars involve a variable-sized bridge along the margin of the physis, which may extend only a few millimeters in from the periphery (Fig. 2.23). This type of arrest may create very severe angular deformation over a short period of time. The clinical deformity is determined by the size, location, and duration of the bar. For example, around the knee, laterally situated bars cause a genu valgum deformity, whereas anterior bars produce genu recurvatum.

Central (type II) bars are the most difficult to treat (Figs. 2.24 and 2.25). A variable-sized bone bridge forms within the central portion of the physis surrounded by normal physis. The peripheral zone is uninvolved. Centrally located bars may cause cupping, tenting, or a dip deformity of the metaphysis and relative shortening of the bone with little, if any, angular deformity, as a result of growth of the periphery. A small central bar may eventually fail in tension because the surrounding healthy physis places it in tension, usually obviating the need for further treatment. The major effect is retardation of longitudinal growth.

Type III or combined bars (elongated) include a bone bridge extending as a linear structure across the physis, connecting two separate segments of the periphery of the physis (Fig. 2.26). The most common site is the medial malleolus. There is normal physis on both sides of the defect, including the periphery. This pattern also may be associated with significant angular deformity. In all three types, it is important to appreciate that the bone bridge usually is comprised of very dense, sclerotic bone that is similar to cortical bone. This is evident at the time of surgery, when it obviously contrasts with the adjacent trabecular bone of the metaphysis and secondary ossification center.

COMPLETE GROWTH ARREST

This is an infrequent sequela of a SH V physeal injury, and its significance depends on the age of the patient at the time of the injury. A younger child is far more likely to develop

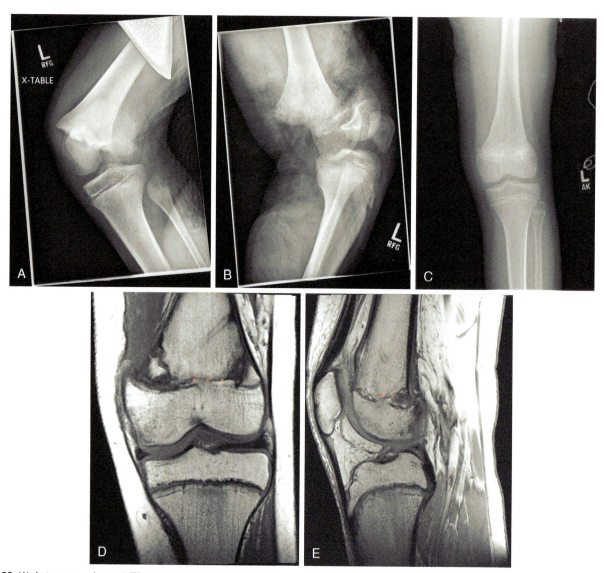

Fig. 2.22 (A) Anteroposterior and (B) lateral x-rays of a severely displaced Salter–Harris type I fracture of the distal femur that was treated by closed reduced and percutaneous pin fixation. Physeal arrest at 6 months is seen on (C) plain radiograph and (D) and (E) MRI. (Images courtesy of the Children's Hospital of Philadelphia.)

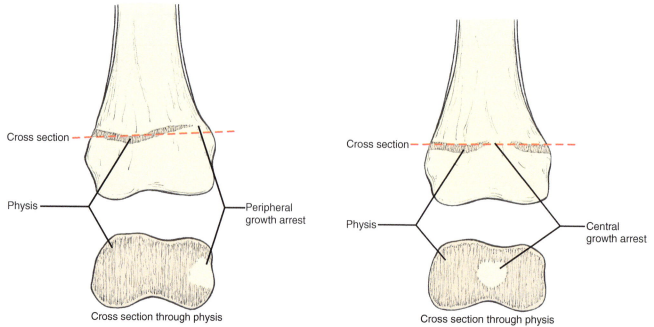

Fig. 2.23 Type I peripheral growth arrest. (Modified from Bright RW: In Rockwood CA Jr, Wilkins KE, King RE, editors: *Fractures in children,* Philadelphia, 1984, JB Lippincott.)

Fig. 2.24 Type II central growth arrest. (Modified from Bright RW: In Rockwood CA Jr, Wilkins KE, King RE, editors: *Fractures in children,* Philadelphia, 1984, JB Lippincott.)

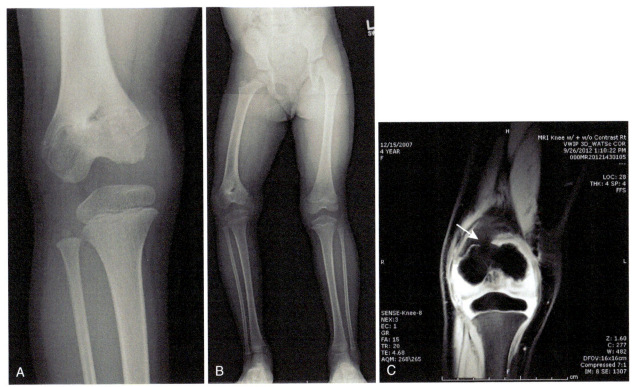

Fig. 2.25 (A) Anteroposterior knee radiograph and (B) a standing hip-to-ankle radiograph of a 4-year-old girl with a history of neonatal septic arthritis of the right knee, demonstrating a central/combined bone bridge associated with significant leg length inequality and angular deformity. (C, *arrow*) The coronal water-only selection (WATS) sequence magnetic resonance image better defines the extent of the bridge. (Images reproduced with permission from Children's Orthopaedic Center, Children's Hospital Los Angeles, Los Angeles, CA.)

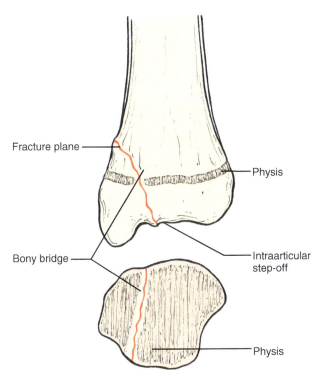

Fig. 2.26 Type III combined growth arrest. (Modified from Bright RW: In Rockwood CA Jr, Wilkins KE, King RE, editors: *Fractures in children*, Philadelphia, 1984, JB Lippincott.)

a significant limb length inequality compared with an adolescent near skeletal maturity. As the arrest is complete, no angular deformity is produced.

CLINICAL AND RADIOGRAPHIC ASSESSMENT

Clinically, growth arrest is noticeable once angular deformity or limb discrepancy develops. Localization of the exact physis involves a thorough history, physical examination, and plain radiographs. It is important to record the severity of limb discrepancy, angular deformity, joint motion, and impairment of function.

Orthogonal radiographs of the involved physis are the first step in the evaluation. Visualization of Harris growth arrest lines may represent an early warning of growth arrest. Asymmetric or oblique line to the physis is suggestive of partial growth arrest (see Fig. 2.11). If the line is parallel to the physis in both planes, no growth arrest is expected (Fig. 2.27).

Tomography, CT, and MRI scanning can be used to further delineate the exact location, size, and contours of the bar, especially when surgical excision is planned. Tomography was traditionally the most common method of localizing bars, but the high amount of radiation exposure required, the time-consuming nature of the investigation, and the propensity for interpretation errors led to its disuse.

CT scanning is often used to plan bar excision (Fig. 2.28). Helical CT is of greater use in preparing physeal maps to determine the extent and location of physeal bony bars because of excellent bony detail, radiation doses one-half to one-quarter those of conventional tomography, and rapid scanning, bypassing the need for sedation.[43] Sagittal and frontal plane reconstructions are essential for adequate mapping because the transverse cuts are often within the plane of the physis and are difficult to interpret.

MRI scanning is the best imaging for delineating physeal bars and also has the advantage of no exposure to radiation.[44] Furthermore, MRI can aid in the early diagnosis of bridge formation and fibrous bars and quantify the amount of plate involvement. Early detection can lead to early treatment and better results because of more growth remaining for correction of deformity.[45] When MRI is used to visualize the physis, fat-suppressed three-dimensional, spoiled, gradient-recalled echo sequences provide the best visualization.[46]

If angular deformity or limb length discrepancy has developed, an assessment of skeletal age in comparison with chronologic age should be made. This allows determination of whether sufficient growth potential remains (≥2 years or 2 cm) for bar excision to be a treatment option. Some of the methods for determining skeletal age include comparison of a radiograph of the hand with an atlas or radiographs of the elbow ossification centers, and more recently, an MRI knee bone age atlas has been presented.[47–49]

In addition to routine radiographs, scanograms allow measurement of limb length discrepancy; panoramic limb images will allow adequate measurement of the mechanical and anatomic bone axis. CT scanograms can more accurately assess limb lengths in children with hip or knee contractures.

TREATMENT

PARTIAL GROWTH ARREST

The treatment of partial growth arrest or physeal bar formation depends on the skeletal age of the patient, the specific physis (location), and the area and extent of physeal

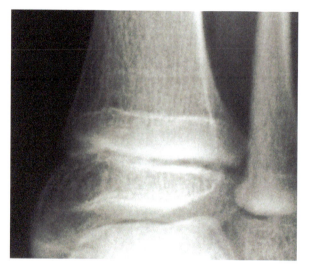

Fig. 2.27 Harris growth line parallel to the physis indicates no growth disruption.

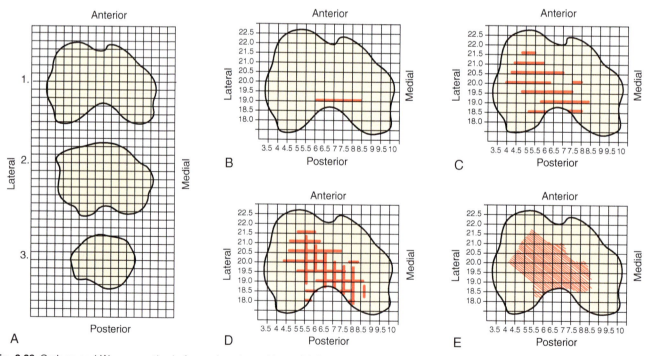

Fig. 2.28 Carlson and Wenger method of mapping physeal bars. (A) Outlines: 1, distal femoral physis; 2, proximal tibial physis; 3, distal tibial physis; (B–E) Distal femoral physeal bar. (B) Anteroposterior projection level indicated by a thick straight line. (C) All anteroposterior levels plotted from tomograms. (D) Lateral projection levels plotted. (E) Final cross-sectional map of the physeal bar. (A–E, Modified from Carlson WO, Wenger DR: A mapping method to prepare for surgical excision of a partial physeal arrest. *J Pediatr Orthop* 4:232–238, 1984.)

involvement. As with complete arrest, no treatment may be required for a child approaching skeletal maturity or if little growth remains in the involved physis.

Treatment options may include the following: use of a shoe lift if not much angular deformity is present and the leg length discrepancy is estimated to be less than 2 cm at maturity; completion of epiphysiodesis of the remaining open physis to avoid angular deformity, especially if only a minor limb length discrepancy is expected; corresponding contralateral bone epiphysiodesis to avoid increasing limb length discrepancy; opening or closing wedge osteotomies to correct angular deformities; lengthening of the involved bone or shortening of the contralateral corresponding bone (only considered for the femur); resection of the bony bar and insertion of interposition material; and various combinations of these techniques.

With respect to surgical bar excision, the aim is to completely remove the bar while preserving the normal remaining physis. Physeal bar resection is only indicated if less than 50% of the physis is involved and if at least 2 years or 2 cm of growth remain.[41] Type I peripheral lesions can be approached directly: the periosteum is elevated over the bridge and resected to prevent subsequent bar reformation. Aggressive periosteal stripping may lead to perichondral ring injury and further growth compromise. The bony bridge is resected through a small window, after which normal physis should be visualized on all sides of the cavity. Optical loupes and dental mirrors can be helpful in visualizing the extent of the bar. Combinations of osteotomes, curettes, rongeurs, and motorized burrs are used to aid resection.

Type II central lesions require a more extensive and difficult approach, because the physis is normal peripherally and a metaphyseal window or osteotomy is performed to reach the area of interest. This approach preserves the perichondral ring and limits further disturbance to the growth plate. The bridge is removed with a curette and dental burr and with the help of headlamps.[41] Visualization of central physeal bars during excision may be aided by the use of arthroscopy, which causes minimal additional morbidity.[50]

Type III arrest is often associated with significant angular deformity and may require osteotomy at the time of bone bar removal. Again, headlamps and/or an arthroscope can be useful in determining the depth of the excision in these cases. There is no firm indication for when angular correction with concomitant bar resection is necessary; in addition, varus or valgus angulation of 15 degrees or less usually does not require corrective osteotomy, especially in young children.[41,42] Angular deformities may correct themselves within a year of restoration of longitudinal growth, and they may do so more quickly if the deformity is in the plane of joint motion. For deformities with an angulation of more than 20 to 30 degrees, spontaneous correction cannot be fully expected.[41,42]

CT navigation has been used with real-time three-dimensional navigation for bar resection as well as MRI-guided bridge resection, which seems to provide excellent results, along with adequate visualization of the bar.[46,51] Metal markers can be placed at the time of surgery in the metaphysis and epiphysis to allow accurate radiographic determination of subsequent growth. They are also

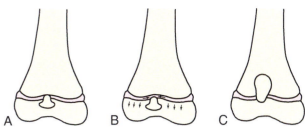

Fig. 2.29 Following successful bar resection, the cavity in the epiphysis and the metaphysis should be filled with fat or Cranioplast (A). It is useful to anchor the interposition material into the epiphysis so that it will migrate distally with the epiphysis during subsequent growth (B). The metaphyseal defect can be packed with local bone graft (C). (From Peterson HA: Partial growth plate arrest and its treatment. *J Pediatr Orthop* 4:246, 1984.)

helpful in differentiating growth at the involved physis from overgrowth at the other end of the same bone. They are placed in cancellous bone away from the area of the excised bar. Ideally, they should be placed in the center of the bone (to prevent extraosseous migration because of growth and metaphyseal remodeling) and in the same longitudinal plane proximal and distal to the defect. The most commonly used metal markers are transversely oriented Kirschner wires.

The major complication of physeal bar excision is bar reformation or recurrence. This complication can be prevented or inhibited by the use of interposition materials. Among the different options for interposition material are fat, methylmethacrylate (commercially available as Cranioplast), bone wax, cartilage, silicone, and muscle.[52] Fat is autologous, readily available, particularly if harvested from the buttock, and has a firm and globular consistency. Its disadvantages are that a separate incision may be required to obtain a graft of adequate size and that the graft may be difficult to contain within the cavity, particularly after tourniquet release. When fat grafts work well, the intraoperative cavity enlarges as the bone and fat graft grow.[53] Cranioplast is radiolucent and thermally nonconductive (in the absence of barium). It has a solid structure that helps to support an epiphysis in compression if a large metaphyseal defect has been surgically created. It is also inexpensive and readily available, and no second incision is required for placement of the product. It is light, easy to handle, moldable, and provides hemostasis because it occupies the entirety of the surgical cavity. It can be poured into a cavity that is gravity dependent in its liquid state; in other cavities, it can be either pushed in through a short polyethylene tube, or it can be allowed to partially set and then can be pushed in like putty. Methylmethacrylate with barium, as used in arthroplasty, is undesirable as an interposition material because it is radiopaque (making detection of recurrent bar formation difficult) and has exothermic properties. The interposition material can be anchored into the epiphysis by contouring the epiphyseal defect or by creating drill holes or "pods" in the epiphysis. This is done to ensure that the interposition material migrates distally with the epiphysis as growth resumes. After insertion of the interposition material, the metaphyseal defect can be packed with local bone graft from the removed bone (Fig. 2.29).

Recurrence is more likely with larger bars, especially the ones occupying 50% or more of the physis. If it occurs soon after surgery and there is a significant amount of growth remaining, reexcision may be attempted and can sometimes be successful. Long-term follow-up is essential in all cases because a bar may reform near skeletal maturity, or the affected physis may cease growth sooner than the contralateral normal physis. In these scenarios, contralateral physeal arrest should be considered.

Several novel approaches to physeal bar treatment have been developed, primarily in small and large animal models. Although some are promising, none is currently in routine clinical use. Tissue engineering has been receiving the most attention; the use of cultured chondrocytes has been shown to potentially allow reconstitution of the growth plate.[54,55]

Knowledge of the underlying physeal anatomy and the relationship of overlying structures is essential for adequate bar excision and for minimizing further damage to the surrounding physis. Birch and colleagues[56] performed anatomic dissection of the most commonly affected physes and described the relevant surgical anatomy as follows:

- **Distal radius physis.** This physis is completely extracapsular and can be easily exposed by any direct approach on its volar, dorsal, or radial aspect; it is obscured by the ulna medially. The volar metaphysis is cloaked by the pronator quadratus and is best exposed through the volar approach of Henry but with the radial artery retracted radially rather than ulnarly.
- **Distal femoral physis.** The synovial reflection of the suprapatellar pouch obscures portions of the anterior, medial, and lateral aspects of the distal end of the femur and must be bluntly dissected anteriorly. The capsular attachment extends to the level of the physis anteriorly and posteriorly. The insertion of the adductor magnus tendon medially and the intermuscular septum laterally serves as a landmark to the level of the physis. This physis is best exposed through a posteromedial approach with direct posterior exposure, which allows mobilization and protection of the neurovascular bundle.
- **Proximal tibial physis.** This physis is completely extracapsular. The medial collateral ligament and tendons of the pes anserinus cover the medial aspect of the physis; in direct exposure, these structures can be mobilized and retracted without difficulty. The anterolateral and anteromedial aspects of the metaphysis are easily accessible, but care must be taken to avoid injury to the apophysis of the tibial tubercle. The posterior aspects of the physis and the metaphysis are obscured in the midline by the popliteus muscle, and this posterolateral region is the least surgically accessible. The posteromedial aspect of the metaphysis can be approached posteromedially in relation to the tibia. After the interval between the semitendinosus and the medial aspect of the gastrocnemius is developed, the popliteus muscle is mobilized and reflected distally and laterally.
- **Distal tibia and fibula physes.** The distal tibial physis is entirely extracapsular. The anterior and posterior tibiofibular ligaments insert across the anterolateral and posterolateral aspects of the physis of the distal end of the fibula. Direct exposure is difficult only on the lateral aspect of the tibia, where the overlying fibula obscures the physis. The distal fibula physis is intracapsular.

COMPLETE GROWTH ARREST

Treatment of complete growth arrest is aimed at limb length discrepancy. The amount of discrepancy is dependent on the physis injured (and its overall contribution to the growth of the involved bone) and the age at which the growth arrest occurred. In children nearing skeletal maturity, where the inequality will be minimal, no treatment is required. In younger children, treatment depends on the expected limb length inequality at skeletal maturity. Upper extremity limb inequality is much better tolerated than limb inequality of the lower extremity; thus, it is less likely that it would need to be addressed. Options for lower limb inequality include an insert or shoe lift, epiphysiodesis of the contralateral or companion (e.g., tibia and fibula or radius and ulna) bone, lengthening of the involved bone, shortening of the contralateral bone, or a combination of these options.

In the upper extremity, humeral growth arrest rarely results in a functional or significant cosmetic deficit and usually only needs intervention when the shortening is significant (e.g., more than 5 cm). For the forearm, if only one of the two bones is involved, changes in distal radial–ulnar variance may develop, and it may lead to wrist pain and deformity. This may require surgical lengthening of the involved bone or shortening of the companion bone.

In general, a lower limb length discrepancy of less than 2 cm causes little functional impairment and can be left untreated or treated with an insert or shoe lift. A discrepancy between 2 and 5 cm is most commonly treated by epiphysiodesis of the contralateral bone, as long as sufficient growth remains, or by shortening of the contralateral bone after skeletal maturity. Ipsilateral bone lengthening is considered when the discrepancy is greater than 5 cm, and may be combined with contralateral epiphysiodesis or shortening. Femoral growth arrest and its resultant leg inequality can be treated by the use of a permanent shoe lift, timed epiphysiodesis of the contralateral distal femoral physis, lengthening of the involved femur, or shortening of the contralateral femur at maturity. Tibial growth arrest is treated in a similar fashion, with the addition of epiphysiodesis of the ipsilateral fibula if significant relative overgrowth of the fibula is likely to occur.[57] Contralateral tibial shortening is not a good option because it can lead to significant weakness of the tibialis anterior muscle and foot drop.

APOPHYSEAL INJURIES

Each apophysis is connected to bone through a histologically recognizable physis. The shape and size of the apophysis are influenced by the forces placed on it by its muscle or tendon attachments. Some apophyses have only a single muscle or tendon attachment, whereas others are attached to whole muscle groups. Initially, the apophyses appear as cartilaginous prominences at the ends of or along the sides of bones; later, centers of ossification develop similar to those of other physes. The ossification centers then either fuse with an associated epiphysis, such as the tibial tubercle fusing with the proximal tibial epiphysis, or remain as isolated centers of ossification. Eventually, the physeal plate between the ossification center and the underlying bone disappears as bony fusion is achieved. Because the attachment of the tendon to the cortex is very strong, excessive force usually causes avulsion or fracture through the apophysis rather than pulling of the tendon from its insertion.

Common problems seen with the apophyses include inflammation or partial avulsion caused by repetitive microtrauma (traction apophysitis). These injuries typically occur in active adolescents between the ages of 8 and 15 years and may manifest as periarticular pain. Common sites of apophyseal injury are the medial epicondyle of the humerus (so-called Little League elbow) and attachments of the sartorius, the direct head of the rectus femoris, and hamstrings to the pelvis. Avulsion fracture of the proximal tibial apophysis occurs most commonly in boys during the eccentric quadriceps contracture of landing from a jump. Displaced injuries with loss of active knee extension require operative fixation.

The two common sites of apophysitis about the hip and pelvis are the iliac crest and the ischial tuberosity. Clancy and Foltz[58] described iliac apophysitis in the adolescent long-distance runner undertaking intensive training programs. Hockey, lacrosse, and football players may also be afflicted. The cause has been attributed to a reaction of the unfused apophysis as a result of repetitive muscular contraction or to a subclinical apophyseal stress fracture. Clinical features include localized tenderness and pain with activity or on resisted hip abduction. Radiographs are often normal but may reveal mild widening of the iliac apophysis. Treatment is nonsurgical and involves rest, ice application, analgesia, and a graded return to sporting activity. Ischial tuberosity apophysitis is less common and presents as a chronic hip or buttock pain with localized tenderness. Hip flexion and knee extension, which stretch the hamstrings, reproduce the pain. Radiographs are often normal but may demonstrate irregularities in the ischial tuberosity contour with rarefaction or fragmentation. Treatment is symptomatic and similar to that used for iliac apophysitis.

Avulsion fractures of the pelvic apophyses are usually caused by sudden contraction of the hamstrings, adductor magnus, iliopsoas, and hip flexors in athletes participating in sports involving a high contraction rate or forceful hamstring stretch, such as sprinting, long jumping, or hurdling. These avulsions have been classified as apophysiolysis (undisplaced), acute avulsion fractures, and old nonunited avulsions (Fig. 2.30).[59] Pain in the groin and buttock is the most common symptom. With separation of the ischial apophysis, the gap is palpable and should be sought after any suspected hamstring injury. Radiographs confirm the diagnosis. These injuries are generally treated nonoperatively (i.e., with rest, ice application, limb positioning to

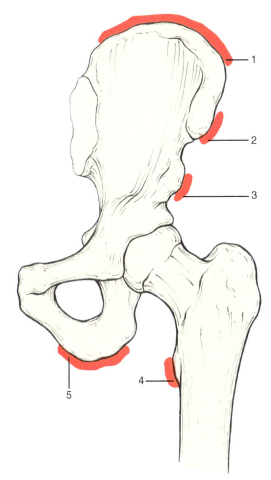

Fig. 2.30 Sites of pelvic avulsion fractures. 1, Iliac crest; 2, anterior superior iliac spine; 3, anterior inferior iliac spine; 4, lesser trochanter; 5, ischium. (From Fernbach SK, Wilkinson RJ: Avulsion injuries of the pelvis and proximal femur. *Am J Roentgenol* 137:581–584, 1981.)

relax the affected muscle group, and a graded rehabilitation program) with no long-term functional limitations. Operative intervention (e.g., open reduction and internal fixation) is only considered when significant fracture displacement is present. The highest rate of nonunion is seen in ischial tuberosity fractures, with as high as 16% seen in one study.[60] Other specific apophyseal avulsion injuries are shown in Table 2.1.

Medial epicondyle apophysitis occurs most frequently in children and adolescents involved in throwing sports, especially baseball, but it has been reported in other sports, including gymnastics, wrestling, and weightlifting. Repetitive microtrauma is caused by tension stress across the medial epicondyle and collateral ligaments. With excessive throwing action, the medial epicondyle may become prominent and painful. Active adolescent baseball pitchers frequently have accelerated growth and widening of the medial epicondylar apophysis; fragmentation of the apophysis is occasionally noted. The pain generally resolves with rest, and there are usually no significant sequelae.

Table 2.1 Specific apophyseal avulsion injuries

Site	Muscle attachment	Clinical information	Management
Anterior inferior iliac spine	Rectus femoris (straight head)	Caused by kicking when hip hyperextended and knee flexed; "sprinter's fracture"; local tenderness and pain on passive hyperextension and active flexion of hip; may be confused with an os acetabuli	Nonsurgical
Anterior superior iliac spine	Sartorius, tensor fascia lata	Caused by forced overpull of sartorius with hip in extension and knee in flexion; most commonly seen in sprinters and hurdlers; local tenderness and pain on passive extension or active flexion of hip	Nonsurgical; rarely, surgical if severe displacement or rotation
Iliac crest	Internal oblique, external oblique, transversus abdominis	Rare; caused by forceful contraction of abdominal musculature; pain on lateral bending of torso and contraction of abdominal muscles	Nonsurgical
Ischial tuberosity	Hamstrings	Caused by sudden forceful eccentric hamstring contraction; seen in hurdlers, long jumpers, and athletes performing splits; local tenderness and pain on passive hip flexion	Nonsurgical if <2 cm; surgical if displacement >2 cm or pain with sitting
Lesser trochanter	Iliopsoas	Most commonly seen in sprinters, jumpers, or kicking athletes; local tenderness and hip held in slight adduction and internal rotation; positive Ludloff sign (inability to flex hip when in seated position)	Nonsurgical
Greater trochanter	Gluteus medius, gluteus minimus, short external rotators	Caused by forceful muscular contraction of hip abductors (e.g., during cutting activities); local tenderness, positive Trendelenburg gait and sign, and pain on resisted abduction and passive adduction	Nonsurgical; consider surgery if >1 cm displacement
Pubic symphysis	Adductor group	Most commonly seen in sprinters; local tenderness along anterior pubis and pain on resisted hip adduction and passive hip abduction	Nonsurgical

REFERENCES

The level of evidence (LOE) is determined according to the criteria provided in the Preface.

1. Guandalini S, Ventura A, Ansaldi N, et al. Diagnosis of coeliac disease: time for a change? *Arch Dis Child*. 1989;64(9):1320–1324. Discussion 1324–1325. **(LOE V)**.
2. Ramachandran M. *Basic Orthopaedic Sciences: the Stanmore Guide*. New York: Oxford University Press. **(LOE N/A)**.
3. Harris HA. The vascular supply of bone, with special reference to the epiphysial cartilage. *J Anat*. 1929;64(Pt 1):3–4.3. **(LOE V)**.
4. Langenskiold A. Role of the ossification groove of Ranvier in normal and pathologic bone growth: a review. *J Pediatr Orthop*. 1998;18(2):173–177 **(LOE V)**.
5. Shapiro F, Holtrop ME, Glimcher MJ. Organization and cellular biology of the perichondrial ossification groove of Ranvier: a morphological study in rabbits. *J Bone Joint Surg Am*. 1977;59(6):703–723. **(LOE N/A)**.
6. Dale GG, Harris WR. Prognosis of epiphysial separation: an experimental study. *J Bone Joint Surg Br*. 1958;40-B(1):116–122. **(LOE N/A)**.
7. Mann DC, Rajmaira S. Distribution of physeal and nonphyseal fractures in 2,650 long-bone fractures in children aged 0-16 years. *J Pediatr Orthop*. 1990;10(6):713–716. **(LOE II)**.
8. Salter R, Harris W. Injuries involving the epiphyseal plate. *J Bone Joint Surg Am*. 1963;45:587–622. **(LOE V)**.
9. Gruber HE, Ashraf N, Cox MD, et al. Experimental induction of physeal injuries by fracture, drill, and ablation techniques: analyses of immunohistochemical findings. *J Pediatr Orthop*. 2017. https://doi.org/10.1097/BPO.0000000000001093. [Epub ahead of print]. **(LOE V)**.
10. Aitken AP. Fractures of the epiphyses. *Clin Orthop Relat Res*. 1965;41:19–23. **(LOE V)**.
11. Li L, Hui JH, Goh JC, et al. Chitin as a scaffold for mesenchymal stem cells transfers in the treatment of partial growth arrest. *J Pediatr Orthop*. 2004;24(2):205–210. **(LOE N/A)**.
12. Ogden JA. *Skeletal Injury in the Child*. 2nd ed. Philadelphia: Saunders. **(LOE N/A)**.
13. Poland J. *Traumatic Separation of the Epiphyses*. London: Smith, Elder, & Co. **(LOE N/A)**.
14. In: Rang M, ed. *The Growth Plate and its Disorders*. Baltimore: Williams & Wilkins. **(LOE N/A)**.
15. Peterson HA. Physeal fractures: part 3. Classification. *J Pediatr Orthop*. 1994;14(4):439–448. **(LOE IV)**.
16. Gufler H, Schulze CG, Wagner S, et al. MRI for occult physeal fracture detection in children and adolescents. *Acta Radiol*. 2013;54(4):467–472. **(LOE III)**.
17. Pai DR, Thapa M. Musculoskeletal ultrasound of the upper extremity in children. *Pediatr Radiol*. 2013;43(suppl 1):S48–S54. **(LOE V)**.
18. Harris HA. Lines of arrested growth in the long bones of childhood: the correlation of histological and radiographic appearances in clinical and experimental conditions. *Br J Radiol*. 1931;4:561–588. **(LOE IV)**.
19. Bright RW. Partial growth arrest: identification, classification, and results of treatment. *Orthop Trans*. 1982;6:65–66. **(LOE IV)**.
20. Gruber H, Phieffer L, Wattenbarger J. Physeal fractures, part II: fate of interposed periosteum in a physeal fracture. *J Pediatr Orthop*. 2002;22(6):710–716. **(LOE V)**.
21. Phieffer L, Meyer R, Gruber H, Easley M, Wattenbarger J. Effect of interposed periosteum in an animal physeal fracture model. *Clin Orthop Relat Res*. 2000;376:15–25. **(LOE V)**.
22. Barmada A, Gaynor T, Mubarak SJ. Premature physeal closure following distal tibia physeal fractures: a new radiographic predictor. *J Pediatr Orthop*. 2003;23(6):733–739. **(LOE III)**.

23. Arkader A, Warner Jr WC, Horn BD, et al. Predicting the outcome of physeal fractures of the distal femur. *J Pediatr Orthop.* 2007;27(6):703–708. **(LOE III)**.

24. Thomson JD, Stricker SJ, Williams MM. Fractures of the distal femoral epiphyseal plate. *J Pediatr Orthop.* 1995;15(4):474–478. **(LOE III)**.

25. Pennock AT, Ellis HB, Willimon SC, et al. Intra-articular physeal fractures of the distal femur: a frequently missed diagnosis in adolescent athletes. *Orthop J Sports Med.* 2017;5(10):2325967117731567. **(LOE IV)**.

26. Abzug JM, Little K, Kozin SH. Physeal arrest of the distal radius. *J Am Acad Orthop Surg.* 2014;22(6):381–389. **(LOE V)**.

27. Golz RJ, Grogan DP, Greene TL, et al. Distal ulnar physeal injury. *J Pediatr Orthop.* 1991;11(3):318–326. **(LOE IV)**.

28. Rhemrev SJ, Sleeboom C, Ekkelkamp S. Epiphyseal fractures of the proximal tibia. *Injury.* 2000;31(3):131–134. **(LOE IV)**.

29. Caterini R, Farsetti P, Ippolito E. Long-term followup of physeal injury to the ankle. *Foot Ankle.* 1991;11(6):372–383. **(LOE IV)**.

30. Anderson AF. Transepiphyseal replacement of the anterior cruciate ligament using quadruple hamstring grafts in skeletally immature patients. *J Bone Joint Surg Am.* 2004;86-A(suppl 1; Pt 2):201–209. **(LOE IV)**.

31. Fabricant PD, Osbahr DC, Green DW. Management of a rare complication after screw fixation of a pediatric tibial spine avulsion fracture: a case report with follow-up to skeletal maturity. *J Orthop Trauma.* 2011;25(12):e115–e119. **(LOE IV)**.

32. Belthur MV, Bradish CF, Gibbons PJ. Late orthopaedic sequelae following meningococcal septicaemia. A multicentre study. *J Bone Joint Surg Br.* 2005;87(2):236–240. **(LOE IV)**.

33. Paulino AC. Late effects of radiotherapy for pediatric extremity sarcomas. *Int J Radiat Oncol Biol Phys.* 2004;60(1):265–274. **(LOE IV)**.

34. Beatty E, Light TR, Belsole RJ, Ogden JA. Wrist and hand skeletal injuries in children. *Hand Clin.* 1990;6(4):723–738. **(LOE IV)**.

35. Silverman FN. Recovery from epiphyseal invagination: sequel to an unusual complication of scurvy. *J Bone Joint Surg Am.* 1970;52(2):384–390. **(LOE IV)**.

36. Steele RG, Lugg P, Richardson M. Premature epiphyseal closure secondary to single-course vitamin A therapy. *Aust N Z J Surg.* 1999;69(11):825–827. **(LOE IV)**.

37. De Luca F. Impaired growth plate chondrogenesis in children with chronic illnesses. *Pediatr Res.* 2006;59(5):625–629. **(LOE V)**.

38. Caine D, Howe W, Ross W, Bergman G. Does repetitive physical loading inhibit radial growth in female gymnasts? *Clin J Sport Med.* 1997;7(4):302–308. **(LOE III)**.

39. Caine D, DiFiori J, Maffulli N. Physeal injuries in children's and youth sports: reasons for concern? *Br J Sports Med.* 2006;40(9):749–760. **(LOE III)**.

40. Pennock AT, Pytiak A, Stearns P, et al. Preseason assessment of radiographic abnormalities in elbows of Little League baseball players. *J Bone Joint Surg Am.* 2016;98(9):761–767. **(LOE III)**.

41. Peterson HA. Partial growth plate arrest and its treatment. *J Pediatr Orthop.* 1984;4(2):246–258. **(LOE IV)**.

42. Ogden JA. The evaluation and treatment of partial physeal arrest. *J Bone Joint Surg Am.* 1987;69(8):1297–1302. **(LOE V)**.

43. Loder RT, Swinford AE, Kuhns LR. The use of helical computed tomographic scan to assess bony physeal bridges. *J Pediatr Orthop.* 1997;17(3):356–359. **(LOE IV)**.

44. Lohman M, Kivisaari A, Vehmas, et al. MRI in the assessment of growth arrest. *Pediatr Radiol.* 2002;32(1):41–45. **(LOE III)**.

45. Wang DC, Deeney V, Roach JW, et al. Imaging of physeal bars in children. *Pediatr Radiol.* 2015;45(9):1403–1412. **(LOE V)**.

46. Blanco Sequeiros R, Vahasarja V, Ojala R. Magnetic resonance-guided growth plate bone bridge resection at 0.23 Tesla: report of a novel technique. *Acta Radiol.* 2008;49(6):668–672. **(LOE IV)**.

47. Diméglio A, Charles YP, Daures JP, et al. Accuracy of the Sauvegrain method in determining skeletal age during puberty. *J Bone Joint Surg Am.* 2005;87(8):1689–1696. **(LOE II)**.

48. Greulich WW, Pyle SI. *Radiographic Atlas of Skeletal Development of the Hand and Wrist.* 2nd ed. Stanford, CA: Stanford University Press. **(LOE N/A)**.

49. Pennock AT, Bomar JD, Manning JD. The creation and validation of a knee bone age atlas utilizing MRI. *J Bone Joint Surg Am.* 2018;100(4):e20. **(LOE III)**.

50. Marsh JS, Polzhofer GK. Arthroscopically assisted central physeal bar resection. *J Pediatr Orthop.* 2006;26(2):255–259. **(LOE IV)**.

51. Kang HG, Yoon SJ, Kim JR. Resection of a physeal bar under computer-assisted guidance. *J Bone Joint Surg Br.* 2010;92(10):1452–1455. **(LOE V)**.

52. Khoshhal KI, Kiefer GN. Physeal bridge resection. *J Am Acad Orthop Surg.* 2005;13(1):47–58. **(LOE V)**.

53. Langenskiold A, Videman T, Nevalainen T. The fate of fat transplants in operations for partial closure of the growth plate. Clinical examples and an experimental study. *J Bone Joint Surg Br.* 1986;68(2):234–238. **(LOE IV)**.

54. Lee EH, Chen F, Chan J, Bose K. Treatment of growth arrest by transfer of cultured chondrocytes into physeal defects. *J Pediatr Orthop.* 1998;18(2):155–160. **(LOE N/A)**.

55. Lee KM, Cheng AS, Cheung WH, et al. Bioengineering and characterization of physeal transplant with physeal reconstruction potential. *Tissue Eng.* 2003;9(4):703–711. **(LOE N/A)**.

56. Birch JG, Herring JA, Wenger DR. Surgical anatomy of selected physes. *J Pediatr Orthop.* 1984;4(2):224–231. **(LOE IV)**.

57. McCarthy JJ, Burke T, McCarthy MC. Need for concomitant proximal fibular epiphysiodesis when performing a proximal tibial epiphysiodesis. *J Pediatr Orthop.* 2003;23(1):52–54. **(LOE III)**.

58. Clancy Jr WG, Foltz AS. Iliac apophysitis and stress fractures in adolescent runners. *Am J Sports Med.* 1976;4(5):214–218. **(LOE IV)**.

59. Fernbach SK, Wilkinson RH. Avulsion injuries of the pelvis and proximal femur. *AJR Am J Roentgenol.* 1981;137(3):581–584. **(LOE IV)**.

60. Schuett DJ, Bomar JD, Pennock AT. Pelvic apophyseal avulsion fractures: a retrospective review of 228 cases. *J Pediatr Orthop.* 2015;35(6):617–623. **(LOE III)**.

Casting Techniques

Steven Lovejoy | Jonathan G. Schoenecker

INTRODUCTION

Immobilization in a cast has been the standard of care for spinal and upper and lower extremity injuries and fractures in children. Techniques were first described in antiquity, and they used a variety of hardening agents. Until the 1900s, plaster-impregnated bandages were used. Today's more common casting material is fiberglass in various forms; it shares some of the same properties of plaster of Paris but is an improvement in other respects.[1]

Casting techniques have evolved over the years. Unfortunately, complications still do occur but can be avoided with careful attention to detail.

Some variation of a body cast can be used to treat spinal fractures in children, of which the most common is a flexion (seat belt) injury treated with a hyperextension cast.[2] Spica hip casting can be used to treat pelvic or femoral fractures. Long arm and short arm casts are routinely used to treat upper extremity fractures from the elbow to the wrist, and long leg and short leg casts are used for fractures of the lower extremities.

GENERAL CAST PRINCIPLES

- Adequate cast padding is three to five layers thick.
- Extra layers should be applied on bony prominences.
- The cast should be molded to fit the anatomy.
- Warm water should be used during application.
- A stretch-relaxation technique should be used for fiberglass casting materials.
- Three-point molding is necessary for long bone fractures.
- The joint should be immobilized in a position to help hold the reduction.

BODY CASTS

The use of fiberglass body casts has dwindled with the increasing use of patient-specific molded braces (thoracic-lumbar-sacral orthoses [TLSOs]) in the treatment of spinal fractures in children. Stable burst fractures, bony Chance fractures, and other stable injuries of the spine in children can typically be treated with body casts and hyperextension molds. These are best applied on a Risser table, which allows total access to the torso for casting. As with all casting techniques, attention to padding over the bony prominences is important for prevention of pressure ulcers.

The typical fiberglass cast has cutouts for the abdomen to allow abdominal distention after eating, as well as molding over the iliac crests to prevent the cast from moving up and down on the patient. Curved cutouts to allow the thighs to flex on the abdomen to at least 90 degrees are also created and well padded. All edges of the body jacket are padded with moleskin, moleskin-like material, or folded stockinette that covers the skin (Fig. 3.1).

SPICA CASTING

Hip spica casting continues to be a mainstay of treatment for fractures of the femur from the hip joint to the knee joint. It is commonly used for fractures that are amenable to closed treatment, and an occasional indication is for fractures that have been treated operatively but require additional immobilization.[3] Spica cast treatment has been used in the operating room and the emergency department successfully.[4]

With the child adequately sedated or fully anesthetized, an underliner of either polypropylene (e.g., Gore-Tex, W.L. Gore Co., Newark, Delaware) or cotton tubular stockinette is applied; two different diameters of stockinette are used.[5] The larger-diameter stockinette is pulled up onto the torso above the nipple line and extended down to midthigh. Appropriate trimming of the stockinette allows the hips to flex as desired. Stockinette of a smaller size is then placed on the extremity to be immobilized. A single-leg spica (Video 3.1) or double-leg spica cast requires one or both legs to be incorporated in the cast. These can extend down past the knee and even out to the toes as deemed necessary for the fracture. Once the stockinette has been applied, the patient is placed on a pediatric spica table, which allows the chest and upper torso to be supported separately from the lower body. The buttocks and pelvis are positioned on a thin, midline extender that attaches to a perineal post, against which gentle traction can be applied by the assistant holding the legs. Placing the table in reverse Trendelenburg position or having a second assistant apply caudally directed, longitudinal pressure on the shoulders helps to keep the child positioned appropriately.

During application of the padding, one or two folds of operative towels are placed underneath the cast padding on the abdomen to allow room for expansion of the abdomen after eating. Synthetic padding material is applied while the limbs are held in the desired position to maintain reduction of the fracture. Moving the extremity after the padding is placed should be avoided so that "binding" by the circumferential padding is prevented. Three to four layers of padding

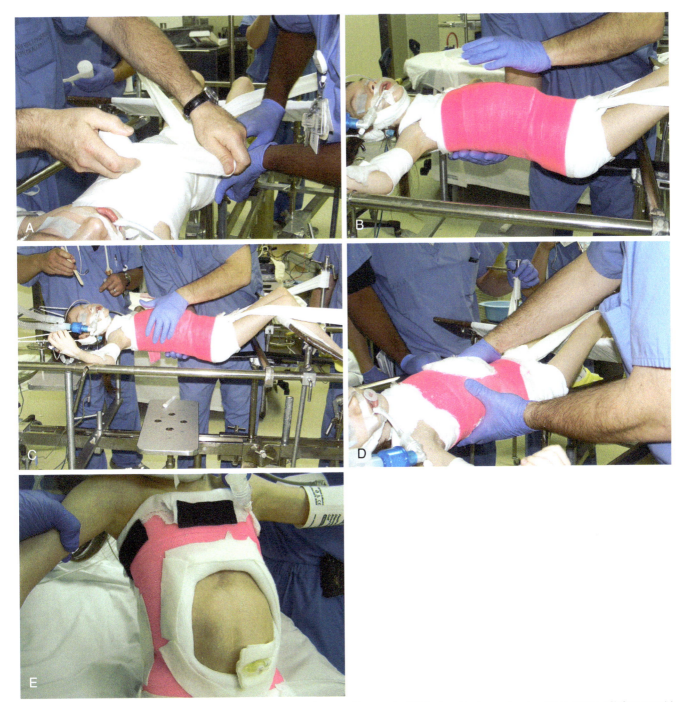

Fig. 3.1 (A) Patient on Risser table with muslin support and molding over iliac crests. (B) Cast molded over chest and iliac crests. (C) Chest mold. (D) Abdominal cutout for breathing comfort. (E) Cast petaled.

are desired. Bony prominences should be protected with extra strips of padding, where needed.

Depending on the fracture type, hip flexion can be incorporated as desired. In general, the more proximal a fracture of the femur, the more hip flexion needed to affect reduction. Once the patient is on the fracture table, fiberglass is applied. The spica cast itself may be applied in one of two ways: proximal-to-distal, or distal-to-proximal. Both require coordination between the holder and the individual placing the cast. In the proximal-to-distal technique, the cast is wrapped by incorporation of the torso first and then extension down onto one or both legs. In

the distal-to-proximal technique, a long leg cast is applied first, supportive traction is applied to the long leg cast, and then the cast is extended proximally onto the torso. As a note of caution, one should avoid using a short leg cast to apply traction before wrapping the upper portion of the spica because this technique has been associated with compartment syndrome.[6,7]

Three to four layers of overlapping fiberglass are typically appropriate, depending on the size of the child. Heat generated by the cast can be reduced with the use of lukewarm water and dissipated further by massaging the water into the pores of the casting material as it hardens. Carefully molding

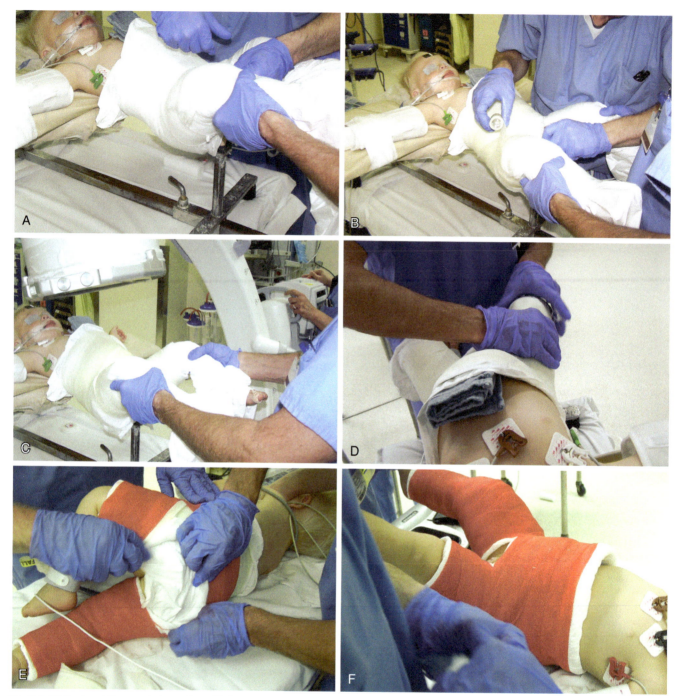

Fig. 3.2 (A) Cast padding applied over liner. (B) Cast built from trunk to legs. (C) Reduction is checked with C-arm. (D) Cast is molded to maintain reduction. (E) Cast is trimmed around buttocks and groin. (F) Edges padded and cast finished.

over the iliac crest, the greater trochanters, and the femoral condyles customizes the fit and allows the best chance for maintenance of fracture reduction. Once the fiberglass has hardened, the cast can be trimmed in the adductor region of the hips and along the buttocks to the top of the gluteal cleft to allow access to the perineum for diapering, toileting, and hygiene. If stiffness of the cast between the leg and torso is a concern, a fiberglass bar can be manufactured from a broomstick or a twisted roll of 3-inch fiberglass and then positioned and overwrapped to span the legs either obliquely from the thigh to the leg or transversely at the level of the distal femur (Fig. 3.2).

UPPER EXTREMITY SPLINTING AND CASTING

Fractures of the upper extremities are often treated by closed reduction and initial splinting, casting, or both. The initial swelling that occurs with early fracture care will dictate which type of immobilization is used. A sugar-tong splint is a safe and effective way to temporarily immobilize fractures of the forearm. Ten thicknesses of plaster of Paris or five thicknesses of 3-inch fiberglass are typically adequate for immobilization of most children's forearm fractures (Fig. 3.3A,B).

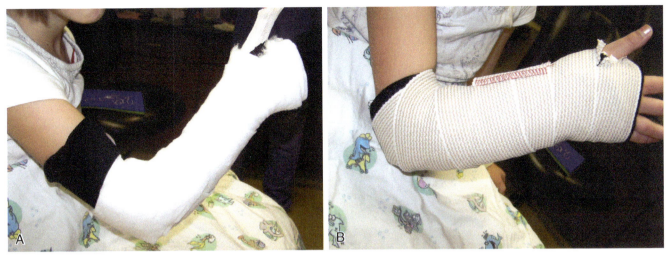

Fig. 3.3 (A) Five thicknesses of fiberglass molded around elbow to forearm. (B) Elastic wrap. Elbow can flex and extend.

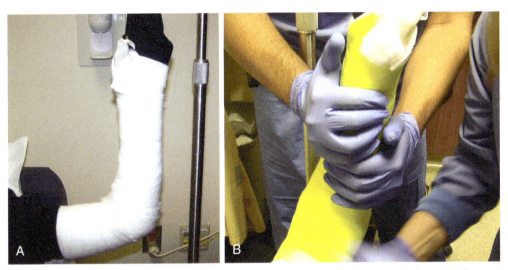

Fig. 3.4 (A) Suspension of forearm by finger traps. (B) Molded dorsal to volar for contouring of the forearm.

Definitive casting is performed in the acute setting or once swelling has resolved. A long arm cast (Video 3.2) is applied with the elbow incorporated for immobilization of forearm fractures. Tubular stockinette is placed at the upper end of the long arm cast and at the wrist and first web space or continuously from top to bottom. If a single continuous piece of stockinette is used, the stockinette should be cut across the antecubital fossa so that the stockinette can layer rather than wrinkle. Rolls of cast padding are then used in three to four layers circumferentially. Fiberglass long arm casting material is then applied with three to four thicknesses of fiberglass. Careful molding is performed at the forearm, flat dorsal to volar, to match the shape of the forearm and interosseous membrane (Fig. 3.4A,B). The ratio of dorsovolar-to-radioulnar distance is the cast index. This ratio should be less than 0.7 in the forearm.[6] The upper arm is molded flat over the triceps and gently shaped triangularly toward the biceps. A recommended method for obtaining this shape is as follows: with the cast hardening and the elbow flexed appropriately, the patient's arm should be slid onto the bed to allow the upper arm to lie flat on the table, forearm to the ceiling, so that the mold will be flat over the triceps. If swelling is anticipated,

the cast padding should be split from the wrist to the upper arm. Noncircumferential layers of padding are placed over the split. The cast is then split and spread over the same area where the cast padding has been split, which then prevents circumferential constriction of either the cast padding or the fiberglass. All sharp edges of the cast are then either covered in folded-down stockinette or petaled with moleskin with an adhesive backing.

Short arm casts (Video 3.3) can be used in the treatment of forearm or wrist fractures deemed stable and amenable to short arm cast treatment.[8] Fingers can be suspended by either finger traps or an assistant. Tubular stockinette can be placed at the most proximal extent of the forearm, at the wrist, and in the first web space. Three to four layers of cast padding should be applied; then the fiberglass casting material should also be applied in three layers. The edges about the hand and proximal extent of the cast are padded with either turndown of the stockinette or petaled with adhesive-backed moleskin. Short arm casts can be split in a similar fashion to long arm casts, either in a volar split that leaves the first web space intact or bivalved in a radial and ulnar direction[9] (Fig. 3.5A,C).

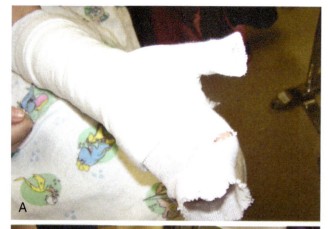

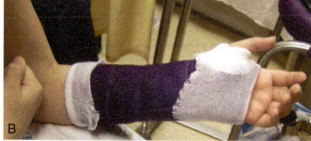

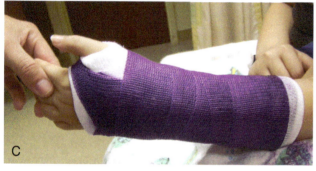

Fig. 3.5 (A) Adequate padding is placed in the thumb web space. (B) Edges of padding are folded down. (C) Molded short arm cast.

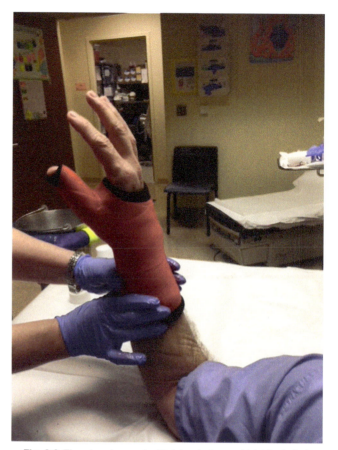

Fig. 3.6 Thumb spica cast with interphalangeal joint included.

A thumb spica cast is used to immobilize the thumb ray. It can incorporate the interphalangeal joint if necessary for distal immobilization. The elbow may be incorporated if needed for more rigid wrist immobilization of the thumb ray including the carpus (scaphoid most commonly) (Fig. 3.6).

A shoulder spica cast is useful for fracture reduction, immobilization, or self-protection in the example shown (Fig. 3.7). This is best placed on a Risser table with all bony prominences well padded and struts placed for support. Iliac crest molding is key to prevent "settling" of the cast with ambulation.

LOWER EXTREMITY SPLINTING

Sugar-tong splints (medial-lateral ankle stirrups) can be used for fractures distal to the proximal tibial metaphysis or for grossly unstable fractures about the ankle. For additional control and stability, a posterior slab can be added to the splint. This type of splint can be either fiberglass or plaster placed over abundant padding held in place with an elastic

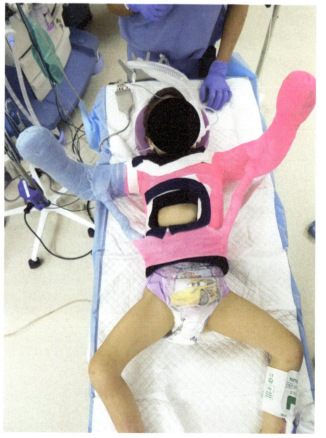

Fig. 3.7 Shoulder spica cast placed under anesthesia.

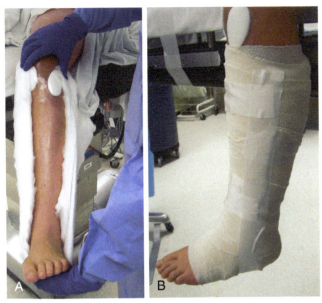

Fig. 3.8 (A) Foot is supported with the stirrup of the casting material. (B) Malleoli should be molded around as the wrap is applied.

bandage or bias-cut stockinette (Fig. 3.8). For metaphyseal and periarticular fractures about the knee, a long posterior splint may be applied from the buttocks to the toes, reinforced with medial and lateral slabs across the knee, until definitive treatment is performed.

SHORT LEG CAST

Short leg casts (Video 3.4) are most often used for immobilizing soft tissue injuries, stable fractures of the distal tibia and fibula, and foot injuries. The cast may be applied with the knee held flexed by an assistant, with the patient sitting with the leg dependent, or with the patient prone with the knee flexed. Three to four layers of cast padding are applied, and additional padding is added over bony prominences such as the malleoli, heel, and metatarsals to prevent skin irritation. The cast is wrapped with three to four overlapping layers of fiberglass and should be molded around the malleoli and be triangular in shape to match the contour of the leg. Extra folds of fiberglass or splints may be added on the bottom of the cast so that it is reinforced for weight-bearing (Fig. 3.9).

LONG LEG CAST

Long leg casts can be applied in the acute care setting for acceptably reduced tibial fractures or nondisplaced supracondylar fractures of the femur. The latter injuries most often occur in younger children.

In smaller children, long leg casts can be applied continuously from the toes to the upper thigh. Three to four layers of cast padding should be applied circumferentially over the stockinette, and extra layers should be added around bony prominences and the heel. The knee should be bent appropriately for the fracture pattern. The foot should not be supported by suspension with traction on the stockinette

because this can lead to pressure on the heel. The use of three to four layers of fiberglass is adequate.

In larger children, adequate cast padding should be applied circumferentially three to four layers thick from the toes to above the knee. The table should be raised to allow the knee to bend over the side of the table. An assistant supports the foot. This allows gravity traction to aid in fracture reduction and eases the job of the assistant. A short leg cast is applied and molds reduction of the fracture. This molding matches the triangular shape of the leg. When the short leg cast is completely applied, the table can be lowered. The foot is placed on the assistant's chest with the hip and knee flexed to the knee position deemed appropriate for the fracture's maintenance of alignment. The thigh portion of the cast is applied with attention to appropriate padding of all bony prominences and molding in the supracondylar and infrapatellar regions to match the anatomy. In very young children with less developed femoral condyles, the cast is molded flat on the quadriceps so that slipping of the cast is avoided. The cast can then be split if concerns about swelling are present, by either bivalving medially and laterally or splitting dorsally and spreading (Fig. 3.10).

CAST WEDGING

At times, even a fracture with the best applied and molded cast loses reduction. Options for regaining alignment include repeated reduction and changing of the cast or cast wedging. A typical fracture amenable to wedging is a long bone fracture in which angulation is the major deformity needing correction. A simple reproducible method of wedging, described by Bebbington and colleagues,[10] is to trace the angulation of the fracture on the cast. With the use of fluoroscopy or plain radiography to mark the apex of the angulation, the cast should be cut circumferentially at this level, and a strip of cast should be left intact on the convex side of the fracture. This strip can be as small as 1 cm or as wide as 5 cm, depending on the size of the cast. Slow opening of the concave cast split using a cast spreader tool allows correction of angulation. Commercially available cast wedges are then placed in the opening until the desired correction is attained. Cast padding is then placed in the split in the cast and overwrapped with casting material. This padding prevents "window edema."

COMPLICATIONS OF CASTING

Whenever a potentially constrictive, circumferential wrap of any type is placed on an injured extremity, soft tissue swelling can lead to pressure elevation within the fascial compartments of the extremity, leading to ischemia and possible neurovascular compromise known as *compartment syndrome*.[11] The risk of applying a fiberglass cast too tightly can be mitigated by use of the "stretch-relax" technique. This technique involves gently stretching out a length of the fiberglass roll by unwinding approximately 4 to 6 inches of the mesh and then laying and contouring the material over the extremity.[12] The process is repeated until the extremity is completely wrapped. Careful molding about bony prominences to keep the cast from pistoning up and down is

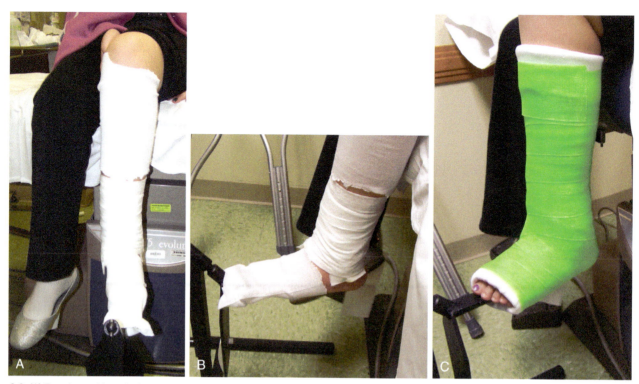

Fig. 3.9 (A) Foot is positioned with the ankle at 90 degrees. (B) Padding should be split on the dorsum of the ankle to prevent wrinkles. (C) Foot should be slid off the support when the cast is finished.

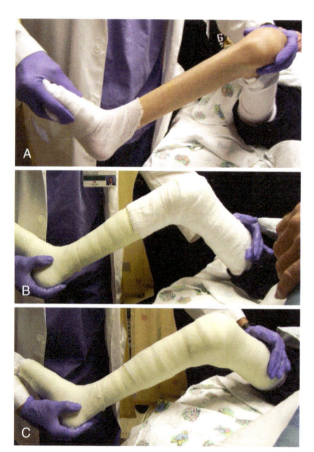

Fig. 3.10 (A) Padding should be applied over bony prominences. (B) The short leg part should be applied next. (C) The cast is then continued up the leg.

important. Splitting the cast in those situations where swelling is anticipated is recommended.[13]

Special consideration and care are needed for high-risk populations treated with casts. These include children with a lack of verbal skills because of incapacity (e.g., cerebral palsy, a genetic disorder, or obtundation because of injury), insensitivity (e.g., a spinal cord injury or myelodysplasia), or young age. Pressure sores underneath casts can occur when padding is inadequate or when the fit is suboptimal because of either too much padding or inadequate molding. These errors in technique allow the cast to shift to a position over unpadded skin or bony prominences where friction or increased pressure can contribute to skin breakdown. This problem is especially worrisome in young children who cannot verbalize their complaint or identify the area of particular concern. When the problem area can be identified (usually designated by the presence of burning or pain), a window may be cut in the cast overlying the area in question to allow the skin to be inspected and problems to be managed. If an area of pain or burning underneath the cast occurs, the area can be "starred," or a window can be cut out over the top of the afflicted area. The piece of the cast that was removed to create the window can then be replaced over a sufficient layer of new cast padding and overwrapped with fiberglass, if the skin does not need to be accessed, or with an elastic bandage if a need exists for ongoing access through the window to address problems with the skin and soft tissues.

Cast burns can occur as a result of the exothermic reaction of the casting material. Several simple practices can help avoid this complication: (1) Lukewarm water should always be used for dipping the cast rolls so that the peak setting temperatures are minimized. Halanski and colleagues[14] have suggested that the water temperature should not exceed 24°C. (2) The cast should be adequately rubbed with water as the material is being applied so that water can reach the interstices of the casting material, which helps dissipate heat. (3) Plastic pillows for propping the extremity after casting or covering the extremity with blankets or other materials that can block dissipation of heat while the cast is curing should be avoided.

CAST SAW BURNS AND CAST REMOVAL

The use of an oscillating saw for cast removal creates the potential for iatrogenic injury. Inadvertent cast saw burns can be attributed to inadequately padded casts, improper technique, or uncooperative patients. Burns and abrasions can occur from direct blade contact and from thermal injury created by frictional forces. Although the oscillating blade is designed to prevent the skin from being cut, proper technique and attention to detail are still a necessity if complications are to be avoided. Shuler and Grisafi[15] have shown that the combination of poor technique (never allowing the blade to leave the cast), fiberglass (as opposed to plaster) casting material, and insufficient cast padding (two layers rather than four) were all factors associated with elevated skin temperatures during cast removal in a cadaveric model. Practical tips for minimizing the risk of cutting or burning the skin during cast removal include the following:

1. Padding should be adequate when the cast is applied.
2. A sharp saw blade should always be used. Dull blades have been shown to generate significantly more heat that sharp ones.[16]
3. The technique of overlapping circles rather than "running" the blade when cutting should be used so that binding, which generates heat, is avoided.
4. Periodically stopping and allowing the blade to leave the cast and cool is recommended, particularly when hard material such as fiberglass is cut and when the cast is thick.[15] Cooling the blade with alcohol, water, or ultrasound gel–soaked sponge will expedite the blade cooling.[17] Commercially available protective strips placed between layers of cast padding shows promise for preventing cast saw injury.[18]
5. When feasible, bony prominences should be cut around rather than over so that the risk of direct blade contact and thermal injury is minimized. It is important to remember that, other than the situation in which a patient is uncooperative, all causes of cast saw injury are physician or equipment dependent and thus are potentially avoidable with attention to technique and detail.
6. Simulated training sessions can and do help prevent cast saw injuries and are a cost-effective tool in preventing litigation associated with these injuries.[19]

REFERENCES

The level of evidence (LOE) is determined according to the criteria provided in the Preface.

1. Wenger DR. *Rang's Children's Fractures*. Lippincott Williams & Wilkins. (**LOE VII**).
2. Gallagher DJ, Heinrich SD. Pediatric chance fracture. *J Orthop Trauma*. 1990;4(2):183–187. (**LOE III**).
3. Allen Jr BL, Schoch EP 3rd, Emery FE. Immediate spica cast system for femoral shaft fractures in infants and children. *South Med J*. 1978;71(1):18–22. (**LOE III**).
4. Mansour AA 3rd, Wilmoth JC, Mansour AS, et al. Immediate spica casting of pediatric femoral fractures in the operating room versus the emergency department: comparison of reduction, complications, and hospital charges. *J Pediatr Orthop*. 2010;30(8):813–817. (**LOE III**).
5. Kruse RW, Fracchia M, Boos M, et al. Goretex fabric as a cast underliner in children. *J Pediatr Orthop*. 1991;11(6):786–787. (**LOE III**).
6. McCarthy RE. A method for early spica cast application in treatment of pediatric femoral shaft fractures. *J Pediatr Orthop*. 1986;6(1):89–91. (**LOE IV**).
7. Mubarak SJ, Frick S, Sink E, et al. Volkmann contracture and compartment syndromes after femur fractures in children treated with 90/90 spica casts. *J Pediatr Orthop*. 2006;26(5):567–572. (**LOE III**).
8. Chess DG, Hyndman JC, Leahey JL, et al. Short arm plaster cast for distal pediatric forearm fractures. *J Pediatr Orthop*. 1994;14(2):211–213. (**LOE III**).
9. Bae DS, Valim C, Connell P, Brustowicz KA, Waters PM. Bivalved versus circumferential cast immobilization for displaced forearm fractures: a randomized clinical trial to assess efficacy and safety. *J Pediatr Orthop*. 2017;37(4):239–246(**LOE II**).
10. Bebbington A, Lewis P, Savage R. Cast wedging for orthopaedic surgeons! *Injury*. 2005;36(1):71–72. (**LOE IV**).
11. Marson BM, Keenan MA. Skin surface pressures under short leg casts. *J Orthop Trauma*. 1993;7(3):275–278. (**LOE II**).
12. Davids JR, Frick SL, Skewes E, et al. Skin surface pressure beneath an above-the-knee cast: plaster casts compared with fiberglass casts. *J Bone Joint Surg Am*. 1997;79(4):565–569. (**LOE II**).
13. Garfin SR, Mubarak SJ, Evans KL, et al. Quantification of intracompartmental pressure and volume under plaster casts. *J Bone Joint Surg Am*. 1981;63(3):449–453. (**LOE III**).
14. Halanski MA, Halanski AD, Oza A, et al. Thermal injury with contemporary cast-application techniques and methods to circumvent morbidity. *J Bone Joint Surg Am*. 2007;89(11):2369–2377. (**LOE N/A**).
15. Shuler FD, Grisafi FN. Cast-saw burns: evaluation of skin, cast, and blade temperatures generated during cast removal. *J Bone Joint Surg Am*. 2008;90(12):2626–2630. (**LOE II**).
16. Ansari MZ, Swarup S, Ghani R, et al. Oscillating saw injuries during removal of plaster. *Eur J Emerg Med*. 1998;5(1):37–39. (**LOE III**).
17. Puddy AC, Sunkin JA, Aden JK, Walick KS, Hsu JR. Cast saw burns: evaluation of simple techniques for reducing the risk of thermal injury. *J Pediatr Orthop*. 2014;34(8):e63–66 (**LOE N/A**).
18. Stork NC, Lenhart RL, Nemeth BA, Noonan KJ, Halanski MA. To cast, to saw, and not to injure: can safety strips decrease cast saw injuries? *Clin Orthop Relat Res*. 2016;474(7):1543–1552 (**LOE N/A**).
19. Bae DS, Lynch H, Jamieson K, Yu-Moe CW, Roussin C. Improved safety and cost savings from reductions in cast-saw burns after simulation-based education for orthopaedic surgery residents. *J Bone Joint Surg Am*. 2017;99(17):e94 (**LOE N/A**).

4 Pathologic Fractures in Children

James P. Norris IV | Herbert S. Schwartz | Ginger E. Holt

INTRODUCTION

Pathologic fractures occur in diseased bone, and, in children, such fractures are caused by a spectrum of conditions different from those in adults. Children's diseases frequently associated with pathologic fractures include noncancerous benign bone tumors and congenital or genetic abnormalities affecting the skeleton. Polyostotic disease with fractures affecting the immature skeleton is often caused by osteomyelitis, histiocytosis, vascular neoplasms, and metastases (neuroblastoma and Wilms tumor). Rarely, sarcomas may initially present with a fracture, and these patients require special consideration in their treatment approach. In contrast, causes of pathologic fractures in the adult skeleton, especially in individuals older than 40 years, include malignancies such as myeloma, metastatic carcinoma, lymphoma, and, rarely, sarcomas of the bone. Occasionally, giant cell tumors and enchondromas are identified. Elderly individuals frequently are seen with pathologic fractures from osteoporosis or Paget disease in addition to metastasis (Table 4.1).

The axial skeleton is frequently the site of metastatic foci because of its rich vascular supply relative to the appendicular skeleton. In general, pathologic fractures create a broad differential diagnosis. As a result, the orthopedic oncologist must approach each case by considering the patient's age, symptoms, image appearance, and an understanding of bone biology. Algorithms rarely suffice in pediatric orthopedics or orthopedic oncology.

The goal of this chapter is to introduce the reader to the multitude of variables involved in the successful treatment of pediatric pathologic fractures. A diagnosis *must* be made before embarking on any treatment strategy. Tissue documentation by biopsy is highly recommended to confirm the underlying diagnosis that lead to the pathologic fracture. Depending on the confidence of the treating surgeon, a radiographic diagnosis may substitute for a tissue one, for example, in unicameral bone cysts (UBCs). After these variables are carefully weighed and balanced, an optimal treatment strategy can be formulated for a particular child. A different child with the same fracture may benefit from a different treatment. Individually, pediatric orthopedics and orthopedic oncology each require a high degree of cognitive decision making. Pediatric pathologic fractures present an intersection of the two, which makes this decision making all the more complex.

BONE PHYSIOLOGY

Bone is a specialized connective tissue with matrix consisting predominantly of type I collagen. It is a dynamic organ that receives one-fifth of the cardiac output and is one of the only organs capable of true regeneration. Shaping of the skeleton and the buildup of bone mass during childhood and adolescence are a result of the constant interplay between bone formation and bone resorption. Bone remodeling continues throughout life. The average individual reaches peak bone mass in the third decade of life, and the adult skeleton contains approximately 2 million bone-remodeling units. Each unit comprises a spatial and temporal group of organized cells responsible for osteoclastic bone resorption and osteoblastic bone formation in response to local and environmental stimuli.

Bone resorption is mediated by the osteoclast, a multinucleated giant cell derived from granulocyte-macrophage precursors. Bone formation requires the presence and function of the osteoblast, which is derived from mesenchymal fibroblast-like cells. Net bone formation occurs by the process of coupling (contiguous and concurrent bone formation and resorption). Under normal circumstances, 88% to 95% of the bone surface area is quiescent, while the remainder is involved in active remodeling. The total time required to complete a remodeling cycle for a typical bone-remodeling unit in a young adult is estimated to be 200 days. One bone-remodeling unit takes approximately 3 weeks to complete bone resorption, whereas it takes 3 months to form bone in an adult. Bone formation is quicker in children. When this balance of resorption and formation is disordered by a pathologic process, the integrity of bone can be compromised.

Bone strength is related to a combination of material and structural properties. The mineral component of bone is responsible for most of its compressive strength, whereas both mineral and protein components are important for strength in tension.[1] Normal activity results in forces of compression, tension, and torsion. However, bone is weakest in torsion, and even a small cortical defect can significantly reduce torsional strength. For example, a 6-mm drill hole in the tibial shaft cortex, such as that generated to obtain a bone biopsy specimen, reduces torsional strength by 50%.[2]

PATHOLOGIC FRACTURE

A tumor present at a fracture delays, alters, or prevents bone healing. In certain instances, the rapid growth of the tumor cells overwhelms the reparative process of bone. In metastatic bone disease, damage to the skeleton is usually much more extensive than can be expected simply from the number of malignant cells present. Much evidence has now shown that most of the tumor-induced skeletal destruction is mediated by osteoclasts. Malignant cells secrete factors that both directly and indirectly stimulate osteoclastic activity.[3] These factors include a variety of cytokines: interleukin-1 (IL-1), IL-6, tumor necrosis factor, IL-11, IL-13, and IL-17. IL-1 is the most powerful stimulator of bone resorption in vitro. Growth factors identified in tumorous bone include transforming growth factor α, transforming growth factor β, and epidermal growth factor. Paracrine factors that also stimulate osteoclastic activity include prostaglandin E and parathyroid hormone–related protein (PTHrP), and these factors are typically produced by malignant cells. PTHrP is immunologically distinct from parathyroid hormone and stimulates osteoblasts and stromal cells to secrete the receptor activator of nuclear factor kB ligand (RANK-L).[4] RANK-L is one of the mechanisms by which osteoblast and osteoclast function is physiologically linked. It binds to osteoclast precursors, leading to osteoclastogenesis and subsequently bone resorption. Because of RANK-L induction by cancer cells, osteoclast activity is elevated leading to resorptive phenomena, like the osteolysis induced by metastatic breast cancer and the hypercalcemia of lung cancer.[5,6] RANK-L production in bone has also been shown to promote cancer cell migration to the local environment, thus creating a positive feedback loop for bone metastases.[7]

What is a pathologic fracture? Is it a radiologic, clinical, or combination diagnosis? Must the bone be completely or incompletely broken or displaced (or both) in one or more planes? Must the patient have symptoms or pain with activity? Can the bone be microscopically but not macroscopically fractured? These questions are pertinent because their answers are vital to the formation of proper treatment strategies. For the purposes of discussion, a pathologic fracture

is defined as a clinically symptomatic interruption in the cortex of a diseased bone—displaced or not. Although fractures are typically macroscopic, they do not necessarily have to be so. A child's bone is much more plastic than that of an adult. Bending without complete fiber separation occurs in a child and may be clinically relevant.

Healing of pathologic fractures has been found to correlate most closely with tumor type and patient survival.[8] Resection of the tumor deposit is an important part of the management of pathologic fractures. Thus, the biology of the bone and its biomechanics in conjunction with tumor pathology are important contributing variables to understand when the overall treatment of pathologic fractures is planned.

The most important task to be performed when a pathologic fracture is first detected is to establish the diagnosis with certainty. Although a radiographic diagnosis can be accurate, especially for UBCs, it is not a substitute for a tissue-confirmed diagnosis. Consequently, the authors recommend that a biopsy be strongly considered for all initial pathologic manifestations and other neoplasms of bone. Biopsy is a complex cognitive skill that depends on a careful history, physical examination, and interpretation of radiographic staging studies, including proper assessment of local, regional, and distant disease. It is crucial to determine whether polyostotic bone involvement is present. The surgeon is best able to interpret the diagnostic, anatomic, and pathologic significance of musculoskeletal disease and should thus review the images personally.

Biopsies are best performed by individuals with frequent experience. Complications from an improperly selected biopsy site can be devastating.[9] Nondiagnostic or nonrepresentative harvesting of lesional tissue delays the diagnosis, and biopsy performed before complete imaging can hamper treatment planning. Care must be taken when choosing image-guided biopsy versus open biopsy, as harm and delay can occur with a seemingly innocuous core/needle biopsy. Only after a tissue diagnosis is made can proper treatment ensue. Treatment must be based on understanding of three key components in each case. The surgeon must understand the relevant bone biology and physiology (component 1) and how this is affected by the pathologic diagnosis obtained (component 2) in order to determine how best to restore function (component 3).

Table 4.1 Age Distribution of Common Orthopedic Bone Tumors

Age (Years)	Tumor	
	Benign	Malignant
0–5	Chondroma Unicameral bone cyst Osteoid osteoma Nonossifying fibroma Fibrous dysplasia	Neuroblastoma (metastatic) Rhabdomyosarcoma (metastatic) Ewing sarcoma Osteosarcoma Lymphoma
10–40	Chondroma Osteoid osteoma Aneurysmal bone cyst Unicameral bone cyst Nonossifying fibroma Fibrous dysplasia Eosinophilic granuloma Chondroblastoma (skeletally immature) Giant cell tumor (skeletally mature)	Osteosarcoma Ewing sarcoma Lymphoma
40+	Chondroma Giant cell tumor Hemangioma	Carcinoma Multiple myeloma Lymphoma Chondrosarcoma Osteosarcoma Chordoma

OUTCOME TRIANGLE

It is an error to treat a pathologic fracture as though it were a fracture through normal bone. Unfortunately, it is far too common for an orthopedic surgeon to emphasize the type and choice of internal fixation implant rather than the timing and planning of surgery for a pathologic fracture. To achieve satisfactory treatment and outcomes in individuals with pathologic fractures, the surgeon must suppress this dangerous reflex. Proper treatment planning depends on weighing all variables about a particular pathologic fracture and the individual patient before developing a treatment strategy. A multitude of treatment variables can be schematically represented in the three points of the outcome triangle (Fig. 4.1). A thorough and properly weighted evaluation of the triad of variables in the outcome triangle is more likely to result in a favorable outcome for a patient with a pathologic fracture than will the more traditional orthopedic surgical approach. Again, these three variables are bone biology and biomechanics (component 1), pathology (component 2), and function (component 3).

OUTCOME, PART I—BONE BIOLOGY

Bone biology, the first part of the triad, includes the cellular makeup of the fractured bone and its biomechanical environment. Each bone is different, and each site within a bone is different, depending on age. The healing potential of a bone is a function of certain variables, including remodeling potential, patient's age, vascularity, position relative to the physis, and the density of bone-remodeling units. Of course, the pathologic process can affect these variables. Osteopetrosis, or marble bone disease, is a congenital disease manifested by deficient or absent osteoclasts. The resultant dense, brittle bone frequently results in pediatric pathologic fractures (Fig. 4.2). The lineage and the sequence of growth and differentiation factors necessary to convert primitive monocyte precursors to functioning osteoclasts were elaborated in an elegant series of experiments.[5,10,11] The first regulating factor converts the primitive monocyte-macrophage stem cell into a macrophage precursor. This transcription factor is labeled PU.1. Experimental knockout mice deficient

in PU.1 lack macrophages and osteoclasts, and the condition is lethal.[12] Mouse mutants deficient in macrophage colony–stimulating factor lack osteoclasts but contain immature macrophages; osteopetrosis develops in these mice but is cured by bone marrow transplantation.

Osteoprotegerin (OPG), a glycoprotein that regulates bone resorption, is a member of the tumor necrosis factor receptor superfamily. It is a decoy receptor that competes with RANK for RANK ligand, which is responsible along with c-*fos* for differentiating the macrophage into an early osteoclast. OPG itself is a macrophage receptor similar to the RANK receptor, and it impedes osteoclastogenesis. Mice lacking αvβ3 integrin or c-*src* have substantial osteoclast numbers, but the cells fail to polarize. It allows conversion of an immature osteoclast into a functioning osteoclast with a ruffled border. *Src* knockout experiments yield nonfunctional osteoclasts lacking cathepsin K, carbonic anhydrase II, or the proton-transporting adenosine triphosphate synthase pump. These nonfunctional osteoclasts are incapable of creating an acidic microenvironment and thus cannot resorb bone. Therefore, overproduction of OPG results in limited osteoclast formation and the clinical syndrome of osteopetrosis. Decreased OPG production results in too many osteoclasts being produced and the clinical syndrome of osteoporosis. Administration of recombinant OPG to normal adult mice causes a profound yet nonlethal form of osteopetrosis. Administration of an OPG analog in humans in the form of denosumab has provided another agent to fight tumor-induced osteolysis and prevent pathologic fracture in metastatic disease.[6] Thus, age and cellular makeup can help in determining the extent and healing potential of the bone and can serve as a guide for treatment.

Fig. 4.2 depicts a subtrochanteric fracture in an osteopetrotic pediatric femur with no evidence of osteoclast function. Marrow formation is absent. A transverse fracture has occurred as a result of the pathologic process and brittleness

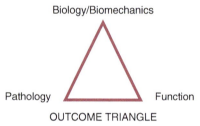

Biology/Biomechanics

Pathology   Function

OUTCOME TRIANGLE

Fig. 4.1 Outcome triangle for pathologic fractures (see text).

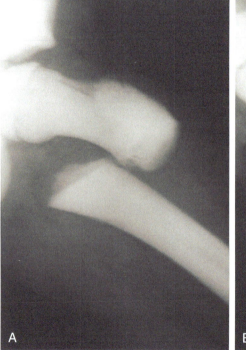
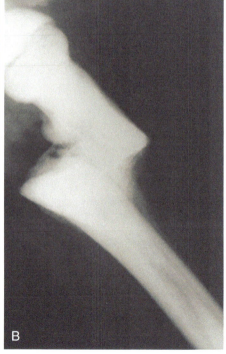

Fig. 4.2 (A) Initial films of a pathologic fracture of the femur of a child with osteopetrosis. (B) The healed fracture shows little remodeling.

A

B

of the bone. The fracture can heal but will not have significant remodeling potential. This outcome can be anticipated by the lack of bone resorption units, or osteoclasts. Understanding the disease process and the healing potential of the bone helps guide the treatment strategy. For instance, intramedullary implants are difficult or impossible to insert because of the lack of a medullary canal, and extramedullary implants create stress risers that increase the risk for additional, delayed fractures. Therefore, biologic manipulation (bone marrow transplantation) of the fracture and secondary bone healing may offer the most advantageous treatment strategy.

Neurofibromatosis provides another example of how understanding bone biology and its relationship to disease affects the healing potential when a physician deals with a pathologic fracture. An anterolateral tibial bow is associated with neurofibromatosis type 1 approximately half the time. The resulting pseudarthrosis is not usually present at birth and therefore not truly congenital, but it occurs during the first decade of life. The dysplastic, hamartomatous bone is poorly vascularized and unable to withstand the continual stresses applied, causing fracture and angulation (Fig. 4.3). Union is compromised, and fracture healing is adversely affected because of the nonanatomic biomechanics and poor

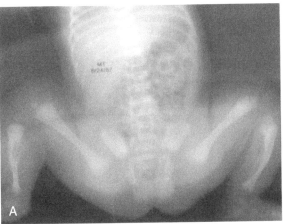

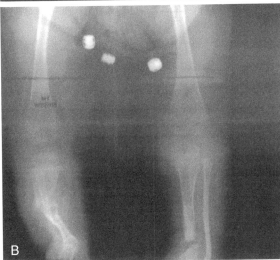

Fig. 4.3 Pseudarthrosis of the tibia from neurofibromatosis. (A) Radiograph of a newborn demonstrating a pathologic fracture of the right tibia and an impending fracture of the left tibia. (B) Radiograph of a 1-year-old demonstrating bilateral pathologic fractures resulting in tibial pseudarthroses.

vascularity at the site. Manifestations of the disease alter with time, thereby limiting the usefulness of many of the morphologic classification systems currently in use. Union is best achieved by correcting the biomechanical and biologic environment because the pathology is of limited consequence in neurofibromatosis. Excision of the pseudarthrosis in conjunction with bone grafting, intramedullary fixation, and occasionally circular external fixation is a common procedure after failure of early treatment, including total contact bracing.[13] Autogenous bone grafting is of assistance. A vascularized fibular graft or distraction osteogenesis can also be considered, depending on the circumstances.[14] Realignment of the limb to create compressive rather than tension forces at the pseudarthrosis site is beneficial. This approach is a good example of a culmination of the three key outcome components: (1) both the biology and biomechanics are altered, (2) the pathology is removed, and (3) function is ultimately restored. A Syme amputation can even result in spontaneous union.[15]

Pathologic fractures of certain bones can help dictate their management. High stress is concentrated on the tension areas of weight-bearing bones, including the femoral neck and diaphysis of the tibia. Far more load is applied to weight-bearing bones than to non–weight-bearing bones. Fractures of vertebral bodies create the potential for spinal cord injuries. Vertebrae plana is caused by localized histiocytosis (eosinophilic granuloma) of the vertebral body. The natural history is one of spontaneous resolution without operative intervention, but a tissue diagnosis is often necessary, especially if monostotic disease is present, to exclude a malignant etiology. Infrequently, vertebrae plana can result in a neurologic deficit.[16] Fig. 4.4 portrays the natural history of vertebrae plana without surgical intervention.

The biology of pathologic fracture healing is affected by the administration of chemotherapy or by irradiation of the injured site, an issue especially important in malignant pathologic fractures. The administration of chemotherapy or radiation therapy to pathologic fractures secondary to sarcoma typically facilitates fracture healing. Although it is generally recognized that chemotherapy and radiation therapy delay the normal bone's cellular response to healing a fracture, in the presence of rapidly dividing malignant cells, cytotoxic therapy provides a net positive result. Chemotherapy or external-beam radiation therapy, by destroying more cancerous than normal cells, creates a more favorable milieu for fracture healing. This effect of therapy on bone is another example demonstrating the need to understand bone biology for facilitation of fracture healing.

OUTCOME, PART II—PATHOLOGY

The pathology component of the outcome triangle is based on an understanding of the disease and its biologic behavior and natural history, factors that are paramount in determining treatment. Treatment also depends on knowing the diagnosis, which can only be established with certainty from a properly obtained and representative biopsy sample. Although myriad pathologic entities may affect bone, thus making it susceptible to fracture, the modes of treatment are far fewer. Groups of pathologic entities that can result in pathologic fracture include (1) genetic or metabolic bone disease abnormalities (e.g., osteogenesis imperfecta [OI] or osteopetrosis), (2) nutritional or environmental disturbances (e.g., rickets), (3) benign bone tumors (e.g., cystic, cartilaginous, and fibrous tumors), (4) skeletal sarcomas (e.g., osteosarcoma and Ewing sarcoma), and (5) skeletal metastases (e.g., neuroblastoma and rhabdomyosarcoma). These five disease categories represent a multitude of diagnoses, both neoplastic and nonneoplastic. Rather than elaborating on each pathologic entity, it is convenient to group them by pathobiologic activity (Table 4.2).

Management of pathologic fractures is predicated on an understanding of the biologic relationship between the pathology and the bone. Both active and inactive UBCs or growing and static cartilage neoplasms of bone may be encountered. Fibrous dysplasia in a femoral neck is not the same as fibrous dysplasia in the diaphysis of a long bone. Despite histologic similarities, a nonossifying fibroma occupying three-quarters of the diameter of a long bone has consequences different from those of a fibrous cortical defect. Hence, the key to understanding neoplastic and non-neoplastic pathologic fractures is to know the effect that the lesion has on a bone and how to best correct the problems caused by it. Treatment is not based on memorizing the textbook definition of a particular tumor. Instead, proper treatment depends on determining the relationship of the pathology to the specific bone and subsequently formulating a method to augment fracture healing for the particular patient.

Pathology alone does not dictate management. Consequently, the plan of this section is to group treatment options into three categories and give appropriate pathologic examples for each. The treatment categories are (1) nonoperative management, (2) intralesional surgery with or without bone grafting or implants, and (3) wide tumor resection with reconstruction of the skeletal defect. Irrespective of the treatment option, strong consideration and respect must be given to the viability and preservation of the physis and epiphysis to avoid the consequences of limb length inequality or deformity. Pathology is but one of the triad of components that compose the outcome triangle and must be weighed in the overall equation for optimal management of a particular pathologic fracture.

NONOPERATIVE MANAGEMENT

Nonoperative management requires that the surgeon who is part of the treatment team be confident in the diagnosis and outcome. Patience and experience result from an understanding of the natural history of the disease and the morbidity associated with surgical intervention. Inherited genetic diseases such as OI or osteopetrosis frequently result in pathologic fractures that are often managed nonoperatively. Fig. 4.2 presents the natural history of pathologic fracture healing managed nonoperatively. Osteopetrotic bone lacks ruffled-bordered osteoclasts; thus, the ability to resorb bone is compromised. Medullary canals are atrophic or absent, but bone formation is not impaired. As a result, fracture healing occurs, but remodeling is slower. The bone is often more brittle than normal bone. Thus, intramedullary or extramedullary implants can create more problems than secondary bone healing alone. Excellent clinical outcomes may result in osteopetrotic pathologic fractures when a conservative management approach is undertaken.

OI is a syndrome resulting from a mutation in one of the two genes controlling type I collagen synthesis, and most fit into four clinical types. Type I OI mutations prematurely terminate the message for 50% of collagen synthesis. Type II OI results from the replacement of a helical glycine with a larger amino acid. The mutant chain interferes with helix formation, and normal collagen falls to 20%. Types III and IV are disruptions in mineralization.[17,18] Hydroxyapatite matrix formation is imperfect, therefore resulting in a structurally weakened bone lattice. The bone fragility in OI has a variable clinical spectrum in terms of the susceptibility to

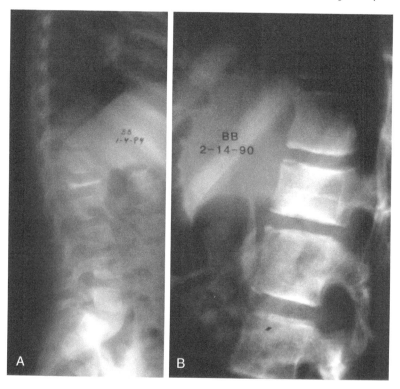

Fig. 4.4 (A) Localized histiocytosis demonstrated as L1 vertebrae plana, and (B) reconstitution of vertebral body height over a 6-year time interval.

Table 4.2   Musculoskeletal-Related Disorders

Disease	Inheritance	Genetics	Defect
Ewing sarcoma	—	t(11,22)	Loss of tumor suppressor gene(s) and creation of a fusion product
Osteosarcoma	—	17p13, p53 13q14	Loss of tumor suppressor gene(s) Retinoblastoma gene type 1
Achondroplasia	AD	4p16	*FGFR-3* gene Abnormal endochondral bone formation
Neurofibromatosis (NF) NF1 NF2	 AD AD	 17q11 22q11	 Neurofibromin Schwannomin
Osteogenesis imperfecta Clinical group I mild Clinical group II lethal Clinical group III deforming Clinical group IV moderate	 AD AR AR AD	 α1, #17 α2, #17	 50% decreased type I collagen Unstable triple helix Abnormal type I Shortened pro-α chains
Osteopetrosis Mild, tarda Malignant, infantile		SRC, OPG, RANK M-CSF; PU.1	Osteoclasts lack complete differentiation Defective osteoclastogenesis
Rickets Vitamin D-deficient Vitamin D-dependent Vitamin D-resistant	 Diet AR X-linked dominant	12q14	Decreased vitamin D intake Leads to secondary hyperparathyroidism Lack of renal 25 (OH)-vitamin $D_1\alpha$-hydroxylase Impaired renal tubular phosphate resorption (*PEX*, cellular endopeptidase)
Fibrous dysplasia	—	20q13.2–13.3	$G_s\alpha$ (receptor-coupled signaling protein for cAMP)
Osteochondromatosis	—	8q24.1/11p11	*EXT1, EXT2* genes

AD, Autosomal dominant; *AR,* autosomal recessive; *cAMP,* cyclic adenosine monophosphate; *M-CSF,* macrophage colony-stimulating factor; *OPG,* osteoprotegerin; *RANK,* receptor for activation of nuclear factor κB; *#,* chromosome number.

fracture and the age at presentation. Weight-bearing bones are treated differently from non–weight-bearing bones. The age of the patient and the proximity of the fracture line to the physis are important considerations in management. Remodeling bone formation and bone resorption both behave and occur in a nearly normal fashion. In Fig. 4.5, nonoperative management and pathologic fracture healing are shown in a patient with OI. Nonoperative management is indicated for upper extremity fractures that can be successfully treated without angular deformity. Lower extremity fractures, especially after deformity has occurred, are best treated with internal fixation and frequently require multiple osteotomies. The Sheffield telescopic intramedullary rod is associated with fewer complications than older rod constructs, but still lacks reliable fixation which can lead to migration.[19] Seen in Fig. 4.6, Fassier telescoping rods offer a single entry point as well as screw thread fixation to prevent migration while achieving comparable or fewer complications.[20] Others have developed interlocking screw constructs to further address the problem of migration.[21] Regardless of implant, the ultimate goal in treatment is to maintain mobility, which is best accomplished by maintaining length and preventing deformity. Fig. 4.5 depicts a fracture that has healed initially by nonoperative treatment, but the deformity of the femur was so great that intramedullary fixation and multiple osteotomies were required. Fracture immobilization in children

with OI can also be a problem because it induces disuse osteoporosis. Therefore, casting of these fractures must emphasize stability.

Nutritional rickets is a condition in which polyostotic pathologic fractures may occur. Fig. 4.7 shows an adolescent with primary hyperparathyroidism and multiple brown tumors, identified on staging radiographic studies. A distal radial pathologic fracture was the presenting symptom, but detection of hypercalcemia and analysis of a bone biopsy specimen were required to establish the diagnosis. Once the diagnosis was determined with certainty, skeletal treatment was clearly best approached in a conservative manner. After removal of the parathyroid adenoma, commencement of skeletal calcium repletion allowed fracture healing to begin. Therefore, the fracture management goals were to maintain alignment while calcium homeostasis normalized. Parathyroidectomy and parenteral calcium repletion over a period of 3 to 4 months were necessary before initiation of fracture healing. Any surgical implant would have served little purpose in this case.

UBCs frequently manifest as pathologic fractures in children and are typically treated nonoperatively. These fractures occur on the metaphyseal side of a long bone, and the cyst abuts the physis. Often, it is not the tumor itself but rather a pathologic fracture that causes pain and prompts the child to complain. The typical radiographic finding is that of a "fallen

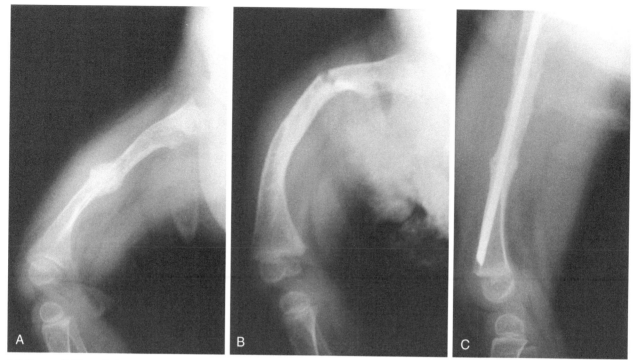

Fig. 4.5 Sequential lateral views of the femur of a child with osteogenesis imperfecta show (A) deformity from sequential fractures and healing, (B) refracture, and (C) healing after shish-kebab realignment osteotomies of the femur.

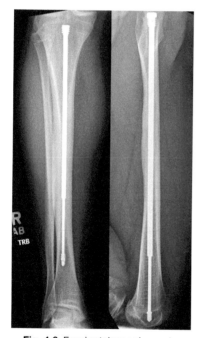

Fig. 4.6 Fassier telescoping rods.

leaf" sign, as noted by the arrows in Fig. 4.8A. One must ask from where the "leaf" falls. In fact, the leaf represents a piece of cortical bone that has fractured, become displaced, and fallen into the fluid-filled cavity inside the bone. The fractures may be displaced, nondisplaced, or shattered like an eggshell. Frequently, UBCs require only nonoperative treatment (Fig. 4.8). Initial fracture healing is likely, but recurrent fractures may occur as a result of the biomechanical inferiority of the hollow cystic bone structure.

The pathogenesis of UBCs remains an enigma. Causes range from the synovial cysts postulated by Mirra and colleagues[22] to dysplastic bone formed in response to trauma.[23] Vascular phenomena have also been attributed to the etiology of UBCs, and vary from venous occlusion of the intramedullary space to the presence of inflammatory cytokine mediators in the cyst fluid that incite osteolysis.[24] Whether the inflammatory mediators are the cause or a result of the bone resorption is unknown. Another possible cause is postulated by the theory that vascular occlusion induces increased venous pressure, which results in bone resorption. These theories all suggest a nonneoplastic origin of UBCs and explain their conservative management strategy.

Nonoperative management should be the first treatment option and has been associated with success rates of 64%.[25] Should this option fail, defined as a persistent cyst and repeated fractures, measures that wash out the inflammatory mediators or lower the interstitial cavity pressure are frequently performed. Trephination procedures involve the insertion of at least two needles into the cavity and injection of methylprednisolone into the cyst, as proposed by Scaglietti and associates,[26] or irrigation with normal saline under fluoroscopic guidance. Additionally, the trocar can be injected with a variety of substances, including autogenous bone marrow, allograft, demineralized bone matrix, or other bone graft substitutes. Older literature suggested a broad range of success with steroid injection, ranging from 15% to 88%, but this required three to four injections on average to achieve healing.[26,27] A more recent analysis suggested pooled success rates of 77% for steroid injections, 78% with bone marrow, and 98.7% with demineralized bone matrix.[25] These outcomes are similar to historical recurrence rates after curettage and filling with various forms of bone graft and bone graft substitutes.[25,27]

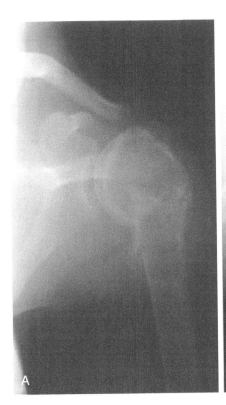
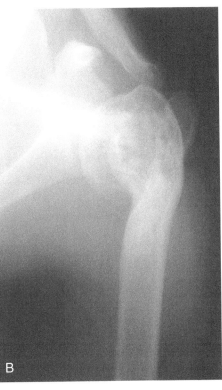

Fig. 4.7 (A) Pathologic fracture of the proximal part of the humerus from rickets of primary hyperparathyroidism. (B) After parathyroidectomy and 14 months of calcium repletion, the fracture has healed.

Because of the lack of a clear advantage to surgical intervention, nonoperative management or injection techniques has been offered preferentially, particularly for non–weight-bearing bones, such as for proximal humeral UBCs. However, several studies have demonstrated that stabilization of UBC pathologic fractures, particularly in weight-bearing bones, such as the proximal femur, offers benefits of prompt mobilization, early weight-bearing without the need of a cast, and avoidance of refracture.[28,29] A proximal femoral UBC warrants caution because intraarticular pathologic neck fractures and their sequelae pose potentially significant long-term orthopedic problems. Fig. 4.9 demonstrates a pathologic fracture in the femoral neck from a UBC.

Fibrous cortical defects are benign bone tumors that are typically incidentally detected on radiographs. Their natural history is one of slow ossification. They are often polyostotic (20%) and are typically located in the long bones of the lower extremities. Until ossification, the cortical lesions may represent stress risers. As a result, they can be the nidus for a fracture line. Fig. 4.10 presents an oblique, low-energy spiral fracture through the distal tibial metaphysis in association with a fibrous cortical defect. The figure demonstrates noneventful healing in a cast in this skeletally immature child. Remodeling has occurred, with subsequent partial obliteration of the benign bone tumor. A fibrous cortical defect appears to be histologically identical to its larger counterpart, nonossifying fibroma. Nonossifying fibromas involve the medullary canal and are typically surgically treatable lesions. They will be discussed later.

Osteochondromas are benign bone tumors with cartilaginous caps. Although fractures through the stalks of these tumors can occur, they seldom, if ever, are associated with pathologic fractures because the bone is often stronger in these areas than the contralateral uninvolved side. They can

result in angular deformities that may require corrective surgery later in childhood.[30]

INTRALESIONAL CURETTAGE

Benign bone tumors with true growth potential are frequently treated operatively with *intralesional curettage*. Such benign bone tumors include nonossifying fibroma, aneurysmal bone cyst, eosinophilic granuloma (monostotic histiocytosis), and chondroblastoma. These lesions have radiographic and clinical features that overlap with those of malignant bone tumors. In addition, osteomyelitis has clinical and radiographic findings in common with malignant bone tumors. Therefore, the reader is reminded that a pathologic diagnosis by biopsy is warranted. Continued neoplastic growth potential is likely for some of these benign bone tumors. Treatment options depend on establishing a diagnosis and involve eradication of the tumor by intralesional resection followed by skeletal reconstruction. Skeletal reconstruction usually entails bone grafting (an autogenous graft or allograft) with or without internal fixation with a metallic implant. Fig. 4.11 depicts a pathologic fracture through a diaphyseal eosinophilic granuloma (localized histiocytosis). The differential diagnosis for this lesion with poor radiographic margins includes Ewing sarcoma and osteomyelitis. The pathologic fracture resulted in displacement and is best managed by biopsy confirmation followed by vigorous (intralesional resection) curettage, bone grafting, and internal fixation with a plate and screws. Occasionally, the trauma of the fracture may be sufficient to disturb the local blood supply and eradicate the neoplasm. However, after a thorough biopsy, it is wise to proceed with complete intralesional resection.

When skeletal reconstruction with a bone graft or bone graft substitute appears to be indicated, many surgeons prefer to avoid the morbidity of iliac bone graft harvesting by

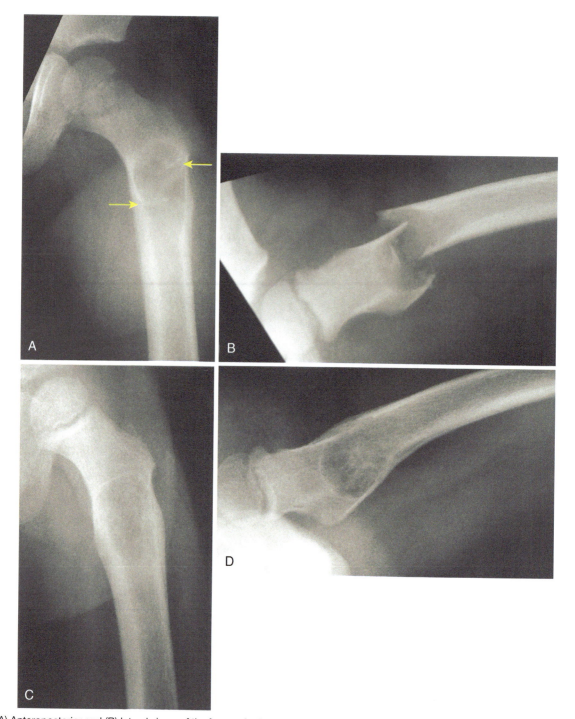

Fig. 4.8 (A) Anteroposterior and (B) lateral views of the femur of a 2-year-old boy who was seen with pain and an inability to bear weight after a fall. After 6 weeks' treatment in a spica cast, the (C) anteroposterior and (D) lateral radiographs show healing of the fracture and early filling of the cyst with bony matrix.

using the variety of bone graft substitutes currently available on the market. However, to date, no reliable, controlled, documented, published series have compared bone graft substitutes with autogenous bone grafts in humans, especially in children, who have the greater potential for bone regrowth. Part of the reason for the paucity of controlled trials is that it is hard to noninvasively measure bone regrowth at the pathologic fracture site. The size of the eradicated tumor cavity and the pathology differ so greatly from patient to patient that uniformity in treatment is hard to achieve.

Nonetheless, it appears that calcium sulfate, allografts with or without demineralized bone matrix, or autogenous bone grafts or bone marrow result in successful bone healing at pathologic fracture sites after curettage in the range of 50% to 80%.[13,31,27] This success rate encourages surgeons to try these measures before proceeding with the separate incision necessary for iliac crest bone graft harvesting.

The use of metallic implants remains controversial. Intramedullary devices offer biomechanical advantages over extramedullary devices. Flexible intramedullary nailing has

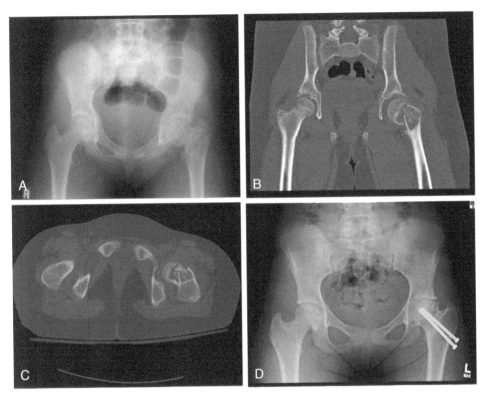

Fig. 4.9 The long-term complications of a pathologic fracture in the femoral neck from a unicameral bone cyst. The femoral head underwent osteonecrosis even though the fracture united. At 3 years postfracture, this teenager remains asymptomatic despite the radiographic appearance of an aspheric noncongruent hip, whose destiny is undoubtedly osteoarthritis. (A) Fracture at age 12 years on standard anteroposterior (AP) plain radiograph. (B) Coronal computed tomographic (CT) reconstruction. (C) Axial CT image. (D) Plain AP radiograph 3 years' postbiopsy, grafting, and pin stabilization.

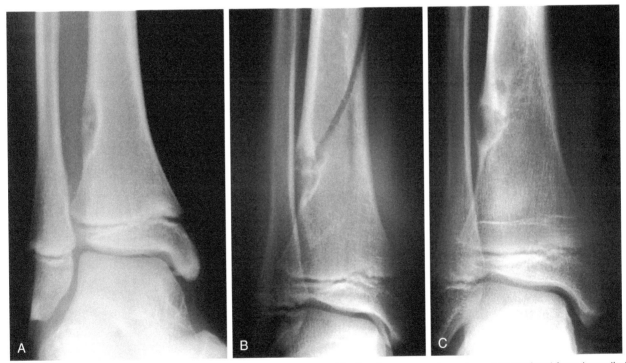

Fig. 4.10 (A) A fibrous cortical defect, which was identified as an incidental finding, becomes a stress riser when torsional force is applied (B). Healing of the fracture and remodeling have partially obliterated the lesion (C).

emerged as an accepted procedure for pediatric long bone fractures. The technique has also been shown to be advantageous in pathologic fractures, providing early stability and mobilization while obviating the need for a cast and potentially decreasing the prevalence of refracture. Rigid intramedullary fixation of skeletally immature long bones is gaining popularity, although the risk of avascular necrosis and alteration of the physis remains real, albeit small.[32,33] Fifty

adolescents from 10 to 16 years of age were treated by inserting antegrade intramedullary devices through the greater trochanteric apophysis for traumatic femoral fractures. A recent review of avascular necrosis rates across 19 studies compared the rate for three separate starting points: piriformis (2%), tip of the greater trochanter (1.4%), and lateral aspect of the trochanter (0%).[32] This issue is better discussed in other chapters in this textbook, but intramedullary devices

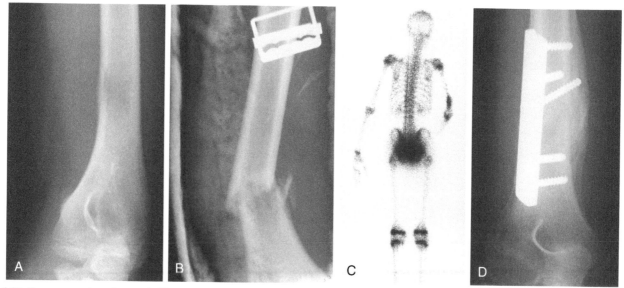

Fig. 4.11 The same male patient as in Fig. 4.4 developed an unrelated lesion of the distal humerus (A). This lesion is purely lytic, with no obvious fracture but with periosteal new bone. After a fracture through this lesion (B), an early bone scan (C) shows increased activity. Bone graft and internal fixation (D) led to good fracture and lesional healing of this eosinophilic granuloma.

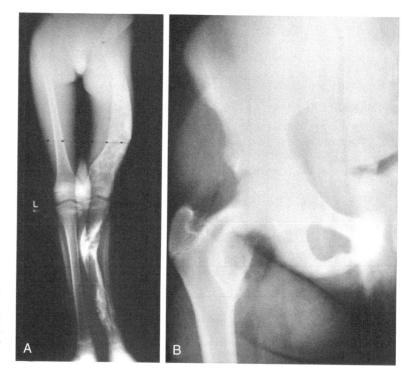

Fig. 4.12 (A) Fibrous dysplasia. A standing anteroposterior view shows the legs of an individual with severe, unilateral fibrous dysplasia. These untreated femoral and tibial deformities result in painful limitation of any weight-bearing activities. (B) Fibrous dysplasia in this proximal femur caused a painful limp and early varus deformity.

appear to be relatively safe, when thoughtfully chosen and carefully placed.[34,35]

Because of the greater reparative capacity of children's fractures, the strength of the implant frequently does not need to be as great as it does in adults. After a pathologic fracture is treated by curettage and bone grafting, it is common to insert internal fixation devices, such as a plate and screws, to prevent a torsional fracture through stress risers created by the bone defect. The typical six to eight cortices required for screw purchase on each side of the fracture site are not indicated, as is dogma for adult fracture osteosynthesis. Children's bones typically withstand earlier loading and are more pliable than those of adults. Early healing and weight-bearing are thus possible.

Fibrous dysplasia and enchondromas are special instances of benign bone tumors that can be associated with pathologic fractures. Their respective polyostotic forms (polyostotic fibrous dysplasia, with or without McCune-Albright syndrome, and Ollier disease, Fig. 4.12) require complex treatment strategies because of the increased tumor burden in the fractured bone or in neighboring bones. Oftentimes, these fibrous and cartilaginous lesions may, in fact, overlap histologically. Malunions, angular deformities, and limb length inequalities present long-term challenges for the orthopedic surgeon. Such reconstruction strategies are best deferred to other chapters. Fibrous dysplasia is not a true bone neoplasm. Rather, it represents the skeletal manifestations of a postzygotic mutation in somatic cells creating an activating gene that encodes the alpha subunit of G protein.[36] The locus of the mutation is chromosome 20q13.2-13.3. As a result, risk of progression is high, and surgical treatment of fibrous dysplasia should not be aimed at removing the entire "tumor."[37] Rather, the surgical goal should be one of skeletal stabilization.

Surgical indications for pathologic fractures in this setting should include fractures causing persistent pain or progressive deformity, as well as the obvious radiographic skeletal fracture. Long-term symptoms are usually the result of multiple and repeated microfractures, which often precede frank fractures. Treatment is best geared toward correcting the biomechanical deformity rather than resecting the entire tumor. Frequently, tumor resection is not advised.[38] The "shepherd's crook" deformity in fibrous dysplasia of the femoral neck is best treated with mechanical implantation (see Fig. 4.12). Enneking and Geran used fibulas or grafts of cortical bone inserted into the intramedullary portion of the head, neck, and shaft, similar to a second-generation intramedullary nail.[38] Twelve of their 15 patients initially were seen with fatigue fractures. No attempt was made to resect the tumors. Osteotomies may be required to restore normal anatomic alignment to the proximal end of the femur. In these situations, intramedullary devices have proved superior to extramedullary devices.[39]

The weight-bearing status of the bone can also affect treatment strategies. Skeletally immature weight-bearing long bones of the lower extremity affected with symptomatic fibrous dysplasia are best treated by open reduction and internal fixation with an intramedullary device.[40] In contrast, upper extremity non–weight-bearing long bones are satisfactorily treated by closed methods. The data imply that continued weight-bearing on a biomechanically deficient pathologic bone results in pain and progressive deformity from repeated microfractures. Eventually, a stress fracture or obvious displaced fracture is radiographically identified. Therefore, internal stabilization with an implant is preferred to minimize pain, deformity, and suffering. The growth potential of these neoplasms remains but is often of a less threatening magnitude. Clinical and radiographic follow-up through at least skeletal maturity is recommended. Malignant transformations of enchondromas in Ollier disease, although technically, *chondrosarcomas* are typically low grade and have a relatively low mortality rate (12%) in comparison to more traditional forms of the disease.[41,42] Therefore, an emphasis on early biomechanical treatment of pathologically weakened bone appears to be a priority.[43]

Nonossifying fibromas, typically when they exceed 50% of the bone's diameter, result in pathologic fractures in weight-bearing long bones. For these reasons, prophylactic fixation after biopsy confirmation and intralesional curettage is indicated for symptomatic lesions.[44] The superiority of autogenous bone grafts over bone graft substitutes in pediatric patients has not been proved.

WIDE TUMOR RESECTION

Wide, margin-free surgical resection of bone tumors is typically reserved for skeletal sarcomas. Pathologic fractures occurring through skeletal sarcomas are complicated orthopedic and oncologic conditions that are best treated by an experienced multidisciplinary management team. This team is large and

encompasses medical and nonmedical professionals who care for children with a pathologic fracture through a malignant bone tumor. Clearly, the method of diagnosis remains of paramount importance because even the placement of a needle puncture or biopsy tract can jeopardize limb survival. Pathologic fractures through skeletal sarcomas such as osteosarcoma come in varied patterns. They can be the initial manifestation of the disease, or they can occur after diagnosis and neoadjuvant chemotherapy. Osteosarcomas that initially manifest as a pathologic fracture frequently do so with displacement and local hemorrhaging (Fig. 4.13). This complication presents the management team with the problem of malignant cell contamination of the fracture hematoma. Pathologic fractures that occur after neoadjuvant therapy are typically those of mechanical insufficiency and result in angular deformity. The risk of tumor seeding is less than after early manifestations. The clinical significance of a pathologic fracture in the setting of a nonmetastatic bone sarcoma has been an issue of debate in the literature over the last two decades. Earlier reports suggested that with standard chemotherapy regimens and appropriate surgical resection margins, local recurrence and survival rates were not significantly lower compared with patients without a fracture.[45,46] More recent meta-analyses have suggested decreased survival with pathologic fractures in the setting of osteosarcoma—an effect that was not seen in chondrosarcoma nor Ewing sarcoma.[47,48] Still yet, a 2016 article considered tumor size and location in a multivariate analysis that appeared to mitigate this worse prognosis.[49] The balance of the literature suggests that survival rates after pathologic fracture can approach those achieved in patients without a fracture. However, such fractures are a serious complication that jeopardize limb salvage and should be prevented as much as is possible. The surgeon should strongly recommend protected weight-bearing and provide appropriate patient teaching.

Wide surgical resection may also be indicated for treating metastatic lesions that are infrequently associated with pathologic fractures in the immature skeleton, including patients with metastatic rhabdomyosarcoma or younger children with metastatic neuroblastoma. Depending on the stage, disease-free interval, and functional condition of the child, variables may dictate whether a wide surgical resection is indicated. Children with an anticipated longer event-free survival period before diagnosis of an isolated metastasis are more likely to require a wide resection margin.

After wide resection, the reconstruction alternatives are more complex than after intralesional or nonoperative management. Large skeletal defects need to be managed with structural allografts or megaprosthesis arthroplasties. Often, composites of the two are indicated. Expandable prostheses offer limb-lengthening options for young children with a large skeletal defect adjacent to a joint. Extra-anatomic reconstructions are also possible, including the Van Nes rotationplasty and the claviculo pro humeri technique. Further discussion of reconstructive options is beyond the scope of this chapter. In short, numerous limb salvage options are available—each with distinct advantages and disadvantages—which must be weighed against those of amputation.

OUTCOME, PART III—FUNCTION

To maximize the return of skeletal function after a pathologic fracture, one must determine how the pathologic

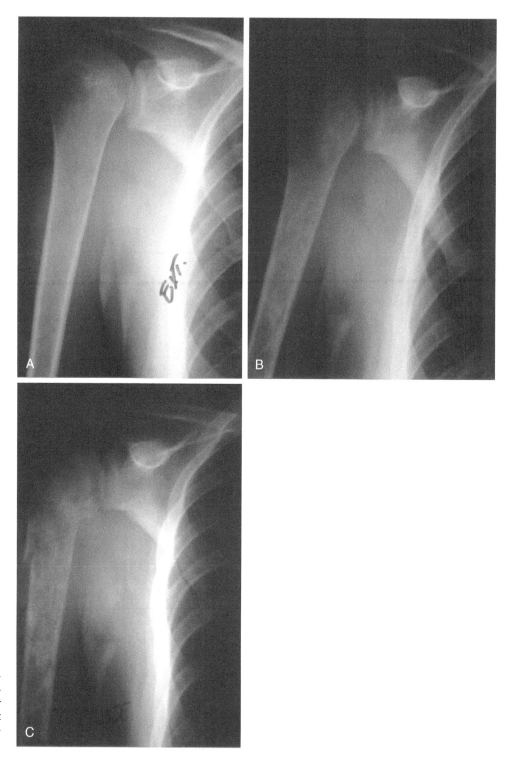

Fig. 4.13 Osteosarcoma of the proximal end of the humerus with a pathologic fracture. (A) Normal, December 1999. (B) Tumor destruction, August 2001. (C) Pathologic fracture, September 2001.

fracture has altered the patient's activity level and lifestyle. Neither radiographic studies nor algorithms are sufficient for determining the next step. Not all pathologic fractures are the same. Rather, each pathologic fracture, especially in a child, is as different as the tumor pathology, stage, age at diagnosis, and the child's needs. The orthopedic surgeon must individualize treatment plans.

The functional condition of the child immediately after a pathologic fracture can help guide the treatment strategy. Pain is frequently the immediate problem and should therefore be the first consideration, provided that neurovascular compromise is not an issue. Whether traction or hospitalization is required needs to be evaluated. Basic orthopedic tenets apply. Often, a sling is all that is necessary, such as after a minimally displaced pathologic fracture in the proximal end of the humerus from a UBC. Perhaps further imaging of the fracture site is indicated if the trauma sustained by the child does not typically result in a fracture or a particular fracture pattern. A high index of suspicion is often necessary when a search for an underlying pathology is undertaken.

After comfort and safety from neurovascular injury are ensured, mobility should be considered next. Pathologic fractures seldom result in open fractures. Will casting allow a child to be mobile? Will the child's mobility alter fracture union rates? Will immobilization produce a decrease in bone mineral density and worsen the child's functional outcome, as is frequently seen in OI? Will surgical intervention diminish the need for a postoperative cast? Will open reduction and internal fixation allow earlier weight-bearing? If return to weight-bearing will not occur sooner with a more aggressive treatment strategy, what are its indications? Is more than one skeletal lesion present? Will the repair of a distal long bone lesion create a secondary lesion more proximally located in the same bone? It is not reasonable to fix one part of the bone if the remaining bone remains structurally compromised.

What is the natural history of a pathologic fracture? Will the fracture spontaneously resolve, as is seen in vertebrae plana (see Fig. 4.4)? Often, an eosinophilic granuloma of a non–weight-bearing bone, such as the clavicle, heals spontaneously after a pathologic fracture.[50] If surgical intervention does not offer significant advantages in terms of functional improvement in the long term or short term, it should not be an option when one is considering only musculoskeletal rehabilitation. Restoration of anatomic alignment and prevention of deformity are important considerations, as are maintenance of the viability of the physis and elimination of future limb length inequality. The likelihood of morbidity associated with surgery may weigh heavier than any proposed benefit.

The psychosocial adaptation of the child or patient reacting to a pathologic fracture and its treatment is another variable to be considered in the functional portion of the outcome triangle. This variable especially comes into play in the management of skeletal sarcomas, when limb salvage versus amputation options frequently present a dilemma to the family and surgeon. Multiple studies have not demonstrated any adverse psychologic outcome from childhood amputation, but clearly, the stigma and fear of amputation are concerns in our society.[51,52] Additionally, long-term financial analyses have demonstrated that the cost of amputation to society is far greater than limb salvage. This difference increases exponentially the younger the children and the longer their survival.[53] The Van Nes rotationplasty offers an alternative to above-knee amputation by providing a more efficient gait. The procedure converts plantar flexion of the ankle to knee extension by transposing the ankle joint to the femur and rotating it 180 degrees. This effectively converts an above-knee amputation to a below-knee amputation. One would think that this would strain the psychosocial adaptation of the child, but studies have not demonstrated any deleterious long-term psychologic sequelae of such procedures.[51,54] Further, patients can achieve good functional outcomes with some expected limitations.[55] Limb salvage with distraction osteogenesis via ring fixators are also a source of stress to children and their family because of the often protracted treatment course. How the child is able to cope with the fixator, adapt in school, and maintain mobility are important considerations to be evaluated. Ultimately, the best treatment strategy will vary from patient to patient and must be individualized to both them and their family.

Functional outcome rating scores for extremities, especially after a large skeletal reconstruction, are not commonly used in everyday practice. Several have been used in the literature, including the Toronto Extremity Salvage Score, the Musculoskeletal Tumor Society score, and the American Academy of Orthopedic Surgeons functional rating system.[56,57] Although these instruments are not directly applicable to most pathologic fractures in children, knowledge of these scores by the treating surgeon can provide a "conscience" that may help direct management strategies toward a more optimal functional result. The components of any validated functional outcome instrument combine objective measures with the subjective perception of the patient. Although possibly difficult in a child, it is important to consider these variables when a treatment strategy is planned. It may often be necessary for the parent's wishes and desires to give way to the priorities of oncologic and orthopedic management. Functional restoration therefore remains a critical component in the overall treatment plan.

CONCLUSION

Pathologic fractures in children occur from a variety of causes. No single approach is best, nor is an algorithm appropriate for every use. One must develop a cognitive treatment strategy that weighs the pros and cons and considers the variables as described by the outcome triangle. The clinician-scientist must consider bone biology and biomechanics at the fracture site. Determining lesional pathology is of paramount importance, whether it be from a neoplastic or non-neoplastic entity, so that bone healing can be maximized. Time-efficient, child-protective skeletal restoration is the measured effect of the surgeon's intervention. This strategy must be individualized for every situation.

Combinations of diseases, fracture sites, and children are many, whereas treatment options are fewer. Options include nonoperative management with observation and intralesional resection with or without bone grafting and with or without internal fixation. Additionally, wide resection with megaprosthetic or biologic reconstruction of skeletal defects may be required. A thoughtful, disciplined, and patterned approach is most often successful.

The goals for treatment of a child's pathologic fracture are all based on the establishment of a diagnosis. Only after establishing the diagnosis with certainty can a proper treatment strategy be formulated. Fracture management is then based on answering the questions posed by the outcome triangle. The goals of treatment are five: (1) pain relief and comfort for the child; (2) achievement of local control or containment of the pathologic entity; (3) skeletal stabilization, preservation of growth, and return to anatomic alignment; (4) fracture union; and (5) restoration of function. Maintaining perspective by "keeping your eye on the ball" facilitates optimal patient care and minimizes the confounding variables that seem to plague the treatment of pathologic fractures.

REFERENCES

The level of evidence (LOE) is determined according to the criteria provided in the Preface.

1. Burstein AH, Zika JM, Heipole KG, et al. Contribution of collagen and mineral to the elastic-plastic properties of bone. *J Bone Joint Surg Am*. 1975;57:956–961. (**LOE N/A**).
2. Brooks DB, Burstein AH, Frankel VH. The biomechanics of torsional fractures: the stress concentration effect of a drill hole. *J Bone Joint Surg Am*. 1970;52:507–514. (**LOE N/A**).

3. Mundy GR. Metastasis to bone: causes, consequences and therapeutic opportunities. *Nat Rev Cancer.* 2002;2(8):584–593. **(LOE V)**.

4. Suva LJ, Winslow GA, Wettenhall RE, et al. A parathyroid hormone-related protein implicated in malignant hypercalcemia: cloning and expression. *Science.* 1987;237:893–896. **(LOE N/A)**.

5. Lacey DL, Timms E, Tan HL, et al. Osteoprotegerin ligand is a cytokine that regulates osteoclast differentiation and activation. *Cell.* 1998;93:165–176. **(LOE N/A)**.

6. Peddi P, Lopez-Olivo Ma, Pratt GF, Suarez-Almazor ME. Denosumab in patients with cancer and skeletal metastases: a systematic review and meta-analysis. *Cancer Treat Rev.* 2013;39(1):97–104. **(LOE II)**.

7. Jones DH, Nakashima T, Sanchez OH, et al. Regulation of cancer cell migration and bone metastasis by RANKL. *Nature.* 2006; 440(7084):692–696. **(LOE N/A)**.

8. Gainor BJ, Buckart P. Fracture healing in metastatic bone disease. *Clin Orthop Relat Res.* 1983;178:297–302. **(LOE IV)**.

9. Mankin HJ, Mankin CJ, Simon MA. The hazards of the biopsy, revisited. *J Bone Joint Surg Am.* 1996;78:656–663. **(LOE IV)**.

10. Bucay N, Sarosi I, Dostan CR, et al. Osteoprotegerin-deficient mice developed early onset osteoporosis and arterial calcification. *Genes Dev.* 1998;12:1260–1268. **(LOE N/A)**.

11. Simonet WS, Lacey DL, Dunstan CR, et al. Osteoprotegerin: novel secreted protein involved in the regulation of bone density. *Cell.* 1997;89:309–319. **(LOE V)**.

12. Trondavi MM, McKercher SR, Anderson K, et al. Osteopetrosis in mice lacking haematopoietic transcription factor PU.1. *Nature.* 1997;386:81–84. **(LOE N/A)**.

13. Zhu GH, Mei HB, He RG, et al. Combination of intramedullary rod, wrapping bone grafting and Ilizarov's fixator for the treatment of Crawford type IV congenital pseudarthrosis of the tibia: midterm follow up of 56 cases. *BMC Musculoskelet Disord.* 2016;17(1):1–8. **(LOE IV)**.

14. Traub JA, O'Connor W, Musso PD. Congenital pseudoarthrosis of the tibia: a retrospective review. *J Pediatr Orthop.* 1999;19:735–740 **(LOE IV)**.

15. Guille JT, Kumar SJ, Shah A. Spontaneous union of a congenital pseudoarthritis of the tibia after Syme amputation. *Clin Orthop Relat Res.* 1998;351:180–185. **(LOE IV)**.

16. Green N, Robertson WW, Kilroy W. Eosinophilic granuloma of the spine with associated neural deficit. *J Bone Joint Surg Am.* 1980;62:1198–1202. **(LOE IV)**.

17. Sillence DO. Osteogenesis imperfecta; an expanding panorama of variance. *Clin Orthop Relat Res.* 1981;159:11–25. **(LOE V)**.

18. Smith R. Osteogenesis imperfecta—where next? *J Bone Joint Surg Br.* 1997;79:177–178. **(LOE V)**.

19. Wilkinson JM, Scott BW, Clarke AM, et al. Surgical stabilisation of the lower limb in osteogenesis imperfecta using the Sheffield telescopic intramedullary rod system. *J Bone Joint Surg Br.* 1998;80:999–1004. **(LOE IV)**.

20. Birke O, Davies N, Latimer M, et al. Experience with the Fassier-Duval telescopic rod: first 24 consecutive cases with a minimum of 1-year follow-up. *J Pediatr Orthop.* 2011;31(4):458–464. **(LOE IV)**.

21. Cho TJ, In HC, Chin YC, Won JY, Ki SL, Dong YL. Interlocking telescopic rod for patients with osteogenesis imperfecta. *J Bone Jt Surg Ser A.* 2007;89(5):1028–1035. **(LOE IV)**.

22. Mirra JM, Bernard GW, Bullough PG, et al. Cementum-like bone production in solitary bone cyst: report of three cases. *Clin Orthop Relat Res.* 1978;135:295–307. **(LOE IV)**.

23. Jaffe HL, Lichtein L. Solitary unicameral bone cyst with emphasis on the roentgen picture. The pathologic picture and the pathogenesis. *Arch Surg.* 1942;44:1004–1025. **(LOE IV)**.

24. Komiya S, Minamitani K, Sasaguri Y, et al. Simple bone cyst: treatment by trepanation and studies on bone resorptive factors in cyst fluid with a theory of its pathogenesis. *Clin Orthop Relat Res.* 1993;287:204–211. **(LOE IV)**.

25. Kadhim M, Thacker M, Kadhim A, Holmes L. Treatment of unicameral bone cyst: systematic review and meta analysis. *J Child Orthop.* 2014;8(2):171–191. **(LOE III)**.

26. Scaglietti O, Marchetti PGM, Bartolozzi P. Final results obtained in the treatment of bone cysts with methylprednisolone acetate (Depo-Medrol) and a discussion of results achieved in other bone lesions. *Clin Orthop Relat Res.* 1982;165:33–42. **(LOE IV)**.

27. Wilkins RM. Unicameral bone cysts. *J Am Acad Orthop Surg.* 2000;8:217–224. **(LOE V)**.

28. Glanzman CG, Campos L. Flexible intramedullary nailing for unicameral cysts in children's long bones. *J Child Orthop.* 2007;1: 97–100. **(LOE IV)**.

29. Roposch A, Saraph V, Linhart WE, et al. Flexible intramedullary nailing for the treatment of unicameral bone cysts in long bones. *J Bone Joint Surg Am.* 2000;82A(10):1447–1453. **(LOE IV)**.

30. Chin KR, Kharrazi FD, Miller BS, et al. Osteochondromas of the distal aspect of the tibia or fibula. Natural history and treatment. *J Bone Joint Surg Am.* 2000;82:1269–1278. **(LOE IV)**.

31. Mirzayan R, Panossian V, Avedian R, et al. The use of calcium sulfate in the treatment of benign bone lesions. *J Bone Joint Surg Am.* 2001;83:355–358. **(LOE IV)**.

32. MacNeil JA, Francis A, El-Hawary R. A systematic review of rigid, locked, intramedullary nail insertion sites and avascular necrosis of the femoral head in the skeletally immature. *J Pediatr Orthop.* 2011;31(4):2009–2012. **(LOE III)**.

33. Momberger N, Stevens P, Smith J, et al. Intramedullary nailing of femoral fractures in adolescence. *J Pediatr Orthop.* 2000;20:182–184. **(LOE IV)**.

34. Beaty JH, Austin SM, Warner WH, et al. Interlocking intramedullary nailing of femoral shaft fractures in adolescents: preliminary results and complications. *J Pediatr Orthop.* 1994;14:178–183. **(LOE IV)**.

35. Crosby SN, Kim EJ, Koehler DM, et al. Twenty-year experience with rigid intramedullary nailing of femoral shaft fractures in skeletally immature patients. *J Bone Jt Surg Am.* 2014;96(13):1080–1089. **(LOE IV)**.

36. DiCaprio MR, Enneking WF. Fibrous dysplasia: pathophysiology, evaluation and treatment. *J Bone and Joint Surg.* 2005;87A: 1848–1864. **(LOE IV)**.

37. Guille JT, Kumar SJ, MacEwen GD. Fibrous dysplasia of the proximal part of the femur. Long-term results of curettage and bone-grafting and mechanical realignment. *J Bone Joint Surg Am.* 1998;80(5):648–658. **(LOE IV)**.

38. Enneking WF, Geran PF. Fibrous dysplasia of the femoral neck. *J Bone Joint Surg Am.* 1986;68:1415–1422. **(LOE IV)**.

39. Freeman B, Bray EW, Meier LC. Multiple osteotomies with Zickel nail fixation for polyostotic fibrous dysplasia involving the proximal part of femur. *J Bone Joint Surg Am.* 1987;69:691–698. **(LOE IV)**.

40. Stephenson B, London MD, Hankin FM, et al. Fibrous dysplasia and analysis of options for treatment. *J Bone Joint Surg Am.* 1987;69:400–409. **(LOE V)**.

41. Schwartz HS, Zimmerman NB, Simon MA, et al. The malignant potential of enchondromatosis. *J Bone Joint Surg Am.* 1987;69:269–274. **(LOE IV)**.

42. Verdegaal SH, Bovee JV, Pansuriya TC, et al. Incidence, predictive factors, and prognosis of chondrosarcoma in patients with Ollier disease and Mafucci syndrome: an international multicenter study of 161 patients. *Oncologist.* 2011;16(12):1771–1779. **(LOE III)**.

43. Shapiro F. Ollier's disease. An assessment of angular deformity, shortening, and pathologic fracture in twenty-one patients. *J Bone Joint Surg Am.* 1982;64:95–103. **(LOE IV)**.

44. Arata MA, Peterson HA, Dahlin DC. Pathologic fractures through non-ossifying fibromas: review of the Mayo Clinic experience. *J Bone Joint Surg Am.* 1981;63:980–988. **(LOE IV)**.

45. Abudu A, Sferopoulos NK, Tillman MR, et al. The surgical treatment and outcome of pathologic fractures in localized osteosarcoma. *J Bone Joint Surg Br.* 1996;78:694–698. **(LOE IV)**.

46. Scully SP, Temple HT, O'Keefe RJ, et al. The surgical treatment of patients with osteosarcoma who have sustained a pathologic fracture. *Clin Orthop Relat Res.* 1996;324:227–232. **(LOE IV)**.

47. Bramer JA, Abudu AA, Grimer RJ, Carter SR, Tillman RM. Do pathological fractures influence survival and local recurrence rate in bony sarcomas? *Eur J Cancer.* 2007;43(13):1944–1951. **(LOE III)**.

48. Salunke AA, Chen Y, Tan JH, Chen X, Khin LW, Puhaindran ME. Does a pathological fracture affect the prognosis in patients with osteosarcoma of the extremities? *Bone Jt J.* 2014;96B(10): 1396–1403. **(LOE III)**.

49. Cates JMM. Pathologic fracture a poor prognostic factor in osteosarcoma: misleading conclusions from meta-analyses? *Eur J Surg Oncol.* 2016;42(6):883–888. **(LOE III)**.

50. DiCaprio MR, Roberts TT. Diagnosis and management of langerhans cell histiocytosis. *J Am Acad Orthop Surg.* 2014;22(10):643–652. **(LOE V)**.

51. Weddington WW, Segraves KB, Simon MA. Psychological outcome of extremity sarcoma survivors undergoing amputation or limb salvage. *J Clin Oncol.* 1985;3:1393–1399. **(LOE III).**

52. Weddington WW, Segraves KB, Simon MA. Current and lifetime incidence of psychiatric disorders among a group of extremity sarcoma survivors. *J Psychosom Res.* 1986;30:121–125. **(LOE IV).**

53. Grimer RJ, Carter SR, Pynsent PR. The cost effectiveness of limb salvage for bone tumors. *J Bone Joint Surg Br.* 1997;79:558–561. **(LOE II).**

54. Forni C, Gaudenzi N, Zoli M, et al. Living with rotationplasty quality of life in rotationplasty patients from childhood to adulthood. *J Surg Oncol.* 2012;105(4):331–336. https://doi.org/10.1002/jso.22088. **(LOE IV).**

55. Benedetti M, Okita Y, Recubini E, Mariani E, Leardini A, Manfrini M. How much clinical and functional impairment do children treated with knee rotationplasty experience in adulthood? *Clin Orthop Relat Res.* 2016;474(4):995–1004. https://doi.org/10.1007/s11999-016-4691-9. **(LOE IV).**

56. Davis AM, Bell RS, Badley EM, et al. Evaluating functional outcome in patients with lower extremity sarcoma. *Clin Orthop Relat Res.* 1999;358:90–100. **(LOE II).**

57. Enneking WF, Dunham W, Gebhardt MC, Malawar M, Pritchard DJ. A system for the functional evaluation of reconstructive procedures after surgical treatment of tumors of the musculoskeletal system. *Class Pap Orthop.* 1993;286:241–246. **(LOE N/A).**

The Multiply Injured Child

Raymond W. Liu | Christina K. Hardesty

INTRODUCTION

Children who are victims of severe trauma often sustain musculoskeletal injuries but may also have injuries to other body areas that can be severe and even life-threatening. Early morbidity and mortality are related to injuries to the nervous system, genitourinary system, abdomen, and thorax,[1] whereas long-term morbidity or disability is caused predominantly by injuries to the central nervous system (CNS) and musculoskeletal system.[1–6] Therefore, careful, coordinated, and integrated management of all injuries is mandatory for minimizing morbidity and mortality.[7] This chapter deals with the assessment of children who have sustained injuries to the musculoskeletal system and other body areas or organ systems. It is not our intent to discuss in detail specific isolated musculoskeletal injuries or their treatment, which are presented in other chapters. Our focus is the evaluation and ranking of treatment options for a multiply injured child who has sustained musculoskeletal trauma; special consideration is given to the aspects of care that may differ as a result of multiple rather than isolated injuries. Much of the material in this chapter is adapted from the American College of Surgeons (ACS) Committee on Trauma, *Advanced Trauma Life Support for Doctors* (ATLS), Ninth Edition.[8]

> ### Key Points: The Multiply Injured Child
>
> - The multiply injured child must be approached with a different mindset than an adult.
> - Early resuscitation is essential.
> - Falls and motor vehicle accidents account for the majority of polytrauma in children.
> - Surgical treatment is more often employed to facilitate overall care of the child.

PATHOLOGY

It has been well documented in both adult and pediatric literature that an individual with multiple injuries must be treated differently from individuals in whom similar injuries have occurred in isolation.[1,3,4] Assessment and treatment of a multiply injured child may also differ from that of an adult. The anatomic, biomechanical, and physiologic differences in the musculoskeletal systems of adults and children have an important influence on orthopedic treatment, as well as injuries to other body areas and organ systems.

ANATOMIC DIFFERENCES

Anatomic differences in the pediatric skeleton are multiple and vary with age and maturity. These differences include the presence of preosseous cartilage, physes, and thicker, stronger periosteum that produces callus more rapidly and in greater amounts than in adults. Because of the effects of age and growth, children vary in body size and proportions.

The size of the child is important not only in the response to trauma but also in the severity and constellation of injuries.[9,10] Being variably smaller, children sustain a different complex of injuries than adults in a similar traumatic situation as well as a higher frequency of polytrauma. An adult pedestrian struck by a motor vehicle is likely to sustain an injury to the tibia or knee because these structures are at the level of the automobile's bumper. In children, depending on their height, the bumper can cause a fracture of the femur or pelvis or, in toddlers, a chest or head injury. Because the mass of a child's body is proportionately less, a child is much more likely to become a projectile when struck and may sustain further injuries caused by secondary contact with the ground or another object. A classic example is the Waddell triad, which consists of an ipsilateral femoral shaft fracture, chest contusion, and contralateral head injury (Fig. 5.1). Because of their smaller size, children are also more likely to be trapped beneath a moving object such as a motor vehicle and sustain crush injuries, fractures, and soft tissue damage. Crush injuries are relatively common in children, and such injuries often result in severe soft tissue loss, which can produce a poorer prognosis.

A child's body proportions, being quite different from those of an adult, can produce a different spectrum of injuries. A child's head is larger in proportion to the body, and the younger the child, the more extreme this disproportion. This comparatively larger head size makes the head and neck much more vulnerable to injury, especially with falls from a height, because the weight of the head often causes it to strike the ground first. In contrast, adults are more likely to protect themselves with their extremities or try to land on their feet. The relative shortness of children's extremities and a lack of strength often prevent them from adequately protecting themselves during a fall. This theory is supported by the high incidence of head injuries sustained by young children as a result of falls[11–14] (Fig. 5.2). Demetriades and colleagues[9] studied pedestrians injured by automobiles and determined that the incidence of severe head and chest trauma increased with age and that femur fractures were more common in the pediatric age groups.

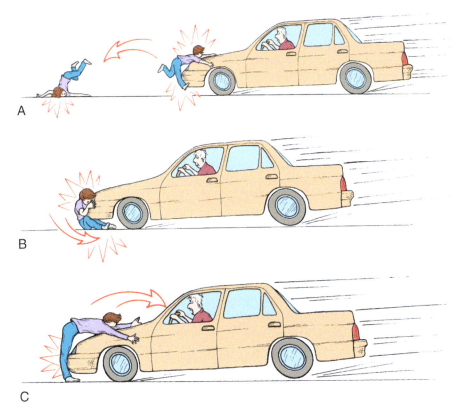

Fig. 5.1 Different injury patterns resulting from a similar car-versus-pedestrian mechanism. (A) A typical Waddell triad in which the child sustains an ipsilateral femoral and chest injury from the initial impact of the car and is then thrown forward and strikes the contralateral side of the head on the ground. (B) A smaller child being struck by the car and sustaining chest and head injuries from a direct blow on the bumper and then sustaining lower extremity crush injuries from being dragged underneath the car. (C) An adolescent being struck, sustaining tibia or knee injuries from the bumper, and then being thrown forward and sustaining chest, head, and neck injuries from impact on the windshield.

BIOMECHANICAL DIFFERENCES

The composition of bone in children is quite different from adult bone. Children, including those who are victims of multiple traumatic injuries, demonstrate unique fracture patterns. These patterns include compression (torus), incomplete tension-compression (greenstick), plastic deformation, complete, and both physeal and epiphyseal fractures. These fracture patterns result from the presence of the physes, the thicker periosteum, and the material properties of the bone itself. Complete fractures occur more commonly in children with multiple injuries because trauma is associated with high-velocity injuries. Biomechanically, the pediatric skeletal system responds differently to an applied force than the adult skeleton does. Pediatric bone has a lower ash content and increased porosity, which are properties indicative of less mineralization. Such bone composition results in increased plasticity and less energy needed for bone failure. This decreases with skeletal maturity.

Bending is the most common mode of failure in long bones. Stress on the tension side of a bone with a low-yield strength initiates a fracture that is followed by compression on the opposite side. As bending continues, the fracture line eventually travels the entire width of the bone. Although pediatric bone is biomechanically weaker, it has a greater capacity to undergo plastic deformation than adult bone. Because pediatric bone yields at a lower force, the stress in the bone is less, and the energy to propagate the fracture is less. These factors account for the compression, greenstick, and plastic deformation fracture patterns. The increased porosity of pediatric bone, which was previously thought to play a major role in the different fracture patterns, is no longer considered a reason for deformation.

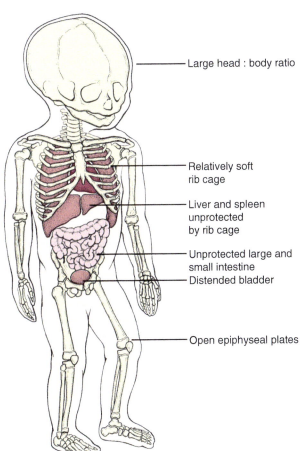

— Large head : body ratio

— Relatively soft rib cage

— Liver and spleen unprotected by rib cage

— Unprotected large and small intestine
— Distended bladder

— Open epiphyseal plates

Fig. 5.2 Anatomic differences predispose a child to injuries different from those of an adult. These differences include a disproportionately large head, pliable rib cage with exposed liver and spleen below its margin, unprotected large and small bowel, distended bladder above the pelvic brim, and open physes.

Ligaments frequently insert into the epiphyses. As a consequence, traumatic forces applied to an extremity may be transmitted to the physis. The strength of the physis is enhanced by the perichondrial ring and, in some cases, by interdigitating mammillary bodies. In spite of this enhanced strength, however, the physis is not as strong biomechanically as the ligaments or metaphyseal or diaphyseal bone. Consequently, physeal fractures are relatively common in multiply injured children, and ligamentous injuries are less common than in adults. Ligamentous injuries, however, do occur and are probably more frequent than previously reported.

Because pediatric bone is more deformable and fractures with less force, it also affords less protection to the internal organs and other structures. The plasticity of bones can allow internal injuries without obvious external trauma, as reflected in the increased incidence of cardiac and pulmonary injuries without apparent damage to the thoracic cage and a high incidence of abdominal injuries without significant injury to the pelvis, abdomen, or lower ribs. Injuries to the liver and spleen are more common in children because of less rib coverage of these structures, as well as the greater pliability of the ribs. Children also have less soft tissue coverage, including muscle mass and strength, to protect their bodies from trauma. The lower mass of soft tissue may contribute to injury to the internal organs.

PHYSIOLOGIC DIFFERENCES

Children respond differently than adults to the metabolic and physiologic stress of trauma. Total blood volume is smaller, depending on the size of the child, so less blood loss can be tolerated; hypovolemia develops more rapidly because the smaller volumes lost represent a larger percentage of the total. Comparison of pediatric versus adult patients in the National Trauma Data Bank (NTDB) found that children have earlier mortality than adults, stressing the importance of early resuscitation.[15] The higher ratio of surface area to volume also makes children more vulnerable to hypothermia. Multisystem organ failure tends to occur early during hospitalization and resuscitation, affecting all organ systems at once. In adults, multisystem organ failure usually happens 48 hours after injury and occurs in a sequential order starting with the lungs.[1] The metabolic response is also significantly different between adults and children. Whereas adults have a significant increase in their metabolic rate from the stress of trauma, children have minimal or no change. This minimal response to stress is believed to be caused by the significantly higher baseline metabolic rate of children, which needs to be increased only a small amount to accommodate the increased metabolic demands. The accelerated metabolic rate, together with the ability to metabolize lipid stores, provides a possible explanation for the increased survival rates in children after severe trauma. Adults also appear to have a significant systemic inflammatory response to trauma that does not occur as severely in children. Conversely, children have a robust local inflammatory response at the tissue level that helps not only with accelerated healing but also with minimizing the systemic insult.[1]

Physiologically, pediatric fractures have the capacity to heal rapidly, remodel, and overgrow if the physis is uninjured, and become progressively deformed or shortened if the physis is injured. For these reasons, pediatric fractures secondary to severe trauma require careful management. Musculoskeletal morbidity is a common sequela of multiple traumatic injuries.[16,17] The ultimate consequences of injury are often not known for many years, and long-term follow-up is recommended.

INCIDENCE

Trauma is the leading cause of death and disability in childhood. It accounts for more than 50% of all deaths in children compared with 10% in the overall population of the United States. More than 10,000 children die in the United States each year from serious injury, and almost one in every four children requires treatment in the emergency department each year for injuries.[18] An epidemiological study investigating from 2000 to 2011 found decreasing mortality rates, decreasing inpatient discharge rates, and increasing injury severity rates with time.[19] Fortunately, most injuries in children are minor; the most common are caused by falls resulting in injury to a single extremity, usually the upper extremity. Chan and associates[20] showed that approximately 13% of the children being evaluated in the emergency department of an urban teaching hospital had serious injuries. There is a bimodal age distribution of traumatic injuries in children: in the first year of life and later through the adolescent years. Although this bimodal distribution holds true for both genders, males have a higher overall incidence of trauma as well as a more dramatic increase in traumatic incidents during adolescence,[21] with motor vehicle accidents a common mechanism in adolescents. The majority of injuries in the earlier years occur where younger children spend the most time, usually in or about the home. It is important to remember that child abuse is also a cause of multiple injuries, particularly in very young children.[22]

MECHANISM OF INJURY

According to the ACS NTDB Report for Pediatrics in 2012, falls and motor vehicle accidents remain the two most common mechanisms of injury in children. Motor vehicle–related deaths are the most common causes of fatality in pediatric trauma. When separated by age group, falls are the most common cause of trauma in children younger than 10 years, whereas at 10 years and older, motor vehicle accidents are much more frequent as a mechanism of injury.[23]

FALLS

Most pediatric injuries are caused by simple falls, which account for approximately half of all injuries. According to 2010 data from the Centers for Disease Control and Prevention, unintentional falls were the leading cause of nonfatal injury in all children younger than 15 years. However, they are not frequently the cause of fatality.[24] Musemeche and associates[25] showed that falls occur predominantly in the younger population; the mean age was 5 years, and there was a 68% male preponderance. Of the falls, 78% occurred from a height of two stories or less at or near the home. Most patients sustained a single major injury that usually involved the head or skeletal system, although the incidence and spectrum of injury may vary with age. Long bone fractures predominate in children, whereas the incidence of spinal injuries and the total number of fractures are increased in adolescents. Fortunately, children can survive falls from significant heights, although serious injuries do occur.[11,14] As would be expected, morbidity and mortality rates increase with the height of the fall. Mortality is usually related to falls of a distance exceeding 10 feet. Pitone and Attia[26] showed that in routine falls, children 2 years or younger fell from a bed or chair and sustained head injuries, whereas those 5 to 12 years of age were likely to fall from playground equipment and fracture an upper extremity.

In the past, falls from windows were noted to be a particular problem in urban areas.[11] Recently, Harris and colleagues[12] demonstrated that there was a decrease in the overall national incidence of falls from windows since 1990, especially in those urban areas in which a prevention program such as "Children Can't Fly" or "Kids Can't Fly" had been implemented. Window-related falls are much more common in children younger than 4 years, who are also more likely to sustain serious injuries as a result of the fall.

MOTOR VEHICLE ACCIDENTS

By far, the most common cause of multiple injuries in children is motor vehicle accidents—accidents in which they are motor vehicle occupants, pedestrians, or cyclists. In a 1989 series of 376 multiply injured children, Kaufmann and colleagues[27] reported that motor vehicle–related accidents accounted for 58% of the overall injuries and 76% of the severely injured children. Marcus and associates[17] reported a 91% incidence of motor vehicle–related mechanisms of injury in their series. Although the mechanism of injury was not analyzed by age, the incidence of motor vehicle–related injuries increases with age. According to the Centers for Disease Control and prevention data from 1999 to 2005, deaths from motor vehicle accidents are lowest from birth to 14 years (3.6–4.4 per 100,000 population), and a peak occurs in the 15- to 24-year-old age group (25.9–28.2 per 100,000).[28] Males in this age group have twice the mortality rate of females. Scheidler and colleagues[29] demonstrated that being an unrestrained child or adolescent and being ejected from the vehicle tripled the risk of mortality and significantly increased injury severity scores. Brown and associates[30] recently demonstrated differences in injury patterns based on the direction at the impact (frontal or lateral) and the position of the patient in the automobile. Lateral impact accidents are characterized by head and chest injuries, whereas front seat passengers had higher trauma scores.

ASSOCIATED INJURIES

By definition, a multiply injured child has injuries involving more than one organ system. It is critical to recognize, evaluate, and treat all injuries sustained. Although many injuries occur in isolation or in random combination, numerous others have been shown to occur in an associated pattern.

One of the more common groups of associated injuries is that described as the Waddell triad—a history of a child being struck by a car and a diagnosis of any one of the triad of injuries (ipsilateral femur and chest injury, contralateral head injury) should alert the physician to evaluate the other associated areas (Fig. 5.1). This admonition holds true for all known injury patterns.

SPINAL INJURIES

A study utilizing the Kid's Inpatient Database from 1997 to 2009 found that the rate of spinal injuries increased, with the majority in the 15- to 19-year-old group and secondary to motor vehicle accidents.[31] The presence of facial injuries, including lacerations, contusions, and fractures, has been shown to be associated with an increased incidence of cervical spine injury in both children and adults.[32,33] The presence of a cervical spine fracture in a multiply injured patient is associated with a 10% increased incidence of a noncontiguous fracture at another level of the spine. Because children are more elastic than adults, the force of injury can be transmitted over multiple segments and result in multiple fractures. In addition, certain anatomic differences have an effect on the type of injury, such as the increased cartilage-to-bone ratio, the presence of secondary ossification centers, variations in the normal planes of the articular facet, and increased laxity. Thus, any child seen with head, facial, or spinal injuries at any level should have a careful evaluation of the entire spinal column, especially a head-injured child who is either comatose or unable to cooperate in the examination. In a multiply injured child, a spinal injury must be assumed to be present until proven otherwise by physical examination and radiographic evaluation. Stabilization of the head and neck should account for the larger head diameter and take care not to place the neck in flexion (Fig. 5.2).

In an automobile accident, the use of a lap belt without shoulder restraint may produce a constellation of injuries referred to as the seat belt syndrome.[34,35] These injuries in children include flexion-distraction injury to the lumbar spine (Chance fracture), small-bowel rupture, and traumatic pancreatitis.[36] Ecchymosis anywhere along the lap belt distribution should alert the physician to search for these injuries. Head and extremity injuries in this circumstance are unusual. Age is a predictor of elevated risk of abdominal injury in seat belt–restrained children. Children ages 4 to 8 years old are at the highest risk of severe abdominal trauma because they are transitioning from child seats to adult seat belts. As a result, the American Academy of Pediatrics and the National Highway Traffic Safety Administration recommend that these children be restrained in a booster seat until they are taller than 4 feet 9 inches. This provides a better fit of the adult seat belt lower on the child's pelvis to help prevent these injuries.[35,37] Booster seat legislation appears to be associated with a decrease in the mortality rate in children ages 4 to 7 years old involved in motor vehicle accidents.[38] The unrestrained passenger, however, is subjected to devastating amounts of energy in the absence of the "ride down" effect afforded by restraints. A recent study reported that two-point and three-point restrained children have an increased likelihood of thoracolumbar and flexion-distraction injuries, whereas car seat, booster, and unrestrained children have an increased likelihood of cervical spine injuries.[39]

RIB FRACTURES

The pediatric thorax has a greater cartilage content and incomplete ossification, which makes fractures of the ribs and sternum uncommon. Severe thoracic injury to the heart, lungs, and great vessels can be present with little external sign of injury or apparent fractures on chest radiographs.[3] Fractures of the first and second ribs are a marker for severe trauma in children.[40] Given the increased energy that is theoretically required to fracture the ribs in children, it is not surprising that a study of the National Trauma Registry found that pediatric patients with rib fractures had higher rates of associated brain injury, hemothorax, pneumothorax, spleen injury, and liver injury as compared with adults.[41]

Multiple rib fractures are also a marker of severe trauma in pediatric patients. Garcia and associates[40] reported a 42% mortality rate in pediatric patients with multiple rib fractures; the risk of mortality increases with the number of ribs fractured. They found that a head injury with multiple rib fractures signified an even worse prognosis: the mortality rate was 71%. Similar results were reported by Peclet and colleagues.[42] Because head injuries are associated with a higher incidence of mortality and long-term disability, it is critical to recognize this relationship. Multiple rib fractures in a child younger than 3 years should also alert the physician to the possibility of child abuse; 63% of the patients in this age group in the series of Garcia and associates[40] were victims of child abuse. Multiple fractures in different stages of healing are also a sign of child abuse and should raise the physician's suspicion accordingly (see Chapter 20).

PELVIC FRACTURES

Pelvic fractures in children are uncommon and, as in adults, usually the result of high-velocity trauma.[43–45] As opposed to adults, children have greater plasticity of the pelvic bones, thicker cartilage, and increased elasticity of the symphysis pubis and sacroiliac joints. Simple or isolated, nondisplaced pelvic fractures have low morbidity and mortality rates and tend not to be associated with other injuries (Fig. 5.3). Silber and Flynn[45] demonstrated that patients with open triradiate cartilages were more likely to sustain pubic rami and iliac wing fractures, whereas those with closed triradiate cartilages were more likely to sustain acetabular fractures and pubic or sacroiliac diastasis. This is secondary to the immaturity of the pelvis early on in life when the pelvic bones are weaker than the more elastic pelvic ligaments. After the triradiate cartilage closes, the bones of the pelvis become stronger than the ligaments. More severe fractures mandate a careful evaluation for other injuries because a great deal of energy is necessary to cause this type of fracture. Compared with adults, pediatric patients have been found to have less severe pelvic fracture patterns despite high frequencies of high-energy mechanisms and high rates of associated injuries[46] and similar overall mortality rates with pelvic fractures.[47] Associated injuries can include head injuries; other fractures, including open fractures; hemorrhage; genitourinary injuries; and abdominal injuries. A sacral fracture, which is common in pelvic fractures, may have associated neurologic deficits. The presence of severe pelvic fractures should alert the physician to possible injuries to the abdominal and pelvic contents, particularly genitourinary injuries such as urethral lacerations (especially in males) and bladder rupture. Abdominal injuries may include rectal lacerations, tears of the small or large intestine, and visceral rupture of the liver, spleen, and kidneys. Blood at the urethral meatus, a high-riding or nonpalpable prostate gland on rectal examination, and blood in the scrotum are indications of serious damage to the genitourinary system. Such genitourinary complications must be investigated further, usually with a retrograde urethrogram, before an attempt is made to insert a Foley catheter. Rectal or vaginal lacerations indicate that the pelvic fracture may be open. A diverting colostomy may be necessary for these individuals so that the risk of infection is decreased. If a pelvic fracture is diagnosed and if it is necessary to perform peritoneal lavage,

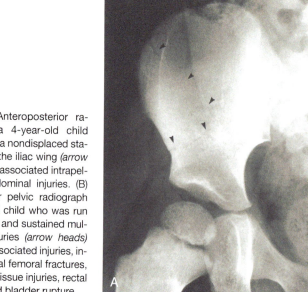
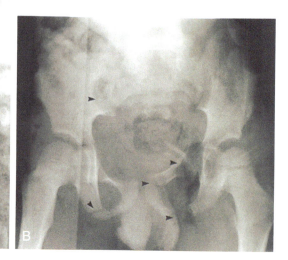

Fig. 5.3 (A) Anteroposterior radiograph of a 4-year-old child demonstrating a nondisplaced stable fracture of the iliac wing *(arrow heads)* with no associated intrapelvic or intraabdominal injuries. (B) Anteroposterior pelvic radiograph of a 5-year-old child who was run over by a truck and sustained multiple pelvic injuries *(arrow heads)* and multiple associated injuries, including proximal femoral fractures, degloving soft tissue injuries, rectal perforation, and bladder rupture.

a supraumbilical approach is recommended instead of the routine infraumbilical approach because the former approach may avoid false-positive findings secondary to pelvic bleeding. Unstable fractures, such as vertical shear or wide pelvic diastasis, are often associated with significant hemorrhaging and hypovolemic shock secondary to retroperitoneal bleeding (see Chapter 11). In general, however, significant hemorrhage requiring transfusion or angiography is rare in children, perhaps because of the ability of their vessels to readily vasoconstrict as well as the smaller caliber of their vessels that contributes to rapid vasoconstriction.[1,48]

OTHER INJURY PATTERNS

Understanding injury patterns and the types of associated injuries can be helpful in evaluating a multiply injured patient. However, almost any combination can occur in a child, and the injury patterns are most closely related to the mechanism, the total force applied, and the age of the patient. According to Peclet and colleagues,[13] head injuries are most common in child abuse victims, occupants in vehicular accidents, and children sustaining falls; nearly 40% of abused children have injuries to the head and face. In their study, thoracic and abdominal injuries were most common in children with penetrating injuries (gunshot and stab wounds), whereas extremity injuries predominate in bicyclists and pedestrians. These investigators also showed that the types of injuries change with age: burns and foreign bodies account for most injuries to children ages 1 to 2 years compared with a median age of 7 years for pedestrian bicycle injuries and 12 years for gunshot and stab wounds. Falls and traffic-related injuries are most common in children 5 to 10 years of age. Children who sustained injuries from falls are significantly younger than those with traffic-related injuries. The pattern of injuries from falls also changes with age. Sawyer and associates[14] found that adolescents sustain a greater number of vertebral fractures and total fractures per fall than do younger children, who have a greater number of long bone fractures. Because the mechanisms of injury change with age, injury patterns and associated injuries also vary accordingly.

OBESITY AND THE PEDIATRIC TRAUMA PATIENT

Childhood obesity is a major public health problem in the United States. Obesity in children is defined as an age- and gender-specific body mass index at or above the 95th percentile. Not only are these children at risk of many short- and long-term health consequences, but several recent studies have also suggested that these children may display different patterns of injury than their peers. In a population-cohort study, Kessler and colleagues[49] demonstrated that overweight, moderately obese, and extremely obese children are at an increased risk of fractures of the foot, ankle, leg, and knee. This association was especially strong in those children 6 to 11 years of age. A recent study of children with tibia and femur fractures 2 to 14 years of age who were treated at a level I trauma center found that compared with nonobese children, obese children had significantly higher injury severity scores, a significantly higher rate of abdominal injury, a significantly higher frequency of pelvic ring injuries, a trend toward more spinal column injuries, and more incidences of bilateral tibia and femur fractures. They were also more likely to be admitted to the intensive care unit and had longer hospital stays and greater mortality when adjusted for age but not injury severity score.[50] Another study completed at a level I trauma center found a higher incidence of extremity fractures and a lower incidence of intraabdominal and intracranial trauma in obese children. They also found an increased rate of deep vein thrombosis and decubitus ulcers in these patients.[51]

The impact of obesity on injuries sustained in motor vehicle collisions was investigated in a retrospective database review in 2009. Among children 2 to 5 years of age who were obese, there was an increased risk of severe head, face, and neck injuries and severe thoracic injuries. Severe thoracic injuries and severe lower extremity injuries were more common in obese children 6 to 13 years of age. In the obese 14- to 17-year-old age group, investigators found an increased risk of severe lower extremity injuries but a decreased risk of severe abdominal, head, face, and neck trauma. Severe upper extremity injuries and spinal cord injuries were not associated with obesity in any age group.[52] Although more prospective data are needed, an increased level of awareness for associated injuries and complications should be present when the physician evaluates and treats obese pediatric trauma patients.

TRAUMA SCORING SYSTEMS

A multiply injured child has a spectrum of injuries of varying degrees of severity. The need for a measure of the severity of trauma is well recognized, both to assist in management and as a predictor of outcome. This need has been documented in adult trauma patients, and several systems have been developed, including the Injury Severity Score, Shock Index, Trauma Score, Revised Trauma Score, Glasgow Coma Scale (GCS),[53] Abbreviated Injury Scale,[54] TRISS-Scan (a combination of the Trauma Score, Injury Severity Score, and patient age), Acute Trauma Index, and Hannover Polytrauma Score. Similar systems have been recommended for pediatric patients, of which the most widely used are the Modified Injury Severity Scale (MISS)[55,56] and the Pediatric Trauma Score (PTS).[57,58]

Significant controversy exists regarding which is the best trauma scoring system and whether specific pediatric scores are needed. Two studies showed that both the Trauma Score and the TRISS-Scan have the greatest accuracy in predicting survival.[59,60] The need for pediatric-specific scores was therefore questioned. Nevertheless, the MISS and PTS can be useful in assessing and monitoring the outcomes of multiply injured children.

MODIFIED INJURY SEVERITY SCALE

The MISS represents an adaptation of the Abbreviated Injury Scale (1980 revision),[54] combined with the GCS for neurologic injuries. The pediatric MISS categorizes injuries into five body areas: (1) neurologic system, (2) face and neck, (3) chest, (4) abdomen and pelvic contents, and (5) extremities and pelvic girdle (Table 5.1).[55,56] The severity of each injury is rated on a scale of 1 to 5: one point for minor injury, two points for moderate injury, three points for severe but not life-threatening injury, four points for severe injury but with probable survival, and five points for critical

TABLE 5.1   The Modified Injury Severity Scale for Multiply Injured Children

Body Area	1: Minor	2: Minor	3: Severe, Not Life-Threatening	4: Severe, Life-Threatening	5: Critical, Survival Uncertain
Neural	GCS Score of 13–14	GCS Score of 9–12	GCS Score of 9–12	GCS Score of 5–8	GCS Score of 4
Face and neck	Abrasions or contusions of the ocular apparatus or lid Vitreous or conjunctival hemorrhage Fractured teeth	Undisplaced facial bone fracture Laceration of the eye, disfiguring laceration Retinal detachment	Loss of an eye, avulsion of the optic nerve Displaced facial fracture Blowout fracture of the orbit	Bone or soft tissue injury with minor destruction	Injuries with airway obstruction
Chest	Muscle ache or chest wall stiffness	Simple rib or sternal fracture	Multiple rib fractures Hemothorax or pneumothorax Diaphragmatic rupture Pulmonary contusion	Open chest wounds Pneumomediastinum Myocardial contusion	Lacerations, tracheal hemomediastinum Aortic laceration Myocardial laceration or rupture
Abdomen	Muscle ache, seat belt abrasion	Major abdominal wall contusion	Contusion of abdominal organs Retroperitoneal hematoma Extraperitoneal bladder rupture	Minor laceration of abdominal organs Intraperitoneal bladder rupture Spine fractures with paraplegia	Rupture or severe laceration of abdominal vessels or organs
Extremities and pelvic girdle	Minor sprains Simple fractures and dislocations	Open fractures of digits Nondisplaced long bone or pelvic fractures	Thoracic or lumbar spine fractures Displaced long bone or multiple hand or foot fractures Single, open long bone fracture Pelvic fractures with displacement Laceration of major nerves or vessels	Multiple closed long bone fractures Amputation of limbs	Multiple open long bone fractures

GCS, Glasgow Coma Scale.
Modified from Mayer T, Matlak ME, Johnson DG, et al. The modified injury severity scale in pediatric multiple trauma patients. *J Pediatr Surg.* 1980;15:719–726.

injury with uncertain survival. The GCS is used for grading neurologic injuries.[53] The usefulness of this scale has been well established in head injuries in both adult and pediatric populations. The verbal component of this score has been modified for children, especially for those younger than 36 months (Box 5.1).[61]

The MISS score is determined by the sum of the squares of the three most severely injured body areas. The MISS has been shown to be an accurate predictor of morbidity and mortality in pediatric trauma. Mayer and colleagues[56] found that scores of 25 points or more were associated with an increased risk of permanent disability. A score of more than 40 points was usually predictive of death. In their initial study, a score of 25 points or more was associated with 40% mortality and 30% disability, whereas a score of 24 points or less was associated with no deaths and only a 1% disability rate. Their mean MISS score for death was 33.4 points; for permanent disability, it was 30.2 points.

Marcus and colleagues[17] used the MISS in their series of 34 multiply injured children and showed a progressive increase in disability and mortality with increasing scores. The mean score was 22 points, with a range of 10 to 34 points. Children with scores of 25 points or less had a 30% incidence of impairment, children with scores of 26 to 40 points had a 33% incidence of impairment, and children with scores of more than 40 points had a 100% incidence of impairment. Contrary to the findings of Mayer and associates, children with scores over 40 were able to survive but with significant disability.

Loder[4] in 1987 also confirmed the relationship of increasing MISS scores with increasing mortality and morbidity in his series of 78 multiply injured children. He reported a mean MISS score of 28 points (range, 10–57 points). No deaths occurred in children with MISS scores of less than 40 points. The mortality rate for those with MISS scores above 40 points was 50%, and above 50 points, it increased to 75%.

BOX 5.1 Glasgow Coma Scale

Eye Opening

1. Spontaneous
2. To speech
3. To pain
4. None

Best Verbal Response

1. Oriented
2. Confused
3. Inappropriate
4. Incomprehensible
5. None

Modified Verbal Response for Children

1. Appropriate words, social smile, fixes and follows
2. Cries, but consolable
3. Persistently irritable
4. Restless, agitated
5. None

Best Motor Response

1. Obeys commands
2. Localizes pain
3. Withdraws
4. Flexes to pain
5. Extends to pain
6. None

From Teasdale G, Bennett B. Assessment of coma and impaired consciousness: a practical scale. *Lancet.* 1974;2:81-84; Hahn YS, Chyung C, Barthel MJ, et al. Head injuries in children under 36 months of age. Demography and outcome. *Childs Nerv Syst.* 1988:4:34-40.

Garvin and colleagues[43] in 1990 demonstrated the accuracy of the MISS in predicting morbidity and mortality after pediatric pelvic fractures. Disrupted pelvic fractures had a higher MISS score than did nondisrupted fractures, and the former were associated with an increased incidence of morbidity and mortality.

Yue and associates[62] in 2000 used the MISS in comparing the extent of injuries and the results of nonoperative versus operative or rigid stabilization in the management of ipsilateral pediatric femur and tibia fractures (i.e., the floating knee). The scores were useful in comparing the severity of injuries in both groups of patients. Loder and associates[63] in 2001 demonstrated an increasing rate of complications related to fracture immobilization in patients 8 years or older with MISS scores of 41 points or greater.

PEDIATRIC TRAUMA SCORE

The PTS can also be used to predict injury severity and mortality in children.[58,64] This score is based on six components: size, airway, systolic blood pressure, CNS injury, skeletal injury, and cutaneous injury. Each category is scored +2 (minimal or no injury), +1 (minor or potentially major injury), or –1 (major or immediately life-threatening injury), depending on severity, and these points are added

(Table 5.2). One major advantage of this system is that it is based on criteria that can be easily obtained either at the scene of the accident or in the emergency department, and it can thus be used for triage purposes. Tepas and associates[58] in 1988 demonstrated an inverse relationship between the PTS and the Injury Severity Score, as well as mortality, and found that the PTS was an effective predictor of both morbidity and mortality. No deaths occurred in children with a PTS greater than 8 points; those with a PTS less than 0 had 100% mortality. The PTS has also been validated in other studies as a tool for predicting mortality in pediatric trauma patients.[3] The PTS allows for rapid assessment of trauma severity in a multiply injured child, which assists in appropriate field triage, transport, and early emergency treatment of these patients. It is recommended that children with a PTS of 8 points or less be transported to a pediatric trauma center for management.

CONSEQUENCES OF INJURY

MORTALITY

Mortality rates in children vary greatly as a result of differences in the mechanism of injury, severity of injury, and age of the patient. A study using the NTDB found that pediatric trauma in children under 13 years of age is associated with higher mortality and complication rates than adults, whereas children from 13 to 17 years of age have lower mortality and complication rates than adults.[65] Unlike adults, who have a trimodal distribution of mortality from trauma, children seem to follow a bimodal curve. Peclet and colleagues[13] in 1990 demonstrated that the majority of deaths in children occurred within the first hour after injury, and another peak occurred at approximately 48 hours. In their series, 74% of deaths occurred within the first 48 hours. Overall, the mortality rate was 2.2% for all patients admitted to the trauma service. Not all the patients in this series were multiply injured, thus explaining the low mortality rate. In series dealing only with multiply injured children, van der Sluis and colleagues,[5] Wesson and colleagues,[6] and Loder[4] reported mortality rates of 20%, 13%, and 9%, respectively. This did not include children who were dead on arrival in the emergency department.

The fact that mortality rates are closely associated with the severity of injury is not surprising. The higher the MISS score or the lower the PTS, the greater the rate of mortality. In spite of significant differences from adults, children tend to have similar outcomes from trauma when equivalent injuries are compared. This finding was supported by the work of Eichelberger and colleagues,[66] who used a statistical method based on the Trauma Score, MISS, and age. These investigators were unable to show statistically significant differences between the various pediatric age groups and the adult population. Other studies have documented higher survival rates in severely injured children than in adults with a similar degree of injury.[4,17] This concept is accepted by many but may not be true. Head injuries are consistently associated with higher mortality rates than are other types of injuries. Acierno and associates[67] showed that children requiring emergent general or neurosurgical intervention were at increased risk of death. Recently, with the use of statistical modeling, Courville and colleagues[68] found that the

TABLE 5.2 Pediatric Trauma Score

Component	Severity Points		
	+2	**+1**	**−1**
Size	>20 kg	10–20 kg	<10 kg
Airway	Normal	Maintainable	Unmaintainable
Central nervous system	Normal	Obtunded	Comatose
Systolic blood pressure	>90 mm Hg	90–50 mm Hg	<50 mm Hg
Open wounds	None	Minor	Major or penetrating
Skeletal	None	Closed fracture	Open or multiple fractures

Modified from Tepas JJ 3rd, Ramenofsky ML, Mollitt DL, et al. The pediatric trauma score as a predictor of injury severity: an objective assessment. *J Trauma.* 1988;28:425–429.

most powerful variables in predicting in-hospital mortality in pediatric trauma were a low GCS score and hypotension in the emergency department.

MORBIDITY

Unlike a child with an isolated injury, which is usually associated with rapid healing, good function, and minimal residual disability, a multiply injured child has a significantly higher risk of residual disability. Morbidity in children is usually related to injuries to the CNS and musculoskeletal system.[2,5,6,17] At a 6-month follow-up in a study by Wesson and associates[6] of severely injured children, 54% still had one or more functional limitations; of these, 4% were in a vegetative state, 11% were severely disabled, 32% were moderately disabled, and 53% were healthy. The cause of the disability at 6 months was head injury in 44% and musculoskeletal injury in 32%. These findings are consistent with other reported series. In the series by Marcus and associates,[17] 10 of the 32 survivors had residual disabilities. Five were related to head injuries with residual seizures and spasticity. The remainder of the disabilities included musculoskeletal injuries associated with nonunion, malunion, and growth disturbances. Feickert and coauthors,[2] in a series of children with severe head injuries, reported that 39% still had severe neurologic impairment at the time of discharge. The incidence and severity of the residual disability increased with the severity of the overall injury, as reflected in a higher MISS score. In children, disability often occurs late and is progressive because of the fact that children are still growing and normal growth patterns have been disrupted. In a study looking at short- and long-term outcomes after trauma, van der Sluis and colleagues[5] found that of 59 survivors, 22% were disabled at 1 year, primarily as a result of severe brain injury. At a 9-year follow-up, 42% of patients had cognitive impairments.

TRAUMA EVALUATION AND MANAGEMENT

FIELD MANAGEMENT BEFORE TRANSPORT

Successful management of a multiply injured child requires rapid, systematic assessment, with early emphasis on the treatment of life-threatening conditions. Treatment is initiated in the field with advanced life support techniques. The importance of treatment in the field or during the prehospital phase is well documented. Because mortality follows a bimodal distribution in pediatric multiple-trauma patients, with most deaths occurring shortly after the accident, an efficient and effective system of prehospital care is mandatory. Delays in treatment can significantly increase mortality rates. Functional recovery is also improved with more rapid surgical care. A delay in diagnosis and treatment has been shown to be particularly detrimental to those with head injuries, and a severely injured child is particularly at risk of delays in diagnosis and treatment. The goal of field treatment is to evaluate the patient rapidly, stabilize life-threatening conditions, prepare the patient for transport by immobilizing injured areas, and deliver the patient to a center equipped for resuscitation and definitive treatment.

Early resuscitation plus stabilization of a pediatric trauma patient requires specialized equipment, including small-diameter airway tubes, small-bore intravenous needles, modified backboards, small cervical collars, and splints of appropriate size. As in adults, it is critical to immobilize the patient properly before transport to avoid further damage, especially when dealing with spinal injuries and extremity fractures. Preventable deaths in multiply injured children are associated with the "golden hour" of trauma resuscitation and occur from such causes as respiratory failure, intracranial hematoma, and inadequately treated hemorrhage. Treatment of respiratory failure and hemorrhage can be safely initiated in the field. Optimal treatment of an intracranial hematoma, however, requires rapid field triage and transport for immediate surgical decompression. Regarding hematomas, a 50% incidence of preventable deaths occur, of which field treatment errors account for one-third of cases and transport errors account for one-fourth. The importance of appropriate field treatment cannot be overemphasized. The American Academy of Pediatrics recommends ongoing education in pediatric trauma care for prehospital care providers.[18]

The use of a pediatric air ambulance should be considered in certain circumstances because a patient's outcome is directly related to the elapsed time between injury and definitive, specialized care.[8]

PEDIATRIC TRAUMA CENTERS

Because most children sustaining multiple injuries require specialized care, they should be rapidly transported to a center that is able to institute the necessary treatment. The ACS has set standards categorizing the level of trauma care that an institution can provide to both adult and pediatric trauma victims. These levels of care are categorized into pediatric trauma centers, adult trauma centers (level I, II, or III), and adult trauma centers with added qualifications to treat children. The ACS has also set guidelines regarding when a patient should be transferred to a pediatric trauma center (Box 5.2). Transport of an injured child to a facility lacking the capability of adequately handling these injuries significantly delays appropriate treatment and may allow inappropriate treatment to be initiated by a well-intentioned but inexperienced physician or staff member. Improved outcomes for trauma victims treated at trauma centers are well documented in both the pediatric and adult literature.[27,69,70] Additionally, it has been demonstrated that younger and more seriously injured children have better outcomes at trauma centers at a children's hospital or at a hospital with integrated adult and pediatric services.[18] Osler and colleagues[70] reported that although pediatric trauma centers have overall higher survival rates for multiply injured children than adult trauma centers do, the difference decreases when controlled for Injury Severity Score, PTS, age, mechanism, and ACS verification status.

TRAUMA TEAM

In a multiply injured child, the complexity and number of injuries mandate a team approach. A multidisciplinary approach with members of specialties working as equal partners usually allows optimal care. In most cases, the team leader should be a pediatric surgeon who specializes in the care of multiply injured children. This person should take primary responsibility for supervising the resuscitation effort, coordinating team members, and making critical decisions regarding treatment priorities. The members of the team are drawn from the pediatric surgical subspecialties and include a thoracic surgeon, cardiovascular surgeon, orthopedic surgeon, neurosurgeon, urologist, pediatric anesthesiologist, and plastic surgeon. Additional members include emergency department physicians and nurses, pediatric intensive care physicians and nurses, respiratory therapists, and physicians and nurses from rehabilitation services. Social workers, psychologists, dieticians, and counselors also have an important role in the treatment of these patients.

Pearls and Pitfalls

- A trauma team is crucial for comprehensive evaluation and management of the multiply injured child.
- Rib or pelvic fractures can be indicative of potentially serious chest or abdominal injury.
- Fracture treatment may be more surgical to facilitate overall care of the child.
- Early fracture management results in better outcomes if the child is stable enough for definitive management.

PRIMARY SURVEY AND RESUSCITATION

The principles of evaluation and stabilization of a pediatric trauma patient have been established as guidelines and protocols by the ACS for ATLS.[8] Although these guidelines are similar to those for adults, pediatric patients require special consideration because of their unique anatomic, physiologic, and pathophysiologic differences. The initial treatment consists of basic resuscitative measures, and the major focus is on diagnosis and treatment of life-threatening injuries. This primary survey consists of the ABCDEs of the initial assessment: Airway, Breathing, Circulation, Disability (consisting of a rapid neurologic examination), and Exposure/Environmental (removing all clothing and then recovering the patient to prevent hypothermia).

AIRWAY AND BREATHING

Assessment of the airway is the first consideration in all trauma patients. Patency of the airway must be assessed from the oral pharynx to the trachea. Evaluation, treatment, and maintenance of the airway must be performed with control and stabilization of the neck because of an increased incidence of cervical spine injuries in these children. All patients should be considered to have a cervical spine injury until proven otherwise. Stabilization of the spine should be provided with a cervical collar and backboard. A modified backboard should be used for young children and infants because of the large size of the head relative to the trunk. Herzenberg and associates[71] demonstrated that the neck is flexed when the child is placed on a standard backboard, thus potentially displacing an unstable cervical spine injury (Fig. 5.4). A backboard with an occipital cutout or a pad under the trunk to elevate it is used to prevent flexion of the cervical spine. Inline traction is used in all patients when trying to establish the airway. Major head and facial injuries should increase the physician's suspicion of potential cervical spine injuries.

BOX 5.2 Guidelines for Pediatric Trauma Center Referral

More than one body system injury
Injuries that require pediatric intensive care
Shock that requires more than one blood transfusion
Fractures with neurovascular injuries
Fractures of the axial skeleton
Two or more major long bone fractures
Potential replantation of an amputated extremity
Suspected or actual spinal cord injury
Head injuries with any of the following:
  Orbital or facial bone fractures
  Altered state of consciousness
  Cerebrospinal fluid leak
  Changing neurologic status
  Open head injury
  Depressed skull fracture
  Requirements of intracranial pressure monitoring
  Ventilatory support required

From American College of Surgeons Committee on Trauma. *Advanced Trauma Life Support for Doctors. Student Course Manual.* 7th ed. Chicago, IL: American College of Surgeons; 2004.

Children have considerable variation in the anatomy of the upper airway, depending on their size and age. The smaller the child, the greater the disproportion between the size of the cranium and the midface. This leads to a propensity of the posterior pharynx to buckle anteriorly as a result of passive flexion of the cervical spine secondary to a large occiput. An inch of padding should be placed beneath the child's torso to improve alignment. The jaw thrust maneuver is best for restoring airway patency; debris can be cleared from the mouth manually or with suction, if available. The neck is stabilized with inline cervical traction. The plane of the face should be kept parallel to the plane of the bed for optimization of the airway. It is important to realize that infants are obligate nasal breathers and that any injury that occludes the nasal passages also occludes the upper airway. These injuries include nasal fractures, foreign material in the nostrils, and bleeding within the nasal passages. Iatrogenically inserted tubes, such as nasogastric tubes, can also contribute to nasal occlusion. Thus, in an infant, both the oral pharynx and the nasal passage need to be cleared to restore the airway.

If a patent airway cannot be guaranteed with these maneuvers, an airway must be established. Before an attempt is made to mechanically establish an airway, the child should be oxygenated, if possible. An oral airway is not recommended in conscious children because it can induce vomiting by the gag reflex.

ENDOTRACHEAL INTUBATION

Endotracheal intubation is indicated in children with severe brain injuries requiring controlled ventilation, in children who cannot maintain an airway, in children exhibiting signs of ventilatory failure, or in children with significant hypovolemia that requires operative intervention. Orotracheal intubation is the most reliable means of a establishing an airway and ventilation in a child.[8] Most trauma centers will have an emergency intubation protocol referred to as drug-assisted intubation (previously known as rapid sequence intubation). Algorithms are available based on the child's weight, vital signs, and level of consciousness.

Because the trachea varies in length and diameter according to the child's size and age, the diameter of the endotracheal tube also varies. A length-based resuscitation tape (Broselow tape) can be used to determine the appropriate size. If this is not available, the size of the tube can be determined based on the size of the external nares or the size of the child's little finger.[8] A full complement of endotracheal tube sizes must be available for dealing with multiply injured children. As of the ninth edition of the ATLS manual, the ACS no longer puts a restriction on the use of cuffed endotracheal tubes in very young children. Because of improvements in cuff design, the concern about tracheal necrosis no longer exists. It is recommended that the cuff pressure be measured as soon as possible and should not exceed 30 mm Hg.

The shortness of the trachea in young children also increases the potential for bronchial intubation. Intubation should be confirmed by auscultation of breath sounds over both lungs and with a secondary confirmatory device such as capnography, end-tidal carbon dioxide detection, or an esophageal detection device. A chest x-ray film should be obtained to document the position of the tube.

CRICOTHYROIDOTOMY

If the upper airway of a child is severely obstructed and ventilation cannot be accomplished either by bag valve mask or endotracheal intubation, a surgical airway must be urgently created. A needle cricothyroidotomy can be performed quickly and safely to establish a temporary airway and is the treatment of choice.[8] A large-bore needle (14 or 16 gauge) can be directly inserted percutaneously into the trachea through the cricothyroid membrane to temporarily create an airway.

Considerations for emergency needle cricothyroidotomy include laryngeal fractures, major foreign bodies that

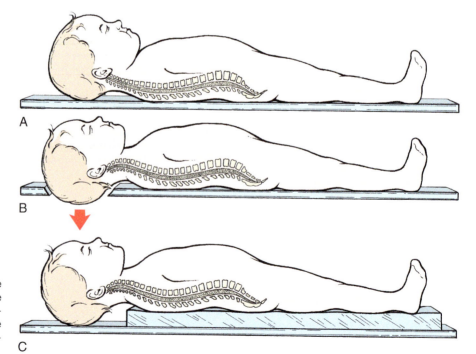

Fig. 5.4 Standard adult backboard. (A) The enlarged occiput causes a child to flex the head forward. (B and C) Appropriate positioning on a modified board with either the occipital area cut out or a pad under the thorax to prevent flexion of the cervical spine.

cannot be removed manually, severe oropharyngeal bleeding prohibiting intubation, edema of the glottis, and facial or mandibular fractures. Because needle cricothyroidotomy with the use of jet insufflation is only a temporary airway, if it is deemed that an oral or nasal airway cannot be achieved rapidly, provision must be made to convert the needle cricothyroidotomy into a surgical cricothyroidotomy. The cricothyroidotomy should be performed in the operating room under controlled conditions to decrease the risk of subglottic tracheal stenosis secondary to damage of the cricoid cartilage. For this reason, surgical cricothyroidotomy is rarely indicated in children younger than 12 years.

Once an airway has been established, adequate ventilation needs to be maintained. The adequacy of ventilation is evaluated both clinically and with arterial blood gas values. A pulse oximeter is also a rapid, noninvasive, and effective means of monitoring ventilation. Symmetric movement of the chest, auscultation for symmetric breath sounds, and palpation for equal chest expansion are necessary to ensure adequate ventilation. A posteroanterior or anteroposterior (AP) radiograph of the chest needs to be obtained so that the position of the endotracheal tube can be evaluated and so that injuries to the thorax (rib fractures), heart, lungs, and great vessels can be assessed. Because the thoracic cage in children is very compliant, pediatric patients can have significant lung and cardiac injuries without obvious external damage to the chest and without rib fractures.[8,30] The presence of a fracture of the first rib or multiple ribs indicates severe trauma and an increased risk of associated injuries.[8,40]

LIFE-THREATENING VENTILATION ABNORMALITIES

Injuries that may have a life-threatening effect on ventilation include tension pneumothorax, open pneumothorax, massive hemothorax, and flail chest. Because infants and small children ventilate primarily with the diaphragm, any injury or condition that compromises diaphragmatic excursion restricts ventilation. Potential injuries that affect diaphragmatic excursion include diaphragmatic rupture and intraabdominal injuries.

GASTRIC DISTENTION

Severe gastric distention can decrease diaphragmatic excursion considerably. Gastric decompression should be performed in all children with signs of ventilatory compromise. Decompression can be achieved easily with the passage of a small nasogastric or orogastric tube. Because of particulate matter, a tube smaller than 10F cannot adequately aspirate the gastric fluid and stomach contents and should not be used.

TENSION PNEUMOTHORAX

Children are more susceptible to pneumothorax secondary to the mobility of their mediastinal structures. A pneumothorax under pressure may initially be managed by the insertion of a large-caliber intravenous catheter, such as a 14- or 16-gauge catheter (Angiocath), just above the third rib in the midclavicular line. Such treatment relieves the pressure and converts it into a simple pneumothorax, which can be managed with the use of a chest tube. In infants and small children, care should be taken not to insert the catheter too deep because this may actually cause a pneumothorax. Large, penetrating chest wounds are initially treated with an occlusive dressing and positive-pressure ventilation. A flail chest is diagnosed by the observation of paradoxical motion with respirations.[67] A child who also exhibits signs of inadequate ventilation should be treated with endotracheal intubation and mechanical ventilation.

CIRCULATION AND RESUSCITATION

The key factors in the evaluation and management of circulation are recognition of shock, fluid resuscitation, blood replacement, venous access, recording of urine output, and thermoregulation.[8]

SHOCK

It is critical to recognize and treat shock in the immediate phases of the primary survey. A child's response to shock is different from that of an adult. A child is often able to maintain normal blood pressure by increasing the heart rate along with significant peripheral constriction while in the supine position. A decrease in blood pressure is not usually seen or is a very late finding; absence of hypotension, however, does not rule out shock. A child can often compensate for a 20% to 30% blood volume loss without a decline in blood pressure. Tachycardia and poor skin perfusion are usually the only signs of early shock. Other more subtle signs include progressive narrowing of pulse pressure, skin mottling, cool extremities, a decreased level of consciousness, and a decreased response to pain. The importance of early resuscitation in children is highlighted by a study demonstrating that admission hypotension and need for trauma bay blood transfusion are both strong predictors of early, intermediate, and late mortality.[72] A guide for normal blood pressure in children is a systolic pressure of 90 mm Hg plus twice the child's age in years and a diastolic pressure that is two-thirds the systolic pressure.[8] Because infants are relatively incapable of increasing their cardiac stroke volume, their only way to increase cardiac output is by increasing the heart rate. Thus, the heart rate must be monitored closely. Normal vital signs by age are presented in Table 5.3. Hypotension in a child represents a state of decompensated shock and severe blood loss. During this stage of shock, tachycardia may also be replaced by bradycardia.

CARDIAC TAMPONADE

Tamponade occurs when the pericardial space surrounding the heart fills with fluid (usually blood) and prevents the normal distention and contractility of the heart. This cardiac compression results in a progressive decrease in cardiac output and, ultimately, heart failure. The clinical findings of cardiac tamponade include the Beck triad: muffled heart sounds, distended neck veins, and pulsus paradoxus. Initial emergency management consists of pericardiocentesis with the use of a long, plastic-sheathed needle that is attached to an electrocardiogram monitor and inserted through a subxiphoid route. The need for emergency surgical drainage of the pericardium can be temporarily delayed by leaving the plastic sheath in place for continued drainage.

HEMORRHAGE

Severe exsanguinating hemorrhage requires prompt identification and treatment, usually by direct pressure. It is not wise to probe wounds and use clamps, which can cause further damage. If direct pressure does not stop the bleeding,

TABLE 5.3   Approximate Weight, Blood Volume, Vital Signs, and Maintenance Fluids by Age

Age	Approximate Weight (kg)	Blood Volume (mL/kg)	Pulse	Systolic Blood Pressure (mm Hg)	Respiration	Maintenance Fluid/24 Hours (D5 ¼ NS)
Birth	3.5	90	140–160	80	40	100 mL/kg
6 months	6.0	90	140–160	80	40	100 mL/kg
1 year	12.0	85	120–160	90	30	1000 mL + 50 mL/kg over 10 kg
4 years	16.0	80	120–140	90	30	1000 mL + 50 mL/kg over 10 kg
10 years	35.0	75	100–120	100	20	1500 mL + 20 mL/kg over 20 kg
15 years	55.0	70	80–100	110	20	1500 mL + 20 mL/kg over 20 kg

the use of a temporary tourniquet is recommended. It is important to note the time of tourniquet application and to plan definitive treatment so that the tourniquet can be removed before permanent ischemic damage occurs. Treatment of shock should proceed concomitantly with an evaluation to determine its cause. If an obvious external source of blood loss is not found, one must assume that the patient is bleeding into a major body cavity. The presence of a head injury or multiple extremity fractures does not usually account for blood loss causing signs of shock; thus, other causes should be investigated. An unstable pelvic fracture can result in significant blood loss and requires urgent reduction and stabilization.[67] A pelvic binder or sheet can also be applied during transport to the hospital and be used during the initial evaluation. Children with displaced pelvic fractures and ongoing hemorrhaging can be treated with an immediate spica cast to close the fracture and decrease transfusion requirements. This technique may be definitive management in certain pediatric pelvic fractures. A simple anterior external fixation frame can be safely and rapidly applied with a single pin (4 or 5 mm, depending on the size of the child) into each anterior iliac crest at the level of the gluteal ridge. These pins are then connected with a single anterior bar that adequately holds the pelvis closed. Sufficient space should be allowed for access to the abdomen. If an emergency laparotomy is needed, a pubic diastasis can be plated through this incision with the use of a two-hole plate. Reduction of a displaced pelvic fracture decreases pelvic volume and hemorrhaging, relieves pain, and provides immobilization.

RESUSCITATION

As in adults, children should have two peripheral percutaneous intravenous lines inserted during the initial survey. These lines should be placed in the upper extremity, although the lower extremities can be used if venous access is inadequate or cannot be achieved. If percutaneous intravenous lines cannot be inserted after two attempts, intraosseous infusion

or insertion of a femoral central line should be considered. Direct venous cutdown is now considered to be a last resort because even in the most experienced hands, it can take more than 10 minutes to perform, whereas an intraosseous line can be placed in less than 1 minute even by providers with limited experience.[8] The preferred site for intraosseous access is the proximal anterior tibia, below the level of the tibial tuberosity. This should not be attempted in a tibia in which a fracture is suspected. Alternatively, the distal femur can be used for access. Complications of intraosseous infusion include compartment syndrome and iatrogenic fractures. This infusion site should be discontinued as soon as other access can be established. After adequate venous access has been achieved, other resuscitative measures can be instituted.

The primary objective of the initial resuscitation of a pediatric patient is to determine the degree of blood loss and the subsequent amount of blood replacement. A child's blood volume is approximately 80 mL/kg body weight. If a child's weight is unknown, it can be estimated with the use of a length-based resuscitation tape. Fluid or blood replacement must be rapid enough to maintain stable vital signs and adequate urinary output. In a child with signs of shock, a bolus of crystalloid solution, such as lactated Ringer solution, should be given at approximately 20 mL/kg body weight. A positive response includes a decrease in heart rate, an increase in systolic blood pressure, improved peripheral circulation, increased urine output, and improved sensorium. If no signs of improvement are apparent, a second bolus of the same volume should be given.[67] If still no obvious improvement is seen after the second bolus, a third bolus of the same volume can be given; further, the physician may consider administering type-specific or type O-negative warmed, packed red blood cells at 10 mL/kg body weight.[8] Blood less than 5 days old is recommended for transfusion because it has higher levels of 2,3-diphosphoglycerate, which improves delivery of oxygen to tissues. When large volumes are required, the blood should be passed through a warming device so that the patient does not become hypothermic. Blood loss replacement in a child is based on the three-for-one rule: 3 mL of crystalloid solution for 1 mL of blood loss. In a child with a severe head injury, fluid administration should be adequate but judicious to avoid overhydration and increased intracranial pressure; monitoring of intracranial pressure is required. After resuscitation, maintenance fluids must be administered (see Table 5.3).

ACID-BASE BALANCE

During resuscitation, pediatric patients may have acid-base complications. Most resolve with adequate ventilation and perfusion. The most commonly encountered abnormality is respiratory acidosis.[8] Without adequate ventilation and perfusion, however, the attempt to correct acidosis with sodium bicarbonate results in further hypercarbia and worsened acidosis. The ninth edition of the ATLS replaces the concept of aggressive resuscitation with the concept of balanced resuscitation, which changes the initial amount of crystalloid used from 2 L to 1 L. Early use of blood products is also emphasized.

URINARY OUTPUT

Urinary output varies with the age of the child (infants up to 1 year: 2 mL/kg/hour; young children 1.5 mL/kg/hour; older children 1 mL/kg/hour). Urinary output and specific gravity is an excellent method for assessing adequacy of volume resuscitation.[8] Insertion of a urinary catheter may help to accurately record and follow urine output.

HYPOTHERMIA

Hypothermia can be a significant problem in a child because of the volume of fluids needed for resuscitation and the high ratio of body surface area to body mass. Every attempt should be made to use warmed fluids. Other means of maintaining body temperature include keeping the child covered, increasing the room temperature, and using overhead heaters and heating blankets. Hypothermia in a small child or infant can significantly complicate resuscitation because it may render the patient refractory to the usual therapy for shock. Hypothermia stimulates catecholamine secretion and muscle shivering, hence resulting in metabolic acidosis with the potential for negative effects on pharmacokinetics. Coagulation disorders may also develop and aggravate the condition. The child's temperature should be maintained at 36°C or 37°C.

SECONDARY SURVEY

In the secondary survey, the history is completed, and a comprehensive physical examination is performed. This should not be completed until the ABCDEs of the primary survey are complete, resuscitation is underway, and vital signs are normalized. A trauma radiographic series is obtained concomitantly. The examination proceeds systematically, with evaluation of the head, spine, chest, abdomen, and extremities so that the extent of the injuries can be determined and subsequent treatment can be prioritized. The secondary survey is followed by definitive management of the injuries.

TRAUMA RADIOGRAPHIC SERIES

During the primary survey, strong consideration should be made for obtaining a radiographic trauma series: a lateral view of the cervical spine, a supine AP view of the chest, and an AP view of the pelvis. These radiographs, however, do not take precedence over the treatment of immediate life-threatening injuries. Depending on the size of the child, the chest and pelvic radiographs may be obtained on a single cassette, thus saving time and reducing the need to move the child. A retrospective study of 176 consecutive children with GCS greater than 12 found a low rate of 6.6% injury on the full trauma series, with no abnormal cervical or chest imaging in children with normal exams, and only two cases of pelvic findings in children both under 3 years of age, suggesting that one can consider skipping imaging in children with reliable physical exams.[73]

LATERAL CERVICAL SPINE RADIOGRAPH

As mentioned previously, a lateral radiograph of the neck is used to screen for cervical spine injuries because this is a common site for injury.[74,75] Although useful as a screen, lateral radiographs cannot be used as the sole measure for determining cervical spine injury in a child who is at high risk of cervical spine injury or in a child who is uncooperative or unresponsive.

Lateral neck radiographs in a young child can be difficult to interpret. An atlantodens interval of up to 5 mm is normal in a child. Displacement of more than 5 mm is considered abnormal and indicative of a tear of the transverse atlantal ligament.[76] In extension, overriding of the anterior arch of the atlas on top of the odontoid can be seen in up to 20% of children.[76] It is not unusual to find slight subluxation in the upper cervical spine, especially at the C2–C3 level and, to a lesser extent, the C3–C4 level.[77] This pseudosubluxation is present in about 40% of children 6 years of age or younger at the C2–C3 level and in about 20% of children 15 years of age or younger.[8,78] The posterior cervical line of Swischuk can help distinguish pseudosubluxation from true pathology. Variations in the curvature and growth of the cervical spine can also resemble an injury. This includes marked angulation at a single cervical interspace, as well as wedging of the C3 vertebral body.[77,79]

The National Emergency X-Radiography Utilization Study (NEXUS) criteria can be used reliably in patients older than 9 years of age to determine whether the child is at low risk of a cervical spine injury. These criteria include no midline cervical tenderness on direct palpation, a normal level of alertness, no evidence of intoxication, no neurologic abnormalities, and no distracting injuries. A Cochrane review found a wide range of sensitivity with NEXUS, suggesting that injuries can be missed with the system.[80] Other criteria that have been added for children that may warrant further imaging include a high-risk mechanism of injury, transient neurologic symptoms, physical signs of neck trauma, head or face trauma, or a child who is inconsolable.[81]

In children who are conscious but who do not meet the aforementioned criteria to be considered low risk, AP, open-mouth odontoid, and oblique views are necessary for completing the radiographic assessment. A computed tomographic (CT) scan should be used as an adjunct when necessary if a fracture is noted or suspected on a plain film, if the plain films are difficult to interpret, or if an injury is highly suspected despite negative radiographs. A recent retrospective study of patients evaluated with radiographs and CT found that radiographs had a 50% sensitivity overall and 62% when only considering significant injuries.[82] Radiographs are more likely to miss injuries in younger children. No clear guidelines exist with respect to patients who are unconscious, but evidence in the literature suggests that obtaining an early CT scan in these patients is advisable.[81]

Magnetic resonance imaging (MRI) is performed if neurologic signs or deficits are noted, and it can also be used as an adjunct in the evaluation of the unconscious child.[81] Flynn and associates[83] outlined the following indications for MRI in children with suspected cervical spine injuries: an obtunded or nonverbal child suspected of having a cervical spine injury; equivocal plain radiographs; neurologic symptoms without radiographic findings; and the inability to clear the cervical spine within 3 days of testing. It must also be remembered that children, because of their elasticity, can sustain a spinal cord injury without radiographic abnormality (SCIWORA).

ANTEROPOSTERIOR CHEST RADIOGRAPH

The supine AP chest radiograph is extremely useful for evaluating whether suspected injuries noted during the primary survey are present, for monitoring the response to any treatment rendered for these conditions, and for assessing whether more subtle, unsuspected injuries are present. Injuries that can be diagnosed on a chest radiograph include pneumothorax, hemopneumothorax, pulmonary contusion, aortic arch injury (mediastinal widening), disruption of the trachea or a bronchus, diaphragmatic rupture, rib fracture or fractures, and thoracic spine injury. As stated previously, because of the compliance of the ribs, a child can sustain significant internal injury without obvious damage to the chest. The diagnosis of a fracture of the first rib or multiple ribs is a marker of severe trauma and warrants further evaluation.[40]

ANTEROPOSTERIOR PELVIC RADIOGRAPH

This radiograph is useful for evaluating injuries to the pelvis. Although minor nondisplaced pelvic fractures may not be associated with significant complications, severe displaced pelvic fractures have an increased risk of associated injuries and therefore a much worse prognosis.[43,44,84] Associated pelvic and extrapelvic injuries must also be suspected and identified, if present.

Fractures and dislocations of the hip and proximal ends of the femurs can also be assessed on a routine AP pelvic radiograph. A pelvic CT is indicated if an injury to the sacrum, sacroiliac joint, or acetabulum is suspected clinically or by standard radiographs (see Chapter 11). Posterior pelvic injuries may not be well visualized on standard radiographs; CT is an excellent radiographic modality for evaluating these types of injuries.[85]

OTHER RADIOGRAPHS

Findings on clinical evaluation of the extremities, including palpation, should be used as the basis for obtaining radiographs of the extremities. These radiographs are of lower priority and should not take precedence over the assessment and treatment of any life-threatening conditions. When radiographs are obtained, they should be orthogonal, with two views 90 degrees apart (anterior-posterior and lateral). They should include the joints above and below if a fracture is present. Comparison views are only occasionally necessary in a child. Appropriate placement of the child or infant on a large plate often gives a single AP view of the entire body (babygram), which can be an extremely helpful screening technique. The use of a technetium bone scan has been recommended by Heinrich and associates[86] for a multiply injured pediatric patient with head injuries to assist in the diagnosis of musculoskeletal injuries.

A study of pediatric fall patients found that the use of CT scans doubled from 2001 to 2010.[87] Recently, radiation exposure in pediatric trauma patients has been a concern. Kharbanda and associates[88] reviewed the radiation exposure of pediatric trauma patients using the NTDB. They concluded that younger children and those with more severe injuries are exposed to the highest levels of radiation, which are well above the yearly background radiation exposure rates. It is unclear what the long-term effects of this level of radiation will have on these children, but efforts should be made to implement programs that will help limit the amount of radiation exposure in these patients.

HEAD INJURIES

A head injury in a child may have a poor prognosis and a high incidence of morbidity and mortality.[2,89] Rapid evaluation and treatment are therefore indicated. Signs of external injury, including scalp lacerations, hematomas, and facial lacerations or fractures, should increase suspicion of potential severe intracranial injury. The eyes should be evaluated both with regard to pupil size and reactivity and for evidence of increased intracranial pressure by funduscopic examination. A neurologic evaluation, including assessment of cranial nerves, motor function, strength, sensation, deep tendon reflexes, and rectal sphincter tone, should be performed and carefully documented. The GCS score should be determined and recorded (see Box 5.1). For children younger than 4 years, the modified verbal score should be used. CT is indicated in any child sustaining a head injury, especially if unconscious or semiconscious. If surgery and thus anesthesia are necessary, CT is required to clear the child for surgery. In a hemodynamically unstable child who warrants emergency surgery to control hemorrhaging, CT may have to be delayed until the patient is stabilized and then performed before surgical treatment is continued. Herniation syndromes and expanding mass lesions must be decompressed urgently. Children with signs of increased intracranial pressure should have direct intracranial pressure measurements routinely. Such measurement can be done safely and greatly aids in the treatment of this condition. Neurosurgery consultation should be obtained early, especially in children with a GCS score of less than 8, multiple injuries with an associated head injury that may require major volume resuscitation, or with a head CT that demonstrates hemorrhaging, cerebral swelling, or herniation.[8]

Remember that uncorrected hypovolemic shock and hypoxemia may further compromise a severe brain injury.[90,91] Hypoxemia must be corrected by intubation, adequate ventilation with supplemental oxygen, and fluid or blood replacement. Restriction of fluids to minimize cerebral edema is not appropriate until after hemodynamic stabilization.

SPINE AND SPINAL CORD INJURIES

Spine fractures in children are relatively rare, making up only 1% to 2% of all pediatric fractures. They may be present with or without spinal cord injury. Injury to the spinal cord is also uncommon, making up 5% of all injuries to the spinal column. In children younger than 10 years, spinal cord injury is most likely the result of a motor vehicle accident, whereas in children ages 10 to 14 years, an equal number of injuries result from motor vehicle accidents and sports-related accidents.[8] In a child who is a victim of multiple traumatic injuries, a spinal column injury should be presumed until ruled out by physical and radiographic evaluation. Information regarding the mechanism of injury, the use of restraints or seat belts (in motor vehicle accidents), the child's neurologic status at the scene of the accident, and any change in neurologic status is important to obtain during the initial evaluation. Any child sustaining an injury above the clavicle or a head injury resulting in loss or alteration of consciousness should be suspected of having a cervical spine injury. Injuries produced by high-velocity accidents should also arouse suspicion of vertebral column injuries. As stated previously, a SCIWORA is also possible. Brown and associates,[32] in a study of 103 consecutive children with cervical spine injuries, reported that almost 75% involved the upper cervical spine (C1 to C4) and that 35% had an associated SCIWORA. Similar results have been reported by others.[75,92] A recent large database study of more than 240,000 pediatric trauma patients found that the incidence of cervical spine injury increases steeply after the age of 9 years. They also noted an increasing amount of lower cervical spine injuries after 9 years of age with a corresponding decrease in upper cervical spine injuries. This is thought to occur because as children approach 9 years old, the vertebrae begin to ossify and mature, which creates a more rectangular shape; the uncinate process begins to protrude; the orientation of the facets become more vertical; and children become less ligamentously lax.[93]

Examination of a child with a suspected spinal injury is carried out with the patient supine, in a neutral position, after the head and neck have been stabilized. In small children, it is appropriate to place a pad beneath the trunk to avoid hyperflexion of the neck because of the disproportion in head size.[94] The child should be protected in this manner until definitive radiographs have been obtained. A careful physical examination should be performed, with particular attention directed to the presence of prominent spinous processes, local tenderness, pain with attempted motion, edema, ecchymoses, visible deformities, and muscle spasms. In suspected cervical spine injuries, it is also important to assess for tracheal tenderness or deviation and the presence of a retropharyngeal hematoma. A careful neurologic examination, including muscle strength, sensory changes, alterations in deep tendon reflex, and autonomic dysfunction, must be performed and accurately recorded. Autonomic dysfunction is identified by the lack of bladder and rectal control.

In spinal cord injuries, it is important to determine whether the lesion is complete or incomplete. The presence of superficial (pinprick) and deep pain discrimination indicates an incomplete lesion and intact lateral column function. Posterior column function is assessed by position and vibratory sensation. Because of the phenomenon of sacral sparing, it is important that sensation to the anal, perianal, and scrotal areas be tested. Evaluation for sacral sparing should include sensory perception and voluntary contraction of the rectum. The presence of sacral sparing indicates that the paralysis is not complete and is a good prognostic sign with respect to neurologic recovery. Detailed sensory examination can be extremely difficult, if possible at all, in younger children.

The evaluation of muscle function and sensation determines the level of spinal cord injury. Sledge and colleagues[95] demonstrated the value of MRI in assessing thoracolumbar fractures, spinal stability, and the spinal cord injury pattern. The latter could be used in predicting the clinical outcome.

Spinal shock may occur after spinal cord injury. The pulse rate is not usually increased with this type of shock, and systolic blood pressure typically falls to approximately 80 mm Hg as blood pools from the dilated visceral vessels. Flaccid muscle paralysis, flaccid sphincters, and absent deep-tendon reflexes are associated with spinal shock. The presence of a bulbocavernosus reflex may be important in distinguishing spinal shock from true spinal cord injury. After completion of a careful neurologic evaluation, spinal radiographs must be obtained.

Lateral cervical spine radiographs are obtained on every patient sustaining multiple traumatic injuries. In the lateral radiograph of the cervical spine, it is important that all seven vertebrae be identified. Occasionally, the patient's shoulders must be pulled down to visualize C6 and C7. Other cervical radiographs include AP, oblique, and odontoid views. Occasionally, CT or MRI may be necessary to confirm a cervical spine injury and to determine its stability. Lateral flexion and extension radiographs can be dangerous and must be performed under appropriate supervision. When injuries to the thoracic and lumbar spine are suspected, AP and lateral radiographs are obtained. Occasionally, oblique radiographs of the lumbar spine may be useful.

Treatment of any vertebral column and associated spinal cord injury is under the direction of the orthopedic surgeon or neurosurgeon (see Chapter 10), preferably at a pediatric trauma center. In unstable cervical spine fractures or fracture-dislocations, stabilization by the application of tongs and traction may be appropriate. However, traction should be used cautiously to avoid distraction. Traction weights should be applied sequentially, and stabilization should be assessed by repeated lateral radiographs. High-dose methylprednisolone given within the first 8 hours of injury for nonpenetrating spinal cord injuries is a currently accepted treatment in adults in North America.[8] However, a recent study of 59 patients found that only 22% followed proper protocol because of the rarity and complexity of methylprednisolone treatment, and also noted a significantly higher complication rate in treated children, calling into question the appropriateness of steroid use in children for spinal cord injury.[96]

CHEST INJURIES

Only 8% of all injuries in children involve the chest, but two-thirds of children who have chest injuries will have multiple injuries.[8] The child's chest is very compliant, and significant intrathoracic injury may occur without obvious external trauma.[97] The chest should be evaluated by palpation, percussion, and auscultation in addition to an AP chest radiograph. The presence of a first-rib fracture or multiple rib fractures is an indicator of severe injury, and other associated injuries must be sought.[40,98] Conditions previously stabilized in the primary survey should undergo definitive treatment during the secondary survey. Definitive treatment may include the insertion of a chest tube for a pneumothorax or drainage of a hemopneumothorax. The diagnosis of blunt cardiac contusion requires a high index of suspicion.[99] It is usually associated with severe trauma to multiple systems. Serial electrocardiograms are indicated. However, serial cardiac enzymes are of questionable utility and presently have no role in monitoring blunt cardiac contusions.

Although rupture of the aorta is rare in children, a widened mediastinum warrants an aortogram. Heckman and associates[100] recognized that older children involved in a motor vehicle accident with severe head, torso, and lower extremity injuries were a group at high risk of injury to the thoracic aorta. Bronchial injuries and diaphragmatic rupture occur more frequently in this group. Pulmonary contusions are quite common with blunt chest trauma in children and may be complicated by aspiration of gastric contents.

Diaphragmatic injuries are fortunately rare but are life-threatening when they occur. According to Brandt and colleagues,[101] they are always associated with either penetrating or high-velocity blunt trauma. Diaphragmatic injuries are usually diagnosed with the trauma chest radiograph, although they can be missed. The incidence of associated injuries is high, and emergency surgical repair is essential.

ABDOMINAL INJURIES

The majority of serious abdominal injuries in children are the result of blunt trauma, although penetrating trauma has an increasing incidence in the inner city population, especially in adolescent males.[102] Approximately 8% of injuries sustained by children involve other children.[103] Serious injuries to the abdominal contents can be inflicted with less force than in an adult because of the anatomic differences in children. The costal margin is higher than in an adult, thus affording less protection to the upper abdominal viscera. In addition, children have less abdominal musculature and a more compliant pelvis.

Routine examination of an injured child's abdomen may be difficult because of the patient's fear, inability to cooperate, and generalized response to pain. In addition, a child's typical response of aerophagia, which results in gastric distention, increases the difficulty of an examination. In an attempt to reduce this problem, all children sustaining blunt abdominal trauma should have a nasogastric tube inserted and the gastric contents aspirated. In the distended state, the bladder in infants and small children can extend up to the umbilicus, and it is helpful to insert a Foley catheter to decompress the bladder, provided that the child has no evidence of a pelvic fracture or genitourinary injury. The presence of gross hematuria after catheterization is more suggestive of urologic injury than is microscopic hematuria, and further investigation of the urinary tract is necessary. Serial abdominal examinations in an injured child in the absence of pelvic or genitourinary injuries are critical.

A child who is seen with signs of peritoneal irritation, a distended abdomen, or signs of hypovolemia without obvious external blood loss needs further urgent diagnostic studies. A child with peritoneal irritation and unstable vital signs requires emergency laparotomy. Those with stable vital signs may undergo further imaging evaluation.

CT is now considered the preferred diagnostic study in most children to detect intraabdominal injury. This has the advantages of being noninvasive and enabling more specific evaluation of solid visceral injuries. Its disadvantages include added time needed for scanning, radiation exposure, expense, and less specificity in evaluating perforations and injuries to the small or large bowel. Focused Assessment Sonography in Trauma (FAST) offers a potentially quick option without radiation exposure for screening for abdominal pathology. However, FAST has been evaluated in pediatric blunt trauma in a large randomized trial and a separate prospective multicenter study, both of which have found that FAST in pediatric trauma does not improve outcomes, reduce CT utilization, or alter emergency room length of stay.[104,105]

Diagnostic peritoneal lavage is a sensitive study for demonstrating intraabdominal bleeding. Peritoneal lavage in a child may be difficult because of a lack of cooperation, distention of the stomach or bladder (or both), and thinness of the abdominal wall, which allows sudden penetrations and iatrogenic visceral injury. This should only be used in children who cannot safely be transported to CT or when a CT scanner is not available.

The spleen is the most commonly injured intraabdominal organ in children, but treatment is quite different from that for adults. Unlike the situation in adults, treatment of splenic injuries in children is initially nonoperative in an attempt to salvage the organ.[69,106] Several considerations influence this nonoperative approach. First, the incidence of late malignant sepsis after splenectomy in children is well documented. Second, the capsule of the pediatric spleen is thicker than that in an adult, which allows for surgical repair. Third, a child's spleen often stops bleeding spontaneously. The spleen is best evaluated with the use of serial CT scans or radioisotope imaging. Children who are seen with evidence of massive bleeding require emergency operative treatment, and every attempt should be made to repair and salvage the spleen. Patients with stable vital signs and hematocrit levels can be observed in the pediatric or surgical intensive care unit and monitored with a repeated CT scan in 5 to 7 days. Surgical intervention is indicated during that time if the patient has signs of continued bleeding, such as a progressive decline in hematocrit level, or shows signs of increasing peritoneal irritation.

The liver is the second most commonly injured abdominal organ in children, and hepatic injuries are also managed nonoperatively, if possible. Close serial clinical examinations and monitoring are indicated in addition to initial and follow-up CT.

Penetrating abdominal injuries such as gunshot or stab wounds should be treated aggressively and require laparotomy. CT and peritoneal lavage are not considered necessary in penetrating trauma. Rupture of hollow viscera also requires early operative intervention.[8]

Other abdominal injuries that are more common in children include duodenal hematomas and pancreatic injuries because of a thin abdominal wall, small-bowel perforations, mesenteric avulsion injuries, and bladder ruptures because of the shallow depth of the pelvis.[8]

EXTREMITY INJURIES

In general, definitive evaluation and management of extremity injuries have a low priority during both the primary and the secondary surveys. Extremity injuries are rarely life-threatening and should rarely take precedence over the evaluation and treatment of other serious injuries. Initial treatment of extremity injuries should include covering all wounds with sterile dressing, realigning deformed extremities, and splinting all potentially injured extremities. A neurovascular examination both before and after splinting is essential. Open wounds of the extremity require débridement of gross contamination, antibiotics, and tetanus prophylaxis when appropriate. Open wounds should never be left uncovered, and multiple inspections of the wounds should be avoided to minimize the chance of iatrogenic infection. These infections are usually with nosocomial organisms, with the added problem of multiple-drug resistance. All wounds in proximity to a fracture should be considered communicating, and the fracture should be treated as an open fracture. Fortunately, the initial use of broad-spectrum antibiotics has been shown to decrease the risk of infection, even if wound débridement and fracture management must be delayed for up to 24 hours.[107]

Assessment of extremity injuries includes visual inspection of the entire extremity, which mandates the removal of all clothing. All extremities should be palpated for evidence of tenderness, swelling, crepitus, and instability, and all joints should be inspected both visually and manually for signs of swelling, effusion, and deformity. Range of motion and ligamentous stability should also be assessed. All major joints should be examined, especially the knees. Ligamentous injury to the knee is commonly associated with other injuries, such as femoral shaft fractures and posterior hip dislocation, and the knee injury can often be missed; instability on examination may represent a physeal injury.

VASCULAR INJURIES

Vascular injury in the pediatric trauma population is very rare overall, occurring in only 0.6% of patients.[108] The most commonly injured arteries are those of the upper extremity, representing 37.9% of all injuries in a database study by Barmparas and associates.[108] However, these injuries had a low mortality rate and were not frequently associated with amputation. Injuries to major arteries in association with extremity fractures are also uncommon in children. Gustilo IIIC fractures, by definition, have an associated vascular injury and may lead to amputation. Vascular injuries can also occur after closed proximal tibial metaphyseal fractures and knee dislocations. Displaced pelvic fractures can result in injuries to the paravaginal, superior gluteal, and internal iliac arteries. These vascular injuries can give rise to large retroperitoneal hematomas. Fortunately, most hemorrhaging from pelvic fractures comes from small arterial injuries rather than major vessels. Prompt clinical recognition, radiographic evaluation, and repair or reconstruction of arterial injuries are necessary for limb salvage. The cardinal signs of arterial injury include the six Ps: pulselessness, pain, pallor, paresthesias, poikilothermia, and paralysis. However, the presence of palpable pulses or Doppler-documented flow does not rule out an arterial injury. Compartment syndromes can have many of the same features as an arterial injury, especially in the forearm and the leg. Thus, careful evaluation is necessary.

Knee dislocation, displaced proximal tibial fractures, and multiple ligamentous injuries are highly associated with injuries to the popliteal artery and warrant further evaluation. Such evaluation can include arteriography, duplex sonography, and the use of the ankle-brachial index (ABI). Measurement of the ABI is accomplished by dividing the Doppler arterial systolic pressure in the injured lower extremity by the corresponding pressure in the uninjured upper extremity. A value of less than 0.90 is indicative of a major arterial injury. This test is rapid and cost-effective and can save valuable time during the secondary survey. However, it does not disclose injuries to the profunda femoris, profunda brachii, and peroneal arteries. It may also not allow recognition of lesions that do not reduce blood flow to the extremity, such as intimal flaps and small pseudoaneurysms.

When an arterial injury is suspected or diagnosed clinically, an arteriogram should be considered. Common indications for arteriographic evaluation of the extremities include dislocation of the knee, absent or asymmetric distal pulses, displaced pelvic fractures with hypotension, signs of peripheral ischemia, and severe open fractures. A formal arteriogram can be performed in injured extremities without significant ischemia. A single-plane, single-bolus arteriogram should be performed in the operating room when the extremity is ischemic and prompt revascularization is essential. In an older child or adolescent, the technique is the same as that used in adults. In an infant or small child, a cutdown is usually necessary for vascular access to avoid iatrogenic injury to the vessels. Angiography and embolization with clotted blood, an absorbable gelatin sponge (Gelfoam), or other material can be effective in controlling hemorrhaging after pelvic fractures. Compartment syndromes can occur after vascular repair, so prophylactic fasciotomies should be performed at the time of repair.

COMPARTMENT SYNDROMES

Compartment syndromes can occur in children and are related to the severity of the trauma (see Chapter 6). The leg and the forearm are the most common sites for compartment syndromes and are usually the result of tibial shaft and supracondylar fractures of the distal portion of the humerus. The presence of a displaced supracondylar fracture and a displaced ipsilateral forearm fracture increases the risk of compartment syndrome. Compartment syndromes can also occur in other areas, such as the ankle (superior retinaculum syndrome) and the foot. The presence of open fractures does not preclude a compartment syndrome. Assuming that an open fracture has decompressed the adjacent compartments is a mistake, considering compartment syndrome develops in approximately 3% of open tibial fractures. In children, the three As have been listed as warning signals of compartment syndrome: increasing anxiety, increasing analgesia needs, and increased agitation. The most important physical examination findings include swelling and tenseness of the compartment and exaggerated pain with passive stretching of the distal joints. Paresthesias, pulselessness, and paralysis are late findings, and the absence of these signs does not rule out this diagnosis. Compartment pressures should be measured in all children with signs consistent with compartment syndrome. Uncooperative children or those with head injuries need to be evaluated very carefully because they will lack the usual symptoms. Rapid surgical treatment with the release of all involved compartments is critical in reducing potential complications.[109] In the forearm, separate incisions are used to decompress the volar or extensor compartment (Fig. 5.5). The Henry approach, which entails division of the lacertus fibrosus, allows excellent exposure and decompression. In the leg, the double-incision technique is commonly utilized to decompress the four compartments (Fig. 5.6), although single-incision approaches are also reasonable.

FRACTURE MANAGEMENT IN THE MULTIPLY INJURED CHILD

Once the extremity injuries have been identified during the secondary survey, definitive treatment needs to be prioritized and planned.[110–112] Extremity injuries that have a high priority include major joint dislocations, open joint injuries, open fractures, fractures associated with vascular injury, and unstable pelvic injuries in children who are hemodynamically unstable. The need for stabilization of long bone fractures, especially the femoral shaft, is probably equally important in adolescents as adults in the scenario of multiple traumatic injuries. Its importance is not as clear in children and infants, although stabilization of these fractures can certainly aid in nursing care, mobility of the child, and control of pain and blood loss. Loder[4] showed that early stabilization of fractures in a multiply injured child reduces the number of days in both the intensive care unit and the hospital. It also decreases the duration of ventilatory support and the overall complication rate in comparison with children with delayed skeletal stabilization. It is important to reemphasize that extremity injuries are not life-threatening and should not supersede intervention for injuries that are life-threatening. They can, however, be limb-threatening and should not be neglected. Long-term morbidity is most frequently associated with inadequate treatment of extremity injuries.[4,109] Because children's fractures tend to heal more rapidly than do similar fractures in adults, plans for surgical intervention need to be completed earlier in the hospital course; otherwise, the option for fracture reduction surgery may be lost, and osteotomies may be required.

> *Reconstruction Tips*
>
> - Trauma scoring systems, including the MISS and the PTS, are useful in managing the overall patient and predicting outcomes.
> - Physeal injuries can begin to heal quickly in children, so early reduction is important.
> - External fixators can be useful for stabilizing long bone fractures in unstable children.
> - Articular and most physeal injuries should be anatomically aligned.

INDICATIONS FOR SURGICAL MANAGEMENT

Most pediatric fractures and dislocations can be managed satisfactorily by closed reduction techniques and cast immobilization or traction with the use of skin or skeletal techniques. However, in specific situations, surgical management may be more advantageous and result in decreased morbidity and better functional results.[110–112] A multiply injured child and skeletally immature adolescent are major examples.

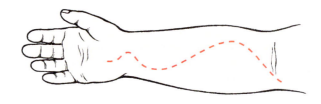
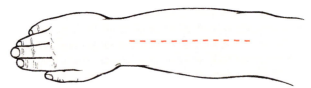

Fig. 5.5 Standard fasciotomy sites for the forearm. The Henry approach is used for the volar surface with a straight dorsal incision.

Indications for operative treatment of pediatric fractures have been outlined by Thompson and associates.[113] These indications include displaced physeal fractures, displaced intraarticular fractures, unstable fractures, multiple injuries, and open fractures. The last indication is frequently present in a multiply injured child. Please refer to the remainder of the text for specific treatment of various pediatric fractures.

Early and definitive management decisions need to take into account several important factors: the prognosis for survival and residual disability; whether standard closed methods of treatment will adversely affect the management of other body area injuries; and whether other body area injuries have a potentially deleterious effect on the musculoskeletal injuries if the latter are managed in a closed fashion. If the prognosis is favorable and either of the last two factors is positive, the surgical option may be advantageous in the overall treatment of the child. Possible examples include a child with a flail chest and a closed femoral shaft fracture. The femoral fracture should not be treated by skeletal traction because of possible compromise in care of the chest. Likewise, a child with a head injury who is combative or spastic may not be a candidate for conservative fracture management, especially a femoral shaft fracture, because of the difficulty in maintaining satisfactory alignment.[111] In both situations, it is more appropriate to surgically stabilize the fractures. It must be remembered that children tend to survive more serious injuries than adults do, and in most cases, survival should be expected.

TIMING OF FRACTURE MANAGEMENT

Severely injured children, as well as adults, are in their best physiologic state immediately after resuscitation. Delaying definitive treatment frequently allows secondary complications to occur, such as pulmonary atelectasis, fat emboli, contamination of abrasions and wounds, fluid and electrolyte imbalances, and deep venous thrombosis, which may preclude surgical management for several weeks. This delay may result in subsequent musculoskeletal complications such as nonunion and malunion.[17] If the musculoskeletal injuries are closed, other body area injuries do not require surgery, and the child's condition is critical, then closed

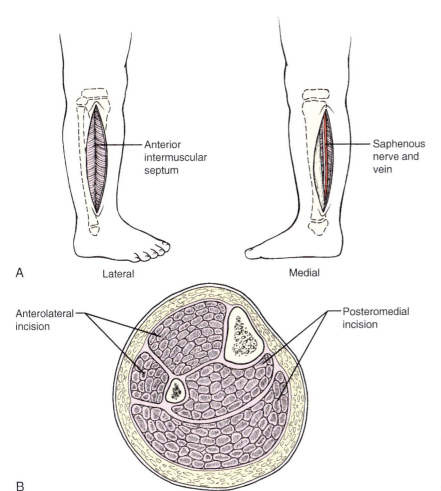

A   Lateral   Medial

B

Fig. 5.6 (A) Double-incision fasciotomies of the leg allow access to all four compartments. Care must be taken on the medial side to avoid injury to the saphenous nerve and vein. (B) Cross section of the lower portion of the leg demonstrating access to the four compartments through the double incisions.

management may be the most appropriate initial method, even if less than optimal alignment is achieved. Definitive management may be delayed several days, pending survival of the child. If surgery for other body areas must be performed on the day of injury, operative fracture management should be performed concomitantly, if possible. Loder[4] showed that children undergoing immediate surgical stabilization of fractures had fewer complications than did those whose stabilization was delayed. Because fractures heal rapidly in children, delays in treatment may significantly increase the difficulty of operative repair. Although multiple studies have been done in the adult population looking at early definitive management versus damage control orthopedics, few similar studies exist in the pediatric trauma population, and prospective studies are still needed. It is recognized, however, that pediatric patients have a decreased risk of multisystem organ failure in the first 48 hours after trauma, so, if possible, extremity injuries should be treated in this period after adequate resuscitation has taken place.[1]

Serious burns are another possible indication for early operative stabilization of associated fractures.[84] Open fractures and periarticular fractures associated with serious burns should be treated as soon as possible. If treatment is initiated within 48 hours, the risk of secondary infection is decreased. After 48 hours, the risk of deep infection about the implant will be high. These fractures are then better managed by external fixation or limited internal fixation.

PHYSEAL FRACTURES

Fractures involving the physeal growth plate are common injuries in children who are victims of multiple traumatic injuries. Upper extremity physeal injuries occur more frequently than those of the lower extremities (1.6:1). The physes of the distal radius, distal tibia, and finger phalanges are most commonly injured. Distal physes of long bones are injured more often than proximal physes, except for the humerus. The peak age of the incidence of physeal injuries is 12 to 13 years, and injuries among males predominate.

The most widely used classification of physeal plate fractures is that of Salter and Harris, and it has been demonstrated to be simple, accurate, and prognostically significant. The Salter-Harris classification differentiates five types of epiphyseal fractures: in type I, the epiphysis is completely separated from the metaphysis without any bone fracture; in type II, the fracture extends partially along the physis and then exits through a portion of the metaphysis and produces the Thurston-Holland fragment; in type III, the fracture extends partially through the physis and then extends through the epiphysis into the joint; in type IV, the fracture extends obliquely across the metaphysis, the physis, and the epiphysis and enters the joint; and in type V, which is a nondisplaced crush injury to the physis, no definite fracture line is visible radiographically.

Type I and type II fractures do not disturb the germinal layer of the physis and do not involve the articular surface;

therefore, they usually have an excellent prognosis after closed reduction and cast immobilization. Displaced type III and type IV fractures violate both the germinal layer and the articular surface, and require anatomic reduction, usually by open reduction and internal fixation (ORIF), to restore alignment of the physis, as well as the articular surface of the joint. The prognosis is usually good, provided that vascularity to the fracture fragment remains intact and the reduction is anatomic. If anatomic alignment of these fractures is not achieved, an osseous bridge may form across the physeal plate and result in premature physeal closure or asymmetric growth; central bridges result in shortening, and peripheral bridges tend to produce angular deformities. These bony bridges can occasionally be resected, and fat or polymethylmethacrylate can be interposed to prevent reformation, thereby restoring longitudinal growth. A type V fracture has a poor prognosis because of the inherent damage to the physis, which leads to a growth disturbance. This injury is typically recognizable only in retrospect and is not usually amenable to resection.

PRINCIPLES OF SURGICAL MANAGEMENT

The principles of surgical management of fractures in a multiply injured child and skeletally immature adolescent are distinctly different from those in a mature adolescent and adult. Spiegel and Mast[114] listed five general principles applicable to the operative management of pediatric fractures; these principles apply to multiple injuries, as well as isolated fractures requiring surgical intervention:

1. Multiple closed reductions of a physeal fracture are contraindicated because they may cause repetitive damage to the germinal cells of the physis, thereby predisposing to premature closure and late deformity.
2. At surgery, anatomic alignment is mandatory, especially for displaced intraarticular and physeal fractures.
3. Internal fixation devices, if used, should be simple when possible, such as K-wires, and should be removed as soon as the fracture has healed.
4. Rigid fixation to allow immediate mobilization of the extremity is not usually the goal; rather, the goal is stability sufficient to hold the fragments in anatomic alignment with a supplemental cast.
5. External fixators, when used, are removed as soon as possible, and cast immobilization is substituted when the soft tissue problems have been corrected or when the fracture is stable. However, in a multiply injured patient, the internal or external fixation must be of sufficient strength to allow for mobilization of the child.

Thus, planning for appropriate surgical procedures is based on the age and size of the child, the bone fractured, and the extent and severity of other injuries.

SURGICAL TECHNIQUES

Three basic surgical techniques are used in the management of pediatric fractures, including multiple traumatic injuries: ORIF, closed reduction and internal fixation, and external fixation.

OPEN REDUCTION AND INTERNAL FIXATION

Displaced physeal fractures, especially Salter-Harris type III and IV fractures, and unstable fractures, such as those involving the forearm diaphysis and the spine, as well as ipsilateral fractures of the femur and tibia (floating knee),[62] may require ORIF. Indications in a multiply injured child include closed fractures, especially of the femoral shaft, and other fractures with neurovascular injuries requiring repair. Fractures are usually stabilized before vascular repair, provided that the ischemia time is not significantly prolonged. However, stabilization should not take precedence over vascular repair if the warm ischemia time is approaching 6 hours because muscle will not tolerate such a deprivation before undergoing necrosis. Occasionally, open or closed femur fractures or open tibia fractures may be candidates for ORIF.

The type of internal fixation used during open reduction depends on the goals of management and the age of the patient. As stated by Spiegel and Mast[114] and by others, the goal of fracture reduction surgery in children is not usually rigid internal fixation but rather attainment and maintenance of acceptable alignment. Thus, most fractures can be managed by simple internal fixation devices such as K-wires, Steinmann pins, cortical screws, and cannulated screws.[113,114] The fractured extremity is protected postoperatively with external immobilization, typically a plaster or fiberglass cast, until satisfactory union is obtained. This type of management usually allows the child sufficient mobilization to enhance overall care.

Compression plates and screws can be used to achieve satisfactory mobilization in children and skeletally immature adolescents to treat unstable diaphyseal fractures, especially those of the femoral shaft. Publications have reported excellent results with the use of compression plates and screws in young children with closed femoral shaft fractures, especially those who are victims of multiple traumatic injuries. In children, internal fixation devices are removed soon after fracture union to minimize the risk of physeal injury and prevent incorporation of the device into the growing bone. They should also be used with caution in highly contaminated open fractures, in which case external fixation should be considered.

CLOSED REDUCTION AND INTERNAL FIXATION

Closed reduction and internal fixation is indicated for certain displaced physeal, intraarticular, and unstable metaphyseal or diaphyseal fractures. In children, this technique generally refers to percutaneous fixation with K-wires or Steinmann pins. Pediatric fractures amenable to closed reduction and percutaneous internal fixation include humeral supracondylar, phalangeal, and femoral neck fractures. Anatomic alignment must be attainable by closed reduction before this method can be used. Failure to obtain anatomic alignment is an indication for open reduction.

Steinmann pins, K-wires, and cannulated screws are the most commonly used devices in closed reduction and internal fixation.[113] They are inserted percutaneously after closed reduction and can either traverse the fracture or be placed above and below the fracture and secured with an external fixation clamp or incorporated into a plaster cast. Smooth pins or wires may be placed across a physis if necessary for fracture fixation. These devices are usually removed as soon as the fracture has healed.

INTRAMEDULLARY NAILING

Certain pediatric fractures, especially those involving the femoral shaft, can be managed by closed intramedullary nailing. Unstable and open forearm or tibia fractures are also a common indication. The most common indication for intramedullary nailing in children is a femoral shaft fracture, especially in victims of multiple traumatic injuries. A recent multicenter study found increased use of locked intramedullary nailing in the 11 year and younger group.[115] The tibia is a much less common indication, although successful results have been reported.

These implants are inserted under fluoroscopy, and prophylactic antibiotics are used in all cases. The results are superior to those of closed management for these fracture types. Two basic techniques may be used: locked and flexible nails. Locked nails are used predominantly in femoral fractures in older adolescents with use of the same technique as in adults, with one important exception: the starting point. The risk of avascular necrosis of the capital femoral epiphysis (femoral head) after reamed intramedullary nailing of the pediatric femur has been well documented. This complication appears to be caused by damage to the anastomotic arterial ring at the base of the femoral neck, by direct damage to the lateral ascending cervical arteries to the femoral head, or by intracapsular tamponade. For this reason, piriformis starting points in patients with open physes are contraindicated. Nails should be introduced through the lateral aspect of the greater trochanter to minimize disruption of the reticular vessels during the initial search for the nail entry point. Premature closure of the greater trochanteric apophysis can also occur after trochanteric femoral nailing. Although it is common to use trochanteric nailing in children 8 years and older, rigorous supportive data for this age cutoff is still lacking. The complication rate is low.

Flexible nailing is performed using small-diameter (2.5-mm–4-mm) flexible rods of titanium or stainless steel. These nails are prebent to conform to the anatomic curves of the involved bone, inserted to provide three-point fixation, and then anchored in the proximal and distal metaphyses. This technique allows end-to-end contact and maintenance of normal bone curvature. The secondary muscles provide additional support. Slight movement occurs at the fracture site and stimulates callus formation. These devices have a high success rate and a low incidence of complications.

EXTERNAL FIXATION

Common indications for external fixation of pediatric fractures include Gustilo type II and III open fractures; fractures associated with severe burns; fractures with bone or extensive soft tissue loss that may require reconstructive procedures, such as free vascularized grafts or skin grafts; fractures requiring distraction, such as those with significant bone loss; unstable pelvic, femoral, and tibial fractures; fractures in children with associated head injuries and spasticity; and fractures associated with vascular or nerve repairs or reconstruction.[112] Open fractures of the femur and tibia are the most common long bones treated by external fixation.

Advantages of external fixation include rigid immobilization of fractures; direct surveillance of the limb and associated wounds; facilitation of wound management, such as repeated débridement, flap procedures, and dressings; patient mobilization for treatment of other injuries and transportation for diagnostic and therapeutic procedures; and possible insertion with local anesthesia in severely injured patients. The major complications of external fixation are pin tract infections and refracture after removal.

A multitude of external fixators are commercially available, and newer multiplane devices are continually being developed. The use of half-pins is preferred for minimizing additional muscle and soft tissue damage and possible neurovascular injury. Ring fixators are not commonly used as an external fixation device in pediatric fractures but can be considered. During the insertion of any external fixation device, care must be taken to avoid the epiphysis and physis. It is recommended that the fixator be removed once satisfactory skin coverage has been obtained or when sufficient callus formation to provide fracture stability is demonstrated radiographically. Protection in a cast after removal of the external fixator may be needed because of the risk of refracture.

OPEN FRACTURES

Open fractures are one of the most serious injuries to the pediatric musculoskeletal system. They are usually caused by high-velocity trauma and are increasing in frequency, especially in multiply injured children. In a series of multiply injured children reported by Marcus and associates,[17] 10% of the fractures were open. Approximately 25% to 50% of children with open fractures have other body area injuries. The objectives of treatment of open fractures in children are the same as for adults: preventing wound sepsis, healing soft tissue injuries, achieving bony union, and returning the patient to optimal function.[7,116,117]

All open fractures are graded according to the size of the wound, the extent of the soft tissue injury, and the degree of contamination because these factors affect the prognosis. The most widely used classification was developed by Gustilo and associates.[7] In a type I open fracture, the wound is less than 1 cm long. It is usually a clean puncture wound from a spike of bone that has pierced the skin. The fracture is generally simple, transverse, or short oblique, with minimal comminution and soft tissue damage. In a type II open fracture, the wound is more than 1 cm in length, but the soft tissue damage is not extensive. A slight or moderate crushing injury, moderate comminution of the fracture site, and moderate contamination may be present. Type III injuries are characterized by extensive damage to the skin and soft tissue, including muscle and possibly neurovascular structures. A significant degree of contamination is present. This type of injury is usually caused by high-velocity trauma and results in considerable fracture comminution and instability.

Type III open fractures are subdivided into three additional categories.[117] In type IIIA, soft tissue coverage of the fractured bone is adequate, despite the extensive soft tissue injury. This group includes segmental or severely comminuted fractures from high-energy trauma, regardless of the size of the wound. Type IIIB open fractures have extensive injury or loss of soft tissue, with periosteal stripping and exposure of bone. Massive contamination and comminution of these fractures are common. After débridement and irrigation are completed, a segment of bone is exposed, and a local or free flap is needed for coverage. A type IIIC injury includes any open fractures associated with arterial injury that must be repaired, regardless of the degree of soft tissue injury. The incidence of wound infection, delayed union, nonunion, amputation, and residual disability is directly related to the classification of the open fracture.

Methods of achieving the goals of management as described by Gustilo and associates include emergency initial care; thorough initial evaluation to diagnose other life-threatening injuries; appropriate antibiotic therapy; extensive and possible repeated wound débridement; fracture stabilization; local wound care; rarely, autogenous cancellous bone grafts; and rehabilitation. Each of these measures is discussed in detail in Chapter 6. Open fractures are frequently managed by external fixation. These devices stabilize the fracture and allow restabilization and access to the associated wounds for repeated débridement and bone grafting procedures. External fixation also allows the child to be more mobile for the evaluation and treatment of other body area injuries. Open fractures of the tibia and fibular shaft are the most common, as well as the most difficult. Open fractures of the pelvis are uncommon but are associated with an approximately 50% mortality rate. The cause of death is either hemorrhage early or sepsis later.

REHABILITATION

Formal physical therapy and rehabilitation are not generally necessary for the majority of injured children. Most of these injuries are simple, low-velocity injuries that heal rapidly because of the resiliency of the child. In a multiply injured child, however, such is not usually the case. Because of the severity and complexity of the injuries, long hospitalization and multiple surgeries are often required. Although it has been shown that a child can tolerate prolonged immobilization without the usual complications (e.g., joint stiffness, severe muscular atrophy, and disuse osteoporosis) seen in an adult, complications can and do occur, and a good result cannot always be assumed. Significant long-term disability, most often related to injuries to the CNS and musculoskeletal system, can occur in children. Aggressive treatment has been shown to decrease these complications and improve the overall result.[4] Further detail is provided in Chapter 22.

PHYSICAL THERAPY

Physical therapy should be initiated as soon as the child's medical condition permits. Early physical therapy consists of gentle range-of-motion exercises of the noninjured or stabilized extremities to avoid soft tissue contractures and joint stiffness. Such therapy is especially important in a head- or spine-injured patient. More physical therapy can be instituted as the child's condition allows, including transfer training, resistive strengthening, and eventually ambulation. Each case must be dealt with individually because the spectrum and severity of injuries dictate the type and level of therapy. Close communication and cooperation between the physician and therapist are extremely important. Physical therapy should be initiated while the child is still in

the trauma center. Once the child's condition no longer requires that level of specialization, transfer to a different facility can be considered; sometimes it is to another acute care facility that is not a trauma center but that is more accessible to the family or a long-term rehabilitation facility if acute care is no longer necessary. Children are often transferred long distances to be treated at trauma centers, and these distances can become a burden for families. Therefore, when the child's condition improves, every effort should be made to transfer the child to a facility closer to home. Some trauma centers are equipped with facilities for both acute care and long-term rehabilitation services. This type of center enables transfer from acute care to long-term care status while maintaining continuity of treatment by many of the same physicians and therapists. Such continuity is desirable because children develop important relationships with and dependencies on the treating physicians and therapists, and severing these relationships can be extremely traumatic to the patient. In a recent study looking at pediatric rehabilitation facilities, Zonfrillo and colleagues[118] found that children with severe injuries have poor function on admission, but most benefit in a substantial way from the care they receive. Children with spinal cord injuries have more comorbidities, longer lengths of stay, and lower physical function at discharge.

Children with severe head, spinal, and musculoskeletal injuries are most often in need of prolonged rehabilitation and are more likely to have permanent disabilities.[4,17] A more detailed discussion of rehabilitation is presented in Chapter 22.

> **Outcomes**
> - Mortality can occur earlier than adults, emphasizing the importance of aggressive resuscitation.
> - Physical therapy and psychologic rehabilitation ensure better outcomes during recovery.
> - Morbidity is often associated with neurologic and orthopedic injuries.

PSYCHOLOGIC REHABILITATION

Psychologic rehabilitation can be as important as physical rehabilitation and should not be overlooked. A more detailed discussion of psychologic rehabilitation is presented in Chapter 22.

REFERENCES

The level of evidence (LOE) is determined according to the criteria provided in the Preface.

1. Pandya NK, Upasani VV, Kulkani VA. The pediatric polytrauma patient: current concepts. *J Am Acad Orthop Surg.* 2013;21:170–179. **(LOE V)**.
2. Feickert H-J, Drommer S, Heyer R. Severe head injury in children: impact of risk factors on outcome. *J Trauma.* 1999;47:33–38. **(LOE II)**.
3. Jakob H, Lustenberger T, Schneidmuller D, et al. Pediatric polytrauma management. *Eur J Trauma Emerg Surg.* 2010;36:325–338. **(LOE V)**.
4. Loder RT. Pediatric polytrauma: orthopaedic care in hospital course. *J Orthop Trauma.* 1987;1:48–54. **(LOE IV)**.

5. van der Sluis CK, Kingma J, Eisma WH, et al. Pediatric polytrauma: short-term and long-term outcomes. *J Trauma*. 1997;43:501–505. **(LOE I)**.

6. Wesson DE, Williams JI, Spence LJ, et al. Functional outcome in pediatric trauma. *J Trauma*. 1989;29:589–592. **(LOE II)**.

7. Gustilo RB, Merkow RL, Templeman D. Current concepts review. The management of open fractures. *J Bone Joint Surg Am*. 1990;72:299–304. **(LOE V)**.

8. American College of Surgeons Committee on Trauma. *Advanced Trauma Life Support for Doctors. Student Course Manual*. Chicago: Pediatric Trauma American College of Surgeons; 2013: Chapter 10. **(LOE N/A)**.

9. Demetriades D, Murray J, Martin M, et al. Pedestrians injured by automobiles: relationship of age to injury type and severity. *Am Coll Surg*. 2004;199:382–387. **(LOE II)**.

10. Ivarsson BJ, Crandall JR, Okamoto M. Influence of age-related stature on the frequency of body region injury and overall injury severity in child pedestrian casualties. *Traffic Inj Prev*. 2006;7:290–298. **(LOE II)**.

11. Benoit R, Watts DD, Dwyer K, et al. Windows 99: a source of suburban pediatric trauma. *J Trauma*. 2000;49:477–481. **(LOE III)**.

12. Harris VA, Rochette LM, Smith GA. Pediatric injuries attributable to falls from windows in the United States in 1990-2008. *Pediatrics*. 2011;128:455–462. **(LOE III)**.

13. Peclet MH, Newman KD, Eichelberger MR, et al. Patterns of injury in children. *J Pediatr Surg*. 1990;25:85–90. **(LOE II)**.

14. Sawyer JR, Flynn JM, Dormans JP, et al. Fracture patterns in children and young adults who fall from significant heights. *J Pediatr Orthop*. 2000;20:197–202. **(LOE II)**.

15. McLaughlin C, Zagory JA, Fenlon M, et al. Timing of mortality in pediatric trauma patients: a national trauma data bank analysis. *J Pediatr Surg*. 2018;53:344–351. **(LOE III)**.

16. Hu X, Wesson DE, Logsetty S, et al. Functional limitations and recovery in children with severe trauma: a one-year follow-up. *J Trauma*. 1994;37:209–213. **(LOE III)**.

17. Marcus RE, Mills M, Thompson GH. Multiple injury in children. *J Bone Joint Surg Am*. 1983;65:1290–1294. **(LOE IV)**.

18. American Academy of Pediatrics and Pediatric Orthopaedic Society of North America. Policy Statement. Management of pediatric trauma. *Pediatrics*. 2008;121:849–854. **(LOE V)**.

19. Oliver J, Avraham J, Frangos S, et al. The epidemiology of inpatient pediatric trauma in United States hospitals 2000 to 2011. *J Pediatr Surg*. 2018;53:758–764. **(LOE III)**.

20. Chan BSH, Walker PJ, Cass DT. Urban trauma: an analysis of 1,116 pediatric cases. *J Trauma*. 1989;29:1540–1547. **(LOE I)**.

21. Nance ML. *National Trauma Date Bank*. Pediatric Report Chicago, IL: American College of Surgeons.

22. DiScala C, Sage R, Li G, et al. Child abuse and unintentional injuries: a 10-year retrospective. *Arch Pediatr Adolesc Med*. 2000;154:16–22. **(LOE III)**.

23. Tracy ET, Englum BR, Barbas AS, et al. Pediatric injury patterns by year of age. *J Pediatr Surg*. 2013;48:1384–1388. **(LOE III)**.

24. National Center for Injury Prevention and Control, Centers for Disease Control and Prevention. *National Estimates of the 10 Leading Causes of Nonfatal Injuries Treated in Hospital Emergency Departments*. United States –; 2010. **(LOE IV)**.

25. Musemeche CA, Barthel M, Cosentino C, et al. Pediatric falls from height. *J Trauma*. 1991;31:1347–1349. **(LOE IV)**.

26. Pitone ML, Attia MW. Patterns of injury associated with routine childhood falls. *Pediatr Emerg Care*. 2006;22:470–474. **(LOE II)**.

27. Kaufmann CR, Rivara FP, Maier RV. Pediatric trauma: need for surgical management. *J Trauma*. 1989;29:1120–1126. **(LOE II)**.

28. Centers for Disease Control and Prevention. Motor-vehicle related death rates – United States, 1999-2005. *MMWR*. 2009;58:161–165. **(LOE IV)**.

29. Scheidler MG, Shultz BL, Schall L, et al. Risk factors and predictors of mortality in children after ejection from motor vehicle crashes. *J Trauma*. 2000;49:864–868. **(LOE II)**.

30. Brown JK, Jing Y, Wang S, et al. Patterns of severe injury in pediatric car crash victims: crash injury research engineering network database. *J Pediatr Surg*. 2006;41:362–367. **(LOE II)**.

31. Mendoza-Lattes S, Besomi J, O'Sullivan C, et al. Pediatric spine trauma in the United States–analysis of the HCUP Kid's Inpatient Database (KID) 1997-2009. *Iowa Orthop J*. 2015;35:135–139. **(LOE III)**.

32. Brown RL, Brunn MA, Garcia VG. Cervical spine injuries in children: a review of 103 patients treated consecutively at a level 1 pediatric trauma center. *J Pediatr Surg*. 2001;36:1107–1114. **(LOE III)**.

33. Lim LH, Lam LK, Moore MH, et al. Associated injuries in facial fractures: review of 839 patients. *Br J Plast Surg*. 1993;46:635–638. **(LOE II)**.

34. Glassman SD, Johnson JR, Holt RT. Seatbelt injuries in children. *J Trauma*. 1992;33:882–886. **(LOE IV)**.

35. Stacey S, Forman J, Woods W, et al. Pediatric abdominal injury patterns generated by lap belt loading. *J Trauma*. 2009;67:1278–1283. **(LOE III)**.

36. Reid AB, Letts RM, Black GB. Pediatric Chance fractures: association with intra-abdominal injuries and seatbelt use. *J Trauma*. 1990;30:384–391. **(LOE IV)**.

37. American Academy of Pediatrics Committee on Injury. Violence and poison prevention, child passenger safety. *Pediatrics*. 2011;127:e1050–e1066. **(LOE V)**.

38. Mannix R, Fleegler E, Meehan WP, et al. Booster seat laws and fatalities in children 4 to 7 years of age. *Pediatrics*. 2012;130:996–1002. **(LOE III)**.

39. Ernat JJ, Knox JB, Wimberly RL et al. The effects of restraint type on pattern of spine injury in children. *J Pediatr Orthop*. 2016;36:594–601. **(LOE III)**.

40. Garcia VF, Gotschall CS, Eichelberger MR, et al. Rib fractures in children: a marker of severe trauma. *J Trauma*. 1990;30:695–700. **(LOE II)**.

41. Kessel B, Dagan J, Swaid F, et al. Rib fractures: comparison of associated injuries between pediatric and adult population. *Am J Surg*. 2014;208:831–834. **(LOE III)**.

42. Peclet MH, Newman KD, Eichelberger MR, et al. Thoracic trauma in children: an indicator of increased mortality. *J Pediatric Surg*. 1990;25:961–966. **(LOE II)**.

43. Garvin KL, McCarthy RE, Barnes CL, et al. Pediatric pelvic ring fractures. *J Pediatr Orthop*. 1990;10:577–582. (LOE IV).

44. Rieger H, Brug E. Fractures of the pelvis in children. *Clin Orthop*. 1997;336:226–239. **(LOE II)**.

45. Silber JS, Flynn JM. Changing patterns of pediatric pelvic fractures with skeletal maturation: implications for classification and management. *J Pediatr Orthop*. 2002;22:22–26. **(LOE III)**.

46. de la Calva C, Jover N, Alonso J et al. Pediatric pelvic fractures and differences compared with the adult population. *Pediatr Emerg Care*. 2018;16 **(LOE III)**.

47. Swaid F, Peleg K, Alfici R, et al. A comparison study of pelvic fractures and associated abdominal injuries between pediatric and adult blunt trauma patients. *J Pediatr Surg*. 2017;52:386–389. **(LOE III)**.

48. Holden CP, Holman J, Herman MJ. Pediatric pelvic fractures. *J Am Acad Orthop Surg*. 2007;15:172–177. **(LOE V)**.

49. Kessler J, Koebnick C, Smith N, et al. Childhood obesity is associated with increased risk of most lower extremity fractures. *Clin Orthop Relat Res*. 2013;471:1199–1207. **(LOE III)**.

50. Backstrom IC, MacLennan PA, Sawyer JR, et al. Pediatric obesity and traumatic lower-extremity long-bone fracture outcomes. *J Trauma Acute Care Surg*. 2012;73:966–971. (LOE III).

51. Rana AR, Michalsky MP, Teich S, et al. Childhood obesity: a risk factor for injuries observed at a level-1 trauma center. *J Pediatr Surg*. 2009;44:1601–1605. **(LOE II)**.

52. Haricharan RN, Griffin RL, Barnhart DC, et al. Injury patterns among obese children involved in motor vehicle collisions. *J Pediatr Surg*. 2009;44:1218–1222. **(LOE III)**.

53. Teasdale G, Bennet B. Assessment of coma and impaired consciousness: a practical scale. *Lancet*. 1974;2:81–84. **(LOE II)**.

54. *Committee on Injury Scaling 1980 The Abbreviated Injury Scale—1980 Revision*. Morton Grove, IL: American Association for Automotive Medicine; 1980. **(LOE N/A)**.

55. Mayer T, Matlak ME, Johnson DG, et al. The modified injury severity scale in pediatric multiple trauma patients. *J Pediatr Surg*. 1980;15:719–726. **(LOE I)**.

56. Mayer T, Walker ML, Clark P. Further experience with the modified abbreviated injury severity scale. *J Trauma*. 1984;24:31–34. **(LOE I)**.

57. Tepas JJ 3rd, Mollitt DL, Talbert JL, et al. The pediatric trauma score as a predictor of injury severity in the injured child. *J Pediatr Surg*. 1987;22:14–18. **(LOE I)**.

58. Tepas JJ 3rd, Ramenofsky ML, Mollitt DL, et al. The pediatric trauma score as a predictor of injury severity: an objective assessment. *J Trauma*. 1988;28:425–429. (**LOE I**).

59. Ott R, Krämer R, Martas P, et al. Prognostic value of trauma scores in pediatric patients with multiple injuries. *J Trauma*. 2000;49:729–736. (**LOE I**).

60. Yian EH, Gullahorn LJ, Loder RT. Scoring of pediatric orthopaedic polytrauma: correlation of different injury scoring systems and prognosis for hospital course. *J Pediatr Orthop*. 2000;20:203–209. (**LOE I**).

61. Hahn YS, Chyung C, Barthel MJ, et al. Head injuries in children under 36 months of age. Demography and outcome. *Child's Nervous System*. 1988;4:34–40. (**LOE II**).

62. Yue JJ, Churchill RS, Cooperman DR, et al. The floating knee in the pediatric patient. Nonoperative versus operative stabilization. *Clin Orthop*. 2000;376:124–136. (**LOE III**).

63. Loder RT, Gullahorn LJ, Yian EH, et al. Factors predictive of immobilization complications in pediatric polytrauma. *J Orthop Trauma*. 2001;15:338–341. (**LOE II**).

64. Kaufmann CR, Maier RV, Rivara FP, et al. Evaluation of the pediatric trauma score. *JAMA*. 1990;263:69–72. (**LOE I**).

65. Marmor M, Elson J, Mikhail C, et al. Short-term pelvic fracture outcomes in adolescents differ from children and adults in the National Trauma Data Bank. *J Child Orthop*. 2015;9:65–75. (**LOE III**).

66. Eichelberger MR, Mangubat EA, Sacco WS, et al. Comparative outcomes of children and adults suffering blunt trauma. *J Trauma*. 1988;28:430–434. (**LOE III**).

67. Acierno SP, Jurkovich GJ, Nathens AB. Patterns of emergent operative intervention in the injured child. *J Trauma*. 2004;56:960–964. (**LOE III**).

68. Courville XF, Koval KJ, Carney BT, et al. Early prediction of posttraumatic in-hospital mortality in pediatric patients. *J Pediatr Orthop*. 2009;29:439–444. (**LOE IV**).

69. Bowman SM, Zimmerman FJ, Christakis DA, et al. Hospital characteristics associated with the management of pediatric splenic injuries. *JAMA*. 2005;294:2611–2617. (**LOE III**).

70. Osler TM, Vane DW, Tepas JJ, et al. Do pediatric trauma centers have better survival rates than adult trauma centers? An examination of the national pediatric trauma registry. *J Trauma*. 2001;50:96–99. (**LOE II**).

71. Herzenberg JE, Hensinger RN, Dedrick BK, et al. Emergency transport and positioning of young children who have an injury to the cervical spine. *J Bone Joint Surg Am*. 1989;71:15–22. (**LOE III**).

72. Leeper CM, McKenna C, Gaines BA. Too little too late: hypotension and blood transfusion in the trauma bay are independent predictors of death in injured children. *J Trauma Acute Care Surg*. 2018;85(4):674–678. (**LOE III**).

73. Alam Khan T, Jamil Khattak Y, Awais M, et al. Utility of complete trauma series radiographs in alert pediatric patients presenting to emergency department of a tertiary care hospital. *Eur J Trauma Emerg Surg*. 2015;41:279–285. (**LOE III**).

74. Brown RL, Koepplinger ME, Mehlman CT, et al. All-terrain vehicle and bicycle crashes in children: epidemiology and comparison of injury severity. *J Pediatr Surg*. 2002;37:375–380. (**LOE III**).

75. Carreon LY, Glassman SD, Campbell MJ. Pediatric spine fractures: a review of 137 hospital admissions. *J Spinal Disord Tech*. 2004;17:477–482. (**LOE IV**).

76. Pennecot GF, Gouraud D, Hardy JR, et al. Roentgenographical study of the stability of the cervical spine in children. *J Pediatr Orthop*. 1984;4:346–352. (**LOE III**).

77. Swischuk LE. Anterior displacement of C2 in children: physiologic or pathologic? *Radiology*. 1977;122:759–763. (**LOE V**).

78. Cattell HS, Filtzer DL. Pseudosubluxation and other normal variation in the cervical spine in children: a study of one hundred and sixty children. *J Bone Joint Surg Am*. 1965;47:1295–1298. (**LOE IV**).

79. Swischuk LE, Swischuk PN, John SD. Wedging of C-3 in infants and children: usually a normal finding and not a fracture. *Radiology*. 1993;188:523–526. (**LOE II**).

80. Slaar A, Fockens MM, Wang J, et al. Triage tools for detecting cervical spine injury in pediatric trauma patients. *Cochrane Database Syst Rev*. 2017;12:CD011686. (**LOE II**).

81. Hutchings L, Willett K. Cervical spine clearance in pediatric trauma: a review of current literature. *J Trauma*. 2009;67:687–691. (**LOE V**).

82. Hale AT, Alvarado A, Bey AK, et al. X-ray vs. CT in identifying significant C-spine injuries in the pediatric population. *Childs Nerv Syst*. 2017;33:1977–1983. (**LOE III**).

83. Flynn JM, Skaggs DL, Sponseller PD, et al. The surgical management of pediatric fractures of the lower extremity. *Instr Course Lect*. 2003;52:647–659. (**LOE V**).

84. Blasier RD. Treatment of fractures complicated by burn or head injuries in children. *J Bone Joint Surg Am*. 1999;81:1038–1043. (**LOE V**).

85. Silber JS, Flynn JM, Katz MA, et al. Role of computed tomography in the classification and management of pediatric pelvic fractures. *J Pediatr Orthop*. 2001;21:148–151. (**LOE III**).

86. Heinrich SD, Gallagher D, Harris M, et al. Undiagnosed fractures in severely injured children and young adults: identification with technetium imaging. *J Bone Joint Surg Am*. 1994;76:561–572. (**LOE I**).

87. Shahi V, Brinjikji W, Cloft HJ, et al. Trends in CT utilization for pediatric fall patients in US emergency departments. *Acad Radiol*. 2015;22:898–903. (**LOE III**).

88. Kharbanda AB, Flood A, Blumberg K, et al. Analysis of radiation exposure among pediatric trauma patients at national trauma centers. *J Trauma Acute Care Surg*. 2013;74:907–911. (**LOE III**).

89. Tepas JJ 3rd, DiScala C, Ramenofsky ML, et al. Mortality and head injury: the pediatric perspective. *J Pediatr Surg*. 1990;25:92. (**LOE III**).

90. Chestnut RM, Marshall LF, Klauber MR, et al. The role of secondary brain injury in determining outcome from severe head injury. *J Trauma*. 1993;43:216–222. (**LOE I**).

91. Pigula FA, Wald SL, Shackford SR, et al. The effect of hypotension and hypoxia on children with severe head injuries. *J Pediatr Surg*. 1993;28:310–316. (**LOE I**).

92. Cirak B, Ziegfeld S, Knight VM, et al. Spinal injuries in children. *J Pediatr Surg*. 2004;39:607–612. (**LOE III**).

93. Mohseni S, Talving P, Castelo Branco B, et al. Effect of age on cervical spine injury in pediatric population: a National Trauma Data Bank review. *J Pediatr Surg*. 2011;46:1771–1776. (**LOE II**).

94. Dietrich AM, Ginn-Pease ME, Bartkowski HM, et al. Pediatric cervical spine features: predominantly subtle presentation. *J Pediatr Surg*. 1991;26:995–1000. (**LOE II**).

95. Sledge JB, Allred D, Hyman J. Use of magnetic resonance imaging in evaluating injuries to the pediatric thoracolumbar spine. *J Pediatr Orthop*. 2001;21:288–293. (**LOE III**).

96. Caruso MC, Daugherty MC, Moody SM, et al. Lessons learned from administration of high-dose methylprednisolone sodium succinate for acute pediatric spinal cord injuries. *J Neurosurg Pediatr*. 2017;20:567–574. (**LOE III**).

97. Bliss D, Silen M. Pediatric thoracic trauma. *Crit Care Med*. 2002;30:S409–S415. (**LOE V**).

98. Harris GJ, Soper RT. Pediatric first rib fractures. *J Trauma*. 1990;30:343–345. (**LOE IV**).

99. Dowd MD, Krug S. Pediatric blunt cardiac injury: epidemiology, clinical features, and diagnosis. *J Trauma*. 1996;40:61–67. (**LOE IV**).

100. Heckman SR, Trooskin SZ, Burd RS. Risk factors for blunt thoracic aortic injury in children. *J Pediatr Surg*. 2005;40:98–102. (**LOE II**).

101. Brandt ML, Luks FI, Spigland NA, et al. Diaphragmatic injury in children. *J Trauma*. 1992;32:298–301. (**LOE IV**).

102. Centers for Disease Control and Prevention. Injury Mortality Atlas of the United States, 1979–1987. Atlanta, GA, 1991, U.S. Centers for Disease Control and Prevention. (**LOE IV**).

103. Cooper A, Barlow B, DiScala C, et al. Mortality and truncal injury. The pediatric perspective. *J Pediatr Surg*. 1994;29:33–38. (**LOE II**).

104. Calder BW, Vogel AM, Zhang J, et al. Focused assessment with sonography for trauma in children after blunt abdominal trauma: a multi-institutional analysis. *J Trauma Acute Care Surg*. 2017;83:218–224. (**LOE II**).

105. Holmes JF, Kelley KM, Wootton-Gorges SL, et al. Effect of abdominal ultrasound on clinical care, outcomes, and resource use among children with blunt torso trauma: a randomized clinical trial. *JAMA*. 2017;317:2290–2296. (**LOE I**).

106. Davis DH, Localio AR, Stafford PW, et al. Trends in operative management of pediatric splenic injury in a regional trauma system. *Pediatrics* 2005;115 89–94. (2005). (**LOE III**).

107. Skaggs DL, Kautz SM, Kay RM, et al. Effect of delay of surgical treatment on rate of infection in open fractures in children. *J Pediatr Orthop.* 2000;20:19–22. (**LOE III**).

108. Barmparas G, Inaba K, Talving P, et al. Pediatric vs adult vascular trauma: a national trauma databank review. *J Pediatr Surg.* 2010;45:1404–1412. (**LOE III**).

109. Mubarak SJ, Carroll NC. Volkmann's contracture in children: aetiology and prevention. *J Bone Joint Surg Br.* 1979;61:285–293. (**LOE IV**).

110. Flynn JM, Sarwark JF, Waters PM, et al. The surgical management of pediatric fractures of the upper extremity. *Instr Course Lect.* 2003;52:635–645. (**LOE V**).

111. Flynn JM, Schwend RM. Management of pediatric femoral shaft fractures. *J Am Acad Orthop Surg.* 2004;12:347–359. (**LOE V**).

112. Tolo VT. Orthopaedic treatment of fractures of the long bones and pelvis in children who have multiple injuries. *Instr Course Lect.* 2000;49:415–423. (**LOE V**).

113. Thompson GH, Wilber JH, Marcus RE. Internal fixation of fractures in children and adolescents. a comparative analysis. *Clin Orthop.* 1984;188:10–20. (**LOE III**).

114. Spiegel PG, Mast JW. Internal and external fixation of fractures in children. *Orthop Clin North Am.* 1980;11:405–421. (**LOE V**).

115. Roaten JD, Kelly DM, Yellin JL, et al. Pediatric femoral shaft fractures: a multicenter review of the AAOS clinical practice guidelines before and after 2009. *J Pediatr Orthop.* 2017:10 (**LOE III**).

116. Gustilo RB, Anderson JT. Prevention of infection in treatment of 1025 open fractures of long bones: retrospective and prospective analysis. *J Bone Joint Surg Am.* 1976;58:453–458. (**LOE II**).

117. Gustilo RB, Mendoza RM, Williams DN. Problems in the management of type II (severe) open fractures: a new classification of type III open fractures. *J Trauma.* 1984;24:742–746. (**LOE II**).

118. Zonfrillo MR, Durbin DR, Winston FK, et al. Physical disability after injury-related inpatient rehabilitation in children. *Pediatrics.* 2013;131:e206–e213. (**LOE II**).

6 Fractures with Soft Tissue Injuries

Kristin Livingston | Sanjeev Sabharwal

CHARACTERISTICS

It is generally accepted that open fractures among children have better clinical outcomes than similar injuries in adults,[1,2] but high-level comparative studies are lacking.[3,4] Although skeletal maturity and preexisting conditions (such as osteogenesis imperfecta) influence the injury patterns of open fractures, it is primarily the kinetic energy $E_k = mv^2/2$ that determines the severity of bone and soft tissue damage of a particular injury. Thus, closed pediatric fractures are largely caused by low-energy domestic activities and play, whereas over 80% of open fractures in children over 2 years are caused by violent accidents.[5] Even in adolescents, athletic activities account for less than 5% of open fractures. Although some open fractures occur through the physes, the majority are located in the diaphyses. Open fractures in children younger than school age are rare because of their small body mass, the large amount of protective subcutaneous fat, and their limited exposure to high-risk activities.

CLASSIFICATION

Most classifications of open musculoskeletal injuries account for the size, severity, and extent of the soft tissue lesion but neglect such modifying factors as wound contamination, fracture pattern, and associated injuries. The open fracture classification that is still most popular for both children and adults was developed by Gustilo and Anderson in 1976 and divides open fractures into three types according to the severity of the soft tissue injury. It was further refined in 1984 to allow for better differentiation of the most severe injuries (Table 6.1).[6] The Gustilo classification continues to be widely used and does help guide treatment and predict clinical outcomes such as risk of wound infections.[1] However, the interobserver reliability and reproducibility of this classification system has been an area of some debate.[7–9]

In type I open fractures, the wound is less than 1 cm long. It is often a clean puncture wound in which a spike of bone has pierced the skin. These fractures are accompanied by minimal soft tissue damage and no sign of crushing injury. The fracture pattern is typically transverse, or short oblique, with little comminution, if any (Fig. 6.1), and this most commonly occurs with a both bone forearm fracture in the skeletally immature patients.

In type II open fractures, the laceration is greater than 1 cm in length, but no extensive soft tissue damage is present. These fractures are associated with a slight or moderate crushing injury, moderate comminution at the fracture site, and moderate contamination.

Type III injuries are characterized by extensive damage to skin, muscle, bone, and, possibly, neurovascular structures. A high degree of contamination may be present. Type III injuries are divided into three subgroups. In type IIIA, soft tissue coverage of the fractured bone is adequate, despite the extensive injury. This subtype includes segmental and severely comminuted fractures from high-energy trauma, regardless of the size of the wound. A type IIIB injury has extensive soft tissue disruption or loss, with periosteal stripping and exposure of bone. Massive contamination and comminution of the fractures are common. A local rotational or free flap is needed to obtain satisfactory wound coverage. Type IIIC includes any open fractures associated with an arterial injury that needs repair, regardless of the extent of soft tissue damage. The incidence of wound infection, delayed union, nonunion, amputation, and residual

TABLE 6.1 Classification of Open Fractures

Type	Description
I	Skin opening of ≤1 cm, quite clean; most likely from inside to outside; minimal muscle contusion; simple transverse or short oblique fractures
II	Laceration >1 cm long, without extensive soft tissue damage, flaps, or avulsion; minimal to moderate crushing component; simple transverse or short oblique fractures with minimal comminution
III	Extensive soft tissue damage, including muscles, skin, and neurovascular structures; often a high-velocity injury with a severe crushing component
IIIA	Usually results from high-energy trauma; however, soft tissue coverage of the fractured bone still adequate, despite extensive soft tissue laceration or flaps
IIIB	More extensive soft tissue injury (than type IIIA) with periosteal stripping and bone exposure; usually associated with massive contamination
IIIC	Any open fracture associated with arterial injury requiring repair, independent of the fracture type

Modified from Gustilo RB, Mendoza R, Williams D. Problems in the management of type III (severe) open fractures: a new classification of type III open fractures. *J Trauma.* 1984;24:742–746.

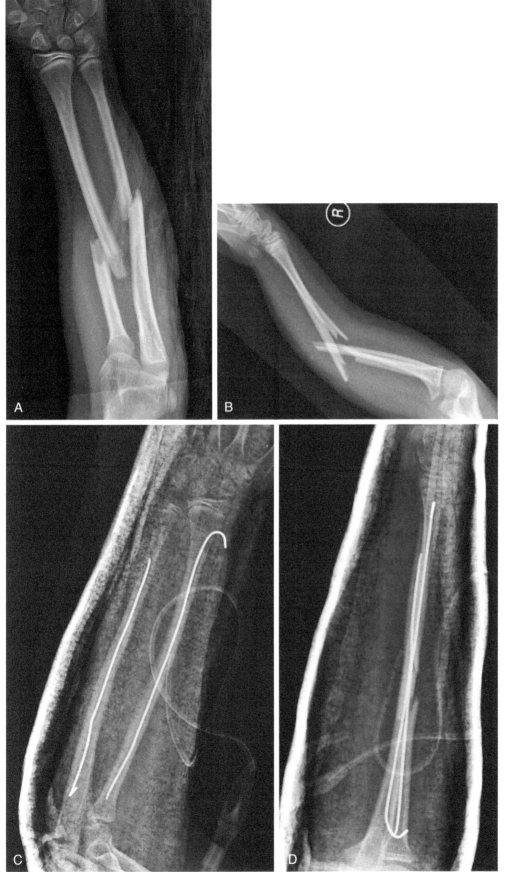

Fig. 6.1 Anteroposterior (A) and lateral (B) radiographs of an 8-year-old female who sustained a type I open fracture of both bones of the right forearm. She underwent urgent irrigation and débridement of the open fracture and elastic intramedullary nailing of both bones with the use of 1.5-mm nails. A prophylactic volar compartment fasciotomy of the forearm was also performed along with insertion of a surgical drain. Postoperative anteroposterior (C) and lateral (D) radiographs with an overlying splint demonstrate the aforementioned findings.

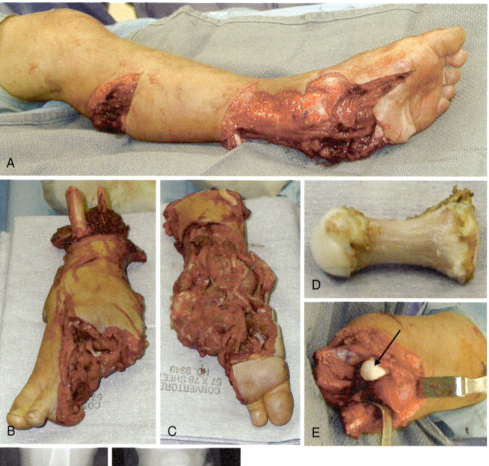

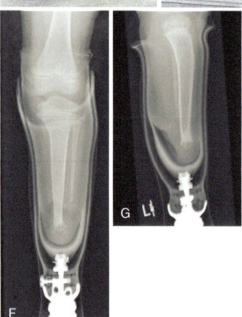

Fig. 6.2 A 6-year-old boy after a severe lawn mower injury to his left leg (A). This injury was not suitable for reconstruction. He underwent a below-knee amputation. Dorsal (B) and plantar (C) views of a portion of the amputated specimen are seen. The first metatarsal retrieved from the amputated foot was placed into the intramedullary canal of the tibial stump to function as an osteochondral graft (D) so that stump overgrowth would be prevented. Osteochondral graft positioned in tibia during below-knee amputation below-knee amputation (E). He required a split-thickness skin graft. Anteroposterior (F) and lateral (G) radiographs of the amputation stump 1 year later demonstrating complete incorporation of the intramedullary graft. He did not have any stump overgrowth over the next few years.

disability is directly related to the type of soft tissue injury. The more severe the injury, the greater the risk of complications.[6,10,11] Based on a systematic review of the literature related to open tibial fractures in children and adolescents, age older than 10 years and type III open fractures were associated with complications and outcomes similar to those reported in adults.[12]

SPECIFIC MECHANISMS OF INJURY

Open fractures inflicted by lawn mowers (Fig. 6.2) and farm machinery deserve particular attention because both generate highly contaminated open injuries, mainly through the impact of debris or through the direct force of the cutting blades, which can rotate at 3000 rpm and generate about 2100 foot-pounds of kinetic injury. This amount of kinetic energy creates trauma analogous to a blast injury,[13] leads to amputation in up to 82% of cases,[14] and is often associated with compartment syndrome.[15] Such injuries most commonly afflict children younger than 14 years (median age 6 years old), with younger children having a higher Injury Severity Score.[16] Farm and lawn mower injuries are often complicated by posttraumatic infections with mixed flora, mostly gram-negative bacilli.[17]

Another unique class of injuries includes those sustained from earthquakes, because the vast majority (87%) of survivable injuries from earthquakes are orthopedic in nature.[18] More than half of these fractures are of the lower extremity, most commonly diaphyseal tibia (27%) and femur (17%). These injuries often have associated severe soft tissue crush or open injuries from falling debris along with extensive fracture comminution. Damage control orthopedics is the treatment of choice, especially when resources are limited, and initial management should focus on hemorrhage control, wound débridement, infection control, and soft tissue stabilization. Where contamination is severe, multiple débridements should be performed before definitive fixation.

Unfortunately, blast and land mine injuries related to acts of terrorism can also affect children and have grave consequences,[19–22] including a 7% mortality rate.[23] Modern low-intensity warfare in conflict regions has resulted in more children experiencing battlefield injuries.[24] Compared with adolescents and adults, young children exposed to terror explosions tend to have greater injury severity, including traumatic brain injury, but may have a lower prevalence of open wounds and lower extremity injuries.[25,26] That said, in the setting of severe traumatic wounds, hemorrhage control, either with tourniquet or hemostatic dressing, is the most common and effective prehospital (PH) intervention. Sokol et al emphasized the importance of training of PH personnel in application of hemorrhage control techniques in pediatric casualties.[24]

THE MANGLED EXTREMITY

With advances in PH resuscitation and the development of free flaps and microvascular reconstruction,[27–29] many limbs with extensive open fractures that involve vascular compromise or partial amputation can now be salvaged. However, despite the great potential for healing that is typical in children, some of the more severe open fractures are better managed with primary amputation (Figs. 6.2 and 6.3) rather than with extensive reconstructive procedures that leave the patient with a dubious cosmetic result and only marginal function.[30] To provide some guidance when deciding between limb salvage and amputation, a number of investigators have developed severity indices, although their applicability and translation to pediatric injuries is controversial. In 1990, Johansen and associates[31] developed the Mangled Extremity Severity Score (MESS), a rating scale for lower extremity trauma based on skeletal and soft tissue damage, limb ischemia, shock, and age of the patient (Table 6.2). The evidence for using MESS in children suffers from low numbers of patients because of the rarity of these injuries. In a series of type III open lower extremity fractures, the MESS accurately predicted successful limb salvage in 93% and amputation in 63% of

children.[32] In a review of pediatric open fractures of the lower extremity, a MESS of 6.5 or greater was a reasonable predictor of the need for amputation.[33] In a rebuttal to that article, Stewart et al describe few failures of limb salvage in children and caution against using MESS, particularly for a score of 6.5, which is lower than the adult standard, or any severity score, as an indication for primary amputation in the pediatric population, as children tend to have better clinical outcome with nerve repair, more likelihood of fracture union, lower wound infection rates, and better use of injured limbs because of neural plasticity.[34] They present their experience showing lack of specificity and low positive predictive value of multiple scoring systems in children, which suggest that strict adherence to scoring systems may lead to unnecessary amputations.[34] The Ganga Hospital Open Injury Severity Score (GHOISS, which includes scoring for skin and fascia, bone and joint, musculotendinous and nerve units, and comorbid conditions) was published recently and has been applied to type IIIB open fractures in children with open physes.[35] A GHOISS of greater than or equal to 17 was found to be a better predictor of amputation as compared with a MESS of greater than 7.

Regardless of decision-making modalities, there is no substitute for evaluation by experienced surgeons with widespread consultation from multiple individuals including orthopedic surgeons, plastic surgeons, anesthesiologists, and critical care specialists. It is also imperative to ensure that parents are counseled that salvage in the setting of severe injury and high injury severity scores may be a long process with uncertain outcome, and some of these children may ultimately need a secondary amputation.

CLOSED FRACTURES WITH SEVERE SOFT TISSUE INJURIES

It has become increasingly clear that some closed fractures caused by violent force may result in extensive destruction of the soft tissue sleeve surrounding the leg and pelvis without resulting in an open lesion.[36–39] These closed fractures with severe soft tissue injury are characterized by skin contusions, deep abrasions, burns, or frank separation of the cutis from the subcuticular tissue. Even in children, these lesions can result in partial or full tissue loss and secondary infection of the fracture site. To avoid catastrophes, surgeons must treat these lesions as open fractures, which facilitates repeated injury evaluation and decreases complications. Tscherne and Gotzen[37] provided a classification that describes four grades of these treacherous injuries that may prove useful in choosing among different treatment options (Table 6.3).

A unique class of these injuries includes concealed degloving injuries, the Morel-Lavallée lesion, which is rare in children but can be seen in fractures (usually peripelvic) caused by motor vehicle, train, and ATV accidents as well as lower-energy sports mechanisms. Hallmark physical findings include a soft fluctuant area caused by collection of blood and lymphatic fluid, and the diagnosis is best confirmed with magnetic resonance imaging. Management of these lesions can include compressive bandages and bedrest in mild lesions, or percutaneous drainage with or without sclerotherapy. In acute lesions with underlying fractures, surgical débridement is usually necessary.[38,40]

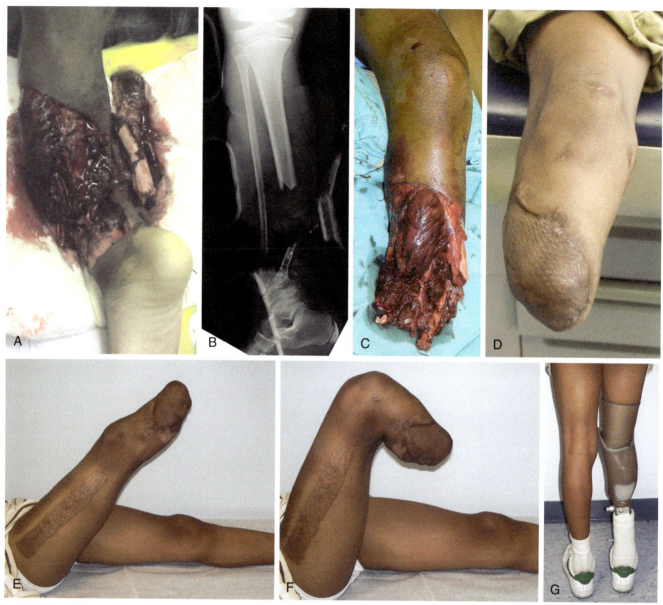

Fig. 6.3 Clinical photograph of a 10-year-old male pedestrian who sustained a type IIIC open tibial shaft fracture with segmental bone loss (A). An anteroposterior radiograph demonstrating the segmental fracture of the tibia and fibula with severe rotational deformity (B). Because of the severe nature of the soft tissue injury, a below-knee amputation (C) with delayed skin grafting (D) was performed. A portion of the amputated first metatarsal was used as an osteochondral intramedullary plug so that stump overgrowth of the tibia would be avoided. Despite the use of the skin graft (E), he regained functional mobility (F) of his knee and was able to tolerate a prosthesis without any major stump-related issues (G). (From Bloom T, Sabharwal S. Tibial shaft fractures. In: Herman M, Horn D, eds. *Contemporary Surgical Management of Fractures and Complications in Children*. New Delhi, India: Jaypee Publishers; 2013.)

TREATMENT PLAN

OVERVIEW

Although most bony and soft tissue disruptions in children have a greater healing potential, the treatment goals and principles of open musculoskeletal injuries in children are the same as those for adults. The principal goals in managing open fractures are restoration and preservation of vital functions,[41] prevention of wound infection,[42] healing of the soft tissue injuries,[43] restoration of bony anatomy and bone union, and recovery of optimal physical and psychosocial function.

These objectives are best attained by prompt initial resuscitation,[41] thorough and complete evaluation of life-threatening injuries followed by a detailed assessment of the fracture site,[42] appropriate antimicrobial therapy at presentation,[43] extensive and possibly repeated wound débridement followed by wound coverage, fracture stabilization, autogenous bone grafting when needed, restoration of major bony defects, and comprehensive functional and psychosocial rehabilitation. These interventions often overlap or occur in a modified temporal sequence, depending on age, injury pattern, and associated lesions. They are also highly interdependent; the type and timing of wound closure, for instance, may affect the choice of fracture fixation.

TABLE 6.2   Mangled Extremity Severity Score

Variable	Points
Skeletal/Soft Tissue Injury Low energy (stab, simple fracture, "civilian" gunshot wound)	1
Medium energy (open or multiple fractures, dislocation)	2
High energy (close-range shotgun or "military" gunshot wound, crush injury)	3
Very high energy (same as high energy plus gross contamination, soft tissue avulsion)	4
Limb Ischemia Pulse reduced or absent but perfusion normal	1[a]
Pulseless; paresthesias, diminished capillary refill	2[a]
Cool, paralyzed, insensate, numb	3[a]
Shock Systolic blood pressure always >90 mm Hg	0
Hypotensive transiently	1
Persistent hypotension	2
Age (Years) <30	0
30–50	1
>50	2

[a]Score doubled for ischemia duration longer than 6 hours.
From Johansen K, Daines M, Howey T, et al. Objective criteria accurately predict amputation following lower extremity trauma. *J Trauma.* 1990;30:568–572.

TABLE 6.3   Classification of Closed Fractures With Soft Tissue Injuries

0	Minimal soft tissue damage; indirect violence; simple fracture patterns (e.g., torsion fracture of the tibia in skiers)
I	Superficial abrasion or contusion caused by pressure from within; mild to moderately severe fracture configuration (e.g., pronation fracture-dislocation of the ankle joint with a soft tissue lesion over the medial malleolus)
II	Deep contaminated abrasion associated with localized skin or muscle contusion; impending compartment syndrome; severe fracture configuration (e.g., segmental "bumper" fracture of the tibia)
III	Extensive skin contusion or crush; underlying muscle damage may be severe; subcutaneous avulsion; decompensated compartment syndrome; associated major vascular injury; severe or comminuted fracture configuration

From Tscherne H, Oestern H-J. [A new classification of soft-tissue damage in open and closed fractures (author's transl)]. *Unfallheilkunde.* 1982;85:111–115.

Acute care follows the general guidelines that have been established for similar injuries in adults. In addition to appropriate and timely acute intervention, the final clinical outcome of these injuries depends on a comprehensive plan of rehabilitation that includes physical therapy as well as educational and socioeconomic support for the family.

INITIAL CARE

PH care of a trauma patient with severe fracture and soft tissue injury follows the ABCD algorithm with attention to cervical spine immobilization.[44] After assessment and initial management of airway and breathing, bleeding, disability, and deformity should be addressed. At the scene of the injury, the open wound is covered with a sterile dressing, if available. Profuse bleeding such as with vascular injury or amputation is controlled by local compression or preferably a tourniquet. PH intervention with a tourniquet is an active area of military training that even prioritizes hemorrhage control over airway issues.[45,46] Tourniquets have been shown to be safe and effective in severely injured pediatric patients.[24] With bleeding under control, a fracture may be managed by gentle traction, manipulation, and splinting in a comfortable position for transport to the emergency department.

In the emergency department, an Advance Trauma Life Support protocol is followed. One or more intravenous lines are established. Tetanus prophylaxis[47] and the first intravenous dose of appropriate antibiotic(s) are administered upon arrival to the emergency department for an open fracture.[1,11,48] After the history is taken and the physical examination is completed, including inspection of wounds (although dressings should be taken down as few times as needed for appropriate decision-making in the emergency department), pertinent radiographs are obtained, and blood is drawn for a complete blood count, typing, and cross-matching and for determination of serum electrolyte levels. Severely displaced fractures, especially when compromising the integrity of the overlying skin or associated with neurovascular deficits, should be realigned and splinted in the emergency department. Any patient with a suspected dysvascular limb is transferred to the operating room without delay for further assessment and possible vascular exploration and repair. Preoperative angiography is not routinely recommended because it further prolongs the warm ischemia time.[49] At some pediatric trauma centers, instituting a lower extremity vascular trauma protocol has been shown to improve the timeliness of vascular care to ensure that ischemia time does not exceed the critical period of 6 to 8 hours.[49]

WOUND CONTAMINATION

It is prudent to assume that all open fractures and closed lesions covered with devitalized tissue are contaminated.[1] Frank infections are more likely to develop if necrotic tissue remains in the wound.[50,51] The infection rates in open pediatric fractures are somewhat lower than adults.[52] Patzakis and Wilkins[1] reported only one infection (1.8%) in 55 open fractures in children. In contrast, they had an overall infection rate of 7.2% in 1049 open adult fractures. In a series of 554 open pediatric fractures, Skaggs and colleagues[11] reported a 3% overall infection rate, and the incidence was 2% in type I and II injuries and 8% in type III fractures. Typically, the infecting organisms are *Staphylococcus aureus* and aerobic or facultative gram-negative rods in fractures with less severe soft tissue injury, whereas mixed flora prevails in type IIIB and IIIC lesions.[1] Among all open fractures, Patzakis and Wilkins[1] found the highest infection rate in tibial lesions, presumably caused by the limited soft tissue envelope and relatively poor vascularity.[53] In two studies of open tibial fractures in children, the overall infection rates were 10% and 11%, similar to those reported in adults.[10,54] No infections developed in type I fractures, whereas infection rates were approximately 12% in type II injuries and 21% to 33% in type III fractures.[10,54]

CLOSTRIDIAL INFECTIONS

TETANUS

Tetanus is a rare but potentially fatal disease.[55,56] Wounds that are deemed tetanus prone include those contaminated with dirt, saliva, or feces; puncture wounds, including nonsterile injections; missile injuries; burns; frostbite; avulsions; crush injuries; and wounds undergoing delayed débridement. The causative organism is *Clostridium tetani*, a gram-positive rod that grows best under anaerobic conditions and in necrotic tissue. The clinical manifestations are caused by the effects of a neurotoxin on skeletal muscle, peripheral nerves, and the spinal cord. Generalized tetanus starts with cramps in the muscles surrounding the wound, neck stiffness, hyperreflexia, and changes in facial expression. Later, contractions of whole muscle groups cause opisthotonos and acute respiratory failure.

Tetanus is preventable through active immunization with a formaldehyde-treated tetanospasmin known as tetanus toxoid. The Immunization Practices Advisory Committee recommends routine active immunization for infants and children against diphtheria, tetanus toxoids, and pertussis at the ages of 2 months, 4 months, 6 months, 15 to 18 months, and 4 to 6 years. Completion of a primary dose series confers humoral immunity to tetanus for at least 10 years in the majority of those who receive the vaccine. A child or adolescent with an open fracture who has not completed the primary series of immunizations or who has not received a booster dose in 10 years should receive tetanus toxoid, which is administered as a 0.5-mL intramuscular injection for patients of all ages. As has been shown in a population-based study, immunity cannot be presumed.[57] Administration of tetanus toxoid immunizes the patient against the next wounding event but does not ensure tetanus prophylaxis for the acute injury.[47] If the child has never received primary immunization against tetanus, passive immunization with human tetanus immune globulin is added. The intramuscular dose varies with age: those older than 10 years receive 250 units, those 5 to 10 years old receive 125 units, and those younger than 5 years receive 75 units. Tetanus immune globulin and tetanus toxoid should not be administered at the same site but may be administered on the same day. Vigorous débridement of open wounds and resection of all nonviable tissue are an integral part of tetanus prevention.

GAS GANGRENE

Gas gangrene is most frequently caused by *Clostridium perfringens* or *Clostridium septicum*, anaerobic gram-positive spore-forming bacteria that produce numerous exotoxins. Gas gangrene is most frequently seen after primary wound closure, after open crush injuries, and in wounds contaminated by bowel contents or soil.[1,58] The exotoxins produced by these organisms create local edema, muscle and fat necrosis, and thrombosis of local vessels. The clostridia also generate several gases that dissect into the surrounding tissue and facilitate rapid spread of the infection. In the terminal stages, clostridial infections cause hemolysis, tubular necrosis, and renal failure.[58,59]

The early clinical manifestations of gas gangrene after an open fracture include excruciating pain in the affected area followed by high fever, chills, tachycardia, convulsions, and evidence of toxemia. Initially, the skin about the wound is very edematous and cool but without crepitation. Later, the skin has a brown or bronze coloration, crepitation, and drainage of a thin brownish fluid with a pungent odor. Radiographs demonstrate gas formation within the muscle and intrafascial planes. Gram stain of the exudate reveals gram-positive rods with spores. However, not all posttraumatic crepitation is caused by gas gangrene. It may also be caused by mechanical introduction of air related to trauma or surgery, especially in the first 12 hours after injury. Crepitation from gas gangrene usually occurs between 12 and 60 hours after injury. The crepitus is initially minimal but progresses with time.

The crucial steps in the treatment of early gas gangrene are emergent radical débridement with removal of all necrotic muscle and fasciotomies of all compartments to relieve pressure from the edema and enhance blood flow. Repeated débridement is usually necessary. In addition, the patient should receive intravenous penicillin. In patients allergic to penicillin, intravenous clindamycin or metronidazole are acceptable substitutes. Because wounds with clostridial contamination are often associated with a mixed flora, additional coverage against such organisms with additional antibiotics such as a cephalosporin and an aminoglycoside is typically necessary. The efficacy of polyvalent gas gangrene serum, which can cause sensitivity reactions, remains unproven. Administration of hyperbaric oxygen may be beneficial because elevated tissue oxygen tension appears to inhibit clostridial growth and the production of exotoxins.[58,59] This technology, however, is no substitute for meticulous surgical débridement.

ANTIMICROBIALS

SYSTEMIC ANTIBIOTICS

The majority of open fractures are contaminated with bacteria at the time of injury. Aerobic gram-positive and gram-negative bacteria are the major pathogens of infections associated with fractures.[1,52] The risk of development of an infection in an open fracture depends on the location of the fracture (lower extremity higher risk than upper extremity), severity of the soft tissue injury, the extent of the contamination, the virulence of the involved flora, timely administration of appropriate antibiotics, and the adequacy of surgical débridement.

Timely administration of antibiotics has been demonstrated to be effective in decreasing the risk of infection in open fractures.[1,11] Administration of appropriate antibiotics as soon as possible after an open fracture is currently considered best practice.[3] The effectiveness of early administration of appropriate antibiotics was confirmed in a large multicenter study of pediatric open fractures.[11] Intravenous antibiotics delivered within 3 hours of injury was the single most important factor in reducing the infection rate in these children. Patzakis and Wilkins[1] found the infection rate to be 13.9% in 79 patients who received no antibiotics versus 5.5% in 815 patients who were treated with broad-spectrum antibiotics (cephalothin alone or cefamandole plus tobramycin). Antibiotics are restarted when another procedure such as delayed primary or secondary wound closure or delayed internal fixation related to the open fracture is performed. For a grade III injury, some authors recommend stopping antibiotics 72 hours after injury, or 24 hours after the wound is surgically covered, whichever occurs first.[60] Although robust clinical trials to establish clear guidelines for duration of antibiotics are currently not available, it does seem clear that prolonged antibiotic therapy, beyond 48 to 72 hours postoperatively, does not reduce the rate of wound infections and may promote the development of resistant organisms[1] or increase the risk of *Clostridium difficile*–related diarrhea.[61]

A cephalosporin (100 mg/kg/day cefazolin divided into doses given every 8 hours, to a maximum dose of 2 g every 8 hours) is currently recommended as baseline therapy for all grade I and II open fractures.[6,53] In the setting of cephalosporin allergy, clindamycin may be used (15 to 40 mg/kg/day divided into doses given every 8 hours, up to a maximum dose of 2.7 g/day). For Gustilo type I and II lesions, this therapy is initially continued for 24 to 48 hours. Although lacking robust studies, Gustilo type III open fractures are treated with a cephalosporin and an aminoglycoside (5–7.5 mg/kg/day gentamicin divided into doses given every 8 hours) to cover both gram-positive and gram-negative bacteria. Alternatively, some protocols recommend Ceftriaxone (50mg/kg/day intravenous [IV] not to exceed 1 g) for grade III injuries. Penicillin (150,000 units/kg/day divided into doses given every 6 hours, to a maximum of 24 million units/day) is added if the patient is at risk of a clostridial infection (e.g., with farm injury). Resection of all devitalized soft tissue, copious irrigation, and the use of systemic antibiotics remain the principal tools in preventing posttraumatic wound infection.

WOUND MANAGEMENT

IRRIGATION AND DÉBRIDEMENT

The dogma of irrigating all pediatric open fractures, especially type I injuries, in the operating room within 6 hours of occurrence has been recently questioned.[11, 62–64] Several retrospective case series have reported satisfactory clinical outcomes, including a less than 5% infection rate, with type I open pediatric fractures that were treated nonoperatively with wound irrigation and cast immobilization in the emergency department in addition to intravenous or oral antibiotics.[62,65,66] Although this option for nonoperative treatment is slowly becoming more popular, until more robust evidence confirms these findings, such clinical practice should not be considered "routine" at this time, particularly in lower extremity long bone fractures, which may be more prone to infection and acute compartment syndrome. When surveyed, 31% of Pediatric Orthopaedic Society of North America (POSNA) members would elect to treat a grade I open forearm fracture in a child with incision and drainage in the emergency room followed by closed reduction and cast/splint with 1 week of antibiotics and close follow-up (19% of POSNA members would opt for similar management for a grade I open tibia fracture and 27% for a grade I open humerus shaft fracture in children).[67] When these injuries are treated without surgical irrigation and débridement in the operating room, there is no consensus on the type and duration of antibiotics. Some treatment protocols include admitting the child for 24 hours of IV antibiotics, while other centers discharge patients from the emergency department on oral antibiotics (usually for 5–7 days).[65] One must use caution if considering a discharge from the emergency department after an open fracture, as acute compartment syndrome is a possible complication in such injuries.

On the basis of a multicenter retrospective cohort study of 554 open pediatric fractures, Skaggs and colleagues[11] have suggested that irrigation and débridement of certain pediatric open fractures can be delayed up to 24 hours after the injury without any adverse effects as long as intravenous antibiotics are administered on arrival in the emergency department. However, these recommendations remain controversial.[68,69] A web-based survey of accredited orthopedic residency program directors in the United States reported that the majority of responders were not willing to wait 6 or more hours when managing type III pediatric open fractures.[70] A recent animal study noted that earlier irrigation in a contaminated wound model resulted in superior bacterial removal.[71]

In the operating room, after induction of anesthesia, the injured extremity is prepared and draped with the use of sterile technique with a chlorhexidine or betadine solution.[72] Avoiding contamination of the fracture site requires that a separate set of instruments be used for the initial part of the procedure, the débridement. Once débridement is completed, the surgical team changes gloves and gowns along with redraping of the operative site before proceeding with fracture fixation and applying the final wound dressing. A sterile pneumatic tourniquet is usually applied as a safety measure but is not inflated unless massive bleeding occurs. The most important process in the management of an open fracture then begins: a search for the extent of the "real injury," which often exceeds the apparent injury by a factor of 2 to 3. Many clues alert the surgeon to the true size of the injury zone, including an estimate of the energy dissipated at the fracture site at the time of injury, the size and location of bruises and secondary skin openings, and such radiographic features as degree of comminution, air pockets extending along tissue planes, and the relationship of bony fragments to neurovascular structures.

This information is used to guide the initiation of débridement: a carefully planned and systematic process that removes all foreign and nonviable material from the wound. As the first step, the wound edges are liberally extended to allow unobstructed access to the entire injury zone (Fig. 6.4). These incisions should be extensile, should not create superficial skin flaps, and should respect vascular and neurologic territories. All nonviable and necrotic skin is resected to a bleeding edge, and necrotic or contaminated

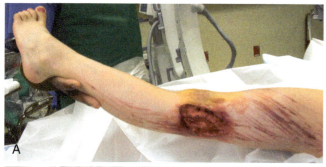

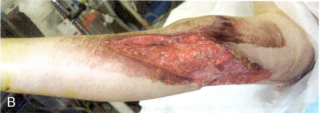

Fig. 6.4 An 8-year-old female pedestrian sustained a traumatic arthrotomy of her knee with a severe laceration and road rash (A). Because of the extent of her soft tissue injury underlying the road rash, the laceration was extended proximally and distally so that adequate débridement of the underlying soft tissues would be ensured (B). This wound was treated with delayed primary closure, and it healed uneventfully.

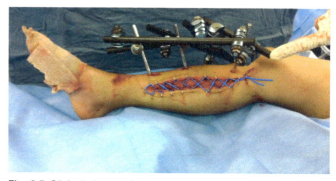

Fig. 6.5 Clinical picture of a 9-year-old female pedestrian who sustained a proximal tibial fracture with compartment syndrome. She was treated urgently with a four-compartment fasciotomy and stabilization of the fracture with the use of an external fixator. A "laced" elastic band was used to prevent retraction of the skin edges. The fasciotomy wounds were closed a few days later with delayed primary closure, and they healed uneventfully.

subcutaneous tissue and fat are sharply débrided. Contaminated fascia is resected, and prophylactic fasciotomies and epimysiotomies are commonly performed to allow the injured tissue to swell without causing secondary vascular compromise and tissue necrosis. Ischemic muscle is the principal culture medium for bacteria and is resected where compromised. The four Cs—consistency, contractility, color, and capacity to bleed—are classic guides to viability but are, unfortunately, not always reliable. The capacity to contract after a gentle pinch with forceps and the presence of arterial bleeding seem to be the best signs of viability.

The intramedullary canal of the principal fracture fragments is carefully inspected and cleansed of any contaminated material. Blood supply to cortical fragments is dependent on soft tissue attachments, and thus, bone fragments without soft tissue attachments should be débrided. Large cortical fragments with limited soft tissue attachments are often retained, especially if they provide intrinsic skeletal stability. Even if major cortical fragments need to be discarded because of gross contamination or lack of any soft tissue attachment, an attempt should be made to preserve the surrounding periosteum because this can contribute to subsequent reconstitution of the missing bone in children. Major neurovascular structures in the surgical field must be carefully identified and preserved. Débridement is completed when all contaminated and nonviable tissues are resected and the remaining wound cavity is lined by viable and well-perfused soft tissues.

Along with débridement, the wound is irrigated with ample amounts of isotonic saline solution. Investigators have questioned the significance of solution type in open fracture wound irrigation, but so far, no clear answer has been reached.[42,73] Optimal delivery pressure of the irrigant solution has been a focus of many studies, but a recent multicenter, blinded, randomized controlled trial showed no clinically important difference in outcomes between very low-, low-, and high-pressure irrigation, in addition to finding no difference between saline and soap solutions.[74] Another study of wound irrigation in open fractures similarly found no difference in reoperation rates among high, low, or very low pressure but did find higher reoperation rate for soap compared with saline irrigant.[75]

WOUND CARE

Nerves, vessels, tendons, articular cartilage, and bone, if exposed, are covered with local soft tissue or skin. The surgical extension of the wound is usually closed, and the remainder of the wound cavity can either be closed loosely over drains, "laced" with the use of rubber bands (Fig. 6.5) so that retraction of the skin edges is prevented, or dressed with a bandage soaked in isotonic saline or an antiseptic. Antibiotic-impregnated beads may be used in extremely contaminated wounds so as to deliver a high local concentration of antibiotics and help lower the infection rate, and also facilitate dead space management.[76,77] The use of negative pressure wound therapy (NPWT) (Fig. 6.6) for providing temporary wound coverage after surgical débridement of open fractures is gaining popularity, especially in children who may have difficulty tolerating frequent dressing changes. NPWT, often referred to as vacuum-assisted closure (VAC), helps stabilize the local wound environment, decreases edema, improves tissue perfusion, lowers the bacterial load, and stimulates formation of healthy granulation tissue. One study noted a decreased need for eventual flap coverage in pediatric open fractures when using a VAC.[78] In a prospective randomized study comparing traditional wet-to-dry dressing changes with NPWT in 62 type II or higher open fractures in adults, the wet-to-dry group had a higher deep infection rate (28% vs. 5.4%, $P = .024$).[79] Based on a review of literature dealing specifically with the use of NPWT in children, there was no consensus regarding the frequency of dressing changes, optimum amount of negative pressure, and selection of interposing contact layer in these younger patients.[80] Irrespective of the choice of such ancillary measures, thorough surgical débridement and removal of all devitalized and contaminated tissues are critical before application of any type of wound dressing.

Because the extent of soft tissue necrosis can be underestimated, injuries with extensive contamination, soft tissue trauma, or both are reevaluated in the operating room within 48 to 72 hours. At that time, it may be necessary to resect more necrotic tissue. The process of débridement is repeated at intervals of 2 to 3 days or less until all underlying tissues appear viable and wound coverage is achieved. Although obtaining perioperative cultures when débriding open fractures has been largely abandoned because of concerns regarding their sensitivity and cost-effectiveness,[50,81,82] a recent study of open fractures in adults suggested that waiting to perform soft tissue coverage until postdébridement wound culture results become negative may be associated with a lower infection rate than that of historical controls.[83]

WOUND COVERAGE

As soon as possible, the surgeon must determine the means through which soft tissue coverage will eventually be achieved. Complex wounds are best assessed early, in conjunction with an expert in soft tissue and microvascular techniques, so that satisfactory wound coverage is completed within 5 to 7 days after the injury and before secondary wound colonization has occurred.[1,84,85] Between débridement sessions, the wound is kept moist with dressings soaked in saline or an antiseptic or with the use of adjuvants such as an antibiotic bead pouch or NPWT. Most open fractures of type I to type IIIA severity in children are covered routinely by delayed primary wound closure or a split-thickness skin graft (see Fig. 6.6).[86] The use of the Allgöwer-Donati suture pattern may compromise cutaneous blood flow less than the more traditional skin closure techniques and can be used to close traumatized soft tissue wounds.[87] For moderate soft tissue defects with exposed bones, nerves, vessels, tendons, or ligaments, local fasciocutaneous and muscle flaps can be ideal.[84,85,88] For larger soft tissue defects and injuries to the most distal part of the leg, microvascular free flaps may be required. Muscle or composite free flaps are indicated for large, combined soft tissue and bone defects.[28] In addition to giving excellent coverage, free flaps may diminish low-grade bacterial colonization in the recipient bed and facilitate fracture union. In a series of 70 open pediatric tibial fractures, greater than 98% of limbs were salvaged with a multidisciplinary approach including early wound coverage.[84]

COMPARTMENT SYNDROME

Although the diagnosis, management, and long-term effects of compartment syndromes in children have been well delineated, the perception persists that compartment syndromes in open fractures are rare. In fact, increased compartment pressure is most commonly seen in type III open fractures, and adolescent boys have the highest risk of acute compartment syndrome of any demographic group.[54,89,90] It is also important to maintain a high suspicion for acute compartment syndrome in the setting of a crush injury with significant soft tissue damage even in the absence of fracture.[91] Because of their limited ability to communicate, young children with a compartment syndrome are prone to a delay in diagnosis,[92,93] particularly when they are intubated or have a head injury, a peripheral neurologic lesion, or mental impairment. The diagnosis of compartment syndrome is predominantly a clinical one. The three As—agitation, anxiety, and increasing analgesic requirement—are helpful indicators that may precede the classic presentation of compartment syndrome in children by several hours.[94] Abnormally elevated compartment pressures must be viewed along with the clinical setting, and checking compartment pressures may be difficult in the scared, uncooperative, or preverbal child. Although it is generally thought that distal limb viability following a warm ischemia time of greater than 8 hours is irreversible, the time course of acute compartment syndrome in children is not well established.[93] Children may take longer to develop peak compartment pressures and may tolerate peak pressures longer than adults. Children can develop compartment syndrome several hours to days after the inciting trauma and recover with minimal sequelae after appropriate decompressive fasciotomies.[92,95] If in doubt, it is safer to decompress all compartments of the injured portion of the extremity. Débridement of ischemic muscle is approached cautiously, recognizing the potential for recovery in initially dusky appearing muscle in children.[93] For the majority of cases (80%–90%), delayed primary closure of all compartment incisions without any need for skin grafting is possible in children. Techniques such as dermatotraction and NPWT can also aid in bringing the skin edges together and minimize the need or extent of skin grafting required.[96]

VASCULAR INJURY

Traumatic vascular injuries to the extremity are rare in children, and there is little high-level evidence to guide management in these often emergent, life- and limb-threatening complex situations. These injuries are particularly challenging in children because of increased risk of vasospasm and smaller diameter of vessels compared with adults.[97] When they do occur, usually in the setting of penetrating trauma, primary repair of the injured vessel is the most preferred and commonly employed strategy, with autogenous vein grafting a reasonable alternative when primary repair is not possible. With appropriate and timely management of the vascular injury, a high rate of limb salvage has been reported in children, although short- and long-term complications are common.[97]

TRAUMATIC AMPUTATIONS AND RELATED INJURIES

Trauma is the leading cause of amputations in children, and pediatric traumatic limb amputations are more common and often more extensive compared with adults.[16,98,99] The majority of these occur in boys between 1 to 5 years and 13 to 17 years of age. Although finger and toe amputations are the most common type and usually caused when a digit gets caught between objects, more proximal and severe amputations are usually caused by powered lawn mowers in the younger group and by motor vehicle and pedestrian accidents amongst adolescents (see Fig. 6.2).[100] In the United States, approximately 68,000 pediatric lawnmower injuries occur annually.[101] Other causes of amputation include farm

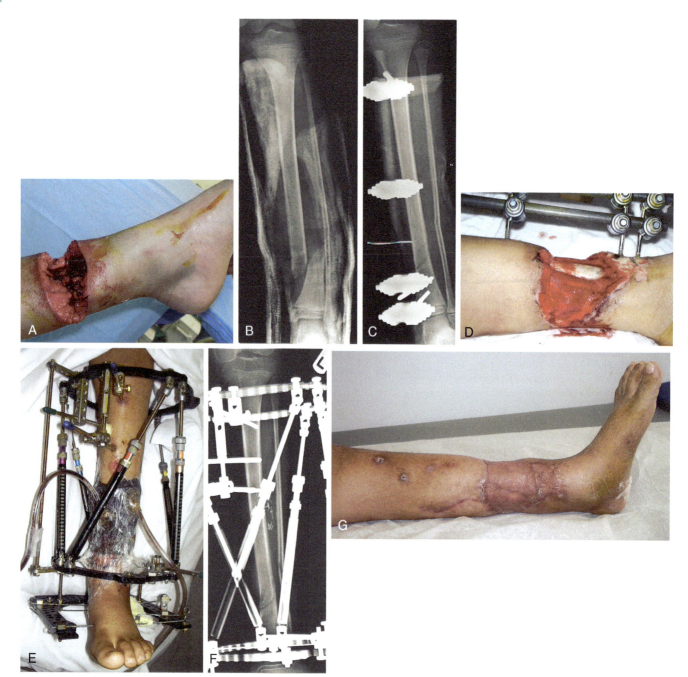

Fig. 6.6 A 10-year-old male pedestrian was struck by a high-speed motor vehicle and sustained a type IIIB open fracture of the distal third of the tibia with a circumferential soft tissue wound of the lower leg. Clinical appearance (A) and anteroposterior radiograph (B) of the left leg at initial presentation. He was treated with urgent irrigation and débridement of the open wound and application of a monolateral external fixator (C). Because the exposed bone was in close proximity to the infected distal pin sites (D), the fixation was changed to a circular external fixator with application of a negative pressure dressing (E and F). The patient subsequently had an attempt at free-flap coverage that failed. He then underwent skin grafting over a granulating wound, and his fracture healed in satisfactory alignment. Clinical appearance of the injured extremity approximately 9 months after the trauma demonstrating healed soft tissues and removal of the external fixator (G). (From Bloom T, Sabharwal S. Tibial shaft fractures. In: Herman M, Horn D, eds. *Contemporary Surgical Management of Fractures and Complications in Children*. New Delhi, India: Jaypee Publishers; 2013.)

injuries,[102,103] all-terrain vehicles,[104] burns, land mines,[19] gunshots, and blast injuries.[23] At one Midwest center, over a 20-year period, 256 traumatic amputations were seen in 235 children.[16] Of these, lawnmower injuries were responsible for 29%, farm machinery for 24%, motor vehicle accidents for 16%, train accidents for 9%, and other mechanisms for the remaining 22% of cases. Seasonal variation in the types

of injuries was noted in that lawnmower injuries were more common in the summer months and farming injuries were common in the spring and fall. The mean age at the time of injury also varied; amputations related to burns occurred most often in younger children, and boating injuries were primarily seen in adolescents. In fact, in children younger than 10 years, power lawn mowers accounted for 42% of all amputations.[105] If children younger than 14 years had not been permitted around lawn mowers, approximately 85% of the injuries would have been prevented. In another study of 74 children who sustained traumatic amputations, 53% were unsupervised at the time of the accident.[106] Better public education is needed to lessen the frequency of these preventable injuries with devastating consequences.[107,108] The American Academy of Pediatrics has recommended that children under 6 should be kept inside during lawnmower use, children should be at least 12 years old before they operate any lawnmower and at least 16 years old for a ride-on mower, and that children should never be passengers on ride-on mowers.[109]

Although no definite guidelines for amputations in children are available, findings that strongly suggest the need for an amputation include an unrestorable perfusion to the injured extremity, warm ischemia time exceeding 6 hours, substantial loss of viable muscle that cannot be replaced with a free flap, the presence of serious secondary bone or soft tissue injuries involving the same extremity, and, possibly, a MESS of 6.5 or higher or GHOISS of 17 or higher.[33,35,110] In the past, the loss of protective plantar sensation was an additional indication to amputate the foot.[110] However, if the lesion is because of neurapraxia of the posterior tibial nerve, it will likely recover over time. Whenever possible, the decision to amputate should be made at the initial débridement because, at least in adults, primary amputation leads to better long-term results.[30] It is prudent to get another orthopedic surgeon or general surgeon, if available, to confirm the need for such ablative reconstruction.

The management of a child with a traumatic amputation is different from that of an adult with a similar injury. The potential for future growth, better healing ability, possibility of stump overgrowth, and psychologic and emotional factors all require special consideration. When possible, preservation of the chondroepiphysis and growth plate of the injured segment should be considered. The distal femoral growth plate, for example, provides 70% of the growth of the femur, and an above-knee amputation done at an early age can lead to an inappropriately short amputation stump that can cause problems with prosthetic fitting as an adult. An estimate of the growth remaining in the residual limb is required to make a decision on the length of the amputated segment. For instance, an ideal tibial length for an adult below-knee amputation is 12.5 to 17.5 cm, depending on body height. In children, a reasonable rule of thumb is to allow for 2.5 cm (1 inch) of proximal tibial stump length for each 30 cm (1 foot) of standing height. In the case of a transfemoral amputation, the ideal level of amputation would allow a stump length of 14 cm proximal to the medial knee joint line at skeletal maturity. For an upper limb amputation, the optimal level of bone cut is 10 cm above elbow joint line for transhumeral amputation, and 14 cm from olecranon for transradial amputation.[111] If length is insufficient, stumps can be lengthened by distraction osteogenesis techniques at a later date.[112,113] Likewise, if stump length is too long (many high-performance prosthetic feet require 13–15 cm), stump epiphysiodesis may be performed at the appropriate time.[114] Skin grafts, especially those involving a limited surface area, can often be used successfully in children to conserve limb length without compromising wound healing or prosthetic fitting (see Fig. 6.3).[86]

If possible, the articular cartilage at the end of the residual bony segment should be preserved so that potential problems with terminal bony overgrowth are avoided. This overgrowth phenomenon is commonly seen after diaphyseal and metaphyseal amputations in children and may require multiple revision operations.[115] The tibia/fibula, humerus, and femur are prone to stump overgrowth in decreasing order of frequency. Occlusion of the medullary canal by a biologic cap consisting of an osteocartilaginous plug can prevent terminal overgrowth. For below-knee amputations, the first metatarsal, talar dome, iliac crest, or ipsilateral fibular head can be used as a biologic cap (see Figs. 6.2 and 6.3).[116] Such capping is recommended at the time of amputation in children younger than 12 years who are undergoing trans-metaphyseal or transdiaphyseal amputations of the tibia or humerus.

A child's rapid growth and high demand on the prosthetic device make frequent repair and replacement necessary. Moreover, the need for appropriate psychologic and emotional support for the child and family needs to be addressed. The management of children who have undergone amputation is often best accomplished by a multidisciplinary team at a tertiary care center.

ACHIEVING BONE UNION

On the basis of a systematic review of 54 children with type IIIB pediatric open tibial fractures, Glass et al[117] noted a longer healing time and higher rate of complications among adolescents (similar to rates noted in adults) compared with younger children. In children, nonunion of open fractures may occur after substantial bone loss or after major bone resection. However, the thick, active, and highly vascularized periosteum of young children makes bony union possible even in the setting of substantial bone loss. Segmental bone loss in younger children, particularly when most of the periosteum has remained intact, may be adequately managed with external fixation and a variety of auxiliary techniques (see Table 6.4). There are case reports of large defects (up to 10 cm in the humerus) filling in completely when a periosteal sleeve is intact.[118] This underscores the importance of maintaining periosteum and soft tissues if at all possible during surgical débridement with large bone defects. Other authors describe treating a bone defect with external fixator with addition of autogenous cancellous bone graft.[119–121] For larger defects in older children, distraction osteogenesis techniques may be more reliable. The use of bone transport over elastic nails has been reported.[122] Additionally, one case series of type IIIB and IIIC open tibia fractures recommended stabilization with circular external fixator and acute shortening across the injured segment to minimize the need for free-flap coverage.[123] In cases where the soft tissues do not allow enough shortening to create bone apposition, then the limb is shortened as much as possible with subsequent bone transport. Use of transverse incisions and close monitoring of distal circulation when performing acute shortening is recommended. Other methods to help achieve union in patients with segmental bone loss include the recently popularized induced membrane method by Masquelet and others,[119,124] along with more traditional vascularized and nonvascularized structural grafts.[119] In a series

TABLE 6.4   Managing Bone Defects Different Techniques for Management of Bone Defects in Children According to Clinical Variables

	Technique	Common Methods of Skeletal Stabilization	Common Indications
Without supplemental bone graft	Expectant (bone defect fills in via secondary new bone formation)	External or internal fixation	Preserved periosteum overlying the skeletal defect in upper extremity[118]
Bone grafting	Autograft structural (vascularized fibula vs. nonvascularized)	External or internal fixation	Typically for defects 6–10 cm [165]
	Autograft nonstructural (cancellous)	External or internal fixation	Intact periosteum to contain graft
	Masquelet-induced membrane method	External or internal fixation	Periosteum deficient, large defect [125]
Shortening	Acute shortening and stabilization	External fixation (circular preferred)	Soft tissues allow acute shortening. Defect is small, typically <3 cm.[123]
Distraction osteogenesis	Acute shortening, stabilization, with immediate or delayed remote lengthening	External fixation/lengthening nail	Soft tissues allow shortening. Defect is large.[123]
	Stabilization with external fixator and bone transport	External fixation/customized lengthening nail	Soft tissues do not allow complete shortening.[123]

of 27 patients (mean age, 11.4 years; range, 3–16 years) with traumatic diaphyseal bone defects, union was achieved in all patients at a mean of 12.3 months.[119] A systematic review of these procedures showed a 91% rate of bone healing; however, this success is tempered by a 54% complication rate.[125]

FRACTURE FIXATION

GENERAL CONCEPTS

Fixation of the principal fracture fragments reduces pain, prevents additional injuries to surrounding soft tissue, decreases the spread of bacteria, and allows for early soft tissue and bone repair.[1,121,126] With few exceptions, indications for the use of particular fixation methods in open fractures are similar to those for closed injuries. However, when compared with closed fractures, those with severe soft tissue injury are generally less stable, demand prolonged observation, require repeated wound débridement, and are commonly associated with injuries elsewhere. Operative fixation of open fractures is therefore more often indicated than similar fracture patterns that are closed. External and internal fixation techniques allow for easier wound and limb access, facilitate earlier joint mobility and weight-bearing, and reduce the length of the hospital stay as well as the frequency of clinic visits and radiographic evaluation when compared with fracture care in casts or traction. Once a clean wound and a viable soft tissue sleeve have been established, definitive stabilization with a cast, K-wires, a plate (Fig. 6.7), intramedullary fixation, or an external fixator (see Fig. 6.6) should follow.

OPERATIVE METHODS

The broad principles that govern the use of internal and external fixation techniques are similar in children and adults.[120,127,128] However, differences such as open growth plates, an increased capability of remodeling, a faster healing rate, and a diminished ability to cooperate, which are typical in children, clearly affect the choice of an optimal implant for a particular injury. In fact, an implant such as an antegrade piriformis entry interlocked femoral nail that may be optimal for an adult can be entirely unsuitable for a similar fracture in children.[129]

PLATES

The large incisions that are often needed for plate application tend to leave unsightly scars and continue to detract from the use of this technique in children. Increased infection rates are also a persistent concern with the use of plates.[130] These concerns, along with the fact that pediatric fractures may not demand the stability, compression, and anatomic fixation that open plating offers, confer greater popularity to other fixation methods. Less invasive means of plate insertion and newer plate designs for fixation of long bone fractures are gaining popularity[129,131–133] and may avoid some of the disadvantages associated with classic open techniques of plate fixation. Minimally invasive plate osteosynthesis with limited contact locking plates has been an effective treatment for certain open pediatric tibia fractures.[134] Internal fixation may be preferable to external fixation or a cast for unstable open humeral and femoral shaft fractures, particularly in children older than 10 years (see Fig 6.7). Submuscular plating is a reliable technique for treatment of complex, high-energy, length-unstable diaphyseal femur fractures of fractures of the proximal or distal shaft where titanium elastic nails may not confer adequate stability.[135] However, difficulty with plate removal[136] and the possibility of progressive valgus deformities in distal diaphyseal femur fractures treated with submuscular plating[137] should be considered when the fixation implant is chosen.

INTRAMEDULLARY NAILS

In children, elastic intramedullary nails are most often used to stabilize long bone shaft fractures. Flexible stainless steel or titanium rods 1.5 to 4.0 mm in diameter (or 0.4 x diameter of intramedullary canal) are best suited for stable mid-diaphyseal fractures in younger children (see Fig. 6.1).[138,139] Elastic intramedullary nailing of diaphyseal fractures of the femur and tibia allows rapid mobilization, faster return to school, and faster healing than cast immobilization, and is generally well tolerated by the child.[140–142] Compared with plating, use of titanium elastic nails for midshaft femur fractures is associated with shorter operating time, with less blood loss and lower overall cost.[143] However, elastic nails do not provide rigid fixation,[144] especially in older and heavier children, and the extremity may need further protection with a cast or splint. The use of immediate elastic nailing for pediatric open tibial fractures does not appear to increase the rate of postoperative infection or wound complications. However, a prolonged period to bone healing compared with closed fractures has been noted.[145] Pediatric far lateral entry locking nails inserted through the greater trochanteric apophysis are an option for unstable femoral shaft fractures in older children and adolescents, particularly those weighing over 45 kg.[146,147] Far lateral entry nailing does not seem to be associated with avascular necrosis or other growth abnormalities around the proximal femur.[147] Standard locking nails that are inserted through the piriformis fossa, however, are contraindicated in those with open proximal femoral physis because of the potential risk of avascular necrosis of the femoral head.[129] In a retrospective cohort study comparing intramedullary nailing and external fixation of 35 open pediatric femur fractures, the external fixator group had a higher refracture rate (26% vs. 0%, $P = .062$) and a greater overall prevalence of complications.[142]

The use of elastic intramedullary nails for managing open forearm fractures (see Fig. 6.1) is also gaining popularity. Whereas Luhmann et al[148] demonstrated superior outcome with elastic nailing compared with cast immobilization after irrigation and débridement for open forearm fractures in children, Greenbaum et al[149] were unable to demonstrate a statistically significant difference between the two groups.

EXTERNAL FIXATION

The well-established principles of damage-control orthopedics can also be applied to children sustaining open long bone fractures.[149,150] External fixators are ideal for managing a variety of open shaft fractures in the immature skeleton, especially in low-resource environments.[151] The pins can be placed away from the injury site and thus do not interfere with débridement or soft tissue reconstruction. Even simple uniplanar fixator constructs are often rigid enough to maintain anatomic alignment and can allow for early weight-bearing. The fast healing times typical of children, application of hydroxyapatite coated half-pins, and judicious use of oral antibiotics for early pin site inflammation have made pin tract complications substantially less frequent. In the early treatment period, the fixator can be replaced by a plate (see Fig. 6.7) or an intramedullary nail, although the possible increased risk of infection needs to be considered.

In older children and adolescents, devices and components designed for adults are well tolerated. However, for smaller children, fixators used for adult wrist fractures or a combination of smaller pins with adult-sized clamps and connecting rods have been useful. The pin diameter should

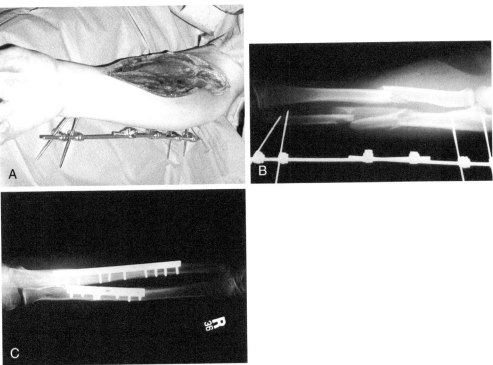

Fig. 6.7 Clinical (A) and radiographic (B) status after initial débridement, right forearm fasciotomies, and restoration of ulnar length and alignment with a temporary external fixator. Three days after the injury, the patient's forearm wound is reevaluated and found to be clean. The right ulna and radius are plated, and the external fixator is removed (C).

not exceed one-third of the diameter of the underlying bone. Pins with diameters ranging from 2.5 to 6.0 mm are commonly used (Fig. 6.8).

Concern about fixator strength and rigidity often leads to oversized two-plane unilateral and two-plane bilateral frame designs.[120,127,152] However, with the exception of obese teenagers, simple one-plane unilateral frames routinely achieve sufficient rigidity for early unsupported weight-bearing.[144] Ring fixators using wires under tension are occasionally indicated for periarticular fractures or comminuted tibial shaft lesions (see Fig. 6.6). At times, they are best applied in delayed fashion after the soft tissue wounds have been covered. The fixators should be kept in place until the fractures have fully healed. Premature removal of the external fixator often leads to secondary angular deformities and should be avoided.[153]

The provision of optimal function and prevention of serious side effects requires consideration of three basic criteria when external fixators are applied: they should not damage vital anatomy,[41] they should provide sufficient

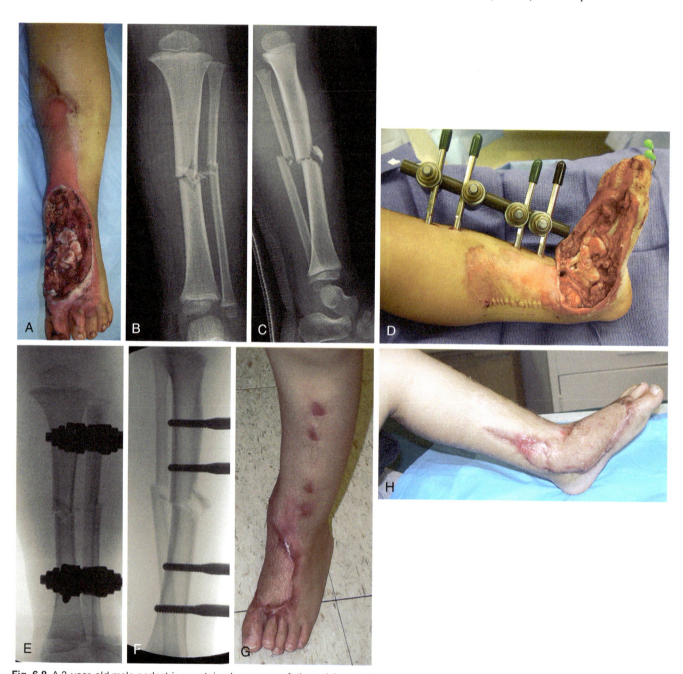

Fig. 6.8 A 3-year-old male pedestrian sustained a severe soft tissue injury to the left foot with exposed bone (A) along with an ipsilateral closed tibial shaft fracture (B and C). Because of the adjacent soft tissue injury, a monolateral external fixator was applied to the tibial fracture so that management of the distal wound would be facilitated. Clinical appearance immediately after application of the external fixator and stabilization of the foot injuries with K-wires (D). Fluoroscopic anteroposterior (E) and lateral (F) views demonstrating placement of the 4.5-mm diameter hydroxyapatite-coated half-pins with satisfactory fracture alignment. Approximately 4 months later, after soft tissue coverage and removal of the external fixator (G and H). (From Bloom T, Sabharwal S. Tibial shaft fractures. In: Herman M, Horn D, eds. *Contemporary Surgical Management of Fractures and Complications in Children.* New Delhi, India: Jaypee Publishers; 2013.)

wound access for the initial débridement and secondary procedures, and the frame should be appropriate to the mechanical demands of the patient and the injury. Simple means of increasing frame stiffness include using larger-diameter pins, spreading the pins in each main bony fragment farther apart, placing the longitudinal rods closer to the bone, double-stacking the rods, and establishing a second pin plane.[152]

As a limb segment in which the principal long bone lies eccentrically, the tibia is ideally suited for the application of an external frame. The safe corridors[127,154] and technique of proper pin insertion for the tibia and femur are well documented.[154] To avoid causing septic arthritis, surgeons should ensure that pins and wires do not penetrate the joint capsule.

External fixators are applied in the operating room under sterile conditions and general anesthesia. The most proximal and distal pins are inserted first under image intensification so that injury to the physes is avoided. This step is followed by insertion of the remaining half-pins, including those for a segmental fragment. An image intensifier is used routinely to check pin location and depth of penetration and overall limb alignment.[41,121,128] The pin holes are predrilled with a sharp drill bit, and a trocar sleeve is inserted to help protect the soft tissue and facilitate accurate placement. Universal articulations that allow for easy alignment are often used. If a simple fixator device with independent articulations is chosen, care must be taken to avoid malrotation, which is difficult to correct after all the pins have been inserted.[41] Once the frame is applied, final fracture alignment is documented on full-length biplanar radiographs of the affected bone. The pin sites are kept clean by washing the leg once daily with warm, soapy water. For younger children, such cleansing is done by the parents, but responsible teenagers can handle this task independently. Unless bone loss has occurred, most patients progress to full weight-bearing and gradually wean off walking aids by 4 to 6 weeks postoperatively.

If healing of a diaphyseal fracture is delayed or a pin becomes infected before the fracture is fully consolidated, one might be tempted to remove the external frame and place the limb in a cast. Unfortunately, this approach frequently leads to secondary deformation of the fracture in the cast and the development of malunion.[153] When faced with delayed union, one option is to keep the fixator in place and support the healing process with an autologous bone graft. Inflamed or infected pins should be managed with improved pin care and a short-term course of oral antibiotics. If this strategy is unsuccessful, the pin should be exchanged, and the frame should be left in place until the fracture has healed. In this author's hands, the use of hydroxyapatite pins and oral antibiotics at the first signs of pin tract infection, along with a simple regimen of washing the pin sites with soap and water once daily, has led to a substantial reduction in pin tract complications. By avoiding oversized and eccentrically placed pins, allowing appropriate dynamization, waiting for clear evidence of union before fixator removal, and protecting the extremity after removal, the orthopedist can minimize the incidence of secondary fractures.[154,155] Monsell et al[156] recently reported on 10 children with high-energy open tibial shaft fractures treated with a programmable circular external fixator.

The mean time in the frame was 16 weeks, and all fractures healed with acceptable alignment and without any deep infections.

SPECIFIC FRACTURE PATTERNS AND LOCATIONS

PERIARTICULAR AND INTRAARTICULAR FRACTURES

After adequate débridement, open intraarticular fractures and epiphyseal injuries are anatomically reduced and stabilized with K-wires or screws. The extremity is then protected with a well-padded splint so that undue force at the fracture site is prevented. Once the soft tissue wound has been closed, a cast is applied until the bone has healed, at which time active range-of-motion exercises are initiated. In the face of a more extensive soft tissue lesion that needs prolonged observation and care, a uniplanar transarticular external fixator is preferable to a splint or cast.

Severe degloving injuries or deep abrasions close to a joint can result in unrecognized injury to the perichondrium with occult physeal injury and peripheral growth arrest causing subsequent angular deformities in young children (Fig. 6.9). Such partial injury to the open growth plate (e.g., type VI physeal fracture) may cause angular deformities with subsequent growth; these children often need further intervention with close follow-up until skeletal maturity (Figs. 6.9 and 6.10).[157,158]

DIAPHYSEAL FRACTURES

In the upper extremity, open shaft fractures with significant soft tissue injury are typically stabilized with skeletal fixation after adequate débridement. In the forearm, insertion of elastic intramedullary nails (see Fig. 6.1) or K-wires have been shown to achieve more anatomic alignment than cast treatment.[148,149] One center reported a 6% incidence of compartment syndrome associated with intramedullary fixation of open forearm fractures in children.[148,149,159] For prevention of infection at the insertion site and refracture, these devices should be buried under the skin and not removed before the underlying bone has fully healed.[160] Although plates can also be used, the need for extensive exposure for hardware insertion and removal, along with the possibility of refracture, make this a less attractive option, especially in children younger than 10 years.

Although open femoral fractures can be managed in traction, this approach is generally inadequate for polytrauma patients and requires a prolonged hospital stay. In most circumstances, operative fracture fixation is preferable in school-age children and adolescents. Based on the extent of soft tissue injury, location of the fracture, comminution, patient's age, and surgeon's experience, a variety of internal and external fixation devices can be used. External fixators that control length, rotation, and angulation can be used reliably for the majority of diaphyseal and metadiaphyseal fractures in all pediatric age groups.[43,128]

Open tibial shaft fractures may be treated with a variety of means, including external fixation, internal fixation, or cast immobilization.[138,161] Although surgery is the mainstay of treatment, some have suggested that a type I open fracture

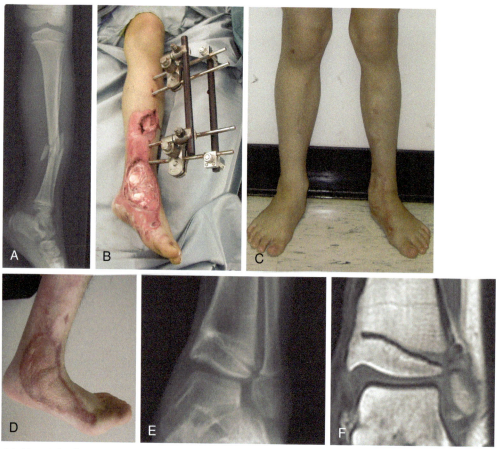

Fig. 6.9 A 5-year-old girl sustained a type IIIA open, comminuted tibial shaft fracture (A) along with severe, deep abrasions of the medial foot and ankle. She underwent an urgent irrigation and débridement of the open wounds and placement of an external fixator for the tibial fracture (B). The medial wound was covered with skin graft 5 days later. The tibial shaft fracture and skin graft healed uneventfully. Clinical appearance of the limb 9 months after injury (C and D). Plain radiograph (E) and MRI (F) 1 year later demonstrating the peripheral bony bar with angular deformity related to the distal tibial physeal injury involving the perichondrium.

with an amenable fracture pattern may be safely treated with irrigation and débridement, and closed reduction and casting with sedation in the emergency department followed by oral antibiotics.[65,162] Children with high-grade open tibial fractures, especially adolescents, have a significantly slower healing rate, a higher complication rate, and high rate of acute compartment syndrome.[10,163] External fixation is particularly helpful in managing high-grade open tibial shaft fractures with extensive comminution and segmental bone loss and degloving injuries around the foot and ankle. Intramedullary fixation with titanium nails is becoming increasingly popular for tibial shaft fractures, and one study showed faster healing with better functional results than external fixation.[141]

PSYCHOSOCIAL FACTORS

Although appropriate orthopedic care of a child with an open fracture or severe extremity injury is of crucial importance, the treating physician must also be aware of the significant psychosocial implications of such an injury. In a study of children sustaining mutilating traumatic injuries, 44% of them continued to experience symptoms of posttraumatic stress disorder, depression, or anxiety 1 year after the incident.[164] Appropriate support services and counseling to the patient and caretakers should be offered in such cases.

> ### Key Points
> Lawn mowers, farm machinery, and ATVs are common causes of mangled extremities in children, and use of these should be discouraged in children.
>
> Even closed fractures may have severe soft tissue injuries.
>
> Thorough treatment of fractures with severe soft tissue injuries includes complete assessment of the injury, timely administration of appropriate antibiotics, fracture stabilization, extensive/repeated wound débridement, soft tissue coverage, and restoration of any bone defects.
>
> High-energy injuries require a high level of suspicion for acute compartment syndrome, which can be difficult to assess in a child.
>
> Depending on the size of the skeletal defects and viability of the surrounding soft tissues, bone defects may fill in with intact periosteum in a young child, or may be managed with autogenous bone grafting, acute shortening, or distraction osteogenesis techniques.

ACKNOWLEDGMENT

The author would like to acknowledge Fred F. Behrens, MD (deceased), for his contributions to earlier versions of this chapter.

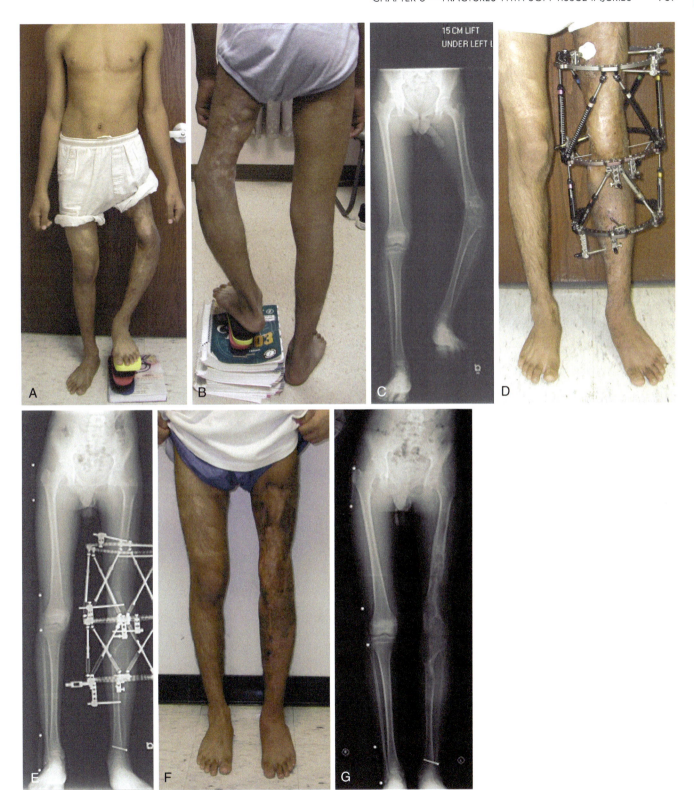

Fig. 6.10 A 15-year-old male was seen from overseas with a severe angular deformity, leg-length discrepancy, and a stiff knee (A–C). At the age of 5 years, he had sustained extensive "deep abrasions" to the thigh in a motor vehicle accident. No obvious fractures were noted at that time. He had subsequently undergone multiple surgeries including several osteotomies for recurrent varus deformity and a knee arthrodesis. The perichondrial injury to the distal femoral growth plate had been unrecognized. He underwent gradual realignment and limb lengthening with the use of a multiplanar external fixator (D) and (E) with substantial improvement of his leg-length discrepancy and limb malalignment (F) and (G).

REFERENCES

1. Patzakis MJ, Wilkins J. Factors influencing infection rate in open fracture wounds. *Clin Orthop Relat Res.* 1989;243:36–40. (**LOE IV**).
2. Skaggs DL, Kautz SM, Kay RM, Tolo VT. Effect of delay of surgical treatment on rate of infection in open fractures in children. *J Pediatr Orthop.* 2000;20(1):19–22. (**LOE III**).
3. Pace JL, Kocher MS, Skaggs DL. Evidence-based review: management of open pediatric fractures. *J Pediatr Orthop.* 2012;32(suppl 2):S123–127. (**LOE IV**).
4. Gougoulias N, Khanna A, Maffulli N. Open tibial fractures in the paediatric population: a systematic review of the literature. *Br Med Bull.* 2009;91:75–85. (**LOE IV**).
5. Hansen ST. Internal fixation of children's fractures of the lower extremity. *Orthop Clin North Am.* 1990;21(2):353–363. (**LOE IV**).
6. Gustilo RB, Mendoza RM, Williams DN. Problems in the management of type III (severe) open fractures: a new classification of type III open fractures. *J Trauma.* 1984;24(8):742–746. (**LOE IV**).
7. Brumback RJ, Jones AL. Interobserver agreement in the classification of open fractures of the tibia. The results of a survey of two hundred and forty-five orthopaedic surgeons.[see comment]. *J Bone Joint Surg Am.* 1994;76(8):1162–1166. (**LOE IV**).
8. Faraj AA. The reliability of the pre-operative classification of open tibial fractures in children a proposal for a new classification. *Acta Orthop Belg.* 2002;68(1):49–55. (**LOE IV**).
9. Horn BD, Rettig ME. Interobserver reliability in the Gustilo and Anderson classification of open fractures. *J Orthop Trauma.* 1993;7(4):357–360. (**LOE IV**).
10. Hope PG, Cole WG. Open fractures of the tibia in children. *J Bone Joint Surg Br.* 1992;74(4):546–553. (**LOE IV**).
11. Skaggs DL, Friend L, Alman B, et al. The effect of surgical delay on acute infection following 554 open fractures in children. *J Bone Joint Surg Am.* 2005;87(1):8–12. (**LOE III**).
12. Gougoulias NE, Khanna A, Maffulin N. Open tibial fractures. Are children small adults? *Hippokratia.* 2009;13(3):147–153. (**LOE IV**).
13. Garay M, Hennrikus WL, Hess J, Lehman EB, Armstrong DG. Lawnmowers versus children: the devastation continues. *Clin Orthop Relat Res.* 2017;475(4):950–356. (**LOE IV**).
14. Laing TA, O'Sullivan JB, Nugent N, O'Shaughnessy M, O'Sullivan ST. Paediatric ride-on mower related injuries and plastic surgical management. *J Plast Reconstr Aesthet Surg.* 2011;64(5):638–642. (**LOE IV**).
15. Park WH, DeMuth WE Jr. Wounding capacity of rotary lawn mowers. *J Trauma.* 1975;15(1):36–38. (**LOE IV**).
16. Loder RT. Demographics of traumatic amputations in children. Implications for prevention strategies. *J Bone Joint Surg Am.* 2004;86-A(5):923–928. (**LOE IV**).
17. Millie M, Senkowski C, Stuart L, Davis F, Ochsner G, Boyd C. Tornado disaster in rural Georgia: triage response, injury patterns, lessons learned. *Am Surg.* 2000;66(3):223–228. (**LOE IV**).
18. MacKenzie JS, Banskota B, Sirisreetreerux N, Shafiq B, Hasenboehler EA. A review of the epidemiology and treatment of orthopaedic injuries after earthquakes in developing countries. *World J Emerg Surg.* 2017;12:9. (**LOE IV**).
19. Bilukha OO, Brennan M, Anderson M. Injuries and deaths from landmines and unexploded ordnance in Afghanistan, 2002-2006. *JAMA.* 2007;298(5):516–518. (**LOE IV**).
20. Bilukha OO, Brennan M, Anderson M. The lasting legacy of war: epidemiology of injuries from landmines and unexploded ordnance in Afghanistan, 2002-2006. *Prehosp Disaster Med.* 2008;23(6):493–499. (**LOE IV**).
21. Can M, Yildirimcan H, Ozkalipci O, et al. Landmine associated injuries in children in Turkey. *J Forensic Leg Med.* 2009;16(8):464–468. (**LOE IV**).
22. Weil YA, Petrov K, Liebergall M, Mintz Y, Mosheiff R. Long bone fractures caused by penetrating injuries in terrorists attacks. *J Trauma.* 2007;62(4):909–912. (**LOE IV**).
23. Edwards MJ, Lustik M, Eichelberger MR, Elster E, Azarow K, Coppola C. Blast injury in children: an analysis from Afghanistan and Iraq, 2002-2010. *J Trauma Acute Care Surg.* 2012;73(5):1278–1283. (**LOE IV**).
24. Sokol KK, Black GE, Azarow KS, Long W, Martin MJ, Eckert MJ. Prehospital interventions in severely injured pediatric patients: rethinking the ABCs. *J Trauma Acute Care Surg.* 2015;79(6):983–989; discussion 9-90. (**LOE IV**).
25. Bendinelli C. Effects of land mines and unexploded ordnance on the pediatric population and comparison with adults in rural Cambodia. *World J Surg.* 2009;33(5):1070–1074. (**LOE IV**).
26. Jaffe DH, Peleg K, Israel Trauma Group. Terror explosive injuries: a comparison of children, adolescents, and adults. *Ann Surg.* 2010;251(1):138–143. (**LOE IV**).
27. Iwaya T, Harii K, Yamada A. Microvascular free flaps for the treatment of avulsion injuries of the feet in children. *J Trauma.* 1982;22(1):15–19. (**LOE IV**).
28. Meland NB, Fisher J, Irons GB, Wood MB, Cooney WP. Experience with 80 rectus abdominis free-tissue transfers. *Plast Reconstr Surg.* 1989;83(3):481–487. (**LOE IV**).
29. Gopal S, Majumder S, Batchelor AG, Knight SL, De Boer P, Smith RM. Fix and flap: the radical orthopaedic and plastic treatment of severe open fractures of the tibia.[see comment]. *J Bone Joint Surg Br.* 2000;82(7):959–966. (**LOE IV**).
30. Georgiadis GM, Behrens FF, Joyce MJ, Earle AS, Simmons AL. Open tibial fractures with severe soft-tissue loss. Limb salvage compared with below-the-knee amputation. *J Bone Joint Surg Am.* 1993;75(10):1431–1441. (**LOE III**).
31. Johansen K, Daines M, Howey T, Helfet D, Hansen ST Jr. Objective criteria accurately predict amputation following lower extremity trauma. *J Trauma.* 1990;30(5):568–572. discussion 72-3. (**LOE IV**).
32. Fagelman MF, Epps HR, Rang M. Mangled extremity severity score in children. *J Pediatr Orthop.* 2002;22(2):182–184.(**LOE IV**).
33. Behdad S, Rafiei MH, Taheri H, et al. Evaluation of mangled extremity severity score (MESS) as a predictor of lower limb amputation in children with trauma. *Eur J Pediatr Surg.* 2012;22(6):465–469. (**LOE IV**).
34. Stewart D, Coombs C, Graham H. Evaluation of mangled extremity severity score (MESS) as a predictor of lower limb amputation in children with trauma. *Eur J Pediatr Surg.* 2013;23(4):333–334. (**LOE IV**).
35. Venkatadass K, Grandhi TSP, Rajasekaran S. Use of Ganga Hospital Open Injury Severity Scoring for determination of salvage versus amputation in open type IIIB injuries of lower limbs in children-An analysis of 52 type IIIB open fractures. *Injury.* 2017;48(11):2509–2514. (**LOE IV**).
36. Anakwenze OA, Trivedi V, Goodman AM, Ganley TJ. Concealed degloving injury (the Morel-Lavallée lesion) in childhood sports: a case report. *J Bone Joint Surg Am.* 2011;93(24):e148. (**LOE IV**).
37. Tscherne H, Gotzen L, eds. *Fractures with Soft Tissue Injuries.* Berlin: Springer-Verlag; 1984.
38. Tseng S, Tornetta P 3rd. Percutaneous management of Morel-Lavallee lesions. *J Bone Joint Surg Am.* 2006;88(1):92–96. (**LOE IV**).
39. Tull F, Borrelli J Jr. Soft-tissue injury associated with closed fractures: evaluation and management. *J Am Acad Orthop Surg.* 2003;11(6):431–438. (**LOE IV**).
40. Rha EY, Kim DH, Kwon H, Jung SN. Morel-lavallee lesion in children. *World J Emerg Surg.* 2013;8(1):60. (**LOE IV**).
41. Alonso JE, Horowitz M. Use of the AO/ASIF external fixator in children. *J Pediatr Orthop.* 1987;7(5):594–600. (**LOE IV**).
42. Anglen JO. Comparison of soap and antibiotic solutions for irrigation of lower-limb open fracture wounds. A prospective, randomized study. *J Bone Joint Surg Am.* 2005;87(7):1415–1422. (**LOE I**).
43. Aronson J, Tursky EA. External fixation of femur fractures in children. *J Pediatr Orthop.* 1992;12(2):157–163. (**LOE IV**).
44. Brown J, Sajankila N, Claridge JA. Prehospital assessment of trauma. *Surg Clin North Am.* 2017;97(5):961–983. (**LOE IV**).
45. Butler FK. Tactical combat casualty care: update 2009. *J Trauma.* 2010;69(suppl 1):S10–13. (**LOE IV**).
46. Butler FK Jr, Blackbourne LH. Battlefield trauma care then and now: a decade of Tactical Combat Casualty Care. *J Trauma Acute Care Surg.* 2-012;73(6 suppl 5):S395–402. (**LOE IV**).
47. Rhee P, Nunley MK, Demetriades D, Velmahos G, Doucet JJ. Tetanus and trauma: a review and recommendations. *J Trauma.* 2005;58(5):1082–1088. (**LOE IV**).
48. Gustilo RB, Merkow RL, Templeman D. The management of open fractures. *J Bone Joint Surg Am.* 1990;72(2):299–304. (**LOE IV**).
49. Gans I, Baldwin KD, Levin LS, et al. A lower extremity musculoskeletal and vascular trauma protocol in a children's hospital may improve treatment response times and appropriate microvascular coverage. *J Orthop Trauma.* 2015;29(5):239–244. (**LOE II**).
50. Merritt K. Factors increasing the risk of infection in patients with open fractures. *J Trauma.* 1988;28(6):823–827. (**LOE IV**).
51. Suedkamp NP, Barbey N, Veuskens A, et al. The incidence of osteitis in open fractures: an analysis of 948 open fractures (a review of the Hannover experience). *J Orthop Trauma.* 1993;7(5):473–482. (**LOE IV**).
52. Stewart DG Jr, Kay RM, Skaggs DL. Open fractures in children. Principles of evaluation and management. *J Bone Joint Surg Am.* 2005;87(12):2784–2798. (**LOE IV**).

53. Rodriguez L, Jung HS, Goulet JA, Cicalo A, Machado-Aranda DA, Napolitano LM. Evidence-based protocol for prophylactic antibiotics in open fractures: improved antibiotic stewardship with no increase in infection rates. *J Trauma Acute Care Surg.* 2014;77(3):400–407; discussion 7-8; quiz 524. **(LOE IV)**.

54. Irwin A, Gibson P, Ashcroft P. Open fractures of the tibia in children. *Injury.* 1995;26(1):21–24. **(LOE IV)**.

55. Centers for Disease Control. Tetanus–United States, 1987 and 1988. *MMWR Morb Mortal Wkly Rep.* 1990;39(3):37–41.

56. Centers for Disease Control and Prevention. Tetanus surveillance–United States, 2001-2008. *MMWR Morb Mortal Wkly Rep.* 2011;60:365–369.

57. Gergen PJ, McQuillan GM, Kiely M, Ezzati-Rice TM, Sutter RW, Virella G. A population-based serologic survey of immunity to tetanus in the United States. *N Engl J Med.* 1995;332(12):761–766. **(LOE IV)**.

58. Brown PW, Kinman PB. Gas gangrene in a metropolitan community. *J Bone Joint Surg Am.* 1974;56(7):1445–1451. **(LOE IV)**.

59. Fee NF, Dobranski A, Bisla RS. Gas gangrene complicating open forearm fractures. Report of five cases. *J Bone Joint Surg Am.* 1977;59(1):135–138. **(LOE IV)**.

60. Jaeger M, Maier D, Kern WV, Sudkamp NP. Antibiotics in trauma and orthopedic surgery – a primer of evidence-based recommendations. *Injury.* 2006;37(suppl 2):S74–80. **(LOE IV)**.

61. Isaac SM, Woods A, Danial IN, Mourkus H. Antibiotic prophylaxis in adults with open tibial fractures: what is the evidence for duration of administration? A systematic review. *J Foot Ankle Surg.* 2016;55(1):146–150. **(LOE II)**

62. Iobst CA, Tidwell MA, King WF. Nonoperative management of pediatric type I open fractures. *J Pediatr Orthop.* 2005;25(4):513–517. **(LOE IV)**.

63. Schlitzkus LL, Goetler CE, Waibel BH, et al. Open fractures: it doesn't come out in the wash. *Surg Infect (Larchmt).* 2011;12(5):359–363. **(LOE IV)**.

64. Werner CM, Pierpont Y, Pollak AN. The urgency of surgical débridement in the management of open fractures. *J Am Acad Orthop Surg.* 2008;16(7):369–375. **(LOE IV)**.

65. Bazzi AA, Brooks JT, Jain A, Ain MC, Tis JE, Sponseller PD. Is nonoperative treatment of pediatric type I open fractures safe and effective? *J Child Orthop.* 2014;8(6):467–471. **(LOE IV)**.

66. Doak J, Ferrick M. Nonoperative management of pediatric grade 1 open fractures with less than a 24-hour admission. *J Pediatr Orthop.* 2009;29(1):49–51. **(LOE IV)**.

67. Wetzel RJ, Minhas SV, Patrick BC, Janicki JA. Current practice in the management of type I open fractures in children: a survey of POSNA membership. *J Pediatr Orthop.* 2015;35(7):762–768. **(LOE IV)**.

68. Khatod M, Botte MJ, Hoyt DB, Meyer RS, Smith JM, Akeson WH. Outcomes in open tibia fractures: relationship between delay in treatment and infection. *J Trauma.* 2003;55(5):949–954. **(LOE IV)**.

69. Kreder HJ, Armstrong P. A review of open tibia fractures in children. *J Pediatr Orthop.* 1995;15(4):482–488. **(LOE IV)**.

70. Lavelle WF, Uhl R, Krieves M, Drvaric DM. Management of open fractures in pediatric patients: current teaching in Accreditation Council for Graduate Medical Education (ACGME) accredited residency programs. *J Pediatr Orthop B.* 2008;17(1):1–6. **(LOE IV)**.

71. Owens BD, Wenke JC. Early wound irrigation improves the ability to remove bacteria. *J Bone Joint Surg Am.* 2007;89(8):1723–1726. **(LOE IV)**.

72. Yammine K, Harvey A. Efficacy of preparation solutions and cleansing techniques on contamination of the skin in foot and ankle surgery: a systematic review and meta-analysis. *Bone Joint J.* 2013;95-B(4):498–503. **(LOE I)**.

73. FLOW Investigators, Petrisor B, Sun X, et al. Fluid lavage of open wounds (FLOW): a multicenter, blinded, factorial pilot trial comparing alternative irrigating solutions and pressures in patients with open fractures. *J Trauma.* 2011;71(3):596–606. **(LOE I)**.

74. Sprague S, Petrisor B, Jeray K, et al. Wound irrigation does not affect health-related quality of life after open fractures: results of a randomized controlled trial. *Bone Joint J.* 2018;100-B(1):88–94. **(LOE IV)**.

75. FLOW Investigators, Bhandari M, Jeray KJ, et al. A trial of wound irrigation in the initial management of open fracture wounds. *N Engl J Med.* 2015;373(27):2629–2641. **(LOE I)**.

76. Decoster TA, Bozorgnia S. Antibiotic beads. *J Am Acad Orthop Surg.* 2008;16(11):674–678. **(LOE IV)**.

77. Ostermann PA, Seligson D, Henry SL. Local antibiotic therapy for severe open fractures. A review of 1085 consecutive cases. *J Bone Joint Surg Br.* 1995;77(1):93–97. **(LOE IV)**.

78. Halvorson J, Jinnah R, Kulp B, Frino J. Use of vacuum-assisted closure in pediatric open fractures with a focus on the rate of infection. *Orthopedics.* 2011;34(7):e256–e260. **(LOE IV)**.

79. Stannard JP, Volgas DA, Stewart R, McGwin G Jr, Alonso JE. Negative pressure wound therapy after severe open fractures: a prospective randomized study. *J Orthop Trauma.* 2009;23(8): 552–527. **(LOE I)**.

80. Contractor D, Amling J, Brandoli C, Tosi LL. Negative pressure wound therapy with reticulated open cell foam in children: an overview. *J Orthop Trauma.* 2008;22(suppl 10):S167–S176. **(LOE IV)**.

81. Kreder HJ, Armstrong P. The significance of perioperative cultures in open pediatric lower-extremity fractures. *Clin Orthop Relat Res.* 1994;(302):206–212. **(LOE IV)**.

82. Valenziano CP, Chattar-Cora D, O'Neill A, Hubli EH, Cudjoe EA. Efficacy of primary wound cultures in long bone open extremity fractures: are they of any value? *Arch Orthop Trauma Surg.* 2002;122(5):259–261. **(LOE IV)**.

83. D'Souza A, Rajagopalan N, Amaravati RS. The use of qualitative cultures for detecting infection in open tibial fractures. *J Orthop Surg (Hong Kong).* 2008;16(2):175–8. **(LOE IV)**.

84. Rao P, Schaverien MV, Stewart KJ. Soft tissue management of children's open tibial fractures–a review of seventy children over twenty years. *Ann R Coll Surg Engl.* 2010;92(4):320–325. **(LOE IV)**.

85. Stewart KJ, Tytherleigh-Strong G, Bharathwaj S, Quaba AA. The soft tissue management of children's open tibial fractures. *J R Coll Surg Edinb.* 1999;44(1):24–30. **(LOE IV)**.

86. Dedmond BT, Davids JR. Function of skin grafts in children following acquired amputation of the lower extremity. *J Bone Joint Surg Am.* 2005;87(5):1054–1058. **(LOE IV)**.

87. Sagi HC, Papp S, Dipasquale T. The effect of suture pattern and tension on cutaneous blood flow as assessed by laser Doppler flowmetry in a pig model. *J Orthop Trauma.* 2008;22(3):171–175. **(LOE IV)**.

88. Glass GE, Pearse MF, Nanchahal J. Improving lower limb salvage following fractures with vascular injury: a systematic review and new management algorithm. *J Plast Reconstr Aesthet Surg.* 2009;62(5):571–579. **(LOE IV)**.

89. DeLee JC, Stiehl JB. Open tibia fracture with compartment syndrome. *Clin Orthop Relat Res.* 1981;160:175–184. **(LOE IV)**.

90. McQueen MM, Duckworth AD, Aitken SA, Sharma RA, Court-Brown CM. Predictors of compartment syndrome after tibial fracture. *J Orthop Trauma.* 2015;29(10):451–455. **(LOE IV)**.

91. Livingston K, Glotzbecker M, Miller PE, Hresko MT, Hedequist D, Shore BJ. Pediatric nonfracture acute compartment syndrome: a review of 39 cases. *J Pediatr Orthop.* 2016;36(7):685–690. **(LOE IV)**.

92. Flynn JM, Bashyal RK, Yeger-McKeever M, Garner MR, Launay F, Sponseller PD. Acute traumatic compartment syndrome of the leg in children: diagnosis and outcome. *J Bone Joint Surg Am.* 2011;93(10):937–941. **(LOE IV)**.

93. Livingston KS, Glotzbecker MP, Shore BJ. Pediatric acute compartment syndrome. *J Am Acad Orthop Surg.* 2017;25(5):358–364. **(LOE IV)**.

94. Noonan KJ, McCarthy JJ. Compartment syndromes in the pediatric patient. *J Pediatr Orthop.* 2010;30(suppl 2):S96–S101. **(LOE IV)**.

95. Ferlic PW, Singer G, Kraus T, Eberl R. The acute compartment syndrome following fractures of the lower leg in children. *Injury.* 2012;43(10):1743–1746. **(LOE IV)**.

96. Potter BK, Freedman BA, Shuler MS. Fasciotomy wound management and closure. *Tech Orthop.* 2012;27:62–66. **(LOE IV)**.

97. Kirkilas M, Notrica DM, Langlais CS, Muenzer JT, Zoldos J, Graziano K. Outcomes of arterial vascular extremity trauma in pediatric patients. *J Pediatr Surg.* 2016;51(11):1885–1890. **(LOE IV)**.

98. Letton RW, Chwals WJ. Patterns of power mower injuries in children compared with adults and the elderly. *J Trauma.* 1994;37(2):182–186. **(LOE IV)**.

99. Letts M, Davidson D. Epidemiology and prevention of traumatic amputations in children. *Child with a Limb Deficiency.* 1998:235–251. **(LOE IV)**.

100. Borne A, Porter A, Recicar J, Maxson T, Montgomery C. Pediatric traumatic amputations in the United States: a 5-year review. *J Pediatr Orthop.* 2017;37(2):e104–e107. **(LOE IV)**.

101. Hill SM, Elwood ET. Pediatric lower extremity mower injuries. *Ann Plast Surg.* 2011;67(3):279–287 **(LOE IV)**.

102. Conway AE, McClune AJ, Nosel P. Down on the farm: preventing farm accidents in children. *Pediatr Nurs.* 2007;33(1):45–48. **(LOE IV)**.

103. Gilliam JM, Jones PJ, Field WE, Kraybill DB, Scott SE. Farm-related injuries among Old Order Anabaptist children: developing a baseline from which to formulate and assess future prevention strategies. *J Agromedicine.* 2007;12(3):11–23. **(LOE IV)**.

104. Kellum E, Creek A, Dawkins R, Bernard M, Sawyer JR. Age-related patterns of injury in children involved in all-terrain vehicle accidents. *J Pediatr Orthop.* 2008;28(8):854–858. **(LOE IV).**

105. Loder RT, Brown KL, Zaleske DJ, Jones ET. Extremity lawn-mower injuries in children: report by the Research Committee of the Pediatric Orthopaedic Society of North America. *J Pediatr Orthop.* 1997;17(3):360–369. **(LOE IV).**

106. Trautwein LC, Smith DG, Rivara FP. Pediatric amputation injuries: etiology, cost, and outcome. *J Trauma.* 1996;41(5):831–838. **(LOE IV).**

107. Lovejoy S, Weiss JM, Epps HR, Zionts LE, Gaffney J. Preventable childhood injuries. *J Pediatr Orthop.* 2012;32(7):741–747. **(LOE IV).**

108. Nguyen A, Raymond S, Morgan V, Peters J, Macgill K, Johnstone B. Lawn mower injuries in children: a 30-year experience. *ANZ J Surg.* 2008;78(9):759–763. **(LOE IV).**

109. American Academy of Pediatrics. Lawn mower safety tips from the American Academy of Pediatrics. https://www.aap.org/en-us/about-the-aap/aap-press-room/news-features-and-safety-tips/Pages/Lawn-Mower-Safety-Tips-from-the-AAP.aspx. Accessed August 16, 2019. **(LOE V).**

110. Bondurant FJ, Cotler HB, Buckle R, Miller-Crotchett P, Browner BD. The medical and economic impact of severely injured lower extremities. *J Trauma.* 1988;28(8):1270–1273. **(LOE IV).**

111. Khan MA, Javed AA, Rao DJ, Corner JA, Rosenfield P. Pediatric traumatic limb amputation: the principles of management and optimal residual limb lengths. *World J Plast Surg.* 2016;5(1):7–14. **(LOE IV).**

112. Bowen RE, Struble SG, Setoguchi Y, Watts HG. Outcomes of lengthening short lower-extremity amputation stumps with planar fixators. *J Pediatr Orthop.* 2005;25(4):543–547. **(LOE IV).**

113. Mertens P, Lammens J. Short amputation stump lengthening with the Ilizarov method: risks versus benefits. *Acta Orthop Belg.* 2001;67(3):274–278. **(LOE IV).**

114. Osebold WR, Lester EL, Christenson DM. Problems with excessive residual lower leg length in pediatric amputees. *Iowa Orthop J.* 2001;21:58–67. **(LOE IV).**

115. Davids JR, Meyer LC, Blackhurst DW. Operative treatment of bone overgrowth in children who have an acquired or congenital amputation. *J Bone Joint Surg Am.* 1995;77(10):1490–1497. **(LOE IV).**

116. Fedorak GT, Watts HG, Cuomo AV, et al. Osteocartilaginous transfer of the proximal part of the fibula for osseous overgrowth in children with congenital or acquired tibial amputation: surgical technique and results. *J Bone Joint Surg Am.* 2015;97(7):574–581. **(LOE IV).**

117. Glass GE, Pearse M, Nanchahal J. The ortho-plastic management of Gustilo grade IIIB fractures of the tibia in children: a systematic review of the literature. *Injury.* 2009;40(8):876–879. **(LOE IV).**

118. Wimberly RL, Wilson PL, Ezaki M, Martin BD, Riccio AI. Segmental metadiaphyseal humeral bone loss in pediatric trauma patients: a case series. *J Pediatr Orthop.* 2014;34(4):400–404. **(LOE IV).**

119. Sales de Gauzy J, Fitoussi F, Jouve JL, et al. Traumatic diaphyseal bone defects in children. *Orthop Traumatol Surg Res.* 2012;98(2):220–226. **(LOE IV).**

120. Tolo VT. External skeletal fixation in children's fractures. *J Pediatr Orthop.* 1983;3(4):435–442. **(LOE IV).**

121. Behrens F. External fixation in children: lower extremity. *Instr Course Lect.* 1990;39:205–208. **(LOE IV).**

122. Popkov D, Popkov A, Haumont T, Journeau P, Lascombes P. Flexible intramedullary nail use in limb lengthening. *J Pediatr Orthop.* 2010;30(8):910–918. **(LOE IV).**

123. Laine JC, Cherkashin A, Samchukov M, Birch JG, Rathjen KE. The Management of soft tissue and bone loss in type IIIB and IIIC pediatric open tibia fractures. *J Pediatr Orthop.* 2016;36(5):453–458. **(LOE IV).**

124. Taylor BC, French BG, Fowler TT, Russell J, Poka A. Induced membrane technique for reconstruction to manage bone loss. *J Am Acad Orthop Surg.* 2012;20(3):142–150. **(LOE IV).**

125. Morelli I, Drago L, George DA, Romano D, Romano CL. Managing large bone defects in children: a systematic review of the 'induced membrane technique'. *J Pediatr Orthop B.* 2017. **(LOE IV).**

126. Merritt K, Dowd JD. Role of internal fixation in infection of open fractures: studies with Staphylococcus aureus and Proteus mirabilis. *J Orthop Res.* 1987;5(1):23–28. **(LOE IV).**

127. Behrens F, Searls K. External fixation of the tibia. Basic concepts and prospective evaluation. *J Bone Joint Surg Br.* 1986;68(2):246–254. **(LOE IV).**

128. Sabharwal S. Role of Ilizarov external fixator in the management of proximal/distal metadiaphyseal pediatric femur fractures. *J Orthop Trauma.* 2005;19(8):563–569. **(LOE IV).**

129. Flynn JM, Schwend RM. Management of pediatric femoral shaft fractures. *J Am Acad Orthop Surg.* 2004;12(5):347–359. **(LOE IV).**

130. Song KM, Sangeorzan B, Benirschke S, Browne R. Open fractures of the tibia in children. *J Pediatr Orthop.* 1996;16(5):635–639. **(LOE IV).**

131. Hedequist DJ, Sink E. Technical aspects of bridge plating for pediatric femur fractures. *J Orthop Trauma.* 2005;19(4):276–279. **(LOE IV).**

132. Kanlic EM, Anglen JO, Smith DG, Morgan SJ, Pesantez RF. Advantages of submuscular bridge plating for complex pediatric femur fractures. *Clin Orthop.* 2004;426:244–251. **(LOE IV).**

133. Sink EL, Faro F, Polousky J, Flynn K, Gralla J. Decreased complications of pediatric femur fractures with a change in management. *J Pediatr Orthop.* 2010;30(7):633–637. **(LOE III).**

134. Ozkul E, Gem M, Arslan H, Alemdr C, Azboy I, Arslan SG. Minimally invasive plate osteosynthesis in open pediatric tibial fractures. *J Pediatr Orthop.* 2016;36(4):416–422. **(LOE IV).**

135. Abdelgawad AA, Sieg RN, Laughlin MD, Shunia J, Kanlic EM. Submuscular bridge plating for complex pediatric femur fractures is reliable. *Clin Orthop Relat Res.* 2013;471(9):2797–2807. **(LOE IV).**

136. Pate O, Hedequist D, Leong N, Hresko T. Implant removal after submuscular plating for pediatric femur fractures. *J Pediatr Orthop.* 2009;29(7):709–712. **(LOE IV).**

137. Heyworth BE, Hedequist DJ, Nasreddine AY, Stamoulis C, Hresko MT, Yen YM. Distal femoral valgus deformity following plate fixation of pediatric femoral shaft fractures. *J Bone Joint Surg Am.* 2013;95(6):526–533. **(LOE IV).**

138. Flynn JM, Skaggs D, Sponseller PD, Ganley TJ, Kay RM, Leitch KK. The operative management of pediatric fractures of the lower extremity. *J Bone Joint Surg Am.* 2002;84(12):2288–2300. **(LOE IV).**

139. Heinrich SD, Drvaric DM, Darr K, MacEwen GD. The operative stabilization of pediatric diaphyseal femur fractures with flexible intramedullary nails: a prospective analysis. *J Pediatr Orthop.* 1994;14(4):501–507. **(LOE IV).**

140. Bar-On E, Sagiv S, Porat S. External fixation or flexible intramedullary nailing for femoral shaft fractures in children. A prospective, randomised study.[see comment][erratum appears in *J Bone Joint Surg Br.* 1998 Jul;80(4):749]. *J Bone Joint Surg Br.* 1997;79(6):975–978. **(LOE I).**

141. Kubiak EN, Egol KA, Scher D, Wasserman B, Feldman D, Koval KJ. Operative treatment of tibial fractures in children: are elastic stable intramedullary nails an improvement over external fixation? *J Bone Joint Surg Am.* 2005;87(8):1761–1768. **(LOE III).**

142. Ramseier LE, Bhaskar AR, Cole WG, Howard AW. Treatment of open femur fractures in children: comparison between external fixator and intramedullary nailing. *J Pediatr Orthop.* 2007;27(7):748–750. **(LOE III).**

143. Allen JD, Murr K, Albitar F, Jacobs C, Moghadamian ES, Muchow R. Titanium elastic nailing has superior value to plate fixation of midshaft femur fractures in children 5 to 11 years. *J Pediatr Orthop.* 2018;38(3):e111–e117. **(LOE III).**

144. Mani US, Sabatino CT, Sabharwal S, Svach DJ, Suslak A, Behrens FF. Biomechanical comparison of flexible stainless steel and titanium nails with external fixation using a femur fracture model. *J Pediatr Orthop.* 2006;26(2):182–187. **(LOE III).**

145. Pandya NK, Edmonds EW. Immediate intramedullary flexible nailing of open pediatric tibial shaft fractures. *J Pediatr Orthop.* 2012;32(8):770–776. **(LOE III).**

146. Gordon JE, Khanna N, Luhmann SJ, Dobbs MB, Ortman MR, Schoenecker PL. Intramedullary nailing of femoral fractures in children through the lateral aspect of the greater trochanter using a modified rigid humeral intramedullary nail: preliminary results of a new technique in 15 children. *J Orthop Trauma.* 2004;18(7):416–422; discussion 23-24. **(LOE IV).**

147. Miller DJ, Kelly DM, Spence DD, Beaty JH, Warner WC Jr, Sawyer JR. Locked intramedullary nailing in the treatment of femoral shaft fractures in children younger than 12 years of age: indications and preliminary report of outcomes. *J Pediatr Orthop.* 2012;32(8):777–780. **(LOE IV).**

148. Luhmann SJ, Schootman M, Schoenecker PL, Dobbs MB, Gordon JE. Complications and outcomes of open pediatric forearm fractures. *J Pediatr Orthop.* 2004;24(1):1–6. **(LOE IV).**

149. Greenbaum B, Zionts LE, Ebramzadeh E. Open fractures of the forearm in children. *J Orthop Trauma.* 2001;15(2):111–118. **(LOE IV).**

150. Mooney JF. The use of 'damage control orthopedics' techniques in children with segmental open femur fractures. *J Pediatr Orthop B*. 2012;21(5):400–403. **(LOE IV)**.

151. Eichinger JK, McKenzie CS, Devine JG. Evaluation of pediatric lower extremity fractures managed with external fixation: outcomes in a deployed environment. *Am J Orthop (Belle Mead NJ)*. 2012;41(1):15–19. **(LOE IV)**.

152. Behrens F, Johnson W. Unilateral external fixation. Methods to increase and reduce frame stiffness. *Clin Orthop Relat Res*. 1989;241:48–56. **(LOE IV)**.

153. Holbrook JL, Swiontkowski MF, Sanders R. Treatment of open fractures of the tibial shaft: ender nailing versus external fixation. A randomized, prospective comparison. *J Bone Joint Surg Am*. 1989;71(8):1231–1238. **(LOE II)**.

154. Sabharwal S, Kishan S, Behrens F. Principles of external fixation of the femur. *Am J Orthop*. 2005;34(5):218–223. **(LOE IV)**.

155. Skaggs DL, Leet AI, Money MD, Shaw BA, Hale JM, Tolo VT. Secondary fractures associated with external fixation in pediatric femur fractures. *J Pediatr Orthop*. 1999;19(5):582–586. **(LOE IV)**.

156. Monsell FP, Howells NR, Lawniczak D, Jeffcote B, Mitchell SR. High-energy open tibial fractures in children: treatment with a programmable circular external fixator. *J Bone Joint Surg Br*. 2012;94(7):989–993. **(LOE IV)**.

157. Abbo O, Accadbled F, Laffosse JM, De Gauzy JS. Reconstruction and anticipatory Langenskiöld procedure in traumatic defect of tibial medial malleolus with type 6 physeal fracture. *J Pediatr Orthop B*. 2012;21(5):434–438. **(LOE IV)**.

158. Havranek P, Pesl T. Salter (Rang) type 6 physeal injury. *Eur J Pediatr Surg*. 2010;20(3):174–177. **(LOE IV)**.

159. Yuan PS, Pring ME, Gaynor TP, Mubarak SJ, Newton PO. Compartment syndrome following intramedullary fixation of pediatric forearm fractures. *J Pediatr Orthop*. 2004;24(4):370–375. **(LOE IV)**.

160. Shoemaker SD, Comstock CP, Mubarak SJ, Wenger DR, Chambers HG. Intramedullary Kirschner wire fixation of open or unstable forearm fractures in children. *J Pediatr Orthop*. 1999;19(3):329–337. **(LOE IV)**.

161. Buckley SL, Smith GR, Sponseller PD, Thompson JD, Robertson WW Jr, Griffin PP. Severe (type III) open fractures of the tibia in children. *J Pediatr Orthop*. 1996;16(5):627–634. **(LOE IV)**.

162. Godfrey J, Choi PD, Shabtai L, et al. Management of pediatric type I open fractures in the emergency department or operating room: a multicenter perspective. *J Pediatr Orthop*. 2017. **(LOE III)**.

163. Grimard G, Naudie D, Laberge LC, Hamdy RC. Open fractures of the tibia in children. *Clin Orthop*. 1996;(332):62–70. **(LOE IV)**.

164. Rusch MD, Grunert BK, Sanger JR, Dzwierzynski WW, Matloub HS. Psychological adjustment in children after traumatic disfiguring injuries: a 12-month follow-up. *Plast Reconstr Surg*. 2000;106(7):1451–1458; discussion 9-60. **(LOE IV)**.

165. El-Sayed M, El-Hadidi M, El-Adl W. Free non-vascularised fibular graft for treatment of post-traumatic bone defects. *Acta Orthop Belg*. 2007;73(1):70–76. **(LOE IV)**.

7 Complications of Fractures in Children

Elizabeth W. Hubbard | Anthony I. Riccio

VASCULAR INJURIES

Overall, vascular trauma is relatively uncommon in pediatric patients. One study reviewed all pediatric patients who presented to a level 1 trauma institution over a 6-year period and found that only 23 presented with a major arterial injury.[1] Other studies have shown that these admissions account for less than 1% of all pediatric trauma admissions. However, 58% of neurovascular injuries in children are associated with orthopedic injuries.[2] Typically, the artery involved is near the fracture. For example, the common femoral artery is at risk with intertrochanteric fractures of the hip and hip dislocation, and the superficial and profunda femoral arteries are at risk with subtrochanteric and midshaft fractures.[3] The femoral artery can be injured at the adductor hiatus by a supracondylar femoral fracture.[4] Injury to the popliteal artery or to a combination of the anterior and posterior tibial arteries is usually associated with fracture of the distal femoral (Fig. 7.1) or proximal tibial epiphysis, or a knee dislocation (32%–64%).[3,5] It is critical that the orthopedist have a high index of suspicion for vascular injury in pediatric trauma patients, because of the association between vascular injury and orthopedic trauma as well as the potentially devastating complications associated with delayed treatment of a vascular injury.

As in adults, massive bleeding and arterial hemorrhaging can occur in children with pelvic fractures. In one study, the mortality rate was 5% in children and 17% in adults. The fracture patterns are usually a combination of anterior and posterior injuries to the pelvic ring, either unilateral or bilateral.[6–8] O'Neill and colleagues noted that posterior arterial bleeding (internal iliac and posterior branches) was more common in patients with unstable posterior pelvic fractures, whereas anterior arterial bleeding through the pudendal and obturator arteries was more often associated with lateral compression injuries.[9] Injury to the superior gluteal artery was the most common injury associated with posterior pelvic fractures. Angiography to identify the arterial hemorrhage and embolization to control bleeding have been helpful.[8,10] Similarly, skeletal fixation to reduce the fracture can help control bleeding in pediatric patients at high risk of life-threatening hemorrhages.[8]

One typically associates vascular injuries with extremity or pelvic trauma. However, Tolhurst and colleagues documented an 11% incidence of cervical vascular injury in 61 patients evaluated for blunt cervical trauma.[11] Central thoracic and abdominal vascular injuries have also been associated with blunt motor vehicle trauma.[12]

The usual signs of vascular compromise are (1) absent distal pulses, (2) decreased skin temperature, and (3) poor skin circulation with diminished capillary and venous filling distal to the injury.[13] In the setting of lower extremity trauma, particularly knee dislocations or severely displaced distal femoral and/or proximal tibial physeal fractures, the ankle brachial index (ABI) is a critical component of the physical examination in the trauma bay. In this setting, palpable distal pulses and an ABI of 0.9 or higher has been shown to be 100% sensitive for detecting an arterial injury.[14] Displaced fracture and/or joint dislocations associated with suspected vascular injury should be emergently and safely reduced, either in the emergency department or in the operative theater. Angiogram or vascular ultrasound studies should be considered whenever vascular injury is suspected, especially if concerns for vascular injury persist after fracture and/or joint reduction. Absolute indications for vascular imaging are a diminished or absent pulse, a large or expanding hematoma, external bleeding, unexplained hypotension, or a bruit. Evidence of a peripheral nerve injury should also raise suspicion for an associated vascular insult.[15] If the period of extremity ischemia approaches 6 hours, operative exploration should proceed immediately, and it may be necessary to obtain vascular imaging in the operating room.[16]

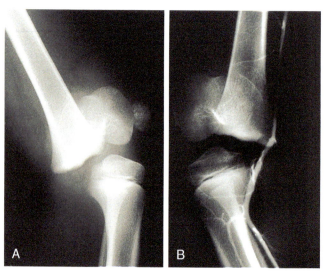

Fig. 7.1 (A) Supracondylar fracture of the femur in an 8-year-old boy with complete displacement of the distal femoral epiphysis. Decreased pulses and this fracture pattern are suggestive of a vascular injury. (B) An arteriogram demonstrates attenuation of the popliteal artery, but it is still intact. The fracture was reduced and fixed with crossed pins; subsequent premature growth arrest occurred.

Pulses may initially be palpable and then disappear (delayed loss of pulse). Such delayed loss is usually caused by damage to the intima with subsequent development of thrombosis.[4] Damage to the popliteal artery from a knee dislocation is commonly limited to the intima.[3,17,18] In children, intimal damage is often more extensive than apparent on simple inspection.[19] Children are particularly prone to ischemia because of arterial spasm, which is less common in adults. The patient should undergo further evaluation for vascular injury if the pulse does not return after reduction of the fracture or dislocation (Fig. 7.2).[4] One study of 116 patients with knee dislocations found that 90% of those who had abnormal pulses after joint reduction had associated vascular injuries found on arteriography.[20] Observation of a warm, pulseless leg after dislocation of the knee is insufficient. Frequently, these patients have good capillary flow because the amount of flow required to maintain viability of the skin and subcutaneous tissue is much less than that required by muscle.[3] In these circumstances, Green and Allen reported that 90% of the limbs either eventually underwent amputation or had claudication or incapacitating muscle fibrosis and contracture.[3]

In general, the indications for limb salvage are extended in children because of their greater capacity for healing; however, no data have established the limits of salvage. Of all limbs, 90% can be salvaged if the circulation is reestablished within 6 hours, whereas revascularization after 8 hours from the time of injury can result in an amputation rate of 72% to 90%.[3,17] With massive crush injuries and collateral vessel damage, the 6-hour period of warm ischemia may be too long because of the risk for associated muscle injury and rhabdomyoloysis.[13] One must also consider the seriousness of associated polytrauma, the degree of damage to the ipsilateral foot, the time required to obtain soft tissue coverage and bone healing, and the potential for rehabilitation.[13] The Mangled Extremity Severity Score can be helpful in determining prognosis of limb salvage in pediatric patients.[21]

In children, autogenous vein grafts are recommended rather than synthetic or bovine material because these types of grafts have been shown to not work well over long-term follow-up in children.[1,22] Spatulation of the ends of the vessels and using interrupted rather than running suture repair techniques allow for a longer suture line that will accommodate a later increase in vessel size without stricture.[1] In contradistinction to proximal injuries, isolated single vessel injuries distal to the elbow or knee may, on occasion, be treated by vessel ligation.[23]

Distal compartment syndromes are common after late diagnosis or repair of vascular injuries. Fasciotomy should be considered after vascular repair so that a late compartment syndrome is avoided. Patients should be monitored in the early postoperative period for myoglobinuria or a rise in creatinine or phosphokinase levels. Signs and symptoms of renal insufficiency should also be sought because both are consistent with the diagnosis of rhabdomyolysis.[23] In the lower extremity, repair of a proximal artery may not result in saving the entire limb but may preserve the knee, which has important functional implications when considering walking speed and energy cost of ambulating with a prosthesis.[24]

Fracture stabilization can be accomplished by a variety of means. Ideally, if time permits, reduction and fixation of the fracture should precede vascular repair. Initial bony fixation provides maximal skeletal stability and reduces further trauma to the soft tissues, nerves, and collateral blood vessels. Similarly, surgical repair of nerve lacerations is facilitated by bony stabilization. If soft tissue coverage can be achieved, internal fixation is preferred.[25] External fixation, particularly in a severely traumatized limb, has many advantages, including a short operative time. Zehntner and colleagues found that complications were less frequent with initial external fixation of lower extremity fractures than with internal fixation.[26] Indwelling arterial and venous shunts can be helpful in selected cases for reduction of the risk of further vessel damage and compartment syndrome.[2,13] Similarly, temporary shunting can provide a satisfactory solution to the clinical problem of whether an ischemic limb should be revascularized before fracture fixation.[2,16,27] Surgical shortening of the bone may facilitate vascular repair, and the leg length discrepancy can be resolved at a later time.

Early complications include wound infection, below-knee amputation, deep vein thrombosis, and motor and sensory deficits.[17] Revascularization does not eliminate the possibility of abnormal growth (i.e., overgrowth and undergrowth). All children should be monitored for limb length discrepancy until limb lengths stabilize.[22] Discrepancies that do not stabilize over time can be addressed through either a contralateral properly timed epiphysiodesis, ipsilateral limb lengthening, or a combination of the two to achieve equal limb lengths at skeletal maturity. In addition, as the child ages, the collateral circulation may not be adequate to meet the increased physiologic demands, ischemia-like symptoms may be triggered by activity, and subsequent arterial reconstruction for chronic vascular insufficiency is sometimes required.[28]

VASCULAR INJURIES ASSOCIATED WITH SUPRACONDYLAR FRACTURES OF THE HUMERUS

Vascular injury is the most serious complication associated with supracondylar fractures; fortunately, it is

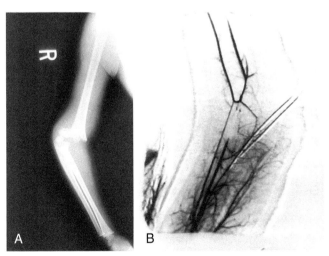

Fig. 7.2 (A) Supracondylar fracture of the humerus in a 7-year-old patient with absent pulses despite satisfactory reduction and pinning. (B) Arteriogram demonstrating good collateral circulation but a complete block of the brachial artery. The artery was explored, an intimal flap was found and resected, and a successful end-to-end anastomosis was performed.

uncommon.[29–31] If the child has a pulseless extremity, the fracture should be reduced immediately in an attempt to restore blood supply and avoid compartmental ischemia (see Fig. 7.2).[4] Campbell and colleagues found a brachial artery injury in 38% of patients who had severe posterior lateral displacement of their supracondylar fracture.[29] Because children are uniquely susceptible to vasospasm, the pulse may not be restored to normal, and a Doppler waveform analysis may be helpful. Many recent technologic improvements, such as color flow duplex scanning and magnetic resonance imaging (MRI), are now available.[32] These techniques are noninvasive and safe for evaluation of the patency of the brachial artery, but they need further study to assess their applicability in clinical practice.[32] Children may have very good secondary capillary perfusion, which can lead to the false assumption that the vascularity is intact. The collateral circulation may be sufficient to maintain a pulse in the distal circulation but not sufficient to maintain perfusion through specific muscle groups. Sabharwal and associates recommended that if the collateral circulation across the elbow is satisfactory, revascularization is not indicated in an otherwise well-perfused hand.[32] They concluded that revascularization of a pulseless but otherwise well-perfused limb with a type III supracondylar fracture, although technically feasible and safe, has a high rate of asymptomatic reocclusion and residual stenosis of the brachial artery.[32] However, a recent meta-analysis was performed, reviewing the relevant observational studies concerning neurovascular injuries in supracondylar humerus fractures; it suggested that the incidence of brachial artery injuries in patients with pulseless but perfused hands is consistently underestimated by treating surgeons.[33] The use of a basilic vein graft from the zone of injury has been shown to be an acceptable arterial conduit in patients requiring grafting.[34]

With more frequent use of fixation for supracondylar fractures, the incidence of vascular injury seems to have decreased, thus suggesting that some of the previous vascular problems were caused by the flexed position required to maintain the reduction. If the vascular status of the limb is questionable, Doppler studies and/or vascular imaging studies should be performed promptly.[4] Similarly, children should have frequent vascular examinations after reduction for signs of vascular insufficiency from intimal tears and brachial artery stenosis. Blakemore and colleagues found that one-third of the children who had displaced supracondylar fractures associated with an ipsilateral forearm fracture (the floating elbow) developed a compartment syndrome.[35] Ring and colleagues found that floating elbows are associated with substantial swelling and increased potential for a compartment syndrome, particularly when they are immobilized in a circumferential cast.[36] Other reports of pediatric patients with floating elbow injuries have described a significantly increased rate of acute neurologic injury in this population but have not demonstrated an increased risk of associated compartment syndrome when compared with isolated supracondylar humerus fractures.[37,38] Loss of reduction is common, and traditionally, it has been recommended that both fractures be stabilized. However, Blumberg et al suggest that forearm fixation is not always essential in these patients, and the decision to stabilize the forearm should be made on a case-by-case basis.[38]

NERVE INJURIES

Nerve injuries are associated with approximately 2.5% of extremity fractures in children and are more than twice as likely to be found with upper extremity fractures than with lower extremity fractures. Displaced supracondylar fractures are often associated with acute neurologic injury, with studies reporting an overall incidence as high as 12% to 16%.[39–41] Campbell and colleagues found that posterior lateral displacement of a type III supracondylar fracture was associated with a higher incidence of median nerve injuries (52%).[29] If the injury is closed and the reduction satisfactory, the child can be treated expectantly, and most will recover, usually in the first 2 months.[30,41–44] One of the more subtle median nerve injuries is injury to the anterior interosseous branch from either traction or contusion.[30,45] Posterior lateral fracture displacement was correlated with the median nerve and vascular compromise, whereas posteromedial fracture displacement is strongly correlated with radial nerve injuries. Medial pinning for supracondylar fractures has been known to place the ulnar nerve at risk of injury.[46] Fortunately, simple removal of the medial pin results in complete recovery in the vast majority of patients.[47] The American Academy of Orthopedic Surgeons Clinical Practice Guidelines for the Treatment of Pediatric Supracondylar Humerus Fractures makes a limited-strength recommendation for the use of two or three lateral pins so that potential harm caused by medial pin placement is avoided.[48]

The ulnar nerve can be injured in the initial trauma, during reduction, or later as a result of progressive elbow deformity.[49,50] The ulnar nerve is often damaged early by posterior dislocation of the elbow, particularly if associated with a medial epicondylar fracture.[49] However, ulnar nerve damage has also been reported with condylar and supracondylar fractures, particularly flexion-type supracondylar fractures, and acute ulnar neuropraxia has been tied to an increased need for open reduction in these injuries.[49,51] Tethered by the cubital tunnel, the ulnar nerve is also at risk of injury in Monteggia fracture variants involving the proximal end of the ulna and has also been reported with radial head fractures and with chronic radial head dislocations.[45,52]

Both valgus and, less frequently, varus deformity that may occur after a lateral condylar fracture can lead to delayed development of ulnar neuropathy.[53–55] Late ulnar nerve lesions at the elbow have been divided into three main categories based on the mechanism of injury: traction such as occurs in a valgus deformity, compression within the limited space of the cubital tunnel, and friction from bone fragments or osteophytes in close proximity to the nerve.[49,50] Symptoms of ulnar nerve neuropathy include paresthesias, intrinsic muscle weakness, and wasting.[56] An electromyogram can be helpful in establishing the diagnosis.[57] Treatment usually consists of surgical decompression of the nerve, correction of the angular deformity of the elbow, or both.[55] Transposition is recommended if the ulnar nerve appears normal, if the symptoms are intractable, or if a valgus deformity of the elbow is present. If the condition has been of long duration, the pain and paresthesias should resolve, but weakness and muscle wasting may persist.[49,58]

Posterior interosseous nerve (PIN) injury is well associated with fractures around the elbow. Li et al described eight cases of acute PIN entrapment in the radiocapitellar joint after Monteggia fracture-dislocations.[59] Acute PIN entrapment into the radiocapitellar joint has also been described after the repair of a Monteggia fracture with an ulnar osteotomy.[45,60] Closed and open reduction of radial neck fractures are also associated with PIN injuries because of the close proximity of the nerve to the fracture site. Choi et al reported excellent results with percutaneous reduction of radial neck fractures without associated PIN palsy and recommend a stepwise approach to minimize the risk of nerve injury.[61]

Median and ulnar nerve injuries are common in physeal and metaphyseal fractures of the distal radius. The mechanism of injury includes direct contusion from the displaced fragment, traction, and ischemia.[45] Waters and associates recommend that if a patient has a normal vascular examination but persistent neurologic symptoms and significant soft tissue swelling, closed reduction and percutaneous pinning may be indicated so that the need for a constrictive cast is eliminated.[62]

Because most pediatric nerve injuries resolve with expectant management after fracture treatment, an initial period of observation is recommended. If no signs of nerve recovery are present 4 months after the injury, then electromyography and nerve conduction studies are recommended. If the electromyographic and nerve conduction studies show no sign of recovery, then exploration and possible repair or grafting of the nerve should be considered. Bolitho and colleagues recommended early repair of ulnar nerve injuries in young children.[63] Distal injuries had a better outcome than proximal ones, but satisfactory function of the intrinsic hand muscles occurred in both groups. Veldman and Goris found that repair of the transected nerve in young children (younger than 13 years) leads to good motor and sensory recovery.[64] Amillo and Mora assessed neural injuries associated with elbow fractures in 25 children (average age at injury, 9.4 years).[58] Eight had discontinuity of the nerve trunk, and 17 had constrictive lesions around the nerve. In those with constrictive lesions, 80% had good results after neurolysis. In those who had disruption, 66% had good results after grafting. The prognosis was poor if surgery was performed more than a year after the injury. They recommended surgical exploration and neural lysis or repair with a graft for open neural injuries.[58] Grafts longer than 10 cm had a poor prognosis.

Under very unusual circumstances, the median and ulnar nerves can become entrapped after dislocation of the elbow.[65,66] When entrapment occurs, the diagnosis is often delayed. Early signs of entrapment are the persistence of a significant median nerve deficit and pain greater than expected after reduction of the elbow dislocation.[65,67] Later signs include a severe elbow flexion contracture and, radiographically, a bony depression in the distal medial humeral cortex corresponding to the location at which the median nerve travels posterior to the humerus and enters the elbow joint.[65,67] The brachial artery and vein and the median nerve can also be trapped between the fracture fragments in a widely displaced supracondylar fracture. Attempts at closed reduction usually lead to vascular compromise, which necessitates open surgical reduction.

Secondary nerve injuries can result from simple positioning, particularly in children in a coma or in those with head

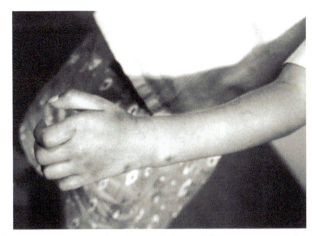

Fig. 7.3 Volkmann ischemic contracture of the forearm after treatment of a both-bones fracture and unrecognized compartment syndrome. Note the contracture of the fingers, which are partially insensate.

injuries.[66,67] The ulnar nerve is very susceptible to compression at the elbow, and the radial nerve is susceptible at the midportion of the humerus if the arm is not properly positioned. Patients with these neurapraxias, if recognized early, have a good chance of recovery. The peroneal nerve may be compressed as it passes over the neck of the fibula. Frequent examination of the extremity for neurovascular status is essential, particularly in the immediate postinjury and early recovery periods or until the child is alert enough to report any changes. Obviously, in children with head injuries, casts should be well padded over these susceptible areas.

COMPARTMENT SYNDROMES

Pediatric acute compartment syndromes (PACS) can occur in a multiply injured child with the same frequency as in an adult. The condition is caused by swelling and increased pressure in a closed space, such as a fascial compartment, but it can also occur from tight skin or a circumferential cast. If not treated promptly, it leads to tissue ischemia, myonecrosis and contractures (Fig. 7.3). The most common anatomic locations for PACS include the leg, forearm, hand, foot, and thigh.[68,69]

The causes of PACS have evolved with time. Initially, fractures of the forearm and femur were associated with the greatest rates of compartment syndrome. As fracture management has evolved, more recent evidence has shown that most common long bone fracture associated with PACS is the tibia. Although tibia fractures account for only 15% of all pediatric long bone fractures, they are associated with 40% of all acute compartment syndrome cases in children.[70,71] PACS may occur after simple Salter-Harris type I or II fracture of the distal end of the radius or proximal part of the tibia and in both open and closed injuries.[72–74] A common misconception is that an open injury will decompress the compartment. However, not all compartments are successfully relieved by an open injury.[75,76] Regardless of fracture location, studies have shown that patients who require longer operative times and more intraoperative fluoroscopy are at greater risk of developing compartment syndrome, which likely reflects the difficulty of the reductions and more manipulation of the fractures intraoperatively.[77–79]

Children with femoral shaft fractures treated by skin traction or early spica cast use have been shown to be at risk for PACS of the thigh and leg.[80,81] When placing a child in a 90/90 spica cast, applying the body and thigh portion of the spica cast before placing the short leg component and minimizing traction through the leg while applying the cast can reduce this risk.[82]

Early operative stabilization of fractures does not eliminate the risk of compartment syndrome. Femoral fractures that are treated with closed intramedullary fixation are also susceptible to compartment ischemia.[78,79,83,84] In restoring femoral length, the muscles are pulled to length, and the integrity of the compartments is restored; however, a compartment syndrome can occur.[76] As flexible intramedullary nailing of forearm and tibia fractures has become more popular, a corresponding rise has been seen in the number of patients experiencing PACS with this technique.[77,85–88] PACS of the foot are most commonly associated with a Lisfranc fracture-dislocation but have also been reported with fractures of the metatarsals and phalanges. They may also occur in the setting of a crush injury, even in the absence of a fracture.[89,90]

In addition to fractures, PACS are associated with severe contusion, crush injuries, vascular injury resulting in prolonged tissue ischemia, prolonged limb compression, burns, and vigorous exercise.[91] Multiple traumatic injuries predispose a child to PACS because of additional high-risk factors such as hypotension, vascular injury, and high-energy blunt trauma, which increase tissue necrosis.[19] PACS in the thigh have been reported in teenagers after blunt trauma and because of systemic hypertension, external compression with antishock trousers, and vascular injury with or without fracture of the femur.[76] Nonfracture-related episodes of PACS have been shown to have longer time to diagnosis and worse outcomes compared with fracture-related compartment syndrome cases, emphasizing the importance of early recognition and treatment of this condition.[92]

Children may be at increased risk for compartment syndrome compared with adults because of (1) predisposition to vasospasm, (2) smaller vessel diameter, (3) greater resting compartment pressures, and (4) atypical presentation compared with adults.

As the pressure increases within the space, one of the early findings or complaints in adults may be a decrease in sensation, or paresthesia.[91] Pain, swelling, and tenseness of the compartment are found on physical examination. These symptoms may be difficult to recognize in children who are too young to cooperate with the examination or in those who have a head injury.[70] Bae and colleagues found that pain, pallor, paresthesia, paralysis, and pulselessness were relatively unreliable signs and symptoms.[70] An increasing analgesia requirement in combination with clinical symptoms was a more sensitive indicator. All 10 of their patients who had access to patient-controlled or nurse-administered analgesia had an increasing requirement for pain medication that preceded other clinical signs or symptoms by an average of 7 hours.[70] Noonan and McCarthy have stressed the importance of recognizing the three As of pediatric compartment syndrome—agitation, anxiety, and increasing analgesic requirement—which often precede the classic presentation by several hours.[93] Pulse oximetry is not helpful in the diagnosis of compartment syndrome because a normal reading does not imply adequate tissue perfusion.[94]

With continued ischemia, voluntary use of the muscles is decreased, and eventually complete paralysis ensues. Pain on stretching the involved muscles is a common finding but is subjective and may be the result of trauma. Early ischemia of the nerve may cause anesthesia and obscure this very sensitive finding.[91] An excellent example of this diagnostic dilemma is the loss of toe dorsiflexion after a metaphyseal fracture of the proximal end of the tibia, which may be caused by a direct injury to the peroneal nerve or anterior tibial artery or by an anterior compartment syndrome.[68]

Compartment pressures are seldom high enough to occlude a major artery, so the peripheral pulses are often palpable, and capillary filling is routinely demonstrated in the skin of the hand or foot.[91] With a tissue pressure exceeding 30 mm Hg, capillary pressure is not sufficient to maintain blood flow to the muscles, and necrosis results.[91] With severe intercompartmental edema, the nerves show a gradual decline in action potential amplitude. A complete conduction block can be obtained with a pressure as low as 50 mm Hg and after 6 to 8 hours of sustained pressure of 30 or 40 mm Hg.

Diagnosis or exclusion of compartment syndrome on clinical grounds alone may be impossible.[68] The most objective method of making the diagnosis is by measuring compartment pressure. Because of the invasive nature of the test, this is not used as routinely in children as in adults. Nonetheless, it is mandatory that anyone who is managing trauma in children be able to determine these values. Generally, a pressure greater than 30 mm Hg is considered abnormal, as muscle damage has been shown to be significant when intercompartmental pressures are greater than 30 mm Hg for a period of 6 to 8 hours.[95]

Although some authors have promoted using pressure readings greater than 30 mm Hg as an absolute threshold for diagnosis of compartment syndrome, there is data to suggest that this value may not always be appropriate. The tissue ischemia caused by PACS is a result of an imbalance between arterial inflow and venous outflow from a myofascial compartment. The patient's mean arterial (MAP) and diastolic blood pressures need to be considered in establishing the diagnosis. In a clinical situation in which a myofascial compartment pressure is less than 30 mm Hg but still within either 30 mm Hg of the MAP or 20 mm Hg of the diastolic blood pressure, there may be an imbalance of arterial inflow and venous outflow within the compartment. This results in vascular congestion, edema, and, ultimately, tissue necrosis.[71,82,87,91] Children have also been shown to have higher resting compartment pressures than adults.[96,97] In combination with a pediatric patient's lower resting blood pressure, the higher resting compartment pressures may predispose children to developing PACS compared with adult patients.

Battaglia and associates measured compartment pressure in children with supracondylar fractures before and after reduction.[98] They found that pressure is greatest in the deep volar compartment and closest to the fracture site. Fracture reduction did not have a consistent or immediate effect on reducing pressure. They recommended that the elbow not be flexed beyond 90 degrees, which was associated with significant (the greatest) pressure elevation. If a fasciotomy is necessary, one must adequately decompress the deep volar musculature. None of their patients exhibited signs and symptoms of compartment syndrome, which suggests that absolute pressure thresholds, no matter how great, are inadequate as indicators of impending compartment syndrome, and they support the concept that the absence of clinical indications alone is insufficient as an indication for fasciotomy.[98]

Initial treatment should include splitting a tight cast and removal of occlusive dressing material and cast padding, all of which will decrease compartment pressure. Univalving the cast and adding spacers of 3 mm to 12 mm in width have been shown to decrease pressure in a cast by as much as 50% to 80%.[99] Elevation of the limb may increase compartment pressure and may be counterproductive if coupled with a decrease in perfusion; this combination may be the mechanism by which ischemic contractures occur after femoral fractures in children.[68,100] Placing the limb at approximately the same level as the heart may be optimal.

Compartment syndrome does not seem to affect healing of the fracture, and nonunion or delayed union is seldom associated with it. However, the healing time for closed fractures associated with compartment syndrome was noted by Turen and associates to be longer, 30.2 versus 17.3 weeks.[101] Interestingly, compartment syndrome lengthens the time for healing of closed fractures, but the healing time was approximately the same as for an open fracture. The method of fixation does not affect the healing time.[101]

The duration of the compartment syndrome before definitive surgical decompression is the most important factor in determining functional outcome.[68] If decompression is accomplished during the early swelling phase of compartment syndrome, most patients will have normal function.[68,85] In the upper extremity, Ziolkowski et al demonstrated that increased time to surgical decompression in PACS resulted both in increased risk of significant functional deficit and need for reconstructive surgery, including flap reconstruction.[102] Livingston et al also found that delayed diagnosis of PACS resulted in a high incidence of myonecrosis noted during surgery and a significant impairment of function postoperatively, with only 56% of patients returning to full function by final follow-up.[92] More than 44% of patients in this study had persistent pain, contractures, limited motor function, and/or paresthesias postoperatively at final follow-up.[92] Late surgical decompression exposes devitalized muscles, which require débridement, and, in some instances, infection can ensue and necessitate multiple débridement procedures and antibiotics. When diagnosis of an upper extremity PACS is delayed, Chuang and colleagues recommended exploration and excision of the infarcted muscle within 3 weeks of injury.[103] They found that such a time frame preserves intrinsic hand function and sensation by removing the ischemic environment and preventing the fibrosis that may add to nerve compression and damage.[103]

Neonatal compartment syndrome is a distinct form of PACs. It is uncommon, and reported causes include disseminated intravascular coagulation and spontaneous arterial thrombosis.[104–106] Neonatal PACS is associated with significant swelling of the limb, and sentinel skin lesions and blisters have been reported.[107,108] Although it is not strictly associated with skeletal trauma, the orthopedist must be familiar with this condition, as early diagnosis and immediate full fasciotomy of the affected extremity is critical for preserving tissue and function of the limb. Immediate recognition can be the difference between limb preservation or amputation and reconstructive surgery in this population.[108,109]

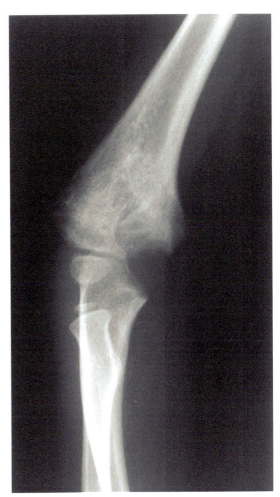

Fig. 7.4 A 4-year-old patient with a supracondylar fracture of the humerus that healed with a cubitus varus deformity.

MALUNION

The most common malunion experienced by children occurs after a supracondylar fracture of the humerus, usually resulting in a cubitus varus deformity (Fig. 7.4). In the past, the deformity was attributed to a disturbance in elbow growth. However, clinical and experimental evidence indicate that the more common cause is an initial unsatisfactory reduction or early loss of reduction. Unfortunately, the cross section of the proximal humeral fragment is narrow, and unless the distal fragment is reduced anatomically, it is easy for this fragment to rotate and tilt medially, causing subsequent cubitus varus deformity and limitation of elbow flexion. Growth at the distal end of the humerus contributes only 10% of the length of the upper extremity, and as a consequence, the potential for subsequent remodeling is limited. The recent popularity of closed reduction with exact anatomic alignment maintained by pin fixation has lessened the frequency of this complication.

Most children do not have a functional deficit but may have a significant cosmetic deformity. If the deformity is present after 1 year and is posing problems, it may be managed by corrective osteotomy. Several authors have described a variety of ways to achieve angular correction.[110] It is not necessary to correct all the deformity of the

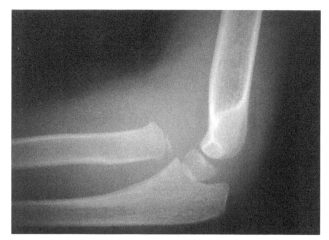

Fig. 7.5 A 6-year-old patient with a Monteggia fracture. Note the anterior dislocation of the radiocapitellar joint.

supracondylar region.[111] Correction of the rotation, however, is much more difficult though the shoulder usually adequately compensates for it. Most authors prefer a lateral closing wedge to correct only the angular alignment and are not concerned about the rotation or flexion-extension aspects of the deformity.[111,112] Barrett and associates, in their review of this procedure, found that patients were generally pleased with this approach.[112] Fixation of the osteotomy is a problem because of the small size and peculiar shape of the distal end of the humerus, which does not lend itself to standard fixation methods.[110] Blasier recommended a triceps-splitting approach to the supracondylar region that provides excellent visualization and facilitates the osteotomy.[113] Pin fixation can be done under direct visualization with greater ease than with a lateral approach. Herzenberg et al have reported successful reconstruction of cubitus varus using gradual correction with external fixation.[114] The advantage of a gradual correction with a hexapod frame is that it minimizes risk of acute vascular and neurologic injury during correction and, by reassessing the osseous alignment and adjusting the hexapod "prescription" during treatment, the surgeon is able to precisely correct all aspects of the deformity.

Unrecognized angular malunion of the ulna in Monteggia injuries can lead to persistent subluxation or dislocation of the radial head and significant loss of pronation[64] and supination.[115] A Monteggia lesion consists of a fracture of the ulna and dislocation of the ipsilateral radial head. This lesion can be subtle; in a small child, it may be difficult to assess the relationship of the radial head to the capitellum, and associated deformation of the ulna may be subtle. As a consequence, an acute lesion is often misdiagnosed (Fig. 7.5).[116] Similarly, displacement or angulation of the ulna and subluxation of the radial head may occur in the weeks after reduction (approximately 20%), especially when the ulnar fracture is oblique.[116] A recent multicenter study reported a 19% rate of loss of reduction in Monteggia fractures treated nonoperatively.[117] In this study, all patients who had recurrent radial head dislocations presented with Monteggia fractures with a complete ulna fracture. These authors recommended that patients with Monteggia fractures who have complete fractures of the ulna be treated surgically in light of the high risk of loss of reduction with nonoperative treatment.[117]

Rodgers and associates published a review of complications and results of reconstruction of Monteggia lesions in children.[116] Attempts at late repair of this lesion were met with considerable problems, including decreased rotation of the forearm, transient motor and sensory ulnar nerve palsies, and residual weakness. However, they believe that the long-term sequelae (pain and weakness) of chronic Monteggia lesions warrant intervention in a skeletally immature patient.[116] If malunion of the ulna prevents reduction, an osteotomy should be performed, preferably one rigidly fixed with a plate (Fig. 7.6). Steinmann pins can be placed antegrade down the ulnar.[112] Inoue and Shionoya recommend overcorrecting the ulna using plate fixation, particularly in situations in which the radial head reduction is unstable.[118] Unrecognized, the deformity of the head caused by growth in a dislocated position makes restoration of the normal radial-ulnar-capitellar relationship difficult. If the radial head is not stable, a temporary pin can be placed to transfix the radiocapitellar joint.[112] If the annular ligament is incompetent, it can be replaced or reconstructed with the use of a strip of triceps fascia as described by Bell Tawse in the article by Rodgers and colleagues.[116]

Fractures of the forearm in children are a common cause of malunion because the reduction can easily be lost and can be difficult to regain (Fig. 7.7).[119,120] Young children can occasionally remodel the fracture dramatically; as a consequence, physicians have a tendency to depend heavily on remodeling and accept a less than adequate reduction. Midshaft fractures are particularly at risk of deformity.[121] Price and colleagues recommend acceptance of up to 10 degrees of angulation, 45 degrees of malrotation, and complete displacement before attempting remanipulation or resorting to open reduction and internal fixation.[122]

Nietosvaara and colleagues found that 48% of distal radial fractures healed in malunion, despite anatomic primary reduction in 85% of the cases.[123] The displacement correlated with marked initial malposition of the fracture (>50% displacement or 20% angulation). An independent risk factor for complications and redisplacement was a nonanatomic reduction of the fracture.[123] In some cases, redisplacement in the cast did not occur until 2 weeks after the injury.[123] They suggested pin fixation should be considered if there is an associated injury, compartment syndrome, or a second fracture in the same extremity (floating elbow), and in children with less than 1 year of growth remaining.[123]

The degree of angular deformity that is acceptable during fracture treatment depends on fracture location and patient age. Remodeling of an angular deformity is better in the distal third of the radius and ulna than in the midshaft or proximal third and is better in younger children.[119,120] A study by Crawford and Lee showed that completely displaced, overriding fractures of the distal radius and ulna could be treated without reduction or sedation in a short arm molded to correct only angulation.[124] Diaphyseal fractures of the forearm with radial or ulnar angulation are less likely to remodel completely. In general, midshaft fractures in children younger than 8 years tend to remodel almost completely; however, in children 11 years or older (particularly girls, who mature earlier), spontaneous correction cannot be anticipated and is unpredictable.[125] Malunion in older patients with diaphyseal forearm fractures may be avoided with the use of intramedullary or plate fixation, and good results have been reported.[126]

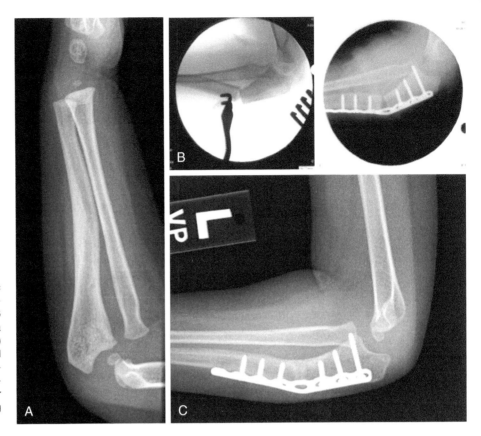

Fig. 7.6 (A) A 6-year old with a chronic Monteggia fracture dislocation who presented with a palpable antecubital mass 6 months after a fall. Note the healed ulna fracture with apex anterior angulation. (B) Intraoperative films following a proximal ulna elongation osteotomy to allow for reduction of the radial head with plate fixation. (C) Congruency of the radiocapitellar joint remains well aligned following healing of the osteotomy.

Price and Knapp have reported a simple method of deformity correction for malunion of forearm shaft fractures.[122] If the deformity is angulated less than 20 degrees and the child is 9 years or younger, the forearm has excellent remodeling potential and generally leads to satisfactory function with an acceptable cosmetic result.[122] Angular deformity of the shaft of the radius-ulna greater than 30 degrees rarely remodels sufficiently in any age group and should be realigned soon after the injury is healed.[122] A brief period of observation (6 months) may be appropriate because of the tremendous ability to remodel.[122] Malunited fractures of the forearm that were surgically corrected less than 1 year after injury had an average improvement of 80 degrees of rotation, whereas those that were managed after 1 year gained only 30 degrees on average.[127]

Although angular deformities have a limited potential for remodeling, rotational deformities do not improve, and they should initially be treated aggressively. A residual rotational deformity can compromise pronation and supination of the forearm, although the clinical significance of this limited rotation has not been clearly established.[128]

Length discrepancy, angulation, and encroachment on the interosseous space are unpredictable indicators of loss of forearm motion. Loss of motion may be caused by soft tissue scarring that produces tension on the interosseous membrane; a few patients with complete remodeling have failed to regain motion.[128] Angulation in the diaphysis is often associated with loss of motion, whereas distal metaphyseal fractures tend to correct themselves, and complete range of motion returns. Similarly, anatomic restoration of alignment by open reduction and internal fixation does not always restore full range of motion. Price and colleagues

suggest that the shortening resulting from fracture displacement allows for relaxation of the interosseous membrane, which preserves motion.[128] The combination of a proximal fracture with angulation, malrotation, and encroachment carries the greatest risk of loss of motion.[128] Price and colleagues recommend open reduction and internal fixation after a refracture because of the greater likelihood in this circumstance of losing forearm rotation.[128]

Much recent attention has been focused on clavicular fracture malunion. A randomized prospective study performed by the Canadian Trauma Society demonstrated significantly improved outcome scores in adult patients treated with open reduction and internal fixation of clavicular fractures when compared with nonoperative treatment.[129] However, Bae and colleagues have questioned whether similar outcomes can be expected in pediatric and adolescent patients.[130] In their study, 16 pediatric patients with fracture displacement greater than 2 cm treated nonoperatively subsequently developed malunion but showed no meaningful loss of shoulder motion or strength.[130]

In the lower extremity, malunion has the potential to lead to degenerative arthritis.[131] In a study of 74 pediatric and adolescent femur fractures followed for a mean of 21 years, Palmu and associates noted a positive correlation between knee arthritis and angular deformity in children older than 10 years at the time of their fractures.[131] Several factors have been associated with femoral or tibial fracture malunion. If comminution of more than 25% is present and the femoral fracture is stabilized with intramedullary nails, an increased risk of shortening, angulation, and loss of reduction has been reported.[132] In length-unstable fractures, locked stainless steel flexible nails may be a better treatment

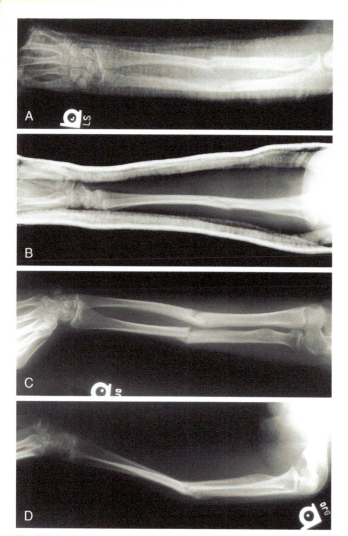

Fig. 7.7 Fracture of the radius and ulna in a 12-year-old girl. Antero-posterior (A) and lateral (B) views of the injury after satisfactory reduction and cast immobilization. (C and D) Fracture reduction was lost because of early removal of the cast, and open reduction plus plate fixation was required to restore satisfactory alignment. In a girl of this age, spontaneous correction cannot be expected.

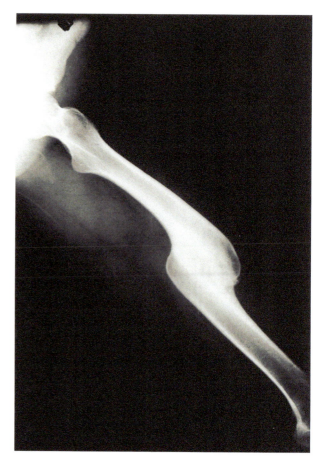

Fig. 7.8 A 15-year-old boy with a serious head injury treated with traction for a femoral shaft fracture. Note the shortening and overriding. The patient has recovered and walks with a cane. The leg-length discrepancy has caused numerous problems.

choice, as these have been shown to have reduced rates of fracture malunion and implant complications compared with nonlocked flexible nail constructs. Malunion or loss of reduction requiring reoperation was strongly associated with the mismatched diameter of flexible nails.[132] Femoral fractures in the subtrochanteric and supracondylar region are less ideally suited to flexible intramedullary fixation and may have a higher malunion rate.[133] Injury severity should also be considered a risk factor for malunion. Bohn and Durbin called attention to the problem of the floating knee, or ipsilateral fracture of the femur and tibia.[134] In this group, operative stabilization of the femoral fracture was associated with fewer complications and better results. Pandya and Edmonds reported the use of flexible intramedullary nails in the treatment of open tibial fractures and described a high union rate but increased incidence of bone healing complications.[135]

Malunion may also occur in children with head or spinal cord injuries.[134,136,137] Ninety percent of head-injured children recover from coma in less than 48 hours. In long-term follow-up, 84% of children who were initially in deep coma (score of 5 to 7 on the Glasgow Coma Scale) were eventually able to walk freely.[136] Rigid fixation of long bone fractures aids in nursing care and rehabilitation efforts. Muscle spasticity in the first few days often displaces or angulates fractures immobilized in casts or leads to overriding of fractures in traction (Fig. 7.8).[134,136] Nonoperative management of fractures in these children results in healing but also produces an unacceptable incidence of malunion, angulation, and shortening (Fig. 7.9).[136,138] Skin insensitivity combined with disorientation may result in skin breakdown with the potential for secondary osteomyelitis.[136] If the child must be moved for special studies, such as computed tomography (CT) or MRI, or requires extensive dressing changes, multiple débridement in the operating room, or whirlpool treatments for burns, the fracture should be stabilized because manipulation of the fracture may increase intracranial pressure. In children with acute quadriplegia or paraplegia, fracture fixation decreases the incidence of skin problems and pressure sores from cast immobilization and the need for external support, which may compromise nursing and rehabilitative efforts.

SYNOSTOSIS (CROSS UNION)

Cross union is a rare and serious complication of fractures of the forearm. Rotation of the forearm is impossible and may

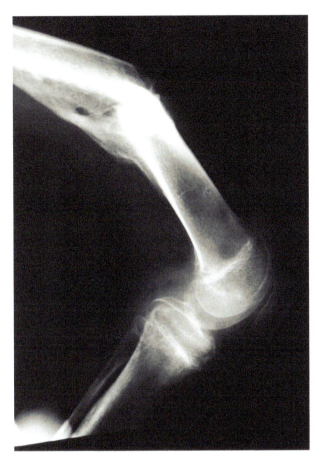

Fig. 7.9 Angulation of a femoral shaft fracture in a 13-year-old head-injured patient who was treated with skeletal traction.

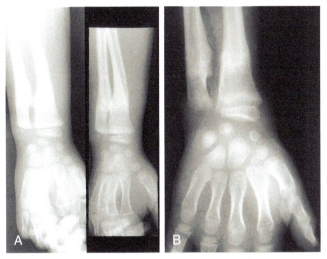

Fig. 7.10 (A) Anteroposterior and oblique views of the distal end of the forearm and wrist of a 7-year-old boy who sustained a fracture of both bones of the forearm. The fracture healed in a malrotated and angulated position with subsequent synostosis that is easily seen on the oblique view. (B) The traumatic synostosis was resected with interposition of fat. Preoperatively, the patient had no forearm rotation; postoperatively, he regained 50 degrees of forearm rotation. (Courtesy of Dr. Neil E. Green. Vanderbilt University, Nashville, TN.)

lead to a serious compromise in function. Cross union must be distinguished from myositis ossificans, which is more common and typically less disabling. Most cross unions are confined to the proximal third of the radius and ulna.[139] Most authors recommend that if open reduction of forearm fractures is required, the surgery be performed through two incisions; however, this technique does not necessarily prevent cross union.[140] Similarly, synostosis has been reported after intramedullary fixation of fractures.[141] Other predisposing factors include severe initial displacement, fracture comminution, residual displacement, periosteal interposition, delayed surgery, remanipulation, and fracture at the same level of the radius and ulna.[140,142]

Early studies of management of synostosis recommended delaying surgical intervention for 1 to 2 years after onset for best results.[140,143] However, surgical intervention has been demonstrated to be safe if there is radiographic evidence consistent with maturation of the synostosis, such as a well-marginated edge and no evidence of bridging trabeculae.[144] A bone scan may be useful for establishing that the healing reaction is complete and that isotope uptake has returned to the same level as that in the surrounding bone, consistent with a mature synostosis. When a synostosis is excised, it is important that the bone bridge and its periosteum be removed intact to lessen the chance of recurrence. Several authors suggest interposing fat, muscle, or silicone elastomer (Silastic) between the radius and ulna to prevent recurrence; however, only a few patients had a recurrence, and follow-up data are limited.[140,145,146] If surgery is delayed

too long, soft tissue contractures may preclude recovery of maximal range of pronation and supination (Fig. 7.10).

The same problem can develop between the tibia and the fibula.[147] Tibial-fibular synostosis is associated with high-energy trauma that results in displaced fractures of the distal tibia and fibula at the same level.[147] In a child, this may lead to disproportionate growth.[148] One should allow 3 months to 1 year for the synostosis to mature before excision.[147] A similar surgical recommendation could be considered to keep the fibula moving freely at the ankle joint. Another alternative is resection of a portion of the fibula and screw fixation of the distal end of the fibula to the tibial epiphysis.

NONUNION

Nonunion of fractures is rare in children (Fig. 7.11).[149] In two large series from the Mayo Clinic, the tibia was the most common diaphyseal region involved, and fractures about the elbow accounted for the largest number of metaphyseal and epiphyseal nonunions.[149,150] Generally, nonunion is associated with high-energy trauma and open fractures with extensive soft tissue disruption and infection.[42,149,151,152] A recent retrospective review of adolescents who sustained diaphyseal fracture nonunions found that soft tissue injury, older patient age, and insufficient fracture fixation were the strongest predictors for nonunion.[153] These findings have been supported by multiple studies. Open reduction and internal fixation may contribute if the fixation is inadequate or holds the fracture fragments apart.[154–157] Nonunion is more likely in an older child who is approaching maturation. An open fracture in children older than 11 or 12 years significantly increases the risk of nonunion when compared with the same injury in children younger than 6 years.[158] Perioperative use of ketorolac has not been associated with an increased risk of nonunion.[159–161]

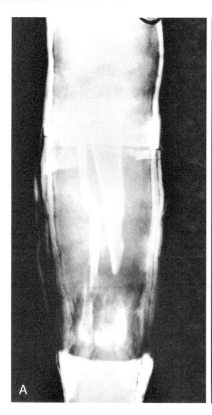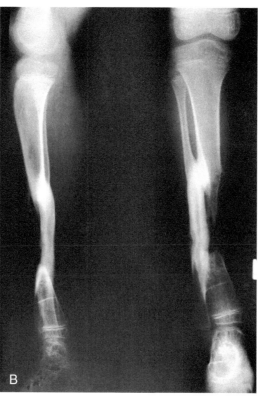

Fig. 7.11 (A) Nonunion of the tibia after a lawn mower injury with extensive soft tissue loss and infection. (B) After the soft tissue problems and infection were resolved, adequate skin coverage was obtained, and a bone graft from the fibula to the proximal and distal ends of the tibia was performed to achieve stability of the leg.

The same treatment techniques for nonunion that have been successful in adults can be used in children. The endosteal response can be improved if the dense fibrous tissue and subchondral bone is resected so that the marrow spaces are communicating. Internal fixation and autogenous bone graft are recommended.[149,162] Intramedullary fixation may be preferable for an unstable fracture. Fixation plates provide more rigid fixation, but great care should be exercised to minimize dissection that may further compromise blood flow to the bone.[163] An Ilizarov fixator may improve results in the lower extremities, in addition to treating pseudarthrosis, and the discrepancy in length or angulation can be corrected at the same time.[163]

Fractures of the femoral neck are associated with a high incidence of nonunion because of failure to achieve and maintain adequate initial anatomic reduction.[154,156] Similarly, loss of reduction can occur because of failure of fixation such as from screw breakage.[154,156] These fractures are usually transcervical and may be associated with avascular necrosis.[154,156] In Morsy's group of 53 children, 36% developed nonunion, the majority of whom had transcervical fractures. Only 2 (8%) of the 26 patients who had anatomic reductions developed a nonunion compared with 9 (64%) of the 14 patients whose fractures were not anatomically reduced.[156] A systematic review of femoral neck fracture outcomes also found that transcervical fractures posed the greatest risk for nonunion, but the authors cited a slightly lower nonunion incidence of 17.4%.[164]

Nonunion of a displaced fracture of the lateral humeral condyle (Fig. 7.12) is a common problem. Among 530 patients treated with lateral condyle fractures, Pace et al reported a 1.4% rate of fracture nonunion with fractures displaced more than 2 mm at the cartilaginous surface at the time of injury having a nonunion rate as high as 3%.[165] Such fractures must be watched closely for displacement if

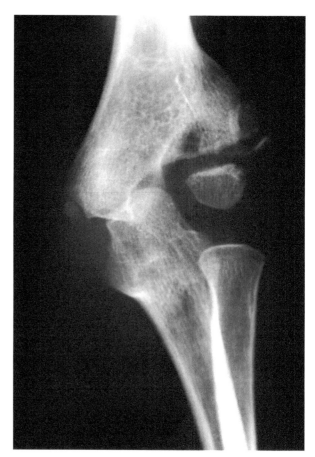

Fig. 7.12 Nonunion of the lateral humeral condyle. The fracture fragment can easily become displaced if the cartilage hinge is broken. If cast immobilization is used, this fracture must be watched closely for displacement. Early recognition leads to salvage by early stabilization. This nonunion healed after bone grafting.

nonoperative treatment is elected. If the fracture becomes displaced, it has a great propensity for nonunion because the fracture surface of the condyle rotates away from the metaphysis.[166] Flynn recommends that when the distance is 2 mm or greater, these fractures should be surgically reduced and pinned to prevent further displacement and possible nonunion.[167]

Early recognition of nonunion should be treated by early stabilization and bone grafting if the fragment is in an acceptable position and the growth plate of the condyle is open.[166,167] Procrastination may allow the physis of the condylar fragment to close prematurely, and a golden opportunity to salvage the elbow would be lost. If the fragment is not rotated or displaced too much, either in situ screw fixation or removal of the fibrous tissue and bone grafting usually suffice.[166–168] Greater displacement requires reattachment of the fragment with a screw or threaded pin; however, some loss of elbow motion may occur.[168,169] Every effort should be made to avoid further stripping of soft tissue to prevent avascular necrosis of the fragment.[170] In late cases in which anatomic reduction is not possible, the fragment is stabilized in the position that yields the greatest range of motion (i.e., functional reduction). If necessary, supracondylar osteotomy can be performed to restore alignment.[170]

A carpal scaphoid nonunion typically occurs in adolescents in whom the injury was originally unrecognized. If the fracture is initially treated by cast immobilization, nonunion is rare. Treatment of the nonunion is similar to that in an adult.[171,172]

REFRACTURE

Refracture suggests accidental repetition of the original injury—probably a combination of a fragile union and reckless physical activity.[173] It can occur after fractures of any bones but is particularly common in forearm fractures. Because healing is rapid in children, immobilization is often discontinued early. Schwarz and colleagues, in their review of 28 forearm refractures, found that 84% were associated with incomplete healing of greenstick fractures. Refracture can occur as late as 12 months after the original injury.[174] In a review of 760 fractures, Bould and Bannister found a refracture rate of 4.9%, usually within the first 9 months.[175] Fracture immobilization for 6 weeks was shown to reduce refracture risk by a factor between 4 and 6.[175] As refracture led to complete displacement in most patients, Bould and Bannister tended to treat them with operative reduction using plates or pins.[175] More recently, Tisosky et al reported a significantly lower refracture rate of only 1.4% over 10 years but did find that residual angulation of more than 10 degrees increased the likelihood of refracture.[176] Refracture occurred an average of 15 weeks after initial injury, but more than 90% of patients with refracture were successfully treated through closed management.[176] Diaphyseal and proximal one-third fractures are significantly more likely to refracture than distal one-third fractures.[177] In a study by Vopat and colleagues, pediatric forearm fractures initially treated with plate fixation had a refracture rate of 7%, slightly higher than the refracture rate associated with cast immobilization.[178] Makki et al reported refracture rates of 8.5% and 16.7% after implant removal from pediatric

forearm fractures treated with primary plate and titanium intramedullary nail fixation, respectively.[179] Refracture rates were higher if implant removal was performed less than 12 months after injury, leading authors to recommend delaying implant removal for at least 12 months after the initial surgery.[179] Children who have osteopenic conditions such as osteogenesis imperfecta, myelodysplasia, paraplegia, or quadriplegia are at great risk of secondary fractures in the extremity that has been immobilized. In this group, immobilization should be of short duration and as little as necessary to keep the bone aligned, such as splints and soft dressings. Typically, exuberant callus formation splints the fracture and allows early removal of the cast.

Refracture can be a complication of external fixation of long bone fractures; the reported rate ranges from 3% to 21% and is most commonly at the original fracture site or less often through a pin site.[180–183] To some degree, this wide range implies that refracture risk is technique dependent, surgeon dependent, or both. Several authors found that refracture correlated with open fractures, bilateral fractures, and a longer time in the fixator.[180] Transverse fractures treated by external fixation have an increased risk of refracture.[180] This increased risk is likely because the fracture ends held in anatomic alignment heal with primary bone formation rather than a large callus.[180] There is a "spot weld" between the bone ends over relatively little surface area, unlike oblique and spiral fractures, which have much greater surface area to promote rapid and strong healing. Kesemenli and colleagues reported that refracture occurred an average of 8 days after fixation was removed.[180] They treated the refractures with closed reduction and spica cast immobilization, and, at follow-up, they were only a centimeter short and had satisfactory function. The authors believe that surgical treatment should be considered when satisfactory anatomic reduction cannot be achieved.[180]

Skaggs and associates[182] found a correlation between refracture and the number of cortices demonstrating bridging callus on the anteroposterior and lateral views at the time of fixator removal. Those with three or four cortices of bridging had a 4% refracture rate. In their report, this rate was not influenced by dynamization, fracture configuration, or alignment. Narayanan and associates reported refractures after elastic stable intramedullary nail fixation, which was associated with removing the nails too early or a second injury in which they were bent and had to be replaced.[132]

GROWTH DISTURBANCES

PHYSEAL INJURY

One of the unique complications of juxtaphyseal injuries is the interruption of normal growth of the physis. This disturbance poses a wide range of problems, from complete arrest with no further growth to partial arrest and gradual slowing or progressive angulation. Typically, the injury results in a bridge of bone from the metaphysis to the epiphysis, commonly referred to as a bony bar. If the injury is at the periphery, the bar acts as a tether leading to an angular deformity with some decreased growth. If allowed to persist, it will eventually result in complete closure. Central arrest leads to slowing of growth; radiographically, it appears as

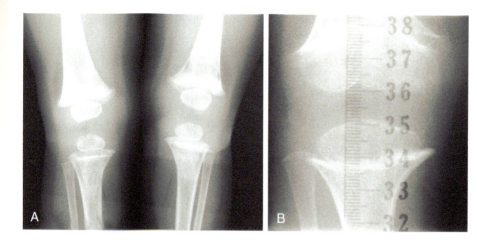

Fig. 7.13 Central growth arrest after severe meningococcemia at 2 years of age. (A) Initial normal appearance of the knees. (B) Two years later: right distal femoral and proximal tibial central growth arrest is apparent. Note that the metaphysis appears to cup the epiphysis and that the epiphyseal plate is tented.

tenting of the epiphyseal plate with cupping of the epiphysis by the metaphysis. The epiphysis appears to be sucked up into the metaphysis (Fig. 7.13). This situation is more commonly associated with a vascular injury, infection such as meningococcemia, or thermal injury such as frostbite.

A decision to resect the bar or to arrest the remaining growth in the physis must be made. The choice is based on the potential of the bar to cause further length discrepancy or angular deformity and the technical problems involved in removing it.[184] The general recommendation is that if less than 50% of the growth plate is involved and the child has 2 years of growth remaining, resection should be considered.[73,185] In general, a leg length discrepancy of 1 inch or less represents little functional impairment, and many discrepancies of up to 2 inches can be adequately compensated by growth arrest of the opposite physis. The decision is further dependent on the percentage of growth contributed by the individual physis to the length of the lower extremity. For example, the distal tibial epiphysis accounts for only 18%, so complete arrest in a teenager is less of a problem; a contralateral epiphysiodesis may be appropriate, which would not be the case in a young child. The decision is much less problematic in the upper extremity because length discrepancy seldom causes functional impairment; many authors recommend that discrepancies of 4 inches or less are best left untreated. Vocke and Von Laer found that fractures of the radial neck frequently lead to radial head deformity (82%) but to functional problems in only 11%.[186]

If the bar is to be resected, it is important to prevent reformation. A number of methods that use interposing material to block the healing reaction have been described. Materials include fat, bone wax, silicone elastomer, and methyl methacrylate. Langenskiöld first popularized bar excision in the 1960s when he resected the bar and filled the space with autogenous fat.[187,188] He subsequently reported that over the long term, the fat functions as a satisfactory material; it generally prevented bar reformation and continued to grow with the patient.[188] Silicone elastomer was popular but is a controlled substance that cannot be used without investigational permission from the US Food and Drug Administration. Methyl methacrylate has been popularized by Peterson.[184] It is helpful in larger resections, particularly when the bone is structurally weakened, because it is a solid substance that fills the cavity, aids in hemostasis, and decreases the need for postoperative protection.[184] The use

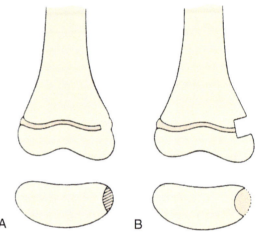

Fig. 7.14 Drawing of peripheral growth arrest shown in an anteroposterior view and transverse section through the physis below. (A) Map of the bar composed from tomograms. (B) Bar excised by a direct approach. (From Peterson HA. Partial growth plate arrest and its treatment. *J Pediatr Orthop.* 1984;4:246.)

of cultured chondrocytes or mesenchymal cells as interpositional material after physeal bridge resection is an area of active research.[189–192] It is important that whatever material is interposed remains in the area of the resection to prevent late bar reformation.

Peripherally located bars are approached directly, and the periosteum is excised to prevent reformation (Fig. 7.14). The bar is removed under direct visualization with a motorized bur because the bony bar is extraordinarily hard. Magnification and a headlamp may be helpful. Curettes are used as one nears the normal physis. Physeal cartilage is usually straighter and wider, often with a blue tinge.[193] Epiphyseal bone feels spongy as though it were floating.[193] It is important to undermine both the metaphysis and the epiphysis so that the physis is sufficiently exposed to prevent bar formation but not so much that its vascularity is jeopardized.[184]

Centrally located bars are difficult to resect (Fig. 7.15). They are approached through the metaphysis and generally require a wide metaphyseal window. These bars can be anatomically confusing because they have a volcanic appearance, and resecting the interior can be difficult. The entire circumference of the physis must be visualized to adequately remove the bar. Dental mirrors and arthroscopes have been

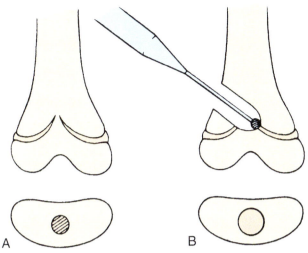

Fig. 7.15 (A) A central bar with growth peripherally results in tenting of the physis. (B) Excision of the central bone through a window in the metaphysis. (From Peterson HA. Partial growth plate arrest and its treatment. *J Pediatr Orthop.* 1984;4:246.)

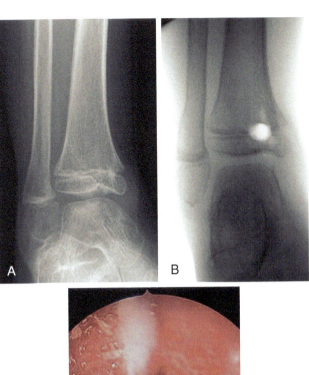

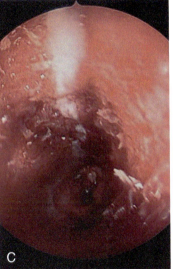

Fig. 7.16 (A) A physeal bar following fixation of a displaced medial malleolus fracture in a 7-year-old male. (B) Intraoperative imaging following resection of the bar. (C) An ankle arthroscope within the resection cavity demonstrates healthy physeal tissue and thus adequacy of the resection.

used to better visualize the normal physis (Fig. 7.16). To prevent migration of the material, the surgeon may stabilize it with a pin or design the resection so that a cavity is created in the epiphysis for the material to be held within the substance of the epiphysis as the child grows (Fig. 7.17). An innovative suggestion is to use the Ilizarov apparatus to distract the epiphysis and cause epiphysiolysis, then resect the bony bridge and fill it with methyl methacrylate, and correct any angular deformity at the same time. These preliminary results are encouraging but need further investigation.[185] It is common to use metal markers for both the epiphysis and the metaphysis to facilitate documentation of continued growth in the postoperative period.

In a young child, angular deformity of up to 15 degrees may correct spontaneously as a result of catch-up growth after bar resection.[184,185] An accompanying corrective osteotomy may be considered when angular deformities are greater than 10 degrees. Near-normal longitudinal growth and correction of moderate angular deformities can be expected when the bridge is less than 25%; most poor results occur in those with very large growth arrest.[185] In total physeal arrest, there is no growth recovery line. Williamson and Staheli recommend that resection be considered in all young children who have considerable growth remaining, even if the bar is large.[185] They reported resection of 48% in a 2-year-old and 54% in another that resulted in excellent growth for 2 years before recurrence.

Children should be monitored until maturity with scanograms; wire markers are helpful to assess growth. Successful results in resections as great as 50% have been reported: 84% of anticipated growth was achieved.[184,185] Most grow vigorously in the beginning, but some close prematurely and may require epiphysiodesis of the contralateral physis toward the end of growth.[194]

DISTAL FEMUR

The complex physeal geometry, large cross-sectional area, and force required for fractures all contribute to a high incidence of growth disturbance after a fracture of the distal

femoral physis, even after relatively simple type I and type II Salter-Harris fractures.[195–197] In contrast, growth disturbance is a rare occurrence after injury in smaller physes, such as the distal end of the radius. The proximal part of the tibia and distal end of the femur account for only 3% of all physeal injuries but account for the greatest incidence of posttraumatic physeal arrest.[194] This finding is particularly troublesome because they account for 60% to 70% of the growth of the respective bones.[184] Riseborough and colleagues found an alarmingly high rate of complications after femoral physeal injury: growth arrest and a limb length discrepancy of more than 2.4 cm developed in 56%, and angular deformities greater than 5 degrees requiring osteotomy developed in 26%.[198] Growth problems correlate well with the severity of the injury and were seen in all the Salter-Harris types. Salter-Harris type III and IV fractures of the distal tibia have also been identified as being especially troublesome: open, anatomic reduction and internal fixation are recommended for prevention of premature physeal

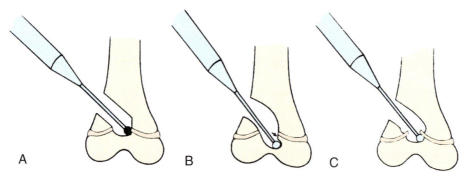

Fig. 7.17 Contour of the cavity. (A) The physis is exposed as usual. The adjacent metaphyseal bone surface should be smooth to help prevent the plug from staying with the metaphysis. (B) Bone in the epiphysis is undermined in an attempt to allow the plug to stay with the epiphysis. A small rim of epiphyseal bone should be preserved to maintain viability of the physis. (C) Undermining of bone away from the physis should be avoided because the protruding physis would be deprived of its blood supply and prevented from growing inward over the plug as the physis grows distally. (From Peterson HA. Partial growth plate arrest and its treatment. *J Pediatr Orthop.* 1984;4:246.)

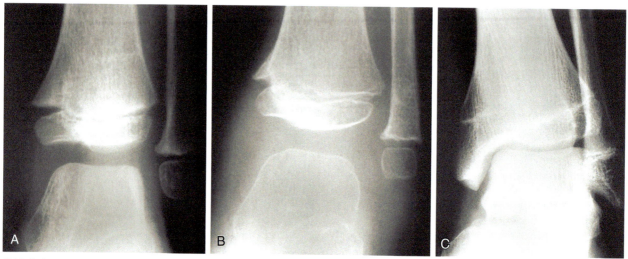

Fig. 7.18 A 4-year-old sustained a distal tibial fracture, Salter-Harris type IV. (A) Six months after initial healing. (B) Two years after injury. (C) Follow-up at 12 years of age. Note the development of angulation and deformity of the ankle joint with overgrowth of the fibula. (Courtesy of Dr. Herman D. Hoeksema. Grand Rapids, MI.)

closure.[199,200] Physeal fractures in children younger than age 11 years have the poorest prognosis; growth problems develop in 83% of these children (Fig. 7.18).[201]

Riseborough and colleagues recommend anatomic reduction and greater use of internal fixation, but this technique is not guaranteed to restore normal growth in those who have sustained a severe injury to the growth plate.[198] With a type II fracture-separation, internal fixation of the large metaphyseal fragment provides better results. Because the potential for growth arrest is so high, children should be monitored closely over the period of remaining growth. Imaging for growth arrest has evolved: initially, trispiral tomograms were preferred, then MRI, and now high-resolution helical CT scanning with coronal and sagittal reconstruction imaging is the preferred imaging modality.[202] If the resultant bridge is of moderate size, less than 40% of the cross-sectional area, and surgically accessible, it can be excised. Scanograms should be taken to determine the precise length of the extremities and to evaluate the hand and wrist for bone age before planning surgical resection. Physeal bars that span greater than 40% to 50% do not typically respond well to bar resection, and completion epiphysiodesis is typically recommended. Management of subsequent limb length inequality should be based on the projected limb length difference at skeletal maturity as well as a discussion with the patient and family regarding the risks and benefits of observation, contralateral epiphysiodesis, and ipsilateral limb lengthening.

Growth arrest can occur after adjacent fractures in the metaphysis or, less often, the diaphysis, especially with fractures above the femur and near the knee.[203–206] Such injury often results in delayed recognition of the physeal injury until a gross angular deformity develops.[201] Berson and colleagues and Hresko and Kasser recommend that all adolescents' injuries be monitored expectantly so that a physeal injury can be detected early.[201,206]

DISTAL TIBIA/ANKLE

Changes in the tibiofibular relationship because of growth disturbances after ankle fractures are frequent in children.[201,207] Fortunately, most occur near the end of growth and, as a consequence, cause only minor problems. Growth arrest of the distal end of the fibula and continued growth of the tibia may initially be compensated for by distal sliding of the fibula as a result of traction from the ankle ligaments.

If the deformity is of long duration, a valgus deformity will occur. Growth arrest of the distal end of the tibia may cause lateral impingement (Fig. 7.19) or a varus deformity if the fibula continues to grow (Fig. 7.20). However, the fibula may slide proximally to compensate for tibial overgrowth; thus, the fibular head may become more prominent at the knee. Distal fibular growth arrest may be necessary.

PROXIMAL TIBIA

Late angulation is a common problem with fractures of the proximal tibial metaphysis in a young child.[208] Typically, the fracture is a relatively nondisplaced or easily reducible fracture of the proximal tibial metaphysis.[209,210] It heals uneventfully, but over the ensuing months, progressive valgus angulation develops in the limb and can be alarming in its appearance (Fig. 7.21).[209,210] Many improve spontaneously, and one should wait at least 18 months to 2 years to be confident that maximal improvement has occurred (Fig. 7.22).[211] Usually, this condition is not associated with a fracture of the fibula, but it has been reported with fractures of both bones. Although many theories have been advanced, the most likely mechanism is an increased vascular response leading to stimulation of growth of the medial metaphysis of the proximal end of the tibia.[209–212]

Interestingly, proximal metaphyseal osteotomy of the tibia and fibula for correction of the deformity can also initiate a progressive valgus deformity with an unacceptably high rate of recurrence of the angulation.[210] Guided growth techniques with the use of a staple or small plate are less morbid and have largely replaced tibial osteotomy as treatment for this condition in the growing child.

PELVIS

Traumatic disruption of the acetabular triradiate physeal cartilage occurs infrequently. However, children whose bones are fractured during the active growth phase have a great potential for early closure and development of a shallow acetabulum.[213,214] Experimentally induced triradiate cartilage closure in rabbits further supports this paradigm.[215] This problem is more common in children younger than 10 years, and in this situation, it can lead to incongruity of the hip joint and progressive subluxation requiring acetabular reconstruction.[213,214,216,217] In older children with less growth potential, this pattern is not as troublesome. Simple displacement of the triradiate cartilage has a more favorable prognosis. In contrast, severe crushing frequently ends in early closure and the worst prognosis. A severe, more crushing type of injury may be difficult to detect on initial radiographs, in which case CT scans are helpful.[213] If a definite osseous bridge can be identified, resection with fat or methyl methacrylate (Cranioplast) interposition is recommended, and small reports have shown that patients can have continued acetabular development without apparent dysplasia at skeletal maturity.[213,218] However, the problem is often not discovered until complete closure of the triradiate cartilage has occurred.[217]

Acetabular injury may be suspected with indirect signs such as concurrent fracture of the neck of the femur, detachment of the proximal femoral epiphysis, traumatic dislocation of the hip, or other pelvic fractures. CT scanning can be helpful in the assessment of pelvic fractures, particularly in patients who may have an osteochondral injury with a retained fragment. Persistent joint widening should arouse suspicion, even in the absence of a clear history of hip dislocation. An arthrogram may not always be diagnostic. Surgical reduction of pelvic fractures should be considered only in cases of hip instability and severe displacement of the femoral head.

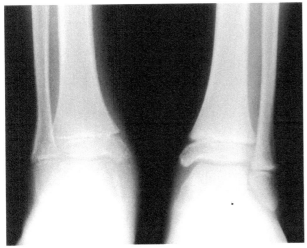

Fig. 7.19 Complete closure of the right distal tibial epiphyseal plate occurred in an 11-year-old boy after a direct impact from a fall. Note that the distal fibular growth plate has not closed and that further growth may pose a problem at the ankle.

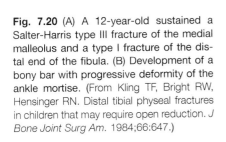

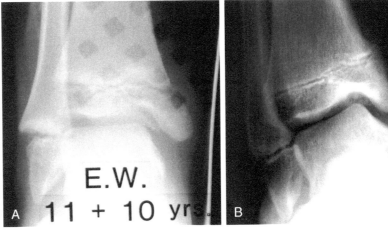

Fig. 7.20 (A) A 12-year-old sustained a Salter-Harris type III fracture of the medial malleolus and a type I fracture of the distal end of the fibula. (B) Development of a bony bar with progressive deformity of the ankle mortise. (From Kling TF, Bright RW, Hensinger RN. Distal tibial physeal fractures in children that may require open reduction. *J Bone Joint Surg Am.* 1984;66:647.)

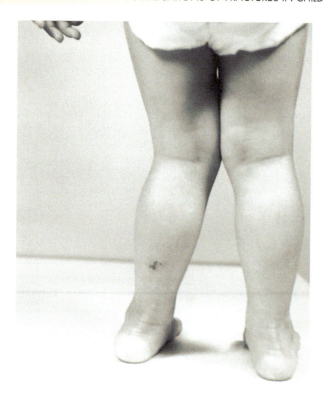

Fig. 7.21 Clinical appearance of a 2.5-year-old patient in whom valgus angulation developed secondary to a fracture of the proximal tibial metaphysis.

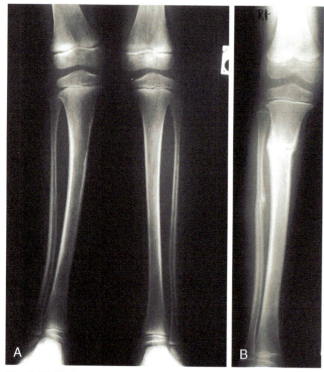

Fig. 7.22 (A) A 7-year-old patient with persistent valgus deformity several years after sustaining a fracture of the proximal tibial metaphysis. Spontaneous remodeling has not occurred. (B) Radiograph after a proximal tibial osteotomy to correct the deformity.

THE OVERGROWTH PHENOMENON

It is well known that a fracture of the femur may lead to overgrowth averaging 1 cm (range, 0.4–2.7 cm).[219] Femoral overgrowth has been shown to occur regardless of the child's age, level of the fracture, or position of the fracture at the time of healing (shortened, lengthened, or distracted).[220,221] Interestingly, it involves the entire limb, with overgrowth of the ipsilateral tibia often present. This phenomenon has been reported to occur in 82% of patients, and 78% of overgrowth occurs in the first 18 months after a fracture.[221] In 9%, overgrowth continued throughout the period of remaining growth, although at a slower rate. Staheli noted slightly greater overgrowth in children 4 to 8 years of age.[222] The available evidence suggests that such overgrowth is caused by an increase in vascularity to the bone as a result of the healing reaction and that it is an obligatory phenomenon rather than a mechanism to compensate for shortening.[221] This phenomenon has led to the clinical suggestion that the fracture fragments be overlapped approximately 1 to 1.5 cm in a young child, with the expectation that such overlapping will lessen the problem of overgrowth. It may become more troublesome as more femoral shaft fractures are managed by intramedullary fixation or external fixation, which restores the fracture to length.[223–225] Submuscular plating has recently gained popularity as an effective treatment for length-unstable femur fractures. A recent report suggests the potential for overgrowth resulting in length discrepancy and valgus alignment in a small percentage of patients treated with this technique.[226,227] Implant removal 6 to 9 months after injury is recommended to prevent this deformity.

Overgrowth is infrequently reported in the upper extremity. In a large study of forearm fractures, overgrowth in the radius or ulna is infrequent and averages 0.44 cm.[228] Davids and colleagues noted that lateral condylar fractures of the humerus can, on occasion, be complicated by lateral bony overgrowth and an unsightly appearance sometimes referred to as "pseudovarus."[229]

LIGAMENTOUS INSTABILITY

Although ligamentous injury can occur in any joint in children, certain problems are often undetected at the time of injury, particularly in the cervical spine and knee. In the cervical spine, teenagers seem to be particularly susceptible to soft tissue and ligamentous disruption between the posterior elements.[230] Such disruption frequently follows a hyperflexion injury. Typically, the initial radiographs appear satisfactory; however, with resolution of the pain and swelling, flexion views reveal posterior widening between the spinous processes. This widening is commonly associated with injuries in the lower portion (C4–C5, C5–C6, and C6–C7).[231] The lesion will not heal spontaneously, and the loose segments should be stabilized by a simple one-level or, occasionally, a two-level posterior spinal fusion.

Ligamentous injuries about the knee are frequently not recognized, particularly in those with an associated fracture of the femur, tibia, or both (floating knee). Injury can occur to the collateral ligaments or the anterior cruciate and, less commonly, the posterior cruciate. Whether the incidence of this injury is increasing or recognition of it is improving is difficult to determine.[134,230,232,233] Arslan and colleagues, in their study of 18 children with floating knees, found five children who had associated knee ligament injuries and meniscal tearing.[232] The children in the follow-up period were often asymptomatic, and the ligamentous injury did not affect the outcome of the floating knee; however, they were undiagnosed at the time of the injury.[232] MRI is the best way to find these injuries because a physical examination can be very difficult.[232] Even after the fracture has been fixed, there is a long period before one can perform a satisfactory physical examination.[134,233] Arslan and colleagues encouraged a late-stage MRI to determine ligamentous and meniscal injuries because a physical examination was only positive in two of their patients.[232] Frequently, the associated knee ligament will benefit from surgical treatment, typically in a staged fashion after femur and tibia fractures have been stabilized and knee range of motion has normalized. Tibial spine fractures may also be associated with an anterior cruciate ligament stretch injury. Even when anatomically reduced, displaced tibial spine fractures may result in persistent anteroposterior laxity, suggesting concurrent intrasubstance ligamentous injury despite gross continuity.[234]

Farley and colleagues reported on ultrasound examination of ankle injuries in children.[235] In children who had ankle injuries but normal radiographs, 10 of 14 had significant ligamentous injuries, including the anterior talofibular ligament and anterior tibiofibular ligament.[235] Previously, many authors had suggested that children were more likely to have physeal injuries (Salter-Harris type I fractures) and, less commonly, ankle sprains and ligamentous injuries. Farley and colleagues recommended that if there was a question about the differentiation on clinical examination, an ultrasound examination can be very helpful.[235]

Kocher and colleagues found that fracture dislocation of the shoulder and elbow can be associated with significant ligamentous injuries, particularly in the adolescent nearing skeletal maturity.[236] Elbow dislocations are often accompanied by ligamentous injuries and muscular avulsions, particularly with a medial epicondylar avulsion. The ulnar collateral ligament may be disrupted in almost 50%.[236]

SPONTANEOUS DEEP VEIN THROMBOSIS

This complication is very uncommon in childhood; only scattered reports exist in the literature. A recent report of pediatric patients with lower extremity trauma cited an incidence of 0.058%, which is similar to the reported rate of 0.0515% among pediatric patients undergoing elective orthopedic surgery.[237,238] Generally, the clinical findings are similar to those found in adults and consist of local discomfort, tenderness and warmth, and, often, swelling of the extremity.[239,240] Deep vein thrombosis should be confirmed by appropriate noninvasive testing and perhaps venograms. The majority of children who develop thrombophlebitis or have a pulmonary embolism have an inherited or congenital thrombophilia.[239] Activated protein C–resistant antithrombin III deficiency, dysfibrinogenemia, impaired fibrolysis, protein C deficiency, protein S deficiency, and factor V Leiden are the more common conditions associated with the increased incidence of thrombophlebitis in children.[239,241] When a child is identified with this condition, the near relatives should be screened because they may also have the condition and require prophylaxis. A serum lipoprotein(a) (Lp(a)) concentration greater than 30 mg/dL is an important risk factor for thromboembolism in childhood.[242] Children who have venous thromboembolic events should be screened for elevated serum Lp(a).[242] It is likely that many cases go unrecognized. Most children respond to routine treatment, similar to adults.[239,240,243] Initial treatment consists of heparin followed by warfarin (Coumadin) or a Factor Xa inhibitor over an appropriate period. The problem occurs more often in older teenagers, the obese, adolescent females on oral contraceptives, and those with local infection in the extremity.[244–248] Critically ill children and those requiring a central venous catheter have been shown to be at increased risk.[240,249]

Acute pulmonary embolism is extremely rare, but it has been reported and should be managed with the same caution as for an adult.[250] Pulmonary angiography is still the gold standard in diagnosing pulmonary embolism. Several other examinations are useful for detecting the presence of a pulmonary embolism; for instance, ventilation-perfusion lung scanning can allow the diagnosis to be made 85% of the time.[240] Helical CT with contrast agents has recently gained popularity.[240]

FAT EMBOLISM

Fat embolism is a syndrome associated with long bone fractures in which fat emboli to the lungs lead to respiratory problems. It is believed to be caused by dissolution of normal circulating fat; however, the exact mechanism is still unexplained.[251,252] This condition may be caused by actual leaking of fat into the bloodstream or a metabolic change that allows normal circulating fat to become free fatty acids.[252] Mudd and associates examined patients who died of fat embolism syndrome after blunt trauma.[253] They found no particular source of the fat, nor was evidence of bone marrow or myeloid tissue seen in the lung sections. Many children have fat emboli after injury, but the clinical syndrome develops in very few.[251,254] Fabian and colleagues found the incidence of fat emboli in pediatric and adolescent long bone fractures to be as high as 10%.[255] Fat embolism is more often seen in teenagers and late adolescents, and the onset is usually shortly after the injury (within the first 2–3 days). Mudd and colleagues found no correlation with the number or severity of fractures; rather, fat embolism syndrome was more likely to be related to the extensive nature of the soft tissue injuries.[253] The pulmonary changes prevent exchange of oxygen across the alveolar-capillary membrane. In adults, this condition is referred to as acute respiratory distress syndrome. The incidence of fat embolism syndrome is markedly decreased by immediate internal stabilization of long bone fractures as opposed to treatment by traction or late reduction.[252,256–258] Intramedullary fixation of long bones (particularly diaphyseal fractures of the femur) is preferred because it reduces the risk of fat embolism syndrome. However, reaming for the nail can cause an increase in circulation and can potentially increase the risk of a fat embolism to the lung.[259] Fat embolism syndrome has been reported in children with muscular dystrophy and as a complication of closed femoral shortening.[260] Patients who are at risk of developing fat embolism syndrome should be monitored with pulse oximetry.[260]

With the full-blown syndrome, children have respiratory distress, tachypnea, and a deterioration in blood gas values, particularly O_2 saturation.[254] Clinically, the child may appear restless and confused; if untreated, stupor and coma may ensue. Petechiae may develop on the skin of the chest, axilla, and base of the neck, but they may be transient and are frequently missed.[251] The most significant laboratory finding is a decrease in arterial oxygen tension. Examination for fat in urine and sputum is of little value relative to more modern diagnostic measures. Recently, bronchoalveolar lavage for detection of fat-containing cells and retinal examination for cotton-wool spots and retinal hemorrhages have been reported to be helpful in early diagnosis.[261,262] A chest radiograph classically demonstrates interstitial edema and increased peripheral vascular markings.[251]

If untreated, fat embolism can be lethal; however, early diagnosis and prompt management can usually sustain the patient until the problem clears. Treatment consists of supportive measures for the respiratory problem, including improvement in oxygen saturation (70 mm Hg), and may require endotracheal positive-pressure breathing. The blood volume should be restored, and fluid and electrolyte balance should be maintained. Adequate oxygenation is the most important part of treatment because respiratory failure is the most common cause of death. Treatment with steroids and heparin remains controversial.

HYPERCALCEMIA OF IMMOBILIZATION

Many children exhibit hypercalcemia after immobilization of a fracture. Cristofaro and Brink reported that 7 of 20 children demonstrated increased serum calcium levels of 10.7 to 13.2 dL (normal, 8.5–10.5 dL).[263] Urinary excretion of calcium peaks approximately 4 weeks after immobilization begins and can be expected to return to normal levels with activity.[264] This increased urinary calcium excretion is believed to be part of the normal reparative process. In those who have preexisting metabolic bone disease, such as rickets or parathyroid disease, immobilization can further increase serum calcium levels.[264] Similarly, for unexplained reasons, some young patients, usually those 9 to 14 years of age, may have significantly high calcium blood levels and systemic symptoms.[264]

Symptoms include anorexia, nausea, vomiting, and increased irritability; if the condition is severe, generalized seizures, pain with movement, flaccid paralysis, muscle hypertonia, and blurred vision can occur. If hypercalcemia is not controlled, renal calculi can develop.[263] The serum alkaline phosphatase concentration is usually normal, unlike in the case of hyperparathyroidism, in which the serum level is generally high. However, to definitively distinguish the two conditions, a parathyroid hormone assay should be performed.[263]

Intravenous administration of fluids and corticosteroids has been reported to be successful in lowering the serum

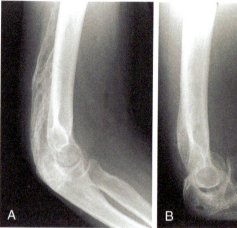
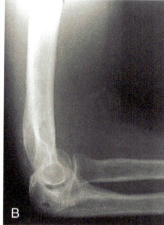

Fig. 7.23 Ectopic bone formation leading to complete elbow ankylosis. Radiographs were obtained before surgery (6 months after a head injury) (A) and 6 months after surgical excision (B). (From Mital MA, Garber JE, Stinson JT. Ectopic bone formation in children and adolescents with head injuries: its management. *J Pediatr Orthop.* 1987;7:83.)

calcium level until mobilization can be accomplished.[264] Usually, a low-calcium diet is recommended. Plicamycin (also known as mithramycin) also effectively lowers calcium, either by direct antagonism of bone resorption or by interference with the metabolism of parathyroid hormone. In addition, calcitonin has been reported to be effective in immediately lowering serum calcium levels by inhibiting bone resorption.[265–267] Finally, bisphosphonates have also been used to successfully treat hypercalcemia of immobilization.[268,269] Appropriate hydration and diuresis can help, as can immediate weight-bearing and movement.[264]

Another problem that is similar in nature is acute hypercalcemia after quadriplegia.[265,266,270] Particularly in young people, this condition can be troublesome and should be routinely evaluated during the first 6 weeks after the onset of paralysis.

ECTOPIC BONE FORMATION

Ectopic bone has been reported to appear around all major joints, most often the hip, elbow, and knee (Fig. 7.23).[271] The condition is more common in teenagers, but any age group is at risk. Ectopic bone formation is typically associated with head injuries and burns.[271,272] Myositis ossificans is associated with burns about the shoulder, distal end of the femur, elbow, and proximal part of the tibia, usually within 4 months after a thermal injury.[273] Mital and colleagues found that heterotopic bone developed in 15% of head-injured children and that coma and spasticity were the most commonly related factors.[271] Fractures about the pelvis and extensive surgical approaches to repair pelvic fractures increase the risk of myositis ossificans.

The process is usually preceded by an inflammatory response and tenderness near the affected joint in an area of soft tissue and bone trauma. Elevated levels of serum alkaline phosphatase usually precede ossification and remain elevated during active bone formation.[271,272] Radiographic evidence is apparent within 3 to 4 weeks after the injury.[271] MRI may be helpful in the early diagnosis of this condition. A rim with low signal intensity is a common finding, but no unique pattern characterizes myositis ossificans.[274] Initially, the process lacks definable borders and then progresses to a more focal mass with a high central intensity that eventually becomes bone.[274,275] This pattern is common in the intramuscular type and less so with the periosteal type. Involution is more evident in the intramuscular type.[275] Some resorption may occur after joint movement has begun. Attempts to excise the heterotopic bone should be delayed until the process is completely mature, usually about a year after injury.[272] Some reports have indicated that pharmacologic agents can reduce the incidence of ectopic bone formation. Mital and colleagues found that in head-injured children, salicylates can help minimize or eliminate ectopic bone, particularly after excision.[271] Similarly, indomethacin has been reported to be helpful.[271,276,277] Diphosphonates have been used, but because of problems with bone metabolism, they are not currently recommended.[272,278] Most children can be treated successfully by observation, and the condition can be allowed to run its course because few children have long-term problems.[278]

SUPERIOR MESENTERIC ARTERY SYNDROME (CAST SYNDROME)

Superior mesenteric artery syndrome consists of acute gastric dilatation and vomiting. In the past, this syndrome was most often recognized in those treated with a hip spica or body cast, hence the older name *cast syndrome*.[279] However, in more recent times, it has been reported to occur in the absence of a cast, such as after traction for extended periods, after spine surgery with instrumentation, particularly after correction of kyphosis, and after a severe traumatic brain injury.[280–283] The problem is caused by mechanical obstruction of the third portion of the duodenum by the superior mesenteric artery (Fig. 7.24).[280] It can be caused by hyperlordosis positioning in the cast, but more often it is associated with weight loss and a decrease in the fat protecting the superior mesenteric artery from the duodenum.[279–281] The angle between the superior mesenteric artery and the aorta becomes more acute and compresses the duodenum. Those with an asthenic body habitus and those who have an alteration in spinal curvature are at greatest risk.[280,281] If this condition is not treated aggressively, the problem becomes difficult to manage, and patients are subject to progressive weight loss, hypokalemia, and life-threatening dehydration and electrolyte abnormalities.[279]

The syndrome can be reversed by increasing the bulk of retroperitoneal fat. Treatment consists of passing a feeding tube beyond the obstruction or intravenous hyperalimentation plus repositioning (side lying) to encourage appropriate duodenal drainage.[282,283] If a cast is hyperextending the spine, it should be modified. Medical treatment duration of 6 weeks may be necessary.[284] In extreme cases that do not resolve with conservative treatment, complete derotation of the duodenum and colon with stabilization of the mesenteric artery (Ladd procedure) can resolve the obstruction.[280,281]

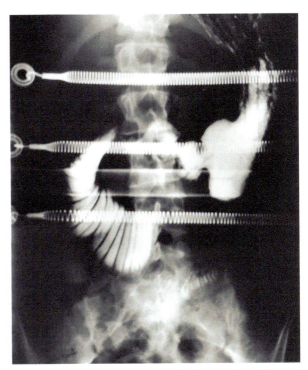

Fig. 7.24 An upper gastrointestinal series in a patient with superior mesenteric artery syndrome (cast syndrome) demonstrates compression of the fourth portion of the duodenum from the superior mesenteric artery as reflected by the abrupt cessation of flow of contrast beyond that point. Complete resolution followed aggressive intravenous hyperalimentation.

TRACTION-INDUCED HYPERTENSION

An uncommon event is hypertension associated with traction for a long bone fracture. Hypertension has also been reported to occur during limb lengthening as a result of traction on the bone and its adjacent soft tissue.[285,286] It may be caused by tension on the sciatic nerve, activation of the renin-angiotensin system, or prolonged immobilization.[285,287] Hamdan and colleagues noted elevated blood pressure in 68% of patients undergoing traction, three of whom required treatment.[285] This problem can be controlled by modification of the traction and by hypertension medication until the primary condition has resolved.[285,288]

REFLEX SYMPATHETIC DYSTROPHY

This condition is believed to be caused by dysfunction of the autonomic nervous system, usually after an injury to the ankle and foot, knee, or shoulder and hand.[289] It occurs more often in the lower extremities in children, in contrast to the shoulder and hand in adults.[290] Many terms have been used in the past to describe the condition, including *causalgia, posttraumatic pain syndrome, shoulder-hand syndrome*, and *Sudeck atrophy*. Reflex sympathetic dystrophy is also known as type I complex regional pain syndrome and is distinguished from type II complex regional pain syndrome by the absence of any direct peripheral nerve injury associated with the onset of symptoms. The onset is heralded by severe pain

Box 7.1   Pediatric Reflex Sympathetic Dystrophy: Diagnostic Criteria

1. Continuing pain, disproportionate to any inciting event
2. Patient reports least 1 symptom from each of the following categories:
   a. Sensory: Hyperalgesia and/or allodynia
   b. Vasomotor: Temperature asymmetry and/or skin color changes and/or skin color asymmetry
   c. Sudomotor/edema: Edema and/or sweating changes and/or sweating asymmetry
   d. Motor/trophic: Decreased range of motion and/or motor dysfunction (weakness, tremor, dystonia) and/or trophic changes (hair, nail, skin)
3. Must display at least one sign[a] at the time of evaluation in two or more categories:
   a. Sensory: Evidence of hyperalgesia and/or allodynia
   b. Vasomotor: Evidence of temperature asymmetry and/or skin color changes and/or skin color asymmetry
   c. Sudomotor/edema: Evidence of edema and/or sweating changes and/or sweating asymmetry
   d. Motor/trophic: Evidence of decreased range of motion and/or motor dysfunction (weakness, tremor, dystonia) and/or trophic changes (hair, nail, skin)
4. There is no other diagnosis that better explains the signs and symptoms

[a]A sign is counted only if it is displayed at the time of evaluation/diagnosis
From: Harden RN, Oaklander AL, Burton AW, et al. Complex regional pain syndrome: practical diagnostic and treatment guidelines, 4th edition. *Pain Med.* 2013;14:180–229.

and exquisite tenderness to light touch, including that from clothing.[289–291] Symptoms are intensified by weight-bearing and relieved by keeping the involved areas as motionless as possible.[289] The extremity is usually swollen and exhibits vasomotor instability (83%), including skin discoloration, swelling with dependency, and decreased peripheral pulses; the skin temperature is usually warmer with increased sweating.[290,292] The diagnostic criteria for reflex sympathetic dystrophy include signs of vasomotor instability and abnormal sensory response to stimuli (Box 7.1).[293–295]

Dietz and associates found a helpful clinical sign of autonomic dysfunction (tache cerebrale) not previously described in the diagnosis of childhood reflex sympathetic dystrophy.[290] Tache cerebrale is elicited by stroking the skin in the affected area with a blunt object such as the head of a safety pin, and the contralateral limbs are used as a control. Autonomic dysfunction is demonstrated by the appearance of an erythematous line 15 to 30 seconds after the stimulus. It may persist as long as 15 minutes. The line was present in all five of the authors' patients.[290]

The onset of symptoms may follow a trivial injury, such as a simple twisted ankle or sprain (52%), or it may not be associated with a definite event.[290,296] Reflex sympathetic dystrophy is usually seen in adolescents, most commonly preadolescent girls, but it has been described in children as young as 3 years.[290,291,297,298] A variety of theories have been proposed, but no satisfactory explanation exists as to the cause of its onset.

Typically, the condition is present for an extended period before the diagnosis is made (average, 8–16 weeks; range, 1 week to 26 months).[299,300] The differential diagnosis includes juvenile rheumatoid arthritis, polymyositis, rheumatic fever, systemic lupus erythematosus, neoplasia, gout, and thrombophlebitis. Symptoms may sometimes be confused with psychiatric conditions such as conversion disorder or malingering.[298] The results of laboratory studies are usually within normal limits.[289] Radiographs may reveal diffuse osteoporosis of the involved part. Bone scan findings have been inconsistent and show both increased uptake when the vasomotor phase is strong and decreased uptake with marked osteoporosis.[289]

Most pediatric patients are found to have psychologic problems, usually a pronounced indifference to the implications of the illness.[289,298,299,301] Such children have a tendency to accept responsibility beyond their years and are very involved in school and extracurricular activities, sports, or social functions.[289,302] They have difficulty expressing anger or being assertive on their own behalf.[289,302] Their strength is in doing rather than saying; this manner of expression is consistent with how these children best approach their environment.[302] The condition may serve a functional role by allowing them to slow down gracefully and affords a safe means of frustrating their parents' demands for performance without having to take responsibility for their behavior.[289] Most (83%) have emotional problems, and treatment must take these psychologic factors into account.[301,302] Marital discord was present in about half the families of these patients, and the child often had the burden of keeping peace in the household. Many families show inappropriately high levels of enmeshment between parents and the child; because of high levels of stress in the parental relationship, the child consciously or unconsciously attempts to alleviate the problem.

The primary emphasis in management is to make the diagnosis and exclude other potential problems. Prompt diagnosis and therapy are directed at alleviating the symptoms quickly, thereby significantly improving the chance for permanent relief.[291,298] Successful management often requires a multidisciplinary approach involving medical management, physical therapy, and psychological support. Most authors suggest that narcotic analgesics be avoided in children.[299] A calcium channel blocker (nifedipine) and a sympathetic blocker (phenoxybenzamine) have been reported to be effective in children.[303] Neuromodulating agents such as gabapentin or pregabalin have also been used with success. Immobilization must be avoided, as this can prolong the problem. Rather, vigorous active exercises, weight-bearing activities, and direct stimulation of the skin are usually successful therapies.[290] Corticosteroid therapy and sympathetic blockade are seldom necessary in children; most respond to continued positive reinforcement by a multidisciplinary team.[289–291,298–300] Recovery occurs in 7 to 8 weeks, but relapse is common (27%).[64,296,299,304]

Occasionally, children will have a much more persistent, severe problem that does not respond to outpatient management. It may require admission for more intensive inpatient therapy.[299] Similarly, in recalcitrant cases, more invasive measures are required, including continuous peripheral nerve blockade used over extended periods, sympathetic blockade, or administration of bisphosphonates.[296,305,306]

Surgical treatment such as sympathectomy is seldom required in children.[290]

The condition is more benign in children than in adults.[289,304] Children seldom have the chronic atrophic changes found in adults.[289,304] In follow-up, few children have long-term problems; most continue to function normally.[289,296,304]

ACKNOWLEDGMENT

The authors would like to acknowledge and thank Dr. Anthony A. Stans and Dr. Robert N. Hensinger, MD, for their contributions to the previous versions of this chapter.

REFERENCES

The level of evidence (LOE) is determined according to the criteria provided in the Preface.

1. Kirkilas M, Notrica DM, Langlais CS, Muenzer JT, Zoldos J, Graziano K. Outcomes of arterial vascular extremity trauma in pediatric patients. *J Pediatr Surg.* 2016;51(11):1885–1890. **(LOE IV).**
2. Harris LM, Hordines J. Major vascular injuries in the pediatric population. *Ann Vasc Surg.* 2003;17(3):266–269. **(LOE IV).**
3. Green NE, Allen BL. Vascular injuries associated with dislocation of the knee. *J Bone Joint Surg Am.* 1977;59(2):236–239. **(LOE IV).**
4. Copley LA, Dormans JP, Davidson RS. Vascular injuries and their sequelae in pediatric supracondylar humeral fractures: toward a goal of prevention. *J Pediatr Orthop.* 1996;16:99–103. **(LOE IV).**
5. Klineberg EO, Crites BM, Flinn WR, Archibald JD, Moorman CT 3rd. The role of arteriography in assessing popliteal artery injury in knee dislocations. *J Trauma.* 2004;56(4):786–790. **(LOE IV).**
6. Bond SJ, Gotschall CS, Eichelberger MR. Predictors of abdominal injury in children with pelvic fracture. *J Trauma.* 1991;31(8):1169–1173. **(LOE IV).**
7. Garvin KL, McCarthy RE, Barnes CL, Dodge BM. Pediatric pelvic ring fractures. *J Pediatr Orthop.* 1990;10(5):577–582. **(LOE IV).**
8. McIntyre Jr RC, Bensard DD, Moore EE, Chambers J, Moore FA. Pelvic fracture geometry predicts risk of life-threatening hemorrhage in children. *J Trauma.* 1993;35(3):423–429. **(LOE IV).**
9. O'Neill PA, Riina J, Sclafani S. Angiographic findings in pelvic fractures. *Clin Orthop Relat Res.* 1998;329:60–67. **(LOE IV).**
10. Vo NJ, Althoen M, Hippe DS, Prabhu SJ, Valji K, Padia SA. Pediatric abdominal and pelvic trauma: safety and efficacy of arterial embolization. *J Vasc Interv Radiol.* 2014;25(2):215–220. **(LOE IV).**
11. Tolhurst SR, Vanderhave KL, Caird MS, Garton HL, Graziano GP, Maher CO, et al. Cervical arterial injury after blunt trauma in children: characterization and advanced imaging. *J Pediatr Orthop.* 2013;33(1):37–42. **(LOE IV).**
12. Milas ZL, Dodson TF, Ricketts RR. Pediatric blunt trauma resulting in major arterial injuries. *Am Surg.* 2004;70(5):443–447. **(LOE IV).**
13. Lange RH, Bach AW, Hansen Jr ST, Johansen KH. Open tibial fractures with associated vascular injuries: prognosis for limb salvage. *J Trauma.* 1985;25(3):203–208. **(LOE IV).**
14. Weinberg DS, Scarcella NR, Napora JK, Vallier HA. Can vascular injury be appropriately assessed with physical examination after knee dislocation? *Clin Orthop Relat Res.* 2016;474(6):1453–1458. **(LOE III).**
15. Mills WJ, Barei DP, McNair P. The value of the ankle-brachial index for diagnosing arterial injury after knee dislocation: a prospective study. *J Trauma.* 2004;56(6):1261–1265. **(LOE III).**
16. Johansen K, Bandyk D, Thiele B, Hansen ST Jr. Temporary intraluminal shunts: resolution of a management dilemma in complex vascular injuries. *J Trauma.* 1982;22(5):395–402. **(LOE IV).**
17. Fabian TC, Turkleson ML, Connelly TL, Stone HH. Injury to the popliteal artery. *Am J Surg.* 1982 Feb;143(2):225–228. **(LOE IV).**
18. Fainzilber G, Roy-Shapira A, Wall MJ Jr, Mattox KL. Predictors of amputation for popliteal artery injuries. *Am J Surg.* 1995;170(6):568–570; discussion 70-71. **(LOE IV).**
19. Cole WG. Arterial injuries associated with fractures of the lower limbs in childhood. *Injury.* 1981;12(6):460–463. **(LOE IV).**
20. Stannard JP, Sheils TM, Lopez-Ben RR, McGwin G Jr, Robinson JT, Volgas DA. Vascular injuries in knee dislocations: the role of physical examination in determining the need for arteriography. *J Bone Joint Surg Am.* 2004;86-A(5):910–915. **(LOE II).**
21. Mommsen P, Zeckey C, Hildebrand F, Frink M, Khaladj N, Lange N, et al. Traumatic extremity arterial injury in children: epidemiology, diagnostics, treatment and prognostic value of mangled extremity severity score. *J Orthop Surg Res.* 2010;5:25. **(LOE IV).**
22. Cardneau JD, Henke PK, Upchurch GR Jr, Wakefield TW, Graham LM, Jacobs LA, et al. Efficacy and durability of autogenous saphenous vein conduits for lower extremity arterial reconstructions in preadolescent children. *J Vasc Surg.* 2001;34(1):34–40. (LOE IV).
23. Rozycki GS, Tremblay LN, Feliciano DV, McClelland WB. Blunt vascular trauma in the extremity: diagnosis, management, and outcome. *J Trauma.* 2003;55(5):814–824. **(LOE IV).**
24. Jeans KA, Browne RH, Karol LA. Effect of amputation level on energy expenditure during overground walking by children with an amputation. *J Bone Joint Surg Am.* 2011;93(1):49–56. **(LOE II).**
25. Starr AJ, Hunt JL, Reinert CM. Treatment of femur fracture with associated vascular injury. *J Trauma.* 1996;40(1):17–21. **(LOE IV).**
26. Zehntner MK, Petropoulos P, Burch H. Factors determining outcome in fractures of the extremities associated with arterial injuries. *J Orthop Trauma.* 1991;5(1):29–33. **(LOE IV).**
27. Bach A, Johansen K. Limb salvage using temporary arterial shunt following traumatic near-amputation of the thigh. *J Pediatr Orthop.* 1982;2:187–190. **(LOE IV).**
28. Eliason JL, Coleman DM, Gumushian A, Stanley JC. Arterial reconstructions for chronic lower extremity ischemia in preadolescent and adolescent children. *J Vasc Surg.* 2018;67(4):1207–1216. **(LOE IV).**
29. Campbell CC, Waters PM, Emans JB, Kasser JR, Millis MB. Neurovascular injury and displacement in type III supracondylar humerus fractures. *J Pediatr Orthop.* 1995;15(1):47–52. **(LOE IV).**
30. Dormans JP, Squillante R, Sharf H. Acute neurovascular complications with supracondylar humerus fractures in children. *J Hand Surg Am.* 1995;20(1):1–4. **(LOE IV).**
31. Lyons ST, Quinn M, Stanitski CL. Neurovascular injuries in type III humeral supracondylar fractures in children. *Clin Orthop Relat Res.* 2000;376:62–67. **(LOE IV).**
32. Sabharwal S, Tredwell SJ, Beauchamp RD, Mackenzie WG, Jakubec DM, Cairns R, et al. Management of pulseless pink hand in pediatric supracondylar fractures of humerus. *J Pediatr Orthop.* 1997;17(3):303–310. **(LOE IV).**
33. White L, Mehlman CT, Crawford AH. Perfused, pulseless, and puzzling: a systematic review of vascular injuries in pediatric supracondylar humerus fractures and results of a POSNA questionnaire. *J Pediatr Orthop.* 2010;30(4):328–335. **(LOE IV).**
34. Lewis HG, Morrison CM, Kennedy PT, Herbert KJ. Arterial reconstruction using the basilic vein from the zone of injury in pediatric supracondylar humeral fractures: a clinical and radiological series. *Plast Reconstr Surg.* 2003;111:1159–1163. **(LOE IV).**
35. Blakemore LC, Cooperman DR, Thompson GH, Wathey C, Ballock RT. Compartment syndrome in ipsilateral humerus and forearm fractures in children. *Clin Orthop Relat Res.* 2000;376:32–38. **(LOE IV).**
36. Ring D, Waters PM, Hotchkiss RN, Kasser JR. Pediatric floating elbow. *J Pediatr Orthop.* 2001;21(4):456–459. **(LOE IV).**
37. Muchow RD, Riccio AI, Garg S, Ho CA, Wimberly RL. Neurological and vascular injury associated with supracondylar humerus fractures and ipsilateral forearm fractures in children. *J Pediatr Orthop.* 2015;35(2):121–125. **(LOE IV).**
38. Blumberg TJ, Bremjit P, Bompadre V, Steinman S. Forearm fixation is not necessary in the treatment of pediatric floating elbow. *J Pediatr Orthop.* 2018;38(2):82–87. **(LOE IV).**
39. Barrios C, de Pablos J. Surgical management of nerve injuries of the upper extremity in children: a 15-year survey. *J Pediatr Orthop.* 1991;11(5):641–645. **(LOE IV).**
40. Kiyoshige Y. Critical displacement of neural injuries in supracondylar humeral fractures in children. *J Pediatr Orthop.* 1999;19(6):816–817. **(LOE IV).**
41. McGraw JJ, Akbarnia BA, Hanel DP, Keppler L, Burdge RE. Neurological complications resulting from supracondylar fractures of the humerus in children. *J Pediatr Orthop.* 1986;6(6):647–650. **(LOE IV).**

42. Haasbeek JF, Cole WG. Open fractures of the arm in children. *J Bone Joint Surg Br.* 1995;77(4):576–581. **(LOE IV).**

43. Brown IC, Zinar DM. Traumatic and iatrogenic neurological complications after supracondylar humerus fractures in children. *J Pediatr Orthop.* 1995;15(4):440–443. **(LOE IV).**

44. Shore BJ, Gillespie BT, Miller PE, Bae DS, Waters PM. Recovery of motor nerve injuries associated with displaced, extension-type pediatric supracondylar humerus fractures. *J Pediatr Orthop.* 2017;2. **(LOE IV).**

45. Hosalkar HS, Matzon JL, Chang B. Nerve palsies related to pediatric upper extremity fractures. *Hand Clin.* 2006;22(1):87–98. **(LOE IV).**

46. Skaggs DL, Hale JM, Bassett J, Kaminsky C, Kay RM, Tolo VT. Operative treatment of supracondylar fractures of the humerus in children. The consequences of pin placement. *J Bone Joint Surg Am.* 2001;83-A(5):735–740. **(LOE III).**

47. Ozcelik A, Tekcan A, Omerolu HJ. Correlation between iatrogenic ulnar nerve injury and angular insertion of the medial pin in supracondylar humerus fractures. *J Pediatr Orthop.* 2006;15(1):58–61. **(LOE IV).**

48. Mulpuri K, Hosalkar H, Howard A. AAOS clinical practice guideline: the treatment of pediatric supracondylar humerus fractures. *J Am Acad Orthop Surg.* 2012;20(5):328–330. **(LOE IV).**

49. Royle SG, Burke D. Ulna neuropathy after elbow injury in children. *J Pediatr Orthop.* 1990;10(4):495–496. **(LOE IV).**

50. Hyatt BT, Schmitz MR, Rush JK. Complications of pediatric elbow fractures. *Orthop Clin North Am.* 2016;47(2):377–385. **(LOE IV).**

51. Flynn K, Shah AS, Brusalis CM, Leddy K, Flynn JM. Flexion-type supracondylar humeral fractures: ulnar nerve injury increases risk of open reduction. *J Bone Joint Surg Am.* 2017;99(17):1485–1487. **(LOE IV).**

52. Nishimura M, Itsubo T, Horii E, Hayashi M, Uchiyama S, Kato H. Tardy ulnar nerve palsy caused by chronic radial head dislocation after Monteggia fracture: a report of two cases. *J Pediatr Orthop B.* 2016;25(5):450–453. **(LOE IV).**

53. Toh S, Tsubo K, Nishikawa S, Inoue S, Nakamura R, Harata S. Long-standing nonunion of fractures of the lateral humeral condyle. *J Bone Joint Surg Am.* 2002;84-A(4):593–598. **(LOE IV).**

54. Abe M, Ishizu T, Shirai H, Okamoto M, Onomura T. Tardy ulnar nerve palsy caused by cubitus varus deformity. *J Hand Surg Am.* 1995;20(1):5–9. **(LOE IV).**

55. Mortazavi SM, Heidari P, Asadollahi S, Farzan M. Severe tardy ulnar nerve palsy caused by traumatic cubitus valgus deformity: functional outcome of subcutaneous anterior transposition. *J Hand Surg Eur.* 2008;33(5):575–580. **(LOE IV).**

56. Stutz CM, Calfee RP, Steffen JA, Goldfarb CA. Surgical and nonsurgical treatment of cubital tunnel syndrome in pediatric and adolescent patients. *J Hand Surg Am.* 2012;37(4):657–662. **(LOE IV).**

57. Karakis I, Liew W, Fournier HS, Jones Jr HR, Darras BT, Kang PB. Electrophysiologic features of ulnar neuropathy in childhood and adolescence. *Clin Neurophysiol.* 2017;128(5):751–755. **(LOE IV).**

58. Amillo S, Mora G. Surgical management of neural injuries associated with elbow fractures in children. *J Pediatr Orthop.* 1999;19(5):573–577. **(LOE IV).**

59. Li H, Cai QX, Shen PQ, Chen T, Zhang ZM, Zhao L. Posterior interosseous nerve entrapment after Monteggia fracture-dislocation in children. *Chin J Traumatol.* 2013;16(3):131–135. **(LOE IV).**

60. Osamura N, Ikeda K, Hagiwara N, Tomita K. Posterior interosseous nerve injury complicating ulnar osteotomy for a missed Monteggia fracture. *Scand J Plast Reconstr Surg Hand Surg.* 2004;38(6):376–378. **(LOE IV).**

61. Choi WS, Han KJ, Lee DH, Lee GE, Kweon HJ, Cho JH. Stepwise percutaneous leverage technique to avoid posterior interosseous nerve injury in pediatric radial neck fracture. *J Orthop Trauma.* 2017;31(5):e151–e157. **(LOE IV).**

62. Waters PM, Kolettis GJ, Schwend R. Acute median neuropathy following physeal fractures of the distal radius. *J Pediatr Orthop.* 1994;14(2):173–177. **(LOE IV).**

63. Bolitho DG, Boustred M, Hudson DA, Hodgetts K. Primary epineural repair of the ulnar nerve in children. *J Hand Surg Am.* 1999;24(1):16–20. **(LOE IV).**

64. Veldman PH, Goris RJ. Multiple reflex sympathetic dystrophy. Which patients are at risk for developing a recurrence of reflex sympathetic dystrophy in the same or another limb. *Pain.* 1996;64(3):463–466. **(LOE IV).**

65. Green NE. Entrapment of the median nerve following elbow dislocation. *J Pediatr Orthop.* 1983;3(3):384–386. **(LOE IV).**

66. Pritchett JW. Entrapment of the median nerve after dislocation of the elbow. *J Pediatr Orthop.* 1984 Nov;4(6):752–753. **(LOE IV).**

67. Hallett J. Entrapment of the median nerve after dislocation of the elbow. A case report. *J Bone Joint Surg Br.* 1981;63-B(3):408–412. **(LOE IV).**

68. Matsen FA. Compartmental syndromes in children. *J Pediatr Orthop.* 1981:33–41. **(LOE IV).**

69. Rooser B, Bengtson S, Hagglund G. Acute compartment syndrome from anterior thigh muscle contusion: a report of eight cases. *J Orthop Trauma.* 1991;5(1):57–59. **(LOE IV).**

70. Bae DS, Kadiyala RK, Waters PM. Acute compartment syndrome in children: contemporary diagnosis, treatment, and outcome. *J Pediatr Orthop.* 2001;21(5):680–688. **(LOE IV).**

71. Mashru RP, Herman MJ, Pizzutillo PD. Tibial shaft fractures in children and adolescents. *J Am Acad Orthop Surg.* 2005;13(5):345–352. **(LOE IV).**

72. De Aerts P, Boeck H, Casteleyn PP. Case report: deep volar compartment syndrome of the forearm following minor crush injury. *J Pediatr Orthop.* 1989;9:69–71. **(LOE IV).**

73. Hernandez J, Peterson HA. Case report: fracture of the distal radial physis complicated by compartment syndrome and premature physeal closure. *J Pediatr Orthop.* 1986;6:627–630. **(LOE IV).**

74. Peters CL, Scott SM. Compartment syndrome in the forearm following fractures of the radial head or neck in children. *J Bone Joint Surg Am.* 1995;77(7):1070–1074. **(LOE IV).**

75. Grottkau BE, Epps HR, Di Scala C. Compartment syndrome in children and adolescents. *J Pediatr Surg.* 2005;40(4):678–682. **(LOE IV).**

76. Schwartz JT Jr, Brumback RJ, Lakatos R, Poka A, Bathon GH, Burgess AR. Acute compartment syndrome of the thigh. A spectrum of injury. *J Bone Joint Surg Am.* 1989;71(3):392–400. **(LOE IV).**

77. Blackman AJ, Wall LB, Keeler KA. Acute compartment syndrome after intramedullary nailing of isolated radius and ulnar fractures in children. *J Pediatr Orthop.* 2014;34:50–54. **(LOE III).**

78. Court-Brown CM, Byrnes T, McLaughlin G. Intramedullary nailing of tibial diaphyseal fractures in adolescents with open physes. *Injury.* 2003;34(10):781–785. **(LOE IV).**

79. Yuan PS, Pring ME, Gaynor TP, Mubarak SJ, Newton PO. Compartment syndrome following intramedullary fixation of pediatric forearm fractures. *J Pediatr Orthop.* 2004;24(4):370–375. **(LOE IV).**

80. Large TM, Frick SL. Compartment syndrome of the leg after treatment of a femoral fracture with an early sitting spica cast. A report of two cases. *J Bone Joint Surg Am.* 2003;85-A(11):2207–2210. **(LOE IV).**

81. Janzing H, Broos P, Romnens P. Compartment syndrome as complication of skin traction, in children with femoral fractures. *Acta Chir Belg.* 1996;96:135–137. **(LOE IV).**

82. Mubarak SJ, Frick S, Sink E, Rathjen K, Noonan KJ. Volkmann contracture and compartment syndromes after femur fractures in children treated with 90/90 spica casts. *J Pediatr Orthop.* 2006;26(5):567–572. **(LOE IV).**

83. Kapoor V, Theruvil B, Edwards SE, Taylor GR, Clarke NM, Uglow MG. Flexible intramedullary nailing of displaced diaphyseal forearm fractures in children. *Injury.* 2005;36(10):1221–1225. **(LOE IV).**

84. Spiguel L, Glynn L, Liu D, Statter M. Pediatric pelvic fractures: a marker for injury severity. *Am Surg.* 2006;72(6):481–484. **(LOE IV).**

85. Flynn JM, Jones KJ, Garner MR, Goebel J. Eleven years' experience in the operative management of pediatric forearm fractures. *J Pediatr Orthop.* 2010;30:313–319. **(LOE III).**

86. Martus JE, Preston RK, Schoenecker JG, Lovejoy SA, Green NE, Mencio GA. Complications and outcomes of diaphyseal forearm fracture intramedullary nailing: a comparison of pediatric and adolescent age groups. *J Pediatr Orthop.* 2013;33(6):598–607. **(LOE III).**

87. Pandya NK, Edmonds EW, Mubarak SJ. The incidence of compartment syndrome after flexible nailing of pediatric tibial shaft fractures. *J Child Orthop.* 2011;5(6):439–447. **(LOE IV).**

88. Shore BJ, Glotzbecker MP, Zurakowski D, Gelbard E, Hedequist DJ, Matheney TH. Acute compartment syndrome in children and

teenagers with tibial shaft fractures: incidence and multivariable risk factors. *J Orthop Trauma.* 2013;27(11):616–621. **(LOE II).**

89. Livingston KS, Glotzbecker MP, Shore BJ. Pediatric acute compartment syndrome. *J Am Acad Orthop Surg.* 2017;25(5):358–364. **(LOE IV).**

90. Wallin K, Nguyen H, Russell L, Lee DK. Acute traumatic compartment syndrome in pediatric foot: a systematic review and case report. *J Foot Ankle Surg.* 2016;55(4):817–820. **(LOE IV).**

91. Mubarak SJ, Owen CA, Hargens AR, Garetto LP, Akeson WH. Acute compartment syndromes: diagnosis and treatment with the aid of the wick catheter. *J Bone Joint Surg Am.* 1978;60(8):1091–1095. **(LOE IV).**

92. Livingston K, Glotzbecker M, Miller PE, Hresko MT, Hedequist D, Shore BJ. Pediatric nonfracture acute compartment syndrome: a review of 39 cases. *J Pediatr Orthop.* 2016;36(7):685–690. **(LOE IV).**

93. Noonan K, McCarthy JJ. Compartment syndromes in the pediatric patient. *J Pediatr Orthop.* 2010;30:S96–S101. **(LOE IV).**

94. Mars M, Hadley GP. Failure of pulse oximetry in the assessment of raised limb intracompartmental pressure. *Injury.* 1994;25(6):379–381. **(LOE IV).**

95. Hargens AR, Akeson WH, Mubarak SJ. Fluid balance within the canine anterolateral compartment and its relationship to compartment syndromes. *J Bone Joint Surgery Am.* 1978;60:499–505. **(LOE N/A).**

96. Mars M, Hadley GP. Raised compartmental pressure in children: a basis for management. *Injury.* 1998;29(3):183–185. **(LOE IV).**

97. Staudt JM, Smeulders MJ, van der Horst CM. Normal compartment pressures of the lower leg in children. *J Bone Joint Surg Br.* 2008;90(2):215–219. **(LOE IV).**

98. Battaglia TC, Armstrong DG, Schwend RM. Factors affecting forearm compartment pressures in children with supracondylar fractures of the humerus. *J Pediatr Orthop.* 2002;22(4):431–439. **(LOE IV).**

99. Kleis K, Schlechter JA, Doan JD, Farnsworth CL, Edmonds EW. Under pressure: the utility of spacers in univalved fiberglass casts. *J Pediatr Orthop.* 2017;24. **(LOE IV).**

100. Matsen FA. Compartment syndrome: a unified concept. *Clin Orthop.* 1975;113:8–14. **(LOE IV).**

101. Turen CH, Burgess AR, Vanco B. Skeletal stabilization for tibial fractures associated with acute compartment syndrome. *Clin Orthop Relat Res.* 1995;(315):163–168. **(LOE IV).**

102. Ziolkowski NI, Zive L, Ho ES, Zuker RM. Timing of presentation of pediatric compartment syndrome and its microsurgical implication: a retrospective review. *Plast Reconstr Surg.* 2017;139(3):663–670. **(LOE IV).**

103. Chuang DC, Carver N, Wei FC. A new strategy to prevent the sequelae of severe Volkmann's ischemia. *Plast Reconstr Surg.* 1996;98(6):1023–1031; discussion 32-3. **(LOE IV).**

104. Badawy SM, Gust MJ, Liem RI, Ball MK, Gosain AK, Sharathkumar AA. Neonatal compartment syndrome associated with disseminated intravascular coagulation. *Ann Plast Surg.* 2016;76(2):256–258. **(LOE IV).**

105. Bekmez S, Beken S, Mermerkaya MU, Ozkan M, Okumus N. Acute forearm compartment syndrome in a newborn caused by reperfusion after spontaneous axillary artery thrombosis. *J Pediatr Orthop B.* 2015;24(6):552–555. **(LOE IV).**

106. Goubier JN, Romana C, Molina V. [Neonatal Volkmann's compartment syndrome. A report of two cases]. *Chir Main.* 2005;24(1):45–47. **(LOE IV).**

107. Martin B, Treharne L. Neonatal compartment syndrome. *Ann R Coll Surg Engl.* 2016;98(7):e111–e113. **(LOE IV).**

108. Agrawal H, Dokania G, Wu SY. Neonatal Volkmann ischemic contracture: case report and review of literature. *AJP Rep.* 2014;4(2):e77–e80. **(LOE IV).**

109. Plancq MC, Buisson P, Deroussen F, Krim G, Collet LM, Gouron R. Successful early surgical treatment in neonatal compartment syndrome: case report. *J Hand Surg Am.* 2013;38(6):1185–1188. **(LOE IV).**

110. Carlson Jr CS, Rosman MA. Cubitus varus: a new and simple technique for correction. *J Pediatr Orthop.* 1982;2(2):199–201. **(LOE IV).**

111. Papandrea R, Waters PM. Posttraumatic reconstruction of the elbow in the pediatric patient. *Clin Orthop Relat Res.* 2000;370:115–126. **(LOE IV).**

112. Barrett IR, Bellemore MC, Kwon YM. Cosmetic results of supracondylar osteotomy for correction of cubitus varus. *J Pediatr Orthop.* 1998;18(4):445–447. **(LOE IV).**

113. Blasier RD. The triceps-splitting approach for repair of distal humeral malunion in children. A report of a technique. *Am J Orthop (Belle Mead NJ).* 1996;25(9):621–624. **(LOE IV).**

114. Belthur MV, Iobst CA, Bor N, Segev E, Eidelman M, Standard SC, et al. Correction of cubitus varus after pediatric supracondylar elbow fracture: alternative method using the Taylor Spatial Frame. *J Pediatr Orthop.* 2016;36(6):608–617. **(LOE IV).**

115. Whitehouse WM, Coran AG, Stanley JC, Kuhns LR, Weintraub WH, Fry WJ. Pediatric vascular trauma. Manifestations, management, and sequelae of extremity arterial injury in patients undergoing surgical treatment. *Arch Surg.* 1976;111(11):1269–1275. **(LOE IV).**

116. Rodgers WB, Waters PM, Hall JE. Chronic Monteggia lesions in children. Complications and results of reconstruction. *J Bone Joint Surg Am.* 1996;78(9):1322–1329. **(LOE IV).**

117. Ramski DE, Hennrikus WP, Bae DS, Baldwin KD, Patel NM, Waters PM, et al. Pediatric Monteggia fractures: a multicenter examination of treatment strategy and early clinical and radiographic results. *J Pediatr Orthop.* 2015;35(2):115–120. **(LOE III).**

118. Inoue G, Shionoya K. Corrective ulnar osteotomy for malunited anterior Monteggia lesions in children. 12 patients followed for 1-12 years. *Acta Orthop Scand.* 1998;69(1):73–76. **(LOE IV).**

119. Creasman C, Zaleske DJ, Ehrlich MG. Analyzing forearm fractures in children. The more subtle signs of impending problems. *Clin Orthop Relat Res.* 1984;188:40–53. **(LOE IV).**

120. Davis DR, Green DP. Forearm fractures in children: pitfalls and complications. *Clin Orthop Relat Res.* 1976;120:172–183. **(LOE IV).**

121. Younger ASE, Tredwell SJ, Mackenzie WG. Factors affecting fracture position at cast removal after pediatric forearm fracture. *J Pediatr Orthop.* 1997;17:332–336. **(LOE IV).**

122. Price CT, Knapp DR. Osteotomy for malunited forearm shaft fractures in children. *J Pediatr Orthop.* 2006;26(2):193–196. **(LOE IV).**

123. Nietosvaara Y, Hasler C, Helenius I, Cundy P. Marked initial displacement predicts complications in physeal fractures of the distal radius: an analysis of fracture characteristics, primary treatment and complications in 109 patients. *Acta Orthop.* 2005;76(6):873–877. **(LOE IV).**

124. Crawford SN, Lee L, Izuka BH. Closed treatment of overriding distal radial fractures without reduction in children. *J Bone Joint Surgery Am.* 2012;94:246–252. **(LOE II).**

125. Vittas D, Larsen E, Torp-Pedersen S. Angular remodeling of midshaft forearm fractures in children. *Clin Orthop Relat Res.* 1991;265:261–264. **(LOE IV).**

126. Teoh KH, Chee YH, Shortt N, Wilkinson G, Porter DE. An age- and sex-matched comparative study on both-bone diaphyseal paediatric forearm fracture. *J Child Orthop.* 2009;3(5):367–373. **(LOE III).**

127. Trousdale RT, Linscheid RL. Operative treatment of malunited fractures of the forearm. *J Bone Joint Surg Am.* 1995;77(6):894–902. **(LOE IV).**

128. Price CT, Scott DS, Kurzner ME. Malunited forearm fractures in children. *J Pediatr Orthop.* 1990;10:705–712. **(LOE IV).**

129. Canadian Orthopaedic Trauma Society. Nonoperative treatment compared with plate fixation of displaced midshaft clavicular fractures. A multicenter, randomized clinical trial. *J Bone Joint Surg Am.* 2007;89(1):1–10. **(LOE I).**

130. Bae DS, Shah AS, Kalish LA, Kwon JY, Waters PM. Shoulder motion, strength, and functional outcomes in children with established malunion of the clavicle. *J Pediatr Orthop.* 2013;33(5):544–550. **(LOE IV).**

131. Palmu SA, Lohman M, Paukku RT. Childhood femoral fracture can lead to premature knee-joint arthritis. *Acta Orthop.* 2013;84:71–75. **(LOE IV).**

132. Narayanan UG, Hyman JE, Wainwright AM. Complications of elastic stable intramedullary nail fixation of pediatric femoral fractures, and how to avoid them. *J Pediatr Orthop.* 2004;24:363–369. **(LOE IV).**

133. Parikh SN, Nathan ST, Priola MJ, Eismann EA. Elastic nailing for pediatric subtrochanteric and supracondylar femur fractures. *J Bone Joint Surgery Am.* 2014;472(9):2735-2744. **(LOE IV).**

134. Bohn WW, Durbin RA. Ipsilateral fractures of the femur and tibia in children and adolescents. *J Bone Joint Surg Am*. 1991;73(3): 429–439. **(LOE IV)**.

135. Pandya NK, Edmonds EW. Immediate intramedullary flexible nailing of open pediatric tibial shaft fractures. *J Pediatr Orthop*. 2012;32:770–775. **(LOE III)**.

136. Hoffer MM, Garrett A, Brink J, Perry J, Hale W, Nickel VL. The orthopaedic management of brain-injured children. *J Bone Joint Surg Am*. 1971;53(3):567–577. **(LOE IV)**.

137. Kirby RM, Winquist RA, Hansen ST. Femoral shaft fractures in adolescents: a comparison between traction plus cast treatment and closed intramedullary nailing. *J Pediatr Orthop*. 1981;1:193–197. **(LOE III)**.

138. Loder RT. Pediatric polytrauma: orthopaedic care and hospital course. *J Orthop Trauma*. 1987;1(1):48–54. **(LOE IV)**.

139. Nenopoulos SP, Beslikas TA, Gigis JP. Long-term follow-up of combined fractures of the proximal radius and ulna during childhood. *J Pediatr Orthop B*. 2009;18(5):252–260. **(LOE IV)**.

140. Vince KG, Miller JE. Cross-union complicating fracture of the forearm. Part II: Children. *J Bone Joint Surg Am*. 1987;69:654–661. **(LOE IV)**.

141. Cullen MC, Roy DR, Giza E, Crawford AH. Complications of intramedullary fixation of pediatric forearm fractures. *J Pediatr Orthop*. 1998;18(1):14–21. **(LOE IV)**.

142. Bergeron SG, Desy NM, Bernstein M, Harvey EJ. Management of posttraumatic radioulnar synostosis. *J Am Acad Orthop Surg*. 2012;20(7):450–458. **(LOE IV)**.

143. Failla JM, Amadio PC, Morrey BF. Post-traumatic proximal radio-ulnar synostosis. Results of surgical treatment. *J Bone Joint Surg Am*. 1989;71(8):1208–1213. **(LOE IV)**.

144. Jupiter JB, Ring D. Operative treatment of post-traumatic proximal radioulnar synostosis. *J Bone Joint Surg Am*. 1998;80(2):248–257. **(LOE IV)**.

145. Fernandez DL, Joneschild E. "Wrap around" pedicled muscle flaps for the treatment of recurrent forearm synostosis. *Tech Hand Up Extrem Surg*. 2004;8:102–109. **(LOE IV)**.

146. Jones ME, Rider MA, Hughes JJ. The use of a proximally based posterior interosseous adipofascial flap to prevent recurrence of synostosis of the elbow joint and forearm. *Surg*. 2007;32B:143–147. **(LOE IV)**.

147. Munjal K, Kishan S, Sabharwal S. Posttraumatic pediatric distal tibiofibular synostosis: a case report. *Foot Ankle Int*. 2004;25(6):429–433. **(LOE IV)**.

148. Frick SL, Shoemaker S, Mubarak SJ. Altered fibular growth patterns after tibiofibular synostosis in children. *J Bone Joint Surg Am*. 2001;83-A(2):247–254. **(LOE IV)**.

149. Lewallen RP, Peterson HA. Nonunion of long bone fractures in children: a review of 30 cases. *J Pediatr Orthop*. 1985;5(2):135–142. **(LOE IV)**.

150. Shrader MW, Stans AA, Shaughnessy WJ, Haidukewych GJ. Nonunion of fractures in pediatric patients: 15-year experience at a level I trauma center. *Orthopaedics*. 2009;410. **(LOE IV)**.

151. Buckley SL, Smith GR, Sponseller PD, Thompson JD, Robertson WW Jr, Griffin PP. Severe (type III) open fractures of the tibia in children. *J Pediatr Orthop*. 1996;16(5):627–634. **(LOE IV)**.

152. Cullen MC, Roy DR, Crawford AH, Assenmacher J, Levy MS, Wen D. Open fracture of the tibia in children. *J Bone Joint Surg Am*. 1996;78(7):1039–1047. **(LOE IV)**.

153. Yeo JH, Jung ST, Kim MC, Yang HY. Diaphyseal nonunion in children. *J Orthop Trauma*. 2018;32(2):e52–e58. **(LOE IV)**.

154. Bagatur AE, Zorer G. Complications associated with surgically treated hip fractures in children. *J Pediatr Orthop B*. 2002;11(3):219–228. **(LOE IV)**.

155. Caglar O, Aksoy MC, Yazici M, Surat A. Comparison of compression plate and flexible intramedullary nail fixation in pediatric femoral shaft fractures. *J Pediatr Orthop B*. 2006;15(3):210–214. **(LOE IV)**.

156. Morsy HA. Complications of fracture of the neck of the femur in children. A long-term follow-up study. *Injury*. 2001;32(1):45–51. **(LOE IV)**.

157. Ogonda L, Wong-Chung J, Wray R, Canavan B. Delayed union and non-union of the ulna following intramedullary nailing in children. *J Pediatr Orthop B*. 2004;13(5):330–333. **(LOE IV)**.

158. Grimard G, Naudie D, Laberge LC, Hamdy RC. Open fractures of the tibia in children. *Clin Orthop Relat Res*. 1996;(332):62–70. **(LOE IV)**.

159. Kay RM, Directo MP, Leathers M, Myung K, Skaggs DL. Complications of ketorolac use in children undergoing operative fracture care. *J Pediatr Orthop*. 2010;30(7):655–658. **(LOE III)**.

160. Kay RM, Leathers M, Directo MP, Myung K, Skaggs DL. Perioperative ketorolac use in children undergoing lower extremity osteotomies. *J Pediatr Orthop*. 2011;31(7):783–786. **(LOE III)**.

161. Donohue D, Sanders D, Serrano-Riera R, Jordan C, Gaskins R, Sanders R, et al. Ketorolac administered in the recovery room for acute pain management does not affect healing rates of femoral and tibial fractures. *J Orthop Trauma*. 2016;30(9):479–482. **(LOE III)**.

162. Ippolito E, Tudisco C, Farsetti P, Caterini R. Fracture of the humeral condyles in children: 49 cases evaluated after 18-45 years. *Acta Orthop Scand*. 1996;67(2):173–178. **(LOE IV)**.

163. Ebraheim NA, Skie MC, Jackson WT. The treatment of tibial nonunion with angular deformity using an Ilizarov device. 38:111–117. **(LOE IV)**.

164. Yeranosian M, Horneff JG, Baldwin K, Hosalkar HS. Factors affecting the outcome of fractures of the femoral neck in children and adolescents: a systematic review. *Bone Joint J*. 2013;95-B(1):135–142. **(LOE IV)**.

165. Pace JL, Arkader A, Sousa T, Broom AM, Shabtai L. Incidence, risk factors, and definition for nonunion in pediatric lateral condyle fractures. *J Pediatr Orthop*. 2018;38(5):e257–e261. **(LOE IV)**.

166. De Boeck H. Surgery for non-union of the lateral humeral condyle in children: 6 cases followed for years. *Acta Orthop Scand*. 1995;402:1–9. **(LOE IV)**.

167. Flynn JC. Nonunion of slightly displaced fractures of the lateral humeral condyle in children: an update. *J Pediatr Orthop*. 1989;9(6):691–696. **(LOE IV)**.

168. Inoue G, Tamura Y. Osteosynthesis for longstanding nonunion of the lateral humeral condyle. *Arch Orthop Trauma Surg*. 1993;112(5):236–238. **(LOE IV)**.

169. Masada K, Kawai H, Kawabata H, Masatomi T, Tsuyuguchi Y, Yamamoto K. Osteosynthesis for old, established non-union of the lateral condyle of the humerus. *J Bone Joint Surg Am*. 1990;72(1):32–40. **(LOE IV)**.

170. Roye DP, Bini SA, Infosino A. Late surgical treatment of lateral condylar fractures in children. *J Pediatr Orthop*. 1991;11:195–199. **(LOE IV)**.

171. Masquijo JJ, Willis BR. Scaphoid nonunions in children and adolescents: surgical treatment with bone grafting and internal fixation. *J Pediatr Orthop*. 2010;30(2):119–124. **(LOE IV)**.

172. Mintzer CM, Waters PM, Simmons BP. Nonunion of the scaphoid in children treated by Herbert screw fixation and bone grafting. A report of five cases. *J Bone Joint Surg Br*. 1995;77(1):98–100. **(LOE IV)**.

173. Arunachalam VS, Griffiths JC. Fracture recurrence in children. *Injury*. 1975;7(1):37–40. **(LOE IV)**.

174. Schwarz N, Pienaar S, Schwarz AF, Jelen M, Styhler W, Mayr J. Refracture of the forearm in children. *J Bone Joint Surg Br*. 1996;78(5):740–744. **(LOE IV)**.

175. Bould M, Bannister GC. Refractures of the radius and ulna in children. *Injury*. 1999;30(9):583–586. **(LOE IV)**.

176. Tisosky AJ, Werger MM, McPartland TG, Bowe JA. The factors influencing the refracture of pediatric forearms. *J Pediatr Orthop*. 2015;35(7):677–681. **(LOE IV)**.

177. Baitner AC, Perry A, Lalonde FD, Bastrom TP, Pawelek J, Newton PO. The healing forearm fracture: a matched comparison of forearm refractures. *J Pediatr Orthop*. 2007;27(7):743–747. **(LOE III)**.

178. Vopat BG, Kane PM, Fitzgibbons PG, Got CJ, Katarincic JA. Complications associated with retained implants after plate fixation of the pediatric forearm. *J Orthop Trauma*. 2014;28(6):360–364. **(LOE IV)**.

179. Makki D, Kheiran A, Gadiyar R, Ricketts D. Refractures following removal of plates and elastic nails from paediatric forearms. *J Pediatr Orthop B*. 2014;23(3):221–226. **(LOE IV)**.

180. Kesemenli CC, Necmioglu S, Kayikci C. Treatment of refracture occurring after external fixation in paediatric femoral fractures. *Acta Orthop Belg*. 2004;70(6):540–544. **(LOE IV)**.

181. Miner T, Carroll KL. Outcomes of external fixation of pediatric femoral shaft fractures. *J Pediatr Orthop*. 2000;20(3):405–410. **(LOE IV)**.

182. Skaggs DL, Leet AI, Money MD, Shaw BA, Hale JM, Tolo VT. Secondary fractures associated with external fixation in pediatric femur fractures. *J Pediatr Orthop.* 1999;19(5):582–586. **(LOE IV)**.

183. Wani MM, Dar RA, Latoo IA, Malik T, Sultan A, Halwai MA. External fixation of pediatric femoral shaft fractures: a consecutive study based on 45 fractures. *J Pediatr Orthop B.* 2013;22(6):563–570. **(LOE IV)**.

184. Peterson HA. Partial growth plate arrest and its treatment. *J Pediatr Orthop.* 1984;4(2):246–258. **(LOE IV)**.

185. Williamson RV, Staheli LT. Partial physeal growth arrest: treatment by bridge resection and fat interposition. *J Pediatr Orthop.* 1990;10(6):769–776. **(LOE IV)**.

186. Vocke AK, Von Laer L. Displaced fractures of the radial neck in children: long-term results and prognosis of conservative treatment. *J Pediatr Orthop B.* 1998;7(3):217–222. **(LOE IV)**.

187. Langenskiold A. Surgical treatment of partial closure of the growth plate. *J Pediatr Orthop.* 1981;1(1):3–11. **(LOE IV)**.

188. Langenskiold A, Osterman K, Valle M. Growth of fat grafts after operation for partial bone growth arrest: demonstration by computed tomography scanning. *J Pediatr Orthop.* 1987;7(4):389–394. **(LOE IV)**.

189. Lee EH, Chen F, Chan J. Treatment of growth arrest by transfer of cultured chondrocytes into physeal defects. *J Pediatr Orthop.* 1998;18:155–160. **(LOE IV)**.

190. Tobita M, Ochi M, Uchio Y, Mori R, Iwasa J, Katsube K, et al. Treatment of growth plate injury with autogenous chondrocytes: a study in rabbits. *Acta Orthop Scand.* 2002;73(3):352–358. **(LOE IV)**.

191. Yoo WJ, Choi IH, Chung CY, Cho TJ, Kim IO, Kim CJ. Implantation of perichondrium-derived chondrocytes in physeal defects of rabbit tibiae. *Acta Orthop.* 2005;76(5):628–636. **(LOE N/A)**.

192. Yoshida K, Higuchi C, Nakura AJ. Treatment of partial growth arrest using an in vitro-generated scaffold-free tissue-engineered construct derived from rabbit synovial mesenchymal stem cells. *J Pediatr Orthop.* 2012;32:314–321. **(LOE N/A)**.

193. Vickers DW. Premature incomplete fusion of the growth plate: causes and treatment by resection (physolysis) in fifteen cases. *Aust N Z J Surg.* 1980;50(4):393–401. **(LOE IV)**.

194. Peterson HA, Madhok R, Benson JT, Ilstrup DM, Melton LJ 3rd. Physeal fractures: Part 1. Epidemiology in Olmsted County, Minnesota, 1979-1988. *J Pediatr Orthop.* 1994;14(4):423–430. **(LOE IV)**.

195. Arkader A, Warner WC Jr, Horn BD, Shaw RN, Wells L. Predicting the outcome of physeal fractures of the distal femur. *J Pediatr Orthop.* 2007;27(6):703–708. **(LOE III)**.

196. Basener CJ, Mehlman CT, DiPasquale TG. Growth disturbance after distal femoral growth plate fractures in children: a meta-analysis. *J Orthop Trauma.* 2009;23(9):663–667. **(LOE IV)**.

197. Wall EJ, May MM. Growth plate fractures of the distal femur. *J Pediatr Orthop.* 2012;32(suppl 1):S40–S46. **(LOE IV)**.

198. Riseborough EJ, Barrett IR, Shapiro F. Growth disturbances following distal femoral physeal fracture-separations. *J Bone Joint Surg Am.* 1983;65(7):885–893. **(LOE IV)**.

199. Leary JT, Handling M, Talerico M, Yong L, Bowe JA. Physeal fractures of the distal tibia: predictive factors of premature physeal closure and growth arrest. *J Pediatr Orthop.* 2009;29(4):356–361. **(LOE III)**.

200. Luhmann SJ, Oda JE, O'Donnell J, Keeler KA, Schoenecker PL, Dobbs MB, et al. An analysis of suboptimal outcomes of medial malleolus fractures in skeletally immature children. *Am J Orthop (Belle Mead NJ).* 2012;41(3):113–116. **(LOE IV)**.

201. Berson L, Davidson RS, Dormans JP, Drummond DS, Gregg JR. Growth disturbances after distal tibial physeal fractures. *Foot Ankle Int.* 2000;21(1):54–58. **(LOE IV)**.

202. Smith BG, Rand F, Jaramillo D, Shapiro F. Early MR imaging of lower-extremity physeal fracture-separations: a preliminary report. *J Pediatr Orthop.* 1994;14(4):526–533. **(LOE IV)**.

203. Aminian A, Schoenecker PL. Premature closure of the distal radial physis after fracture of the distal radial metaphysis. *J Pediatr Orthop.* 1995;15(4):495–498. **(LOE IV)**.

204. Bowler JR, Mubarak SJ, Wenger DR. Tibial physeal closure and genu recurvatum after femoral fracture: occurrence without a tibial traction pin. *J Pediatr Orthop.* 1990;10(5):653–657. **(LOE IV)**.

205. Cramer KE, Limbird TJ, Green NE. Open fractures of the diaphysis of the lower extremity in children. Treatment, results, and complications. *J Bone Joint Surg Am.* 1992;74(2):218–232. **(LOE IV)**.

206. Hresko MT, Kasser JR. Physeal arrest about the knee associated with non-physeal fractures in the lower extremity. *J Bone Joint Surgery Am.* 1989;71(5):698–703. **(LOE IV)**.

207. Karrholm J, Hansson LI, Selvik G. Changes in tibiofibular relationships due to growth disturbances after ankle fractures in children. *J Bone Joint Surgery Am.* 1984;66:1198–1210. **(LOE IV)**.

208. Cozen L. Fracture of the proximal portion of the tibia in children followed by valgus deformity. *Surg Gynecol Obstet.* 1953;97(2):183–188. **(LOE IV)**.

209. Green NE. Tibia valga caused by asymmetrical overgrowth following a nondisplaced fracture of the proximal tibial metaphysis. *J Pediatr Orthop.* 1983;3(2):235–237. **(LOE IV)**.

210. Robert M, Khouri N, Carlioz H, Alain JL. Fractures of the proximal tibial metaphysis in children: review of a series of 25 cases. *J Pediatr Orthop.* 1987;7(4):444–449. **(LOE IV)**.

211. Zionts LE, Harcke HT, Brooks KM. Posttraumatic tibial valga: a case demonstrating asymmetric activity at the proximal growth plate on technetium bone scan. *J Pediatr Orthop.* 1987;7:458–462. **(LOE IV)**.

212. Jordan SE, Alonso JE, Cook FF. The etiology of valgus angulation after metaphyseal fractures of the tibia in children. *J Pediatr Orthop.* 1987;7(4):450–457. **(LOE IV)**.

213. Bucholz RW, Ezaki M, Ogden JA. Injury to the acetabular triradiate physeal cartilage. *J Bone Joint Surg Am.* 1982;64(4):600–609. **(LOE IV)**.

214. Scuderi G, Bronson MJ. Triradiate cartilage injury. Report of two cases and review of the literature. *Clin Orthop Relat Res.* 1987;217:179–189. **(LOE IV)**.

215. Hallel T, Salvati EA. Premature closure of the triradiate cartilage. A case report and animal experiment. *Clin Orthop Relat Res.* 1977;124:278–281. **(LOE IV)**.

216. Heeg M, Visser JD, Oostvogel HJ. Injuries of the acetabular triradiate cartilage and sacroiliac joint. *J Bone Joint Surg Br.* 1988;70(1):34–37. **(LOE IV)**.

217. Holden CP, Holman J, Herman MJ. Pediatric pelvic fractures. *J Am Acad Orthop Surg.* 2007;15(3):172–177. **(LOE IV)**.

218. Badina A, Vialle R, Fitoussi F, Damsin JP. Case reports: treatment of traumatic triradiate cartilage epiphysiodesis: what is the role of bridge resection? *Clin Orthop Relat Res.* 2013;471:3701–3705. **(LOE IV)**.

219. Kregor PJ, Song KM, Routt Jr ML, Sangeorzan BJ, Liddell RM, Hansen ST Jr. Plate fixation of femoral shaft fractures in multiply injured children. *J Bone Joint Surg Am.* 1993;75(12):1774–1780. **(LOE IV)**.

220. Nork SE, Bellig GJ, Woll JP, Hoffinger SA. Overgrowth and outcome after femoral shaft fracture in children younger than 2 years. *J Bone Joint Surgery Am.* 1998;(357):186–191. **(LOE IV)**.

221. Shapiro F. Fractures of the femoral shaft in children. The overgrowth phenomenon. *Acta Orthop Scand.* 1981;52(6):649–655. **(LOE IV)**.

222. Staheli LT. Femoral and tibial growth following femoral shaft fracture in childhood. *Clin Orthop Relat Res.* 1967;55(1):159–163. **(LOE IV)**.

223. Aronson J, Tursky EA. External fixation of femur fractures in children. *J Pediatr Orthop.* 1992;12(2):157–163. **(LOE IV)**.

224. Beaty JH, Austin SM, Warner WC, Canale ST, Nichols L. Interlocking intramedullary nailing of femoral-shaft fractures in adolescents: preliminary results and complications. *J Pediatr Orthop.* 1994;14(2):178–183. **(LOE IV)**.

225. Blasier RD, Aronson J, Tursky EA. External fixation of pediatric femur fractures. *J Pediatr Orthop.* 1997;17(3):342–346. **(LOE IV)**.

226. Kelly B, Heyworth B, Yen YM, Hedequist D. Adverse sequelae due to plate retention following submuscular plating for pediatric femur fractures. *J Orthop Trauma.* 2013;27(12):726–729. **(LOE IV)**.

227. May C, Yen YM, Nasreddine AY, Hedequist D, Hresko MT, Heyworth BE. Complications of plate fixation of femoral shaft fractures in children and adolescents. *J Child Orthop.* 2013;7(3):235–243. **(LOE IV)**.

228. de Pablos J, Franzreb M, Barrios C. Longitudinal growth pattern of the radius after forearm fractures conservatively treated in children. *J Pediatr Orthop.* 1994;14(4):492–495. **(LOE IV)**.

229. Davids JR, Maguire MF, Mubarak SJ, Wenger DR. Lateral condylar fracture of the humerus following posttraumatic cubitus varus. *J Pediatr Orthop.* 1994;14(4):466–470. **(LOE IV)**.

230. Buckley SL, Sturm PF, Tosi LL, Thomas MD, Robertson WW Jr. Ligamentous instability of the knee in children sustaining fractures of the femur: a prospective study with knee examination under anesthesia. *J Pediatr Orthop.* 1996;16(2):206–209. **(LOE III)**.

231. Pennecot GF, Leonard P, Peyrot Des Gachons S, Hardy JR, Pouliquen JC. Traumatic ligamentous instability of the cervical spine in children. *J Pediatr Orthop.* 1984;4:339–345. **(LOE IV).**

232. Arslan H, Kapukaya A, Kesemenli C, Subasi M, Kayikci C. Floating knee in children. *J Pediatr Orthop.* 2003;23(4):458–463. **(LOE IV).**

233. Yue JJ, Churchill RS, Cooperman DR, Yasko AW, Wilber JH, Thompson GH. The floating knee in the pediatric patient. Nonoperative versus operative stabilization. *Clin Orthop Relat Res.* 2000;376:124–136. **(LOE III).**

234. Kocher MS, Mandiga R, Klingele K, Bley L, Micheli LJ. Anterior cruciate ligament injury versus tibial spine fracture in the skeletally immature knee: a comparison of skeletal maturation and notch width index. *J Pediatr Orthop.* 2004;24(2):185–188. **(LOE III).**

235. Farley FA, Kuhns L, Jacobson JA, DiPietro M. Ultrasound examination of ankle injuries in children. *J Pediatr Orthop.* 2001;21(5):604–607. **(LOE IV).**

236. Kocher MS, Waters PM, Micheli LJ. Upper extremity injuries in the paediatric athlete. *Sports Med.* 2000;30(2):117–135. **(LOE IV).**

237. Murphy RF, Naqvi M, Miller PE, Feldman L, Shore BJ. Pediatric orthopaedic lower extremity trauma and venous thromboembolism. *J Child Orthop.* 2015;9(5):381–384. **(LOE III).**

238. Georgopoulos G, Hotchkiss MS, McNair B, Siparsky G, Carry PM, Miller NH. Incidence of deep vein thrombosis and pulmonary embolism in the elective pediatric orthopaedic patient. *J Pediatr Orthop.* 2016;36(1):101–109. **(LOE IV).**

239. Babyn PS, Gahunia HK, Massicotte P. Pulmonary thromboembolism in children. *Pediatr Radiol.* 2005;35(3):258–274. **(LOE IV).**

240. Van Ommen CH, Peters M. Acute pulmonary embolism in childhood. *Thromb Res.* 2006;118:13–25. **(LOE IV).**

241. Sabharwal S, Zhao C, Passanante M. Venous thromboembolism in children: details of 46 cases based on a follow-up survey of POSNA members. *J Pediatr Orthop.* 2013;33(7):768–774. **(LOE IV).**

242. Nowak-Göttl U, Junker R, Hartmeier M, et al. Increased lipoprotein(a) is an important risk factor for venous thromboembolism in childhood. *Circulation.* 1999;100:743–748. **(LOE IV).**

243. Manco-Johnson MJ, Nuss R, Hays T, Krupski W, Drose J, Manco-Johnson ML. Combined thrombolytic and anticoagulant therapy for venous thrombosis in children. *J Pediatr.* 2000;136(4):446–453. **(LOE IV).**

244. Letts M, Lalonde F, Davidson D, Hosking M, Halton J. Atrial and venous thrombosis secondary to septic arthritis of the sacroiliac joint in a child with hereditary protein C deficiency. *J Pediatr Orthop.* 1999;19(2):156–160. **(LOE IV).**

245. Rana AR, Michalsky MP, Teich S. Childhood obesity: a risk factor for injuries observed at a level-1 trauma center. *J Pediatr Surg.* 2009;44:1601–1605. **(LOE III).**

246. Copley LA, Barton T, Garcia C, Sun D, Gaviria-Agudelo C, Gheen WT, et al. A proposed scoring system for assessment of severity of illness in pediatric acute hematogenous osteomyelitis using objective clinical and laboratory findings. *Pediatr Infect Dis J.* 2014;33(1):35–41. **(LOE II).**

247. Hollmig ST, Copley LA, Browne RH, Grande LM, Wilson PL. Deep venous thrombosis associated with osteomyelitis in children. *J Bone Joint Surg Am.* 2007;89(7):1517–1523. **(LOE III).**

248. McDonald JE, Copley LA. Upper-extremity deep venous thrombosis associated with proximal humeral osteomyelitis in a child: a case report. *J Bone Joint Surg Am.* 2010;92(11):2121–2124. **(LOE IV).**

249. Hanson SJ, Punzalan RC, Greenup RA, Liu H, Sato TT, Havens PL. Incidence and risk factors for venous thromboembolism in critically ill children after trauma. *J Trauma.* 2010;68(1):52–56. **(LOE III).**

250. Greenwald LJ, Yost MT, Sponseller PD, Abdullah F, Ziegfeld SM, Ain MC. The role of clinically significant venous thromboembolism and thromboprophylaxis in pediatric patients with pelvic or femoral fractures. *J Pediatr Orthop.* 2012;32(4):357–361. **(LOE II).**

251. Limbird TJ, Ruderman RJ. Fat embolism in children. *Clin Orthop Relat Res.* 1978;136:267–269. **(LOE IV).**

252. White T, Petrisor BA, Bhandari M. Prevention of fat embolism syndrome. *Injury.* 2006;37(suppl 4):S59–S67. **(LOE IV).**

253. Mudd KL, Hunt A, Matherly RC, Goldsmith LJ, Campbell FR, Nichols GR 2nd, et al. Analysis of pulmonary fat embolism in blunt force fatalities. *J Trauma.* 2000;48(4):711–715. **(LOE IV).**

254. Carty JB. Fat embolism in childhood: review and case report. *Am J Surg.* 1957;94(6):970–973. **(LOE IV).**

255. Fabian TC, Hoots AV, Stanford DS, Patterson CR, Mangiante EC. Fat embolism syndrome: prospective evaluation in 92 fracture patients. *Crit Care Med.* 1990;18(1):42–46. **(LOE IV).**

256. Lozman J, Deno DC, Feustel PJ, Newell JC, Stratton HH, Sedransk N, et al. Pulmonary and cardiovascular consequences of immediate fixation or conservative management of long-bone fractures. *Arch Surg.* 1986;121(9):992–999. **(LOE IV).**

257. Pell AC, Christie J, Keating JF, Sutherland GR. The detection of fat embolism by transoesophageal echocardiography during reamed intramedullary nailing. A study of 24 patients with femoral and tibial fractures. *J Bone Joint Surg Br.* 1993;75(6):921–925. **(LOE III).**

258. ten Duis HJ, Nijsten MW, Klasen HJ, Binnendijk B. Fat embolism in patients with an isolated fracture of the femoral shaft. *J Trauma.* 1988;28(3):383–390. **(LOE IV).**

259. Giannoudis PV, Tzioupis C, Pape HC. Fat embolism: the reaming controversy. *Injury.* 2006;37(suppl 4):S50–S58. **(LOE IV).**

260. Edwards KJ, Cummings RJ. Case report: fat embolism as a complication of closed femoral shortening. *J Pediatr Orthop.* 1992;12:542–543. **(LOE IV).**

261. Chastre J, Fagon JY, Soler P, Fichelle A, Dombret MC, Huten D, et al. Bronchoalveolar lavage for rapid diagnosis of the fat embolism syndrome in trauma patients. *Ann Intern Med.* 1990;113(8):583–588. **(LOE IV).**

262. Chuang EL, Miller FS 3rd, Kalina RE. Retinal lesions following long bone fractures. *Ophthalmology.* 1985;92(3):370–374. **(LOE IV).**

263. Cristofaro RL, Brink JD. Hypercalcemia of immobilization in neurologically injured children: a prospective study. *Orthopedics.* 1979;2(5):485–491. **(LOE III).**

264. Winters JL, Kleinschmidt AG Jr, Frensilli JJ, Sutton M. Hypercalcemia complicating immobilization in the treatment of fractures. A case report. *J Bone Joint Surg Am.* 1966;48(6):1182–1184. **(LOE IV).**

265. Carey DE, Raisz LG. Calcitonin therapy in prolonged immobilization hypercalcemia. *Arch Phys Med Rehabil.* 1985;66(9):640–644. **(LOE IV).**

266. Kaul S, Sockalosky JJ. Human synthetic calcitonin therapy for hypercalcemia of immobilization. *J Pediatr.* 1995;126(5 Pt 1):825–827. **(LOE III).**

267. Meythaler JM, Tuel SM, Cross LL. Successful treatment of immobilization hypercalcemia using calcitonin and etidronate. *Arch Physical Med Rehab.* 1993;74(3):316–319. **(LOE IV).**

268. Lteif AN, Zimmerman D. Bisphosphonates for treatment of childhood hypercalcemia. *Pediatrics.* 1998;102(4 Pt 1):990–993. **(LOE IV).**

269. Massagli TL, Cardenas DD. Immobilization hypercalcemia treatment with pamidronate disodium after spinal cord injury. *Arch Phys Med Rehabil.* 1999;80(9):998–1000. **(LOE IV).**

270. Claus-Walker J, Carter RE, Compos RJ, Spencer WA. Hypercalcemia in early traumatic quadriplegia. *J Chronic Dis.* 1975;28(2):81–90. **(LOE IV).**

271. Mital MA, Garber JE, Stinson JT. Ectopic bone formation in children and adolescents with head injuries: its management. *J Pediatr Orthop.* 1987;7(1):83–90. **(LOE IV).**

272. Kaplan FS, Glaser DL, Hebela N, Shore EM. Heterotopic ossification. *J Am Acad Orthop Surg.* 2004;12(2):116–125. **(LOE IV).**

273. Koch BM, Wu CM, Randolph J, Eng GD. Heterotopic ossification in children with burns: two case reports. *Arch Phys Med Rehabil.* 1992;73(11):1104–1106. **(LOE IV).**

274. De Smet AA, Norris MA, Fisher DR. Magnetic resonance imaging of myositis ossificans: analysis of seven cases. *Skeletal Radiol.* 1992;21(8):503–507. **(LOE IV).**

275. Ehara S, Shiraishi H, Abe M, Mizutani H. Reactive heterotopic ossification. Its patterns on MRI. *Clin Imaging.* 1998;22(4):292–296. **(LOE IV).**

276. Johnson EE, Kay RM, Dorey FJ. Heterotopic ossification prophylaxis following operative treatment of acetabular fracture. *Clin Orthop Relat Res.* 1994;305:88-95. **(LOE IV).**

277. Moed BR, Maxey JW. The effect of indomethacin on heterotopic ossification following acetabular fracture surgery. *J Orthop Trauma.* 1993;7(1):33–38. **(LOE IV).**

278. Carlson WO, Klassen RA. Myositis ossificans of the upper extremity: a long-term follow-up. *J Pediatr Orthop.* 1984;4(6):693–696. **(LOE IV).**

279. Berk RN, Coulson DB. The body cast syndrome. *Radiology.* 1970;94(2):303–305. **(LOE IV).**

280. Amy BW, Priebe CJ Jr, King A. Superior mesenteric artery syndrome associated with **(LOE IV)**

281. Dabney KW, Miller F, Lipton GE, Letonoff EJ, McCarthy HC. Correction of sagittal plane spinal deformities with unit rod instrumentation in children with cerebral palsy. *J Bone Joint Surg Am.* 2004;86-A(suppl 1(Pt 2):156–168. (**LOE IV**).

282. Philip PA. Superior mesenteric artery syndrome: an unusual cause of intestinal obstruction in brain-injured children. *Brain Inj.* 1992;6(4):351–358. (**LOE IV**).

283. Walker C, Kahanovitz N. Recurrent superior mesenteric artery syndrome complicating staged reconstructive spinal surgery: alternative methods of conservative treatment. *J Pediatr Orthop.* 1983;3(1):77–80. (**LOE IV**).

284. Shin MS, Kim JY. Optimal duration of medical treatment in superior mesenteric artery syndrome in children. *J Korean Med Sci.* 2013;28(8):1220–1225. (**LOE IV**).

285. Hamdan JA, Taleb YA, Ahmed MS. (**LOE IV**).

286. Turner MC, Ruley EJ, Buckley KM, Strife CF. Blood pressure elevation in children with orthopedic immobilization. *J Pediatr.* 1979;95(6):989–992. (**LOE IV**).

287. Talab YA, Hamdan J, Ahmed M. Orthopaedic causes of hypertension in pediatric patients. Case report and review of the literature. *J Bone Joint Surg Am.* 1982;64(2):291–292. (**LOE IV**).

288. Linshaw MA, Stapleton FB, Gruskin AB, Baluarte HJ, Harbin GL. Traction-related hypertension in children. *J Pediatr.* 1979;95(6):994–996. (**LOE IV**).

289. Bernstein BH, Singsen BH, Kent JT, Kornreich H, King K, Hicks R, et al. Reflex neurovascular dystrophy in childhood. *J Pediatr.* 1978;93(2):211–215. (**LOE IV**).

290. Dietz FR, Mathews KD, Montgomery WJ. Reflex sympathetic dystrophy in children. *Clin Orthop Relat Res.* 1990;258:225–231. (**LOE IV**).

291. Wilder RT, Berde CB, Wolohan M, Vieyra MA, Masek BJ, Micheli LJ. Reflex sympathetic dystrophy in children. Clinical characteristics and follow-up of seventy patients. *J Bone Joint Surg Am.* 1992;74(6):910–919. (**LOE IV**).

292. Chelmisky TC, Low PA, Naessens JM. Value of autonomic testing in reflex sympathetic dystrophy. *Mayo Clin Proc LOE IV.* 1995;70:1029–1040. (**LOE IV**).

293. Stanton RP, Malcolm JR, Wesdock KA, Singsen BH. Reflex sympathetic dystrophy in children: an orthopedic perspective. *Orthopedics.* 1993 Jul;16(7):773–779; discussion 779-80. (**LOE III**).

294. Bayle-Iniguez X, Audouin-Pajot C, Sales de Gauzy J, Munzer C, Murgier J, Accadbled F. Complex regional pain syndrome type I in children. Clinical description and quality of life. *Orthop Traumatol Surg Res.* 2015;101(6):745–748. (**LOE IV**).

295. Harden RN, Oaklander AL, Burton AW, Perez RS, Richardson K, Swan M, et al. Complex regional pain syndrome: practical diagnostic and treatment guidelines, 4th edition. *Pain Med.* 2013;14(2):180–229. (**LOE IV**).

296. Barbier O, Allington N, Rombouts JJ. Reflex sympathetic dystrophy in children: review of a clinical series and (**LOE IV**).

297. Bukhalo Y, Mullin V. Presentation and treatment of complex regional pain syndrome type 1 in a 3 year old. *Anesthesiology.* 2004;101(2):542–543. (**LOE IV**).

298. Silber TJ, Majd M. Reflex sympathetic dystrophy syndrome in children and adolescents. Report of 18 cases and review of the literature. *Am J Dis Child.* 1988;142(12):1325–1330. (**LOE IV**).

299. Maillard SM, Davies K, Khubchandani R, Woo PM, Murray KJ. Reflex sympathetic dystrophy: a multidisciplinary approach. *Arthritis Rheum.* 2004;51(2):284–290. (**LOE IV**).

300. Pawl RP. Controversies surrounding reflex sympathetic dystrophy: a review article. *Curr Rev Pain.* 2000;4(4):259–267. (**LOE IV**).

301. Cimaz R, Matucci-Cerinic M, Zulian F, Falcini F. Reflex sympathetic dystrophy in children. *J Child Neurol.* 1999;14(6):363–367. (**LOE IV**).

302. Sherry DD, Weisman R. Psychological aspects of childhood reflex neurovascular dystrophy. *Pediatric.* 1988;81:572–578. (**LOE IV**).

303. Muizelaar JP, Kleyer M, Hertogs IA. Complex regional pain syndrome (reflex sympathetic dystrophy and causalgia): management with the calcium channel blocker nifedipine and/or the alpha-sympathetic blocker phenoxybenzamine in 59 patients. *Clin Neurol Neurosurg LOE IV.* 1997;99:26–30. (**LOE IV**).

304. Ruggeri SB, Athreya BH, Doughty R, Gregg JR, Das MM. Reflex sympathetic dystrophy in children. *Clin Orthop Relat Res.* 1982;163:225–230. (**LOE IV**).

305. Dadure C, Motais F, Ricard C. Continuous peripheral nerve blocks at home for treatment of recurrent complex regional pain syndrome I in children. *Anesthesiology.* 2005;102:387–391. (**LOE IV**).

306. Petje G, Radler C, Aigner N. Treatment of reflex sympathetic dystrophy in children using a prostacyclin analog: preliminary results. *J Bone Joint Surgery Am.* 2005;433:178–182. (**LOE IV**).

8 Nerve Injury and Repair in Children

Scott H. Kozin | Dan A. Zlotolow

The following videos are included with this chapter and may be viewed at ExpertConsult:
Video 8.1 Tinel sign.
Video 8.2 Desensitization.
Video 8.3 Follow-up clinical examination.

INTRODUCTION

Nerve injuries in children are relatively uncommon; however, children tend to put their hands in all sorts of unexpected places with sharp objects. Garbage disposals, conveyer belts, and dishwashers are uninteresting to adults but are a fascinating source of curiosity for children (Fig. 8.1). Reaching into a nest of sharp surfaces can lead to varying degrees of damage to the pediatric hand, including nerve injury. In emerging countries, childhood labor is common and occupational safety is lacking, which leads to dangerous conditions (Fig. 8.2). In addition, the advent of high-velocity sporting events like the X Games has resulted in an increasing incidence of severe, high-energy fractures in children, with periosteal disruption and marked fracture displacement. The surrounding nerve(s) are in jeopardy from sharp, bony fragments unchecked by the normal encompassing periosteum. Even if the nerves are not lacerated from the fracture fragments, traction on the nerves and swelling may result in nerve injury and compartment syndrome. Lastly, although iatrogenic nerve injuries are uncommon, surgeons unfamiliar with the idiosyncrasies of the pediatric musculoskeletal system can make the operating room a less safe place for children. Regardless of the cause, iatrogenic nerve injuries are distressing to the physician, child, and family. This chapter will discuss the prevention, diagnosis, and treatment of upper extremity nerve injuries in children.

CHILDREN ARE NOT SMALL ADULTS

Infants, young children, teenagers, and adolescents are not only distinctly different than adults in their ability to provide an accurate history and comply with a thorough examination, but are also distinctly different from each other. Infants cannot provide a history at all, and young children are notoriously poor historians. Teenagers have a difficult time expressing their symptoms, expectations, and concerns, whereas adolescents tend to perseverate on factors that may be peripheral to the central problem. Parents are often unclear about the onset of symptoms or the severity of the injury, and family dynamics can introduce stress and frustration for both the child and the physician. The musculoskeletal and neurovascular evaluation, made difficult by the suboptimal available history, is further complicated by an often-limited examination. One cannot approach an infant or young child and expect to have them sit still and cooperate with an examination. The examination of young children is relegated to playtime and requires gentle encouragement. The authors' office is replete with age-appropriate toys that allow the surgeon and occupational therapists to interact and observe the child in a less threatening environment. The authors spend a lot of time observing patterns of hand usage, looking for clues that signal potential nerve injuries.

The sensory examination in children is fraught with error. Children are unable to reliably participate in two-point discriminatory assessment until about 8 years of age.[1] Any attempt at pinprick examination will quickly end the examination. A subtler and less invasive test is to evaluate for moistness or dryness of the fingers compared with the unaffected hand. Fingers without sensory innervation will be dry compared with uninjured digits. Another test is submersing the hand in warm water and checking for pruning of the digits, which also requires innervation. However, the classic sign of a sensory nerve injury in children is neglect of the insensate digit(s). In other words, a 3-year-old who has injured his median nerve will revert to an ulnar grasp pattern with his ring and small fingers, avoiding the thumb, index, and long fingers in pinch and grasp. The sine qua non finding of reinnervation is similar because hypersensitivity during nerve regeneration is painful, again leading to avoidance.

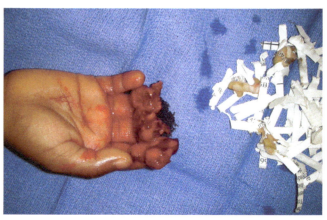

Fig. 8.1 A 7-year-old child could not resist reaching into a paper shredder. (Courtesy of Shriners Hospital for Children, Philadelphia Unit.)

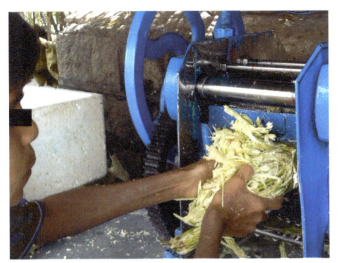

Fig. 8.2 Young Cambodian child placing hands dangerously close to sugar cane–squeezing machine. (Courtesy of Shriners Hospital for Children, Philadelphia Unit.)

The authors have seen children with such intense hypersensitivity during nerve recovery that they avoid washing or cutting their nails on that part of the hand.

The motor examination can also be frustrating to the examiner and the child, particularly if the child is tired, hungry, teething, or ill. The examination should initially gain the confidence and trust of the child and the parents. The child must be comfortable with the physician being in the room before the physician can place hands on the child for an examination. Subsequently, the examination should be succinct with a focus on determination of the motor status of the nerve(s) in question. The examiner should begin with the most important and least painful or disruptive tests, reserving anything that requires restraining the child or causing the child discomfort for last. A slow, deliberate, and detailed examination is impractical in the infant and child. A comprehensive knowledge of the anatomy of the peripheral nervous system is critical for facilitating an accurate and swift diagnosis. From a practical standpoint, the authors assess peripheral nerves according to Table 8.1 and Fig. 8.3. Adolescents can be examined in a manner similar to adults, both for motor and sensory determination.

TYPES OF NERVE INJURY/WHAT HAPPENS AFTER NERVE INJURY

Nerve conduction, the nerve's primary function, can be compromised by ischemia or necrosis, distraction or stretch injuries, and laceration. Ischemia is, by definition, reversible, whereas necrosis is not. Early or mild ischemia can lead to focal demyelination, with characteristic slowing of nerve conduction across the lesion on electrodiagnostic studies. Prolonged ischemia can result in a complete conduction block, but the nerve distal and proximal to the lesion typically has normal conduction. Severe compression, devascularization, or tenting of a nerve over a bony prominence or hardware can eventually lead to nerve necrosis. The necrotic nerve becomes "woody," with localized fibrosis in the necrotic segment. Distally, the axons degenerate (Wallerian degeneration), but the neural architecture remains intact.

TABLE 8.1 Tests for Assessment of Major Peripheral Nerve Function

Nerve	Assessment	Favorite Test (Age Dependent)
Radial	Wrist extension Digital extension (metacarpophalangeal joint) Elbow extension	"Hook em horns" "Thumbs up"
Median	Thumb and index finger distal interphalangeal joint flexion (anterior interosseous nerve) Flexor digitorum superficialis via proximal interphalangeal joint flexion Thumb palmar abduction Forearm pronation	OK sign Thumb palmar abduction
Ulnar	Digital abduction and adduction ring and small distal interphalangeal joint flexion	Cross fingers
Musculocutaneous	Elbow flexion	"Make a muscle"
Axillary	Shoulder-forward flexion and abduction	"Reach for the sky"

Spontaneous neurologic recovery is limited because the fibrotic scar blocks axonal sprouting.

Lacerations can be complete or incomplete. Partial lacerations can partly recover spontaneously if the distal and proximal lacerated segments continue to line up with each other. Imperfect coaptation or gapping can lead to the formation of a neuroma-in-continuity. Complete lacerations have poor potential for spontaneous recovery. Traction injuries can similarly show a variable degree of recovery potential based on the amount of disruption of the axons and the supporting neural architecture.

The severity of a traumatic nerve injury begins with neuropraxia, extends to axonotmesis, and concludes in neurotmesis.[2,3] *Neuropraxia* is a segmental demyelination with maintenance of intact nerve fibers and the axonal sheath. A temporary localized conduction block follows, without axonal damage or Wallerian degeneration. Nerve conduction in the segments proximal to or distal to the site of demyelination is unaffected. Complete recovery follows over the subsequent days to weeks as remyelination is completed. Electrodiagnostic studies demonstrate either a decrease in nerve conduction velocity or a complete conduction block across the area of demyelination, but no electromyographic (EMG) changes of denervation are seen within the muscle.[4] Conduction velocities and amplitudes across nerve segments outside of the zone of injury are usually normal.

Axonotmesis is a disruption of nerve fiber integrity with conservation of the architecture of the axonal sheath. Wallerian degeneration and subsequent nerve fiber regeneration are necessary for recovery. Retrograde degeneration is limited to the next more proximal node of Ranvier. Distal antegrade degeneration continues down the entire length of the nerve to the motor end plate. The cell bodies (dorsal root ganglion

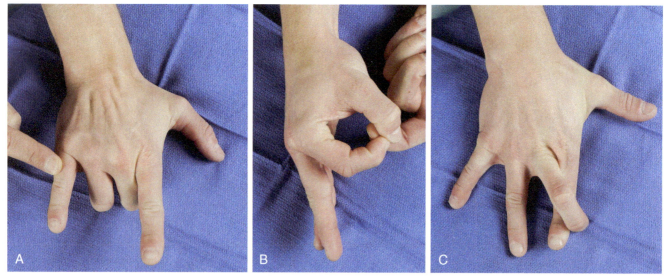

Fig. 8.3 Favorite tests for nerve function. (A) Hook 'em horns for posterior interosseous nerve (radial nerve). (B) OK sign for anterior interosseous nerve (median nerve). (C) Crossing fingers (ulnar nerve). (Courtesy of Shriners Hospital for Children, Philadelphia Unit.)

and anterior horn cells) switch from regulatory bodies to renewal centers. Axonal sprouting into the retained axonal sheath and framework occurs at a slow rate of 1 mm/day, or approximately 1 inch/month, but may be faster in younger children and infants. Electrodiagnostic studies exhibit loss of nerve conduction distal to the lesion and EMG changes of muscle denervation (i.e., insertional activity, fibrillations, and positive sharp waves).[4] Partial axonotmetric injuries where part of the nerve is intact or just demyelinated will show a normal conduction velocity distal to the lesion but a decrease in amplitude relative to the degree of axonal loss. Prolonged denervation (>18–24 months) results in irreversible motor end-plate degradation with fatty degeneration and fibrosis of the target muscle (Fig. 8.4). In contrast, the encapsulated sensory receptors retain their capacity for reinnervation for many years. Considering all these factors, the outcome after axonotmesis is variable. Distal injuries closer to the end plates recover better than proximal injuries. Sensory recovery is also possible long after the possibility of motor recovery has passed. This information regarding recovery should be conveyed to the patient and family.

Neurotmesis is an interruption of the nerve fiber and axonal sheath. Transection is the common example of this injury, but severe traction or contusion can produce similar disruption of nerve integrity. The prognosis is bleak without surgical intervention. Nerve repair or reconstruction is necessary to restore axonal inflow to the downstream muscles and sensory receptors. After restoration of nerve continuity, the same process ignites as described for axonotmesis. In other words, axonal sprouting into the retained axonal sheath and framework occurs at a slow rate of 1 mm/day or 1 inch/month. Electrodiagnostic studies cannot distinguish between a neurotmetric and an axonotmetric injury. Imaging studies that are currently available are likewise of little help. Unfortunately, the only way to distinguish between these two injury types is to observe for spontaneous recovery. An axonometric injury will exhibit an advancing Tinel sign and recovery of the muscle most proximal to the nerve injury.

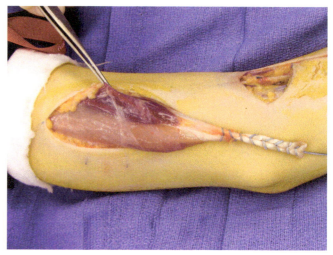

Fig. 8.4 Biceps muscle demonstrating innervation of the anterior portion and denervation of the posterior portion. (Courtesy of Shriners Hospital for Children, Philadelphia Unit.)

DIAGNOSTIC STUDIES

Peripheral nerve imaging is still in its infancy. Magnetic resonance neurography and its related techniques for imaging neural tracts in the brain and spinal cord (tractography or diffusion tensor imaging) are still under development for imaging nerve continuity.[5] Ultrasound is also undergoing technical modifications and software updates for improved nerve imaging.[6] Currently, these imaging studies are unable to accurately discriminate an axonotmesis from a neurotmesis unless there is a clear gap between the nerve ends.

Electrodiagnostic studies also have a limited role in the treatment algorithm of children with peripheral nerve injuries. EMG can discriminate neuropraxia from axonotmesis or neurotmesis. Because neuropraxia represents segmental demyelination with preservation of intact axons, EMG results will remain normal except for decreased recruitment.

In contrast, axonotmesis and neurotmesis interrupt axonal integrity and lead to fibrillation potentials in the affected muscles. One potential benefit of EMG is the ability to detect reinnervation before it is evident on clinical examination, which allows an earlier diagnosis of axonotmesis. Reinnervation findings include active polyphasic motor units, the emergence of nascent potentials, and a decrease in the number of fibrillation potentials.[4] However, the lack of early detection of reinnervation on EMG does not exclude the possibility of later recovery and does not definitively diagnose neurotmesis. In other words, the presence of reinnervation makes everyone feel better sooner, but its absence does not guide treatment.

DEMYSTIFYING TREATMENT OF NERVE INJURIES

The treatment algorithm of nerve injuries may seem overwhelming to those physicians unaccustomed to managing nerve problems. The basic tenets guiding all treatment decisions are based on the slow rate of nerve regeneration (1 mm/day) and the need to save the motor end plate from irreversible end-plate demise 18 to 24 months after an injury.[7] The hardest part of the algorithm is discriminating axonotmesis from neurotmesis. Currently, no available electrodiagnostic or imaging test can accurately distinguish between the two injuries. Ultimately, a modality will be developed to precisely identify a neurotmetric injury, which will allow for immediate surgical intervention. However, for now, the diagnosis is based on history and examination findings alone, which often leads to delays in treatment and inexact surgical indications.

The timing of recovery is the most reliable marker of the type of injury. A patient will recover from neuropraxia days to weeks after an injury, and motor and sensory deficits will resolve. A patient will show signs of recovery from axonotmesis within the first few months as the axons grow down the nerve, reach their target organs, and the most proximal muscle that is distal to the injury is reinnervated. Reinnervation occurs in a segmental fashion from distal to proximal. For example, an axonotmetric injury to the radial nerve in the midhumerus should be assessed for reinnervation of the brachioradialis muscle and not for the wrist or digital extensor muscles. The pathognomonic finding of early regeneration in axonotmesis is the advancing Tinel sign. Tapping on the regenerating axons leads to paresthesias in the sensory distribution of the regenerating nerve (Video 8.1). Pain on tapping on the nerve is not an indication of regeneration. In children, the test is more difficult because paresthesias are difficult for children to describe. Tapping on the regenerating nerve may produce an exaggerated withdrawal response as paresthesias travel down the arm. Older children describe the sensation as "electric shocks," "fire ants," or "zingers." An advancing Tinel sign is an encouraging prognostic factor.

A neurotmetric injury will not demonstrate an advancing Tinel sign and will not lead to reinnervation of the most proximal muscle. Neurotmetric injuries require timely surgical intervention so that the motor end plates will survive. Unnecessary delays in surgical reconstitution of nerve continuity can make the difference between a near-full recovery and lifelong disability. Far too often, the authors see children past the point of meaningful intervention.

TREATMENT OPTIONS

Prompt diagnosis of a nerve laceration allows for primary repair. Discourse about the merits of group fascicular repair versus epineurial repair continues, but evidence to suggest that group fascicular repair is superior is scarce. Therefore, the authors perform an epineurial repair with direct coaptation of the nerve ends. Alignment is achieved by matching the sizes of the group fascicles and aligning the vaso nervosum. Loupe or microscopic magnification is necessary depending on the size of the lacerated nerve. The repair is performed with microsutures, fibrin glue, or both. Animal and clinical outcome studies have reported similar results comparing sutures and glue unless underlying tension is present.[8] Sutures are better at resisting tension, although any tension across a nerve repair is detrimental.[9] In cases with slight tension, the authors prefer a few sutures followed by fibrin glue. The authors believe that glue is less disruptive to the nerve than suture placement, especially by surgeons or trainees less experienced in nerve surgery. If there is too much tension for a primary repair, a small gap may be bridged by a conduit.

Delayed recognition or presentation of a nerve laceration usually negates the possibility of direct repair. In children, neuroma formation and nerve retraction are exaggerated (Fig. 8.5). Once the neuroma has been resected, a considerable gap is often present. Options for overcoming the gap are numerous, including conduits and nerve grafts. The gold standard remains autologous nerve grafting with a series of grafts bridging the deficit (i.e., cable grafting). This technique alleviates any tension and allows early revascularization of the autografts via imbibition, which preserves some of the cellular nerve elements within the graft. There are numerous potential donor nerves, although the sural nerve remains the preferred choice for any substantial deficit because of its length, caliber, and minimal donor site deficit.[10] The sural nerve can be harvested with use of a long longitudinal incision, a series of transverse incisions, or endoscopy.[11] Transverse incisions heal better with less incidence of hypertrophic scarring.

Another option for treating a nerve injury is a nerve transfer.[7,12] This technique involves circumventing the injury altogether. Motor and/or sensory deficits can be overcome by direct transfer downstream to the injury with motor or sensory nerves harvested from intact, functioning nerves. The nerves harvested must be expendable such that the gains outweigh any potential loss. This expendability can take various forms, depending on the situation. Proximal nerves have inherent redundancy, and harvesting a group fascicle has only subclinical deficits. For example, a carefully selected group fascicle transferred from the median and/or ulnar nerves (donor nerves) to the motor nerves of the biceps and brachialis (recipient nerves) results in no clinical deficit in the donor nerves.[13] Distal nerve transfers follow the tenets of tendon transfers. The donor nerve must be available and expendable. For example, transfer

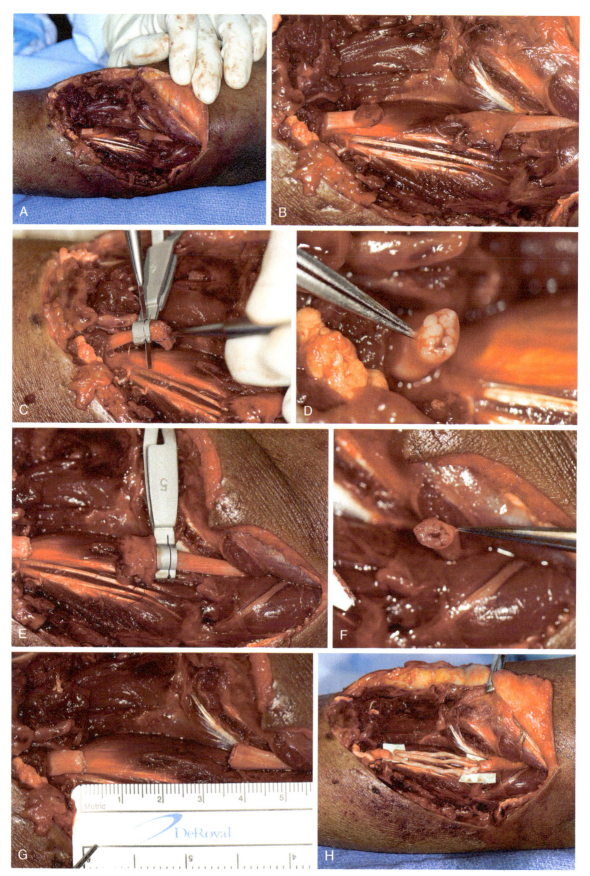

Fig. 8.5 A 15-year-old male patient 1 month after ulnar nerve laceration. (A) Large laceration across left forearm. (B) Large neuromas and extensive retraction between nerve ends. (C) Resection of distal neuroma. (D) Good viable axons after neuroma excision. (E) Resection of proximal neuroma. (F) Good viable proximal axons. (G) A 4-cm gap after neuroma resections. (H) Sural nerve cable grafting. (Courtesy of Shriners Hospital for Children, Philadelphia Unit.)

of the motor nerve from the flexor digitorum superficialis and/or flexor carpi radialis to an injured radial nerve must have intact flexor digitorum profundus and flexor carpi ulnaris to avoid loss of finger flexion and wrist flexion, respectively.[14]

NERVE INJURIES AFTER A FRACTURE

Nerve injuries secondary to a fracture are infrequent but routinely seen in the authors' clinical practice. Fractures of any bone about the arm, elbow, forearm, and wrist can injure adjacent nerves. However, the classic fractures that present with nerve injuries are the mid- to distal humeral diaphyseal fracture and the supracondylar elbow fracture. Less commonly, a nerve can be injured after fractures involving the forearm.

DIAPHYSEAL HUMERAL FRACTURES

The radial nerve travels from the posterior cord of the brachial plexus along subcutaneous fat of the posteromedial brachium and the lateral and long heads of the triceps muscle until it reaches the spiral groove at about the midhumerus.[15] The nerve is held tightly against the humerus in the spiral groove by a fascial band connecting the lateral and medial heads of the triceps. The nerve then travels along the lateral humerus, becoming an anterior structure at the level of the metaphyseal flare just proximal to the origin of the brachioradialis muscle. Therefore, from the spiral groove and distal, the radial nerve resides immediately adjacent to the humerus and is at highest risk of injury from a fracture. The injury can vary from a neuropraxia to a neurotmesis. In the majority of pediatric cases, the injury is an axonotmesis. Recovery takes time because subsequent Wallerian degeneration and regeneration is a slow, arduous process. The key muscle that allows detection of regeneration and reinnervation is the most proximal muscle to be reinnervated. In cases of radial nerve injury, the brachioradialis muscle is the harbinger of recovery. On physical examination, one can palpate the brachioradialis by asking the patient to flex his or her elbow against resistance with the forearm in neutral position (Fig. 8.6). Absence of recovery by 3 to 4 months may indicate neurotmesis. EMG of the brachioradialis muscle may detect evidence of reinnervation before recovery is clinically evident. No recovery by 6 months warrants surgical exploration and nerve reconstruction. The nerve may be lacerated with the proximal and distal segments retracted. The nerve may also be compressed or entrapped in the bone with a necrotic and fibrosed segment. Either way, treatment requires dissecting the proximal and distal nerve ends back to healthy-appearing fascicles and grafting across the gap. Entrapped nerves require extirpation before grafting. The surgeon can easily be lured into neurolysis without resecting a fibrosed segment if the nerve appears to be in continuity. The authors use intraoperative stimulation with a Checkpoint device (Checkpoint Surgical LLC, Cleveland, Ohio) at a maximum of 2 mA to determine whether there is conduction across a questionable segment. Their bias is to resect a nerve segment that is pale and feels firm ("woody") unless a robust muscle contraction is seen in the brachioradialis.

ELBOW FRACTURES

Pediatric extension supracondylar fractures are notorious for injuring adjacent nerves. The distal humerus is displaced and/or angulated in a posterior direction whereas the proximal fragment is thrust in an anterior direction (Fig. 8.7). The proximal fragment can tent or penetrate the overlying brachialis muscle. The radial and median nerves lie anterior to the brachialis muscle and can be injured by the proximal fracture fragment. The anterior interosseous branch of the median nerve resides in the posterior aspect of the nerve and is most susceptible to injury in these cases.[16] The radial nerve also resides in harm's way during anterior displacement of the proximal fragment. After a pediatric supracondylar fracture, the child's intense pain and panic make the examination difficult to obtain. The examiner must be patient and assess these critical nerves (see Table 8.1) along with the circulation of the limb. The status of the pulses and the circulation within the hand (capillary refill) are critical elements in the treatment algorithm. A limb without palpable pulses or with a neurologic deficit requires prompt reduction. Reduction often leads to restoration of palpable pulses without the need for additional vascular treatment. If pulses are not restored, an assessment of limb perfusion is required. The treatment of a well-perfused but pulseless hand, the so-called pink pulseless hand, remains controversial. Although data exist that support observation in this setting based on the persistence of adequate perfusion in these cases, it is unclear whether these pulseless hands will demonstrate signs and symptoms of arterial insufficiency in the long term.[17] A white dysvascular hand requires immediate exploration of the brachial artery.

The majority of nerve injuries are axonotmetric in nature. Recovery is prolonged because Wallerian degeneration is followed by slow nerve regeneration (1 mm/day). In cases of median nerve injury, the pronator teres muscle is

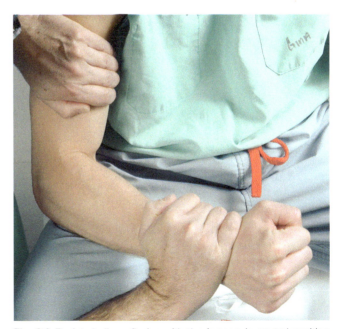

Fig. 8.6 Resisted elbow flexion with the forearm in neutral position allows palpation of the brachioradialis muscle. (Courtesy of Shriners Hospital for Children, Philadelphia Unit.)

the first to be reinnervated (Fig. 8.8). One can palpate the muscle by asking the patient to pronate against resistance. In cases of high radial nerve injury, the crucial muscle is the brachioradialis, as described for humeral fractures (see Fig. 8.6). In cases of low radial nerve injury (posterior interosseous nerve), the key muscle is the supinator, which can be palpated deep during effortless forearm supination with the elbow flexed to 90 degrees to negate the effects of the biceps muscle.[18] The extensor digitorum communis is also evaluated for recovery by assessment of metacarpophalangeal joint extension with the wrist in neutral or slight flexion

(see Fig. 8.3A). Absence of any recovery by 3 to 4 months may indicate neurotmesis. EMG of the appropriate muscles may detect evidence of reinnervation before clinical appreciation. No recovery of motor function by 6 months warrants surgical exploration and nerve reconstruction via nerve grafting or nerve transfers. Early recovery of sensation is heralded by hypersensitivity in the reinnervating dermatome. As previously discussed, in young children, hyperpathia leads to avoidance. Patients may refuse to wash their hand or have their nails cut. Therapy focused on desensitization is beneficial for decreasing the hyperpathia (Video 8.2).

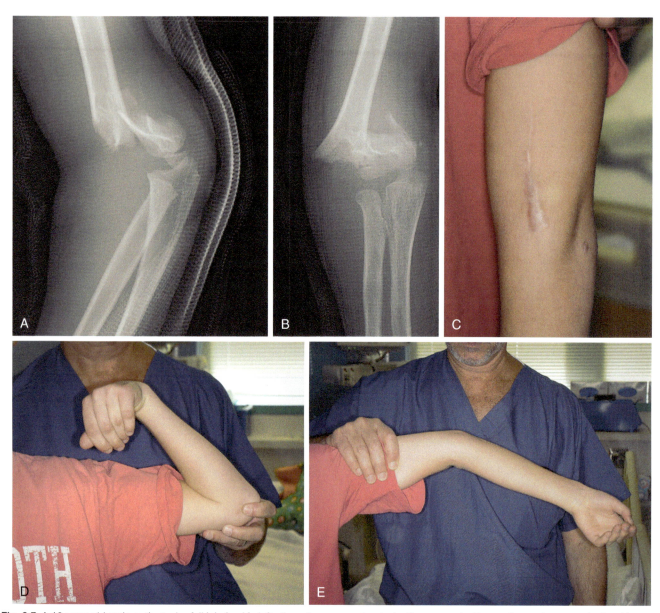

Fig. 8.7 A 13-year-old male patient who fell injuring his left elbow 5 years ago treated with open reduction and percutaneous pinning. He presents with inability to extend his wrist, fingers, and thumb. (A) Injury lateral x-ray demonstrates extension type supracondylar humerus fracture with distal fragment in extension and the proximal fragment thrust in an anterior direction toward the radial and median nerves. (B) Anteroposterior x-ray reveals posteromedial displacement of distal fracture fragment. (C) Hypertrophic lateral incision. (D) Elbow flexion. (E) Elbow hyperextension.

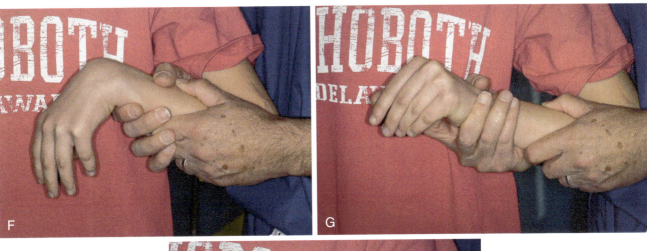

Fig. 8.7, cont'd (F) Absent wrist extension. (G) Absent finger metacarpophalangeal joint extension with the wrist held in extension. (H) Absent thumb extension. (Courtesy of Shriners Hospital for Children, Philadelphia Unit.)

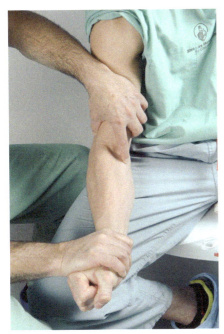

Fig. 8.8 Palpation of the pronator teres during resisted forearm pronation. (Courtesy of Shriners Hospital for Children, Philadelphia Unit.)

FOREARM FRACTURES

Fractures of the radius, ulna, or both can injure the adjacent nerves. The fractures are usually widely displaced and require closed reduction and fixation. Determining whether the nerve function was intact before surgery is a difficult task. Pain and apprehension may preclude an adequate physical examination. Late presentation is common. Radiographs taken in multiple views may reveal a clue to the diagnosis (Fig. 8.9). Radiographic examination can be accomplished with the use of pain radiographs or minifluoroscopy. A "hole in the bone" indicates bony entrapment that requires exploration, extirpation, and possible grafting. Absence of any recovery by 3 to 4 months may indicate neurotmesis. Lack of recovery of sensory and motor function by 6 months warrants surgical exploration and nerve reconstruction (Fig. 8.10).

NERVE INJURIES AFTER A DISLOCATION

Nerves that are vulnerable to injury after dislocation tend to be in close proximity to the joint and tethered proximal and distal to the joint. The axillary nerve is particularly susceptible to injury after anterior shoulder dislocation.

The axillary nerve is tethered between the posterior cord and the deltoid muscle, which limits its mobility and

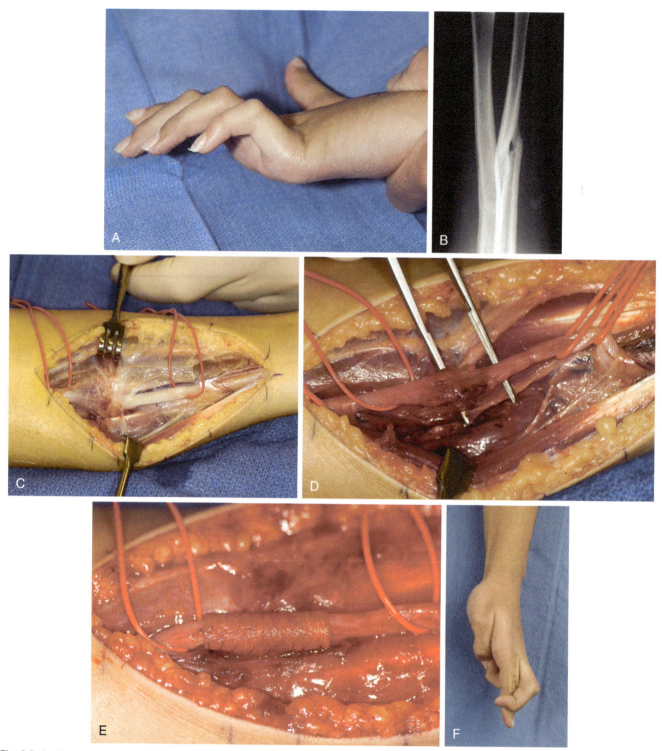

Fig. 8.9 An 11-year-old female patient 4 months after closed reduction and casting of a displaced both-bone forearm fracture. (A) Ulnar neuropathy with clawing. (B) Radiograph reveals bony hole within the ulna consistent with ulnar nerve entrapment. (C) Ulnar nerve found entrapped in healed ulna. (D) Ulnar nerve extricated from fracture site. (E) Nerve wrapped with conduit. (F) Clinical recovery 3 months after surgery with ability to cross fingers and resolution of clawing. (Courtesy of Shriners Hospital for Children, Philadelphia Unit.)

increases its susceptibility to injury. In addition, the nerve is directly adjacent to the inferior capsule, which places it in harm's way during anterior-inferior dislocation of the humeral head. The head impacts the nerve and continues to apply pressure if a reduction is delayed. The injury is frequently an axonotmesis requiring Wallerian degeneration and regeneration for recovery. In children, the examination

must be comprehensive to make the correct diagnosis. In contrast to adults, children and adolescents can exhibit full range of motion despite complete axillary neuropathy (Fig. 8.11). Their main complaint is either a small area of numbness about the lateral aspect of the shoulder or decreased endurance during repetitive overhead activities (Fig. 8.11B). Therefore, delayed presentation is common.

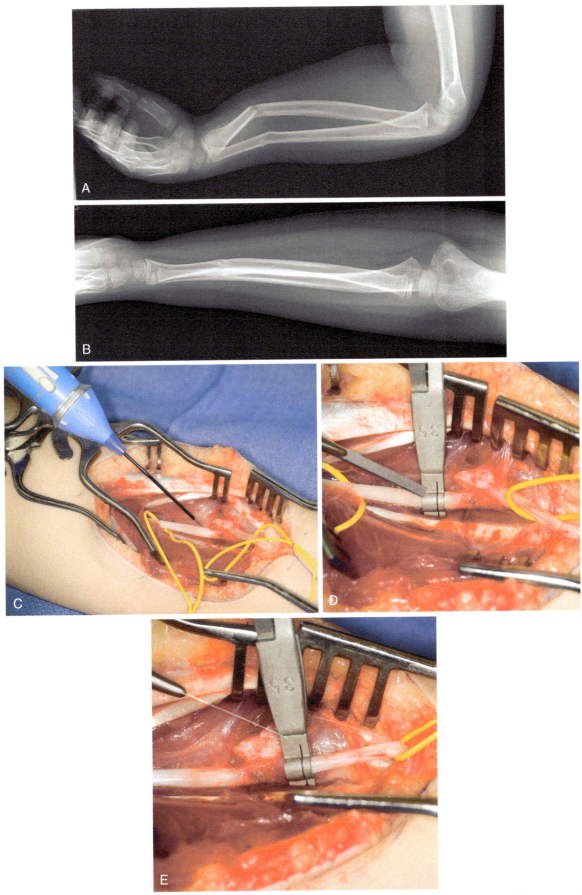

Fig. 8.10 A 9-year-old male who fell off a slide 6 months ago, sustaining a left both-bone forearm fracture. Treated with hematoma block and closed reduction. Absent median motor and sensation in hand. Absent sensory and motor conduction on nerve conduction studies. (A) Prereduction x-ray. (B) Recent x-rays. (C) Nerve exploration revealing nerve entering and exiting fracture site. Checkpoint stimulator showed no distal response. (D) Nerve cut proximal with nerve-cutting device. (E) Nerve cut distal with nerve cutting device.

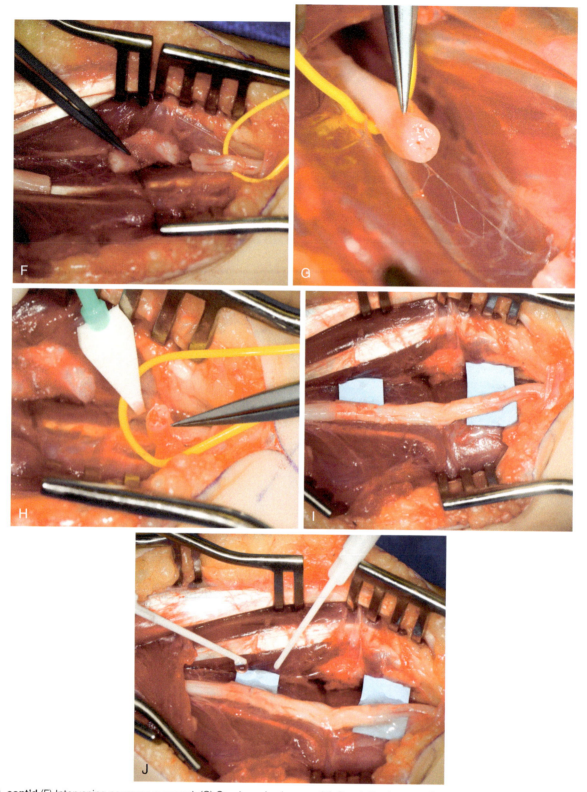

Fig. 8.10, cont'd (F) Intervening neuroma removed. (G) Good proximal axons. (H) Good distal axons. (I) A 3-cm defect bridged with sural nerve cable grafts augmented by nerve connectors to facilitate alignment. (J) Fibrin glue applied to secure coaptation sites.

The initial treatment is directed at maintaining shoulder motion while awaiting spontaneous nerve regeneration. Controversy exists regarding the appropriate time for surgical exploration after an isolated axillary nerve injury. Considering the location of injury and distance from the motor end plates, one should expect signs of reinnervation about 3 to 4 months after an axonotmetric nerve injury. EMG of the deltoid muscle may detect findings of reinnervation before clinical detection. No recovery by 6 months warrants surgical exploration and nerve reconstruction.

Two primary treatment options are available for axillary neurotmesis. Nerve grafting has been the preferred

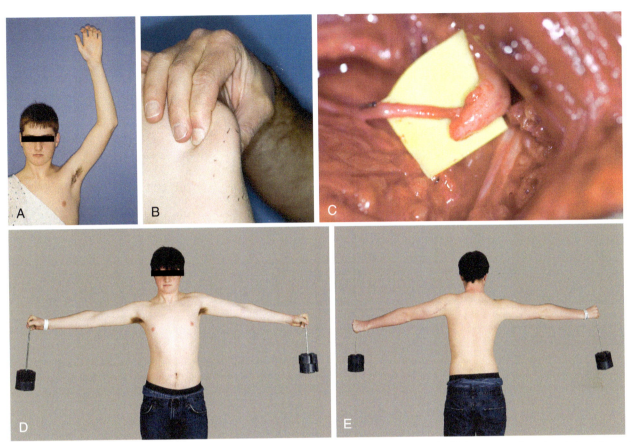

Fig. 8.11 A 15-year-old status post–shoulder dislocation with complete left axillary neuropathy. (A) Maintenance of overhead shoulder motion. (B) Absent deltoid contraction and area of numbness about the left shoulder. (C) Nerve transfer (radial to axillary) via posterior approach. (D) Frontal view with restoration of deltoid contour. (E) Healed posterior incision with adequate strength. (Courtesy of Shriners Hospital for Children, Philadelphia Unit.)

method of surgical treatment for isolated axillary nerve disruption.[19–22] Nerve grafting through the quadrilateral space is a difficult procedure that requires an anterior and a posterior exposure to the shoulder. A deltopectoral incision is performed, and the pectoralis minor is released from the coracoid process. The underlying brachial plexus and axillary vessels are isolated and mobilized. The axillary nerve is identified by its course over the subscapularis and into the quadrilateral space. The axillary nerve must be dissected in a proximal direction until normal nerve is encountered. Distal dissection toward the quadrilateral space will reveal dense scar formation about the nerve, indicative of injury and loss of viable fascicles. The neuroma is resected until viable fascicles are encountered. A posterior shoulder incision from the acromion to the posterior axillary crease is also performed so that the axillary nerve exiting from the quadrilateral space can be identified. A viable axillary nerve distal to the quadrilateral space is then identified. The defect between the axillary nerve in the anterior and posterior incisions is measured for graft distance. This distance is calculated with the arm in abduction and external rotation to grafting without tension. The defect is bridged by cable grafting with the use of multiple strands of sural nerve.

Over the past few years, the authors have preferred a nerve transfer to restore axillary nerve continuity (Fig. 8.11C).[7,11,23,24] The procedure is easier and more straightforward, negates sural nerve harvesting, and avoids the dual incisions necessary for nerve grafting. However, the results

of nerve grafting and nerve transfer are similar.[22] A longitudinal incision is performed from the posterior border of the deltoid to a line between the long and lateral heads of the triceps muscles. The authors have also used an axillary incision with distal extension for donor harvest. The quadrangular space and axillary nerve are identified. The axillary nerve is traced proximal to the nerve branch to the teres minor and is cut. The sensory branch is separated from the motor components and not included in the transfer. The radial nerve is isolated exiting the triangular space and traced in a distal direction to identify its branches to the lateral, long, and medial heads. Electric stimulation is helpful. Any one of the branches to the triceps muscle can be used as a donor. The authors typically use the medial head branch because this nerve can be dissected quite distal and provides ample length for nerve coaptation.[7,11] The donor nerve is reflected in a proximal direction and directly coapted to the axillary nerve under magnification. Microsutures, fibrin glue, or both can be used to secure the repair site. Clinical recovery occurs over the ensuing 6 to 12 months (Fig. 8.11D–E).

NERVE INJURY AFTER A LACERATION OR PENETRATING TRAUMA

Pediatric nerve injuries can also occur secondary to penetrating trauma, such as a stab wound, glass cut, or gunshot wound (see Fig. 8.5). Sharp trauma requires immediate diagnosis and urgent management. Lacerations directly over nerves are best explored so that nerve continuity is ensured. The rationale for exploration has been equated to the general surgery approach toward an appendectomy. The surgeon should not be afraid of a negative exploration because early detection allows for a primary repair and a superior outcome. Unfortunately, the difficulty in examining young children confounds many physicians and practitioners. Therefore, delayed presentation is fairly common because detection is delayed.

The treatment of delayed nerve injuries depends on the timing of presentation. Most children are seen in the subacute phase (weeks or months) from injury. Because children produce larger neuromas and the cut nerve ends retract further than adults, the surgeon must be prepared to perform a primary repair or reconstruction using nerve grafts. The decision is made during surgery with an assessment of the injury, quality of the nerve ends, and tension required for primary repair. Tension is deleterious for nerve recovery and should be minimized.

IATROGENIC NERVE INJURIES

Surgical mishaps occur even in the best of hands and can result in nerve injury. The offending agent is variable, and multiple potential culprits include the scalpel, drill, saw, burr, or arthroscopic equipment (e.g., punch, shaver, or thermal probes). Intraoperative recognition permits the most expedient treatment with the best outcome. As soon as the injury is recognized, a frank conversation should be had with the family and the patient. This requires extreme care and compassion, and ample time should be planned to answer all questions. Despite being informed of the potential for nerve injury, no patient or family imagines that occurrence. The family may be distressed and angry. Poignant questions are asked, and respectful, honest answers are expected. The "blame game" should not be played. The surgeon should explain that all surgery has inherent risks and that unexpected events do occur from time to time. The discussion should also stress that no malice was involved and that the immediate concern is rectifying the problem. It is important for the family to believe that their surgeon is sorry for what has happened and is taking every step to optimize the outcome. Furthermore, the family must appreciate that the surgeon is available to them for practical and emotional support. The family and patient also need to feel empowered and involved in the decision-making process.

Exploration of the nerve is compulsory following direct trauma. The assessment of damage dictates the necessary method for restoration of nerve continuity. A sharp laceration can undergo immediate nerve repair, whereas a more diffuse injury (e.g., high-speed burr or shaver) may require primary nerve grafting (Fig. 8.12). If the surgeon is unfamiliar with nerve repair techniques or if the appropriate equipment is unavailable, the nerve ends should be tagged with a small suture, and the patient should be referred urgently to an experienced nerve surgeon. A poorly performed nerve repair should be avoided because this will lead to further damage of the nerve ends.

By contrast, observation is appropriate for iatrogenic nerve injuries from positioning or traction. Neuropraxia will resolve over the ensuing weeks. Axonotmesis will require substantial time for axonal regeneration. On rare occasions, a permanent nerve injury occurs secondary to a long surgery and prolonged nerve compression (e.g., ulnar nerve injury after spinal surgery). Decompression may be warranted after 3 months of observation without signs of recovery.

NERVE INJURY SECONDARY TO COMPARTMENT SYNDROME

Compartment syndrome in children is a dreaded outcome after skeletal trauma. Certain fracture patterns are notorious for causing a compartment syndrome. In the upper extremity, the supracondylar humeral fracture coupled with a both-bone forearm fracture (i.e., floating elbow) is such an injury (Fig. 8.13). The biggest hurdle in the treatment of children with a compartment syndrome is making the diagnosis. The five Ps of symptoms/signs of adult compartment syndrome (i.e., pain, pallor, paresthesia, paralysis, and pulselessness) do not apply to young children. Children have trouble quantifying pain and do not understand paresthesias or numbness. Pulselessness and pallor are very late signs and imply a missed opportunity. The authors teach their trainees to look for the As and not the Ps.[25] The As stand for analgesia, agitation, and anxiousness. In children who have undergone fracture stabilization, their pain and anxiety decrease rapidly, often to the point of not requiring narcotics for pain relief. A child with increasing pain heralds an impending problem. In addition, a child who has undergone fracture stabilization should be resting comfortably and be neither anxious nor agitated. A restless child who is squirming and uncomfortable signals an underlying problem. A child with the As requires prompt evaluation and intervention. Assessment of nerve function and circulation is mandatory. Splitting any circumferential dressing is compulsory. Inability to alleviate the problem requires emergent fasciotomies to preserve muscle and nerve integrity. The authors do not use compartment pressure measurements because the diagnosis of compartment syndrome is based on clinical findings.

Untreated compartment syndrome results in Volkmann ischemic contracture. Volkmann ischemic contracture is especially prevalent in developing countries without assess to orthopedic care (Fig. 8.14). In these countries, bone setters are prevalent who tightly wrap fractured limbs, producing the ideal scenario for compartment syndrome. The extent of muscle necrosis and nerve damage is variable. Typically, the deep forearm volar compartment is the most severely affected, followed by the superficial volar compartment, and lastly the dorsal compartments. An inventory of each individual muscle and nerve is necessary. Ongoing cicatrix formation can further compress and compromise nerves situated between contracting muscles. The timing of muscle release is controversial and ranges from immediate to delayed. Partial forearm ischemia may benefit from therapy with a focus on resolving joint contractures. Nerve recovery should be assessed at regular intervals. Intervention is indicated when therapy or neurologic recovery has plateaued at an unacceptable level. Persistent symptomatic contracture will improve after release of the contracted forearm muscles. The authors prefer the ulnar-based flexor-pronator muscle slide popularized by Stevanovic and Sharpe.[26] Via a

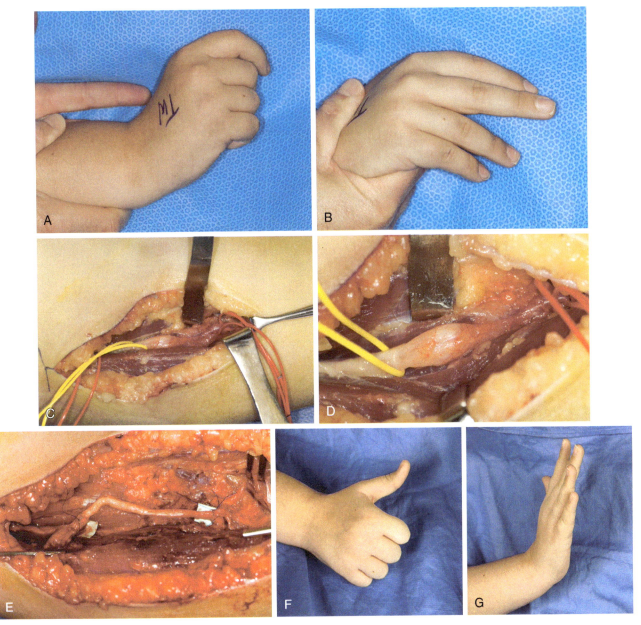

Fig. 8.12 A 12-year-old male status post–right elbow arthroscopy with absent posterior interosseous nerve function. (A) Weak wrist extension. (B) Absent finger metacarpophalangeal joint extension. (C) Anterolateral surgical approach. (D) Large neuroma and zone of injury. (E) Dorsal radial sensory nerve used to span 4.5-cm defect. (F) Outcome with full thumb extension. (G) Mild extension lag at finger metacarpophalangeal joints. (Courtesy of Shriners Hospital for Children, Philadelphia Unit.)

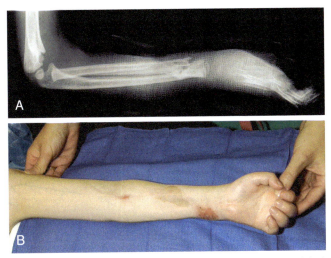

Fig. 8.13 A 5-year-old boy fell from the monkey bars. (A) Radiograph of floating elbow with supracondylar humerus fracture coupled with a both-bone forearm fracture. (B) Unrecognized compartment syndrome with substantial muscle loss and contracture. (Courtesy of Shriners Hospital for Children, Philadelphia Unit.)

longitudinal ulnar incision, the ulnar nerve is transposed, and a complete release of the volar compartment muscle origins is performed from ulnar to radial. The dissection proceeds across the interosseous membrane; care should be taken to preserve the anterior interosseous neurovascular structures. The release is sufficient when the wrist and digits can be extended completely (Fig. 8.14). Subsequently, the child is immobilized with the wrist and digits in maximal extension for a month. An Orthoplast splint is used thereafter for 2 months, during which range of motion and strengthening exercises are initiated.

In children with extensive muscle involvement, the timing of intervention is also controversial. The authors believe that if no signs of muscle or nerve recovery are present by 3 months, then a muscle slide and nerve decompression are warranted. A similar surgical approach is used, although any nonviable muscle is excised. The dissection is quite tedious because differentiating muscle from fat from nerve is quite difficult. Occasionally, a nonviable attenuated nerve will be encountered, and nerve grafting will be necessary. A completely ischemic volar compartment is reconstructed by free muscle transfer performed at the time of muscle release or

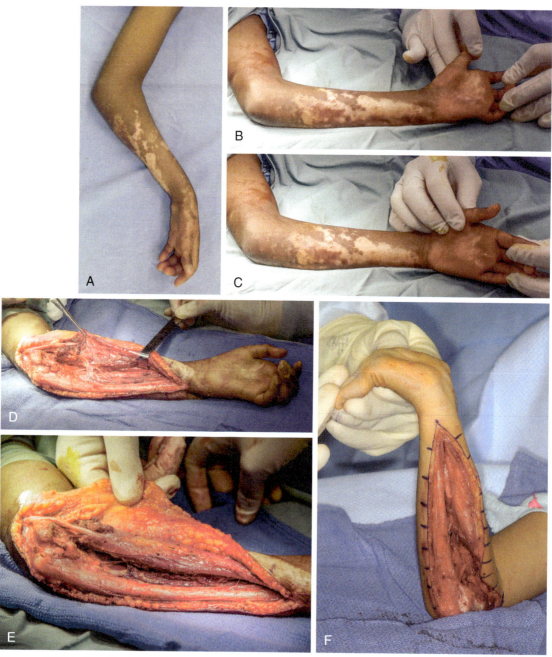

Fig. 8.14 A 12-year-old Ethiopian girl who sustained a left forearm fracture treated by liniment application and tight wrapping. (A) Left forearm with resting posture and caustic skin changes. (B) Limited passive finger extension with wrist held in extension consistent with ischemic contracture of the deep flexor compartment (flexor digitorum profundus). (C) Wrist flexion allows complete finger extension by relaxing the flexor compartment. (D) Complete release of the volar muscle compartment. (E) Close-up view of the ulnar release and the infarcted flexor muscle. (F) Full finger extension with wrist in extension.

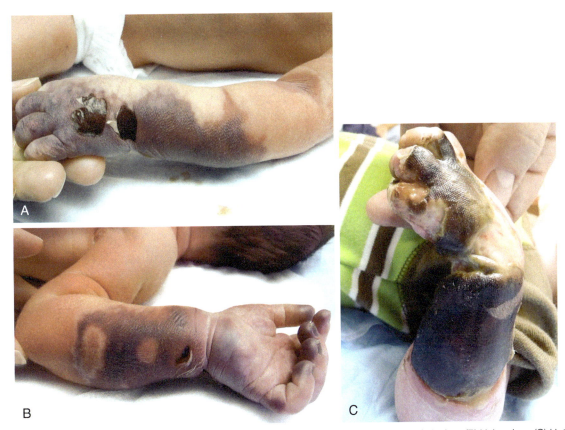

Fig. 8.15 Newborn with left neonatal or intrauterine forearm compartment syndrome. (A) Sentinel skin lesion. (B) Volar view. (C) Untreated with resultant ischemia and limb loss. (Courtesy of Shriners Hospital for Children, Philadelphia Unit.)

as a delayed procedure. The selection of vascular inflow and donor nerve is variable and is dependent on the injury pattern and remaining viable structures.

A less understood phenomenon is neonatal or intrauterine compartment syndrome.[27] This is a rare event, but it occurs most commonly in the forearm (Fig. 8.15). A skin lesion over the area of ischemia is pathognomonic (sentinel skin lesion). This lesion may be secondary to exuberant edema and fetal skin rupture. The child will present at birth in variable stages of a compartment syndrome, depending on the acuity of the event before birth. As with all compartment syndromes, an emergent fasciotomy is mandatory to preserve limb viability. Observation results in tissue loss and possible limb loss.

CONCLUSION

The moment a nerve injury occurs, the clock starts running. Because motor end plates suffer irreversible demise at 18 to 24 months after denervation, diagnostic and treatment strategies should focus on delivering viable axons to the most distal end plates before that window closes. Neuropraxias from traction or temporary compression typically resolve by 6 to 8 weeks because they only require remyelination of intact axons. More severe injuries such as axonotmesis will have some level of spontaneous recovery, but the timing of recovery is directly proportional to the distance that the regenerating axon has to travel to reach its target

organ. In addition, the recovery process is slow (1 mm/day) and prolonged. A patient will not recover from neurotmesis. At this time, there is no diagnostic test capable of distinguishing between an axonotmesis and neurotmesis, which complicates the decision process regarding timing of treatment. When in doubt, it is better to err on the side of exploring a nerve injury that is not recovering (Video 8.3). The timing should allow for reconstruction and recovery to reach the nerve's most distal innervated muscle. Managing these injuries can be exceedingly complex, and even surgeons at referral centers often phone a friend or colleague for advice.

REFERENCES

The level of evidence (LOE) is determined according to the criteria provided in the Preface.

1. Ashworth S, Kozin SH. Brachial plexus palsy reconstruction: tendon transfers, osteotomies, capsular release and arthrodesis. In: Skirven TM, Osterman AL, Fedorczyk JM, Amadio PC, eds. *Rehabilitation of the Hand and Upper Extremity.* Philadelphia, Mosby;792–812. (**LOE V**).
2. Seddon HJ. *Surgical Disorders of Peripheral Nerve Injuries.* 2nd ed. Edinburgh: Churchill-Livingstone. (**LOE V**).
3. Seddon HJ. Nerve grafting. *J Bone Joint Surg Br.* 1963;45:447–461. (**LOE IV**).
4. Campion D. Electrodiagnostic testing in hand surgery. *J Hand Surg Am.* 1996;21:947–956. (**LOE V**).

5. Gasparotti R, Lodoli G, Meoded A, et al. Feasibility of diffusion tractography of brachial plexus injuries at 1.5 T. *Invest Radiol.* 2013;48:1–9. **(LOE II).**

6. Cartwright MS, Yoon JS, Lee KH, et al. Diagnostic ultrasound for traumatic radial neuropathy. *Am J Phys Med Rehabil.* 2011;90(4):342–343. **(LOE II).**

7. Kozin SH. Nerve transfers in brachial plexus birth palsies: indications, techniques, and outcome. *Hand Clin.* 2008;24:363–376. **(LOE V).**

8. Feldman MD, Sataloff RT, Epstein G, Ballas SK. Autologous fibrin tissue adhesive for peripheral nerve anastomosis. *Arch Otolaryngol Head Neck Surg.* 1987;113(9):963–967. **(LOE II).**

9. Temple CL, Ross DC, Dunning CE, Johnson JA. Resistance to disruption and gapping of peripheral nerve repairs: an in vitro biomechanical assessment of techniques. *J Reconstr Microsurg.* 2004;20(8):645–650. **(LOE II).**

10. Kozin SH. Injuries of the brachial plexus. In: Iannotti JP, Williams GR, eds. *Disorders of the Shoulder: Diagnosis and Management.* 2nd ed. Philadelphia: Lippincott Williams & Wilkins;1087–1134. **(LOE V).**

11. Malessy MJA, Pondaag W. Obstetric brachial plexus injuries. *Neurosurg Clin N Am.* 2009;20:1–14. **(LOE III).**

12. Colbert SH, Mackinnon S. Posterior approach for double nerve transfer for restoration of shoulder function in upper brachial plexus palsy. *Hand.* 2006;1:71–77. **(LOE III).**

13. Teboul F, Kakkar R, Ameur N, et al. Transfer of fascicles from the ulnar nerve to the biceps in the treatment of upper brachial plexus palsy. *J Bone Joint Surg Am.* 2004;86:1485–1490. **(LOE II).**

14. Ray WZ, Mackinnon SE. Clinical outcomes following median to radial nerve transfers. *J Hand Surg Am.* 2011;36(2):201–208. **(LOE IV).**

15. Zlotolow DA, Catalano LW, Barron OA, Glickel SZ. Surgical exposures of the humerus. *J Am Acad Orthop Surg.* 2006;14:754–765. **(LOE III).**

16. Zhao X, Lao J, Hung LK, et al. Selective neurotization of the median nerve in the arm to treat brachial plexus palsy: an anatomic study and case report. *J Bone Joint Surg Am.* 2004;86-A(4):736–742. **(LOE II).**

17. Choi PD, Melikian R, Skaggs DL. Risk factors for vascular repair and compartment syndrome in the pulseless supracondylar humerus fracture in children. *J Pediatr Orthop.* 2010;30:50–56. **(LOE III).**

18. LeClerq C, Hentx VR, Kozin SH, Mulcahey MJ. Reconstruction of elbow extension. *Hand Clin.* 2008;24:185–201. **(LOE V).**

19. Coene LN, Narakas AO. Operative management of lesions of the axillary nerve, isolated or combined with other lesions. *Clin Neurol Neurosurg.* 1992;94(suppl):S64–S66. **(LOE III).**

20. Petrucci FS, Morelli A, Raimondi PL. Axillary nerve injuries: 21 cases treated by nerve graft and neurolysis. *J Hand Surg.* 1982;7:271–278. **(LOE III).**

21. Wehbe J, Maalouf G, Habanbo J, et al. Surgical treatment of traumatic lesions of the axillary nerve. A retrospective study of 33 cases. *Acta Orthop Belg.* 2004;70:11–18. **(LOE III).**

22. Wolfe SW, Johnsen PH, Lee SK, Feinberg JH. Long-nerve grafts and nerve transfers demonstrate comparable outcomes for axillary nerve injuries. *J Hand Surg Am.* 2014;39(7):1351–1357. **(LOE III).**

23. Bertelli JA, Ghizoni MF. Nerve transfer from triceps medial head and anconeus to deltoid for axillary nerve palsy. *J Hand Surg Am.* 2014;39(5):940–947. **(LOE IV).**

24. Chaung DCC, Lee GW, Hashem F, Wei FC. Restoration of shoulder abduction by nerve transfer in avulsed brachial plexus injury: evaluation of 99 patients with various nerve transfers. *Plast Reconstr Surg.* 1995;96:122–128. **(LOE III).**

25. Bae DS, Kadiyala RK, Waters PM. Acute compartment syndrome in children: contemporary diagnosis, treatment, and outcome. *J Pediatr Orthop.* 2001;21(5):680–688. **(LOE IV).**

26. Stevanovic M, Sharpe F. Management of established Volkmann's contracture of the forearm in children. *Hand Clin.* 2006;22:99–111. **(LOE V).**

27. Ragland III R, Maukoko D, Ezaki M, et al. Forearm compartment syndrome in the newborn: report of 24 cases. *J Hand Surg Am.* 2005;30(5):997–1003. **(LOE III).**

Outcomes Assessment of Fractures in Children

9

Unni G. Narayanan

INTRODUCTION

How do we know that our interventions have been successful? The success or *effectiveness* of an intervention is best defined in terms of whether or not it consistently achieves the goal(s) for which the intervention is intended. Outcomes research is the science of measuring effectiveness. Wennberg, one of the pioneers of the outcomes research movement, defined the imperative to "sort out what works in medicine and to learn how to make clinical decisions that reflect more truly the needs and wants of individual patients."[1] This philosophy is embodied in the definition of evidence-based medicine (EBM) that is characterized by the "… conscientious, explicit and judicious use of the current best evidence (derived from systematic research) in making decisions about the care of individual patients."[2] The spirit of EBM requires that the effectiveness of the intervention(s) of interest should be judged using meaningful, validated outcome measures that reflect the goals and expectations of patients. These goals may seem self-evident, but too often the perspectives of individual patients are not taken into sufficient consideration during clinical decision-making, much less measuring their outcomes.

Outcomes assessment has come a long way from its origins exemplified by Codman[3] to the era of comparative effectiveness research (CER) of today.[4] This chapter provides an overview of outcomes assessment to provide a context for the measurement of conventional and patient-reported outcomes (PROs) in the management of pediatric fractures. Some of the limitations of current assessments will be highlighted and a framework suggested for conceptualizing "meaningful" outcomes and developing instruments to measure such outcomes.

WHAT ARE OUTCOMES?

Outcomes can be defined as the effects of health care on the health status of patients and populations and are one of the three dimensions of care, along with process and structure, in Donabedian's framework for evaluating the quality of care.[5] An outcome is what happens to a patient as a consequence of an intervention or the passage of time (natural history).[6] An intervention can be associated with multiple outcomes. Outcomes can be desirable (*benefits*) or undesirable (*harms*). An outcome is desirable when the intended *goal* has been achieved. The goals of an intervention can be *reactive*, aiming to eliminate a symptom (e.g., pain) or correct a recognizable impairment or problem (e.g., limb lengthening procedure to correct an acquired limb length inequality from a growth arrest). The goal of an intervention can be *preventative* or *prophylactic*, intended to prevent some future harm (e.g., contralateral epiphysiodesis following a high-risk physeal injury). Consequently, some outcomes occur early, whereas others become evident only after a period of time. Outcomes may not come to light for many years (e.g., open reduction of an intraarticular fracture to prevent osteoarthritis in adulthood). An undesirable outcome can be expected and inevitable (e.g., an incisional scar after surgery); expected some of the time, such as a known side effect of the treatment (e.g., pin site infection of external fixation); or unexpected, when it is considered an *adverse event*. A *complication* is an undesirable outcome associated with an injury or its treatment, occurring some of the time (e.g., avascular necrosis following a femoral neck fracture). The likelihood (probability) or *risk* of such a complication may not always be reliably quantifiable, and there may be measures that can be taken to reduce or prevent such risks. Undesirable outcomes can be transient or reversible, or permanent.

An understanding of these concepts is essential for shared decision-making, the central tenet of patient-centered clinical care. Most clinicians recognize these as key elements to be considered during discussions with patients about treatment recommendations and the process for obtaining *informed consent*. The evidence to guide these discussions must be derived from high-quality research that measures these harms and benefits. CER is involved in the generation and synthesis of evidence that compares the benefits and harms of alternative methods to prevent, diagnose, treat, and monitor a clinical condition or to improve the delivery of care.[4] The purpose of CER is to assist patients, clinicians, purchasers, and policy makers to make informed decisions that will improve health care at both the individual and population levels.[4]

FRAMEWORKS OF HEALTH AND DISEASE AND THE EVALUATION OF OUTCOMES

An evolution has occurred in the conceptualization of health since the traditional medical model, in which health was characterized merely by the absence of disease, to more complex models that take a more holistic account of the human experience.[7] This evolution has been accompanied by changes in the way we measure health and disease, reflected by an array of outcome measures that quantify a wide range of health-related phenomena, including physical, mental, and social status and quality of life (QOL).[8]

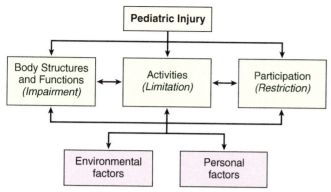

Fig. 9.1 The International Classification of Functioning, Disability and Health model. (Modified from the World Health Organization)

INTERNATIONAL CLASSIFICATION OF FUNCTIONING, DISABILITY AND HEALTH

The *International Classification of Functioning, Disability and Health (ICF)*, developed by the World Health Organization (WHO), provides a unified, standard language that classifies health and health-related domains of individuals or populations, and provides a framework to measure health and disability associated with any health condition.[9] The ICF complements the International Classification of Diseases (ICD) system, which codifies these conditions.[10,11] The model has been adapted for children to develop the ICF for Children and Youth.[12,13] The ICF list of domains includes a list of body structures and functions and a list of activities and participation, which can be influenced by contextual factors such as the environment and personal characteristics (Fig. 9.1).[12]

In the ICF framework, the term *body structures* refers to the anatomic parts of the body affected by the health condition of interest (e.g., effect of an injury on bones, muscles, and neurovascular structures), and the term *body functions* refers to physiological and psychological functions of various body systems (e.g., range of motion). Intact body structures and body function allow for *activities.* An activity refers to the completion of a specific task or action (e.g., throwing, running), which, when performed for a particular purpose or role, is referred to as *participation* (e.g., playing baseball). Participation implies doing things that one wants to do. Participation in life roles is a key component of QOL. Disruption of body structures and body functions, associated with a health condition, results in *impairments.* For instance, pediatric injury may be associated with impairments of the body structure, specifically the musculoskeletal system (e.g., femur fracture) and body function (e.g., joint range of motion). Impairments of body structures and body functioning may lead to *limitation* in activities. Limitation in an activity (e.g., inability to run) can result in *restriction* of participation (e.g., being dropped from the soccer team). The impact of a health condition and its treatment on activities and participation constitute what are often called "functional" outcomes. The ICF framework includes the consideration of *contextual factors* that can be strong determinants, either as facilitators or barriers, of functional outcomes. These include external *environmental factors,* such as home/school/community, socioeconomic status, access to health care, as well as *personal factors,* such as demographic characteristics, culture and

upbringing, lifestyle preferences, motivation, and personality traits.[14] Contextual factors are important to consider, as they can explain the gap between what one *can* do (capacity) and what one actually *does* do in daily life (performance).[15]

TECHNICAL VERSUS FUNCTIONAL OUTCOMES[16]

In the management of fractures, the immediate objective of interventions is to restore and maintain alignment and length until the fracture unites and consolidates. In the ICF framework, these are outcomes at the level of impairments of body structures and body functions. Goldberg refers to these as *technical (or clinical) outcomes.*[16] These are important indicators of the success of the intervention in achieving its "technical" objectives (e.g., anatomic alignment and bony union after open reduction and internal fixation). However, there is an expectation that these will lead to the *functional outcomes* that patients and parents ultimately want, which is to return to full activities and participation without restrictions (e.g., return to playing soccer). It is important to measure functional outcomes separately because these are related to the ultimate goals of the patient. A technically successful outcome cannot always be assumed to result in a functionally successful outcome. A functionally successful outcome may not always require technical perfection. Indeed, more harm than good might arise from one's pursuit, and even achievement, of technical perfection. For example, an open reduction of a radial neck fracture to restore anatomic alignment might lead to a worse functional outcome than accepting some magnitude of malalignment that is completely compatible with a perfect functional result. Functional outcomes are more meaningful indicators of effectiveness than technical/clinical outcomes.

THE PRIORITY FRAMEWORK FOR OUTCOMES EVALUATION[17]

Outcomes are most meaningful when they are aligned with *patient priorities.* Living with a health condition is associated with a set of experiences that include current symptoms or "complaints" and/or potential future consequences related to the natural history of that condition. These experiences and the knowledge of future consequences can be associated with a set of *concerns* about the health condition and/ or its treatment, resulting in certain *desires (wishes)* and *expectations* of these treatments and outcomes.[18,19] Concerns, desires, and expectations can be collectively considered as patient priorities. Elicitation of these priorities enables a patient to define a set of *goals* related to their priorities, which can influence their choice (or preference) for specific treatment options.[20] The elicitation of patients' priorities might provide important insight into hitherto unknown patient preferences, which, in turn, might influence the process of informed choice, decision-making, and true informed consent, and facilitate the evaluation of outcomes that matter most to patients.[21] PRO instruments will only be meaningful if the questions asked of patients reflect what is relevant and important to them.[22,23]

These concepts have been incorporated in a priority framework for evaluation of outcomes.[17] In the center of the framework is the health condition of interest (e.g., pediatric fractures). Living with the health condition leads to a set of

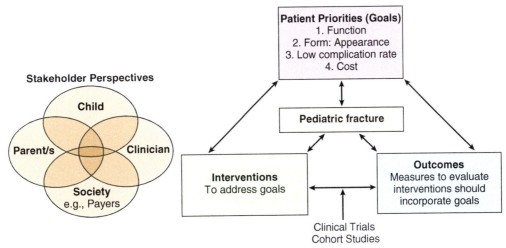

Fig. 9.2 The Priority Framework for Outcomes Assessment.

priorities (concerns, needs, desires, and expectations), which are fundamental to defining the *goals* that are derived from these priorities. Different stakeholders might have different priorities (e.g., child, parent[s], family, surgeon, societal) which might overlap but may not be concordant. Understanding priorities and goals is crucial for making decisions about *interventions* that will best address these priorities and goals, or for developing new treatments/interventions where these do not exist or are insufficiently effective in addressing the priorities and goals. Interventions must be held accountable in terms of achievement of these goals. Their effectiveness is evaluated (e.g., in clinical trials or cohort studies or at the level of the individual patient) using *outcome measures* that specifically incorporate the goals and priorities of the patient population. In this framework, defining goals, choosing interventions, and evaluating outcomes or developing valid measures to do so all come back to and depend on an understanding of patient priorities and the goals that arise from these priorities (Fig. 9.2).[17]

In the management of fractures, achieving anatomic alignment and bony union are a means to an end. The ultimate goal is to ensure that the injured patient is restored to the preinjured state. If the desired goals include that the injured limb should look, feel, and work as well as it did before the injury, these goals should be embedded in any outcome measure that purports to evaluate effectiveness in terms that are meaningful for patients.

OUTCOME MEASURES: GENERAL CONSIDERATIONS

WHOSE PERSPECTIVE PREVAILS?

Outcome measures are tools used to assess a change in particular attributes that are deemed meaningful to a person's life over time.[24] To the extent that the patient's perspective is recognized to be preeminent in making judgments about effectiveness, the use of *PRO* measures is now considered the standard when the effectiveness of interventions is evaluated. PROs should be derived from patients themselves, particularly for outcomes that pertain to personal experience (e.g., pain, body image, and self-esteem). This is challenging in the

context of pediatric conditions. When children are too young or too cognitively immature to respond, one has to rely on the report of the child's parent(s). A parent(s)' report must be recognized to be a proxy for what the child might report. The views of older children can and must be taken into consideration, but their perspective might differ from those of their parents. Parents may or may not recognize that their priorities might be different from those of their children, and parents may not agree with each other. The level of agreement between parents and children is usually good for domains reflecting physical activity, functioning, and symptoms, but poorer for domains reflecting more social or emotional issues.[25] Proxies and children may not agree about many issues, but both perspectives may be valid and should be considered during decision-making, as well as in measuring outcomes.

Some outcomes are more important than others, and different stakeholders will have different perspectives on the relative importance of different outcomes. Clinical outcomes are more relevant to patients; nonclinical outcomes (e.g., length of stay, cost) are of interest to hospital administrators, payers, and health policy makers.

GENERIC VERSUS CONDITION-SPECIFIC MEASURES

Outcome measures can be generic or disease- or condition-specific.[26] *Generic* outcome measures include those that measure general physical function, health status, and well-being. These have the advantage of comparing outcomes across different clinical conditions and interventions and are particularly useful to policy makers who might be interested in understanding the relative value of some types of interventions over others for purposes of health care utilization, planning, and resource allocation. However, generic outcome measures may assess some things that are not relevant to the condition and may neglect to include other issues of crucial importance. Generic measures are usually less sensitive to change than *condition-specific* measures that are designed to focus on issues relevant to the condition of interest. Condition-specific measures have more limited applicability. For instance, an outcome measure designed to evaluate outcomes of lower extremity (LE) fractures in children may not be relevant for other musculoskeletal conditions in children, let alone nonmusculoskeletal pediatric conditions.

MORTALITY, HEALTH, AND QUALITY OF LIFE

When the primary goal of an intervention is to save or extend life, measuring *mortality* (survival) must be the primary outcome. However, every life saved ought to be a life worth living, and who best to make that judgment than the person whose life has been prolonged? *QOL* is defined as "individuals' perceptions of their position in life in the context of the culture and value systems in which they live, and in relation to their goals, expectations, standards and concerns."[27] *Health-related quality of life* (HRQL) refers to the health-related factors that contribute toward the goodness and meaning of life, and how one perceives one's ability to fulfill certain life roles. *Health* itself is defined as "a state of complete physical, mental and social well-being, and not merely the absence of disease or infirmity."[28] HRQL is therefore a multidimensional construct that encompasses physical, mental, and social well-being as well as role attainment, daily functioning, and participation in community life.[29,30] HRQL measures provide a more complete picture of an individual, and are complementary to traditional biomedical measures and functional assessments.[31] Functional status refers to the degree to which an individual is able to perform socially allocated roles without physical or mental limitations.

CAPACITY AND PERFORMANCE

Capacity is the term used to describe an activity or task that an individual *can* do in a standardized environment, whereas *performance* refers to tasks or activities that the individual actually carries out or *does* do in daily life.[15] Some outcome instruments are measures of capacity or capability, whereas others are measures of performance.

PROPERTIES OF A GOOD OUTCOME MEASURE

There are several factors to consider in the selection of an outcome measure.[32,33] The outcome measure must be relevant to the goals of the intervention. It should measure issues that are important to the children being evaluated and to their parents, and in a format that is accessible, comprehensible, and not unduly burdensome. The purpose of the selected outcome measure must be considered. There are three main types of outcome measures.[34,35] *Discriminative measures* are able to distinguish patients from each other, for instance, those with a disorder from those without, and those with more severe involvement from those less severely involved. *Predictive measures* provide some indication of a future outcome (e.g., Stulberg criteria of the morphology of the femoral head and acetabulum at skeletal maturity predict the risk of osteoarthritis of the hip in the future). Prediction is also concerned with classifying patients. For example, outcome measures may be used in diagnosis and screening to identify individuals for suitable forms of treatment. *Evaluative measures* are designed to measure change over time, such as after an intervention.[36] Any measurement tool must be shown to be psychometrically sound (reliable and valid) to achieve the purpose for which the measure is intended.[33]

Reliability is a fundamental requirement of any valid measure. This is the property of *reproducibility* or *consistency*. A reliable measure is one that produces the same result when it is administered repeatedly, provided there has been no change in the subject or attribute that is being measured. Reliability reflects the amount of error that is inherent in any measurement.[35] Reliability can be assessed between repeated administrations over a time frame in which one would not expect to observe a change (test-retest reliability), by the same rater (intrarater reliability), and between different raters of the same subjects (interrater reliability). Reliability is usually measured using statistical tests of concordance or agreement, rather than just correlation. The two common measures of reliability are the intraclass correlation coefficient used for continuous data and the weighted kappa for ordinal data. Reliability is expressed as a numeric value between 0 and 1, where 1 represents perfect agreement or concordance.[37,38] *Internal consistency* refers to a special type of reliability to assess how well the items within a scale correlate with each other to measure a single dimension (e.g., physical function).[32] The most common way of measuring internal consistency is by Cronbach's alpha.[39]

Reliability and consistency do not ensure *accuracy*. A measure can be perfectly reliable but very inaccurate. For instance, a patient might be asked to recall the maximum distance he has walked in the last week. He may consistently (reliably) report this to be 100 meters, when in fact if it was to be measured objectively, the distance is only 50 meters. Many factors play a role in influencing the accuracy of a measure, including the ability to recall or to make estimates accurately.

A measure is *valid* when it measures what it was intended to measure. The validity of a scale is the degree of confidence one can place on inferences about people based on their scores from that scale.[35] An outcome measure has *face validity* when the items in the measure appear to be measuring what they are supposed to.[32] It is an indication of the *sensibility* of the measure.[40] *Content validity* examines the extent to which the attribute of interest is comprehensively sampled by the items or questions in the instrument so that all the relevant and important content or domains are represented. Face and content validity reflect a judgment about whether an outcome measure is reasonable and appropriate for the purpose it was intended. These judgments are usually sought during the development of the measure from patients with the condition and experts who work with these patients. *Criterion validity* is assessed when an instrument correlates with another instrument or measure that is regarded as a more accurate measure (gold standard) of the "criterion." *Concurrent validity* is one type of criterion validity in which an outcome measure (new) is compared with another criterion measure by administering both at the same time. Often, such a gold standard measure does not exist, particularly for subjective attributes like pain or measures of health. Validation then takes through a process of hypothesis testing.[35] *Construct validity* examines the logical relations that should exist between a measure and characteristics of patients and patient groups.[35] For example, an outcome measure can be tested on two groups of patients, one known to have the condition and the other not, or one known to be the more severely involved and the other group just mildly involved. One would test the hypothesis that these groups would be rated differently on the outcome measure, thereby demonstrating *known groups* or *extreme groups validity*. *Convergent validity*, another type of construct validity, is shown when the scales of a measure correlate as expected with the related scales of another measure, but not to unrelated scales (*divergent validity*). When applied to the population of interest, a *discriminative* instrument is sufficiently *sensitive* to detect small (but meaningful) differences between patients. An instrument should be free from *ceiling effects,* which occur when many subjects of the population of interest rate the highest possible score on the measure because it is not sensitive enough to be able to discriminate or distinguish higher-functioning subjects from each other. When an instrument is less discriminative of lower-functioning subjects and rates them all at the lowest end of the scale, it suffers from *floor effects.*

An outcome instrument that is intended to measure effectiveness (*evaluative measure*) must possess the property of *responsiveness* or *sensitivity to change,* which is the ability to measure change over time or following interventions.[34,36] Responsiveness must be tested in longitudinal studies and can be quantified by the standardized response mean, which is the ratio of the mean change to the standard deviation of that change, or the effect size, which is the ratio of the mean change to the standard deviation of the initial measurements.[36]

OUTCOME MEASURES FOR PEDIATRIC FRACTURES

The ultimate goals of fracture management are to restore *form* and *function*. Restoration of function generally requires the fracture to unite and soft tissues (e.g., muscles and ligaments) to heal en route to the resolution of pain, stiffness, weakness, and fatigue; restoration of range of motion and strength; and return to full use. Bones are the lever arms upon which the muscles act, and bone alignment and length influences lever arm function. Form (appearance) is influenced by alignment, length, and (absence of) atrophy and scarring. Restoration of alignment and length is common to both goals and is therefore the most common outcome measured when the effectiveness of fracture treatments is evaluated. These are outcomes at the level of body structures and body functions in the ICF framework, or the technical outcomes of Goldberg.[16]

RADIOGRAPHIC OUTCOMES OF ALIGNMENT AND LENGTH

Alignment and length outcomes are measured on radiographs, recorded at some sufficiently elapsed time point after the injury to allow for remodeling. Conventionally, alignment has been reported in terms of *residual angulation at the fracture site,* which is by far the most common outcome reported in fracture studies. In these studies, *malalignment* is typically defined based on some threshold magnitude of angulation that is believed to be clinically significant either in terms of its physiologic and biomechanical impact now or in the future, or its external visibility (appearance). For example, in a multicenter randomized trial comparing early spica cast with external fixation of femur fractures in children, the primary outcome measure reported was (the rate of) fracture malunion at 2 years after the fracture, defined as any of the following: limb length difference of greater

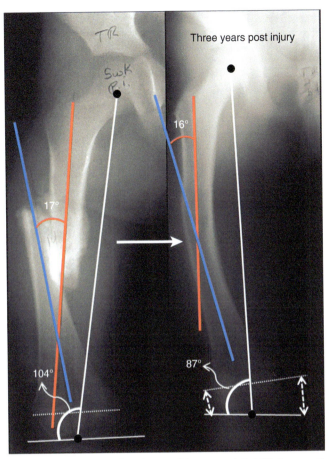

Fig. 9.3 Femur fracture in a 4-year-old was angulated 17 degrees at the fracture site at the time of cast removal, with a mechanical lateral distal femoral angle (mLDFA) of 104 degrees (normal is 87 degrees). Three years later, the mLDFA has normalized, even though there has been little change at the fracture site. This child would be labeled with a malunion based on the residual angulation at the fracture site of 16 degrees varus.

than 2 cm, more than 15 degrees of anterior or posterior angulation, or more than 10 degrees of varus or valgus angulation.[41]

A number of serious limitations are associated with the use of residual angulation at the fracture site as a valid primary outcome measure of fracture management, particularly in children. First, the remodeling of long bone fractures occurs predominantly at the physes by asymmetric growth to correct the alignment, and less so at the fracture site.[42,43] In femur fractures, Wallace and Hoffman demonstrated that 85% of angular deformity had corrected at an average of 45 months, of which only about 26% of the remodeling occurred at the fracture site.[44] This would imply that measuring residual angulation at the fracture site will not take into account where most of the remodeling and correction has occurred, which will potentially lead to overreporting of "malunions." This problem will be especially true for fractures treated by nonoperative or closed methods, as these are less likely to achieve anatomic alignments at the outset (Fig. 9.3). For instance, in the pediatric femur fracture trial of early spica cast with external fixation femur fractures in children, the rate of malunions was reported to be 45% and 16% in the spica cast and external fixation groups, respectively.[41] The majority of these malunions were caused by residual angulation at the fracture site. The authors concluded that early spica casting was associated with a three times greater rate of malunion than external fixation. However, there were no corrective osteotomies or other corrective procedures reported to address these malunions for either group. Furthermore, there was no difference in functional outcomes or parental and child satisfaction, which were excellent in both groups. One possible explanation for this wide gap between the radiographic outcomes and PROs might be that the measurement of residual angulation at the fracture site is misleading because it fails to account for correction that has occurred at the physes. This might also explain why the rate of surgery to correct these "malunions" is usually far lower than the rate of reported malunions in these studies.

There are several other limitations of using residual angulation at the fracture site as the measure of alignment that would apply to fractures in adults as well. The angulation thresholds used to define a malunion are arbitrary and not evidence based. Angulation will have a different impact on the mechanical axis deviation of the limb depending on the level of the fracture. Twenty degrees of angulation in the proximal femur will have a different impact on the mechanical axis than a 20-degree angular deformity in the distal femur. Reporting just the magnitude of the angulation without taking into account the location of the angulation will completely disregard this. There is also more to malalignment than angulation. Translations can have an impact on the mechanical axis and are generally ignored in reports of fracture alignment at union. Different permutations and combinations of coronal (or sagittal) plane translations with angulation and shortening (transverse plane translation) will have a different impact on the appearance and mechanical axis of the limb, and these combinations are seldom taken into account in outcomes reporting, even though they are fundamental to the analysis of deformities for the purpose of correcting these.

Current-day deformity correction uses a framework that is based on the overall mechanical axis of the lower limb and each limb segment to quantify the magnitude of overall deformity.[45–47] Each long bone segment is defined by the fixed (angular) relationship between its own mechanical axis (drawn from proximal to distal joint centers) with the respective proximal and distal joint lines (Fig. 9.4).[48] This representation takes into account all the above factors contributing to the (mal)alignment and its impact on the overall mechanical axis deviation. Although this is a more valid model of alignment and is the standard framework used in analysis of deformity for deformity correction, fracture studies seldom report radiographic outcomes in these terms. Inferences about alignment based solely on the residual angulation at the fracture site are simplistic at best and often flawed and potentially misleading.

Our current concepts of mechanical axis deviation and its measurement are also associated with some limitations. There is a lack of evidence for the long-term clinical significance of mechanical axis deviation and the magnitude of acceptable deviation that might still be compatible with an excellent long-term outcome.[49] The mechanical axis model is based on two-dimensional imaging in orthogonal planes. Malrotations are harder to measure and tend to be underreported. Future models are likely to provide valid three-dimensional representations of the mechanical axis and length, taking into consideration all three planes. For instance, imaging

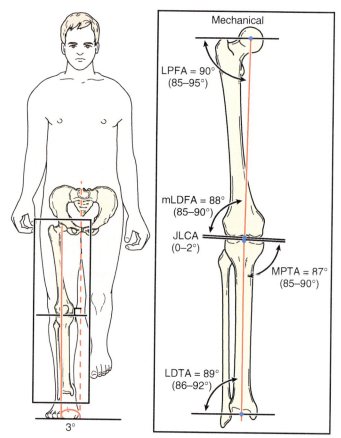

Fig. 9.4 Mechanical axis of the lower limb and each limb segment in the coronal plane. The mechanical axis of the femur has a fixed relationship between the proximal femoral joint line (lateral proximal femoral angle [*LPFA*]) and the distal femoral joint line (lateral distal femoral angle [*LDFA*]). The mechanical axis of the tibia has a fixed relationship between the proximal tibial joint line (medial proximal tibial angle [*MPTA*]) and the distal tibial joint line (lateral distal tibial angle [*LDTA*]). The angle between the distal femoral and proximal tibial joint lines is the joint line convergent angle (*JLCA*). Modified from Paley D. Normal lower limb alignment and joint orientation. In: *Principles of Deformity Correction*. 1st ed. Berlin, Germany: Springer Verlag; 2005.[61]

technology such as the EOS system allows for simultaneous biplanar imaging with very low radiation and combines the accuracy (minimal distortion) of CT with the advantage of upright weight-bearing positioning to capture more valid measurements of length and alignment and has the capacity to render three-dimensional images based on these.[50]

Other radiographic measures include time to healing (based on some subjective assessment of callus formation and consolidation) and markers of complications (e.g., avascular necrosis, hardware failure, delayed or nonunion, and refracture). Time to healing/radiographic union is neither reliable nor accurate because this outcome is based typically on radiographs obtained at standardized follow-up visits separated typically by at least a few weeks, which makes it impossible to ascertain with any precision when these radiographic outcomes occurred.

CLINICAL MEASUREMENTS

These include measures of body structure and function such as limb lengths, limb appearance, and symmetry compared with the uninjured limb, joint range of motion, ligamentous stability, torsional profile, and measures of muscle strength. Lower limb lengths are clinically best recorded in the standing position to assess the level of the pelvis using anatomic landmarks such as the anterior superior iliac spine and the use of blocks underfoot on the short side to level the pelvis. The level of the pelvis can be more objectively quantified, and the source of differences confirmed with full-length standing radiographs. Coronal plane alignment of the upper extremity (UE) can be quantified by measuring the carrying angle with a goniometer and comparing it to the uninjured side. Range of motion can be recorded using traditional goniometers or electronically, using applications available on mobile devices. The reliability, accuracy, and validity of these measurements have not been reported. Clinical measures in the activity domain of the ICF include assessment of gait, which can be recorded objectively by video or motion analysis; however, this is seldom done (nor necessary) in the context of pediatric fractures. Other clinical measures include complications such as wound infections, loss of reduction or clinical malunions requiring secondary interventions, and refracture rates.

PATIENT-REPORTED OUTCOME MEASURES FOR PEDIATRIC FRACTURES

Clinical outcomes in the domains of participation in the ICF model (e.g., resolution of pain and restoration of full function) are related to the ultimate goals of fracture management and are more relevant to the patient and their families. These are best measured using PRO measures. The following are a sample of generic health status or functional patient- or parent-reported outcome measures that have been used for pediatric fracture outcomes evaluations.

PEDIATRIC OUTCOMES DATA COLLECTION INSTRUMENT[51]

The *Pediatric Outcomes Data Collection Instrument* (PODCI) was developed jointly by the American Academy of Orthopaedic Surgeons, the Pediatric Orthopaedic Society of North America, the American Academy of Pediatrics, and the Shriners Hospitals as a measure of musculoskeletal-related functional and health outcomes in children and adolescents.[51] The PODCI comprises 115 items that cover the dimensions of UE function, transfers and mobility, sports and physical function, comfort/pain, global function (mean of the mean scores for the previous four dimensions), happiness and satisfaction with physical condition, and expectations of treatment. The PODCI is self-reported (by parents of children <10 years of age and by both parents and adolescents from 11–18 years). It has been shown to have good reliability, construct validity, and sensitivity to change when tested in a large sample of children (and parents) over a range of ages (2–18 years) and diagnoses and has been used to evaluate pediatric fracture management.[52,53]

ACTIVITIES SCALE FOR KIDS[41]

The *Activities Scale for Kids* (ASK) is a reliable and valid, self-reported measure of physical function in children.[54,55] It was designed to measure physical disability arising from musculoskeletal disorders in children (5–15 years of age). The current ASK comprises 30 items spanning the following dimensions: locomotion, standing skills, transfers, play, personal care, dressing, and other skills. There is a capability version (ASK Capability) that asks kids what they *could have* done, and a performance version (ASK Performance) that asks kids about what they *did* in the past week. It has been used as a measure of functional outcome in studies of fractures of the UE and LE in children.[56–59]

CHILD HEALTH QUESTIONNAIRE[60]

The *Child Health Questionnaire* (CHQ) is a generic measure of the physical and psychosocial well-being of children (5–18 years of age). It has been extensively validated in children with conditions such as asthma, epilepsy, and attention deficit disorder and musculoskeletal disorders such as juvenile rheumatoid arthritis and pediatric injury.[60–62] The CHQ has an 87-item child self-reported version (CHQ-CF87) and two parental versions (CHQ-PF50 and CHQ-PF28) comprising 50 and 28 items, respectively. The items of the CHQ span 14 unique physical and psychosocial constructs. The results of the CHQ can be reported at the scale or concept level (CHQ Profile Scores). The scales can also be combined appropriately to provide a summary score for overall physical and overall psychosocial health, respectively. This is a generic measure for which normative values and benchmarks of the parent-reported versions are available for the United States. The CHQ is useful for comparing the impact of outcomes across different health conditions but might be less useful as a primary outcome measure of pediatric fracture management because it is less likely to be responsive in evaluating change after interventions.[54,63]

PEDIATRIC QUALITY OF LIFE INVENTORY[64]

The *Pediatric Quality of Life Inventory* (PedsQL) is a generic, multidimensional measure of HRQL in children and adolescents. The 23 items of this questionnaire cover the core dimensions of health delineated by the WHO (physical, social, and emotional functioning), as well as role (school) functioning. The questions are phrased in terms of frequency of problems experienced over the past month. The PedsQL generates a total summary score and summary scores for physical health and psychosocial health, respectively. The PedsQL includes three self-reported children's versions for age groups 5 to 7 years, 8 to 12 years, and 13 to 18 years, and separate parent proxy reports for age groups 2 to 4 years, 5 to 7 years, 8 to 12 years, and 13 to 18 years.[64] To be more responsive and relevant, the creators of the PedsQL also developed condition-specific modules for different pediatric health conditions, but one does not exist for musculoskeletal injury. Nevertheless, the PedsQL has been used as a primary outcome measure in some fracture studies.[65]

DISABILITIES OF THE ARM, SHOULDER AND HAND[66]

The *Disabilities of the Arm, Shoulder and Hand* (DASH) outcome measure is a 30-item self-reported questionnaire that was designed to measure physical function and symptoms arising from musculoskeletal disorders of the UE.[67] Both the DASH and its shorter version, the *QuickDASH* (11 items), have been shown to be reliable, valid, and responsive for this purpose.[67,68] The items include questions that refer to the degree of difficulty in accomplishing a particular task in the previous week, the impact of the UE on social function and work activity, the severity of symptoms, and the impact on sleep and self-confidence. In addition, the DASH includes separate optional modules for work and sports/performing arts. Although developed for adults, it has been used for pediatric conditions, including fractures of the upper limb.[69,70]

PROMIS: ITEM RESPONSE THEORY AND COMPUTER ADAPTIVE TESTING

PROMIS, which stands for *Patient Reported Outcome Measurement Information System*, is an initiative funded by the National Institutes of Health to establish a system of reliable, valid, flexible, precise, and responsive assessment tools that measure PROs of health status.[71,72] PROMIS measures cover physical, mental, and social health and can be used across chronic conditions. PROMIS establishes a standard set of methods to develop PRO measures and provides a large number of PRO measures of health in multiple languages for adults and children that can be accessed with PROMIS-developed software called the "Assessment Center." The PROs were developed with the use of *item response theory* (IRT), which is a psychometric method commonly used in educational testing.[73] Statistical models based on IRT produce scores or calibrations associated with answers to each question that allow the computer software, called *Computer Adaptive Testing*, to select the most informative follow-up question to an initial question. This allows the creation of a large bank of items *(item bank)* to evaluate the full spectrum of a particular domain or aspect of health (e.g., 124 items in the physical functioning item bank).[74] These items will have been ordered and calibrated on a scale using IRT methodology (e.g., Rasch scaling). Although an item bank provides a common metric for all, each respondent will only have to complete or respond to a minimum set of items based on responses to a prior question, which will appropriately and precisely place them along the continuum of that domain, corresponding to their level of physical function.[35] This is not only efficient in terms of reducing respondent burden; it also avoids creating frustration that might arise from being administered a large number of inappropriate items that are beyond the respondent's ability.

Currently, a number of child or proxy item banks are available for pediatric health domains, with new ones under development.[75–77] The following are item banks in pediatric health domains that are relevant to pediatric fractures and injury. The *PROMIS Pediatric Mobility* item bank assesses activities of physical mobility (such as getting out of bed or a chair) to activities such as running. The *PROMIS Pain Intensity* item pool assesses how much a person hurts. The *PROMIS Pain Interference* item bank assesses the consequences of pain on relevant aspects of persons' lives and may include the impact of pain on social, cognitive, emotional, physical, and recreational activities, as well as on sleep and enjoyment in life. The *PROMIS Pediatric Upper Extremity* item bank assesses activities that require use of the UE, including shoulder, arm, and hand activities. The *Peer Relationships* item bank assesses the quality of relationships with friends and other acquaintances.

PATIENT SATISFACTION

Derived from the consumer literature, the construct of *satisfaction* has been widely adopted in health care. Achieving patient satisfaction is not only an important goal but is also considered one of the key indicators of the quality of care received.[5,78,79] Satisfaction is believed to be related to meeting patient expectations with respect to treatment goals.[80] There are many factors that influence patient satisfaction besides the actual outcomes, and in studies that have measured this construct, most patients are satisfied, even when they have experienced a poor outcome.[81] If patients are seldom dissatisfied with outcomes, measuring patient "satisfaction" may not be a useful measure of effectiveness of outcomes, even though it might be an important indicator of the quality of care and processes associated with care.[82]

NONCLINICAL MEASURES

Nonclinical outcomes are of interest to hospital administrators, payers, and health policy makers. These include outcomes such as length of stay, readmission rates, and costs.

COSTS: HEALTH ECONOMIC EVALUATIONS

An intervention should not only be effective but also affordable. As the demand for health care grows and the cost of health care rises in an environment of finite resources, it is imperative that health economic issues be considered. Economic evaluation is a comparison of two or more treatments in terms of costs and benefits. Different approaches exist for the analysis of costs of treatments relative to the benefits.[83] *Costs* are the resources consumed by and associated with a particular intervention (or healthcare program). Costs can be *direct* (e.g., radiographs, laboratory tests, drugs, implants, cast material, physician services, and physical therapy) or *indirect* (e.g., overhead costs to run a facility, time off work or school, and lost wages) and are typically expressed in monetary units (e.g., dollars). *Benefits* can be measured in one of three ways. *Effectiveness* is expressed in terms of units of meaningful outcomes (e.g., life years gained, time to return to full function, malunions, or reoperations avoided). *Cost-effectiveness analysis* (CEA) is expressed as cost per unit effect. When two interventions are being compared, the *incremental CEA ratio* is defined as the incremental cost per incremental health benefit, that is, ratio of the difference in costs between the two treatments (cost of treatment A – cost of treatment B) to the difference in outcomes between each treatment.[84]

Utilities are a quantitative representation of patients' preferences for a particular health state and reflect their perceptions of HRQL. Each health state (e.g., painful nonunion, incisional scar, angular deformity) associated with a health outcome is placed on a scale of 0 (equivalent to death) to 1 (perfect health). Many methods are available for generating utilities for different health states, including visual analog scales, time trade-off, and the standard gamble. In the time trade-off method, the utility of a particular health state is quantified by evaluating how many years of life a subject is willing to give up (trade) in exchange for a life unencumbered by that health outcome. The *Health Utilities Index* is a generic, multiattribute outcome measure that rates the composite health state of the respondent to generate a utility score.[85] The utility measurement can be used to weight life expectancy to generate *quality-adjusted life years* (QALYs). For example, if after an intervention, one's life expectancy is 50 years, but the (chronic) health state one has to live in because of the outcome of the intervention is associated with a utility of 0.8, then living 50 years with that health state is considered equivalent to living (0.8 × 50) 40 years in perfect health, or 40 QALYs. *Cost-utility analysis* (CUA) is expressed as cost per unit of effect (e.g., dollars per QALY gained).[86] CUA has the benefit of allowing comparisons to be made across diseases because the unit of effect or consequences is common to all. In *cost-benefit analysis*, the health outcomes are expressed in monetary units.

When two interventions are being compared, the intervention that is more effective *and* cheaper (win-win) is a clear winner or *dominant*; similarly, an intervention that is more harmful (or less effective) *and* more expensive (lose-lose) should be abandoned.[84] It also stands to reason that when outcomes of two interventions are equivalent, the less expensive intervention ought to be the preferred option. In practice, however, it is more commonplace to encounter interventions that might be more effective but that are also more expensive. The difficult question of how much some, often small, difference in effectiveness is worth is important for policy makers, payers, and to the society at large that ultimately bears the cost. In general, CEA ratios of less than $20,000 per QALY are considered worthwhile, whereas a CEA ratio of $100,000 per QALY is considered poor.[87]

DEVELOPMENT OF GOAL-BASED OUTCOME MEASURES FOR PEDIATRIC FRACTURES

Few condition-specific PRO measures evaluate outcomes of pediatric fractures. Consequently, most studies of pediatric fracture management use radiographic measures of alignment as the primary outcome, as currently available PROs are not as discriminative or sensitive to change. Consequently, there is an imperative to develop more meaningful outcome measures for children's fractures. Development of any outcome measure requires *item generation* as the first step.[35] This requires direct input from a sufficient sample of the primary stakeholders—children with fractures and their parents—acquired using qualitative methods such as open-ended or structured interviews or focus groups so that their perspectives on their experiences with a fracture and its management are understood. Understanding patients' priorities is essential for the development of meaningful patient-based outcome measures.[23] The patient priority model, previously described, provides a useful framework to identify patient goals that are derived from their priorities and must be included in any measure of treatment outcomes. For instance, some of the ultimate goals of long bone fracture management will likely relate to how well the limb looks (appearance), how well it feels (with respect to comfort, strength, endurance, and agility), and how well it works (ability to use limb for daily activities, sports, and recreation). All things being equal, the differences between two interventions might be in the treatment-specific recovery experience associated with each intervention (method or extent of immobilization, time for healing, and need for secondary procedures to remove implants). The purpose of the item generation exercise is to identify how children and their parents conceptualize these goals and ensure that these goals are represented in specific items of the questionnaire. There follows an iterative process using additional patients and their parents to confirm that these items are indeed important to them and are easily and consistently understood. During the next step of *item reduction*, redundant and less important items are discarded, and the initial list is reduced to a manageable number of items that make the outcome measure more practical and feasible. Involving healthcare professionals in the latter stages of item generation and item reduction is also useful to ensure sensibility, face, and content validity. Then the outcome measure must be tested for its reliability, internal consistency, validity, and responsiveness to ensure that it is psychometrically sound.[35] Finally, an outcome measure developed in one language needs to undergo a formal process of translation and back-translation and cross-cultural adaptation before it can be adopted in a different language.[88]

A new PRO for pediatric fractures has recently been developed using the framework described above. Iterative interviews of patients (and their parents) with a spectrum of fractures generated the items for the Patient/Parent Report of Outcomes of Fracture Healing (PROOF) Questionnaire for UE and LE fractures, respectively. These were subsequently evaluated for their sensibility by additional sets of patients and parents until saturation was reached about the content and the format. An online international survey of pediatric orthopedic experts in children's fractures was conducted to evaluate the sensibility of the PROOF UE and LE, respectively. The content of the PROOF-UE (37 items) and PROOF-LE (27 items) questionnaires spans four domains: (1) how it looks (appearance), (2) how it feels, (3) how it works (function), and (4) how it recovered.[89] The short form version of the PROOF-UE was used along with photographs as the primary outcome measure in a prospective study of supracondylar fractures to evaluate what is an acceptable magnitude of residual displacement following closed reduction and percutaneous wire fixation that remains compatible with a perfect outcome on all four domains.[90] The PROOF will become available for wider use following further psychometric testing to establish reliability, construct validity, and responsiveness.[89]

OTHER CONSIDERATIONS

Although the "final" outcomes are the most important in selecting the "best" treatment, there are many situations where different management options are associated with similar treatment outcomes, but the choice of a specific intervention may be influenced by other considerations. The desired outcome should ideally be achieved in the shortest time possible and be associated with the least number of complications or adverse events and the lowest costs. Some outcomes are more important than others, and each set of patients or parents might have different perspectives on the relative importance of different outcomes, making the case for shared decision-making.

Consider the example of two competing options to manage an isolated femur fracture in a 7-year-old girl: closed reduction and immobilization with a spica cast, and elastic intramedullary nailing.[91] With the use of the goal-based framework discussed previously, either treatment might be expected to yield the desired outcomes. Yet each intervention is associated with a different set of advantages and disadvantages. The spica cast can be cumbersome for the child and creates some challenges with hygiene, daily care, positioning, transportation, and attending school. There is a higher risk of loss of reduction, necessitating more frequent monitoring and potentially a second procedure to address the loss of reduction.[58,92] On the other hand, there is no scarring, no risk of infection, and in the event of a loss of reduction, the option of switching to an operative approach remains viable and still effective, provided the loss of reduction was detected sufficiently early.[93,94] Elastic nailing, by comparison, is more invasive, entailing some, albeit minor, scarring, some symptoms at the nail insertion site,[95] and possibly a second operation to remove the nails, which some surgeons believe is routinely necessary.[96] However, fracture alignment and length is easier to obtain and more assuredly maintain, and leaves the child unencumbered to move about more freely, bathe, even swim, and attend school while the fracture is healing. For an identical injury, two different patients and their families might (legitimately) choose different options, based on their individual circumstances, preferences, values, and judgments of the risks and benefits of each of these options. For instance, if both parents work outside the home and are unable to take time off work to look after the child at home, this would be an important contextual factor that influences choice of treatment and judgment of outcomes. Assuming the treating surgeon is competent with either treatment strategy, discussing these pros and cons would allow children or their parents to make more informed choices about the treatment that would be most appropriate for them.[97]

As the number, diversity, complexity, and costs of treatment options grow, the imperative to evaluate outcomes and the adverse events associated with interventions becomes even more compelling. This evidence must be generated from high-quality research, clinical trials, and prospective comparative cohort studies. These trials will be of little value without the appropriate means to measure effectiveness, using outcome measures that are meaningful and valid.

REFERENCES

The level of evidence (LOE) is determined according to the criteria provided in the Preface.

1. Wennberg JE. Outcomes research, cost containment, and the fear of health care rationing. *N Engl J Med.* 1990;323(17):1202–1204. **(LOE N/A)**.
2. Sackett DL, Rosenberg WM, Gray JA, et al. Evidence based medicine: what it is and what it isn't. *BMJ.* 1996;312(7023):71–72. **(LOE N/A)**.
3. Codman EA. The classic: the registry of bone sarcomas as an example of the end-result idea in hospital organization. 1924. *Clin Orthop Relat Res.* 1924;467(11):2766–2770. **(LOE N/A)**.
4. Institute of Medicine. Initial national priorities for comparative effectiveness research; 2009. Available from http://www.iom.edu/Reports/2009/ComparativeEffectivenessResearchPriorities.20%aspx. Accessed December 10, 2013. **(LOE N/A)**.
5. Donabedian A. Evaluating the quality of medical care. 1966. *Milbank Q.* 2005;83(4):691–729. **(LOE N/A)**.
6. Natsch S, Kullberg BJ, Hekster YA, et al. Selecting outcome parameters in studies aimed at improving rational use of antibiotics—practical considerations. *J Clin Pharm Ther.* 2003;28(6):475–478. **(LOE N/A)**.
7. Larson JS. The conceptualization of health. *Med Care Res Rev.* 1999;56(2):123–136. **(LOE N/A)**.
8. Greenfield S, Nelson EC. Recent developments and future issues in the use of health status assessment measures in clinical settings. *Med Care.* 1992;30(suppl 5):MS23–MS41. **(LOE N/A)**.
9. WHO. International Classification of Functioning, Disability and Health (ICF); 2001. Available from www.who.int/classifications/icf/en/. Accessed December 10, 2013. **(LOE N/A)**.
10. Simeonsson RJ, Scarborough AA, Hebbeler KM. ICF and ICD codes provide a standard language of disability in young children. *J Clin Epidemiol.* 2006;59(4):365–373. **(LOE N/A)**.
11. WHO. International. Classification of Diseases (ICD-10); 2010. Available from: https://www.who.int/browse10/2016/en/. Accessed December 10, 2013. **(LOE N/A)**.
12. Simeonsson RJ, Leonardi M, Lollar D, et al. Applying the International Classification of Functioning, Disability and Health (ICF) to measure childhood disability. *Disabil Rehabil.* 2003;25(11-12):602–610. **(LOE N/A)**.
13. WHO. International Classification of Functioning, Disability and Health – children and youth. Geneva: World Health Organization; 2007. Available from http://apps.who.int/classifications/icfbrowser/20%Default.aspx. Accessed December 10, 2013. **(LOE N/A)**.
14. Majnemer A, ed. *Measures for Children With Developmental Disabilities: an ICF-CY Approach.* London: Mac Keith Press; 2012. **(LOE N/A)**.
15. Young NL, Williams JI, Yoshida KK, et al. The context of measuring disability: does it matter whether capability or performance is measured? *J Clin Epidemiol.* 1996;49(10):1097–1101. **(LOE N/A)**.
16. Goldberg MJ. Measuring outcomes in cerebral palsy. *J Pediatr Orthop.* 1991;11(5):682–685. **(LOE N/A)**.
17. Narayanan UG. *Concerns, Desires and Expectations of Surgery for Adolescent Idiopathic Scoliosis: A Comparison of Patients', Parents' and Surgeons' Perspectives. Health Policy Management & Evaluation.* Toronto: University of Toronto; 2008. Available from https://tspace.library.utoronto.ca/bitstream/1807/11155/1/Narayanan_Unni_G_2008June_MSc_thesis.pdf. Accessed December 10, 2013. **(LOE N/A)**.
18. Kravitz RL, Callahan EJ, Paterniti D, et al. Prevalence and sources of patients' unmet expectations for care [see comments]. *Ann Intern Med.* 1996;125(9):730–737. **(LOE N/A)**.
19. Uhlmann RF, Inui TS, Carter WB. Patient requests and expectations. Definitions and clinical applications. *Med Care.* 1984;22(7):681–685. **(LOE N/A)**.
20. Bowling A, Ebrahim S. Measuring patients' preferences for treatment and perceptions of risk. *Qual Health Care.* 2001;10(suppl 1):i2–i8. **(LOE N/A)**.
21. Entwistle VA, Renfrew MJ, Yearley S, et al. Lay perspectives: advantages for health research. *BMJ.* 1998;316(7129):463–466. **(LOE N/A)**.
22. Amadio PC. Outcomes measurements. *J Bone Joint Surg Am.* 1993;75(11):1583–1584. **(LOE N/A)**.
23. Wright JG, Rudicel S, Feinstein AR. Ask patients what they want. Evaluation of individual complaints before total hip replacement. *J Bone Joint Surg Br.* 1994;76(2):229–234. **(LOE N/A)**.
24. Majnemer A, Limperopoulos C. Importance of outcome determination in pediatric rehabilitation. *Dev Med Child Neurol.* 2002;44(11):773–777. **(LOE N/A)**.
25. Eiser C, Morse R. Can parents rate their child's health-related quality of life? Results of a systematic review. *Qual Life Res.* 2001;10(4):347–357. **(LOE N/A)**.
26. Patrick DL, Deyo RA. Generic and disease-specific measures in assessing health status and quality of life. *Med Care.* 1989;27(suppl 3):S217–S232. **(LOE N/A)**.
27. WHO. The World Health Organization Quality of Life assessment (WHOQOL): position paper from the World Health Organization. *Soc Sci Med.* 1995;41(10):1403–1409. **(LOE N/A)**.
28. WHO. 19-22 June, 1946. *WHO Definition of Health in Preamble to the Constitution of the World Health Organization as Adopted by the International Health Conference.* New York: Official Records of the World Health Organization; 1948,2:100. **(LOE N/A)**.
29. Rosenbaum PL, Livingston MH, Palisano RJ, et al. Quality of life and health-related quality of life of adolescents with cerebral palsy. *Dev Med Child Neurol.* 2007;49(7):516–521. **(LOE N/A)**.
30. Measuring health-related quality of life in pediatric populations: conceptual issues. In: Rosenbaum PL, Saigal S, eds. *Quality of Life and Pharmacoeconomics in Clinical Trials.* Philadelphia: Lippincott-Raven; 1996. **(LOE N/A)**.

31. Understanding and using health-related quality of life instruments within clinical research studies. In: Berzon RA, ed. *Quality of Life Assessment in Clinical Trials*. New York: Oxford University Press; 1998. **(LOE N/A)**.

32. Fitzpatrick R, Davey C, Buxton MJ, et al. Evaluating patient-based outcome measures for use in clinical trials. *Health Technol Assess*. 1998;2(14):i–iv. 1–74. **(LOE N/A)**.

33. Jerosch-Herold C. An evidence-based approach to choosing outcome measures: a checklist for the critical appraisal of validity, reliability and responsiveness studies. *Br J Occup Ther*. 2005;68:347–353. **(LOE N/A)**.

34. Kirshner B, Guyatt G. A methodological framework for assessing health indices. *J Chronic Dis*. 1985;38(1):27–36. **(LOE N/A)**.

35. Streiner DL, Norman GR. *Health Measurement Scales: A Practical Guide to their Development and Use*. Oxford: Oxford University Press; 2008. **(LOE N/A)**.

36. Guyatt G, Walter S, Norman G. Measuring change over time: assessing the usefulness of evaluative instruments. *J Chronic Dis*. 1987;40(2):171–178. **(LOE N/A)**.

37. Bland JM, Altman DG. Statistical methods for assessing agreement between two methods of clinical measurement. *Lancet*. 1986;1(8476):307–310. **(LOE N/A)**.

38. Landis JR, Koch GG. The measurement of observer agreement for categorical data. *Biometrics*. 1977;33(1):159–174. **(LOE N/A)**.

39. Cronbach LJ. Coefficient alpha and the internal structure of tests. *Psychometrika*. 1951;16:297–334. **(LOE N/A)**.

40. Feinstein AR. *Clinimetrics*. New Haven: Yale University Press; 1987. **(LOE N/A)**.

41. Wright JG, Wang EE, Owen JL, et al. Treatments for paediatric femoral fractures: a randomised trial. *Lancet*. 2005;365(9465):1153–1158. **(LOE I)**.

42. Irwin DE, Gross HE, Stucky BD, et al. Development of six PROMIS pediatrics proxy-report item banks. *Health Qual Life Outcomes*. 2012;10:22. **(LOE N/A)**.

43. Ryoppy S, Karaharju EO. Alteration of epiphyseal growth by an experimentally produced angular deformity. *Acta Orthop Scand*. 1974;45(4):490–498. **(LOE N/A)**.

44. Wallace ME, Hoffman EB. Remodelling of angular deformity after femoral shaft fractures in children. *J Bone Joint Surg Br*. 1992;74(5):765–769. **(LOE IV)**.

45. Paley D, Herzenberg JE, Tetsworth K, et al. Deformity planning for frontal and sagittal plane corrective osteotomies. *Orthop Clin North Am*. 1994;25(3):425–465. 1994. **(LOE N/A)**.

46. Paley D, Tetsworth K. Mechanical axis deviation of the lower limbs. Preoperative planning of multiapical frontal plane angular and bowing deformities of the femur and tibia. *Clin Orthop Relat Res*. 1992;280:65–71. **(LOE N/A)**.

47. Paley D, Tetsworth K. Mechanical axis deviation of the lower limbs. Preoperative planning of uniapical angular deformities of the tibia or femur. *Clin Orthop Relat Res*. 1992;280:48–64. **(LOE N/A)**.

48. Paley D. Normal lower limb alignment and joint orientation. Chapter 1. In: *Principles of Deformity Correction*. Berlin: Springer-Verlag; 2002. **(LOE N/A)**.

49. Tetsworth K, Paley D. Malalignment and degenerative arthropathy. *Orthop Clin North Am*. 1994;25(3):367–377. **(LOE V)**.

50. Escott BG, Ravi B, Weathermon AC, et al. EOS low-dose radiography: a reliable and accurate upright assessment of lower limb lengths. *J Bone Joint Surg Am*. 2013;95:e1831–e1837. **(LOE N/A)**.

51. Daltroy LH, Liang MH, Fossel AH, et al. The POSNA pediatric musculoskeletal functional health questionnaire: report on reliability, validity, and sensitivity to change. Pediatric Outcomes Instrument Development Group. Pediatric Orthopaedic Society of North America. *J Pediatr Orthop*. 1998;18(5):561–571. **(LOE N/A)**.

52. Kubiak EN, Egol KA, Scher D, et al. Operative treatment of tibial fractures in children: are elastic stable intramedullary nails an improvement over external fixation? *J Bone Joint Surg Am*. 2005;87(8):1761–1768. **(LOE III)**.

53. Kunkel S, Eismann E, Cornwall R. Utility of the pediatric outcomes data collection instrument for assessing acute hand and wrist injuries in children. *J Pediatr Orthop*. 2011;31(7):767–772. **(LOE III)**.

54. Pencharz J, Young NL, Owen JL, et al. Comparison of three outcomes instruments in children. *J Pediatr Orthop*. 2001;21(4):425–432. **(LOE N/A)**.

55. Young NL, Williams JI, Yoshida KK, et al. Measurement properties of the activities scale for kids. *J Clin Epidemiol*. 2000;53(2):125–137. **(LOE N/A)**.

56. Boutis K, Willan A, Babyn P, et al. Cast versus splint in children with minimally angulated fractures of the distal radius: a randomized controlled trial. *CMAJ*. 2010;182(14):1507–1512. **(LOE I)**.

57. Boutis K, Willan AR, Babyn P, et al. A randomized, controlled trial of a removable brace versus casting in children with low-risk ankle fractures. *Pediatrics*. 2007;119(6):e1256–e1263. **(LOE I)**.

58. Epps HR, Molenaar E, O'Connor DP. Immediate single-leg spica cast for pediatric femoral diaphysis fractures. *J Pediatr Orthop*. 2006;26(4):491–496. **(LOE IV)**.

59. Silva M, Eagan MJ, Wong MA, et al. A comparison of two approaches for the closed treatment of low-energy tibial fractures in children. *J Bone Joint Surg Am*. 2012;94(20):1853–1860. **(LOE II)**.

60. Landgraf JMAL, Ware JE. *The Child Health Questionnaire User's Manual*. Boston: HealthAct; 1999. **(LOE N/A)**.

61. Aitken ME, Tilford JM, Barrett KW, et al. Health status of children after admission for injury. *Pediatrics*. 2002;110(2 Pt 1):337–342. **(LOE I)**.

62. Willis CD, Gabbe BJ, Butt W, et al. Assessing outcomes in paediatric trauma populations. *Injury*. 2006;37(12):1185–1196. **(LOE N/A)**.

63. Boykin RE, McFeely ED, Shearer D, et al. Correlation between the Child Health Questionnaire and the International Knee Documentation Committee score in pediatric and adolescent patients with an anterior cruciate ligament tear. *J Pediatr Orthop*. 2013;33(2):216–220. **(LOE N/A)**.

64. Varni JW, Seid M, Kurtin PS. PedsQL 4.0: reliability and validity of the Pediatric Quality of Life Inventory version 4.0 generic core scales in healthy and patient populations. *Med Care*. 2001;39(8):800–812. **(LOE N/A)**.

65. Ding R, McCarthy ML, Houseknecht E, et al. The health-related quality of life of children with an extremity fracture: a one-year follow-up study. *J Pediatr Orthop*. 2006;26(2):157–163. **(LOE III)**.

66. Solway SB, McConnell S, Bombardier C. *The DASH Outcome Measure User's Manual*. 3rd ed. Toronto: Institute for Work & Health; 2002. **(LOE N/A)**.

67. Hudak PL, Amadio PC, Bombardier C. Development of an upper extremity outcome measure: the DASH (disabilities of the arm, shoulder and hand). The Upper Extremity Collaborative Group (UECG). *Am J Ind Med*. 1996;29(6):602–608. **(LOE N/A)**.

68. Beaton DE, Wright JG, Katz JN; Upper Extremity Collaborative Group. Development of the QuickDASH: comparison of three item-reduction approaches. *J Bone Joint Surg Am*. 2005;87(5):1038–1046. **(LOE N/A)**.

69. Bae DS, Shah AS, Kalish LA, et al. Shoulder motion, strength, and functional outcomes in children with established malunion of the clavicle. *J Pediatr Orthop*. 2013;33(5):544–550. **(LOE IV)**.

70. Lawrence JT, Patel NM, Macknin J, et al. Return to competitive sports after medial epicondyle fractures in adolescent athletes: results of operative and nonoperative treatment. *Am J Sports Med*. 2013;41(5):1152–1157. **(LOE IV)**.

71. Patient NIH. Reported Outcomes Measurement Information System (PROMIS); 2010. Available from http://www.nihpromis.org/about/overview. Accessed December 10, 2013. **(LOE N/A)**.

72. Gershon RC, Rothrock N, Hanrahan R, et al. The use of PROMIS and assessment center to deliver patient-reported outcome measures in clinical research. *J Appl Meas*. 2010;11(3):304–314. **(LOE N/A)**.

73. Hambleton RKSH, Rogers HJ. *Fundamentals of Item Response Theory*. Newbury Park, NJ: Sage; 1999. **(LOE N/A)**.

74. Cella D, Riley W, Stone A, et al. The Patient-Reported Outcomes Measurement Information System (PROMIS) developed and tested its first wave of adult self-reported health outcome item banks: 2005-2008. *J Clin Epidemiol*. 2010;63(11):1179–1194. **(LOE N/A)**.

75. DeWitt EM, Stucky BD, Thissen D, et al. Construction of the eight-item patient-reported outcomes measurement information system pediatric physical function scales: built using item response theory. *J Clin Epidemiol*. 64(7):794–804. **(LOE N/A)**

76. Irwin DE, Gross HE, Stucky BD, et al. Development of six PROMIS pediatrics proxy-report item banks. *Health Qual Life Outcomes*. 2012;10:22. **(LOE N/A)**.

77. Varni JW, Thissen D, Stucky BD, et al. PROMIS(R) Parent Proxy Report Scales: an item response theory analysis of the parent proxy report item banks. *Qual Life Res*. 2012;21(7):1223–1240. **(LOE N/A)**.

78. Donabedian A. Quality, cost, and clinical decisions. *Ann Am Acad Pol Soc Sci.* 1983;468:196–204. **(LOE N/A)**.
79. Donabedian A. *The Criteria and Standards of Quality.* Ann Arbor, Mich: Health Administration Press; 1982. **(LOE N/A)**.
80. Fitzpatrick R, Hopkins A. Problems in the conceptual framework of patient satisfaction research: an empirical exploration. *Sociol Health Illn.* 1983;5(3):297–311. **(LOE N/A)**.
81. Williams B, Coyle J, Healy D. The meaning of patient satisfaction: an explanation of high reported levels. *Soc Sci Med.* 47(9):1351–1359. **(LOE N/A)**
82. Coyle J, Williams B. Seeing the wood for the trees: defining the forgotten concept of patient dissatisfaction in the light of patient satisfaction research. *Int J Health Care Qual Assur Inc Leadersh Health Serv.* 1999;12:6–7. i-ix. **(LOE N/A)**.
83. Drummond MF, Stoddart GL, Torrance GW. *Methods for the Economic Evaluation of Health Care Progammes.* 2nd ed. Toronto: Oxford Medical Publications; 1997. **(LOE N/A)**.
84. Detsky AS, Naglie IG. A clinician's guide to cost-effectiveness analysis. *Ann Intern Med.* 1990;113(2):147–154. **(LOE N/A)**.
85. Horsman J, Furlong W, Feeny D, et al. The Health Utilities Index (HUI): concepts, measurement properties and applications. *Health Qual Life Outcomes.* 2003;1:54. **(LOE N/A)**.
86. Robinson R. Cost-utility analysis. *BMJ.* 1993;307(6908):859–862. **(LOE N/A)**.
87. Laupacis A, Feeny D, Detsky AS, et al. How attractive does a new technology have to be to warrant adoption and utilization? Tentative guidelines for using clinical and economic evaluations. *CMAJ.* 1992;146(4):473–481. **(LOE N/A)**.
88. Beaton DE, Bombardier C, Guillemin F, Ferraz MB. Guidelines for the process of cross-cultural adaptation of self-report measures. *Spine.* 2000;25:3186–3191. **(LOE N/A)**.
89. Narayanan UG. *The PROOF Questionnaires.* Personal Communication; 2018. **(LOE N/A)**.

90. Wood W, Martinelli, A, Gangwar A, Turner J, Gargan M, Tan T, Narayanan UG. What is an "acceptable reduction" for supracondylar humerus fractures in children? Abstract at the combined annual meeting of the Pediatric Orthopaedic Society of North America (POSNA) & the European Pediatric Orthopaedic Society (EPOS). May 2017. **(LOE II)**
91. Flynn JM, Luedtke LM, Ganley TJ, et al. Comparison of titanium elastic nails with traction and a spica cast to treat femoral fractures in children. *J Bone Joint Surg Am.* 2004;86-A(4):770–777. **(LOE III)**.
92. DiFazio R, Vessey J, Zurakowski D, et al. Incidence of skin complications and associated charges in children treated with hip spica casts for femur fractures. *J Pediatr Orthop.* 2011;31(1):17–22. **(LOE IV)**.
93. Flynn JM, Garner MR, Jones KJ, et al. The treatment of low-energy femoral shaft fractures: a prospective study comparing the walking spica with the traditional spica cast. *J Bone Joint Surg Am.* 2011;93(23):2196–2202. **(LOE II)**.
94. Leu D, Sargent MC, Ain MC, et al. Spica casting for pediatric femoral fractures: a prospective, randomized controlled study of single-leg versus double-leg spica casts. *J Bone Joint Surg Am.* 2012;94(14):1259–1264. **(LOE I)**.
95. Narayanan UG, Hyman JE, Wainwright AM, et al. Complications of elastic stable intramedullary nail fixation of pediatric femoral fractures, and how to avoid them. *J Pediatr Orthop.* 2004;24(4):363–369. **(LOE IV)**.
96. Ligier JN, Metaizeau JP, Prévot J, et al. Elastic stable intramedullary nailing of femoral shaft fractures in children. *J Bone Joint Surg Br.* 1988;70(1):74–77. **(LOE IV)**.
97. Narayanan UG, Phillips JH. Flexibility in fixation: an update on femur fractures in children. *J Pediatr Orthop.* 2012;32(suppl 1):S32–S39. **(LOE N/A)**.

Fractures of the Spine

10

Jeffrey E. Martus | Gregory A. Mencio

Spine injuries in children are fortunately rare, involving only 1% to 4% of children admitted to trauma centers.[1–4] Treating pediatric patients with spine injuries can be challenging. Clinical evaluation is often hampered by an inability to obtain accurate historical information and unreliability of the physical examination. Children are often frightened, usually unable to describe pain, and either unable (altered mental status, age) or unwilling to cooperate with an examiner because of communication issues. Difficulty with the physical examination, anatomic and biomechanical differences of the immature spine, and nuances of normal developmental anatomy further complicate the process. Polytraumatized children are especially susceptible to cervical spine injury because of the unique anatomy and biomechanical characteristics of this region.[5–7]

DEVELOPMENTAL ANATOMY

To evaluate the child's spine, it is critical to have an understanding of the developmental anatomy of the growing spine so as to avoid mistaking normal variations for injury. The first two cervical vertebrae are unique in their development, whereas the remaining cervical, thoracic, and lumbar vertebrae follow a similar pattern of ossification and maturation.

The atlas (C1) is formed by three primary centers of ossification, the anterior arch and the two neural arches[8] (Figs. 10.1A and 10.2A). The primary ossification centers of the two neural arches, which eventually develop into the lateral masses, are visible at birth. The anterior arch is ossified at birth in only 20% of children and, in the remaining infants, ossifies over the subsequent year. Therefore the atlantodens interval (ADI) is unreliable in detecting atlantoaxial instability in children less than 1 year old. The neural arches ossify posteriorly by age 3 years, and the neurocentral synchondroses close by age 7 years.[9] Injuries can occur through these synchondroses before the time of closure, and occasionally closure may not occur. Persistence of these synchondroses can be differentiated from a traumatic injury by the presence of sclerotic, well-corticated borders and absence of soft tissue swelling. Congenital failure of formation can present as an absence of one of the neural arches.

The axis (C2) is formed by five primary centers of ossification (Figs. 10.1B and 10.2B). The odontoid process is formed by two parallel ossification centers that fuse in utero during the seventh fetal month. The os terminale is a secondary ossification center that occurs at the tip of the odontoid, arising between the ages of 3 to 6 years and fusing by age 12 years (seen as the gray region on the schematic in Fig. 10.1B). The remaining primary centers of ossification are the body and two neural arches.[8] The body typically fuses with the odontoid process by 6 years, but the synchondroses may persist until age 11. The neural arches fuse anteriorly to the body by age 6 and posteriorly by age 3, similar to the atlas. Fractures can occur through the synchondroses at the base of the odontoid and may be recognized by soft tissue swelling, asymmetry of the synchondroses, and/or excessive angulation of the dens.[10]

The subaxial cervical spine (C3–C7), thoracic spine, and lumbar spine all develop in a similar fashion. There are three primary ossification centers: the two neural arches and the body (Fig. 10.1C). The lower cervical neural arches have been reported to fuse to the body between ages 3 and 6 years.[8] A magnetic resonance imaging (MRI) study noted closure of the thoracic neurocentral synchondroses between the ages of 11 and 16 years.[11] Edelson et al found that closure of the neurocentral synchondroses begins first in the lumbar and cervical areas, whereas the thoracic region occurs later.[12] The age range of neurocentral closure was 2 to 8 years in the cervical region, 2.5 to 18 years in the thoracic region, and 2 to 12 years in the lumbar region. Occasionally, fusion of the thoracic synchondroses was observed to be incomplete in adulthood. Secondary centers of ossification can exist at the tips of the transverse processes, spinous process, and superior and inferior aspect of the vertebral body (depicted in gray on the schematic in Fig. 10.1). These centers ossify in early adulthood, and can be mistaken for fractures.[8,9] The superior and inferior ring apophyses begin to ossify between ages 8 to 12 years and fuse to the body by ages 21 to 25 years.[13] The vertebral bodies grow in height by endochondral ossification that progresses in a posterior to anterior direction as the child ages, eventually achieving their characteristic rectangular shape by age 7 years. Until that time, the subaxial cervical, thoracic, and lumbar vertebra may appear to have anterior wedging, which may be confused with anterior compression fractures. This "physiologic" wedging can be profound at C3 and may contribute to the appearance of subluxation.[14]

RELEVANT ANATOMY

The articulations and ligamentous supporting structures are as unique in the atlas and axis, as is their respective developmental anatomy. Occipital condyles project downward and articulate with the atlas. The predominant motion of this joint is flexion and extension, and 50% of total cervical spine motion in this plane occurs at this joint. The atlantooccipital joint has more of a horizontal orientation, and the occipital condyles

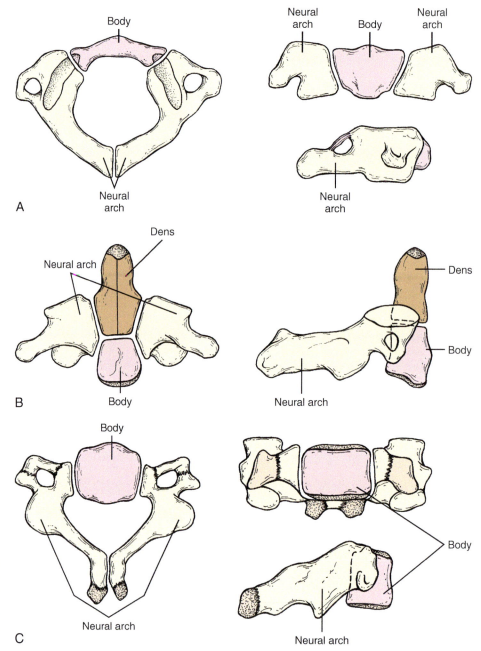

Fig. 10.1 (A) Ossification centers of C1. (B) Ossification centers of C2. (C) Ossification centers of subaxial cervical vertebrae (C3-L5). (From Green NE, Swiontowski M, eds. *Skeletal Trauma in Children*. 3rd ed. Philadelphia: WB Saunders; 2003:345, Fig. 11.1.)

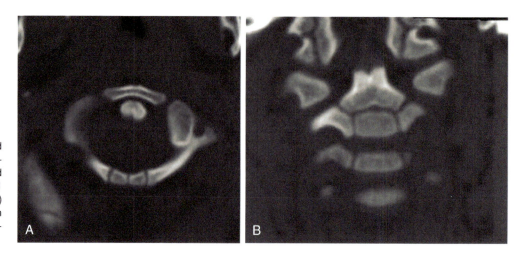

Fig. 10.2 (A) Axial computed tomography (CT) scan demonstrating ossification centers and multiple synchondroses of C1 in a 19-month-old patient. (B) Coronally reformatted CT scan demonstrating ossification centers of C2 in the same patient.

are small relative to adults, perhaps explaining the increased risk (2.5 times) of atlantooccipital dislocation in children as compared with adults.[15,16] The odontoid process projects upward from the body of the axis, articulating with the posterior aspect of the anterior arch of the atlas. The odontoid is secured in this position by the transverse ligament, which spans from one side of the anterior arch of the atlas to the other, passing posterior to the odontoid process. This ligament functions as the primary stabilizer, preventing anterior translation of the atlas and dislocation of the atlantoaxial joint. The secondary stabilizers are the paired alar ligaments, which arise from each side of the dens and attach to the occipital condyles, functioning as checkrein ligaments with head rotation. In addition, the apical ligament arises from the tip of the dens and attaches to the foramen magnum. The facet joints between the atlas and axis are more horizontally oriented to permit rotation of the atlas and head.[17]

The vertebra in the subaxial cervical spine articulate at five points: paired facet and uncovertebral joints and the intervertebral disk. The facet joints in the subaxial cervical spine are relatively horizontal, averaging 30 degrees of inclination at birth and increasing to 60 to 70 degrees at maturity. The thoracic and lumbar vertebrae articulate with one another via paired facet joints and the intervertebral disks. The thoracic vertebrae articulate with ribs through costochondral articulations. Other supporting structures include the interspinous/supraspinous ligament, ligamentum flavum, posterior longitudinal ligament, and anterior longitudinal ligament.

The spine typically assumes adult characteristics by the age of 8 to 10 years, and until that time, children tend to be more susceptible to upper cervical spine (above C3) injuries.[2,5,6,18,19] There are two main reasons for the increased incidence of upper cervical spine injuries in this younger age group. The head is disproportionately large, creating a large bending moment in the upper cervical spine that shifts the fulcrum of motion to the axial (C2-C3) region of the spine as compared with C5-C6 in the older child. The spine is also inherently more mobile in the upper cervical region. The factors unique to younger children that contribute to the increased mobility include the presence of generalized laxity of the interspinous ligaments and joint capsules, underdeveloped neck musculature, thick cartilaginous end plates, incomplete vertebral ossification (wedge-shaped vertebral bodies), and shallow-angled facet joints, particularly in the upper segments (between the occiput and C4). As a consequence, subluxation/dislocation and spinal cord injuries without fracture are more common than fractures in this age group.[2,18,20]

CHARACTERISTICS OF SPINAL INJURY IN CHILDREN AND ADOLESCENTS

INCIDENCE AND PREVALENCE

Analysis of the Kid's Inpatient Database (KID) has noted that the prevalence of spine injuries for children and adolescents has increased from 77 to 108 per million population over the time period from 1997 to 2009.[21] The older adolescent group (15–19 years old) had the highest prevalence at 345 per million population. Approximately 15% of those with spinal injury also sustained neurologic injury, of which 87% occurred in the older adolescent group. In 2009, the incidence of spinal cord injury (SCI) was estimated at 24 per million in the population under 21 years of age.[22] However, the true incidence of pediatric spine injury may be higher than reported because of failure to recognize these injuries. Aufdermaur found evidence of fractures of the spine at autopsy in 12 of 100 children over an 8-year period.[23] Seven injuries occurred in the cervical spine, four in the thoracic spine, and one in the lumbar spine. Importantly, only one of the 12 subjects had been suspected of having a spine fracture before necropsy.

MECHANISM OF INJURY

Although these injuries are rare, a high index of suspicion is warranted in polytraumatized children, especially those with head injuries.[1–3,18] Approximately 25% to 50% of children with a cervical spine injury have associated head trauma,[18,20,24,25] and as a consequence of this comorbidity, the mortality rate is higher in children with spine injuries than their adult counterparts.[18,24,26] Associated injuries most commonly involve the thorax, abdomen, head, and appendicular skeleton, and are present in 42% to 65% of children and adolescents with spinal trauma.[27,1,28]

In older children, sports injuries, diving accidents, and gunshot injuries are the most common causes.[2,4,18,28–32] A review of 300,394 emergency department visits from 1999 to 2008 found that 23% of pediatric cervical spine fractures were sports related.[33] At the 17 Pediatric Emergency Care Applied Research Network (PECARN) hospitals, sports were responsible for as many cervical spine injuries as motor vehicle accidents among children age 8 to 15 years from 2000 to 2004.[34]

The most common mechanisms of injury in young children are motor vehicle accidents, pedestrian-vehicle accidents, falls, or nonaccidental trauma (NAT) (child abuse). Polk-Williams reviewed the National Trauma Data Bank (NTDB) from 2001 to 2005 for patients younger than age 3 years that were injured via blunt trauma. The incidence of cervical spine injury was 1.6%, and the most common mechanisms were motor vehicle crashes (MVCs) (66%) or falls (15%).[35]

In infants and young children, NAT is a significant cause of injury to the spine. NAT was identified in 3.2% of spinal injuries at a level 1 pediatric trauma center over an 8-year period.[36] The mechanism was NAT in 19% of children aged 3 years or younger and 38% for those under the age of 2 years.[36,37] These injuries are often associated with other typical stigmata of child abuse, including fractures of the skull, ribs, or long bones, and cutaneous lesions. The cervical spine is a common location of spine injuries in abused children (73%), and multilevel injuries are frequent.[36] Upper cervical ligamentous injuries, avulsion fractures of the spinous processes, fractures of the pars or pedicles (most commonly C2), or compression fractures of multiple vertebral bodies are common patterns of injury and are thought to result from severe shaking or battering.[36,38–41] Thoracic and lumbar injuries are less common. Displaced fractures through the thoracolumbar (TL) neurocentral synchondroses may occur in young children.[42]

In neonates, birth trauma is the most common cause of injury to the cervical spine. Spinal column and spinal cord injuries occur in approximately 1 in 60,000 births[43] and may be an unrecognized cause of death in newborns, as evidenced by necropsy findings of injury to the spinal cord in 10% to 50% of stillborn babies.[44–46] Excessive distraction and/or hyperextension of the cervical spine are thought to be the most common mechanisms of injury, and may be associated with abnormal intrauterine position (transverse lie) or a difficult cephalic or breech delivery.[47,48] When associated with cephalic delivery, the injuries tend to occur in the upper cervical spine and are caused by rotation.[49] Injuries associated with breech delivery are thought to be caused by traction and occur in the lower cervical and thoracic spine.[46,50] These injuries commonly occur in the absence of osseous injury. The diagnosis of SCI in neonates is often delayed and should always be considered in a neonate with hypotonia or cardiopulmonary instability or in an older infant with decreased tone, a nonprogressive neurological deficit, and no history of familial neurological disorders.[50–52] Diagnosis can be made with either bedside ultrasound or MRI.[53] Prevention of this injury is preferable. Recognition of intrauterine neck hyperextension in association with breech position may allow for a planned caesarean delivery, which may reduce the risk of SCI.[47,54]

DIAGNOSIS

INITIAL EVALUATION AND TRANSPORT

Proper care of pediatric spine injuries begins at the scene of the accident with an appropriate index of suspicion. It should be assumed that a polytraumatized child has a spine injury until proven otherwise and appropriate precautions and immobilization undertaken. Children should be initially placed in a well-fitting cervical collar and immobilized on a spine board. In the event that commercial adult collars do not fit appropriately, sandbags or towel rolls can be placed on each side of the head to prevent motion. The prehospital triage algorithm endorsed by the Center for Disease Control for patients with a suspected cervical spine injury indicates that those with altered mental status (Glasgow Coma Scale [GCS] score <15) or paralysis should be directly transported to a trauma center.[55] Improved neurologic outcomes and reduced mortality have been noted for pediatric patients who were directly transported to a pediatric trauma center following a cervical spine injury, after adjusting for injury severity.[56] However, local hospitals should not be bypassed during transport if supportive care interventions such as airway management are not available from emergency medical services. Once the child arrives in the emergency room, every effort should be undertaken to evaluate the child expeditiously. The spine backboard is for transport/transfers only and should be removed from beneath the patient as soon as possible to prevent skin breakdown.

Herzenberg et al were the first to note that transport of young children (<8 years of age) on a standard adult spine board tended to cause excessive flexion of the cervical spine as a result of the disproportionately large head diameter relative to the chest in this age group. The obvious concern is that the flexed position of the spinal column could

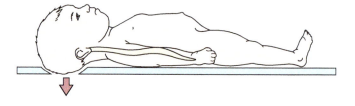

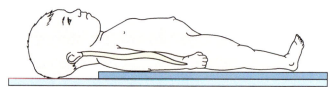

Fig. 10.3 Schematics of two types of spine boards modified for transportation of the year-old child with a suspected cervical spine injury. Note the occipital recess in the top drawing and the extra padding to elevate the torso in the lower to prevent flexion of the spine by the child's head, which is disproportionately larger than the chest in year-old children. (From Dormans JP. Evaluation of children with suspected cervical spine injury. *Instr Course Lect.* 2002;51:403.)

potentially jeopardize the cervical spinal cord, particularly if the mechanism of injury is related to a flexion force, which is often the case in motor vehicle accidents. Therefore, to obtain neutral position during transport, they recommended using a pediatric spine board with a cutout for the occiput or building up the child's torso with blankets on a standard spine board. Alternatively, a standard spine board can be used placing a towel role under the shoulders to allow the head to drop into slight extension[57] (Fig. 10.3).

In a subsequent study, Curran et al prospectively evaluated methods of positioning the child to achieve neutral alignment of the cervical spine after trauma. They measured sagittal alignment on supine lateral radiographs in 118 pediatric trauma patients and determined that only 60% were within 5 degrees of neutral alignment.[58] They suggested that younger children might need more relative chest elevation to avoid flexion of the head and cervical kyphosis following immobilization. These findings were confirmed by Nypaver et al, who determined in their study that children under 4 years old required an average of 5 additional millimeters of elevation of the torso than those older than 4 years to achieve neutral cervical spine alignment.[59]

Although it is not known how alignment of the cervical spine during transport impacts outcome, it seems prudent to avoid flexion of the neck by following the recommendations of Herzenberg et al regarding spine board immobilization, keeping in mind that the very young may need additional elevation to achieve neutral alignment. A pediatric-sized cervical collar and appropriate positioning may not be enough to ensure neutral alignment of the cervical spine in young children. As a practical guideline for proper positioning of a child on the spine board during transport, the external auditory meatus should be aligned with or slightly posterior to the shoulders.

CERVICAL SPINE CONSIDERATIONS

Clinical evaluation of a child suspected of having a spinal injury may be hampered by an inability to obtain accurate

Box 10.1   Risk Factors for Cervical Spine Injury

Concerning injury mechanism
Motor vehicle accident, motorcycle, or all-terrain vehicle accident
Pedestrian- or cyclist-motor vehicle accident
Vehicle crash (bicycle, skateboard, scooter, etc.) when patient is thrown from the vehicle, not a simple fall
Fall from greater than body height
Diving accident
Suspected nonaccidental trauma
Loss of consciousness
Abnormal neurologic exam
Unreliable examination because of intoxication or distracting injury
History of transient neurologic symptoms (concerning for spinal cord injury without radiographic abnormality [SCIWORA])
Neck pain
Signs of neck trauma
    Neck tenderness
    Limited range of motion or torticollis
Ecchymosis, abrasion, deformity, swelling
Head or facial trauma
Inconsolable child

historical information and the unreliability of the physical examination. Children are often frightened, usually unable to describe pain, and either unable (altered mental status, age) or unwilling to cooperate with an examiner. The likelihood of missing a cervical spine injury has been reported to be increased almost 23-fold in children who are incapable of verbal communication for whatever reason, and therefore, a thorough and careful examination is essential when evaluating a polytraumatized child.[60] The PECARN investigators identified eight risk factors for cervical spine injury in children presenting after blunt trauma: altered mental status, focal neurologic findings, neck pain, torticollis or limited range of motion, substantial torso injury, preexisting condition predisposing to cervical spine injury, diving injury mechanism, and high-risk MVC.[61] A high-risk MVC was defined as a head-on collision, rollover accident, ejection from the vehicle, death within the same accident, or speed greater than 55 miles per hour. Historically, several mechanisms of injury are considered to be risk factors for overt or occult injury to the cervical spine: falls from a distance greater than the height of the child, pedestrian- or cyclist-motor vehicle accidents, and unrestrained occupant-motor vehicle accidents. The presence of head or facial trauma or loss of consciousness are also considered to be risk factors. Neck pain, guarding, and torticollis are the most reliable signs of an injury to the cervical spine in children. Extremity weakness, sensory changes (numbness or tingling), bowel and bladder dysfunction, and, less frequently, headaches, seizures, syncope, and respiratory distress are signs heralding injury to the spinal cord (Box 10.1). If any of these conditions are present, immobilization of the cervical spine should be continued or initiated until imaging studies can be completed and the spine cleared.[18,24,29,62]

The entire spine, from occiput to the sacrum, should be palpated while considering that spinal injuries can occur at multiple levels and are noncontiguous in up to 38%.[27,63–67]

Approximately 16% of noncontiguous spinal injuries may be initially overlooked, and one must maintain a high index of suspicious for other injuries.[64] During the examination, the cervical collar should be carefully removed with an assistant stabilizing the head so that the patient or examiner does not inadvertently move the head. Cervical spine injuries often present with torticollis, so it is important to note the position of the head and the presence of asymmetry in alignment. The anterior and posterior neck is examined for lacerations and wounds. The cervical spine is palpated anteriorly and posteriorly for the presence of tenderness or interspinous widening. The collar is reapplied, and attention is directed to the TL spine.

THORACOLUMBAR SPINE CONSIDERATIONS

The possibility of injury to the TL spine should always be suspected in children who are comatose, have a distracting injury, or are not verbal because of age.[68] The thorax and abdomen need to be inspected for signs of trauma. Abdominal injuries, particularly those of the small bowel, are associated with flexion-distraction injuries of the TL spine and are often heralded by the presence of contusions or abrasions caused by lap belts.[62] The patient should be log rolled while keeping the head and neck in alignment with the rest of the spine and trunk. During this maneuver, cervical in-line traction should be avoided, particularly in young children because of the increased risk of ligamentous and atlanto-occipital (A-O) injuries.[69] The TL spine should be palpated along the spinous processes for evidence of tenderness, interspinous widening, or malalignment. The finding on physical examination of midline or paravertebral pain alone is predictive of the presence of a fracture of the TL spine with a sensitivity of 87% and specificity of 75%.[68] Evaluation of the entire TL spine is critical so as not to miss a noncontiguous fracture, and a thorough neurological examination is important, given that 20% to 30% will have a have a deficit.[1,68]

NEUROLOGICAL EXAMINATION

For all suspected spine injuries, an accurate baseline neurological examination should be carefully documented in patients who are conscious and cooperative. The sensory examination should include evaluation of light touch, pain, and proprioceptive function. Pain and temperature sensation are mediated by the spinothalamic tract that traverses the anterolateral column of the spinal cord. This can be assessed by using a clean needle to test pinprick sensation and an alcohol pad for temperature discrimination. Light touch and proprioceptive (position) sensation are functions of the posterior spinal columns. Light touch may be tested by stroking the extremity with a piece of paper and proprioception by asking the patient to determine directional change in the position of a finger or toe.

Dermatomal patterns of sensation correlate with the spinal nerve roots exiting specific anatomic levels of the spinal cord (Fig. 10.4). C1 and C2 innervate the occipital region; C3 and C4, the nape of the neck; C5, the deltoid region; C6, the radial aspect of the forearm; C7, the long finger; C8, the ulnar border of the hand; and T1, the medial border of the arm. The chest and abdomen are innervated by the T2-T12 nerve roots. Specifically, T4 provides sensation at the nipple

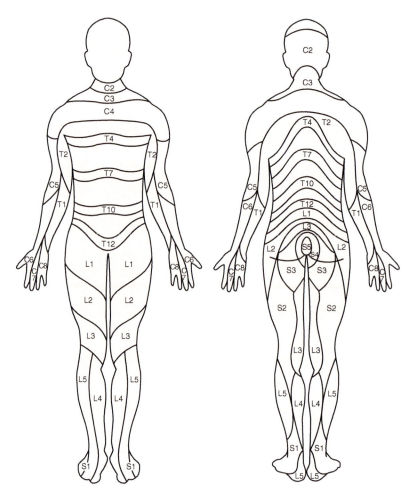

Fig. 10.4 Schematic of sensory dermatomes (From Keenen TL, Benson DR. Initial evaluation of the spine-injured patient. In: Browner BD, Jupiter JB, Levine AM, et al, eds. *Skeletal Trauma: Fractures, Dislocations, Ligamentous Injuries*. Vol. 1. Philadelphia: WB Saunders; 1992:594.)

line; T10, the umbilicus; and T12, the inguinal ligament. In the lower extremities, the pattern of sensory innervation mirrors the embryonic rotational maturation of the limbs. L1 and L2 contribute innervation below the inguinal ligament to medial thigh; L3 provides sensation to the anterior midthigh; L4, to the knee region and medial calf; L5, to the lateral calf and first web space; and S1, to lateral aspect and sole of foot. The perineal region is innervated by the S3-S5 roots. Preservation of function at this level, referred to as "sacral sparing," is important because it indicates that some of the spinal tracts are still intact and that the injury to the spinal cord is incomplete and therefore associated with a better prognosis for neurologic recovery.

Motor function should be graded on a scale of 0 to 5, with grade 0 indicating complete paralysis; grade 1, trace function; grade 2, full range of joint motion with gravity eliminated; grade 3, antigravity function; grade 4, function against slight resistance; and grade 5, normal strength against resistance. The level of SCI can be assessed by the presence or absence of function in key muscle groups. In the upper extremities, C5 innervates the muscles responsible for elbow flexion; C6, wrist extension; C7, wrist flexion; C8, finger flexion; and T1, finger abduction. In the lower extremities, L2 innervates hip flexion; L3, knee extension; L4, ankle dorsiflexion; L5 great, toe extension; and S1, ankle plantar flexion.

Deep tendon reflexes should be graded as absent (0), hypoactive (1), normal (2), or hyperreflexic (3). In the upper extremities, the biceps tendon reflex is mediated by the C5 nerve root, brachioradialis by C6, and the triceps by C7. In the lower extremity, the patellar tendon reflex is mediated by L4 and the Achilles tendon by S1.

The abdominal, Babinski, and bulbocavernosus reflexes should also be assessed. The abdominal reflex is performed by dividing the belly into four quadrants, with the umbilicus at the center. When the skin in each of the quadrants is stroked, the umbilicus should deviate in that direction. Absence of a response may signify an upper motor neuron lesion, whereas asymmetrical loss of the reflex may indicate a localized lower motor neuron lesion. The Babinski test is performed by stroking the lateral plantar aspect of the foot. A pathologic response is indicated by an up-going great toe and is indicative of an upper motor neuron lesion.

The bulbocavernosus reflex is an important test to determine the status of an injury to the SCI. The test is done by performing a digital rectal examination while simultaneously applying traction on an in-dwelling Foley catheter (or squeezing the glans penis or clitoris). Presence of the reflex is indicated by concurrent contraction of the anal sphincter and heralds the end of spinal shock. Spinal shock is a transient phenomenon that occurs within the first 24 hours of SCI and is thought to be caused by swelling about the neural structures within the spinal column. Once spinal shock has passed, as indicated by return of the bulbocavernosus reflex, the status of the SCI can be predictably characterized. This reflex is less reliable with injuries around the conus medullaris (T12-L2), as the afferent nerve fibers that mediate the reflex lie within the zone of injury and may be directly affected. As a consequence, return of the reflex may take much longer in this group of patients.[70] Additionally, all patients with a significant spinal injury should have an evaluation of bladder function using postvoid straight catheterization.

When an accurate neurological examination cannot be obtained because of the child's age or altered mental status, findings that may suggest a SCI in the initial evaluation period include flaccidity, diaphragmatic breathing without the assistance of accessory muscles, priapism, and the presence of clonus.[71.] Evaluation of a patient in this setting should include inspection and palpation of the spine from the occiput to sacrum, assessment of motor and sensory function by ability to withdraw from painful stimuli, and testing of deep tendon, abdominal, Babinski, and bulbocavernosus reflexes.

RADIOLOGY OF THE SPINE

INDICATIONS

The National Emergency X-Radiography Utilization Study (NEXUS) is a decision-making instrument that has been used in adults to determine the need for radiographic imaging of the cervical spine following trauma.[72] The criteria for clinical clearance are absence of neck pain/midline cervical tenderness, neurological symptoms, distracting injuries, or altered mental status (because of injury or intoxication). If any of these conditions are present, the patient is considered to be at high risk for a spine injury and must be evaluated with radiographs. Application of this protocol in the pediatric population was studied by Viccellio et al in a prospective, multicenter study of 3065 patients who were evaluated using the NEXUS instrument before undergoing radiographic imaging.[73] All of those placed in the high-risk group underwent anteroposterior (AP), lateral, and open-mouth odontoid x-rays. The instrument correctly placed all 30 cervical spine injuries into a high-risk group, and imaging confirmed the presence of an injury in each instance. More importantly, there were no cervical spine injuries noted in the low-risk group, giving it a negative predictive value of 100%. One fault of this study is that only four of the injured children were younger than 9 years old, and none were younger than 2 years old. A second concern is the possibility of false-negative x-rays in the low-risk group, given the recognized limitations of plain radiography in detecting injuries of the cervical spine. The authors concluded that application of the NEXUS criteria in an appropriate age group could potentially decrease pediatric cervical spine imaging by nearly 20%. They also cautioned that NEXUS rules should not be applied in a very young child, if an accurate history and examination cannot be obtained, or if there are associated injuries that heighten the suspicion of a spine injury.

Garton et al retrospectively evaluated the NEXUS criteria in 190 pediatric patients with documented cervical spine injury.[74] Utilizing the NEXUS criteria to determine the need for cervical imaging would have resulted in no missed injuries among the 157 patients older than 8 years. However, in the 33 patients aged younger than 8 years, two injuries would have been missed (94% sensitivity). The two missed

injuries were in the upper cervical region and in patients aged younger than 2 years.

The Canadian C-spine (cervical spine) rule (CCR) was designed to guide the decision for cervical imaging in adult trauma patients.[75] Imaging is recommended if the patient is high risk (age ≥65 years, dangerous mechanism, or extremity paresthesias) and if the patient is unable to actively rotate the neck to 45 degrees in each direction (tested only in the presence of low-risk factors). The CCR and NEXUS criteria were retrospectively evaluated by Ehrlich in trauma patients under 10 years of age.[76] Both criteria would have missed important cervical injuries. The sensitivity of the CCR was 86% and specificity was 94%, whereas the NEXUS had a sensitivity of 43% and specificity of 96%. The authors concluded that these criteria are not adequate for the pediatric population as currently designed.

Laham et al defined children at high risk for cervical spine injury as those who were incapable of verbal communication because of young age (<2 years old), those with altered mental status, and those with neck pain. They retrospectively evaluated 268 children with isolated head injuries and, using these criteria, placed 133 in the high-risk group and 135 in the low-risk group. They identified fractures in 10 children in the high-risk group (7.5%) and no fractures in the low-risk group.[60]

In a multicenter review, Pieretti-Vanmarcki evaluated 12,537 blunt trauma patients younger than age 3 years and created a scoring system utilizing four independent predictors of cervical spine injury: (1) GCS score of less than 14 (3 points), (2) GCS eye score of 1 (2 points), (3) motor vehicle accident mechanism (2 points), and (4) age 25 to 36 months (1 point). A total score of 0 or 1 had a negative predictive value of 99.93% for cervical spine injury. The five outliers with injuries despite scores of 0 or 1 had associated facial or skull fractures, loss of consciousness, or neck splinting.[77]

Imaging of the cervical spine after trauma should be undertaken if the mechanism of injury is high risk and if the child is nonverbal because of age or altered mental status, is intoxicated, has a neurologic deficit (persistent or transient), complains of neck pain, exhibits physical signs of neck or lap belt trauma, or has sustained other painful distracting injuries[78] (Box 10.1). Unexplained cardiorespiratory instability can be an indication of a high cervical spine injury and should be evaluated appropriately.[32] Imaging is *not* required for children who are communicative, alert, and nonintoxicated and have no neck pain, neurologic deficit (transient or persistent), mental status change, or painful distracting injury. There is a paucity of literature on clinical clearance of the TL spine. However, if a fracture is found at one level of the spine, the remaining spine should be imaged because of the high risk of noncontiguous injury.[79] Firth et al identified a median divergence of four vertebral segments between noncontiguous spinal injuries, supporting imaging of the entire spinal column after identification of single injured level.[64]

PLAIN RADIOGRAPHY, CERVICAL

Plain radiography of the cervical spine has been studied most extensively because of the length of time it has been available. A single supine lateral cervical radiograph with visualization of all seven cervical vertebrae, including the occipitocervical and cervicothoracic junctions, has a reported sensitivity of approximately 80% in the pediatric population.[80] Lally et al found that all seven cervical vertebrae were seen in only 57% of children on the initial cervical spine series, usually because of difficulty in visualizing the cervicothoracic junction.[81] Visualization of the cervicothoracic junction can be improved with traction or the so-called swimmer's view, in which the arm is extended overhead. The addition of AP and open-mouth odontoid x-rays increases the sensitivity of plain radiography to approximately 94% if adequate images can be obtained.[82] However, the open-mouth odontoid can be especially challenging to obtain in the young child. Buhs et al performed a multiinstitutional retrospective review on children under 16 years old with a documented cervical spine injury. Standard AP and lateral x-rays confirmed the diagnosis in 13 of 15 children younger than 9 years old. In none of the 15 patients did the open-mouth odontoid view provide any additional information. In only one of 36 patients aged 9 to 16 years old was the open-mouth odontoid deemed to be beneficial, identifying a type III odontoid fracture. The authors concluded that the open-mouth odontoid view was not helpful in children less than 9 years old. Instead, they recommended use of computed tomography (CT) to evaluate the upper cervical spine from the occiput to C2.[83] Similarly, Garton et al noted that for children younger than 8 years, the use of CT (occiput to C3) in combination with radiographs was more sensitive (94%) than radiographs with flexion/extension views (81%) or radiographs alone (75%).[74]

The PECARN investigators reviewed a multicenter retrospective cohort of children younger than 16 years who sustained bony or ligamentous cervical spine injury after blunt trauma.[84] Among 186 children with cervical spine injury who had adequate radiographs, 18 injuries were missed for a sensitivity of 90%. Only 4 of the 18 injuries not identified by radiographs would be considered "not clinically significant" by the NEXUS study group criteria; the remainder were clinically important injuries such as multilevel burst fractures and A-O dislocation. (Box 10.3)

NORMAL RADIOGRAPHIC ALIGNMENT

Interpretation of cervical spine x-rays in children requires an understanding of normal anatomy as well as the normal anatomic variants of the immature spine that can sometimes mimic trauma. On the lateral radiograph, the vertebral bodies, lamina, and spinous processes should be aligned in a gentle lordotic contour, and the facet joints should overlap symmetrically (Fig. 10.5). Assessment should proceed methodically in a cephalic to caudal direction so as to not miss an injury. Special attention should be given to evaluating the upper cervical (atlanto-axial) and craniocervical (A-O) region, given the propensity for injuries to this area in children and the subtlety of associated radiographic findings.[85]

Several methods for evaluating alignment at the craniocervical junction using the lateral x-ray have been described. *Wackenheim's line* is drawn along the posterior aspect of the clivus toward the odontoid process and should intersect the superior/posterior aspect of the odontoid process (Fig. 10.6). An anterior or posterior shift of this line relative to the odontoid indicates anterior or posterior displacement, respectively, of the occiput on the atlas. In

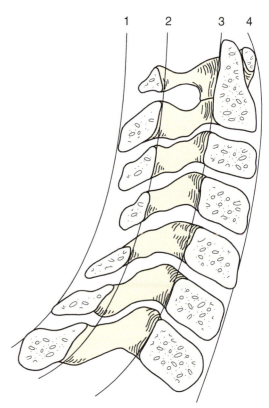

Fig. 10.5 Normal relationships seen on the lateral cervical spine x-ray. 1, spine processes; 2, spinolaminar line; 3, posterior vertebral body line; and 4, anterior vertebral body line. (From Copley LA, Dormans JP. Cervical spine disorders in infants and children. *J Am Acad Orthop Surg.* 1998;6:205.)

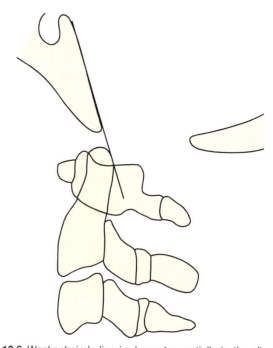

Fig. 10.6 Wackenheim's line is drawn tangentially to the clivus and should intersect the superior/posterior aspect of the odontoid process. A shift of the intersection point anteriorly or posteriorly is indicative of atlanto-occipital displacement in the same direction. In the young child, incomplete ossification of the odontoid can give false impression that there is an anterior translation.

Powers Ratio

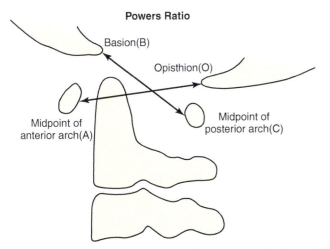

Fig. 10.7 The Powers ratio is determined by drawing a line from the basion (B) to the posterior arch of the atlas (C) and a second line from the opisthion (O) to the anterior arch of the atlas (A). The length of line BC is divided by the length of the line OA. A ratio of more than 1 is diagnostic of anterior atlanto-occipital translation, and a ratio of less than 0.55 is less sensitive for posterior translation. (From Hosalkar HS, Cain EL, Horn D, Chin KR, Dormans JP, Drummond DS. Traumatic atlanto-occipital dislocation in children. *J Bone Joint Surg Am.* 2005;87:2480-2488.)

Harris Method

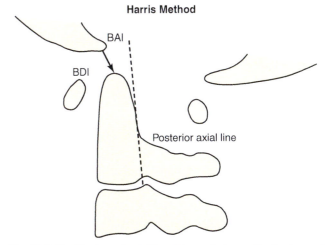

Fig. 10.8 The Harris method. The distance between the basion and the tip of the odontoid (basion-dens interval, BDI) should be less than 12 mm, and the distance from the dens to a line drawn superiorly from the posterior aspect of the body of C2 along the odontoid (basion-axis interval, BAI) should also be less than 12 mm. (From Hosalkar HS, Cain EL, Horn D, Chin KR, Dormans JP, Drummond DS. Traumatic atlanto-occipital dislocation in children. *J Bone Joint Surg Am.* 2005;87:2480-2488.)

Kaufman Method

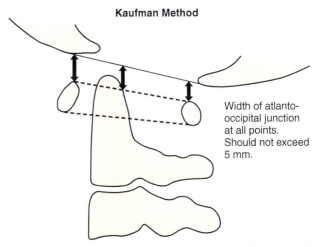

Width of atlanto-occipital junction at all points. Should not exceed 5 mm.

Fig. 10.9 The Kaufman method. The width of the atlanto-occipital junction, including the distance between the occipital condyles and articular surfaces of the lateral masses of C1 (facet-condylar distance), should not exceed 5 mm at any point. (From Hosalkar HS, Cain EL, Horn D, Chin KR, Dormans JP, Drummond DS. Traumatic atlanto-occipital dislocation in children. *J Bone Joint Surg Am.* 2005;87:2480-2488.)

children less than 13 years old, the odontoid may not be completely ossified, giving the false impression that there is an anterior atlantooccipital dislocation. *Powers ratio* is determined by drawing a line from the basion to the posterior arch of the atlas and a second line from the opisthion to the anterior arch of the atlas[86] (Fig. 10.7). A ratio of more than 1.0 or less than 0.55 represents anterior or posterior displacement of the A-O joint, respectively. However, the ratio is much more sensitive for anterior dislocations.[87] The *rule of 12s*, described by Harris, is another method for evaluating instability between the occiput and C1 on a lateral cervical radiograph. In this technique, the distance between the basion and tip of the odontoid process (basion-dens interval [BDI]) should be 12 mm or less, and a line drawn superiorly from the posterior aspect of the body of C2 and odontoid (basion-axis interval [BAI]) should pass within 12 mm of the basion (Fig. 10.8). The BDI is unreliable in children younger than 13 years old because of incomplete ossification of the odontoid; however, the basion-axis interval should still be less than 12 mm.[88] Normal BDI values measured on CT are different than radiographs because of improved resolution; a BDI greater than 9 mm on CT is suggestive of craniocervical junction injury in adults.[89–91] The basion-cartilaginous dens interval (BCDI) has been described for children, identifying the tip of the unossified odontoid on the soft tissue windows of the sagittal CT images.[92,93] The upper limit of normal BCDI varies with age: 4.4 mm for children 0 to 24 months,[92] 5.6 mm for children less than age 6 years, and 7.2 mm in children 6 to 10 years.[93] Distraction at the A-O junction can also be detected measuring the vertical height of the A-O junction. According to Kaufman, this distance should not exceed 5 mm at any point in the normal spine[94] (Fig. 10.9).

Integrity of the atlantoaxial articulation can be evaluated using the ADI. The ADI is measured from the posterior aspect of the anterior ring of C1 to the anterior aspect of the odontoid. The normal distance is less than 3 mm in adults, but in children, the normal ADI can be up to 5 mm. If the ADI exceeds 5 mm on lateral flexion and 4 mm on lateral extension, the transverse atlantal ligament (TAL) is likely to be incompetent.[16,95] When the ADI exceeds 10 to 12 mm, the alar and apical ligaments are probably insufficient as well, and the risk of spinal cord compression from instability of C1 on C2 is high.[96,97] The risk of spinal cord compression as a result of atlantoaxial instability can also be determined by directly measuring the space available for the spinal cord (SAC). Steel's "rule of thirds" states that at the level of the dens, one-third of the anterior-to-posterior diameter of the spinal column extending from inside the anterior ring of C1 to the inside of the ring posteriorly should be occupied by

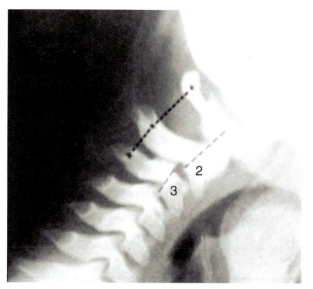

Fig. 10.10 Swischuk described the posterior cervical line (spinolaminar line), which is drawn from the anterior aspect of the spinous process of C1 to the anterior aspect of the spinous process of C3. The line should pass within 1.5 mm of the anterior aspect of the spinous process of C2 on flexion extension radiographs; otherwise, a true injury should be suspected.

the odontoid, one-third by the spinal cord, and one-third by the SAC. When the ring of C1 shifts anteriorly or the dens migrates posteriorly so that the SAC is reduced to less than one-third, the spinal cord is likely to be compressed.[97]

Swischuk described the posterior cervical or spinolaminar line to help diagnose pathologic angulation and translation in the upper cervical spine. This line is drawn from the anterior aspect of the spinous process of C1 to the anterior aspect of the spinous process of C3 and should pass within 1.5 mm of the anterior aspect of the spinous process of C2. If the distance exceeds 1.5 mm, an injury should be suspected[98] (Fig. 10.10).

NORMAL DEVELOPMENTAL ANOMALIES

In the immature spine, there are a number of normal, developmental anatomic variants that may be confused with trauma, and it is important to be aware of these entities when evaluating x-rays (Box 10.2). Persistent synchondroses (delayed closure) and incompletely ossified vertebral bodies (wedge-shaped anteriorly)[14] can simulate fractures. A helpful aid in differentiating a subtle fracture from one of these physiologic entities is the width of the prevertebral soft tissues. In children, the retropharyngeal space (at C2) should be less than 7 mm wide, and the retrotracheal space (at C6) should be less than 14 mm. More simplistically, the retropharyngeal space should be half of the AP width of the C2 vertebral body, and the retrotracheal space as wide as the C6 vertebral body. The retropharyngeal soft tissue can be falsely increased with expiration, as may be the case with a crying child, so it is important to obtain the radiograph during inspiration to determine if a true abnormality exists.[99]

In up to 20% of normal children, the anterior arch of the atlas can appear to override the odontoid on the lateral radiograph, particularly if the neck is extended. This finding is caused by incomplete ossification of the apical portion of

the dens.[16,100] Anterior angulation of the odontoid is a normal variant in approximately 5% of children and can be mistaken for a Salter-Harris type I fracture. Another common finding on x-rays of the immature cervical spine is subluxation of C2 on C3 and, less commonly, C3 on C4. Cattell and Filtzer were the first to note this normal variant in a study involving 160 pediatric patients with no history of cervical spine trauma. Forty-six percent of children younger than 8 years old had up to 4 mm anterior translation of C2 on C3, and 14% of all children had radiographic "pseudosubluxation" of C3 on C4.[100] In a subsequent study, Shaw et al found pseudosubluxation in 22% of all children younger than 16 years old.[101] Based on these studies as well as others, translation up to 4 mm can be considered a normal variant and not pathologic instability.[100–103]

Focal kyphosis of the midcervical spine is another normal variant that can similarly be misinterpreted. The absence of cervical lordosis on static lateral x-rays can be a normal finding in up 30% of children up to age 19 years[16,100,104,105] Been et al noted that 23% of children had straightening of the cervical spine, and 6% had a kyphotic posture.[105] This normal variant can be differentiated from a more ominous posterior ligamentous injury by assessing the posterior interspinous distance. The distance between the tips of the spinous processes should not be more than 1.5 times greater than the interspinous distance directly above and below a given level (Fig. 10.11). The only exception to this rule is the C1-C2 interspinous distance, which can be greater because the posterior ligaments extending from C1 to the occiput are disproportionately stout relative to the C1-C2 ligaments.[80,106] Subaxial cervical instability excluding C2/C3 and C3/C4 should be suspected when lateral x-rays demonstrate sagittal plane angulation between two vertebrae of greater than 11 degrees or translation of one vertebra on an adjacent vertebrae of more than 3.5 mm.[107]

Within the TL spine, differentiation of normal vertebral development and other conditions from fracture may be challenging. Anterior vertebral findings may simulate fracture. There is often mild physiologic wedging of the midthoracic vertebral bodies. At the TL junction, from T10 to L3, there is less than 11% anterior height loss in 95% of children.[108] Wedging in this region of greater than 11% is suspicious for fracture. Before ossification of the ring

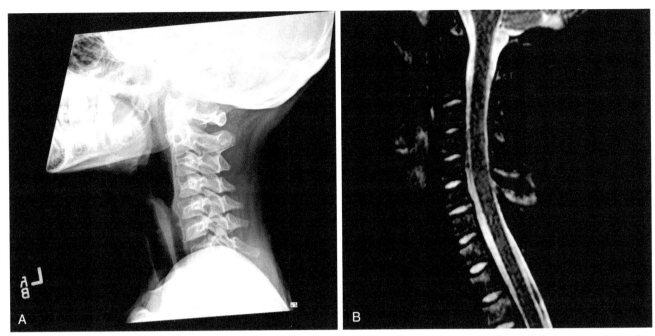

Fig. 10.11 A 9-year-old male sustained multiple injuries in a motor vehicle collision. (A) Lateral cervical radiograph demonstrates interspinous widening at C6-C7. (B) Sagittal magnetic resonance imaging short-TI inversion recovery sequence demonstrates posterior ligamentous injury.

apophysis, there may be a small radiolucent notch at the anterior superior end plate, which may be confused with fracture. Similarly, the anterior vertebral artery impression within the anterior vertebral body cortex may mimic fracture. Anterior vertebral beaking is observed in congenital hypothyroidism and skeletal dysplasias such as the mucopolysaccharidoses, representing an impression in the unossified ring apophysis. These anterior vertebral findings may be differentiated from fracture by the lack of association with anterior wedging.[109]

Central and posterior TL findings may also suggest injury. "Cupid's bow" is a normal variant curved indentation of the posterior third of the end plate, often at L3-L5.[110] "Balloon disk" is similar and noted when both the adjacent end plates demonstrate bowing.[111] These findings can be distinguished from biconcave end plate fractures, which are centered in the middle third. Scheurmann disease may mimic multiple compression fractures because of anterior wedging of adjacent vertebrae. This condition typically manifests with Schmorl nodes, end plate irregularity, and disc space narrowing. Schmorl nodes are defined by areas of focal end plate depression outlined by sclerosis and are common in the lower thoracic and upper lumbar region. A short posterior vertebral wall at L5 is commonly a normal variant, as L5 frequently has a trapezoidal shape.[109] Chronic pars defects, spina bifida occulta, and segmentation anomalies should also not be mistaken for fracture.

DYNAMIC RADIOGRAPHS

Flexion/extension radiographs have been shown to add little diagnostic information to that gleaned from static imaging modalities in the initial evaluation of suspected injuries of the cervical spine. Ralston et al performed a retrospective study in which blinded radiologists compared static and flexion/extension radiographs in 129 children and found that flexion/extension radiographs were confirmatory when the static lateral x-ray was suspicious for an injury. However, if the static x-rays were normal, the flexion/extension views failed to identify any abnormalities.[112] Dwek et al retrospectively evaluated 247 children in whom flexion-extension radiographs failed to demonstrate any cervical injuries when static radiographs of the cervical spine were normal. They did find the dynamic studies to be helpful in ruling out an injury in four patients whose static radiographs were originally thought to be abnormal.[113] Pollack et al evaluated the results of a subset of 86 patients from the NEXUS study who had undergone flexion-extension radiographs, and detected two stable injuries that were not originally detected on static x-rays.[114] The authors concluded that flexion-extension radiographs added little to the evaluation of the cervical spine in the acute trauma setting and that MRI was more sensitive at detecting subtle ligamentous injury.

Although flexion/extension lateral radiographs may not be helpful in the acute period, they can be useful in evaluating for instability after an appropriate period of observation or brace immobilization of a suspected soft tissue injury. In this setting, dynamic images can either confirm healing and resultant stability, or identify the presence of instability and the need for operative treatment.

PLAIN RADIOGRAPHS, THORACOLUMBAR SPINE

Conventional radiography is commonly used for screening of the TL spine. However, the efficacy of this modality is sometimes hindered by the inability to obtain satisfactory views of the upper two or three thoracic vertebrae. The swimmer's view can be helpful in such situations to counter obstruction by the shoulders and improve visualization of this transitional region of the spine. Screening radiographs should be obtained as soon as the initial trauma survey is completed to expedite the process of clearing the TL spine. Radiographs should be evaluated for the presence of fractures, overall alignment of the spine, facet joint symmetry, and interspinous distance. The lines described for evaluating the cervical spine should have a smooth contour in the TL spine. Although burst fractures are best seen on CT scan, subtle findings on conventional radiography include interpedicular widening on the AP projection and small cortical defects at the posterior-superior corner of the vertebral body on the lateral projection.

COMPUTED TOMOGRAPHY, CERVICAL

Inadequate radiographs were the leading cause of missed injury and subsequent neurologic deterioration in large series of trauma patients.[115,116] Having to repeat x-rays when initial studies are suboptimal is also inefficient for patient care and costly. Given these deficiencies of conventional radiographs and the continuing advances in digital cross-sectional imaging, including speed of data acquisition, image resolution, and reformatting capabilities, the use of CT to evaluate spine trauma in children has continued to evolve. In adults, the use of CT has replaced conventional radiography as the screening tool of choice for the cervical spine in the setting of blunt trauma.[117,118] The role of CT in evaluating spine trauma in the pediatric population is controversial. Keenan et al demonstrated that CT of the cervical spine may be especially beneficial in a subgroup of children who were over 8 years old, unrestrained in a motor vehicle accident, with a GCS of greater than 13 and were intubated. They found that a CT scan obtained early in the evaluation process prevented the need for obtaining multiple equivocal radiographs. Link et al[119] reviewed a series of 202 patients with severe cranial trauma in whom CT scans of the head as well as plain radiographs were performed. A total of 28 had fractures of C1 or C2, and plain radiographs failed to identify fractures in 11 of the 28. Another 11 had occipital condyle fractures that were identified only with CT. The authors concluded that routine CT of the craniocervical junction in patients with head trauma is useful to detect occult fractures of C1, C2, or the occipital condyles. Hartley et al[120] proposed an algorithm for cervical spine clearance in children based on a five-view cervical spine x-ray series, consisting of AP, lateral, open-mouth odontoid, and oblique views plus CT of the axial region of the spine, from occiput to C2. The rationale for CT included the preponderance of injuries in the upper cervical region in children less than 8 years old and the technical difficulty imaging this area with plain radiographs. In this study of 112 children, two of six osseous injuries (33%) were diagnosed only by CT scan.

The risk of developing thyroid cancer from exposure to ionizing radiation is a valid concern. Previous estimates have put the radiation dose associated with CT at up to four times that of conventional radiography.[121,122] Muchow et al estimated the radiation exposure of pediatric trauma patients for cervical imaging with plain radiographs (AP, lateral, and open-mouth odontoid) and multidetector CT (MDCT) by calculating absorbed doses based on imaging protocols.[123] The mean absorbed thyroid dose was approximately 0.9 mGy for radiographs and 64 mGy for CT. With this radiation exposure, the median excess relative risk of thyroid cancer induction with CT was 13% in males and 25% in females, compared with 0.24% in males and 0.51% in females for radiographs. This translates to an increased in the absolute risk of thyroid cancer after CT from 5.2 to 5.87/100,000 in males and 15.2 to 19.0/100,000 in females.

> **Box 10.3   Cervical Spine Injuries Documented as Not Clinically Significant by the National Emergency X-Radiography Utilization Study (NEXUS) Study Group**
>
> 1. Spinous process fracture
> 2. Simple wedge compression fracture without loss of 25% or more of vertebral body height
> 3. Isolated avulsion without associated ligamentous injury
> 4. Type 1 (Anderson-D'Alonzo) odontoid fracture
> 5. End plate fracture
> 6. Osteophyte fracture, not including corner fracture or teardrop fracture
> 7. Injury to trabecular bone
> 8. Transverse process fracture
>
> Modified from Hoffman JR, Mower WR, Wolfson AB, et al. Validity of a set of clinical criteria to rule out injury to the cervical spine in patients with blunt trauma. National Emergency X-Radiography Utilization Study Group. *N Engl J Med.* 2000;343(2):94-99.

Actual radiation exposure from a CT is dependent upon the specific scanner technology and imaging protocols. Marin et al documented significant variation in the radiation dose index for pediatric cervical spine CT examination across 296 hospitals, with a 2.5-fold difference between the 25th and 75th percentiles.[124] Pediatric hospitals had the lowest radiation indices and the least amount of variability. At our institution, we have calculated absorbed thyroid doses and whole-body effective doses, utilizing our 64-slice MDCT with age-specific protocols, and found the doses to be only two to three times greater than five cervical spine digital radiographs (AP, lateral, obliques, and open-mouth odontoid). We anticipate that further advances in technology will allow the radiation doses from CT to approximate digital radiography.

The central issue is whether the specificity and sensitivity of CT is sufficiently superior to plain radiographs to justify the higher costs and to offset the risks of increased radiation exposure in children. Rana et al reviewed 318 pediatric trauma patients where 27 cervical injuries were identified. There were five false negatives and five false positives with radiographs. The sensitivity of CT was 100% with a specificity of 98%, whereas the sensitivity of plain radiographs was 62% with a specificity of 1.6%.[125] Hale et al retrospectively studied 1296 pediatric trauma patients who were screened for cervical spine injury and identified 164 who were diagnosed with spinal cord or column injures (12.7%).[126] A total of 75 of the patients were evaluated with both radiographs and CT. Using the NEXUS definitions, 62 patients (78%) had clinically significant injuries, whereas 13 (22%) had nonsignificant injuries[72] (Box 10.3). All injuries were detected by CT. Radiographs had greater sensitivity for significant injuries (62%) in comparison with nonsignificant injuries (0%), which were missed on all x-rays. Radiographs did not identify 24 significant cervical spine injuries (32%) as defined by NEXUS. Operative intervention was required in 34% of those with significant injury; no patient with a nonsignificant injury required an operation.

The utility of CT to detect ligamentous injury when compared with MRI has a reported sensitivity of 23%, specificity of 100%, positive predictive value of 100%, and a negative predictive value of 88%.[127] However, a recent study by Gargas et al suggests that technologic advances allowing greater CT scan resolution may make MRI and CT comparable for the detection of significant ligamentous injury that requires operative treatment. They reviewed 173 pediatric trauma patients with a normal cervical CT who subsequently had an MRI scan. MRI detected five unstable injuries that required operative stabilization in the low-resolution (single-slice) CT group (85 patients), whereas there were no missed unstable injuries (0/88) in the high-resolution (64-slice) CT group (88 patients).[128]

Based on the available data, either conventional radiography or CT may be used effectively to screen for cervical spine injuries. In children less than 8 years old, a soft tissue or chondral injury is more likely than a fracture, and MRI is arguably a more appropriate study, although it may be logistically difficult to use as a screening study.[18] CT with sagittal and coronal reconstructions is our preferred method for initially evaluating the cervical spine in children of all ages in the polytrauma setting. When the CT is normal but there remains concern for an unstable spine injury, we use MRI to evaluate for soft tissue or chondral injuries, particularly in children less than 8 years old.

COMPUTED TOMOGRAPHY, THORACOLUMBAR

There is also growing evidence that CT is superior to plain radiography for evaluating the TL spine in adults. In polytraumatized patients, the use of data reformatted from "traumagrams," which are CT scans of the head to the pelvis intended to evaluate the thoracic and abdominal cavities, has been shown to be very sensitive at screening for injuries of the thoracic, lumbar, and sacral (TLS) spine and, in many centers, has eliminated the need for conventional radiographs. There have been at least five prospective studies that demonstrate a higher sensitivity for CT (93%–100%) when compared with plain radiography (33%–74%) and better interobserver reliability.[129–133] This information can likely be extrapolated to the pediatric population, but further studies need to be performed before CT with sagittal and coronal reconstructions replace conventional radiography for TLS clearance in children.

MAGNETIC RESONANCE IMAGING

MRI is the study of choice to evaluate the spinal cord and soft tissue structures, including ligaments, cartilage, and intervertebral discs. It is useful to assist with cervical spine clearance in the obtunded patient. Young children usually require sedation, so the logistics of performing this study can be cumbersome unless the child is already intubated or obtunded. MRI should be obtained in those with evidence of a neurologic deficit. MRI should also be performed if the neurologic deficit is transient, as this may herald an underlying ligamentous injury that requires immobilization.[28]

Recognizing that spine injuries in young children are more likely to involve the soft tissues or chondral structures, Flynn et al have advocated for the definitive role of MRI, in addition to plain x-rays and CT, in their evaluation protocol. In their study of 74 children, MRI altered the diagnosis in 34%, identifying injuries in 15 patients with normal radiographs and excluding injuries suspected on plain radiographs and CT scans in seven and two patients, respectively. In 25 obtunded or uncooperative children, MRI demonstrated three with significant injuries.[134] Keiper et al obtained MRI studies in 52 children who had clinical findings that were consistent with a cervical spine injury despite having negative plain x-rays and CT studies.[135] The MRI was abnormal in 16 of 52 patients, and posterior soft tissue injury was the most common pathology. Henry et al compared MRI with CT for the detection of osseous and ligamentous/soft tissue injury in 84 pediatric trauma patients. MRI identified all six fractures among these patients as well as an additional compression fracture, whereas CT detected only one of the six ligamentous injuries seen with MRI. Using CT as the standard for osseous injury, MRI had a sensitivity of 100%, specificity of 97%, positive predictive value of 100%, and a negative predictive value of 75%.[127]

MRI can be especially helpful in clearing the cervical spine of possible soft tissue injury in obtunded patients in whom the physical examination may be unreliable or unobtainable. Frank et al evaluated the effectiveness of MRI at decreasing time to cervical spine clearance, length of time in the pediatric intensive care unit (ICU), and length of time in the hospital, and found a statistically significant decrease for all of these outcome measures.[136] In a study of the use of MRI and CT in a clearance protocol for the obtunded trauma patient, Stassen found a significant number of ligamentous cervical spine injuries (25%) identified by MRI that were missed by CT alone.[137]

In the TL spine, MRI also affords effective visualization of injury to the ligaments, intervertebral disks, bones, and spinal cord. Sledge et al found that MRI was capable of determining the fracture classification, spinal stability, and appropriate treatment in 19 children with TL fractures and neurologic deficits. They also found that the pattern of acute cord changes seen on MRI was predictive of the potential for neurological recovery.[138]

SPINE CLEARANCE PROTOCOLS

Cervical

Once a cervical collar has been placed on a child or the neck immobilized, either at the scene of an accident or in the emergency department, formal clearance of the cervical spine is necessary before immobilization may be discontinued. Early cervical spine clearance has multiple benefits and helps avoid known complications including skin breakdown, dysphagia, pulmonary complications, and increased intracranial pressure.[139–141] There are no universally accepted protocols for clearing the cervical spine in children and adolescents. A recent survey of pediatric trauma centers demonstrated considerable variability in the imaging strategy and clinical service responsible for cervical spine clearance. A written, standardized pediatric clearance protocol was used by only 46% of centers.[142]

The goals of a cervical spine clearance protocol are to identify all important cervical spine injuries and to efficiently discontinue cervical spine precautions when appropriate while minimizing radiation exposure and overall associated cost. The protocol must balance the risk of missing a clinically significant injury with excessive imaging studies.

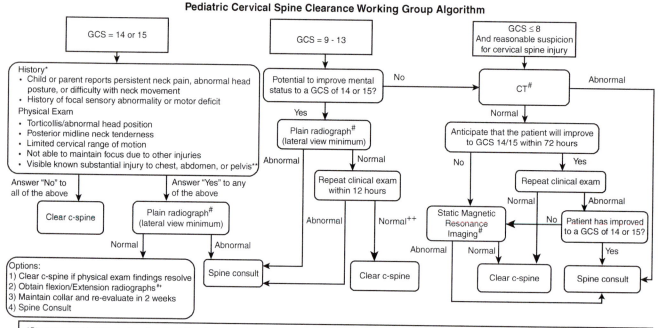

Fig. 10.12 The Pediatric Cervical Spine Clearance Working Group Algorithm for cervical spine clearance. (From Herman MJ, Brown KO, Sponseller PD, et al. Pediatric cervical spine clearance: a consensus statement and algorithm from the Pediatric Cervical Spine Clearance Working Group. *J Bone Joint Surg Am.* 2019;101[1]:e1.)

In comparison with adult trauma centers where imaging is routinely obtained during cervical spine clearance, there has been an increased interest in algorithms that emphasize clearance of the cervical spine based on history and clinical examination alone if the child is awake, alert, communicative, and neurologically normal.

Recognizing high rates of CT scans among pediatric trauma patients, Connelly et al implemented a protocol utilizing NEXUS criteria for clinical clearance in patients age 3 years and greater. AP and lateral cervical radiographs were the initial screening study for patients not meeting NEXUS criteria. After implementation of the protocol, cervical spine CT usage declined from 30% to 13%, with a 54% reduction in the lifetime attributable risk for thyroid cancer.[143] Similarly, Sun et al designed an age-specific algorithm to minimize radiation exposure in children age 10 years and younger.[144] Clinical clearance was possible with normal mental status (GCS = 15) and ability to communicate at a developmentally appropriate level in the absence of neck pain, neurologic deficit, intoxication, or distracting injuries. If clinical clearance was not possible, AP and lateral radiographs of the cervical spine were obtained. If a head CT was to be performed, the scan also included the occiput to C3 region. A full cervical spine CT was not obtained unless the radiographs were concerning for multilevel injury or if requested by the spine consult team. This algorithm reduced the use of full cervical spine CT by 60% and decreased the radiation dose to the thyroid by 80%.

An efficient multidisciplinary approach can facilitate rapid clearance of the cervical spine, decreasing the average time to under 8 hours in the nonintubated patient and 20 hours in the intubated child.[78] The ability to rapidly clear the spine is dependent upon a protocol that is safe and user-friendly enough for the primary team to perform. Anderson et al demonstrated the safety and effectiveness of such protocols, reporting a 60% increase in the number of spines appropriately cleared (no late injuries detected) by nonspine physicians after institution of a spine clearance protocol.[145]

A spine clearance protocol should incorporate a thorough history and physical examination with judicious use of imaging modalities. Clinical clearance can be performed when the following criteria are met: the child is able to effectively communicate pain, the child is fully alert without evidence of intoxication or mental status change, there is no paraspinal or midline cervical tenderness, there is neither evidence of a neurologic deficit nor history of a transient deficit, and there are no other substantial injuries which may distract from examination. If no abnormalities exist, the spine may be cleared without imaging if there is the absence of torticollis and painless, full range of motion out of the collar. However, if any of the above criteria are not met, or if provocative movement causes pain, then spine precautions should be continued.

The multidisciplinary Pediatric Cervical Spine Clearance Working Group (PCSCWG) used the Delphi method to achieve consensus on best practice guidelines, and three cervical spine clearance pathways were devised[146] (Fig. 10.12). Pathway 1, for patients with a GCS of 14 or higher, focuses on clinical clearance for the awake and alert patient when possible. The initial imaging recommendation is a cervical radiograph (lateral view minimum) if the history or physical examination do not allow for clearance. If the imaging is abnormal, consultation with the spine team is recommended. If the imaging is normal, then four options exist: (1) clearance if the physical examination findings resolve, (2) obtain flexion/extension radiographs, (3) maintain collar and reevaluate in 2 weeks, or (4) spine team consultation.

Kavuri et al have demonstrated the value in a "next day" repeat examination in reducing radiation exposure when the initial physical examination is abnormal but the initial radiographs are normal.[147] Upon reexamination, if the physical findings have resolved, then no further imaging is required, avoiding additional imaging with CT or MRI. Dynamic radiographs may also be used acutely to identify potential ligamentous instability if the initial imaging is normal; however, adequacy of the images may be limited by muscular guarding and spasm. An alternative approach for children with neck pain but normal initial imaging is to immobilize with a rigid collar for 10 to 14 days to allow time for paraspinal muscle spasm to resolve and then perform flexion-extension radiographs to rule out instability. Among 289 pediatric trauma patients with persistent cervical tenderness who were discharged from the emergency department with collar immobilization after normal radiographs or CT, only 1.4% were later diagnosed with a clinically significant injury, and no patient required surgical intervention.[148]

Pathway 2, for patients with a GCS of 8 or less, describes the process for clearance when physical examination is limited by neurologic function, such as a traumatic brain injury. The initial imaging recommendation for this population is CT because of the elevated risk for cervical spine injury among patients in this cohort.[77,149] If the patient does not recover to normal mental status within 72 hours of injury, then MRI of the cervical spine is indicated to facilitate clearance so that problems associated with cervical collar immobilization may be avoided. In these patients, expeditious use of MRI has been shown to decrease time spent in the ICU as well as overall hospital stay. For these reasons, MRI should be obtained as early as is reasonably possible.[78,134] If the MRI is normal, the cervical spine can be safely cleared.

Pathway 3 is for patients presenting with an intermediate GCS score of 9 to 13. The initial imaging recommendation is cervical radiographs (lateral view minimum) if the patient is judged to have the potential to return to a GCS score of 14 to 15 within 12 hours of admission. Otherwise, cervical spine CT is the recommended initial imaging. If the altered mental status improves with observation, then clinical clearance may be possible without additional imaging.

The PCSCWG algorithm recommends spine team consultation when initial imaging (radiographs or CT) or subsequent imaging (MRI) is abnormal. In the presence of a neurologic deficit, or a history of transient deficit, an MRI of the entire spine should be obtained. If SCI without radiographic abnormality (SCIWORA) is suspected, then the C-collar should remain in place, spine precautions continued, and the patient admitted for observation, given the risk of delayed neurological deterioration following these injuries.[150,151]

THORACOLUMBAR

Expedient clearance of the TL spine in the polytraumatized child is also very important. The child should be kept supine with spinal precautions until appropriate evaluation has been performed. Clinical clearance of the TL spine can be performed in the alert, cooperative patient without distracting injuries. However, imaging is required for a patient with a substantial injury mechanism if they are obtunded, have a distracting injury, or there are examination findings concerning for injury such as TL spine tenderness, edema, ecchymosis, or deformity.

Frequently, CT is performed from the head to the pelvis as part of the initial evaluation of polytraumatized children, and reformatted images of the thoracic and lumbar spine with sagittal and coronal reconstructions may be used to evaluate the TL spine. Otherwise, conventional radiographs of the thoracic and lumbar spine should be obtained. If the imaging studies are normal and the child is nontender to palpation without evidence of a neurologic deficit, the TL spine can be cleared. If there is continued bony tenderness in the setting of normal or equivocal plain radiographs, a CT scan through the region in question may prove diagnostic. If radiographs and CT are normal and a ligamentous injury is suspected, or if a neurologic deficit is present or there is a history of a transient neurologic deficit, an MRI should be obtained before the TL spine can be cleared.

SPINAL CORD INJURY IN CHILDREN

CHARACTERISTICS OF SPINAL CORD INJURY

The annual incidence of SCI in the pediatric population within the United States is approximately 24 injuries per one million children, representing approximately 1800 new cases per year.[22] In most studies of pediatric spinal trauma, spine fracture without SCI is slightly more common than fracture with SCI.[152,153] Vitale et al reviewed the KID and the NTDB from 1997 to 2000 and noted that spinal cord injuries in children most often occurred as a result of motor vehicle accidents (56%), followed by accidental falls (14%), firearm injuries (9%), and sports (7%).[154] The incidence of SCI was more than twice as common in males. Additionally, alcohol or drugs were involved in 30% of pediatric SCI, and 67% of those injured in motor vehicle accidents were not restrained.[154] Herndon reported diving accidents as causative of 9% of pediatric SCI.[155]

In younger children (<10 years of age), the most common causes are pedestrian-motor vehicle accidents and falls, and in children over 10 years of age, the most common etiologies are passenger-related motor vehicle accidents, diving, and other sports-related injuries (gymnastics, diving, downhill skiing, and contact sports).[63,156] There is a 5% to 10% mortality rate during the first year following SCI in children, and children younger than 11 years old are five times more likely to die within the first year after sustaining an injury to the spinal cord.[31,32]

Because of the anatomic and biomechanical characteristics of the immature spine, spinal cord injuries in children younger than 8 years old usually involve the upper cervical spine, often with no discernable bony injury, and are twice as likely to result in quadriplegia. Children older than 8 years are more likely to have fractures and injury patterns that more closely mirror the injury pattern in adults.[157] Overall, Rang found that paraplegia was three times more common than quadriplegia in his review of spine trauma in children at Toronto Sick Children's Hospital over a 15-year interval.[158] In comparison with adults, multilevel injuries are more likely, occurring in approximately 25% of children with cervical spine fractures, and SCIWORA is much more common than in adults.[24,157,159]

SPINAL CORD INJURY WITHOUT RADIOGRAPHIC ABNORMALITY

This syndrome was first described by Pang et al in 1982 before the use of MRI to describe spinal cord injuries without a discernable fracture on conventional x-rays, CT scans, myelograms, and dynamic flexion/extension radiographs.[160] It excludes injuries caused by penetrating trauma, electrical shock, obstetric complication, or those associated with congenital anomalies. In essence, physiologic disruption of the spinal cord occurs without a demonstrable anatomic lesion. The incidence of SCIWORA in spinal cord injured patients from birth to 17 years is approximately 35%, with the majority occurring in those less than 8 years old.[150] The injury is most common in the cervical region (74%) and may be related to the greater elasticity of the pediatric spinal column, where considerable deformation may occur without disruption.[151]

MRI may be diagnostic in demonstrating spinal cord edema or hemorrhage, soft tissue or ligamentous injury, or apophyseal or disc disruption, but is completely normal in approximately 35% of cases. SCIWORA is the cause of paralysis in approximately 20% to 30% of all children with injuries of the spinal cord. Potential mechanisms of SCIWORA include hyperextension of the cervical spine, which can cause compression of the spinal cord by the ligamentum flavum; followed by flexion, which can cause longitudinal traction; transient subluxation without gross failure; or unrecognized cartilaginous end plate failure (Salter-Harris type I fracture). Regardless of the specific mechanism, injury to the spinal cord occurs because of the variable elasticity of the elements of the spinal column in children.[161] Experimentally, it has been shown that the osteocartilaginous structures in the spinal column can stretch about 2 inches without disruption but that the spinal cord ruptures after only one-quarter inch of elongation.[48,162] A study of the tensile properties of the pediatric cervical spine noted normalized displacements from the occiput to C2 that were six times greater in an infant as compared with an adult.[7] The malleable nature of the spinal column is because of the elasticity of the ligaments and joint capsules,[163] high water content of the intervertebral disc and annulus,[164] horizontal facets and wedge-shaped vertebral bodies (permits translation),[100] underdeveloped uncinate processes (allows excessive rotation), and cartilaginous vertebral end plates.[23] In contrast, the spinal cord is relatively tethered by the horizontally departing spinal nerve roots, the dural attachment to the foramen magnum, and the brachial plexus.[165] SCI occurs when deformation of the musculoskeletal structures of the spinal column exceeds the physiologic limits of the spinal cord.[161] Injury may be complete or incomplete. Partial spinal cord syndromes reported

in SCIWORA include Brown-Séquard, anterior and central cord syndromes, as well as mixed patterns of injury.[150,156,160]

SCIWORA may also occur in the TL spine in association with high-energy thoracic or abdominal trauma. The mechanisms of injury include vascular insult to the "watershed" area of the spine associated with profound and/or prolonged hypotension, distraction mechanism in the seatbelt restrained patient, or hyperextension mechanism following a crush injury, as most often occurs when a child is rolled over by a car while in the prone position, resulting in the spine collapsing into the chest cavity.[150]

Prognosis following SCIWORA is correlated with MRI findings, if any are present, and the severity of neurological injury.[150,156,166–169] The changes seen on MRI are caused by edema and hemorrhage and may involve intra- or extraneural structures. Edema is seen as isointense on T1 and hyperintense on T2. Extracellular methemoglobin, a by-product of hemoglobin and a marker for bleeding in the soft tissues or neural elements, is seen as hyperintense on T1 and hypointense on T2. Findings in the extraneural supporting tissues often tell the story of the mechanism of injury. Injury to the anterior longitudinal indicates a hyperextension mechanism, whereas signal changes in the posterior longitudinal ligament and disc herniation are often caused by a hyperflexion injury. Damage to the tectorial membrane can be a sign of child abuse ("shaken baby" syndrome). These changes in the extraneural tissues can be detected by MRI within hours of injury, given that the blood is quickly metabolized into a form (methemoglobin) easily seen on MRI. Conversely, intraneural changes that are indicative of spinal cord hemorrhage may not be detectable for days as a result of a delay in the metabolism of hemoglobin in the spinal cord.[170,171] For these reasons, it is recommended that an MRI be obtained at the time of presentation to rule out an extraneural compressive lesion that may need to be surgically addressed and then repeated at 6 to 9 days after injury to improve detection of intraneural changes, which may be an important predictor of long-term prognosis.[150] In a recent multicenter review of SCIWORA, 94% of patients with a normal MRI had full neurologic recovery in comparison with 27% with an abnormal MRI.[172]

Grabb identified five patterns of intraneural injury that may be seen on MRI: Complete disruption of the spinal cord and cord hemorrhage involving more than 50% of the cross-sectional area of the cord on axial MRI is usually associated with severe neurologic deficits and a dismal prognosis. Minor cord hemorrhage involving less than 50% of the cross-sectional area of the cord is usually associated with moderate to severe neural deficits and a reasonable chance for partial recovery. Edema, without evidence of hemorrhage, is predictive of a very good outcome. No MRI changes are detectable in up to 35% of patients with electrophysiologically proven SCI, and these injuries are associated with an excellent prognosis for full recovery.[171]

Effective management of SCIWORA demands careful evaluation of the spine to exclude osseous or cartilaginous injury or mechanical instability and stabilization of the spine to prevent recurrent injury.[150,156] Radiographic findings of cervical or thoracic fractures and/or dislocations may be subtle, and there may be up to 10% error on the initial reading of radiographs.[29] Brace immobilization is usually adequate treatment for SCIWORA. The rationale for brace treatment is that the energy responsible for injury to the spinal cord also stressed the restraining structures (interspinous ligaments and facet joint capsules) enough to cause a partial tear or severe sprain and occult instability.[150] This concept of occult instability is strongly suggested by two patterns of injury seen in patients with SCIWORA: delayed-onset neurological deterioration and recurrent SCIWORA. Children with SCIWORA can present without neurologic deficit and subsequently develop symptoms up to 4 days after injury (delayed onset).[153] Recurrent SCIWORA is characterized by neurological deterioration that may occur within the first 2 weeks of injury, following an initial period of neurological stabilization or improvement.[156] Both delayed-onset and recurrent SCIWORA are thought to be caused by repeat injury to a damaged spinal cord that is vulnerable to even minor instability. The incidence of these injury patterns was significantly reduced after initiation of a protocol enforcing strict immobilization of the cervical spine at one institution.[150]

Overall, it is recommended that children with SCIWORA be immobilized for up to 12 weeks and then evaluated with lateral flexion/extension radiographs of the injured region before discontinuing treatment.[150,173] Cervical and upper thoracic injuries may be treated in a cervicothoracic orthosis and lower thoracic and lumbar lesions in a TL orthosis (TLSO). Surgical stabilization is rarely indicated. Following SCIWORA, a 6-month period of activity restriction is a consideration to avoid recurrence. The duration of brace treatment to treat SCIWORA remains a controversial issue. A meta-analysis of the literature by Launay et al showed that there was a 17% chance of recurrent SCIWORA when brace treatment was discontinued at 8 weeks but that no patients immobilized for 12 weeks developed a recurrent SCI.[151] In contrast, in a 34-year review of SCIWORA at a single institution, recurrent injury was uncommon and of uncertain etiology. Immobilization did not prevent recurrent symptoms or improve outcomes.[166]

CLASSIFICATION OF SPINAL CORD INJURY

Functionally, SCI is classified as complete if there is total absence of motor and sensory function below the level of injury or incomplete if any neurologic function remains after resolution of spinal shock. Sacral sparing, evidenced by preservation of sensation in the perianal area (S4-5 dermatome) and intact anal sphincter control, indicates continuity of long tracts and is associated with a 50% likelihood of improved neurologic function.[174] Spinal cord syndromes rarely present as classically described, but being able to define the pattern of neurological injury may be helpful prognostically. Central cord syndrome is not common in children.[175] It is characterized by more pronounced weakness and sensory changes in the upper extremities than in the lower. Bowel and bladder function is usually unaffected. The chance for recovery is variable and generally better in younger children. Brown-Séquard syndrome is characterized by a functional "hemisection" of the spinal cord with ipsilateral loss of motor and proprioceptive function and contralateral loss of pain and temperature below the level of injury. This injury is more likely to be caused by penetrating trauma, although it has been described in children following blunt trauma.[176] The prognosis is better following blunt injury. Anterior cord syndrome is characterized by loss of

> **Box 10.4 American Spinal Injury Association Impairment Scale**
>
> A= **Complete.** No motor or sensory function is preserved in the sacral segments S4-S5.
> B= **Incomplete.** Sensory but no motor function preserved below the neurologic level, including S4-S5.
> C= **Incomplete.** Motor function is preserved below the neurologic level, and more than half of the key muscle below the neurologic level has a muscle grade of <3.
> D= **Incomplete.** Motor function is preserved below the neurologic level, and at least half of the key muscles below the neurologic level have a muscle grade ≥3.
> E= **Normal.** Sensory and motor functions are normal.

motor strength and pain/temperature sensation with preservation of light touch and proprioception. It has the worst prognosis for recovery.[177]

The Frankel classification and American Spinal Injury Association (ASIA) Impairment Scale of traumatic SCI are both based on testing of motor and sensory function. Frankel Grade A is defined by absent motor and sensory function; Grade B, by intact sensation but absent motor; Grade C, intact sensation and motor active but not useful; Grade D, intact sensation and motor active but weak; and Grade E, by normal motor and sensory function.[178] The ASIA Impairment Scale score, which has gained more widespread acceptance, is based on sensory examination of 28 dermatomes and motor testing of 10 key muscle groups bilaterally. A sensory score of 0 (absent), 1 (impaired), or 2 (normal) is assigned to each dermatome and a motor score of 0 to 5 to each key muscle group. The sensory level is defined as the most caudal level with intact (2/2) sensation and the motor level as the lowest muscle group with at least grade 3 (antigravity) strength. The ASIA Impairment Scale further classifies an injury as complete or incomplete (Box 10.4).

MANAGEMENT OF SPINAL CORD INJURY

Following acute SCI, hemodynamic and respiratory monitoring is recommended to detect cardiovascular or respiratory insufficiency.[179] The rationale is that avoidance of hypoxemia may exacerbate spinal cord ischemia following injury. Clinical series of adult patients treated with aggressive management of blood pressure, oxygenation, and hemodynamics suggest improved neurologic outcomes after SCI without negative effect.[180,181] At our institution, we manage acute SCI patients in the intensive care unit with age specific mean arterial pressure (MAP) goals over the first 5 days following injury (Table 10.1). Pharmacologic agents are used to maintain the MAP goals, and respiratory insufficiency is avoided with ventilator support when required.

Pharmacologic treatment of SCI is directed at the secondary injury cascade. The primary insult, usually caused by rapid spinal cord compression in the setting of fracture or dislocation, is irreversible. The hallmarks of the secondary injury cascade include lipid peroxidation, ischemia, and electrolyte derangements. Corticosteroids are stabilizing agents that decrease edema and protect the cell membranes by scavenging oxygen free radicals. Studies in older children (>13 years of age) and adults indicated that methylprednisolone administered in the first 8 hours after injury

Table 10.1   Age-Specific Mean Arterial Pressure Goals for the First 5 Days After Acute Spinal Cord Injury

Age (years)	MAP Goal (mm Hg)
<3	60
3–12	70
13–16	75
>16	80

MAP, Mean arterial pressure.

may improve the chances of recovery.[182–184] However, the outcomes of neurologic improvement have not been reproducible in subsequent studies.[185,186] Additionally, there are significant complications associated with high-dose steroids in this population, including hyperglycemia, gastrointestinal bleeding, sepsis, myopathy, urinary tract infection, wound infection, pneumonia, and respiratory failure.[185,187–191] Within a population of pediatric patients with acute spinal cord injuries, a significantly higher rate of complications was observed among those treated with steroids as compared with those who did not receive steroid therapy.[192] At our institution, we no longer use methylprednisolone in adult or pediatric patients with SCI.

Enhancement of neurologic recovery following acute SCI has also been reported with administration of GM_1 ganglioside. This complex acidic glycolipid found in cell membranes in the central nervous system has been shown to have neuroprotective and neurofunctional restoration potential. Prospective, randomized, placebo-controlled drug studies with GM_1 ganglioside and methylprednisolone have shown improved recovery in patients who were administered both drugs in comparison to those given methylprednisolone alone.[193,194] However, a subsequent multicenter randomized study demonstrated no difference in the primary outcome measures at 1 year between the active and placebo treatment groups.[195] Currently, this type of pharmacologic therapy is not recommended.

Enthusiasm for hypothermic therapy has resurfaced following a well-publicized use of systemic hypothermia in a professional football player.[196] Potential benefits of hypothermia include reduced tissue metabolism and energy requirements, slowing of enzymatic activity, decreased parenchymal and axonal swelling, reduced hemorrhage, and diminished activation of postinjury inflammatory cascades.[197] Levi et al published a retrospective case control study comparing the complications and outcomes of 14 patients with acute cervical SCI treated with moderate (33ºC) intravascular hypothermia to a matched control group of 14 patients.[198] The age range was 16 to 73 years, and all had complete SCI at presentation (ASIA grade A). Six patients in the treatment group (43%) improved by one or more ASIA levels in comparison with three in the control group (21%), a difference that was not statistically significant. The rate of complications was similar in the two groups, although there was a statistically greater incidence of pleural effusions and anemia in the treatment group. A potential confounding

variable within the study was that early surgery was performed in 85% of the hypothermia group as compared with 50% of the control group. Additionally, postinjury hemodynamic control was not compared between the groups. Systemic hypothermia is a potential therapy for acute SCI that deserves further investigation in well-controlled studies that minimize confounding variables.

The indications for operative treatment in children with SCI are the same as in adults: spinal cord compression in the setting of an incomplete or progressive neurologic deficit, open spinal injury, or a grossly unstable injury pattern. Laminectomy alone is not beneficial. Multiple studies have shown it to be potentially harmful because it increases instability of the spinal column and the likelihood of angular deformity at all levels.[158,199–201] The goal of surgical decompression is to prevent or halt the deleterious effects of ischemia, which is an important component of the secondary injury cascade. The standard practice has been to proceed with urgent decompression for incomplete spinal cord injuries or those with progressive neurologic deficits.[202,203] Early decompression (< 24 hours after injury) was compared with late decompression in the Surgical Timing in Acute Spinal Cord Injury (STASCIS) Study.[204] This was a multicenter, prospective cohort study of patients aged 16 to 80 years with traumatic cervical spinal cord injuries (ASIA grade A–D). Improvement of two ASIA grades or greater was noted in 20% of early decompression patients as compared with 9% of the late decompression group (P = .03), whereas the rate of complications was not statistically different between groups. The STASCIS study suggests improved neurologic outcomes with early decompression of both complete and incomplete SCI. The goal of surgical stabilization is to prevent further mechanical injury to the spinal cord that might exacerbate existing SCI and to permit early mobilization of the patient to avoid pulmonary complications, disuse osteopenia, and complications from insensate skin.[174] (Fig. 10.13). In a study by Jacobs comparing operative and nonoperative treatment of spine fractures in patients with SCI, patients who were treated surgically walked 4.6 weeks earlier or used their wheelchair 5.2 weeks earlier than the nonoperative group.[205]

PROGNOSIS AND OUTCOMES OF SPINAL CORD INJURY

Fortunately, children have a greater propensity for useful neurologic recovery after SCI than adults, and younger children have a better prognosis than older ones. The likelihood for patients with SCI to have at least partial recovery after a complete injury has been reported between 10% and 38%.[63,152,153,206] Hadley et al found that 89% of children with incomplete spinal cord injuries showed improvement, and 20% of patients with complete SCI had significant recovery.[63] In Rang's series, children with both complete and incomplete SCI showed some recovery, except when the injuries occurred in the thoracic region, where the prognosis was regarded as hopeless.[158] In the series reported by Wang et al, 64% of their patients demonstrated at least partial recovery after SCI, including 80% with incomplete injuries and 25% with complete injuries who eventually became ambulatory. Early mortality was high among those with complete injuries (35%); if only survivors were analyzed,

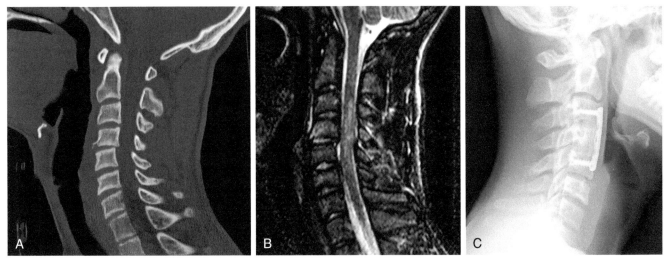

Fig. 10.13 A 14-year-old male, injured when struck by a car while riding his skateboard. He presented with an incomplete spinal cord injury with an extension distraction injury with retrolisthesis of C4 on C5. (A and B) Associated injuries included a skull fracture. Given the canal stenosis to 8 mm, he underwent C5 corpectomy and anterior fusion from C4-C6 with fibular allograft. (C) At 2 years postinjury, he had returned to sports with a remaining residual deficit of mild unilateral wrist weakness.

38% of complete injuries had neurologic improvement and progressed to ambulation. Recovery was seen up to 1 year following the original injury and was postulated to be because of the increased ability of the young nervous system to reroute neural pathways and produce axonal sprouting.[206]

Long-term, functional outcomes are determined by the level of SCI. Patients with injuries above C4 usually have paralysis of the diaphragm and often are ventilator dependent. Patients with injuries above C3 can shrug their shoulders and are only capable of neck motion. They can only operate equipment with sip and puff, voice activation, eyebrow or eye blink, or head or chin controls. Patients with C6 lesions can operate the controls of a motorized wheelchair and may be able propel a manual wheelchair if they have triceps function. Children with acquired quadriplegia and paraplegia require management by a variety of specialties including orthopedics, urology, pediatrics, psychology, social services, physical and occupational therapy, orthotists, and education specialists.

Paralytic, posttraumatic spinal deformity is a complication that is unique to children following an SCI.[207] The combination of spine trauma, paralysis, and growth invariably leads to the occurrence of spinal deformity in a number of ways. The vertebral apophyses in children are functional growth plates that can be injured directly by injury to the spinal column (intrinsic mechanism) or indirectly by factors associated with SCI (extrinsic mechanism). Intrinsic factors such as unstable fractures, loss of ligamentous integrity, and osteochondral (apophyseal) growth plate injuries can contribute to structural incompetence of the spine resulting in acute progressive deformity at the fracture site. This mechanism is more typically seen in children who are injured after their teenage growth spurt.[208,209] Extrinsic factors such as trunk muscle weakness, spasticity, and contractures can cause asymmetric forces to be exerted on the growing vertebral column that result in progressive deformity. This mechanism represents the classic scenario of posttraumatic spinal deformity. A third mechanism by which posttraumatic spinal deformity occurs is iatrogenic and is most often caused by

laminectomy without fusion or improperly instrumented spinal levels. The risk of postlaminectomy kyphosis is about 50%, with a much higher incidence in the cervical and thoracic spine.[201]

Patient age at the time of injury and level of paralysis seem to be the most significant factors in determining who will develop this problem. Mayfield et al reviewed 49 children younger than 18 years old with SCI.[208] Spinal deformities developed in all 28 patients who were injured before their teenage growth spurt had occurred, and the deformities were progressive in 80%. Scoliosis was the most common deformity and was encountered in 93% of patients, followed by kyphosis (57%) and lordosis (18 %). Some 61% of patients required spinal fusion. Conversely, in the group of patients who were injured after the teenage growth spurt, only 38% had a significant, progressive deformity, and only one-third of these patients required stabilization. In two other studies by Betz and associates, 98% of children who sustained SCI more than 1 year before skeletal maturity developed spinal deformity, and 67% of them ultimately underwent spinal fusion. However, if the injury occurred less than 1 year before skeletal maturity, the child had only a 20% risk of developing scoliosis and a 5% risk of requiring surgery.[210,211] In a review of 50 patients, Lancourt et al documented a 100% incidence of scoliosis in children injured before age 10 years old, a 19% incidence in those injured between 10 and 16 years of age, and a 12% incidence in those over 17 years old.[212]

The development of significant spinal deformity can result in pelvic obliquity and difficulty sitting, often requiring the use of the upper extremities for support. Pressure ulcers, pain, and difficulty in proper fit and use of wheelchairs are other significant problems caused by paralytic scoliosis. Orthotic treatment has been shown to be unsuccessful in altering the natural history of these paralytic spinal curves but can be helpful as a temporizing measure to delay surgery during childhood (<11 years of age) to allow adequate spinal growth.[208,211,212,213] However, use of an orthosis adversely impacts independence level and time requirements for functional activities in this population.[214] When curves are very severe (>40 to 45 degrees) and/or stiff, and the patients are over 10 years old, surgical stabilization and fusion is indicated to definitively treat the problem. Although these children experience a high complication rate, over 90% achieve a solid fusion.[208] The goals of surgery are to halt curve progression and obtain curve correction to balance the spine and pelvis to equalize sitting skin pressure and restore functional use of the upper extremities. Anterior release may be needed if the deformity is severe and rigid. Long fusions should be performed to avoid the problem of adjacent segment kyphosis, and sacropelvic fixation is necessary if pelvic obliquity exists.

Long-term outcomes are suboptimal following pediatric SCI. Anderson et al interviewed 161 adults who had sustained a SCI as a child and found that 64% lived independently and approximately 50% reported life satisfaction.[215] In comparison with the general population, they are less likely to live to live independently, drive independently, or be married.[216] At longer-term follow-up, depression is a common problem among adult patients with pediatric-onset SCI and is associated with poorer outcomes and a lower quality of life.[217] The risk of increased annual mortality is 31% higher for pediatric-onset SCI as compared with adult onset. Incomplete injuries with minimal deficits lead to 83% normal life expectancy as compared with 50% of normal for high cervical injuries without ventilator dependence.[218]

SPECIFIC CERVICAL SPINE INJURIES

OCCIPITAL CONDYLE FRACTURES

Fractures of the occipital condyles may occur after high-energy trauma and are often associated with head and neck injuries. Common presenting symptoms include neck pain, headache, and torticollis. Neurologic deficits may be related to concurrent head injury, and cranial nerve deficits are relatively frequent.

Radiologic diagnosis is difficult with plain films. CT is the preferred modality for diagnosis and classification. MRI may define injury to the tectorial membrane and alar ligaments. These injuries are commonly classified by fracture morphology and the mechanism of injury as described by Anderson and Montesano.[219] Type 1 are impaction fractures caused by axial loading of the skull into the atlas. Unilateral fractures are generally stable; however, bilateral fractures may be unstable. Type 2 fractures often are secondary to direct trauma to the skull and represent extension of a basioccipital fracture to the occipital condyle(s) and into the foramen magnum. Type 2 fractures are typically stable. Stable type 1 and 2 fractures are treated with a rigid collar. Type 3 fractures are a result of head rotation and lateral bending, producing an avulsion of the occipital condyle by the alar ligament. Type 3 fractures may be unstable and may require occipitocervical fusion for instability, chronic pain, or neurologic compression. Evidence of craniocervical malalignment indicates the need for arthrodesis.[220,221]

ATLANTO-OCCIPITAL DISLOCATION

Injury to the A-O junction is rare and often fatal. The mechanism of injury is sudden acceleration-deceleration forces, usually caused by severe passenger- or pedestrian-motor vehicle trauma. This injury has been associated with deployment of airbags.[222] The child's head is thrown forward on the relatively fixed trunk, causing sudden craniovertebral separation. Young children are at particular risk of this injury because of the relatively small size of their occipital condyles, the horizontal orientation of the A-O joint, ligamentous laxity, and their relatively large head size. In one study of 26 cervical spine injuries associated with severe trauma, nine involved the A-O junction and occurred primarily in young children.[85] Anatomic studies clearly show that clinical stability of the distance from the opisthion to the anterior arch of the atlas (OA) junction is primarily dependent on the integrity of the A-O capsule and the ligaments bridging the axis to the cranium.[223] There is essentially no inherent chondro-osseous stability of the articulation. The apical dental and alar ligaments run from the tip of the dens to the anterior rim of the foramen magnum and occipital condyles, respectively. The posterior longitudinal ligament continues cephalad from the posterior arch of C1 to the ventral surface of the rim of the foramen magnum as the tectorial membrane. The alar ligaments control and limit lateral bending and axial rotation, whereas the tectorial membrane limits hyperextension and vertical translation of the OA complex.[223,224] A-O dislocation occurs when these soft tissue stabilizers are disrupted.[225] Another pertinent anatomic characteristic of the occipitocervical junction in infants and children is that the foramen magnum is larger and more elliptical than the posterior arch of the atlas.[226] When the neck is hyperextended, the ring of C1 can protrude into the foramen magnum with potential for injury to the brainstem, spinal cord, and vertebral arteries.

Although traditionally thought of as a fatal injury, more patients are surviving this injury, potentially related to improvements in emergency and trauma care.[87,227–233] Recognition and appropriate immobilization of the head and neck without distraction is critical to patient survival. Clinical manifestations of traumatic OA instability include neck or occipital pain, cranial nerve palsy, spasticity, paralysis (usually quadriplegia), and respiratory arrest.[223] Some 80% of patients presenting with an A-O dislocation will have a neurologic deficit.[63] Cranial nerves VI, IX, X, XI, and XII are the most commonly affected in A-O dislocation. Bilateral injury to the ninth cranial nerves causes denervation of the carotid sinuses, which can lead to severe hypertension and circulatory instability. Injury to the vertebral and/or anterior spinal arteries may result in unusual neurological findings characterized by unilateral cranial nerve palsies and contralateral motor and sensory deficits. Difficulty weaning a child with a closed head injury from a ventilator may be attributed to an occult or missed upper cervical spine injury with damage to the respiratory center in the lower brainstem. Additionally, patients who survive an A-O dislocation are at risk for the development of hydrocephalus or syringomyelia.[234,235]

Radiographic diagnosis can be challenging. Spontaneous reduction of the occipital condyles after initial displacement may mask the pathology. Furthermore, the occipitocervical junction is difficult to image, and, because of anatomic vagaries, radiographs are usually hard to interpret. Several radiographic parameters, based on a true lateral x-ray of the cervical spine, have been described to help diagnose this

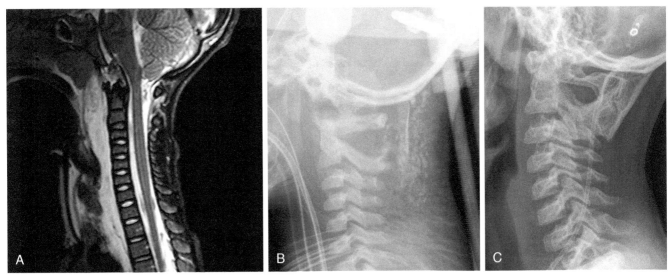

Fig. 10.14 A 4-year-old male victim of a pedestrian-motor vehicle "hit and run" accident. He had a Glasgow Coma Scale score of 3 at the scene. Magnetic resonance imaging demonstrated atlantooccipital and atlantoaxial dissociation. (A) A halo was placed acutely, and then he subsequently underwent in situ O-C2 arthrodesis with an occipital periosteal turndown flap and iliac crest bone graft.(B) Posttraumatic hydrocephalus required ventriculoperitoneal shunting. He was ambulatory by 15 weeks postinjury. A solid arthrodesis is present at 4 years postoperative (C).

injury. As in any injury to the cervical spine, anterior soft tissue swelling may be apparent. Excessive axial displacement of the occiput may be reflected by an abnormal basion-dens distance (>12 mm) (Fig. 10.8) or widened space between the articular surface of the lateral masses and occipital condyles (>5 mm) (Fig. 10.9). Wackenheim's line, drawn along the clivus towards the spinal canal, may be shifted anteriorly so that it intersects or passes anterior to the tip of the odontoid, rather than posterior to it (Fig. 10.6). Powers ratio, calculated by comparing the distance from the basion to the posterior arch of the atlas (BC) to the OA, is useful in diagnosing anterior OA instability (ratio >1.0) but not as helpful in posterior (ratio <0.55) or lateral OA instability (Fig. 10.7). Dynamic analysis by CT with sagittal and coronal reconstructions or flexion-extension-distraction fluoroscopic examination may be helpful to identify the pattern of instability.[223,233,236] Subluxation or distraction of greater than 2 to 3 mm between the occiput and C1 suggests instability. MRI may be helpful in diagnosing soft tissue and ligamentous injuries. The direction of displacement has been classified by Traynelis as type 1 with anterior displacement, type 2 with longitudinal distraction, and type 3 with posterior displacement.[237] Steinmetz defined incomplete (grade 1) and complete (grade 2) injuries based upon the integrity of the tectorial membrane by MRI.[238] Horn defined grade 1 injuries as the presence of no displacement by CT measurements with moderately abnormal MRI findings (abnormal signal within the A-O articulation or posterior ligaments). Grade 2 injuries are displaced by CT measurements with grossly abnormal MRI findings (abnormal signal in A-O joints, tectorial membrane, or alar or cruciate ligaments).[239]

Following diagnosis, the head and neck should be immobilized by a hard collar or halo, securing the torso in the process, so as to prevent inadvertent displacement of the head. If necessary, gentle and appropriately directed halter or skull traction can be used to provide immediate anatomic reduction. Anterior displacement can be reduced by slight extension of the skull and posterior displacement by flexion. Radiographs should be obtained immediately following any manipulation to assess the position of the head following realignment, in particular to guard against axial displacement.[223] Astur et al recommend against preoperative halo vest placement, as the vest may not adequately immobilize the trunk and can lead to inadvertent distraction and displacement.[233]

These injuries usually require surgical stabilization for definitive treatment. Immobilization alone with either halo vest or Minerva cast has been shown to be unpredictable, at best, in restoring ligamentous stability of the A-O junction.[240] Grade 1 injuries (Steinmetz or Horn classification) may be carefully evaluated by fluoroscopic examination. If stable, conservative treatment by immobilization with an external orthosis could be considered. Unstable injuries (grade 2, Steinmetz or Horn classification) require operative stabilization. Posterior arthrodesis from occiput to C1 offers the advantage of preserving C1-C2 motion.[232] Extending the arthrodesis to C2 permits superior fixation and a larger surface area for the fusion mass.[223]

A variety of techniques for occipitocervical arthrodesis are available. In a young child, a periosteal turndown flap with autograft and halo immobilization can be very effective. The periosteal flap is based at the posterior aspect of the foramen magnum and is sutured to the C1 and C2 posterior elements. (Fig. 10.14) Wiring techniques with iliac crest or rib autograft may be used.[241,242] The advantage of rib is that its curve more closely matches the natural lordosis of the occipitoatlantoaxial complex. Internal fixation may be achieved with a contoured rod loop utilizing sublaminar wires and wiring via cranial burr holes.[233] The cranial burr holes must be created below the superior nuchal line to avoid the transverse sinus.[243] Nonscrew fixation options at C2 include wire placed through a drill hole in the base of the spinous process and looped around the caudal aspect of the spinous process. Alternatively, sublaminar wires may be placed at C2. If the osseous anatomy is of sufficient size, internal fixation with occipitocervical plates and screw fixation may be considered. Screws may be placed in the occiput, occipital condyle, C1 lateral mass, C2 pars, or C2 lamina.[244–247]

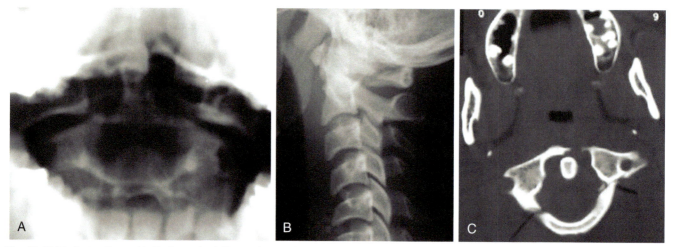

Fig. 10.15 Typical radiographic findings of a Jefferson fracture in a 14-year-old female involved in an all-terrain vehicle accident. (A) Open-mouth odontoid view demonstrates widening of the lateral masses of C1 that overhang the C2 facets. (B) Lateral radiograph demonstrates fracture of the posterior ring of C1. (C) Axial CT scan shows disruption of the ring of C1.

Fixation constructs may also include C1-C2 transarticular screws.[248] A technique for compression of structural bone graft to the occiput and upper cervical spine utilizing rigid internal fixation has been described.[249] Depending on the rigidity of the fixation, immobilization with a hard collar or halo vest is utilized.

FRACTURES OF THE ATLAS

Bursting fractures of the ring of C1, also called a Jefferson fracture, is a relatively uncommon injury in children. The mechanism of injury is an axial load transmitted from the head through the occipital condyles to the lateral masses of C1.[250] Disruption of the ring must, by definition, involve failure at two places and can occur through bone, cartilage (synchondrosis), or both. Most often both the anterior and posterior rings are disrupted. Isolated "single-ring" fractures may occur in children with the second site of failure being a physeal injury through one of the synchondroses.[251,252] SCI is exceptionally rare owing to the large space available for the cord at this level and the fact that disruption of the ring actually results in further expansion.[253] Associated cranial nerve deficits are rare.[254] Head injuries are commonly associated with atlas fractures, and the presence of concomitant cervical fractures is 50%.[255]

Stability of the transverse ligament is usually preserved unless the lateral masses are displaced widely (>6.9 mm) beyond the lateral margin of the body of C2.[256] However, a large clinical series did not demonstrate significant C1-C2 instability in fractures that healed with excessive displacement.[257] Plain radiographs may demonstrate a fracture of the ring of C1, but CT is much more accurate in defining the fracture pattern, extent of displacement, and potential integrity of the TAL (Fig. 10.15).

If the transverse ligament is intact and the lateral masses are minimally displaced, these injuries can usually be treated by immobilization with a hard collar, Minerva cast, or halo vest. When the lateral masses are displaced more than 6.9 mm, 4 to 6 weeks of halo traction is an option to reduce the fracture and obtain early healing with subsequent immobilization in halo vest. Unfortunately, complete reduction with halo traction may only occur in approximately 20% of displaced fractures.[257] Adequate outcomes may be achieved with halo immobilization alone for fractures with more than 6.9 mm of displacement.[258] Healing should be documented radiographically by CT scan, and C1-C2 stability (TAL integrity) documented by flexion-extension lateral radiographs of the cervical spine after discontinuation of immobilization. Residual instability is an indication for posterior fusion of C1-C2.[162]

ATLANTO-AXIAL SUBLUXATION

Excessive mobility of C1 on C2 can be caused by rupture of the restraining ligaments, fracture of the odontoid, or excessive ligamentous laxity.[259] Acute rupture of the TAL is rare and a much less common cause of atlanto-axial subluxation than fracture of the odontoid process.[260] These injuries have been classified by Dickman as type 1 for intrasubstance ruptures and type 2 for avulsion fractures of the TAL insertion from the C1 lateral mass.[261] The TAL is the primary stabilizer of an intact odontoid against forward displacement of C1. The normal distance from the anterior cortex of the dens to the posterior cortex of the anterior ring of C1 is less than 5 mm in children (ADI)[95] Anterior translation of the atlas beyond this distance decreases the SAC and increases the potential for SCI. Diagnosis of C1-C2 instability is suggested by a history of trauma to the cervical spine and the finding of painful torticollis.[250] The diagnosis is confirmed by plain radiographs or CT scan of the cervical spine and flexion-extension views demonstrating an ADI of greater than 5 mm. CT may also show avulsion of the transverse ligament from the C1 ring. Even though soft tissue healing is somewhat unpredictable, a trial of conservative treatment is indicated in a child for type 1 injuries. The subluxation is reduced by extension of the head and immobilized in a halo vest or Minerva cast for 8 to 12 weeks. Type 2 fractures should also be treated with immobilization, and 74% will stabilize without arthrodesis.[261] If, after this period of immobilization, flexion-extension radiographs indicate continued instability of greater than 5 mm, C1-C2 fusion should be performed.

A variety of operative techniques may be used for posterior C1-2 arthrodesis.

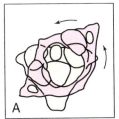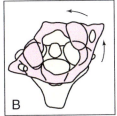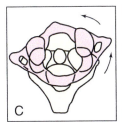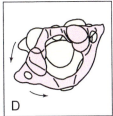

Fig. 10.16 Fielding and Hawkins classification of atlantoaxial rotatory displacement. (A) Type I, no anterior displacement and odontoid acting as pivot. (B) Type II, anterior displacement of 3 to 5 mm and one lateral articular process acting as the pivot. (C) Type III, anterior displacement of more than 5 mm. (D) Type IV, posterior displacement. (From Dormans JP. Evaluation of children with suspected cervical spine injury. *Instr Course Lect.* 2002;51:407.)

Traditional wire fixation with autograft and postoperative halo vest immobilization have fusion rates of 60% to 97%.[262–264] The Magerl technique of C1-C2 transarticular screw fixation has the advantage of not requiring postoperative halo immobilization, with fusion rates up to 100% in pediatric patients.[265,266] The most significant risk associated with this technique is injury to the vertebral artery, which normally lies immediately lateral and slightly anterior to the C2 transverse foramina. In 18% to 23% of individuals, the artery follows an anomalous course on at least one side, making screw passage risky or impossible.[267] CT angiography with sagittal, coronal, and three-dimensional reformatting can help define the vascular anatomy preoperatively. With knowledge of this anatomy, screws can be safely placed using a free hand technique with intraoperative fluoroscopy. Alternatively, image guidance can be used to place the screws. In the series by Gluf et al, the risk of vertebral artery injury in 67 children who had placement of transarticular screws was 1.6%, and none had neurologic deficits.[266] An alternative technique is to use C1 lateral mass and C2 pars or laminar screws for fixation, which circumvents the issues associated with potential variations in the course of the vertebral artery.[246,268,269] However, the size of the pediatric C1 lateral mass may remain a challenge for screw insertion. A "pedicle exposure technique" for insertion of C1 screws via the posterior arch and lateral mass has been described for pediatric patients.[270]

ATLANTOAXIAL ROTARY FIXATION

Atlantoaxial rotary fixation (AARF), also called atlantoaxial rotary subluxation, is a common cause of childhood torticollis that occurs most often as a result of trauma or infection (Grisel syndrome).[271,272] Common traumatic mechanisms include falls, MVC, and clothes lining.[273] Other associations have been noted: postsurgical, juvenile inflammatory arthritis, and congenital abnormalities.[274] The defining feature of AARF is that the C1-C2 joint is actually subluxated, resulting in pain, loss of cervical motion, and abnormal position of the head and neck.[271] Neurological symptoms are infrequent, with 14% reporting paresthesias, sensory loss, motor weakness, or other neurologic findings.[273] Diagnosis is often delayed, perhaps owing to the subtle nature of the mechanisms of injury (minor trauma and upper respiratory infection) and the insidious presentation of the symptoms.[271,272] In Fielding's series, the average delay in diagnosis was 11.6 months. Neck extension was reduced by as much as 50%, and the characteristic position of the head was approximately a 23-degree tilt to one side and 20-degree rotation in the opposite direction. In contradistinction to muscular torticollis, the sternocleidomastoid muscle is contracted on the side to which the chin is rotated, presumably in reactive spasm as an attempt to stabilize or reduce the rotational subluxation. Another characteristic of AARF is the inability to rotate the head past midline in the direction opposite to which the head is turned.[275]

The diagnosis of AARF must be confirmed radiographically. AP and lateral x-rays can be difficult to interpret because of the abnormal positioning of the head and cervical spine.[272] However, these views are helpful to rule out a congenital deformity, obvious trauma that might explain the presentation or evidence of TAL insufficiency. Because of the head tilt, the lateral x-ray needs to be taken with the cassette parallel to the skull and the x-ray beam directed perpendicular to the skull ("lateral of the skull"). On the lateral x-ray, the two halves of the posterior arch will not be superimposed because of tilting of the atlas, and because of forward rotation of one of the lateral masses, the spinal canal can appear to be narrowed. An open-mouth AP x-ray may show asymmetry of the lateral masses of C1 in relation to the odontoid. The lateral mass of C1 that is rotated forward appears wider and closer to the odontoid than the contralateral one that is rotated posteriorly and appears smaller and farther away from the odontoid. Also, on the side on which the lateral mass is rotated posteriorly, the joint space between the lateral masses is obliterated. Fielding and Hawkins developed a classification system for AARF, based on conventional radiographic findings. Type I is unilateral facet subluxation without any anterior displacement of the atlas, implying that the transverse ligament is intact. This is the most common and benign type. Type II is characterized by unilateral facet subluxation with 3 to 5 mm of anterior displacement and implies some deficiency off the TAL. In Type III, the anterior facet displacement is more than 5 mm and is thought to be associated with deficiencies of both the transverse and secondary restraining ligaments. Type IV is rare and characterized by posterior displacement of the atlas caused by a deficient odontoid process[271] (Fig. 10.16). CT scans with coronal and sagittal reconstructions or three-dimensional rendering can be helpful in demonstrating the pattern of subluxation (Fig. 10.17A).

In addition to abnormal alignment, AARF is also characterized by abnormal motion between C1 and C2 that can be demonstrated on dynamic imaging studies in which diagnosis is based on limitation of motion between the C1 and C2 joints. Cineradiography shows that the posterior arches of C1 and C2 move together rather than independently during neck rotation. Dynamic CT, in which 3-mm cuts are taken with the head in neutral position and then with left and right rotation, have been shown to be more sensitive than

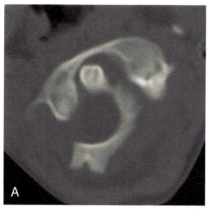
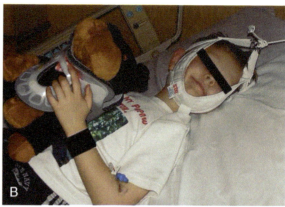

Fig. 10.17 A 7-year-old male presented with painful torticollis of 5 days duration after a minor injury. CT demonstrated Type II atlantoaxial rotatory fixation. (A) He was treated with 2 days of halter traction, pain control, and antispasmodics. (B) The torticollis resolved, and he was immobilized in a hard collar for 6 weeks.

static CT.[276–278] In this study, the angle subtended by lines drawn in an AP direction through the midline of C1 and C2 represents the axial, rotational relationship between C1 and C2. In patients with muscular torticollis, the measured angle reduces to nearly zero, and C1 may even cross over C2 when the head is rotated to the contralateral side. In AARF, this angle never reduces to zero despite maximum contralateral rotation attempting to reduce the subluxation.[279]

The natural history of AARF is a progressive painful deformity that can also affect vision and phonation. The most important aspect influencing outcome is early diagnosis and initiation of treatment. Secondary changes within the atlantoaxial joint and surrounding soft tissues develop the longer the condition goes untreated, and the critical time period seems to be about 3 to 4 weeks. After this interval, incomplete reduction and recurrent subluxation after closed treatment are much more likely.[272,280] Cases that present within the first week after onset of symptoms can be treated with simple cervical immobilization and antiinflammatory medication. If the subluxation fails to reduce, cervical traction in conjunction with benzodiazepines or manipulative reduction should be performed.[279,280] (Fig. 10.17B). Manual reduction should be done with extreme caution, and most recommend doing it with the patient awake with continuous neurologic monitoring.[272] Traction can be performed with either head halter or skeletal skull devices starting with 3.5 kg and increasing by 0.5 kg every 3 days up to a limit of about 7 kg.[271,272,279] Traction can be successful even with neglected AARF of greater than 6 weeks duration.[281] Successful reduction is followed by a 6- to 12-week course of immobilization in a cervical collar or similar orthosis.

Proponents for longer courses of treatment cite the occurrence of worse outcomes if subluxation recurs. Recurrence is thought to occur because of a combination of persistent laxity of the joint capsules and stabilizing ligaments as well as remodeling of the C1-C2 articulation into a downward-slanting orientation that is rotationally unstable.[282,283] Recurrent subluxation should be treated with prompt cervical traction until reduction is achieved, followed by a 3-month course in a halo orthosis.[279] A second recurrence warrants C1-C2 fusion. Before fusion, reduction should be attempted. If unsuccessful, then an in situ C1-C2 fusion should be done.[272] Alternatively, posterior stabilization without arthrodesis using a suture "check ligament" between C1 and C2 has been described.[283] It has been observed that clinical improvement does occur following fusion despite continued malalignment of the atlantoaxial joint because of compensatory

occiput-C1 rotation.[279] Arthrodesis has traditionally been recommended for failed closed reduction of AARF.[272] However, Crossman et al advocated for open reduction of the anteromedial C1-C2 articulation via an extreme lateral approach and then halo vest immobilization.[284] In their series of 13 patients with failed closed treatment of AARF, 11 were successfully managed with open reduction without arthrodesis and halo vest immobilization for 8 to 12 weeks.

ODONTOID FRACTURES

Fractures of the odontoid are among the most common injuries of the cervical spine in children. They occur at an average age of 4 years.[285] In contrast to fractures of the odontoid in adults, which occur at the base of the odontoid, these injuries in children are typically physeal fractures (Salter-Harris type I). These fractures tend to occur at a slightly lower level within the body of C2 through the dentocentral synchondrosis, joining the odontoid process to the body of the axis.[285]

They may occur after minor or major trauma. The dens typically displaces anteriorly in association with a flexion injury; however, hyperextension will produce posterior displacement. The anterior periosteal sleeve usually remains intact, blocking excessive displacement and stabilizing the fracture so that neural injury is unusual.[286] Recognition is the key to successful treatment of odontoid fractures in children. Lateral radiographs often demonstrate this fracture unless spontaneous reduction has occurred, in which case MRI or dynamic (flexion-extension) radiographs may be diagnostic.[287]

Fractures of the odontoid can usually be reduced by simply extending the head. Perfect anatomic reduction is not necessary as long as angulation is corrected and at least 50% apposition achieved. If satisfactory alignment cannot be achieved with simple positioning, head halter or skeletal traction is usually effective before immobilization in a Minerva or halo brace.[288] Healing predictably occurs in 6 to 12 weeks[285,287] (Fig. 10.18). When immobilization has been discontinued, lateral flexion-extension radiographs should be obtained to assess stability. Nonunion of these fractures in children is rare.

Odontoid fractures were classified by Anderson and D'Alonzo, where type 1 fractures are avulsions at the tip of the dens, type 2 fractures occur at the base of the dens, and type 3 fractures extend into the vertebral body.[289] Fractures of the odontoid in older children, after closure of the

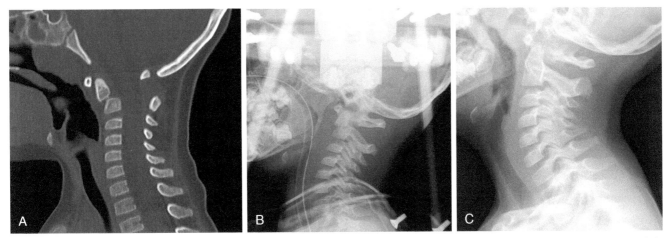

Fig. 10.18 A 3-year-old male, injured in a rollover motor vehicle accident. (A) Evaluation demonstrated a displaced physeal fracture of the odontoid. He was neurologically normal. (B) This was managed with closed reduction and halo vest immobilization. (C) The fracture healed uneventfully.

dentocentral synchondrosis (approximately 3–6 years of age), are more likely to occur at a slightly higher level, within the dens itself. These injuries are more like the type II fractures typically seen in adults. The vast majority of these fractures can be successfully managed nonoperatively by reduction and immobilization in a halo brace. Posterior C1-C2 fusion techniques are employed when external immobilization is unable to maintain acceptable alignment of the odontoid atop the C2 body or after failure of closed treatment, as demonstrated by persistent instability on flexion-extension views. Wang et al have demonstrated successful use of odontoid screw fixation for type II fractures with an intact transverse ligament in children older than 3 years.[290] Nonunions of odontoid fractures of any type treated with closed methods are unusual in children, whereas the nonunion rate in adults is approximately 30% for type 2 fractures and 0% to 8% for type 3 fractures.[291] In adults, risk factors for nonunion of type 2 odontoid fractures include advanced age and greater fracture displacement.[258] In the rare instance of odontoid nonunion in children and adolescents, posterior C1-C2 arthrodesis is indicated.

These acute injuries must be differentiated from os odontoideum. This abnormality of the odontoid is characterized by a hypoplastic apical segment of dens that is separated from the axis by a wide gap. There is debate about whether os odontoideum is a developmental abnormality or an acquired traumatic lesion.[292–294] Fielding reported three patients with normal radiographs of the odontoid who subsequently developed an os odontoideum following trauma.[293] There is an increased incidence of os odontoideum in Down syndrome, Klippel-Feil syndrome, multiple epiphyseal dysplasia, and spondyloepiphyseal dysplasia.[293,295] It is not known whether these conditions are congenitally predisposed to this abnormality or if it develops in these conditions because of altered biomechanics. Schuler has documented the development of an os odontoideum in a young girl who presented with neck pain following a significant fall. Serial radiographs were obtained over a 13-month period. At 4 months after the original injury, the dens had resorbed, and by 13 months, an os odontoideum had developed. The author postulated a vascular insult as the most likely etiology.[296]

Os odontoideum is characterized by a hypoplastic dens that is separated from the body of C2 and is essentially a separate ossicle. Children with os odontoideum may be asymptomatic but can demonstrate myelopathy, vertigo, or cardiorespiratory arrest, depending upon the amount of instability present.[297] A lateral radiograph of the cervical spine demonstrates a well-corticated ossicle above the body of the axis. CT scan with sagittal and coronal reconstructions can be used in the setting of trauma to differentiate an os from a fracture. Instability of the atlantoaxial joint has been reported in up to 83% of cases, and because the os is essentially a free-floating peg that allows C1 to move independently from C2, the instability can occur both anteriorly with flexion and posteriorly with extension.[293] Kinematic MRI of the cervical spine while the head is moved from full extension to flexion can provide a real-time view of the atlantoaxial joint and a more accurate picture of the instability pattern and dynamic spinal cord compression.[298] Neurologic symptoms with radiographic evidence of cord compression are a clear indication for surgical stabilization. Instability is also an indication for surgical treatment, even in the absence of symptoms, because catastrophic neurologic injuries have been reported after minor trauma when an os odontoideum is present.[299–302] C1-C2 fusion can be performed using interspinous wire, transarticular screw fixation, or segmental screw fixation (C1 lateral mass and C2 pars or lamina) (Fig. 10.19). Overreduction must be avoided when using wires because the os can be pulled posteriorly into the spinal canal by overtightening the wires. The fusion may be extended from the occiput to C2 if atlantoaxial fusion is not possible.[303]

HANGMAN FRACTURES

Traumatic spondylolisthesis of C2, also called a hangman fracture, is a relatively rare injury in children.[260] The mechanism of injury may be flexion or extension, combined with an axial or distractive load. Failure of the posterior elements of C2 can occur through the pars interarticularis, the pedicles, or, in younger children, the synchondroses of the pedicles.[304,305] If the forces responsible for disruption of the posterior elements are severe, horizontal tearing of the C2-C3 disk can occur with resultant instability.[250]

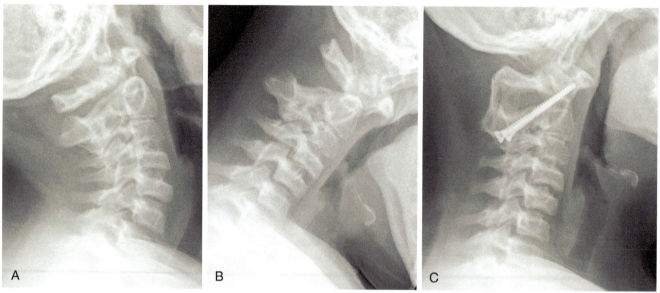

Fig. 10.19 A 9-year-old male with spondyloepiphyseal dysplasia and C1-2 instability secondary to os odontoideum. (A and B) At age 6 years, he had injured his neck in a fall from a slide; however, no imaging was obtained. He was asymptomatic; however, to prevent catastrophic neurologic injury, he was treated with posterior spinal fusion C1-C2 with transarticular screws. Sublaminar suture was used to stabilize iliac crest bone graft between the C1 and C2 posterior elements. (C) Lateral radiograph at 6 months postoperative.

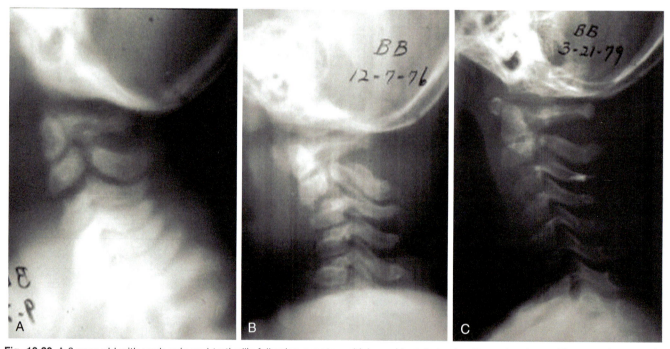

Fig. 10.20 A 3-year-old with neck pain and torticollis following a motor vehicle accident. Lateral radiographs show a Hangman fracture with injury through the synchondroses (A) that was successfully treated in a Minerva cast for 2 months (B) with excellent long-term result (C).

These fractures can be well visualized on a plain lateral radiograph of the cervical spine in approximately 90% of cases.[306] Radiographs show a lucency in the posterior arch of C2 immediately behind the articular surface of the lateral mass. Persistence of the synchondrosis of C2 is a normal developmental variant that can simulate traumatic spondylolisthesis and must be differentiated from this pathologic entity based on clinical criteria[307] (Fig. 10.20).

A modification of the Effendi classification is used to describe these fractures.[308] Type 1 injuries involve a fracture through the pars interarticularis with less than 3 mm of translation and angulation. The intervertebral disc and anterior longitudinal ligament remain intact. Type 2 fractures extend through the bilateral pedicles with greater than 3 mm of translation and angulation and are often associated with disruption of the C2-C3 disc and compression deformities of C2 or C3. Fractures of the type 2A subtype have minimal translation but significant angulation related to disruption of the disc and posterior longitudinal ligament. Type 2 atypical fractures demonstrate extension of the neural arch fracture line into the posterior vertebral body with unilateral or bilateral continuity of the posterior vertebral cortex or pedicle.[309] Type 3 fractures are unstable injuries involving fracture of the neural arch combined with unilateral or bilateral facet dislocation. The posterior longitudinal ligament and C2-C3 disc are disrupted.

Neurologic injury is rare because these fractures actually increase the SAC. The type 2 atypical fracture pattern is an exception, with a 33% incidence of neurologic deficit.[309] The atypical type 2 fractures produce neurologic injury via anterior translation of the anterior column while the spinal cord is compressed against the posterior vertebral body cortex, which remains in continuity with the posterior elements. Type 3 fractures are often associated with neurologic injury, as these unstable injures are produced by a flexion-distraction mechanism followed by hyperextension.

Type 1 injuries can be managed for 8 to 12 weeks with a hard collar. Type 2 fractures may be treated with traction to correct the flexion deformity and then immobilization in a halo vest. However, with type 2A fractures traction is dangerous because of the risk of overdistraction, and this variation should be managed with halo immobilization alone. Type 3 fractures require reduction of the facet dislocation with posterior arthrodesis of C2-C3. Posterior arthrodesis is only indicated for unstable fractures (type 3), or fractures that cannot be controlled by halo or Minerva cast immobilization, delayed union with instability, or established nonunion.[305]

LOWER CERVICAL SPINE INJURIES

Subaxial cervical spine injuries are more common in older children and adolescents as the cervical spine matures and begins to take on adult characteristics.[31] In a study by Evans of 24 consecutive cases of cervical spine injury in older children (average age was 13 years), 71% of the injuries involved C3-C7.[30] Dogan studied pediatric subaxial injuries and found that 80% occurred in children aged 9 to 16 years.[25] Mechanisms, in descending order of frequency, were motor vehicle accidents, sports injuries, falls, motor vehicle versus pedestrian injuries, and motorcycle accidents. Typical injuries in the subaxial cervical spine include both unilateral and bilateral facet subluxations or dislocations and a spectrum of fractures and/or ligamentous injuries with varying degrees of instability.

Ligamentous injuries are more common in children under age 8 years old but also occur, albeit with decreasing frequency, in older children. Flexion is the typical mechanism of injury. Clinically, these injuries present with pain posteriorly and a palpable gap between the spinous processes. Radiographs may show widening of the interspinous distance, loss of cervical lordosis, discontinuity of the spinolaminar line, and subluxation of the facet joints and vertebral bodies (Fig. 10.11). Subluxation of up to 4 mm at C2-C3 and 3 mm below this level may be normal.[100,162,200] MRI will usually demonstrate signal change within the ligament and surrounding soft tissues. These injuries can be treated initially with immobilization and, if continued instability is demonstrated by flexion-extension radiographs, then surgery.[310] Some would argue for direct surgical stabilization of these injuries given the unpredictable nature of ligament healing with nonoperative treatment and the excellent results following surgical stabilization.[19,51]

Compression fractures are the most common injuries of the subaxial spine in children. Flexion is the typical mechanism.

Radiographs show anterior wedging of the vertebral bodies with loss of height. Incomplete ossification of the vertebral bodies is a normal variant that may simulate the wedging associated with compression fractures and needs to be distinguished from the pathologic entity. This phenomenon is most commonly observed at C3.[14] These injuries, by definition, affect only the anterior column of the spine and are stable. They heal rapidly and require only 3 to 6 weeks of immobilization with a hard collar. If there is greater than 50% anterior wedging, disruption of the posterior ligamentous complex should be suspected and an MRI obtained.[250] These more unstable injuries often require a longer period of immobilization and should be given consideration for early surgical stabilization.[51]

Burst fractures occur when the spine is axially loaded in a nonflexed position (straight or lordotic). By definition, this injury must involve the middle column of the spine. These injuries are commonly secondary to motor vehicle accidents, contact or collision sports, falls from a height, or diving accidents. The most commonly injured levels are C6 and C7.[311] Conventional radiographs often underrepresent the extent of injury to the vertebral body and the amount of bone displaced into the spinal canal; therefore, a CT scan is a much more useful study if this injury is suspected. The stability of these fractures is dependent on the status of the posterior ligamentous complex. If there is suspicion of significant posterior ligamentous disruption or a neurologic deficit is present, an MRI should be obtained.

Allen et al have described three stages of vertical compression injuries. Stage 1 involves fracture of the superior or inferior end plate with minimal loss of height and no significant angular or translational deformity. Stage 2 is the same as stage 1, but both end plates are fractured. Stage 3 involves both end plates with fragmentation of the vertebral body, retropulsion, loss of height, and possible posterior ligamentous disruption.[311]

If the spinal canal is minimally compromised and neurologic function intact, these injuries may be treated by immobilization with rigid cervical collar, a sternal-occipital-mandibular immobilizer brace, or a halo vest for 12 weeks. If neurologic deficits or significant canal compromise are present or fracture alignment cannot be maintained, anterior decompression via corpectomy, interbody reconstruction, and plate fixation may be indicated. In a neurologically intact patient, posterior stabilization and arthrodesis alone can be considered. Posterior ligamentous instability is also an indication for operative stabilization (Fig. 10.21).

Flexion teardrop fractures are flexion compression injuries, commonly involving C4, C5, or C6. The mechanism is an axial load combined with a flexion force. These injuries are often the result of diving accidents, football spear tackling, or motor vehicle collisions. Approximately 90% of these fractures are associated with neurologic injury, with a higher rate of anterior cord syndrome as compared with other cervical injury patterns. Some 50% of these injuries produce quadriplegia.[312–314]

The key characteristic separating these fractures from burst fractures is the presence of the "teardrop" fracture line, running from the anterior cortex toward the inferior end plate and disc. Allen has classified these injuries into five stages.[311]

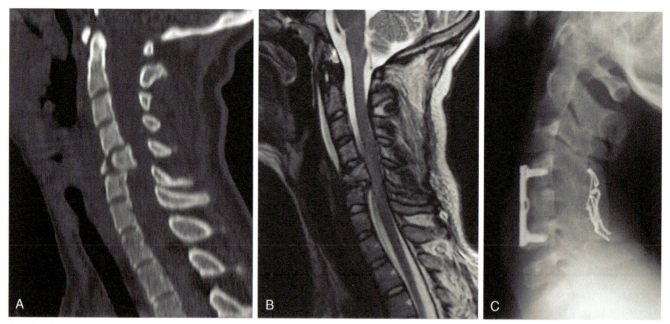

Fig. 10.21 A 13-year-old male who catapulted over the handlebars of his bike, landing on his head in a lake. (A and B) Sagittal computed tomography scan and magnetic resonance imaging show a C5 burst fracture. (C) He was treated with a C5 corpectomy and fusion with instrumentation followed by posterior interspinous process wiring and arthrodesis.

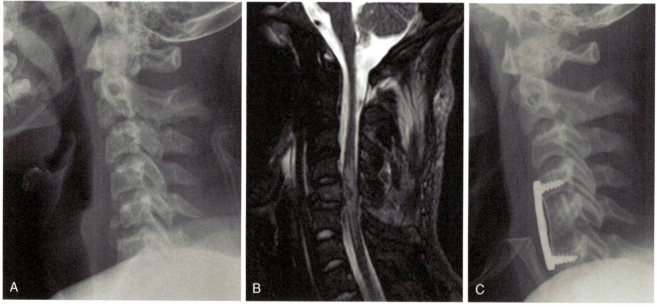

Fig. 10.22 A 14-year-old male injured in a diving accident. He presented with an incomplete spinal cord injury (American Spinal Injury Association [ASIA] B). Imaging demonstrated C5 flexion teardrop fracture with relative canal stenosis and associated intraneural hemorrhage. (A and B) Decompression was performed via C5 corpectomy with iliac crest strut grafting. (C) Over the next year, neurologic function improved to ASIA Impairment Scale C.

Nonoperative treatment may be considered for the neurologically intact patient with posterior ligamentous stability. Stage 1 and 2 fractures, with relatively intact anterior columns, may be managed with a rigid collar. After healing, flexion-extension films should confirm stability. For unstable injuries (most stage 3 and all stage 4 and 5), operative stabilization is recommended. Anterior corpectomy, interbody support, and plate fixation provides direct decompression in the setting of a neurologic deficit (Fig. 10.22). Supplemental posterior fixation may be required for extensive disruption of the posterior ligaments. Posterior instrumented arthrodesis alone may be considered for a neurologically intact patient where traction reduces the vertebral body retrolisthesis.

Vertebral apophyseal injuries are unique to children and adolescents. The usual mechanism is hyperextension, and the injury typically involves the inferior end plate. The uncinate processes are thought to protect the superior end plates from avulsion. In older children, these injuries are typically ring apophyseal fractures with minimal instability or neurologic compromise. They can usually be treated by immobilization and heal very rapidly. In younger children, they can involve a significant portion of the cartilaginous end plate and be associated with severe SCI. These injuries are rarely encountered clinically but have been described extensively at necropsy.[23]

Facet dislocations and fracture dislocations may occur in young children but are more common in older children and adolescents. These injuries are similar to their adult counterparts. The mechanism of injury is flexion and distraction, commonly the result of a fall from a height or other high-energy trauma. Unilateral injuries also involve a rotational force. Bilateral facet dislocations are very unstable and are associated with a higher incidence of neurologic injury than unilateral dislocations. Diagnosis can usually be made on lateral radiographs, which demonstrate anterior displacement of the inferior facet(s) and a variable amount of anterolisthesis (from 25%–50%) of the cephalad vertebral body on the next caudal level.[162] CT scans are useful to delineate an associated fracture. These flexion distraction injuries have been classified into four stages by Allen.[311] Stage 1 is a facet sprain with widening of the facet(s) and interspinous ligament. Stage 2 is a unilateral facet dislocation or fracture-dislocation. Stages 3 and 4 are bilateral facet dislocations or fracture-dislocations, with incomplete anterolisthesis in stage 3 and complete anterolisthesis in stage 4.

The majority of unilateral facet dislocations have a root deficit, and bilateral facet dislocations are frequently associated with complete spinal cord injuries.[162,315] Unilateral and bilateral facet dislocations can be reduced manually or with traction. Because there is a concern that an associated disc herniation can displace into the spinal canal and cause cord compression as the facets are reduced, it is recommended that reduction be performed with the patient awake and able to cooperate with serial neurological exams.[316] If the patient is comatose or has an altered mental status, an MRI should be obtained before reduction is attempted.

Reduction is performed by applying traction with Gardner Wells tongs or a halo ring, starting with 10 pounds of weight and sequentially increasing it in 5- to 10-pound increments. Lateral radiographs are obtained after each change in weight, and neurologic status is closely monitored. In bilateral dislocations, it is usually helpful to flex the neck slightly to unlock the facets and then to alter the traction vector into slight extension to allow the facets to reduce. Unilateral facet dislocations can be unlocked by flexion and rotation away from the dislocated facet followed by traction to reengage the superior facet. Although appropriate closed reduction and immobilization may obviate the need for surgery, the unpredictable nature of soft tissue healing and the risk of persistent instability make a strong argument for operative stabilization following reduction of these injuries.[51,162] The failure rate of halo immobilization for "perched" or locked facet injuries may approach 45%.[317] Facet dislocations that do not reduce by closed methods require open reduction and operative stabilization (Fig. 10.23). Two-level posterior arthrodesis with interspinous wire or lateral mass fixation can be considered and may be preferred if the dislocation was irreducible by closed reduction. Via the posterior approach, reduction may be achieved directly by carefully levering the dislocated cephalad facet over the caudad facet. Reduction may also be facilitated by resection of the superior portion of the caudad facet. Anterior cervical discectomy and fusion (ACDF) is preferred if there is loss of disc integrity and/or significant disc herniation. ACDF may also be advantageous to minimize fusion levels in the presence of a facet fracture that would preclude a two-level posterior arthrodesis.

PEDIATRIC HALO

Halo vest immobilization is being used with increasing frequency in children with cervical spine injuries. It affords superior immobilization to a rigid cervical collar and is easier to apply and more versatile than a Minerva cast. It permits access for skin and wound care while avoiding the skin problems (maceration, ulceration) typically associated with both hard collars and casts.[139–141,318,319] However, complication rates as high as 68% have been reported with pediatric halo use.[318] Similar complication rates have been noted in a younger, toddler-age group of younger than 3 years.[320,321] The most common problems are pin site infections, but skull perforation and brain abscesses have also been reported.[318] The thickness of the skull in children is decreased and, in children under age 6 years old, can vary considerably. Letts et al have suggested that CT scan of the skull to measure calvarial thickness can be helpful in determining optimal sites for pin placement, particularly in children under 6 years old.[322] Halo pin designs with a wide flange and short tip may reduce the risk of skull penetration.[323]

In children over 6 years old, the standard adult halo construct utilizing four pins (two anterolaterally, two posterolaterally) inserted at standard torques of 6 to 8 inch-pounds generally works. The two anterior pins are placed 1 cm above the eyebrow in the outer two-thirds of the orbit. Insertion more medially places the supratrochlear and supraorbital nerves at risk, and placement more laterally puts the pins in the temporalis region where the bone can be very thin. The optimal position for the posterior pins is above the ear approximately in line with the mastoid process. In younger children, more pins (up to 12) placed with lower insertional torques (2 to 4 inch-pounds) have been advocated[319,320] (Fig. 10.24).

In adolescents, pins should be retightened at 24 to 48 hours. Pins should be checked for loosening at each postoperative visit. The most common complication of halo immobilization in children is pin site infection; therefore, meticulous pin care should be performed daily.[318] Standard pediatric halo rings fit most children, but custom rings may be needed for infants and toddlers. Although standard pediatric halo vests are available, custom vests or body casts generally provide superior immobilization, particularly in very young children.[319] In toddlers, activity should be restricted during treatment, as falls in a halo vest are common and may produce injury.[321]

THORACOLUMBAR FRACTURES

Thoracic, lumbar, and sacral fractures are relatively uncommon in children.[324] The majority of these injuries are caused by motor vehicle accidents, pedestrian-vehicular accidents, or falls. The most common injuries are compression fractures and flexion-distraction injuries. Apophyseal

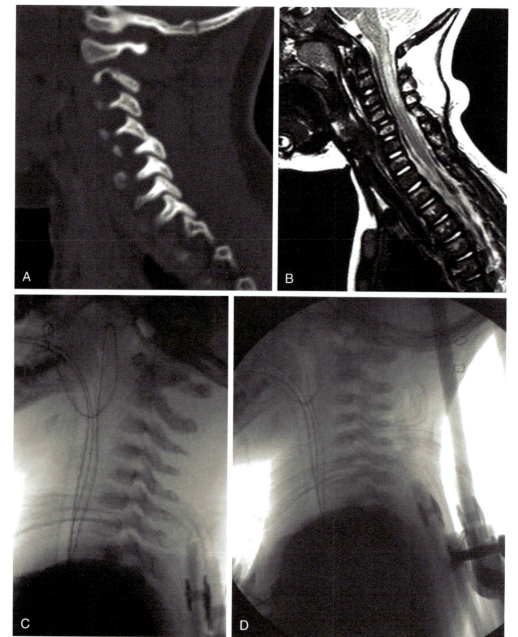

Fig. 10.23 A 19-month-old male struck by a car. He had paresis of his right upper extremity. (A) Computed tomography traumagram sagittal reconstruction shows a unilateral C4/5 facet dislocation on the right side. (B) Magnetic resonance imaging shows significant intraneural signal change. (C) Attempts at closed reduction with halo traction and by manipulation were unsuccessful, as demonstrated under fluoroscopy by the residual anterolisthesis of C4 on C5. (D) Open reduction was performed and stabilization achieved by interspinous fixation with an absorbable suture and halo.

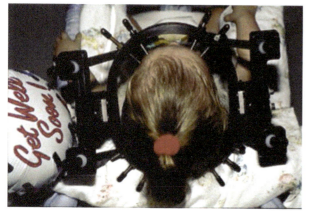

Fig. 10.24 A 2.5-year-old child with halo. A total of 10 pins were placed at a lower insertional torque of 2 to 4 inch-lb.

endplate fractures are injuries that are unique to older children and teenagers whose symptoms mimic disc herniation. In infants and young children, NAT (child abuse) may be a cause of significant spinal trauma.[36,325] Avulsion fractures of the spinous processes, fractures of the pars or pedicles, ligamentous injury, or compression fractures of multiple vertebral bodies are common patterns of injury that usually occur from severe shaking or battering. These injuries may be associated with other signs of child abuse including fractures of the skull, ribs, or long bones and cutaneous lesions.

Patients with thoracic or lumbar fractures often present with midline or paravertebral musculature tenderness, and this physical finding alone has a sensitivity of 87% and a specificity of 75%.[68] Noncontiguous fractures are common, and neurological deficits are present in about 25%.[1,64,68] Associated injuries are common in greater than 50% of patients, particularly extremities, head, neck, and thorax.[27] Close examination of the thorax and abdomen should be performed to rule out possible visceral or mesenteric injuries, particularly when there are chest or abdominal contusions from lap or seat belts.[62]

The classification system most often used to describe thoracic and lumbar spine fractures in children is the one described by Denis for adult fractures.[326] This system introduced the concept of the three-column spine (anterior, middle, and posterior), placing particular emphasis on mode of failure to the middle column to stratify fracture types and risk of neurologic injury. According to this classification system, the four major types of fractures are compression, burst, flexion/distraction (Chance fractures), and fracture-dislocation injuries.

When operative treatment is required for unstable TL fractures, instrumentation and arthrodesis is commonly performed. However, temporary percutaneous pedicle screw stabilization without arthrodesis has been described in adolescents in an effort to minimize long-term morbidity associated with fusion.[327]

Transverse and spinous process fractures of the TL spine are common injuries. Isolated fractures are not associated with neurologic injury or spinal instability, however, but are frequently associated with solid organ injuries. Approximately 95% pediatric and adolescents with isolated fractures have injuries in other systems.[328] These fractures may be managed conservatively with analgesics and short-term bracing if required for comfort.

Compression fractures of the TL spine are relatively common. These injuries are caused by a combination of hyperflexion and axial compression. Because the disk in children is stronger than the cancellous bone, the vertebral body is the first structure in the spinal column to fail. The fractures may be classified by the direction of applied load and resultant deformity (anterior or lateral).[326] It is common for children to sustain multiple compression fractures.[68,324] Most fractures are visible on lateral radiographs, although evidence may be subtle. A difference in height of more than 3 mm between the anterior and posterior cortices of a given vertebral body causes the body to appear wedged and indicates a true fracture.[29] Compression rarely exceeds more than 20% of the vertebral body. The amount of kyphosis can be accurately determined by the Cobb method, which has been shown to be a very reproducible method of quantifying deformity.[329] Based on findings in cadaveric studies, when loss of vertebral body height exceeds 50%, the possibility of injury to the posterior column of the spine should be considered.[330] Integrity of the posterior ligamentous complex can be assessed by looking for interspinous widening or loss of parallelism of the facet joints. If there is any question of an injury, a CT scan or MRI can be helpful in identifying potential bony or soft tissue disruption of the posterior column. When there is concern that osteopenia may be contributing factor to the compression fracture(s), endocrinology evaluation and assessment of bone density is appropriate. Infectious, inflammatory, and neoplastic conditions should also be considered as potential contributors to TL compression deformities, particularly if there is not a history of trauma.

The majority of these fractures can be managed conservatively with rest, analgesics, and possible bracing with a TLSO for 4 to 6 weeks. Upright x-rays should be obtained to confirm stability with closed treatment. Surgical stabilization may rarely be indicated if there is posterior column involvement and instability. Additionally, operative treatment may be considered if there is excessive local kyphosis (30–40 degrees), which more commonly occurs in the setting of multilevel compression fractures.

Age-dependent remodeling of TL compression fractures has been observed.[207,331,332] With nonoperative treatment of stable fractures, vertebral height will more readily reconstitute in the sagittal plane than in the coronal plane in skeletally immature patients, particularly if the Risser sign is 2 or less.[207,333] When the focal deformity caused by the fracture is more than 10 degrees, brace treatment has been found to be more effective than not using a brace with regard to final alignment in children followed to skeletal maturity. When the deformity is less than 10 degrees, bracing makes no difference in the final outcome, although it may still be a valid treatment acutely, from a symptomatic standpoint. In contrast, Singer et al noted that the use of bracing regimen did not influence the remodeling capacity of stable compression fractures.[331] Posttraumatic scoliosis has been noted after TL compression fractures.[334] Risk factors for greater deformity include increased skeletal maturity at the time of injury (Risser grade ≥3), lumbar fracture, and single fractures.

Burst fractures are also rare injuries in children that result from a combination of axial compression and flexion. They are most common in adolescents and often occur at the TL junction or in the lumbar spine.[335–337] These fractures are characterized by disruption of the middle column of the spine and retropulsion of a variable amount of bone into the spinal canal and neural foramina, although the amount of canal compromise does not correlate with neurologic deficit or clinical outcome.[338] Thoracic level burst fractures are more commonly associated with neurologic injury.[339]

Subtle findings on conventional radiography include interpedicular widening on the AP view, loss of posterior height, and small cortical defects at the posterior-superior corner of the vertebral body on the lateral projection. CT has been shown to be superior to conventional radiographs in evaluating these fractures and guiding treatment.[340] Integrity of the posterior ligamentous complex may be assessed with radiographs, CT, or MRI.[341]

The Denis classification of burst fractures includes type A fractures, which involve rupture of both end plates. A single end plate is ruptured in type B (superior end plate) and type C (inferior end plate) fractures.[326,342] Type D combines a type A fracture with rotational deformity, and type E is an eccentrically loaded type A, B, or C fracture with lateral flexion deformity. Fractures may be considered unstable with three-column disruption, anterior cortical collapse greater than 50%, focal kyphosis greater than 20 degrees, and progressive neurologic deficit. Other factors that may predict instability include greater degrees of retropulsion (>50%), laminar fracture, facet subluxation, and disruption of the posterior ligamentous complex.[338,343] Translation of the vertebral body greater than 3.5 mm may predict failure of the posterior ligamentous complex.[344]

The need for operative treatment is determined by the stability of the fracture and the presence of neurologic deficits. In neurologically intact children, nonoperative treatment by

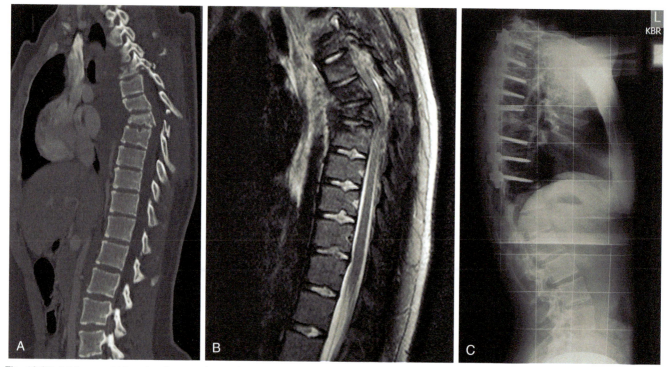

Fig. 10.25 A 14-year-old female who was thrown from a trailer towed behind an all-terrain vehicle. She presented with a complete spinal cord injury. Imaging demonstrated three-column fractures at T4 and T7. (A and B) She underwent urgent reduction and instrumented arthrodesis from T2-T10. (C) Neurologic function gradually normalized, and she has returned to sports.

immobilization in a custom molded TLSO for 8 to 12 weeks is a viable option. Confirmation of stability needs to be done by obtaining upright AP and lateral x-rays after application of the brace. A significant amount of bony remodeling of the vertebral body can be expected, leading to reconstitution of the spinal canal over time; however, it has also been shown that most children will develop a mild progressive angular deformity at the fracture site during the first year after the injury.[15,335] It has been demonstrated that operative stabilization of these fractures prevents this kyphotic deformity from occurring and also decreases the length of hospitalization.[335,339]

Children with neurologic deficits should undergo decompression and stabilization through either an anterior or posterior (transpedicular) approach. All fractures that are mechanically unstable should be treated operatively with posterior instrumentation and fusion (Fig. 10.25). In patients without neurologic deficit, posterior instrumentation *without* arthrodesis is a consideration, functioning as a temporary internal splint to allow fracture healing.[345,346] Unstable fractures should be stabilized one to two levels above and below the site of injury in most instances. In patients with complete neurological injuries, longer constructs should be considered in an attempt to avoid the problem of paralytic deformity.[13]

A higher failure rate may be anticipated if short segment posterior constructs are used without anterior support associated with significant anterior column disruption.[347–349] Circumferential short segment arthrodesis has been successful in adolescents and is beneficial to maintain a greater number of mobile segments in the lumbar spine.[350] This technique uses hybrid posterior instrumentation one level above and below the fractured vertebrae with pedicle screws and sublaminar implants followed by staged anterior structural support. Alternatively, a transforaminal lumbar interbody fusion may be performed to provide anterior structural support with short segment posterior instrumentation. In the setting of a neurologic deficit, the posterior transpedicular approach allows direct neural decompression, anterior column reconstruction with interbody support, and circumferential arthrodesis with posterior instrumentation.[351]

Fracture-dislocations of the spine are unstable injuries that usually occur at the TL junction and often are associated with neurologic deficits. Denis classified three patterns of injury: flexion-rotation, shear, and flexion-distraction.[326] These are rare injuries in children that always require rigid instrumentation and arthrodesis.[15] Instrumentation should extend at least two levels above and below the injury; longer constructs may be considered in the setting of SCI.

Flexion-distraction injuries (or seat belt injuries) occur in the upper lumbar spine in children wearing a seat belt.[352] This injury pattern was first described by G.Q. Chance in 1948.[353] With sudden deceleration, the belt slides up on the abdomen, where it acts as a fulcrum. As the spine rotates around this axis, it fails in tension, resulting primarily in disruption of the posterior column with variable patterns of extension into the middle and anterior column. The upper lumbar spine is commonly involved, particularly L2 and L3.

The "seat belt syndrome" was described in 1962 by Garrett and Braunstein, who recognized the triad of a "seat belt sign" (abdominal wall abrasion, ecchymosis, contusion), visceral injury, and lumbar spine injury.[354] The presence of an abdominal wall contusion is associated with intraabdominal injury in up to 75% and a vertebral fracture in approximately 50%[355] (Fig. 10.26). Up to two-thirds of Chance fractures have associated intraabdominal injuries, which may lead to

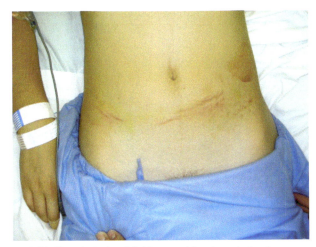

Fig. 10.26 "Seat belt sign." A 16-year-old male restrained passenger involved in a motor vehicle accident sustained a T12/ L1 flexion-distraction injury; physical examination showed contusion of the abdomen from the seatbelt. At laparotomy, he was found to have a mesenteric tear. The fracture was treated by open reduction and fusion with pedicle screw instrumentation.

delayed diagnosis of the vertebral fracture. Commonly injured organs include small bowel, colon, stomach and duodenum, pancreas, and kidney. Ruptures of internal organs, aortic injuries, and mesenteric tears may be life-threatening if not diagnosed and treated appropriately.[356,357] Diaphragmatic avulsion has also been reported.[358]

Neurologic injury with Chance fractures is noted more commonly in children than adults, with reported paraplegia rates of 15%[356] and variable neurologic deficits of 20% to 43%.[359,360] Arkader noted permanent neurologic deficits in 10% of restrained patients and 42% of unrestrained.[359] Blunt abdominal aortic injury uncommon, but has a mortality rate of 18% to 37% and has been associated with pediatric Chance fractures.[357,361,362] If neurovascular abnormalities are incorrectly attributed to the spine fracture, an aortic injury may be overlooked, with potentially devastating consequences. The injury may be recognized by abdominal CT scan or by the presence of lower extremity ischemia with variable neurologic deficit. Early recognition is critical to avoid amputation, paralysis, or mortality.

Chance fractures in children may occur with the use of two-point restraints (lap belt), with improperly applied three-point restraints (misuse of shoulder strap), or even with proper use of a three-point restraint.[363] In a review of seat belt syndrome among Canadian children, only 18% were properly restrained based upon age-specific recommendations.[364] Booster seat use for appropriate-age children may reduce the vulnerability to the seat belt syndrome and decrease the risk of injury by 59%.[365,366]

A lateral radiograph demonstrated widening of the interspinous space is the most helpful study in diagnosing this fracture. An increased distance between the spinous processes may occasionally be seen on the AP x-ray. Because of the transverse plane of orientation of this group of injuries, abnormalities may be missed by thick-section axial CT scanning and may not be detected even with complementary thin sections unless sagittal reconstructions are included (Fig. 10.27). MRI may be the single best imaging modality

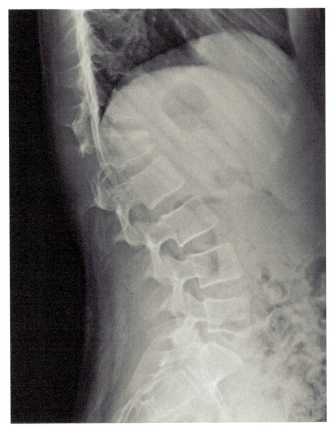

Fig. 10.27 Missed Chance fracture. An 11-year-old female was a backseat restrained passenger in a rollover motor vehicle accident. She was evaluated at an outside hospital with a computed tomography traumagram that was interpreted as normal. The CT scan did not include sagittal reconstructions of the lumbar spine. She presented a week later with persistent back pain and an L1 flexion-distraction injury.

because it can accurately identify the extent of posterior ligament injury and identify disc herniation.[138]

Four patterns of injury have been described by Rumball and Jarvis.[356] In simplistic terms, these injuries can be divided into those that propagate primarily through soft tissue structures and those that occur mostly through bony elements. Type A is a bony disruption of the posterior elements extending to a variable degree into the middle column. Type B is an avulsion of the spinous process with facet joint disruption or fracture and extension into the vertebral apophysis. Type C is a disruption of the interspinous ligament with a fracture of the pars interarticularis extending into the body. Type D is a posterior ligamentous disruption with laminar fracture and disruption of the vertebral apophysis.

Lap belt injuries with mostly osseous involvement and kyphosis less than 20 degrees may be treated nonoperatively with hyperextension casting or bracing for 8 to 12 weeks. A cast may be applied after the concern for ileus has passed.[367] Stability is confirmed with standing radiographs following cast/brace application, and healing is confirmed with flexion and extension radiographs at the termination of treatment. Glassman found that all cases with successful nonoperative management had less than 20 degrees of kyphosis at presentation.[368] LeGay noted that kyphosis of greater than 17 degrees was associated with a poor prognosis.[369]

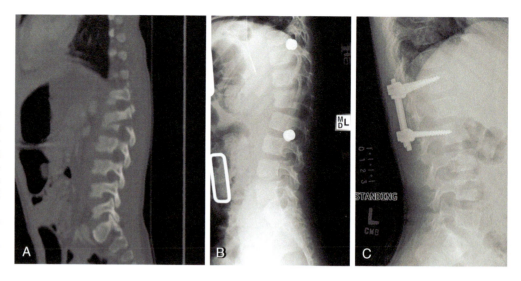

Fig. 10.28 A 5-year-old male injured by a lap belt restraint in a motor vehicle accident. He sustained an L1 flexion-distraction injury without intrabdominal injury. (A) Despite an extension orthosis, upright films demonstrated unacceptable local kyphosis (B). He underwent instrumentation without arthrodesis from T12-L2. (C) Implants were removed after the fracture was healed.

Relative operative indications include associated abdominal injuries, neurologic injury, or patient inability to tolerate an external orthosis or cast. When the injury pattern is predominantly soft tissue with posterior ligamentous disruption, operative stabilization with posterior instrumentation and arthrodesis is recommended. Instrumentation without arthrodesis can be considered in younger patients with subsequent implant removal to preserve lumbar motion (Fig. 10.28). Interspinous process wiring and casting may be sufficient in younger children, whereas hook or pedicle screw constructs are more appropriate in older children.[368] Short-segment constructs may be protected postoperatively with an orthotic. If there is an associated disc herniation, excision may be indicated to minimize the risk of neurologic injury when the fracture is reduced with compression instrumentation.[370]

A multicenter retrospective review of 35 pediatric Chance fractures with mean 3-year follow-up compared outcomes between patients treated operatively and nonoperatively, defining a good outcome as absence of chronic pain or neurologic deficit.[359] Good outcomes were noted in 84% of operatively treated fractures (mean initial kyphosis of 22 degrees) in comparison with 45% of nonoperative fractures (mean initial kyphosis of 11 degrees). The authors concluded that surgical treatment is preferred with significant initial deformity, posterior ligamentous injury, or associated injuries.

Fracture of the vertebral end plate (slipped vertebral apophysis) may occur in adolescents and young adults. It is characterized by traumatic disruption of the vertebral ring apophysis and disk with extrusion into the spinal canal. A number of descriptors for this condition have been used, including "avulsed vertebral rim apophysis," "limbus vertebral fracture," "lumbar posterior marginal node," and "posterior rim apophysis fracture." Younger patients may be more susceptible to this injury, as the fusion of the ring apophysis may remain incomplete until the ages of 18 to 25 years[371]; however, the entity has been reported in patients with an age range from 8 to 69 years and described as "posterior apophyseal ring separation."[372,373] The reported incidence of apophyseal fracture among children and adolescents with lumbar disc herniation is between 5.8% and 38% as compared with 5.4% to 11% in adults.[372,374–376,377,378] The injury occurs at L4-L5 or L5-S1 in 92% of cases, typically involving the superior end plate,

whereas the inferior end plate may be more susceptible in the upper lumbar region.[373] The entity has been noted more commonly in males at a ratio of 2.85 to 1,[373] which may be related to the common mechanisms of injury, including sports, weightlifting, shoveling, gymnastics, and trauma.

The clinical symptoms are essentially the same as a herniated disk and include back and leg pain, muscle spasm, and root tension signs; neurologic signs such as muscle weakness, sensory changes, and absent reflexes may be present as well. Patients with significant stenosis may describe symptoms consistent with neurogenic claudication; however, cauda equina dysfunction is uncommon.[373] These injuries may be purely cartilaginous with herniation of the apophysis and disk, or osseous with fractures of the cortical and cancellous rim of the vertebral body. This injury may be identified on plain radiographs in 16% to 69%; however, the findings may be subtle.[373] Cross-sectional imaging is needed to make the diagnosis. CT and CT-myelography have been found to be the superior study in evaluating this pathology, with intermediate sensitivity for MRI.[379,380] MRI may miss 78% of fractures.[381] The modified Takata classification includes four types: (1) central avulsion of the posterior cortical vertebral rim, (2) central avulsion of the posterior cortical vertebral rim with cancellous fragment, (3) localized lateral teardrop fragment, and (4) central cortical avulsion extending the full length of the posterior vertebral margin from superior to inferior end plate.[382,383] Type 3 fragments have been subclassified into calcified and noncalcified lesions. The noncalcified type 3 fragment may mimic a simple disc herniation on CT and MRI.[381] Another method classification of the apophyseal fracture is based upon location (central or lateral) and size (small or large), where large lesions are greater than 50% of the posterior vertebral body width.[375,377]

Nonoperative management is not always successful, and for intractable pain, dysfunction, or neurologic deficit, the preferred treatment is removal of the bony and cartilaginous fragments. This usually requires a more extensive exposure (bilateral laminotomies, hemilaminectomy, or occasionally a full laminectomy) than a simple disc excision.[379] Removal of the apophyseal fragment is not always required. Epstein advocated for removal of the bone fragment if a neurologic deficit was present, and others have recommended removal of mobile bone fragments; otherwise, decompression with

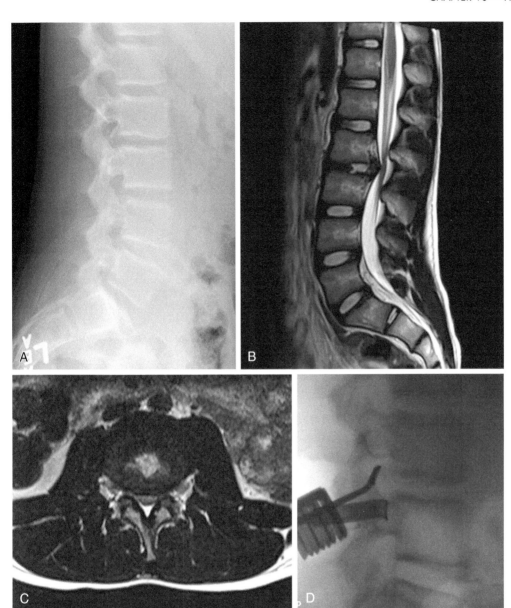

Fig. 10.29 A 14-year-old male experienced acute back pain during a football game and subsequently developed radicular bilateral leg pain without weakness. Three months following the injury, radiographs (A) and magnetic resonance imaging (B) and (C) demonstrate slipped vertebral apophysis at L2-L3. Conservative therapy was unsuccessful because of the significant stenosis, and he underwent bilateral partial laminectomy with excision of the slipped apophysis. Reverse-angled curettes and tamps were used during piecemeal resection of the ossified apophyseal fragment (D). His pain and radicular symptoms resolved.

discectomy may be adequate.[384] In general, the goal should be removal of bone, cartilage, and disc fragments to achieve adequate neural decompression and avoid late spinal stenosis because of retained bone or cartilaginous material. Resection of the apophyseal fragments requires a different technique than standard discectomy with the use of piecemeal resection with reverse angled curettes and tamp and mallet technique[379] (Fig. 10.29). Local arthrodesis may be considered in the setting of preoperative segmental instability, multiple level laminectomy, or if an extended facetectomy is required of greater than 50% of the facet joints.[385-387]

Favorable long-term outcomes after conservative or operative treatment of lumbar apophyseal lesions have been reported.[388] In this series, most patients had no permanent neurologic deficits and returned to sports or normal daily activity; however, 50% developed degenerative changes in the disc and vertebral body on MRI. In those patients initially managed conservatively, resorption of the retropulsed bone fragments did not occur with the concern for eventual symptomatic spinal stenosis. Another long-term follow-up study of adolescent lumbar disc herniation and apophyseal fractures found that patients with large apophyseal lesions managed conservatively had a greater frequency of chronic back pain with limitations of activities of daily living.[377]

REFERENCES

The level of evidence (LOE) is determined according to the criteria provided in the Preface.

1. Cirak B, Ziegfeld S, Knight VM, Chang D, Avellino AM, Paidas CN. Spinal injuries in children. *J Pediatr Surg.* 2004;39(4):607–612. (**LOE IV**).
2. Kokoska ER, Keller MS, Rallo MC, Weber TR. Characteristics of pediatric cervical spine injuries. *J Pediatr Surg.* 2001;36(1):100–105. (**LOE IV**).
3. Patel JC, Tepas JJ 3rd, Mollitt DL, Pieper P. Pediatric cervical spine injuries: defining the disease. *J Pediatr Neurosurg.* 2001;36(2):373–376. (**LOE IV**).
4. Partrick DA, Bensard DD, Moore EE, Calkins CM, Karrer FM. Cervical spine trauma in the injured child: a tragic injury with potential for salvageable functional outcome. *J Pediatr Surg.* 2000;35(11):1571–1575. (**LOE IV**).

5. Nuckley DJ, Ching RP. Developmental biomechanics of the cervical spine: tension and compression. *J Biomech*. 2006;39(16):3045–54. (**LOE N/A**).

6. Ouyang J, Zhu Q, Zhao W, Xu Y, Chen W, Zhong S. Biomechanical assessment of the pediatric cervical spine under bending and tensile loading. *Spine*. 2005;30(24):716–723. (**LOE IV**).

7. Luck JF, et al. Tensile failure properties of the perinatal, neonatal, and pediatric cadaveric cervical spine. *Spine (Phila Pa 1976)*. 2013;38(1):E1–E12. (**LOE N/A**).

8. Bailey DK. The normal cervical spine in infants and children. *Radiology*. 1952;59:712–719. (**LOE III**).

9. Herman MJ, Pizzutillo PD. Cervical spine disorders in children. *Orthop Clin N America*. 1999;30:457–466. (**LOE V**).

10. Bohn D, Armstrong D, Becker L, Humphreys R. Cervical spine injuries in children. *J Trauma*. 1990;30(4):463–469. (**LOE IV**).

11. Yamazaki A, Mason DE, Caro PA. Age of closure of the neurocentral cartilage in the thoracic spine. *J Pediatr Orthop*. 1998;18(2):168–172. (**LOE N/A**).

12. Edelson JG, Nathan H. Stages in the natural history of the vertebral end-plates. *Spine*. 1988;13(1):21–26. (**LOE N/A**).

13. Clark P, Letts M. Trauma to the thoracic and lumbar spine in the adolescent. *Can J Surg*. 2001;44(5):337–345. (**LOE V**).

14. Swischuk LE, Swischuk PN, John SD. Wedging of C-3 in infants and children: usually a normal finding and not a fracture. *Radiology*. 1993;188(2):523–526. (**LOE III**).

15. Akbarnia BA. Pediatric spine fractures. *Orthop Clin N America*. 1999;30:521–536. (**LOE V**).

16. Roche C, Carty H. Spinal trauma in children. *Pediatr Radiology*. 2001;31:677–700. (**LOE V**).

17. Murphy MJ, Ogden JA, Bucholz RW. Cervical spine injury in the child. *Contemp Orthop*. 1981;3:615–623. (**LOE V**).

18. Eleraky MA, Theodore N, Adams M, Rekate HL, Sonntag VK. Pediatric cervical spine injuries: report of 102 cases and review of the literature. *J Neurosurg Spine*. 2000;92(1):12–17. (**LOE IV**).

19. Finch GD, Barnes MJ. Major cervical spine injuries in children and adolescents. *J Pediatr Orthop*. 1998;18(6):811–814. (**LOE IV**).

20. Duhem R, et al. Unstable upper pediatric cervical spine injuries: report of 28 cases and review of the literature. *Childs Nerv Syst*. 2008;24(3):343–348. (**LOE IV**).

21. Mendoza-Lattes S, et al. Pediatric spine trauma in the United States–analysis of the HCUP Kid's Inpatient Database (KID) 1997-2009. *Iowa Orthop J*. 2015;35:135–139. (**LOE III**).

22. Piatt JH Jr. Pediatric spinal injury in the US: epidemiology and disparities. *J Neurosurg Pediatr*. 2015;16(4):463–471. (**LOE IV**).

23. Aufdermaur M. Spinal injuries in juveniles: necropsy findings in twelve cases. *J Bone Joint Surg*. 1974;56(Br):513–519. (**LOE IV**).

24. Givens TG, Polley KA, Smith GF, Hardin WD Jr. Pediatric cervical spine injury: a three-year experience. *J Trauma*. 1996;41(2):310–314. (**LOE IV**).

25. Dogan S, et al. Pediatric subaxial cervical spine injuries: origins, management, and outcome in 51 patients. *Neurosurg Focus*. 2006;20(2). (**LOE IV**).

26. Orenstein JB, Klein BL, Gotschall CS, Ochsenschlager DW, Klatzko MD, Eichelberger MR. Age and outcome in pediatric cervical spine injury: 11-year experience. *Pediatr Emer Care*. 1994;10(3):132–137. (**LOE IV**).

27. Rush JK, et al. Associated injuries in children and adolescents with spinal trauma. *J Pediatr Orthop*. 2013;33(4):393–397. (**LOE IV**).

28. Brown RL, Brunn MA, Garcia VF. Cervical spine injuries in children: a review of 103 patients treated consecutively at a level 1 pediatric trauma center. *J Pediatr Surg*. 2001;36(8):1107–1114. (**LOE IV**).

29. Dietrich AM, Ginn-Pease ME, Bartkowski HM, King DR. Pediatric cervical spine fractures: predominantly subtle presentation. *J Pediatr Surg*. 1991;26(8):995–1000. (**LOE IV**).

30. Evans DL, Bethem D. Cervical spine injuries in children. *J Pediatr Orthop*. 1989;9:563–568. (**LOE IV**).

31. McGrory BJ, Klassen RA, Chao EY, Staeheli JW, Weaver AL. Acute fractures and dislocations of the cervical spine in children and adolescents. *J Bone Joint Surg*. 1993;75A(7):988–995. (**LOE IV**).

32. Niticki S, Moir CR. Predictive factors of the outcome of traumatic cervical spine fracture in children. *J Pediatr Surg*. 1994;29:1409–1411. (**LOE IV**).

33. Meehan 3rd WP, Mannix R. A substantial proportion of life-threatening injuries are sport-related. *Pediatr Emerg Care*. 2013;29(5):624–627. (**LOE IV**).

34. Leonard JR, et al. Cervical spine injury patterns in children. *Pediatrics*. 2014;133(5):e1179–e1188. (**LOE IV**).

35. Polk-Williams A, Carr BG, Blinman TA, et al. Cervical spine injury in young children: a National Trauma Data Bank review. *J Pediatr Surg*. 2008;43(9):1718–1721. (**LOE IV**).

36. Knox J, Schneider J, Wimberly RL, Riccio AI. Characteristics of spinal injuries secondary to nonaccidental trauma. *J Pediatr Orthop*. 2013;29:29. (**LOE IV**).

37. Knox JB, Schneider JE, Cage JM, et al. Spine trauma in very young children: a study of 186 patients presenting to a level 1 pediatric trauma center. *J Pediatr Orthop*. 2014;34(7):698–702.

38. Caffey J. The whiplash shaken infant syndrome. *Pediatrics*. 1974;54:396. (**LOE IV**).

39. Ranjith RK, Mullett JH, Burke TE. Hangman's fracture caused by suspected child abuse. *J Pediatr Orthop*. 2002;11:329–332. (**LOE IV**).

40. Swischuk LE. Spine and spinal cord trauma in the battered child syndrome. *Radiology*. 1969;92:733–738. (**LOE IV**).

41. Rooks VJ, Sisler C, Burton B. Cervical spine injury in child abuse: report of two cases. *Pediatr Radiology*. 1998;28:193–195. (**LOE IV**).

42. Vialle R, et al. Spinal fracture through the neurocentral synchondrosis in battered children: a report of three cases. *Spine*. 1976;31(11):E345–E349. (**LOE IV**).

43. Vogel LC. Unique management needs of pediatric spinal cord injury in patients: etiology and pathophysiology. *J Spinal Cord Med*. 1997;20:10–13. (**LOE V**).

44. Burke DC. Spinal cord trauma in children. *Paraplegia*. 1970;8:1–4. (**LOE IV**).

45. Stein WE, Rand RW. Birth injuries to the spinal cord: a report of two cases and review of the literature. *Am J Ob Gyn*. 1959;78:498–512. (**LOE IV**).

46. Towbin A. Central nervous system damage in human fetus and newborn infants. *American J Dis Child*. 1970;119:529–541. (**LOE IV**).

47. Bresnan MJ, Adams IF. Neonatal spinal cord transection secondary to intrauterine hyperextension of the neck in breech presentation. *J Pediatr*. 1974;84(5):734. (**LOE IV**).

48. Leventhal HR. Birth injuries of the spinal cord. *J Pediatr*. 1960;56:447–453. (**LOE IV**).

49. Shulman ST, Madden JD, Esterly JR, Shanklin DR. Transection of spinal cord. A rare obstetrical complication of cephalic delivery. *Arch Dis Child*. 1971;46:291–294. (**LOE V**).

50. MacKinnon JA, Perlman M, Kirpalani H, Rehan V, Sauve R, Kovacs L. Spinal cord injury at birth: diagnostic and prognostic data in twenty-two patients. *J Pediatr*. 1993;122:431–437. (**LOE IV**).

51. Jones E, Haid R. Injuries to the pediatric subaxial cervical spine. *Seminars in Spine Surgery*. Vol. 3. Philadelphia: W.B. Saunders Company; 1991:61–70.

52. Rossitch E Jr, Oakes WJ. Perinatal spinal cord injury. *Pediatr Neurosurg*. 1992;18:149–152. (**LOE IV**).

53. Fotter R, Sorantin E, Schneider U, Ranner G, Fast C, Schober P. Ultrasound diagnosis of birth-related spinal cord trauma: neonatal diagnosis and follow-up and correlation with MRI. *Pediatr Rad*. 1994;24:241–244. (**LOE IV**).

54. Caird MS, et al. Cervical spine fracture-dislocation birth injury: prevention, recognition, and implications for the orthopaedic surgeon. *J Pediatr Orthop*. 2005;25(4):484–486. (**LOE V**).

55. Sasser SM, et al. Guidelines for field triage of injured patients: recommendations of the National Expert Panel on Field Triage. *MMWR Recomm Rep, 2012*. 2011;61(Rr-1):1–20. (**LOE V**).

56. Anders JF, et al. Comparison of outcomes for children with cervical spine injury based on destination hospital from scene of injury. *Acad Emerg Med*. 2014;21(1):55–64. (**LOE IV**).

57. Herzenberg JE, Hensinger RN, Dedrick DK, Phillips WA. Emergency transport and position of young children who have an injury of the cervical spine. The standard backboard may be hazardous. *J Bone Joint Surg*. 1989;71(1):15–22. (**LOE IV**).

58. Curran C, Dietrich AM, Bowman MJ, Ginn-Pease ME, King DR, Kosnik E. Pediatric cervical spine immobilization: achieving neutral position? *J Trauma*. 1995;39(4):729–732. (**LOE II**).

59. Nypaver M, Treloar D. Neutral cervical spine positioning in children. *Ann Emerg Med*. 1994;23(2):208–211. (**LOE II**).

60. Laham JL, Cotcamp DH, Gibbons PA, Kahana MD, Crone KR. Isolated head injuries versus multiple trauma in pediatric patients: do the same indications for cervical spine evaluation apply? *Pediatr Neurosurg*. 1994;21:221–226. (**LOE IV**).

61. Leonard JC, et al. Factors associated with cervical spine injury in children after blunt trauma. *Ann Emerg Med.* 2011;58(2):145–155. **(LOE IV)**.

62. Mann DC, Dodds JA. Spinal injuries in 57 patients 17 years or younger. *Orthopaedics.* 1993;16:159–164. **(LOE IV)**.

63. Hadley MN, Zabramski JM, Browner CM, Rekate H, Sonntag VK. Pediatric spinal trauma. *J Neurosurg.* 1988;68(1):18–24. **(LOE IV)**.

64. Firth GB, Kingwell SP, Moroz PJ. Pediatric noncontiguous spinal injuries: the 15-year experience at a level 1 trauma center. *Spine (Phila Pa 1976).* 2012;37(10):E599–E608. **(LOE IV)**.

65. Hofbauer M, et al. Spine injuries in polytraumatized pediatric patients: characteristics and experience from a Level I trauma center over two decades. *J Trauma Acute Care Surg.* 2012;73(1):156–161. **(LOE IV)**.

66. Mortazavi MM, et al. Pediatric multilevel spine injuries: an institutional experience. *Childs Nerv Syst.* 2011;27(7):1095–1100. **(LOE IV)**.

67. Kim C, et al. Traumatic spinal injuries in children at a single level 1 pediatric trauma centre: report of a 23-year experience. *Can J Surg.* 2016;59(3):205–212. **(LOE IV)**.

68. Santiago R, Guenther E, Carroll K, Junkins EP Jr. The clinical presentation of pediatric thoracolumbar fractures. *J Trauma.* 2006; 60:187–192. **(LOE III)**.

69. McGuire RA, Neville S, Green BA, Watts C. Spinal instability and the log-rolling maneuver. *J Trauma.* 1987;27(5):525–531. **(LOE N/A)**.

70. Yang CC, Bradley WE. Somatic innervation of the human bulbocavernosus muscle. *Clin Neurophysiolog.* 1999;110(3):412–418. **(LOE N/A)**.

71. Sneed RC, Stover SL. Undiagnosed spinal cord injuries in brain-injured children. *Am J Dis Child.* 1988;142:965–967. **(LOE IV)**.

72. Hoffman JR, et al. Validity of a set of clinical criteria to rule out injury to the cervical spine in patients with blunt trauma. National Emergency X-Radiography Utilization Study Group. *N Engl J Med.* 2000;343(2):94–99. **(LOE II)**.

73. Viccellio P, Simon H, Pressman BD, Shah MN, Mower WR, Hofffman JR. A prospective multicenter study of cervical spine injury in children. *Pediatrics.* 2001;108(2):1–6. **(LOE I)**.

74. Garton HJ, Hammer MR. Detection of pediatric cervical spine injury. *Neurosurgery.* 2008;62(3):700–708; discussion 700-8. **(LOE III)**.

75. Stiell IG, et al. The Canadian C-spine rule for radiography in alert and stable trauma patients. *J Am Med Assoc.* 2001;286(15):1841–1848. **(LOE II)**.

76. Ehrlich PF, et al. Canadian C-spine rule and the National Emergency X-Radiography Utilization Low-Risk Criteria for C-spine radiography in young trauma patients. *J Pediatr Surg.* 2009;44(5):987–991. **(LOE IV)**.

77. Pieretti-Vanmarcke R, et al. Clinical clearance of the cervical spine in blunt trauma patients younger than 3 years: a multi-center study of the American Association for the Surgery of Trauma. *J Trauma.* 2009;67(3):543–549; discussion 549-50. **(LOE IV)**.

78. Lee SL, Sena M, Greenholz SK, Fledderman M. A multidisciplinary approach to the development of a cervical spine clearance protocol: process, rationale, and initial results. *J Pediatr Surg.* 2003;38(2):358–362. **(LOE IV)**.

79. Heilman CB, Riesenburger RI. Simultaneous noncontiguous cervical spine injuries in a pediatric patient. *Neurosurg.* 2001;49:1017–1020. **(LOE V)**.

80. Bonadio WA. Cervical spine trauma in children. I. General concepts, normal anatomy, radiographic evaluation. *Am J Emer Med.* 1993;11:158–165. **(LOE V)**.

81. Lally KP, Senac M, Hardin WD, Haftel A, Kaehler M, Mahour GH. Utility of the cervical spine radiograph in pediatric trauma. *Am J Surg.* 1989;158:540–541. **(LOE IV)**.

82. Baker C, Kadish H, Schunk JE. Evaluation of pediatric cervical spine injury. *Am J Emer Med.* 1999;17:230–234. **(LOE IV)**.

83. Buhs C, Cullen M, Klein M, Farmer D. The pediatric trauma C-spine: is the 'odontoid' view necessary? *J Pediatr Surg.* 2000;35(6):994–997. **(LOE IV)**.

84. Nigrovic LE, et al. Utility of plain radiographs in detecting traumatic injuries of the cervical spine in children. *Pediatr Emerg Care.* 2012;28(5):426–432. **(LOE IV)**.

85. Bucholz RW, Burkhead WZ. The pathological anatomy of fatal atlanto-occipital dislocations. *J Bone Joint Surg.* 1979;61:248–250. **(LOE IV)**.

86. Powers B, Miller MD, Kramer RS, Martinez S, Gehweiler JA. Traumatic anterior atlanto-occipital dislocation. *Neurosurg.* 1979;4:12–17. **(LOE IV)**.

87. Labbe JL, Leclair O, Duparc B. Traumatic atlanto-occipital dislocation with survival in children. *J Pediatr Orthop.* 2001;10:319–327. **(LOE V)**.

88. Harris JH Jr, Carson GG, Wagner LK, Kerr N. Radiologic diagnosis of traumatic occipitovertebral dissociation. Comparison of three methods. *Am J Roentgenol.* 1994;162:887–892. **(LOE IV)**.

89. Gonzalez LF, et al. Vertical atlantoaxial distraction injuries: radiological criteria and clinical implications. *J Neurosurg Spine.* 2004;1(3):273–280. **(LOE II)**.

90. Omercikoglu S, et al. Normal values of cervical vertebral measurements according to age and sex in CT. *Am J Emerg Med.* 2017;35(3):383–390. **(LOE N/A)**.

91. Rojas CA, et al. Reassessment of the craniocervical junction: normal values on CT. *AJNR Am J Neuroradiol.* 2007;28(9):1819–1823. **(LOE N/A)**.

92. Birchansky, S. et al. Pediatric craniocervical metrics revisited: establishing landmark CT measurements of basion-cartilaginous dens interval (BCDI) in infants using soft tissue window. In: *Proceedings of the American Society of Head and Neck Radiology 50th Annual Meeting.* 2016. Washington, D.C.

93. Singh AK, et al. Basion-cartilaginous dens interval: an imaging parameter for craniovertebral junction assessment in children. *AJNR Am J Neuroradiol.* 2017;38(12):2380–2384. **(LOE N/A)**.

94. Kaufman RA, Carroll CD, Buncher CR. Atlantooccipital junction: standards for measurement in normal children. *Am J Neurorad.* 1987;8:995–999. **(LOE IV)**.

95. Locke GR, Gardner JI, Van Epps EF. Atlas-dens interval (ADI) in children: a survey based on 200 normal cervical spines. *Am J Roentgenol Radium Ther Nucl Med.* 1966;97:135–140. **(LOE IV)**.

96. Fielding JW, Cochran GV, Lawsing JF 3rd, Hohl M. Tears of the transverse ligament of the atlas. A clinical and biomechanical study. *J Bone Joint Surg.* 1974;56:1683–1681. **(LOE IV)**.

97. Steel HH. Anatomical and mechanical considerations of the atlanto-axial articulation. *J Bone Joint Surg.* 1968;50:1481–1482. **(LOE IV)**.

98. Swischuk L. Anterior displacement of C2 in children. *Radiology.* 1977;122:759–763. **(LOE IV)**.

99. Ardran GM, Kemp FH. The mechanism of changes in from of the cervical airway in infancy. *Med Radiography Photography.* 1968;44(2):26–38. **(LOE IV)**.

100. Cattell HS, Filtzer DL. Pseudosubluxation and other normal variations in the cervical spine in children. *J BoneJoint Surg.* 1965;47:1295–1309. **(LOE IV)**.

101. Shaw M, Burnett H, Wilson A, Chan O. Pseudosubluxation of C2 on C3 in polytraumatized children: prevalence and significance. *Clin Radiolog.* 1999;54:377–380. **(LOE III)**.

102. Pennecot GF, G.D, Hardy JR. Roentgenographical study for the cervical spine in children. *J Pediatr Orthop.* 1984;4:339–345. **(LOE IV)**.

103. Townsend EH Jr, Rowe ML. Mobility of the upper cervical spine in health and disease. *Pediatrics.* 1952;10:567–573. **(LOE IV)**.

104. Hall DE, Boydston W. Pediatric neck injuries. *Pediatr Rev.* 1999;20(1):13–19. **(LOE IV)**.

105. Been E, Shefi S, Soudack M. Cervical lordosis: the effect of age and gender. *Spine J.* 2017;17(6):880–888. **(LOE N/A)**.

106. Naidich JB, Naidich TP, Garfein C, Liebeskind AL, Hyman RA. The widened interspinous distance: a useful sign of anterior cervical dislocation in the supine frontal projection. *Radiology.* 1977;123:113–116. **(LOE II)**.

107. White AA 3rd, et al. Biomechanical analysis of clinical stability in the cervical spine. *Clin Orthop Relat Res.* 1975;(109):85–96. **(LOE N/A)**.

108. Gaca AM, Barnhart HX, Bisset GS 3rd. Evaluation of wedging of lower thoracic and upper lumbar vertebral bodies in the pediatric population. *AJR Am J Roentgenol.* 2010;194(2):516–520. **(LOE N/A)**.

109. Jaremko JL, et al. Common normal variants of pediatric vertebral development that mimic fractures: a pictorial review from a national longitudinal bone health study. *Pediatr Radiol.* 2015;45(4):593–605. **(LOE V)**.

110. Dietz GW, Christensen EE. Normal "Cupid's bow" contour of the lower lumbar vertebrae. *Radiology.* 1976;121(3 Pt. 1):577–579. **(LOE N/A)**.

111. Tsuji H, Yoshioka T, Sainoh H. Developmental balloon disc of the lumbar spine in healthy subjects. *Spine (Phila Pa 1976).* 1985;10(10):907–911. **(LOE IV)**.

112. Ralston ME, et al. Role of flexion-extension radiographs in blunt pediatric cervical spine injury. *Acad Emerg Med.* 2001;8(3):237–245. **(LOE IV)**.

113. Dwek JR, Chung CB. Radiography of cervical spine injury in children: are flexion-extension radiographs useful for acute trauma? *AJR Am J Roentgenol.* 2000;174(6):1617–1619. **(LOE IV)**.

114. Pollack CV Jr, Hendey GW, Martin DR, Hoffman JR, Mower WR. Use of flexion-extension radiographs of the cervical spine in blunt trauma. *Academic Emergency Med.* 2001;8(5):488. **(LOE IV)**.

115. Davis JW, Phreaner DL, hoyt DB, Mackersie RC. The etiology of missed cervical spine injuries. *J Trauma.* 1993;34:342–346. **(LOE IV)**.

116. Gerrelts BD, Petersen EU, Mabry J, Petersen SR. Delayed diagnosis of cervical spine injuries. *J Trauma.* 1991;31:1622–1626. **(LOE IV)**.

117. Grogan EL, Morris JA Jr, Dittus RS, et al. Cervical spine evaluation in urban trauma centers: lowering institutional costs and complications through helical CT scan. *J Am Col Surg.* 2005;200(2):160–165. **(LOE II)**.

118. Nunez DB Jr, Zuluaga A, Fuentes-Bernardo DA, Rivas LA, Becerra JL. Cervical spine trauma: how much more do we learn by routinely using helical CT? *Radiographics.* 1996;16:1307–1318. **(LOE IV)**.

119. Link TM, Schuierer G, Hufendiek A, Horch C, Peters PE. Substantial head trauma. Value of routine CT examination of the cervicocranium. *Radiology.* 1995;196:741–755.

120. Hartley W, M.G. Green N. *Clinical and radiographic algorithm for acute management of pediatric cervical spine trauma.* In *Scoliosis Research Society,* 32nd Annual Meeting. 1997. St. Louis, MO.

121. Fearon T, Vucich J. Normalized pediatric organ-absorbed doses from CT examinations. *Am J Roentgenol.* 1987;148:171–174. **(LOE N/A)**.

122. Huda W, Bissessur K. Effective dose equivalents, HE, in diagnostic radiology. *Med Phys.* 1990;17:998–1003. **(LOE N/A)**.

123. Muchow RD, et al. Theoretical increase of thyroid cancer induction from cervical spine multidetector computed tomography in pediatric trauma patients. *J Trauma Acute Care Surg.* 2012;72(2):403–409. **(LOE III)**.

124. Marin JR, et al. Variation in pediatric cervical spine computed tomography radiation dose index. *Acad Emerg Med.* 2015;22(12):1499–1505. **(LOE N/A)**.

125. Rana AR, et al. Traumatic cervical spine injuries: characteristics of missed injuries. *J Pediatr Surg.* 2009;44(1):151–155; discussion 155. **(LOE III)**.

126. Hale AT, et al. X-ray vs. CT in identifying significant C-spine injuries in the pediatric population. *Childs Nerv Syst.* 2017;33(11):1977–1983. **(LOE III)**.

127. Henry M, et al. A retrospective comparison of CT and MRI in detecting pediatric cervical spine injury. *Childs Nerv Syst.* 2013;29(8):1333–1338. **(LOE III)**.

128. Gargas J, et al. An analysis of cervical spine magnetic resonance imaging findings after normal computed tomographic imaging findings in pediatric trauma patients: ten-year experience of a level I pediatric trauma center. *J Trauma Acute Care Surg.* 2013;74(4):1102–1107. **(LOE III)**.

129. Gestring ML, Gracias VH, Feliciano MA, et al. Evaluation of the lower spine after blunt trauma using abdominal computed tomographic scanning supplemented with lateral scanograms. *J Trauma.* 2002;53:9–14. **(LOE I)**.

130. Hauser CJ, Visvikis G, Hinrichs C, et al. Prospective validation of computed tomographic screening of the thoracolumbar spine in trauma. *J Trauma.* 2003;55:228–235. **(LOE I)**.

131. Rhea JT, Sheridan RL, Mullins ME, Novelline RA. Can chest and abdominal trauma CT eliminate the need for plain films of the spine? Experience with 329 multiple trauma patients. *Emer Radiolog.* 2001;8:99–104. **(LOE III)**.

132. Sheridan R, Peralta R, Rhea J, Ptak T, Novelline R. Reformatted visceral protocol helical computed tomographic scanning allows conventional radiographs of the thoracic and lumbar spine to be eliminated in the evaluation of blunt trauma patients. *J Trauma.* 2003;55:665–669. **(LOE III)**.

133. Wintermark M, Mouhsine E, Theumann N, et al. Thoracolumbar spine fractures in patients who have sustained severe trauma: depiction with multi-detector row CT. *Radiology.* 2003;227:681–689. **(LOE I)**.

134. Flynn JM, Closkey RF, Mahboubi S, Dormans JP. Role of magnetic resonance imaging in the assessment of pediatric cervical spine injuries. *J Pediatr Orthop.* 2002;22:573–577. **(LOE IV)**.

135. Keiper MD, Zimmerman RA, Bilaniuk LT. MRI in the assessment of the supportive soft tissues of the cervical spine in acute trauma in children. *Neuroradiology.* 1998;40:359–363. **(LOE IV)**.

136. Frank JB, Lim CK, Flynn JM, Dormans JP. The efficacy of magnetic resonance imaging in pediatric cervical spine clearance. *Spine.* 2002;27(11):1176–1179. **(LOE IV)**.

137. Stassen NA, et al. Magnetic resonance imaging in combination with helical computed tomography provides a safe and efficient method of cervical spine clearance in the obtunded trauma patient. *J Trauma.* 2006;60(1):171–177. **(LOE IV)**.

138. Sledge JB, Allred D, Hyman J. Use of magnetic resonance imaging in evaluating injuries to the pediatric thoracolumbar spine. *J Pediatr Orthop.* 2001;21:288–293. **(LOE IV)**.

139. Davis JW, Parks SN, Detlefs CL, Williams GG, Williams JL, Smith RW. Clearing the cervical spine in obtunded patients: the use of dynamic fluoroscopy. *J Trauma.* 1995;39:435–438. **(LOE III)**.

140. Kolb JC, Summers RL, Galli RL. Cervical collar-induced changes in intracranial pressure. *Am J Emer Med.* 1999;17(2):135–137. **(LOE N/A)**.

141. Stambolis V, Brady S, Klos D, Wesling M, Fatianov T, Hildner C. The effects of cervical bracing upon swallowing in young, normal, healthy volunteers. *Dysphagia.* 2003;18(1):39–45. **(LOE N/A)**.

142. Pannu GS, Shah MP, Herman MJ. Cervical spine clearance in pediatric trauma centers: the need for standardization and an evidence-based protocol. *J Pediatr Orthop.* 2017;37(3):e145–e149. **(LOE IV)**.

143. Connelly CR, et al. Performance improvement and patient safety program-guided quality improvement initiatives can significantly reduce computed tomography imaging in pediatric trauma patients. *J Trauma Acute Care Surg.* 2016;81(2):278–284. **(LOE III)**.

144. Sun R, et al. A pediatric cervical spine clearance protocol to reduce radiation exposure in children. *J Surg Res.* 2013;183(1):341–346. **(LOE III)**.

145. Anderson RC, Kan P, Hansen KW, Brockmeyer DL. Cervical spine clearance after trauma in children. *Neurosurg Focus.* 2006;20(2):E3. **(LOE IV)**.

146. Herman MJ, et al. Pediatric cervical spine clearance: a consensus statement and algorithm from the Pediatric Cervical Spine Clearance Working Group. *J Bone Joint Surg Am.* 2019;101(1):e1. **(LOE V)**.

147. Kavuri V, et al. "Next Day" examination reduces radiation exposure in cervical spine clearance at a Level 1 pediatric trauma center: preliminary findings. *J Pediatr Orthop.* 2018. **(LOE IV)**.

148. Dorney K, et al. Outcomes of pediatric patients with persistent midline cervical spine tenderness and negative imaging result after trauma. *J Trauma Acute Care Surg.* 2015;79(5):822–827. **(LOE IV)**.

149. Brockmeyer DL, Ragel BT, Kestle JR. The pediatric cervical spine instability study. A pilot study assessing the prognostic value of four imaging modalities in clearing the cervical spine for children with severe traumatic injuries. *Childs Nerv Syst.* 2012;28(5):699–705. **(LOE II)**.

150. Pang D. Spinal cord injury without radiographic abnormality in children, 2 decades later. *Neurosurg.* 2004;55(6):1325–1342. **(LOE V)**.

151. Launay F, Leet AI, Sponseller PD. Pediatric spinal cord injury without radiographic abnormality: a meta-analysis. *Clin Orthop Relat Res.* 2005;(433):166–170. **(LOE III)**.

152. Hamilton MG, Myles ST. Pediatric spinal injury: review of 174 hospital injuries. *J Neurosurg.* 1992;68:700–704. **(LOE IV)**.

153. Osenbach RK, Menezes AH. Pediatric spinal cord and vertebral column injury. *Neurosurg.* 1992;30:385–390. **(LOE IV)**.

154. Vitale MG, et al. Epidemiology of pediatric spinal cord injury in the United States: years 1997 and 2000. *J Pediatr Orthop.* 2006;26(6):745–749. **(LOE IV)**.

155. Herndon WA. Injuries to the head and neck. In: Sullivan JA, Grana Wa, eds. *The Pediatric Athlete.* Park Ridge, IL: *American Academy of Orthopaedic Surgeons; 1990.*

156. Pang D, Pollack IF. Spinal cord injury without radiographic abnormality in children: the SCIWORA syndrome. *J Trauma.* 1989;29:654–664. **(LOE IV)**.

157. d'Amato C. Pediatric spinal trauma. *Clin Orthop Rel Research.* 2005;432:34–40. **(LOE V)**.

158. Rang MC. *Children's Fractures.* Philadelphia: J.B. Lippincott; 1983.

159. Hadden WA, Gillepsie WJ. Multiple level injuries of the cervical spine. *Injury.* 1985;16:628–633. **(LOE IV).**

160. Pang D, Wilberger JE Jr. Spinal cord injury without radiographic abnormalities in children. *J Neurosurg.* 1982;57:114–129. **(LOE IV).**

161. Kriss V, Kriss T. SCIWORA (spinal cord injury without radiographic abnormality) in infants and children. *Clin Pediatr.* 1996;35(3):119–124. **(LOE V).**

162. Copley L, Dormans J. Pediatric cervical spine problems: developmental and congenital anomalies. *J Am Acad Orthop Surg.* 1998;6(4):204–214. **(LOE V).**

163. Fesmire FM, Luten RC. The pediatric cervical spine: developmental anatomy and clinical aspects. *J Emerg Med.* 1989;7:133–142. **(LOE V).**

164. Henrys P, Lyne ED, Lifton C, Salciccioli G. Clinical review of cervical spine injuries in children. *Clin Orthop Rel Research.* 1977;129:172–176. **(LOE IV).**

165. Kewalramani LS, Tori JA. Spinal cord trauma in children: neurologic patterns, radiologic features, and pathomechanics of injury. *Spine.* 1980;5:11–18. **(LOE IV).**

166. Bosch PP, Vogt MT, Ward WT. Pediatric spinal cord injury without radiographic abnormality (SCIWORA): the absence of occult instability and lack of indication for bracing. *Spine.* 2002;27(24):2788–2800. **(LOE IV).**

167. Dare AO, Dias MS, Li V. Magnetic resonance imaging correlation in pediatric spinal cord injury without radiographic abnormality. *J Neurosurg.* 2002;97(suppl 1):33–39. **(LOE IV).**

168. Davis PC, et al. Spinal injuries in children: role of MR. *AJNR Am J Neuroradiol.* 1993;14(3):607–617. **(LOE IV).**

169. Liao CC, et al. Spinal cord injury without radiological abnormality in preschool-aged children: correlation of magnetic resonance imaging findings with neurological outcomes. *J Neurosurg.* 2005;103(suppl 1):17–23. **(LOE IV).**

170. Flanders AE, Schaefer DM, Doan HT, Mishkin MM, Gonzalez CF, Northrup BE. Acute cervical spine trauma: correlation of MR imaging findings with degree of neurologic deficit. *Radiology.* 1990;177:25–33. **(LOE IV).**

171. Grabb PA, Pang D. Magnetic resonance imaging in the evaluation of spinal cord injury without radiographic abnormality in children. *Neurosurgery.* 1994;35:406–414. **(LOE IV).**

172. Mahajan P, et al. Spinal cord injury without radiologic abnormality in children imaged with magnetic resonance imaging. *J Trauma Acute Care Surg.* 2013;75(5):843–847. **(LOE III).**

173. Rozzelle CJ, et al. Management of pediatric cervical spine and spinal cord injuries. *Neurosurgery.* 2013;72(suppl 2):205–226. **(LOE V).**

174. Marino RJ, Ditunno JF Jr, Donovan WH, Maynard Jr F. Neurologic recovery after traumatic spinal cord injury: data from the Model Spinal Cord Injury Systems. *Arch Phys Med Rehab.* 1999;80(11):1391–1396. **(LOE IV).**

175. Saleh J, Raycroft JF. Hyperflexion injury of the cervical spine and central cord syndrome in a child. *Spine.* 1992;17(2):234–237. **(LOE V).**

176. Oller DW, Boone S. Blunt cervical spine Brown-Séquard injury. A report of three cases. *Am Surg.* 1991;57(6):361–365. **(LOE IV).**

177. Hakimi KN, Massagli TL. Anterior spinal artery syndrome in two children with genetic thrombotic disorders. *J Spinal Cord Med.* 2005;28(1):69–73. **(LOE IV).**

178. Wells JD, Nicosia S. Scoring acute spinal cord injury: a study of the utility and limitations of five different grading systems. *J Spinal Cord Med.* 1995;18(1):33–41. **(LOE N/A).**

179. Ryken TC, et al. The acute cardiopulmonary management of patients with cervical spinal cord injuries. *Neurosurgery.* 2013;72(suppl 2):84–92. **(LOE V).**

180. Levi L, Wolf A, Belzberg H. Hemodynamic parameters in patients with acute cervical cord trauma: description, intervention, and prediction of outcome. *Neurosurgery.* 1993;33(6):1007–1016; discussion 1016-7. **(LOE IV).**

181. Vale FL, et al. Combined medical and surgical treatment after acute spinal cord injury: results of a prospective pilot study to assess the merits of aggressive medical resuscitation and blood pressure management. *J Neurosurg.* 1997;87(2):239–246. **(LOE IV).**

182. Bracken MB, Shepard MJ, Holford TR, et al. Administration of methylprednisolone for 24 or 48 hours or tirilazad mesylate for 48 hours in the treatment of acute spinal cord injury: results of the Third National Acute Spinal Cord Injury Randomized Controlled Trial. National Acute Spinal Cord Injury Study. *J Am Med Assoc.* 1997;277:1597–1604. **(LOE I).**

183. Bracken MB, Shepard MJ, Holford TR, et al. Methylprednisolone or tirilazad mesylate administration after acute spinal cord injury: 1-year follow-up. Results of the third National Acute Spinal Cord Injury randomized controlled trial. *J Neurosurg.* 1998;89:699–706. **(LOE I).**

184. Bracken MB. Pharmacological treatment of acute spinal cord injury: current status and future projects. *J Emerg Med.* 1993;11:43–48. **(LOE V).**

185. Ito Y, et al. Does high dose methylprednisolone sodium succinate really improve neurological status in patient with acute cervical cord injury? A prospective study about neurological recovery and early complications. *Spine.* 2009;34(20):2121–2124. **(LOE II).**

186. Pointillart V, et al. Pharmacological therapy of spinal cord injury during the acute phase. *Spinal Cord.* 2000;38(2):71–76. **(LOE I).**

187. Galandiuk S, et al. The two-edged sword of large-dose steroids for spinal cord trauma. *Ann Surg.* 1993;218(4):419–425; discussion 425-7. **(LOE III).**

188. Gerndt SJ, et al. Consequences of high-dose steroid therapy for acute spinal cord injury. *J Trauma.* 1997;42(2):279–284. **(LOE III).**

189. Lee HC, et al. Pitfalls in treatment of acute cervical spinal cord injury using high-dose methylprednisolone: a retrospect audit of 111 patients. *Surg Neurol.* 2007;68(suppl 1):S37–S41; discussion S41-2. **(LOE III).**

190. Qian T, et al. High-dose methylprednisolone may cause myopathy in acute spinal cord injury patients. *Spinal Cord.* 2005;43(4):199–203. **(LOE II).**

191. Suberviola B, et al. Early complications of high-dose methylprednisolone in acute spinal cord injury patients. *Injury.* 2008;39(7):748–752. **(LOE III).**

192. Caruso MC, et al. Lessons learned from administration of high-dose methylprednisolone sodium succinate for acute pediatric spinal cord injuries. *J Neurosurg Pediatr.* 2017;20(6):567–574. **(LOE IV).**

193. Geisler FH, Dorsey FC, Coleman WP. Recovery of motor function after spinal cord injury-a randomized, placebo-controlled trial with GM-1 ganglioside. *N Engl J Med.* 1991;324:1829–1838. **(LOE I).**

194. Geisler FH, Dorsey FC, Coleman WP. Past and current clinical studies with GM-1 ganglioside in acute spinal cord injury recovery. *Ann Emerg Med.* 1993;22:1041–1047. **(LOE V).**

195. Geisler FH, et al. The Sygen multicenter acute spinal cord injury study. *Spine.* 2001;26(suppl 24):S87–S98. **(LOE I).**

196. Cappuccino A, et al. The use of systemic hypothermia for the treatment of an acute cervical spinal cord injury in a professional football player. *Spine.* 2010;35(2):E57–E62. **(LOE V).**

197. Dietrich WD, et al. Hypothermic treatment for acute spinal cord injury. *Neurotherapeutics.* 2011;8(2):229–239. **(LOE V).**

198. Levi AD, et al. Clinical outcomes using modest intravascular hypothermia after acute cervical spinal cord injury. *Neurosurgery.* 2010;66(4):670–677. **(LOE IV).**

199. Morgan TH, Wharton GW, Austin GN. The results of laminectomy in patients with incomplete spinal cord injuries. *Paraplegia.* 1971;9:14–23. **(LOE IV).**

200. Sherk HH, Schut L, Lane JM. Fractures and dislocations of the cervical spine in children. *Orthop Clin North Am.* 1976;7:593–604. **(LOE V).**

201. Yasuoko F, Peterson HA, MacCarty C. Incidence of spinal column deformity after multiple level laminectomy in children and adults. *J Neurosurg.* 1982;57:441–445. **(LOE IV).**

202. Fehlings MG, Perrin RG. The timing of surgical intervention in the treatment of spinal cord injury: a systematic review of recent clinical evidence. *Spine.* 2006;31:S28–S35. **(LOE III).**

203. Papadopoulos SM, Selden NR, Quint DJ, Patel N, Gillespie B, Grube S. et al. Immediate spinal cord decompression for cervical spinal cord injury: feasibility and outcome. *J Trauma.* 2002;52:223–232. **(LOE II).**

204. Fehlings MG, et al. Early versus delayed decompression for traumatic cervical spinal cord injury: results of the Surgical Timing in Acute Spinal Cord Injury Study (STASCIS). *PLoS One.* 2012;7(2):e32037. **(LOE II).**

205. Jacobs RR, Asher MA, Snider RK. Thoracolumbar spinal injuries: a comparative study of recumbent and operative treatment in 100 patients. *Spine.* 1980;5:463–477. **(LOE III).**

206. Wang MY, Hoh DJ, Leary SP, Griffith P, McComb JG. High rates of neurological improvement following severe traumatic pediatric spinal cord injury. *Spine.* 2004;29(13):1493–1497. **(LOE IV).**

207. Pouliquen JC, Kassis B, Glorion C, Langlais J. et al. Vertebral growth after thoracic or lumbar fracture of the spine in children. *J Pediatr Orthop.* 1997;17:115–120. (**LOE IV**).

208. Mayfield JK, Erkkila JC, Winter RB. Spine deformity subsequent to acquired childhood spinal cord injury. *J Bone Joint Surg.* 1981;63A:1401–1411. (**LOE IV**).

209. Vaccaro AR, Silber JS. Post-traumatic spinal deformity. *Spine.* 2001;26: S111–S118. (**LOE V**).

210. Betz RR, Mulcahey MJ. Spinal cord injury rehabilitation. In: Weinstein SL, ed. *The Pediatric Spine: Principles and Practice.* Vol. 1. New York: Raven Press: 1994: 781–810.

211. Dearolf WW 3rd, Betz RR, Vogel LC, Levin J, Clancy M, Steel HH. Scoliosis in pediatric spinal cord injured patients. *J Pediatr Orthop.* 1990;10:214–218. (**LOE IV**).

212. Lancourt JE, Dickson JH, Carter RE. Paralytic spinal deformity following traumatic spinal cord injury in children and adolescents. *J Bone Joint Surg Am.* 1981;63:47–53. (**LOE IV**).

213. Mehta S, et al. Effect of bracing on paralytic scoliosis secondary to spinal cord injury. *J Spinal Cord Med.* 2004;27(suppl 1):S88–S92. (**LOE IV**).

214. Chafetz RS, et al. Impact of prophylactic thoracolumbosacral orthosis bracing on functional activities and activities of daily living in the pediatric spinal cord injury population. *J Spinal Cord Med.* 2007;30(suppl 1):S178–S183. (**LOE N/A**).

215. Anderson CJ, Vogel LC, Willis KM, Betz RR. Stability of transition to adulthood among individuals with pediatric-onset spinal cord injuries. *J Spinal Cord Med.* 2006;29(1):46–56. (**LOE IV**).

216. Vogel LC, et al. Long-term outcomes of adults with pediatric-onset spinal cord injuries as a function of neurological impairment. *J Spinal Cord Med.* 2011;34(1):60–66. (**LOE IV**).

217. Anderson CJ, et al. Depression in adults who sustained spinal cord injuries as children or adolescents. *J Spinal Cord Med.* 2007;30(suppl 1):S76–S82. (**LOE IV**).

218. Shavelle RM, et al. Long-term survival after childhood spinal cord injury. *J Spinal Cord Med.* 2007;30(suppl 1):S48–S54. (**LOE IV**).

219. Anderson PA, Montesano PX. Morphology and treatment of occipital condyle fractures. *Spine.* 1988;13(7):731–736. (**LOE IV**).

220. Maserati MB, et al. Occipital condyle fractures: clinical decision rule and surgical management. *J Neurosurg Spine.* 2009;11(4):388–395. (**LOE IV**).

221. Vaccaro AR, Lim MR, Lee JY. Indications for surgery and stabilization techniques of the occipito-cervical junction. *Injury.* 2005;36(2):B44–B53. (**LOE V**).

222. Giguere JF, St-Vil D, Turmel A, et al. Airbags and children: a spectrum of C-spine injuries. *J Pediatr Surg.* 1998;33(6):811–816. (**LOE IV**).

223. Pizzutillo P. Pediatric occipitoatlantal injuries. *Seminars Spine Surg.* 1992;3:24–32. (**LOE V**).

224. Dvorak J, Panjabi MM. Functional anatomy of the alar ligaments. *Spine.* 1987;12(2):183–189. (**LOE N/A**).

225. Werne S. Studies in spontaneous atlas dislocation. *Acta Orthop Scan.* 1957;23:1–15. (**LOE IV**).

226. Gilles F, Bina M, Sotrel A. Infantile atlantooccipital instability. *Am J Dis Child.* 1979;133:30–37. (**LOE N/A**).

227. DiBendetto T, Lee CK. Traumatic atlanto-occipital instability: a case report with follow-up and a new diagnostic technique. *Spine.* 1990;15:595. (**LOE V**).

228. Donahue D. Childhood survival of atlantooccipital dislocation: underdiagnosis, recognition, treatment, and review of the literature. *Pediatr Neurosurg.* 1994;21:105. (**LOE IV**).

229. Harmanli O, Koyfman Y. Traumatic atlanto-occipital dislocation with survival. *Surg Neurol.* 1993;39:324. (**LOE V**).

230. Hosalkar HS, Cain EL, Horn D, Chin KR, Dormans JP, Drummond DS. Traumatic atlanto-occipital dislocation in children. *J Bone Joint Surg.* 2005;87:2480–2488. (**LOE IV**).

231. Papadopoulos SM, Dickman CA, Sonntag VK, Rekate HL, Spetzler RF. Traumatic atlantooccipital dislocation with survival. *Neurosurg.* 1991;28:574–579. (**LOE V**).

232. Sponseller P. Atlanto-occipital arthrodesis for instability with neurologic preservation. *Spine.* 1997;22:344. (**LOE IV**).

233. Astur N, et al. Traumatic atlanto-occipital dislocation in children: evaluation, treatment, and outcomes. *J Bone Joint Surg Am.* 2013;95(24):e194. (1–8). (**LOE IV**).

234. Collalto PM, et al. Traumatic atlanto-occipital dislocation. Case report. *J Bone Joint Surg Am.* 1986;68(7):1106–1109. (**LOE V**).

235. Reed CM, et al. Atlanto-occipital dislocation with traumatic pseudomeningocele formation and post-traumatic syringomyelia. *Spine.* 1976;30(5):E128–E133. (**LOE V**).

236. Matava MJ, Whitesides TE Jr, Davis PC. Traumatic atlanto-occipital dislocation with survival. Serial computerized tomography as an aid to diagnosis and reduction: a report of three cases. *Spine.* 1993;18:1897–1903. (**LOE IV**).

237. Traynelis VC, et al. Traumatic atlanto-occipital dislocation. Case report. *J Neurosurg.* 1986;65(6):863–870. (**LOE V**).

238. Steinmetz MP, Lechner RM, Anderson JS. Atlantooccipital dislocation in children: presentation, diagnosis, and management. *Neurosurg Focus.* 2003;14(2). (**LOE V**).

239. Horn EM, et al. Survivors of occipitoatlantal dislocation injuries: imaging and clinical correlates. *J Neurosurg Spine.* 2007;6(2):113–120. (**LOE IV**).

240. Georgopoulos G, Pizzutillo PD, Lee MS. Occipito-atlantal instability in children. A report of five cases and review of the literature. *J Bone Joint Surg.* 1987;69(3):429–436. (**LOE IV**).

241. Cohen MW, Drummond DS, Flynn JM, Pill SG, Dormans JP. A technique of occipitocervical arthrodesis in children using autologous rib grafts. *Spine.* 2001;26:825–829. (**LOE V**).

242. Dormans JP, Drummond DS, Sutton LN, Ecker ML, Kopacz KJ. Occipitocervical arthrodesis in children. *J Bone Joint Surg.* 1995;77:1234–1240. (**LOE IV**).

243. Ebraheim NA, Lu J, Biyani A, Brown JA, Yeasting RA. An anatomic study of the thickness of the occipital bone. Implications for occipitocervical instrumentation. *Spine.* 1996;21:1725–1730. (**LOE N/A**).

244. Bekelis K, et al. Placement of occipital condyle screws for occipitocervical fixation in a pediatric patient with occipitocervical instability after decompression for Chiari malformation. *J Neurosurg Pediatr.* 2010;6(2):171–176. (**LOE V**).

245. Chamoun RB, et al. Use of axial and subaxial translaminar screw fixation in the management of upper cervical spinal instability in a series of 7 children. *Neurosurgery.* 2009;64(4):734–739; discussion 739. (**LOE IV**).

246. Haque A, et al. Screw fixation of the upper cervical spine in the pediatric population. Clinical article. *J Neurosurg Pediatr.* 2009;3(6):529–533. (**LOE IV**).

247. Keen JR, et al. Rigid internal fixation for traumatic cranio-cervical dissociation in infants and young children. *Spine.* 2019;44(1):17–24. (**LOE IV**).

248. Brockmeyer DL, Apfelbaum RI. A new occipitocervical fusion construct in pediatric patients with occipitocervical instability. Technical note. *J Neurosurg.* 1999;90(suppl 2):271–275. (**LOE IV**).

249. Iyer RR, et al. A modified technique for occipitocervical fusion using compressed iliac crest allograft results in a high rate of fusion in the pediatric population. *World Neurosurg.* 2017;107:342–350. (**LOE IV**).

250. Bonadio WA. Cervical spine trauma in children: Part II. Mechanisms and manifestations of injury, therapeutic considerations. *Amer J Emer Med.* 1993;11:256–278. (**LOE V**).

251. Lawson JA, Ogden JA, Bucholz RW, Hughes SA. Physeal injuries of the cervical spine. *J Pediatr Orthop.* 1987;7:428–435. (**LOE IV**).

252. AuYong N, Piatt Jr J. Jefferson fractures of the immature spine. Report of 3 cases. *J Neurosurg Pediatr.* 2009;3(1):15–19. (**LOE IV**).

253. Marlin AE, Williams GR, Lee JF. Jefferson fractures in children. *J Neurosurg.* 1983;58:277–279. (**LOE IV**).

254. Connolly B, et al. Jefferson fracture resulting in Collet-Sicard syndrome. *Spine.* 2000;25(3):395–398. (**LOE IV**).

255. Levine AM, Edwards CC. Fractures of the atlas. *J Bone Joint Surg Am.* 1991;73(5):680–691. (**LOE IV**).

256. Spence Jr KF, Decker S, Sell KW. Bursting atlantal fracture associated with rupture of the transverse ligament. *J Bone Joint Surg Am.* 1970;52(3):543–549. (**LOE V**).

257. Fowler JL, Sandhu A, Fraser RD. A review of fractures of the atlas vertebra. *J Spinal Disord.* 1990;3(1):19–24. (**LOE IV**).

258. Hadley MN, et al. Acute traumatic atlas fractures: management and long term outcome. *Neurosurgery.* 1988;23(1):31–35. (**LOE IV**).

259. Greene KA, et al. Transverse atlantal ligament disruption associated with odontoid fractures. *Spine.* 1994;19(20):2307–2314. (**LOE IV**).

260. Pathria MN, Petersilge CA. Spinal trauma. *Rad Clin North Am.* 1991;29:847–865. (**LOE V**).

261. Dickman CA, Greene KA, Sonntag VK. Injuries involving the transverse atlantal ligament: classification and treatment guide-

lines based upon experience with 39 injuries. *Neurosurgery.* 1996;38(1):44–50. **(LOE IV)**.

262. Brooks AL, Jenkins EB. Atlanto-axial arthrodesis by the wedge compression method. *J Bone Joint Surg.* 1978;60:279–284. **(LOE IV)**.

263. Dickman CA, Sonntag VK, Papadopoulos SM, Hadley MN. The interspinous method of posterior atlantoaxial arthrodesis. *J Neurosurg.* 1991;74:190–198. **(LOE IV)**.

264. Gallie WE. Fracture and dislocations of the cervical spine. *Am J Surg.* 1939;46:495–499. **(LOE V)**.

265. Magerl F, S.P. Spine Cervical, K. P, W. A, eds. *Stable posterior fusion of the atlas and axis by transarticular screw fixation.* Vienna: Springer-Verlag; 1987:322-327.

266. Gluf WM, Brockmeyer DL. Atlantoaxial transarticular screw fixation: a review of surgical indications, fusion rate, complications, and lessons learned in 67 pediatric patients. *J Neurosurg Spine.* 2005;2:164–169. **(LOE IV)**.

267. Paramore CG, Dickman CA, Sonntag VK. The anatomical suitability of the C1-2 complex for transarticular screw fixation. *J Neurosurg.* 1996;85(2):221–224. **(LOE N/A)**.

268. Singh B, Cree A. Laminar screw fixation of the axis in the pediatric population: a series of eight patients. *Spine J.* 2015;15(2):e17–e25. **(LOE IV)**.

269. Yang BW, et al. C2 translaminar screw fixation in children. *J Pediatr Orthop.* 2018;38(6):e312–e317. **(LOE IV)**.

270. Yi P, et al. Clinical application of a revised screw technique via the C1 posterior arch and lateral mass in the pediatric population. *Pediatr Neurosurg.* 2013;49(3):159–165. **(LOE IV)**.

271. Fielding JW, Hawkins RJ. Atlanto-axial rotatory fixation. *J Bone Joint Surg.* 1977;59:37–44. **(LOE IV)**.

272. Phillips WA, Hensinger RN. The management of rotatory atlanto-axial subluxation in children. *J Bone Joint Surg.* 1989;71:664–668. **(LOE IV)**.

273. Powell EC, et al. Atlantoaxial rotatory subluxation in children. *Pediatr Emerg Care.* 2017;33(2):86–91. **(LOE III)**.

274. Beier AD, et al. Rotatory subluxation: experience from the Hospital for Sick Children. *J Neurosurg Pediatr.* 2012;9(2):144–148. **(LOE IV)**.

275. Van Holsbeeck EM, MacKay NN. Diagnosis of acute atlanto-axial rotatory fixation. *J Bone Joint Surg.* 1989;70:90–91. **(LOE IV)**.

276. Kowalski HM, Cohen WA, Cooper P, Wisoff JH. Pitfalls in the CT diagnosis of atlantoaxial rotary subluxation. *Am J Roentgenol.* 1987;149:595–600. **(LOE IV)**.

277. Li V, P.D. ed. *Atlanto-Axial Rotatory Fixation. Disorders of the Pediatric Spine, ed.* P. D. New York: Raven Press; 1995: 531–553

278. Rinaldi I, Mullins WJ Jr, Delaney WF, Fitzer PM, Tornberg DN. Computerized tomographic demonstration of rotational atlanto-axial fixation. *J Neurosurg.* 1979;50:115–119. **(LOE V)**.

279. Pang D, Li V. Atlantoaxial rotatory fixation: Part 3 of a prospective study of the clinical manifestation, diagnosis, management, and outcome of children with atlantoaxial rotatory fixation. *Neurosurg.* 2005;5:954–971. **(LOE II)**.

280. Subach BR, McLaughlin MR, Albright AL, Pollack IF. Current management of pediatric atalantoaxial rotatory subluxation. *Spine.* 1998;23:2174–2179. **(LOE IV)**.

281. Chechik O, et al. Successful conservative treatment for neglected rotatory atlantoaxial dislocation. *J Pediatr Orthop.* 2013;33(4):389–392. **(LOE IV)**.

282. Mihara H, Onari K, Hachiya M, Toguchi A, Yamada K. Follow-up study of conservative treatment for atlantoaxial rotatory displacement. *J Spinal Disord Tech.* 2001;14:494–499. **(LOE IV)**.

283. Crossman JE, et al. Recurrent atlantoaxial rotatory fixation in children: a rare complication of a rare condition. Report of four cases. *J Neurosurg.* 2004;100(3 Suppl Spine):307–311. **(LOE IV)**.

284. Crossman JE, et al. Open reduction of pediatric atlantoaxial rotatory fixation: long-term outcome study with functional measurements. *J Neurosurg.* 2004;100(3 Suppl Spine):235–240. **(LOE IV)**.

285. Odent T, et al. Fractures of the odontoid process: a report of 15 cases in children younger than 6 years. *J Pediatr Orthop.* 1999;19(1):51–54. **(LOE IV)**.

286. Loder R, ed. *The Cervical Spine Lovell and Winter's Pediatric Orthopaedics, ed.* W.S.e. Morrisy RA. Philadelphia: Lippincott Raven; 1996: 739–779.

287. Sherk HH, Nicholson JT, Chung SM. Fractures of the odontoid process in young children. *J Bone Joint Surg.* 1978;60:921–924. **(LOE IV)**.

288. Mandabah M, Ruge JR, Hahn YS, McLone DG. Pediatric axis fractures: early halo immobilization, management and outcome. *Pediatr Neurosurg.* 1993;19:225–232. **(LOE IV)**.

289. Anderson LD, D'Alonzo RT. Fractures of the odontoid process of the axis. *J Bone Joint Surg Am.* 1974;56(8):1663–1674. **(LOE IV)**.

290. Wang J, Vokshoor A, Kim S, Elton S, Kosnik E, Bartkowski H. Pediatric atlantoaxial instability: management with screw fixation. *Pediatr Neurosug.* 1999;30(2):70–78. **(LOE IV)**.

291. Pryputniewicz DM, Hadley MN. Axis fractures. *Neurosurgery.* 2010;66(suppl 3):68–82. **(LOE V)**.

292. Choit RL, Jamieson DH, Reilly CW. Os odontoideum: a significant radiographic finding. *Pediatr Rad.* 2005;35:803–807. **(LOE IV)**.

293. Fielding JW, Hensinger RN, Hawkins RJ. Os odontoideum. *J Bone Joint Surg.* 1980;62:376–383. **(LOE IV)**.

294. Sankar WN, et al. Os odontoideum revisited: the case for a multifactorial etiology. *Spine.* 2006;31(9):979–984. **(LOE IV)**.

295. Nakamura K, et al. Risk factors of myelopathy at the atlantoaxial level in spondyloepiphyseal dysplasia congenita. *Arch Orthop Trauma Surg.* 1998;117(8):468–470. **(LOE IV)**.

296. Schuler TC, Kurz L, Thompson DE, et al. Case report: natural history of os odontoideum. *J Pediatr Orthop.* 1991;11:222–225. **(LOE V)**.

297. Galli J, Tartaglione T, Calo L, Ottaviani F. Os odontoideum in a patient with cervical vertigo. *Am J Otolaryngology.* 2001;22:371–373. **(LOE V)**.

298. Hughes TB Jr, Richman JD, Rothfus WE. Diagnosis of os odontoideum using kinematic magnetic resonance imaging. *Spine.* 1999;24:715–718. **(LOE V)**.

299. Dempster AG, Heap SW. Fatal high cervical spinal cord injury in an automobile accident complication os odontoideum. *Am J Forensic Med Path.* 1990;11:252–256. **(LOE V)**.

300. McGoldrick JM, Marx JA. Traumatic central cord syndrome in a patient with os odontoideum. *Ann Emerg Med.* 1989;18:1358–1361. **(LOE V)**.

301. Sasaki H, Itoh T, Takei H, et al. Os odontoideum with cerebellar infarction: a case report. *Spine.* 2000;25:1178–1181. **(LOE V)**.

302. Zhang Z, Wang H, Liu C. Acute traumatic cervical cord injury in pediatric patients with os odontoideum: a series of 6 patients. *World Neurosurg.* 2015;83(6):1180.e1–6. **(LOE IV)**.

303. Dai L, Yuan W, Ni B, Jia L. Os odontoideum: etiology, diagnosis, and management. *Surg Neurol.* 2000;53:106–108. **(LOE IV)**.

304. Grisoni NE, Ballock RT, Thompson GH. Second cervical vertebrae pedicle fractures versus synchondrosis in a child. *Clin Orthop Relat Res.* 2003;(413):238–242. **(LOE V)**.

305. Pizzutillo PD, et al. Bilateral fracture of the pedicle of the second cervical vertebra in the young child. *J Bone Joint Surg Am.* 1986;68(6):892–896. **(LOE IV)**.

306. Maves CK, Souza A, Prenger EC, Kirks DR. Traumatic atlanto-occipital disruption in children. *Pediatr Radiolog.* 1991;21:504–507. **(LOE IV)**.

307. Smith T, Skinner SR, Shonnard N. Persistent synchondrosis of the second cervical vertebra simulating a hangman's fracture in a child. *J Bone Joint Surg.* 1993;75A:892–893. **(LOE V)**.

308. Levine AM, Edwards CC. The management of traumatic spondylolisthesis of the axis. *J Bone Joint Surg Am.* 1985;67(2):217–226. **(LOE IV)**.

309. Starr JK, Eismont FJ. Atypical hangman's fractures. *Spine (Phila Pa 1976).* 1993;18(14):1954–7. **(LOE IV)**.

310. Harris MB, Waguespack AM, Kranlage S. "Clearing" cervical spine injuries in polytrauma patients: is it really safe to remove the collar? *Orthopaedics.* 1997;20:903–907. **(LOE V)**.

311. Allen BL Jr, Ferguson RL, Lehmann TR, O'Brien RP. A mechanistic classification of closed, indirect fractures and dislocations of the lower cervical spine. *Spine (Phila Pa 1976).* 1982;7(1):1–27. **(LOE IV)**

312. Lee C, Kim KS, Rogers LF. Triangular cervical vertebral body fractures: diagnostic significance. *AJR Am J Roentgenol.* 1982;138(6):1123–1132. **(LOE IV)**.

313. Kim KS, et al. Flexion teardrop fracture of the cervical spine: radiographic characteristics. *AJR Am J Roentgenol.* 1989;152(2):319–326. **(LOE IV)**.

314. Kahn EA, Schneider RC. Chronic neurological sequelae of acute trauma to the spine and spinal cord. I. The significance of the acute-flexion or tear-drop fracture-dislocation of the cervical spine. *J Bone Joint Surg Am.* 1956;38-A(5):985–997. **(LOE IV)**.

315. Anissipour AK, et al. Cervical facet dislocations in the adolescent population: a report of 21 cases at a Level 1 trauma center from 2004 to 2014. *Eur Spine J.* 2017;26(4):1266–1271. **(LOE IV)**.

316. Vaccaro AR, Madigan L, Schweitzer ME, Flanders AE, Hilibrand AS, Albert TJ. Magnetic resonance imaging analysis of soft tissue disruption after flexion-distraction injuries of the subaxial cervical spine. *Spine.* 2001;26:1866–1872. **(LOE IV)**.

317. Bucholz RD, Cheung KC. Halo vest versus spinal fusion for cervical injury: evidence from an outcome study. *J Neurosurg.* 1989;70(6):884–892. **(LOE III)**.

318. Dormans JP, Criscitiello AA, Drummond DS, Davidson RS. Complications in children managed with immobilization in a halo vest. *J Bone Joint Surg.* 1995;77A:1370–1373. **(LOE IV)**.

319. Mubarak SJ, C.J, Vueltich W, et al. Halo application in the infant. *J Pediatr Orthop.* 1989;9:612–614. **(LOE IV)**.

320. Arkader A, et al. Analysis of halo-orthoses application in children less than three years old. *J Child Orthop.* 2007;1(6):337–344. **(LOE IV)**.

321. Caird MS, et al. Complications and problems in halo treatment of toddlers: limited ambulation is recommended. *J Pediatr Orthop.* 2006;26(6):750–752. **(LOE IV)**.

322. Letts M, K.D, Gouw G. A biomechanical analysis of halo fixation in children. *J Bone Joint Surg.* 1988;70B:277–279. **(LOE N/A)**.

323. Copley LA, et al. A comparative evaluation of halo pin designs in an immature skull model. *Clin Orthop Relat Res.* 1998;(357):212–218. **(LOE N/A)**.

324. Reddy SP, J.J, Backsrom JW. Distribution of spinal fractures in children: does age, mechanism of injury, or gender play a significant role? *Pediatr Radiology.* 2003;33(11):776–781. **(LOE IV)**.

325. Dickson RA, L.K. Spinal injuries in child abuse. *J Trauma.* 1978;18:811–812. **(LOE V)**.

326. Denis F. The three column spine and its significance in the classification of acute thoracolumbar spinal injuries. *Spine.* 1983;9:817–831. **(LOE IV)**.

327. Cui S, Busel GA, Puryear AS. Temporary percutaneous pedicle screw stabilization without fusion of adolescent thoracolumbar spine fractures. *J Pediatr Orthop.* 2016;36(7):701–708. **(LOE IV)**.

328. Akinpelu BJ, et al. Pediatric isolated thoracic and/or lumbar transverse and spinous process fractures. *J Neurosurg Pediatr.* 2016;17(6):639–644. **(LOE IV)**.

329. Seel EH, V.C, Mehta RL, Davies EM. Measurement of fracture kyphosis with the Oxford Cobbometer: intra and interobserver reliabilities and comparison with other techniques. *Spine.* 2005;30:964–968. **(LOE II)**.

330. Roaf R. A study of mechanics of spinal injuries. *J Bone Joint Surg.* 1960;42:810–823. **(LOE N/A)**.

331. Singer G, et al. The influence of brace immobilization on the remodeling potential of thoracolumbar impaction fractures in children and adolescents. *Eur Spine J.* 2016;25(2):607–613. **(LOE III)**.

332. Karlsson MK, et al. A modeling capacity of vertebral fractures exists during growth: an up-to-47-year follow-up. *Spine (Phila Pa 1976).* 2003;28(18):2087–2092. **(LOE IV)**.

333. Angelliaume A, et al. Conservative treatment of pediatric thoracic and lumbar spinal fractures: outcomes in the sagittal plane. *J Pediatr Orthop B.* 2017;26(1):73–79. **(LOE IV)**.

334. Angelliaume A, et al. Post-trauma scoliosis after conservative treatment of thoracolumbar spinal fracture in children and adolescents: results in 48 patients. *Eur Spine J.* 2016;25(4):1144–1152. **(LOE IV)**.

335. Lalonde F, L.M, Yang JP, Thomas K. An analysis of burst fractures of the spine in adolescents. *Am J Orthop.* 2001;30:115–120. **(LOE IV)**.

336. Parisini P, Di Silvestre M, Greggi T. Treatment of spinal fractures in children and adolescents: long-term results in 44 patients. *Spine.* 2002;27(18):1989–1994. **(LOE IV)**.

337. Thomas KC, et al. Multiple-level thoracolumbar burst fractures in teenaged patients. *J Pediatr Orthop.* 2003;23(1):119–123. **(LOE IV)**.

338. Wood K, B.G, Mehbod A, Garvey T, Jhanjee R, Sechriest V. Operative compared with nonoperative treatment of a thoracolumbar burst fracture without neurologic deficit. *J Bone Joint Surg.* 2003;85A:773–781. **(LOE II)**.

339. Vander Have KL, et al. Burst fractures of the thoracic and lumbar spine in children and adolescents. *J Pediatr Orthop.* 2009;29(7):713–719. **(LOE IV)**.

340. DeWald R. Burst fractures of the thoracic and lumbar spine. *Clin Orthop Rel Research.* 1984;189:150–161. **(LOE V)**.

341. Vaccaro AR, et al. A new classification of thoracolumbar injuries: the importance of injury morphology, the integrity of the posterior ligamentous complex, and neurologic status. *Spine (Phila Pa 1976).* 2005;30(20):2325–2333. **(LOE V)**.

342. Denis F, et al. Acute thoracolumbar burst fractures in the absence of neurologic deficit. A comparison between operative and nonoperative treatment. *Clin Orthop Relat Res.* 1984;189:142–149. **(LOE IV)**.

343. Daniels AH, Sobel AD, Eberson CP. Pediatric thoracolumbar spine trauma. *J Am Acad Orthop Surg.* 2013;21(12):707–716. **(LOE IV)**.

344. Radcliff K, et al. Correlation of posterior ligamentous complex injury and neurological injury to loss of vertebral body height, kyphosis, and canal compromise. *Spine.* 2012;37(13):1142–1150. **(LOE IV)**.

345. Wang ST, et al. Is fusion necessary for surgically treated burst fractures of the thoracolumbar and lumbar spine? A prospective, randomized study. *Spine (Phila Pa 1976).* 2006;31(23):2646–2652; discussion 2653. **(LOE IV)**.

346. Wild MH, et al. Five-year follow-up examination after purely minimally invasive posterior stabilization of thoracolumbar fractures: a comparison of minimally invasive percutaneously and conventionally open treated patients. *Arch Orthop Trauma Surg.* 2007;127(5):335–343. **(LOE III)**.

347. Carl AL, Tromanhauser SG, Roger DJ. Pedicle screw instrumentation for thoracolumbar burst fractures and fracture-dislocations. *Spine (Phila Pa 1976).* 1992;17(suppl 8):S317–S324. **(LOE IV)**.

348. McLain RF, Sparling E, Benson DR. Early failure of short-segment pedicle instrumentation for thoracolumbar fractures. A preliminary report. *J Bone Joint Surg Am.* 1993;75(2):162–167. **(LOE IV)**.

349. McNamara MJ, Stephens GC, Spengler DM. Transpedicular short-segment fusions for treatment of lumbar burst fractures. *J Spinal Disord.* 1992;5(2):183–187. **(LOE IV)**.

350. Ilharreborde B, et al. Circumferential fusion with anterior strut grafting and short-segment multipoint posterior fixation for burst fractures in skeletally immature patients: a preliminary report. *J Pediatr Orthop.* 2012;32(5):440–444. **(LOE IV)**.

351. Agrawal M, et al. Management of pediatric posttraumatic thoracolumbar vertebral body burst fractures by Use of single-stage posterior transpedicular approach. *World Neurosurg.* 2018;117:e22–e33. **(LOE IV)**.

352. Ebraheim NA, S.E, Southworth SR. Pediatric lumbar seat belt injuries. *Orthopaedics.* 1991;14:1010–1033. **(LOE IV)**.

353. Chance GQ. Note on a type of flexion fracture of the spine. *Br J Radiol.* 1948;21(249):452. **(LOE V)**.

354. Garrett JW, Braunstein PW. The seat belt syndrome. *J Trauma.* 1962;2:220–238. **(LOE V)**.

355. Achildi O, Betz RR, Grewal H. Lapbelt injuries and the seat-belt syndrome in pediatric spinal cord injury. *J Spinal Cord Med.* 2007;30(suppl 1):S21–4. **(LOE V)**.

356. Rumball K, J.J. Seat-belt injuries of the spine in young children. *J Bone Joint Surg.* 1992;74B:571–574. **(LOE IV)**.

357. Choit RL, et al. Abdominal aortic injuries associated with chance fractures in pediatric patients. *J Pediatr Surg.* 2006;41(6):1184–1190. **(LOE IV)**.

358. Couselo M, et al. Diaphragmatic avulsion with chance fracture: a rare association in the seat belt syndrome. *Pediatr Emerg Care.* 2011;27(6):553–555. **(LOE V)**.

359. Arkader A, et al. Pediatric Chance fractures: a multicenter perspective. *J Pediatr Orthop.* 2011;31(7):741–744. **(LOE III)**.

360. Mulpuri K, et al. The spectrum of abdominal injuries associated with chance fractures in pediatric patients. *Eur J Pediatr Surg.* 2007;17(5):322–327. **(LOE IV)**.

361. Swischuk LE, Jadhav SP, Chung DH. Aortic injury with Chance fracture in a child. *Emerg Radiol.* 2008;15(5):285–287. **(LOE V)**.

362. West Jr CA, et al. Acute aortic occlusion in a child secondary to lap-belt injury treated with thromboendarterectomy and primary repair. *J Vasc Surg.* 2011;54(2):515–518. **(LOE V)**.

363. Louman-Gardiner K, et al. Pediatric lumbar Chance fractures in British Columbia: chart review and analysis of the use of shoulder restraints in MVAs. *Accid Anal Prev.* 2008;40(4):1424–1429. **(LOE IV)**.

364. Santschi M, Lemoine C, Cyr C. The spectrum of seat belt syndrome among Canadian children: results of a two-year popula-

tion surveillance study. *Paediatr Child Health*. 2008;13(4):279–283. **(LOE IV)**.

365. Durbin DR, Elliott MR, Winston FK. Belt-positioning booster seats and reduction in risk of injury among children in vehicle crashes. *J Am Med Assoc*. 2003;289(21):2835–2840. **(LOE III)**.

366. Howard A, Snowdon A, Macarthur C. Removing barriers to booster seat use in Canada. *Paediatr Child Health*. 2004;9(5):309–311. **(LOE V)**.

367. Gallagher DJ, Heinrich SD. Pediatric chance fracture. *J Orthop Trauma*. 1990;4(2):183–187. **(LOE V)**.

368. Glassman SD, J.J, Holt RT. Seatbelt injuries in children. *J Trauma*. 1992;33:882–886. **(LOE IV)**.

369. LeGay DA, Petrie DP, Alexander DI. Flexion-distraction injuries of the lumbar spine and associated abdominal trauma. *J Trauma*. 1990;30(4):436–444. **(LOE IV)**.

370. Heller JG, Garfin SR, Abitbol JJ. Disk herniations associated with compression instrumentation of lumbar flexion-distraction injuries. *Clin Orthop Rel Research*. 1992;284:91–98. **(LOE IV)**.

371. Bick EM, Copel JW. The ring apophysis of the human vertebra; contribution to human osteogeny. *II. J Bone Joint Surg Am*. 1951;33-A(3):783–787. **(LOE N/A)**.

372. Akhaddar A, et al. Posterior ring apophysis separation combined with lumbar disc herniation in adults: a 10-year experience in the surgical management of 87 cases. *J Neurosurg Spine*. 2011;14(4):475–483. **(LOE IV)**.

373. Wu X, et al. A review of current treatment of lumbar posterior ring apophysis fracture with lumbar disc herniation. *Eur Spine J*. 2013;22(3):475–488. **(LOE V)**.

374. Bae JS, et al. Clinical and radiologic analysis of posterior apophyseal ring separation associated with lumbar disc herniation. *J Korean Neurosurg Soc*. 2013;53(3):145–149. **(LOE IV)**.

375. Scarfo GB, et al. Posterior retroextramarginal disc hernia (PREMDH): definition, diagnosis, and treatment. *Surg Neurol*. 1996;46(3):205–211. **(LOE IV)**.

376. Yang IK, et al. Posterior lumbar apophyseal ring fractures: a report of 20 cases. *Neuroradiology*. 1994;36(6):453–455. **(LOE IV)**.

377. Chang CH, et al. Clinical significance of ring apophysis fracture in adolescent lumbar disc herniation. *Spine (Phila Pa 1976)*. 2008;33(16):1750–1754. **(LOE IV)**.

378. Singhal A, et al. Ring apophysis fracture in pediatric lumbar disc herniation: a common entity. *Pediatr Neurosurg*. 2013;49(1):16–20. **(LOE IV)**.

379. Epstein NE, Epstein EJ. Limbus lumbar vertebral fractures in 27 adolescents and adults. *Spine*. 1991;16:962–966. **(LOE IV)**.

380. Mendez JS, Huete IL, Tagle PM. Limbus lumbar and sacral vertebral fractures. *Neurologic Research*. 2002;24:139–144. **(LOE IV)**.

381. Epstein NE. Lumbar surgery for 56 limbus fractures emphasizing noncalcified type III lesions. *Spine (Phila Pa 1976)*. 1992;17(12):1489–1496. **(LOE IV)**.

382. Epstein NE, Epstein JA, Mauri T. Treatment of fractures of the vertebral limbus and spinal stenosis in five adolescents and five adults. *Neurosurgery*. 1989;24(4):595–604. **(LOE IV)**.

383. Takata K, et al. Fracture of the posterior margin of a lumbar vertebral body. *J Bone Joint Surg Am*. 1988;70(4):589–594. **(LOE IV)**.

384. Shirado O, et al. Lumbar disc herniation associated with separation of the ring apophysis: is removal of the detached apophyses mandatory to achieve satisfactory results? *Clin Orthop Relat Res*. 2005;(431):120–128. **(LOE IV)**.

385. Asazuma T, et al. Lumbar disc herniation associated with separation of the posterior ring apophysis: analysis of five surgical cases and review of the literature. *Acta Neurochir*. 2003;145(6):461–466; discussion 466. **(LOE IV)**.

386. Baba H, et al. Posterior limbus vertebral lesions causing lumbosacral radiculopathy and the cauda equina syndrome. *Spinal Cord*. 1996;34(7):427–432. **(LOE IV)**.

387. Dang L, Liu Z. A review of current treatment for lumbar disc herniation in children and adolescents. *Eur Spine J*. 2010;19(2):205–214. **(LOE V)**.

388. Higashino K, et al. Long-term outcomes of lumbar posterior apophyseal end-plate lesions in children and adolescents. *J Bone Joint Surg Am*. 2012;94(11):e74. **(LOE III)**.

11 Fractures and Dislocations about the Hip and Pelvis

John B. Erickson | Walter Samora | Kevin E. Klingele

FRACTURES AND DISLOCATIONS OF THE PELVIS AND ACETABULUM

INTRODUCTION/PATHOLOGY

INCIDENCE

The overall incidence of pediatric pelvic fractures is 1 per 100,000 children per year.[1,2] Although rare, these fractures are identified in pediatric trauma patients at a reported rate between 2.4% and 7.5%.[3–8] This rate increases to nearly 20% in polytraumatized patients.[9] There is a male predominance with a male-to-female ratio of 1.4:1 and an average age of 9 years.[10] Sacral fractures are present in 0.16% of pediatric trauma and 4.76% of pediatric pelvic fractures.[11] Acetabular fractures constitute 0.8% to 15% of fractures of the pelvis in children.[6,12–16]

RELEVANT ANATOMY

The immature pelvic bone consists of three primary ossifications centers along with their corresponding physes undergoing endochondral ossification.[17,18] These ossifications centers represent the developing ilium, ischium, and pubis. The physeal portion of the ilium, ischium, and pubic bones converge at the immature acetabulum and form the Y-shaped triradiate cartilage (Fig. 11.1). The triradiate cartilage typically closes at 12 to 14 years of age and is a reliable predictor of skeletal maturity.[7] In addition to these primary ossification centers, a number of secondary ossifications centers arise in the pelvis as development continues (Fig. 11.2). It is important for treating clinicians to be familiar with these structures, as it is key to accurately interpreting radiographic studies of the immature pelvis. Children also have thicker periosteum and more elastic pubic symphyseal and sacroiliac (SI) joints compared with adults. For this reason, multifocal pelvic ring fractures and ligament ruptures are rare in children as compared with adults. The high cartilaginous volume and thick periosteum found in the immature pelvis provides a greater capacity for energy absorption and helps mitigate fracture displacement. However, fractures occurring within the cartilaginous regions of the pelvis can often make diagnosis more difficult. Furthermore, fractures in these regions can result in growth disturbances that may lead to deformity or secondary dysplasia.[19]

In addition to their more durable pelvic rings, children also have a more effective hemostatic response to pelvic trauma. Children have smaller, more compliant blood vessels, allowing better vasoconstriction in response to pelvic hemorrhage. Furthermore, their thick periosteum reduces fracture displacement and has a tamponade effect on bleeding from osseous surfaces. For these reasons, pelvic fractures in children rarely lead to life-threatening arterial hemorrhage, which has been reported in 10% to 20% of adult pelvic fracture cases.[20–22]

MECHANISM OF INJURY/BIOMECHANICS

Because the pediatric pelvis is more resilient to sustaining a fracture, pelvic and acetabular fractures in children are generally the result of high-energy trauma.[23–25] The majority of pediatric pelvic fractures are the result of pedestrian versus motor vehicle accidents. This mechanism accounts for 39% to 78% of cases in the pediatric population, whereas the majority of adult pelvic fractures are the result of motor vehicle accidents (passenger injuries). Motor vehicle passenger injuries are the second most common cause of pediatric pelvic fractures, accounting for 10% to 30% of cases.[26–30] Other common mechanisms include falls from height, bike and motorbike accidents, and high-energy sports injuries.[30–34] These differences in mechanism of injury also play a role in the different mortality rates from pelvic injury seen between these two populations.[35,36] Children are more likely to be struck on the side, resulting in lateral compression–type injuries, which typically reduce pelvic volume and blood loss. Adults often sustain head-on motor vehicle collisions, resulting in anterior-posterior compression injuries, which can result in life-threatening hemorrhage and mortality.[37]

Avulsion fractures of the pediatric pelvis are much more common than pelvic ring and acetabular fractures.[38–44] They typically occur as the result of traction from an attached muscle on secondary ossification centers, including the ischial tuberosity, anterior-superior iliac spine (ASIS), anterior-inferior iliac spine (AIIS), and iliac apophysis. These injuries are often the result of low-energy mechanisms and often occur during athletic participation.[45] The vast majority of these injuries can be treated nonoperatively—a period of protected weight-bearing followed by gradual strengthening and return to activities.[46] Avulsion fractures displaced greater than 2 cm have a higher rate nonunion and may be treated with open reduction internal fixation.[47–49]

ASSOCIATED INJURIES

Pelvic fractures are associated with additional injuries in approximately 58% to 87% of cases.[9,50] These injuries include both visceral and additional skeletal injuries. The most commonly associated fractures include femur, skull, ribs, tibia and fibula, clavicle, facial bones, and humerus in decreasing order of incidence.[51] Children with at least one other associated fracture have a significantly higher incidence of

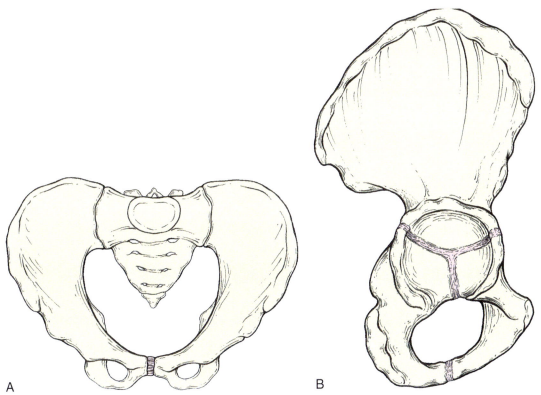

Fig. 11.1 Pediatric pelvic osseous anatomy. (A) The inlet orientation illustrates the two innominate bones, the sacrum, and the pubic symphysis. (B) The lateral orientation reveals the triradiate cartilage as the confluence of the iliac, ischial, and pubic apophyses.

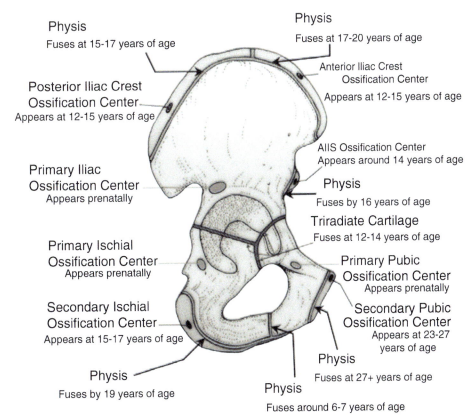

Fig. 11.2 The location of ossification centers in the pelvic bone, noting when they appear and when physes fuse. Note the Y-shaped triradiate cartilage at the acetabulum. (From Scheuer L, Black SM. *The Juvenile Skeleton*. London: Elsevier Academic Press; 2004.)

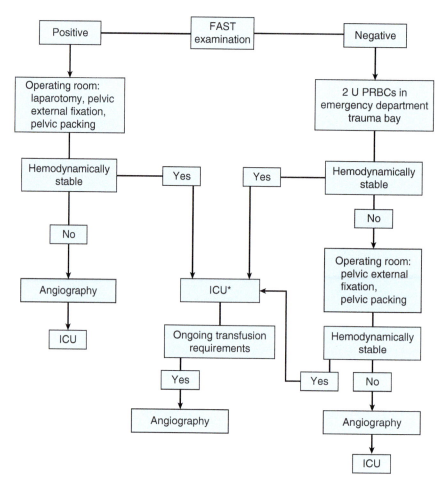

Fig. 11.3 Algorithm for the treatment of patients with pelvic fracture who present with hemodynamic instability. *Patients in whom a laparotomy was not done usually have an abdominal computed tomography scan en route to the intensive care unit (*ICU*). In the ICU, the patient receives further fluid resuscitation and is warmed; attempts are made to normalize the coagulation status. Recombinant factor VIIa should be considered if the patient is recalcitrant to all other interventions. Abbreviations: *FAST*, focused abdominal sonography for trauma; *PRBCs*, packed red blood cells. (From Hak DJ, Smith WR, Suzuki T. Management of hemorrhage in life-threatening pelvic fracture. *J Am Acad Orthop Surg.* 2009;17(7):447-457. With permission.)

head and abdominal injuries, as well as an associated need for blood transfusions.[52,53] The visceral injuries directly related to the pelvic injury include bladder and urethral injuries, traction or avulsion injuries of the lumbosacral plexus, and injury to the major and minor arterial and venous systems, with resultant hemorrhage.[54,55] Injuries associated with high-energy blunt trauma may involve the pulmonary, cardiac, gastrointestinal, and central nervous systems. Lateral compression (LC)–type pelvic injuries are associated with neurologic injury, including closed head injuries, with up to 57% of pediatric pelvic fracture patients sustaining a concomitant neurologic injury. Head trauma has been reported to be responsible for 75% of deaths seen in children with traumatic pelvic fractures.[3,56] Identification of a pelvic injury in the primary phase of the resuscitation and injury survey should alert the physician to the possibility of these associated injuries. The associated injuries are often more difficult to treat and generally have a greater effect on the patient's overall outcome than does the pelvic fracture.[57]

EVALUATION

The evaluation of the pediatric trauma patient must be systematic and multidisciplinary, including the surgical trauma team, emergency medicine personnel, and orthopedic specialists.

HISTORY

As mentioned, pelvic and acetabular fractures in the pediatric population typically occur secondary to children being struck by automobiles or as a result of their being unrestrained passengers in motor vehicle accidents. A history of high-energy trauma should direct the emergency medical service team to an appropriate response in the field and during transfer of the patient to a regional trauma center. The history of high-energy injury mechanism dictates full-scale primary and secondary surveys, institution of large-bore venous access, and other resuscitative measures as outlined in previous chapters. Apophyseal avulsion injuries are generally caused by lower-energy athletic injuries and typically do not require trauma system activation.

PHYSICAL EXAM

The evaluation procedure for a pediatric trauma patient suspected of having pelvic trauma should follow Advanced Trauma Life Support (ATLS) guidelines beginning with primary survey, including airway, breathing, and circulatory status. Special attention should then be given to injuries of the head, chest, abdominal viscera, spine, and pelvis to evaluate for potential life-threatening injuries. Hemodynamically unstable patients with suspected pelvic injury should be promptly evaluated with an anteroposterior (AP) pelvis radiograph and stabilized with a sheet or pelvic binder as dictated by radiographic findings. Concurrently, the trauma team should evaluate the patient for other sites of hemorrhage and treat accordingly. An algorithm for the trauma bay treatment of these patients has been proposed by Hak et al (Fig. 11.3).[21]

Once the primary survey is completed and the patient is found to be hemodynamically stable, attention may be

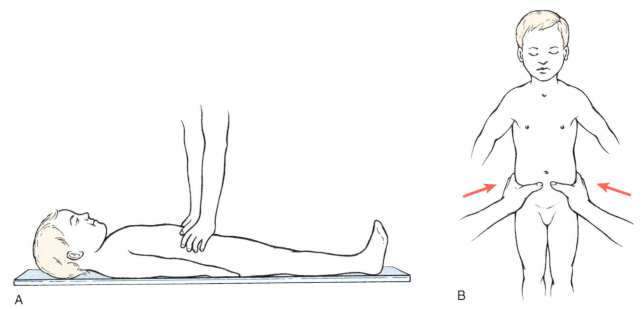

A   B

Fig. 11.4 Clinical examination of pelvic stability. (A) Examining for anteroposterior instability by applying posteriorly directed force on the anterior iliac crests. The examination is most effective when done early, while the patient is in the emergency department and still on the backboard used for transport. (B) Examination for external rotation stability (such as that occurring in an open-book fracture, type B1) by applying force on the external aspect of the pelvis and directing it toward the midline.

turned to the secondary survey, including evaluation for potential pelvic injury. Visual inspection of the pelvic region, including the scrotum, vagina, urethra, and perineal region, is necessary to rule out potential injury. Contusions, abrasions, and areas of degloving are identified and recorded. Although Morel-Lavallee (internal degloving) lesions are uncommon in children, they can be seen in overweight children and adolescents.[58] In the perineum, lacerations are often the result of open fractures.[59] Vaginal lacerations are not unusual,[60,61] and a digital pelvic examination should be performed in all female patients with a displaced anterior ring fracture; preferably, this examination is done with the patient under sedation or with the use of an anesthetic in prepubescent children.[62] Similarly, a digital rectal examination is done to check for gross blood or boney fragments, indicative of a rectal perforation or sphincter injury.[25]

When the inspection is completed, pelvic stability is evaluated, preferably while the patient is still on the backboard. AP stability is assessed by the clinician, placing the palms of the hands on the anterior iliac crests and applying posteriorly directed pressure (Fig. 11.4). By placing the palms on the lateral aspect of the anterior crests and applying pressure directed toward the midline, the examiner can check for rotational instability (Fig. 11.4). Pain on AP or medially directed pressure in a conscious patient is carefully documented. In addition, the examiner uses palpation along the posterior iliac spine, SI joint, and sacrum to look for pain consistent with a posterior pelvic ring injury. A final check on vertical or rotational instability can be made by assessment of the relative height of the anterior superior iliac spine and relative leg lengths.

After the inspection and palpation phases are completed, a thorough evaluation of the arterial circulation is made. The femoral, popliteal, dorsalis pedis, and posterior tibial pulses are palpated. If nonpalpable, a Doppler ultrasound

examination is done for determination of biphasic pulsatile flow. Limb temperature is assessed by palpation. Finally, in an alert and cooperative patient, a gross motor examination of all major muscle groups in the lower extremity is completed bilaterally, as well as a sensory examination with light touch and pinprick. The latter should include the perirectal area because of the frequent involvement of the sacral plexus with sacral fractures. This is not possible in younger children who are unable to cooperate with the demands of this type of evaluation. Rectal tone should be assessed and documented during the digital rectal examination.

IMAGING

An important part of the initial evaluation of a multiply injured child is an AP radiograph of the pelvis. Gonadal shielding should not be used because it may obscure the anterior pelvic ring.[63] It is important to note that the pubic symphysis in very young children may be 10 mm to 12 mm wide as compared with 2 mm to 4 mm wide in adult patients.[16] It is important to thoroughly evaluate all obtained imaging studies, as the presence of one injury can often interfere with the detection of additional injuries.[64,65] Two additional views are indicated if a fracture of the pelvic ring is identified on the initial radiograph: a 30- to 45-degree (aimed distally) inlet view or "down shot," which will demonstrate a posterior pelvic ring injury and any anterior/posterior displacement more clearly, and a 40- to 45-degree (aimed toward the head of the patient) "tangential," outlet, "brim shot," or "up view," which will delineate the anterior pelvic ring and help assess vertical stability (Figs. 11.5 and 11.6).[66,67] Both are helpful for identifying internal or external rotation of one of the hemipelves relative to the other. These three radiographs can help determine the mechanism of injury and the form of treatment for most fractures.[68] Sacral fractures and SI joint injuries are frequently missed with standard plain

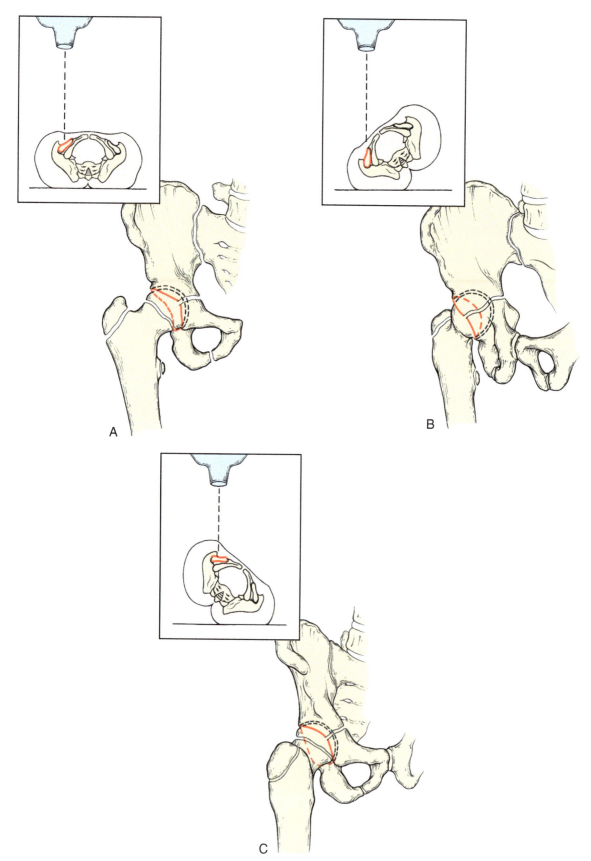

Fig. 11.5 Schematics of three radiographic views necessary for assessment of acetabular fractures. (A) The anteroposterior pelvis (or hip) view allows assessment of the iliopectineal line, the ilium, the anterior and posterior walls, and the pubis. (B) The iliac oblique view of Judet allows optimal assessment of the ischial spine, the posterior column and anterior wall, and the iliac fossae. (C) The obturator oblique view of Judet allows optimal assessment of the iliac wing, anterior column and posterior wall, and the obturator foramen.

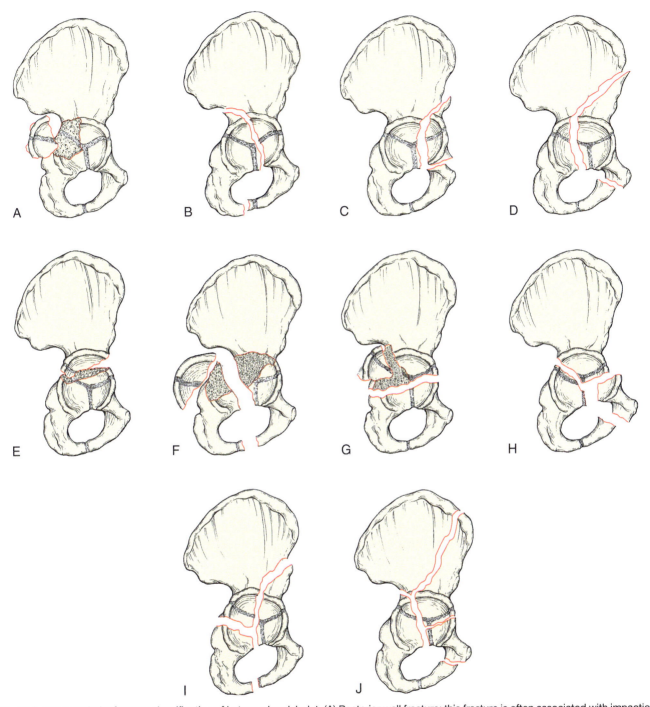

Fig. 11.6 The acetabular fracture classification of Letournel and Judet. (A) Posterior wall fracture; this fracture is often associated with impaction of the intact side of the fracture margin. (B) Posterior column fracture. (C) Anterior wall fracture; an atypically large fragment size is shown. (D) Anterior column fracture; the most posterior location of the fracture line through the acetabulum is shown. (E) Transverse fracture pattern; this location is transtectal. The fracture may cross the acetabulum either higher (juxtatectal) or lower (infratectal). (F) Associated posterior column and posterior wall fractures. (G) Associated transverse and posterior wall fractures. (H) T-shaped fracture. (I) Associated anterior column and posterior hemitransverse fractures. (J) A both-column fracture; note that no segment of the acetabulum remains attached to the intact ilium.

radiographs and may require computed tomography (CT) for further evaluation. CT is also helpful in diagnosing pelvic hematoma, an important factor in the initial treatment of the patient. Cut intervals of 2 to 3 mm are generally sufficient for delineating the skeletal injury.[69] Images should be obtained from the L5 vertebral body to the lower pelvic region in the axial plane with the use of contiguous sections and soft tissue and bone window techniques.[70] Because CT

is becoming more widely used to screen for abdominal injuries, the images should be scrutinized by the treating orthopedist.[71] These images can be useful for detecting fracture or SI joint disruption. CT has been shown to have greater sensitivity than the AP pelvic radiograph in children; however, the radiation dose exposure to children should prompt careful consideration of the value of treatment implications from the information gleaned.[71]

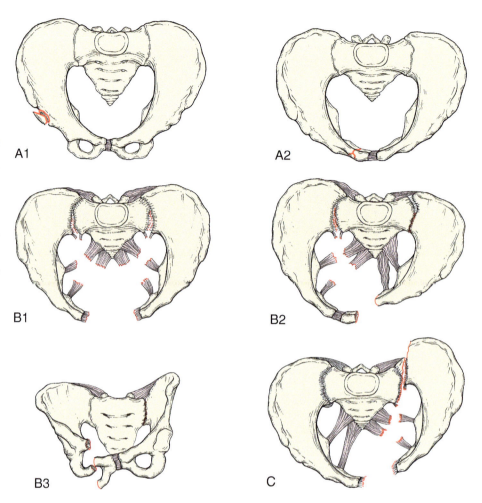

Fig. 11.7 The Pennal-Tile classification of pelvic fractures as applied to children. Type A1: An avulsion fracture of the anterior inferior iliac spine (the straight head of the rectus femoris muscle). Type A2: A minimally displaced fracture of the ischium and pubis without posterior ring injury. Type B1: An anteroposterior force has produced an open-book injury with more than 3 cm of symphyseal disruption. By definition, the anterior portion of the sacroiliac joints has been disrupted. Type B2: A lateral compression mechanism has produced an ipsilateral anterior sacral alar crush and displaced ischial and pubic ramus fractures. Type B3: The same force vector (laterally applied, oriented toward the midline in the coronal plane) has produced contralateral disruption of the sacroiliac joint (with a minor ipsilateral anterior sacral impaction) and displaced pubic and ischial ramus fractures. Type C: A Pennal-Tile IIIC1 injury with total disruption of the sacroiliac joint and posterior vertical and rotational displacement of the hemipelvis associated with symphyseal disruption.

Because of the complex anatomy of the innominate bone, fractures of the acetabulum require a different approach for radiographic evaluation. The 45-degree oblique views described by Letournel and associates[72] are indicated when the scout AP pelvic film demonstrates involvement of the acetabulum. The iliac oblique view shows the posterior column in profile, as well as the iliac ring and anterior wall. The obturator oblique view places the anterior column in profile and shows the obturator foramen clearly, as well as the posterior wall. The two views, combined with the AP pelvic view, allow the physician to classify the fracture according to the scheme of Letournel and Judet (Fig. 11.7).[72] CT is an important adjunct to these conventional radiographic views but is not a substitute.[69] It is especially helpful for detecting intraarticular loose fragments, which occur commonly in patients with associated hip dislocation.[27] CT also helps define fragments impacted in the acetabular margin (posterior wall), as well as occult posterior pelvic ring fractures.[73] Sacral fractures can easily be missed without CT imaging.[74]

When evaluating radiographic studies of the pediatric trauma patient, it is important to pay special attention to the status of the triradiate cartilage, as this has been shown to be a reliable indicator of skeletal maturity.[7] A number of studies have found differences in pelvic fracture patterns based on the status of the triradiate cartilage.[288] Both Silber et al and Shaath et al found higher rates of unstable pelvic ring injuries, acetabular fractures, and sacral fractures in patients with closed triradiate cartilages.[281] Furthermore, patients with

closed triradiate cartilage lack the elasticity and remodeling potential seen in patients with an immature pelvis and should therefore be treated similar to the adult patients.[1]

SPECIAL STUDIES

In the case of suspected hip dislocation or injury to cartilaginous structures (triradiate cartilage), hip arthrography or magnetic resonance imaging (MRI) may be useful.[59] Although MRI can provide valuable information in regard to cartilage injury in the immature pelvis, it is often difficult to obtain in the acute setting and is contraindicated in the unstable patient. Further information can be found in the section entitled "Hip Dislocations".

When injury to the lower urinary tract is suspected, either by blood at the urethral meatus or by widely displaced anterior ring fractures, a retrograde urethrogram should be performed.[75–79] Once a Foley catheter has been definitively placed, a cystogram can be performed to exclude bladder rupture. A urine specimen can be sent for laboratory evaluation for occult hematuria.

CLASSIFICATION

The Tile-Pennal (Fig. 11.7) and Young-Burgess (Fig. 11.8) classification systems have historically been used to classify pelvic ring fractures in adults.[80–82] These classifications systems divide pelvic ring injury–based mechanism of injury and pelvic ring stability. Anterior-posterior compression–type injuries are seen in cases of frontal impacts (head-on

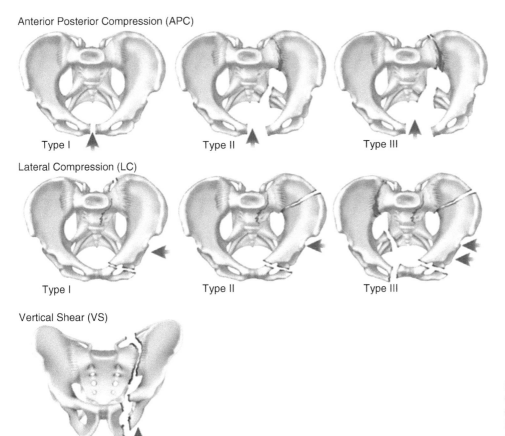

Anterior Posterior Compression (APC)

Type I   Type II   Type III

Lateral Compression (LC)

Type I   Type II   Type III

Vertical Shear (VS)

Fig. 11.8 The classification of pelvic disruptions as described by Young et al. (Published with permission from Kate Sweeney, UW Creative, University of Washington, Seattle, WA, USA.)

MVCs [motor vehicle crashes]) and are associated with higher risk for vascular injury and hemorrhage. LC injuries typically result from side-on collisions (pedestrian versus motor vehicle) and are associated with high rates of abdominal and head injuries. Vertical shear injuries typically result from falls from height. These classification systems are useful in patients with a mature pelvis, including adolescents with a closed triradiate cartilage.

Pediatric patients with an immature pelvis are better described using the Torode and Zieg classification system. The system was originally described in 1985 and classifies pediatric pelvic fractures into four categories (I–IV).[56] The system was further modified by Shore et al in 2012, creating the Modified Torode and Zieg (MTZ) classification, which created two subgroups for type III fractures. This modification reclassified multifocal but stable pelvic ring fractures from type IV fractures, reserving type IV classification for unstable pelvic ring injures (Fig. 11.9).[83] Fracture stability is typically assessed using combined clinical and radiographic examination. Stable fractures demonstrate stability to clinical compression and less than 2 mm of displacement on CT imaging of the anterior and posterior ring injuries. Unstable fractures demonstrate gross clinical instability and/or greater than 2 mm of displacement of both anterior and posterior ring fractures on CT imaging.

MTZ type I fractures represent avulsion fractures of the immature pelvis. These typically involve separation of bony elements of the pelvis through or adjacent to a cartilaginous growth plate at the site of muscular attachments. Common pediatric pelvic avulsion injuries include the ischial

tuberosity, ASIS, and AIIS. Type II fractures involve fractures of the iliac wing and do not disrupt pelvic ring stability. These injuries can be either bony or apophyseal, and are typically the result of a direct blow to the lateral aspect of the pelvis. Type III fractures involve fractures of the pelvic ring but do not result in clinical instability. Type IIIa fractures include simple anterior pelvic ring fractures involving the pubic rami or pubic symphysis disruption. Type IIIb fractures include multifocal pelvic ring injuries with fractures of both the anterior and posterior structures. Although both represent clinically stable fracture patterns, it is important to distinguish between type IIIa and IIIb fractures. Patients with type IIIb fractures exhibit characteristics similar to type IV fractures in regard to length of stay, number of concomitant injuries, and need for blood product transfusion, with type IIIb fractures requiring blood products greater than 2.5 times more frequently than type IIIa fracture.[83] Type IV fractures include unstable pelvic ring injuries, straddle injuries (bilateral superior and inferior pubic rami fractures), pelvic fractures with associated hip dislocation, and pelvic ring injuries with extension into the acetabulum, or combined injuries of the pelvic ring and acetabulum.

For acetabular fractures, the classification of Letournel and Judet is the most universally used system.[72] This system is typically used for skeletally mature patients (closed triradiate cartilage). For skeletally immature patients, the Bucholz classification for acetabular fractures can be used (Fig. 11.10). This system describes the injury to the immature acetabulum using the Salter-Harris classification system and is based on the mechanism of injury and direction of force

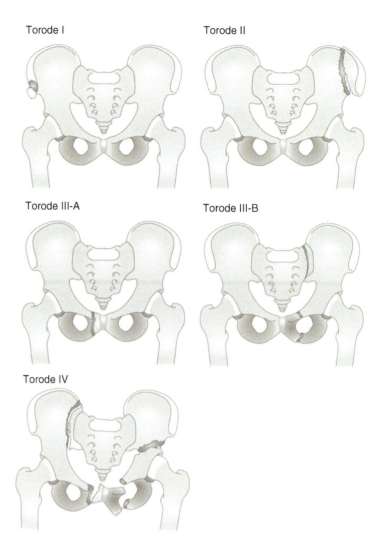

Fig. 11.9 The modified Torode classification. Torode I (avulsion fractures): avulsion of the bony elements of the pelvis, invariably a separation through or adjacent to the cartilaginous growth plate. Torode II (iliac wing fractures): resulting from a direct lateral force against the pelvis, causing a disruption of the iliac apophysis or an infolding fracture of the wing of the ilium. Torode III-A (simple anterior ring fractures): this group involved only children with stable anterior fractures involving the pubic rami or pubic symphysis. Torode III-B (stable anterior and posterior ring fractures): this new group involved children with both anterior and posterior ring fractures that were stable. Torode IV (unstable ring disruption fractures): this group of children had unstable pelvic fractures, including ring disruptions, hip dislocations, and combined pelvic and acetabular fractures. (From Shore BJ, Palmer CS, Bevin C, Johnson MB, Torode IP. Pediatric pelvic fracture: a modification of a preexisting classification. *J Pediatr Orthop.* 2012;32(2):162-168. With permission.)

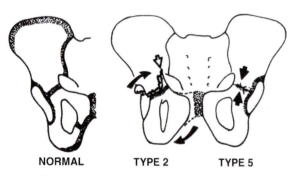

Fig. 11.10 Schematic drawing of type II and type V growth-mechanism injuries. A type II injury is often associated with a rotatory disruption of the ischiopubic unit (curved arrows). A Thurston-Holland fragment *(open arrow)* occurs along the medial wall of the pelvis. Type V is a crushing injury *(arrows)*. (From Bucholz RW, Ezaki M, Ogden JA. Injury to the acetabular triradiate physeal cartilage. *J Bone Joint Surg Am.* 1982;64(4):600-609. With permission.)

across the physes of the triradiate cartilage. A shearing-type injury occurs as a result of a blow to the pubis, ischial ramus, or proximal femur and results in an injury between the two superior arms of the triradiate cartilage and the metaphysis of the ilium. This results in a Salter-Harris type I or II fracture. This fracture pattern splits the acetabulum into the superior one-third (weight-bearing) and inferior two-thirds (minimal weight-bearing) portions and is associated with a lower rate of growth disturbance. The second fracture type results from a crushing- or impaction-type injury across the triradiate cartilage and results in a Salter-Harris type V injury. This injury may be difficult to detect on plain imaging and may only become clinically evident after growth arrest has occurred.[19]

TREATMENT

PELVIC FRACTURES

EMERGENT TREATMENT

Emergency treatment follows the same protocols established in adult patients and focuses on restoration of hemodynamic stability and damage-control orthopedic surgery.[84,85] Emergent pelvic bleeding control, provisional pelvic ring fixation, and prompt treatment of life-threatening additional pelvic injuries are the measures necessary for achieving hemodynamic stability. Pelvic fractures associated with significant hemorrhage or concomitant intraabdominal injury requiring laparotomy may benefit from more aggressive emergency treatment. This situation is rare in children.[5]

Direct retroperitoneal or preperitoneal packing has been shown to be effective in stabilizing hemodynamically unstable pediatric pelvic fractures.[86–88] Embolization should be considered in the setting of patients not responding to direct packing, although the survival rate is not significantly improved in those cases.[89] Pelvic hemorrhaging frequently responds to closing down the pelvic volume. This may be accomplished using a pelvic binder or sheeting technique. Recently, pelvic straps have been developed that are placed at the level of the trochanters and can be tightened and held with Velcro, closing down the pelvic volume. Caution with other compressive techniques, such as antishock trousers, should be used, as they can cause more harm than benefit to the patient.[90] Open fractures require intravenous (IV) antibiotics and urgent irrigation and débridement. After appropriate resuscitation, definitive fracture management is initiated after the full diagnostic evaluation is complete.

NONOPERATIVE TREATMENT

INDICATIONS

It is estimated that between 77% and 94% of all pediatric pelvic fracture patients can be successfully treated nonoperatively.[5,8,91,92] Indications for nonoperative treatment of skeletally immature pelvic fractures and ring injuries include minimally displaced modified Torode and Zeig type I to III fractures in patients without evidence of hemodynamic instability. Straddle injuries, although considered type IV injuries, can typically be treated nonoperatively, as only the anterior ring is disrupted.

TECHNIQUE

Methods of nonoperative treatment have historically included bed rest, protected weight-bearing, immobilization, skeletal traction, and pelvic sling or binder. However, long periods of bed rest and immobilization have fallen out of favor because of the additional risks this places on the polytrauma patient with multiorgan system injuries. For this reason, a short period of immobilization and/or non-weight-bearing, followed by early rehabilitation and mobilization, has become common place in nonoperative treatment of children with pelvic fractures. Typically, the patient is initially kept non-weight-bearing on the affected side. Spica cast immobilization maybe useful in young children during the early immobilization period.[93–95]

The patient is followed radiographically on a weekly basis to monitor for fracture displacement and callus formation. Once callus formation has begun, the patient may be progressed to partial weight-bearing and begin the rehabilitation process with isometric muscle exercises. Fracture union can be expected between 6 and 8 weeks, depending on the patient's age, at which time, the patient may be progressed to weight-bearing as tolerated. The patient should be followed clinically and radiographically periodically in the first 1 to 2 years after injury to monitor for signs of pelvic growth arrest.[1]

SKELETAL TRACTION

INDICATIONS

Indications for distal femoral pin traction include a vertical shear injury through the iliac wing, SI joint, or sacrum that is shown to be reduced in traction.[96] This injury generally occurs in children younger than 8 to 10 years. Contraindications to skeletal traction treatment include lateral compression injuries, open-book A2 injuries, and stable avulsion-type fractures.[83] In addition, fractures that do not achieve reduction in traction should not be definitively managed with this form of treatment because leg-length discrepancy may result.

TECHNIQUE

A distal femoral Steinmann pin is inserted approximately 2 to 3 cm proximal to the distal femoral physis under fluoroscopic control.[97] A traction bow is applied and weight added. As much as 10 to 20 kg may be necessary for reduction of the fracture, depending on the child's age and body habitus. The opposite leg may be held in skin traction so that significant abduction does not occur; this is more often necessary in children younger than 8 years. If reduction to within 2 mm is not obtained within 5 days, despite increasing weight, traction should be discontinued and consideration given to reduction and fixation. Traction should continue for 4 weeks in children younger than 10 years and for 6 weeks in those ages 10 to 14 years. Strong consideration should be given to open surgical treatment of displaced vertical shear fractures in adolescents 12 years and older. As previously mentioned, skeletal traction typically requires prolonged bed rest and may not be the best option in trauma patients with multisystem injuries.

OPERATIVE TREATMENT

In the literature, treatment of pediatric pelvic fractures has been nearly universally conservative until the past decade.[2,63,98–108] However, more recent evidence suggests that the outcome of unstable pelvic fractures in pediatric patients are poor with conservative treatment. Schwarz et al reported on 17 skeletally immature patients with unstable pelvic fractures treated nonoperatively. At final follow-up ranging from 2 to 25 years, all patients demonstrated poor clinical outcomes, including low back pain and pelvic asymmetry with varying degrees of functional impairment.[109] Similarly, Smith et al retrospectively reviewed 20 patients with open triradiate cartilage treated for unstable pelvic fractures. They defined pelvic instability as displacement of the pelvic ring that occurs with normal weight-bearing. In their review, patients with pelvic asymmetry greater than 1 cm demonstrated poor outcomes associated with low back pain, compensatory scoliosis, SI pain, and Trendelenburg gait. For this reason, the authors recommended operative treatment of all unstable pelvic fractures with greater than 1 cm of pelvic asymmetry.[110] A number of authors have proposed several other indications for operative fixation of pediatric pelvic fractures. These include fractures with concomitant soft tissue injures requiring open wound treatment, need for additional stabilization during resuscitation of a hemodynamically unstable patient, and optimization of patient mobility.[12,109,111–113]

In skeletally immature patients, Torode and Zeig type IV fractures comprise the majority of operatively treated pelvic fractures. Further indications include displaced vertical sacral fractures, displaced and unstable SI joint dislocations, and displaced iliac wing fractures with extension into the SI joint or acetabulum.[1] In patients with a closed triradiate cartilage, pelvic fractures behave very similar to those seen in adults and should therefore be classified and treated in a such a manner. This may include consultation with an adult orthopedic trauma specialist, depending on the resources of the treating facility. The goals of operative treatment are anatomic reduction with stable fixation. Techniques for operative treatment of pediatric pelvic fractures typically include closed reduction and external fixation versus open reduction and internal fixation.

EXTERNAL FIXATION

INDICATIONS

The indications for external fixation include stabilization of anterior pelvic ring instability, hemodynamic instability, patients with open pelvic fractures, and in polytrauma situations.[1] Although external fixation may provide definitive stability for anterior ring disruptions, this method of treatment cannot hold reductions of displaced posterior ring injuries.[15,25,66] A pelvic C-clamp may be useful in these situations.[114,115] An external fixator with a modular frame can be used to treat an open-book pelvic ring fracture or can be used as a supplemental anterior fixation for Tile B2, B3, and C fractures after a posterior SI injury has been stabilized (Figs. 11.11 and 11.12).

ANESTHESIA AND POSITIONING

General anesthesia is the technique of choice for either resuscitative application or definitive reduction. The patient is positioned supine for application of the frame.

TECHNIQUE

Before frame placement, open wounds should be irrigated and débrided.[116–122] Pins of appropriate diameter are selected for the patient's age and size.[123] For children older than 8 years, standard 5-mm pins are appropriate. In children younger than 8 years old, 4-mm pins can be used. Fixation can be obtained with either iliac crest or supra-acetabular pins. Supra-acetabular pins have been shown to be biomechanically superior to iliac crest pins in adult patients.[1,124,125] When placing iliac crest pins, smooth pins are preferred to treaded Steinmann pins to decrease the risk for iatrogenic injury to the apophysis.[123] When placing iliac crest pins, one or two pins in each ilium are introduced through 1-cm stab incisions (Fig. 11.13). The pins are introduced through predrilled holes of slightly smaller diameter, and are placed by hand chuck to minimize the chance of perforation of the inner or outer table of the ilium. This is typically performed under fluoroscopic guidance. Smooth K-wires can be placed on the inner and outer cortices of the iliac ring as directional guides. Supra-acetabular pins are placed in a similar fashion. The obturator oblique fluoroscopic view is used to obtain the appropriate starting point and trajectory, and the iliac oblique view used to judge depth of pin placement. Pins are placed in the bone cephalad to the hip joint and triradiate cartilage to avoid iatrogenic injury.[1,126,127] Once the pins are placed on both sides of the pelvis, the pelvic ring injury is reduced and stabilized by application of the frame to the pins. Reduction and pin placement should be confirmed fluoroscopically. Adequate room should be left between the bars and the abdomen to allow patient mobility and repeated abdominal examinations.[128–131] Regular radiographs are used to monitor for loss of reduction and fracture healing. External fixation frames may be removed once sufficient callus formation is observed, which typically occurs by 4 to 6 weeks in pediatric patients.[1,16]

OPEN REDUCTION INTERNAL FIXATION

INDICATIONS

Indications for open reduction and internal fixation of pediatric pelvic fractures include open fractures, displaced fractures with greater than 1 cm of pelvic asymmetry, and injuries with posterior ring instability. These typically include displaced Tile-Pennal types A2, B1, B2, C1, and C2 fractures, as well as most Torode and Zieg type IV fractures and displaced vertical shear injuries. Inadequate closed reduction or failure to maintain reduction with immobilization or external fixation are relative indications for open reduction internal fixation. This often occurs in fractures treated more than 5 days from time of injury.[120]

TIMING

Operative treatment of displaced pelvic fractures in the hemodynamically stable patient is optimally done 48 to 72 hours after injury. Active hemorrhaging will have ceased by then, and preoperative studies such as CT scans can be obtained and carefully reviewed. Delaying operative reduction more than 5 to 7 days increases the difficulty of obtaining anatomic reduction.

PREOPERATIVE PLANNING

Selection of the surgical approach is based on the location of the posterior ring injury. The plain radiographs and CT scans are studied for determination of optimal positioning of the implants. In patients younger than 10 years, 3.5- or 4.5-mm cannulated or 3.5-mm cortical screws are the optimal implants. Screws up to 100 mm in length should be available.

ANESTHESIA AND POSITIONING

A general anesthetic is appropriate for all closed or open pelvic reductions. The patient is positioned supine for anterior ring approaches. Sacroiliac joint or posterior iliac ring injuries can be addressed with the iliac fossae portion of the ilioinguinal approach.[6] For posterior approaches to the SI joint and for displaced sacral fractures, the patient may be positioned supine or prone. In both instances, the patient should be on a radiolucent table with C-arm available to confirm placement of the hardware intraoperatively.

TECHNIQUE

For anterior ring injuries, a modified Stoppa approach can be used to gain access to the pubic symphysis, the pubic rami, the quadrilateral surface, the pubic eminence, and the infrapectineal surface. It also allows visualization of posterior structures, including the sciatic buttress, sciatic notch, and the anterior SI joint.[132] For symphysis disruptions, fracture fixation should be accomplished utilizing the smallest footprint possible. A simple two-hole one-third tubular plate or two- to four-hole small fragment or reconstruction plate may be used for fixation (Fig. 11.14). Longer reconstruction plates may be used when increased stability is required.

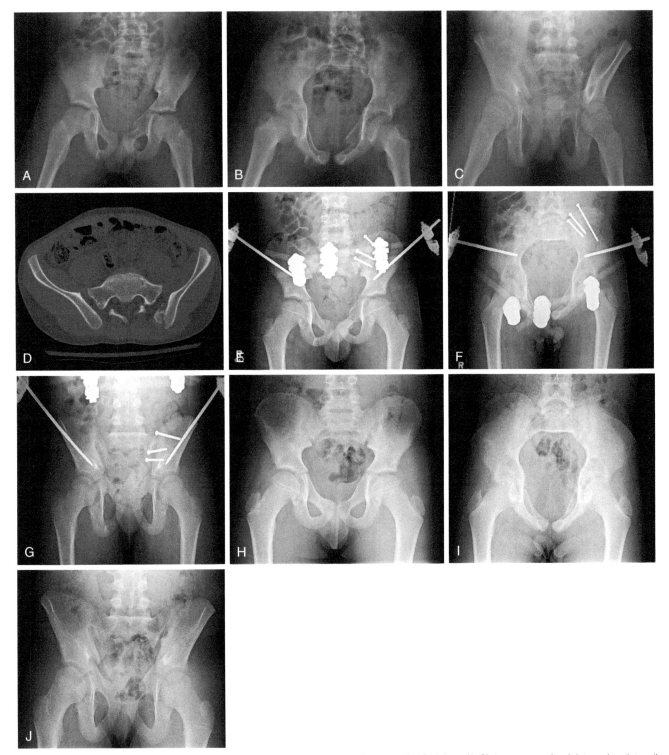

Fig. 11.11 An 8-year-old boy run over by a pickup truck sustaining a highly displaced Tile C2 injury. (A-C) Anteroposterior, inlet, and outlet radiographs demonstrate disrupted bilateral anterior rami and posterior arch. (D) Computed tomographic scan confirms left-sided crescent fracture dislocation and right-sided anterior sacroiliac joint diastasis. (E-G) Open reduction of left posterior crescent fracture dislocation with supplemental anterior pelvic external fixation on anteroposterior, inlet, and outlet views. (H-J) At 2 years, there were no concerns of complications, and the bilateral sacroiliac joint and acetabular apophyses remained open. Hardware was removed 1 year after the index procedure.

Alternatively, in very young patients, transosseous suturing of the pubic symphysis may be performed. This allows safe fixation without disruption of the symphyseal physes, and may obviate the need for subsequent implant removal.[1,133]

Sacral fractures, crescent fractures, and disruptions of the SI joint in children can often be stabilized with 3.5- or 4.5-mm cannulated screws placed percutaneously under fluoroscopic control and the patient in the supine position (Fig. 11.15).[134–137] Experience with this technique is required because of the high frequency of sacral anatomic variations and the technical difficulty of this procedure. A preoperative CT scan should be obtained and analyzed to

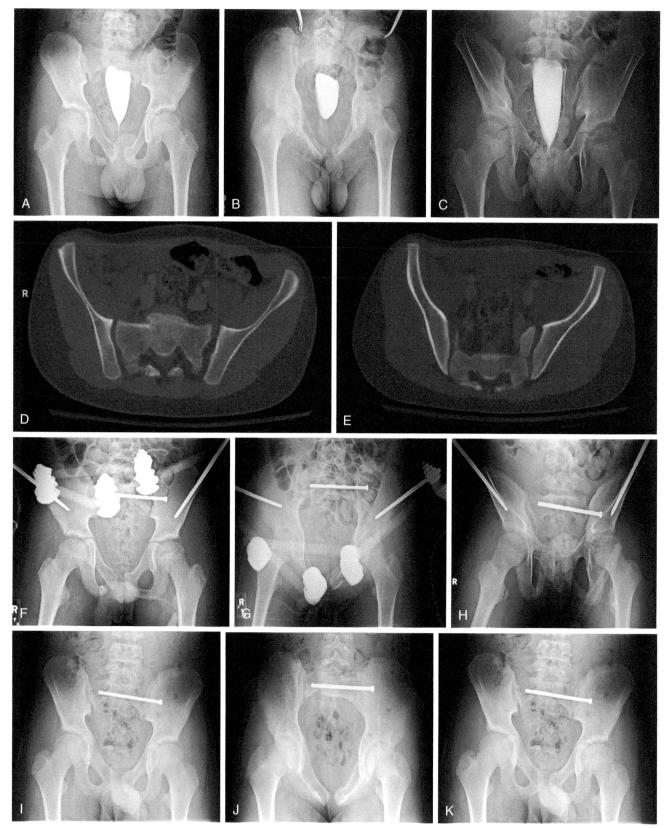

Fig. 11.12 A 12-year-old boy run over by a bus sustaining a moderately displaced Tile B3 injury. (A-C) Anteroposterior, inlet, and outlet radiographs demonstrate a right-sided zone 3 sacral fracture and left-sided anterior sacroiliac diastasis with bilateral anterior rami fractures. (D-E) Computed tomographic scans confirm bilateral posterior arch disruption with left open-book external rotation and right lateral compression sacral fractures. (F-H) Left-sided percutaneous sacroiliac screw placement with supplemental anterior external fixation. (I-K) External fixation was removed at 6 weeks, and the patient regained full function when followed up at 6 months after injury with healed fractures.

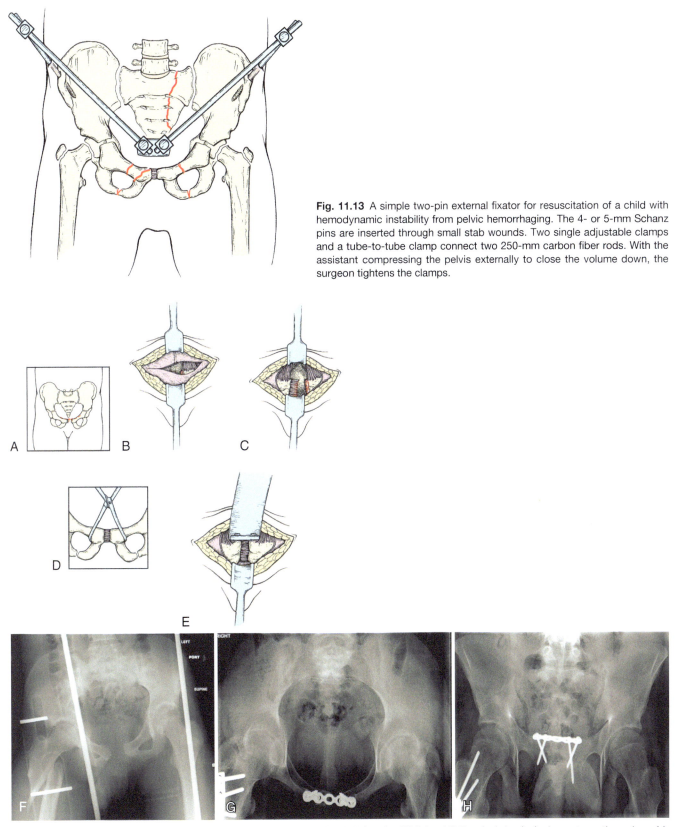

Fig. 11.13 A simple two-pin external fixator for resuscitation of a child with hemodynamic instability from pelvic hemorrhaging. The 4- or 5-mm Schanz pins are inserted through small stab wounds. Two single adjustable clamps and a tube-to-tube clamp connect two 250-mm carbon fiber rods. With the assistant compressing the pelvis externally to close the volume down, the surgeon tightens the clamps.

Fig. 11.14 A simple two-hole plate may be used for closing an open-book deformity. (A) If the child has (or is having) a laparotomy through a midline incision, this plate is easily applied by exposing the superior aspect of the pubis bilaterally. If not, the Pfannenstiel approach is preferred. (B) With this approach, one side of the rectus abdominis is generally seen to be avulsed from the pubis. (C) With a periosteal elevator, the opposite pubis is exposed. (D) A reduction forceps is then applied to the anterior aspect of the pubis bilaterally to close the deformity. A Schanz pin 4 or 5 mm in diameter can be inserted through a percutaneous incision into the iliac crest to help with this reduction. (E) Generally, 3.5-mm cortical screws with a four- or five-hole 3.5-mm reconstruction plate are recommended for children younger than 12 years. (F) A 12-year-old victim of blunt trauma with an open-book injury and subtrochanteric femur fracture. (G and H) Open reduction with internal fixation of the pelvic ring as described above as rod and plate fixation of the subtrochanteric femur fracture.

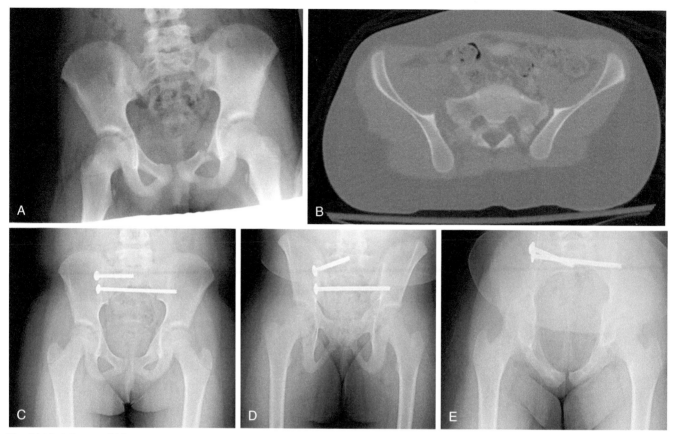

Fig. 11.15 A 9-year-old female was injured in a motor vehicle accident. (A) Anteroposterior (AP) pelvis radiograph demonstrating bilateral SI disruption and multiple pubic rami fractures. (B) Axial computed tomography image demonstrating significant displacement of the right SI joint. Postoperative AP (C), outlet (D), and inlet (E) radiographs reveal dysmorphic sacrum and enlarged S2 corridor, therefore requiring the shorter screw construct.

map the size and trajectory of the S1 and S2 corridors and determine if safe screw passage is possible. Burn et al recently evaluated the safety of placing iliosacral and transiliosacral screws in pediatric patients aged 2 to 16 years. Their results demonstrated a safe corridor for placement of S1 iliosacral screws (99%) and S2 transiliosacral screws (89%) in nearly all patients. However, only 51% of patients demonstrated a safe corridor for S1 transiliosacral screw placement.[138] Furthermore, safe placement of percutaneous iliosacral screws has been described in children as young as 20 months of age.[139] Recently, some authors have advocated for placement of percutaneous SI screws under CT guidance.[140–142] The use of intraoperative CT scanners and combined computer-assisted navigation has been validated and is being used with increased frequency. A number of studies have demonstrated the safety and accuracy of these systems, even in the hands of less experienced surgeons.[143–145] In cases with a comminuted sacral fracture, it is very important to not overcompress the fracture. This may lead to compression of the sacral foramina and result in sacral nerve root injury. To avoid this, a full-threaded positional screw may be placed across the fracture.[135,137]

Often, reduction of the anterior ring injury results in indirect reduction of the posterior ring. However, in unstable injuries, this may not be the case. In such cases, the operative approach and fixation are often dictated by a number of factors including location of the fracture/dislocation,

amount of displacement, and concomitant soft tissue injury. The SI joint can be stabilized in an open fashion with one or more two-hole 3.5-mm dynamic compression plates, with one screw placed in the sacrum and the other one is in the iliac wing.[146,147] Transiliac fracture dislocation, also known as a crescent fracture, can typically be treated with posterior screw fixation of the iliac fracture with 3.5-mm or 4.5-mm lag screws. This can be combined with anterior ring external fixation when needed (Fig. 11.11).

POSTOPERATIVE CARE AND REHABILITATION

IMMOBILIZATION

The duration and type of immobilization depend on the fracture type and method of treatment. Typical healing time for pediatric pelvic and acetabular fractures ranges from 6 to 8 weeks. However, this may be as short as 4 to 6 weeks for children younger than 7 years, or as long as 10 to 12 weeks for adolescents older than 14 years. Surgically treated pelvic fractures can be mobilized with a walker or crutches. The patient may be full weight-bearing on the intact side of the pelvis and non-weight-bearing on the injured side. Once radiographic evidence of fracture healing is seen, the patient's weight bearing status may be progressed. Caution must be exercised in patients who have significant posterior pelvic ring displacement, and frequent radiographs are recommended.

PHYSICAL THERAPY

Other than for crutch ambulation instruction, physical therapy is not generally required for children with pelvic or acetabular fractures. Swimming is excellent rehabilitative therapy for both pelvic and acetabular fractures and can be initiated 6 to 8 weeks after injury.[148]

IMPLANT REMOVAL

Removal of implants is necessary only in children with significant growth remaining. Children younger than 10 years with implants transfixing the SI joint or symphysis pubis implant removal 6 to 12 months after injury is recommended. Removal of implants placed in the ilium, ischium, or pubis to fixate anterior ring or acetabular fractures in children younger than 8 to 10 years old is also recommended. This is done to decrease risk of growth restriction and to allow for further corrective procedures as needed.

ACETABULAR FRACTURES

EMERGENT TREATMENT

Acetabular fractures should be managed after achieving hemodynamic stability. Reduction of concomitant hip dislocation should occur urgently in the emergency department under conscious sedation. Skeletal traction may be required to maintain reduction and take pressure off of the cartilage in fracture-dislocation cases.

NONOPERATIVE TREATMENT

BED REST/NON-WEIGHT-BEARING

Bed rest or non-weight-bearing ambulation with crutches is appropriate only for nondisplaced or fractures with less than 2 mm of displacement. The patient must be closely supervised so that weight-bearing ambulation is prevented. Similarly, patients allowed touchdown weight-bearing with crutches on the injured side must be carefully supervised to avoid weight-bearing forces being transmitted across the fracture surface and subsequent displacement. Such treatment is appropriate only for older children who can be relied on to cooperate with these instructions. Regular imaging is required to monitor for fracture displacement.

SKELETAL TRACTION

Traction treatment is appropriate only for acetabular fractures that are reducible to less than 1 to 2 mm of displacement. However, because of the elastic nature of skeletal tissue in children, this is rarely the case. A traction pin should be inserted in the distal end of the femur under fluoroscopic control and with the patient under anesthesia so that physeal injury is avoided. The fracture must be followed with regular radiographs to monitor for maintained reduction. Fracture patterns that may be reducible with traction include two-column fractures and associated variants. Isolated columnar injuries or posterior wall fractures are not generally reducible with traction.

OPERATIVE TREATMENT

OPEN REDUCTION INTERNAL FIXATION

All acetabular fractures with 2 mm or greater of displacement documented on CT or MRI should undergo operative reduction and internal fixation. Additional indications for operative treatment include nonconcentric hip joint reduction (fracture dislocations), incarcerated fragments in the hip joint, and acetabular fractures with associated unstable pelvic ring injury. The surgical approach varies according to the fracture pattern and the nature and direction of the displacement. Preoperative CT scans and radiographs are used to determine the optimal approach and fixation techniques.[69,71] Posterior fractures, including those of the posterior wall and posterior column, are generally accessible through the Kocher-Langenbeck approach. During this approach, it is important to protect and preserve the blood supply to the femoral head. The Kocher-Langenbeck approach may be performed with the patient in the prone or lateral decubitus position. When the approach is being performed for a fracture involving the posterior column, it is typically done with the patient prone, as described by Letournel and colleagues.[72] Anterior column injuries are optimally managed with the ilioinguinal or modified Stoppa approaches.[1] Some transverse fractures and transverse fractures with associated posterior wall injuries may require the extended iliofemoral approach or combined anterior and posterior approaches. However, this is rarely necessary and is associated with greater blood loss and a higher incidence of heterotopic ossification.[149]

Internal fixation is typically performed with 2.0-mm, 2.4-mm, 2.7-mm, or 3.5-mm screws and reconstruction plates, depending on the size of the patient and size of the fracture fragments (Fig. 11.16). As previously mentioned, children have thicker periosteum than in adults. This thick periosteum can become entrapped in the fracture site and must be removed to facilitate accurate fracture reduction. Fracture fragments that are too small for fixation may be excised as needed to allow for concentric hip reduction. Multiple assistants, Schanz pins, femoral distractors, specialized pelvic clamps, and long screws should be available as needed. A surgeon experienced in acetabular fracture approaches and fixation in adults should be consulted for all operative pediatric acetabular fractures.[67,150]

TRIRADIATE CARTILAGE INJURIES

Injuries to the triradiate cartilage are rare, and available evidence to guide their treatment is limited.[151] Historically, nonoperative treatment of triradiate cartilage injuries was recommended. Bucholz and colleagues provided the original classification for triradiate cartilage injuries based on nine skeletally immature patients with such injuries (Fig. 11.10). In their series, all four patients that sustained type V crush injuries went on to experience growth arrest of the triradiate cartilage. Of the five patients who sustained type I and II injuries, only one went on to premature growth arrest of the triradiate cartilage.[19] Heeg et al reported on two patients with type I injury, one patient with a type II injury, and three patients with type V injury. All patients with type I and II injury were treated nonoperatively and went on to uneventful healing without radiographic growth arrest or functional limitations. However, all three patients with type V injury developed growth arrest requiring corrective osteotomies in adulthood.[1,14] Additional studies have noted the increased rate of growth arrest in cases of combined triradiate cartilage and SI injuries, regardless of the type of triradiate cartilage fracture.[1,15]

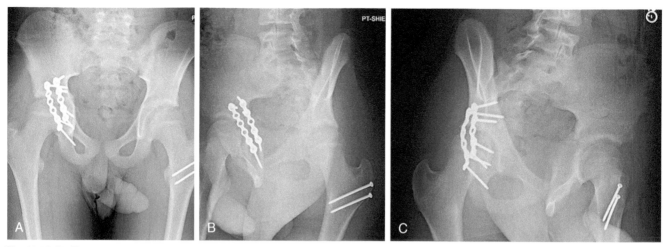

Fig. 11.16 (A-C) The same patient as in Fig. 11.15, post–open reduction and internal fixation, transverse acetabulum fracture via plating pattern used for isolated posterior column fracture. The patient underwent staged left hip surgical dislocation and reduction and repair of posterior labral osteochondral avulsion.

Some authors recommend initial nonoperative treatment of all triradiate cartilage injuries, instead choosing to correct any growth arrest that does occur. Some recommend early intervention with removal of osseous bridge, whereas others choose to perform a corrective periacetabular osteotomy after pelvic growth has completed.[1,31,152,153] Triradiate cartilage injuries that are significantly displaced should be reduced. If reduction cannot be obtained by closed means, operative intervention should be performed. These fractures may be approached via the ilioinguinal or modified Stoppa approach, being cautious to preserve the overlying periosteum and perichondrium.[1,19,154] When concomitant SI joint dislocation is present, it should be reduced and fixated when unstable. Reduction of the SI joint will often indirectly reduce the triradiate cartilage. When fixation of the triradiate cartilage is necessary, it should be performed with mini-fragment or small-fragment plates placed in buttress fashion. This is done to avoid placement of screws across the cartilage and prevent iatrogenic injury to the physes.[1] All patients with triradiate cartilage injuries should be followed with yearly clinical and radiographic examination to monitor for posttraumatic acetabular dysplasia. Younger children have greater remaining growth and are therefore at increased risk of developing dysplasia if growth arrest does occur[30] (Fig. 11.17).

POSTOPERATIVE CARE AND REHABILITATION

IMMOBILIZATION

Patients with acetabular fractures typically require 6 to 8 weeks of healing time before weight-bearing is allowed. Younger children may be mobilized at 5 to 6 weeks if adequate healing is noted radiographically. Adolescents older than 12 years should be treated with partial weight-bearing for an additional 3 to 4 weeks (for a total of 10–12 weeks). Fractures that are minimally displaced and those treated with internal fixation can tolerate partial weight-bearing on the injured side with a walker or crutches beginning 2 to 3 weeks after the injury. Fractures reduced in traction should be held there for 5 to 6 weeks. Minimally displaced or operatively fixed acetabular fractures can be mobilized with partial weight-bearing on the injured side 4 to 5 weeks after injury. Posterior hip precautions should be followed when the Kocher-Langenbeck approach is used.

PHYSICAL THERAPY

See the "Physical Therapy" section under "Fractures and Dislocations of the Pelvis and Acetabulum."

IMPLANT REMOVAL

See the "Implant Removal" section under "Fractures and Dislocations of the Pelvis and Acetabulum."

COMPLICATIONS

Complications in the early phase of pediatric pelvic fracture management include bladder rupture, urethral injury, vaginal or rectal laceration, vascular injury, lumbosacral plexus injury, deep venous thrombosis, hemorrhage, and death. Long-term complications of pelvic fractures include delayed union, nonunion, malunion, fusion of the SI joint, and leg-length inequality. Delayed union and malunion can generally be prevented by an adequate reduction and period of immobilization. Nonunion of pediatric pelvic fractures is rare, whereas malunion is far more common.[155,156] Symptomatic nonunion is best managed by stabilization with internal fixation and bone grafting. Malunion of the anterior pelvic ring may require osteotomy and stabilization if it proves to be disabling.[67,97] Fusion of the SI joint is likely a result of the severe trauma that produced the injury. However, the rate of this complication may be favorably influenced by anatomic reduction of the joint. Appropriate reduction and stabilization of pelvic asymmetry are key to preventing leg-length inequality. Treatment of leg-length inequality is typically based on the patient's age and degree of leg-length inequality predicted at skeletal maturity. Treatment options for leg-length inequality are numerous and include contralateral epiphysiodesis, contralateral femoral shortening, and ipsilateral femoral lengthening procedures.

Long-term complications of acetabular fractures include posttraumatic hip arthritis and premature closure of the triradiate cartilage with resultant posttraumatic acetabular

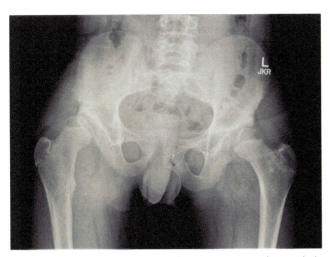

Fig. 11.17 A 16-year-old male with bilateral posttraumatic acetabular dysplasia secondary to pelvic ring injury at age 4 resulting in triradiate closure.

dysplasia. Anatomic reduction of the acetabulum and triradiate cartilage with careful surgical exposure can minimize this incidence.[157–159] The most severe long-term complications of acetabular fractures (i.e., avascular necrosis [AVN], loss of joint space, and degenerative arthritis) are treatable only with drastic surgical measures. When these complications occur, temporizing measures including weight loss, activity modification, and antiinflammatory medications are typically used. Ultimately, the choice in most cases comes down to arthrodesis versus arthroplasty, with the latter being delayed as long as possible. Premature closure of the triradiate cartilage may be optimally managed by bridge resection and fat interposition. However, these procedures are technically challenging and have varying degrees of clinical success.[1,31,153] For these reasons, many authors recommend delayed treatment with corrective acetabular osteotomy after skeletal maturity is reached.[1,152]

OUTCOMES

An appropriate functional assessment for both pelvic and acetabular fractures in children includes an evaluation of pain, gait, hip motion, leg-length inequality, activities of daily living, and sports performance.[136,160] Both males and females can have residual genitourinary, reproductive, and sexual problems in rare instances.[161] A recent assessment of functional outcomes, at a mean of 6.5 years after injury, supports open reduction and internal fixation in patients with greater than 1 cm of pelvic asymmetry after closed reduction.[110] Furthermore, numerus studies have demonstrated a correlation between fracture malunion and pelvic asymmetry with poor clinical outcomes.[109,110]

Mortality rates for children with pelvic fractures range from 2% to 12%, which is not significantly different from figures published for adults with pelvic fractures. However, children are more likely to die from their associated head, thoracic, and abdominal injuries, rather than their pelvic fracture. Open pelvic fractures and those with significant major vascular injury carry the highest risk.[162,163] Patients with avulsion injuries and minor anterior pelvic disruption can be expected to have no residual disability, although

nonunion can rarely result. On follow-up at maturity, two-thirds of patients with serious pelvic displacement have no significant functional disability, and half have normal radiographic results that accompany their functional outcomes. One-third have residual limping and pain and have had to alter their activities.[164] Growth arrest deformities may be related to triradiate cartilage injury, but these deformities are seen much more rarely than growth arrest resulting from proximal femoral physeal injury.[165,166]

CONCLUSION

Pediatric pelvic fractures are the result of high-energy injuries and are rare. Significant hemorrhaging and associated visceral injuries should be prioritized and treated aggressively with the goal of achieving hemodynamic stability. Pelvic fractures can be provisionally stabilized and definitively treated 3 to 5 days later. Open pelvic fractures have a high mortality rate and should be considered an orthopedic emergency. Thorough débridement and irrigation plus appropriate antibiotic coverage and tetanus shots can help to lower the rate of complications. The majority of pelvic fractures can be managed closed, and most complications and poor outcomes are related to unstable pelvic fractures. A trend toward definitive fixation with either a closed or open approach has been seen in multiple case series. However, no current consensus exists on the indications for definitive surgical management of pediatric pelvic fractures. External fixation, percutaneous SI screw fixation, anterior pelvic ring plating, posterior SI plating, or combined approaches have all been reported with good outcomes. Acetabular fractures are caused by high-energy trauma and are even more rare in the pediatric population. Associated injuries must be scrutinized and treated. Displacement of more than 2 mm requires open reduction and internal fixation. There is good correlation between the clinical and radiologic result.

PROXIMAL FEMUR FRACTURES

INCIDENCE

Fractures of the proximal femur in children are rare and represent less than 1% of all pediatric fractures.[28,167–175] Avulsion fractures of the proximal femur tend to occur in athletes and are more common in the lesser trochanter than in the greater trochanter.[148]

RELEVANT ANATOMY

The anatomy of the proximal femur in children is typically divided into osseous and vascular anatomy. Knowledge of the anatomy of the proximal femur is important in influencing the treatment options and outcomes after traumatic injury.

At birth, the proximal femur consists of a single growth plate (physis) that separates into two distinct physes, the femoral head and greater trochanter. The development of the ossific nucleus of the femoral head occurs between 4 and 6 months of age, with the greater trochanteric apophysis appearing at age 4 years old. The closure of the proximal

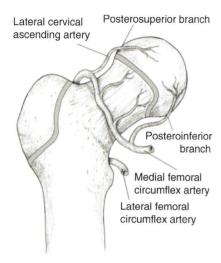

Fig. 11.18 The blood supply of the femoral head. (From Beaty JH. Fractures of the hip in children. *Orthop Clin North Am.* 2006;37:223-232. With permission.)

femoral physis occurs earlier in girls than in boys and contributes 30% of the length of the femur and 13% of the growth of the entire lower extremity.[176] The apophysis of the greater trochanter contributes to the growth and development of the femoral neck up to age 8 and is thought to transition to apophyseal growth thereafter until it closes around 16 to 18 years of age. Damage to the femoral head physis can cause leg-length discrepancies and differences in the neck-shaft angle, anteversion, or trochanteric height, depending on the age of the child at the time of the trauma. Damage of the greater trochanteric apophysis before age 8 typically causes a narrow, valgus femoral neck.[165,177]

Advanced imaging studies, as well as elaborate injection studies, have greatly contributed to our current knowledge of the vascular anatomy of the proximal femur.[178–184] At birth, both the medial and lateral circumflex arteries combine to provide vascularity to the greater trochanter and femoral head. The artery of the ligamentum teres, as well as small penetrating vessels that cross the physis, are thought to contribute the vascularity of the femoral head. After 18 months of age, passage of blood vessels through the physis ceases. By 3 years of age, the contribution of the lateral femoral circumflex artery begins to diminish, and the main blood supply to the proximal femur comes from the medial circumflex artery via the lateral ascending branches. After 10 years of age, the artery of the ligamentum teres begins to contribute to the blood supply of the femoral head and vascular anastomoses that form between these vessels, and the lateral ascending branches of the medial circumflex artery are thought to explain the lower incidence of AVN in adults after fractures of the proximal femur[185–188] (Fig. 11.18).

MECHANISM OF INJURY/BIOMECHANICS

Fractures of the proximal femur typically represent high-energy injuries.[189–191] These include falls from heights, MVCs, motor vehicle versus pedestrian, or bicycle crashes.[192–195] In the setting of low-energy injuries or minimal trauma, pathologic fractures should be suspected and evaluated

accordingly. Cases of traumatic proximal femur epiphyseal separation in newborns and infants have also be described.[196–198]

ASSOCIATED INJURIES

These injuries can be seen in the setting of multisystem trauma 30% of the time, most commonly abdominal, pelvic, or neurological.[199,200] In this setting, it is important to adhere to ATLS protocols before proceeding with treatment of the orthopedic injuries. Occasionally, traction or external fixation can be used to temporize the injuries.

EVALUATION

The majority of fractures of the proximal femur are seen in the setting of high-energy trauma and are initially evaluated in the emergency department. A thorough history and physical examination is necessary to adequately evaluate the child.

HISTORY

In the setting of high-energy trauma, the relevant history of the injury can usually be obtained from either the child, caregiver, or emergency services personnel. Because pathologic injuries can occur in the setting of minimal trauma, a past medical history of conditions that affect bone quality should be obtained. Some examples include osteogenesis imperfecta, Ollier disease, or polyostotic fibrous dysplasia.

PHYSICAL EXAM

The child will typically hold the lower extremity in the position of greatest comfort, which is usually slight flexion, abduction, and external rotation of the hip.

IMAGING

In the setting of severe trauma, ATLS protocols include x-rays of the cervical spine, chest, and pelvis. However, more recent literature favors the use of CT scanning in lieu of plain radiographs. Injuries to the proximal femur can be seen on the AP pelvis. In the setting of shortening or pathologic fracture, a gentle traction radiograph can be obtained to better define the fracture pattern. Because the child will usually not tolerate movement in the extremity, a cross-table lateral is performed to obtain the orthogonal image.

TREATMENT

The Delbet classification, first described in the early 1900s, was not widely recognized until Colonna's description of 12 cases published in 1929.[31,201] The Delbet system is simple and predictive (Fig. 11.19).[201] This classification system divides the proximal femur into four distinct anatomical areas. The type I fracture is through the proximal femoral physis, the type II fracture is through the femoral neck, and the type III fracture occurs through the base of the femoral neck. Because these fractures are intracapsular, they represent orthopedic emergencies and should be treated as such. There is some controversy as to whether the type I fracture represents an unstable slipped capital femoral epiphysis (SCFE).[202,203] Other factors, such as the mechanism of injury and prodromal symptoms, can help to distinguish between these two entities. The type

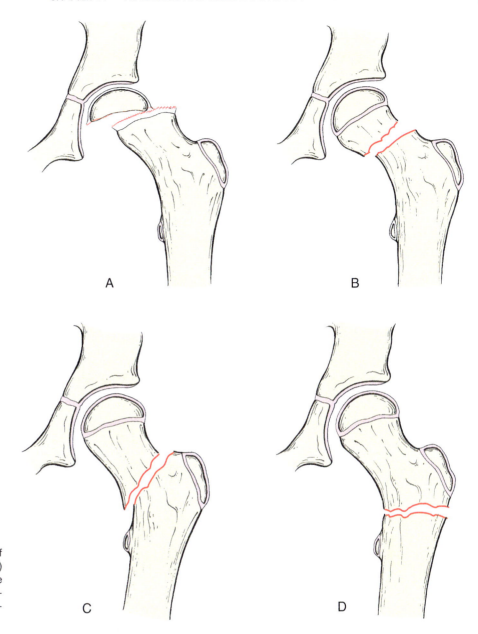

Fig. 11.19 The Delbet classification of proximal femoral fractures in children. (A) Type I: transepiphyseal fracture. (B) Type II: transcervical fracture. (C) Type III: cervicotrochanteric fracture. (D) Type IV: intertrochanteric fracture.

IV fracture occurs through the intertrochanteric region. Although not intracapsular, this fracture patterns still represents an orthopedic emergency and should be treated promptly once the patient has been medically stabilized. Moon and Mehlman reported on 25 femoral neck fractures over a 24-year period and performed a meta-analysis of 360 patients to evaluate the risk of AVN. Based on their results, only age and fracture type were found to be independent predictors of AVN in this trauma population. Based on the fracture type, there was a 38% risk of AVN with type I fractures, 28% rate with type II fractures, 18% rate with type III fractures, and 5% rate with type IV fractures.[204]

FEMORAL NECK FRACTURES

NONOPERATIVE

Nonoperative treatment of femoral neck fractures is rarely indicated because of the increased risk of complications.[189,205–212] Stress fractures of the femoral neck, if nondisplaced and on the compression (inferior) side, may be treated with limited weight-bearing until healing is seen on radiographs.

OPERATIVE

Most femoral neck fractures should be treated operatively.[174,175,190,191,213–217] Once the child has been stabilized, definitive treatment of the fracture can be performed.

SKELETAL TRACTION

Skeletal traction is rarely used for proximal femur fractures. Current indications would include patients who are too medically unstable to undergo definitive surgical treatment.

CLOSED REDUCTION AND INTERNAL FIXATION

Closed reduction and internal fixation is indicated in displaced type I fractures, displaced type II fractures in children older than 8 or failure of closed reduction in a younger child, displaced type III fractures, failure to maintain reduction in traction or a spica cast, or an irreducible type IV fracture in a child between 6 and 12 years of age.[218] Closed reduction techniques should aim for a neck-shaft angle of within 3 to 5 degrees of the opposite hip and avoid varus.

ANESTHESIA AND POSITIONING

The child should be positioned supine on a radiolucent table or fracture table. General endotracheal anesthesia will facilitate muscle relaxation and is preferred.

TECHNIQUE

For a type I fracture, closed reduction can be obtained with gentle traction and external rotation. Fluoroscopy is then used to verify the reduction on the AP and lateral planes. Fixation is typically performed with cannulated screws or Steinmann pins, taking great care to avoid penetration into the hip joint. If performed through a small incision, capsulotomy can also be performed with a #10 blade or tissue elevator, or aspiration can be performed via large bore needle.

For a type II fracture, a similar closed reduction is performed and verified fluoroscopically. Fixation is typically performed with screws, either cortical or cannulated. A minimum of two screws should be used to allow for fixation and derotation. If possible, the screws should stop short of the physis to prevent premature physeal closure (PPC), especially in children younger than 4 to 6 years of age. Fixation into the femoral head should be performed if adequate stability cannot be maintained without crossing the physis. Boardman et al demonstrated superior fracture stability when using transphyseal screws in Delbet type II fractures.[169] As with type I fractures, a capsulotomy/aspiration can be performed through the same small incision used to place the screws.

Type III fractures usually allow more stable fixation without the need to cross the proximal femoral physis. Cheng et al demonstrated excellent results with closed reduction and stable internal fixation with cannulated screws and capsular decompression via aspiration.[219]

Type IV fractures are the most amenable to closed reduction and stable internal fixation. Typically, up to 5 degrees of malalignment is acceptable with this fracture pattern. Fixation can be performed with screws or pediatric hip plate/proximal femoral locking plate. Pediatric hip screw/side plate devices can provide excellent fixation and compression across the fracture site and are the implant of choice for Delbet type IV fractures.[169]

OPEN REDUCTION INTERNAL FIXATION

Open reduction internal fixation is indicated in displaced type I, II, III, or IV fractures in which anatomic or near-anatomic reduction is not attainable via closed means.[173,220–224]

ANESTHESIA AND POSITIONING

Anesthesia and positioning are similar to those used in closed reduction and internal fixation.

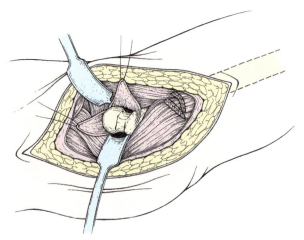

Fig. 11.20 The Watson-Jones approach for open reduction of femoral neck fractures. The incision curves gently toward the interval between the tensor fasciae lata and the gluteus medius muscles from the tip of the greater trochanter and extends distally along the midlateral line of the femur. The vastus lateralis is elevated off the intertrochanteric ridge, and a T-shaped capsulotomy is performed by elevation of the anterior hip capsule off the intertrochanteric ridge and extension of the capsulotomy toward the center of the acetabulum to expose the femoral neck fracture. Placing sutures in the edges of the capsulotomy and inserting a Hohmann retractor along the anterior aspect of the acetabulum allows excellent visualization of the femoral neck fracture.

TECHNIQUE

For a type I fracture, reduction can be performed via closed means and verified with an open approach, or treated initially with an open approach. The Watson-Jones approach is most commonly used for the approach to the femoral head and neck (Fig. 11.20). This allows for the reduction to be visualized directly, as well as evacuation of any intracapsular hematoma.[225] Once the fracture is adequately reduced, fixation can be performed with pins or screws. Reduction can be facilitated by placing a bone hook around the medial femoral neck while traction is applied to control the head/neck junction. During this approach, it is important to protect the ascending branch of the medial femoral circumflex artery, which sits on the superolateral aspect of the posterior femoral head/neck junction.

Special consideration should be given to the treatment of the type I fracture associated with a low-energy injury seen in the adolescent patient. In this circumstance, it may be difficult to differentiate a Delbet type I fracture from an acute, unstable SCFE. Treatment of acute, unstable SCFE is evolving, and open subcapital realignment via surgical hip dislocation (modified Dunn procedure) has recently become a popular treatment option in the acute, unstable SCFE patient (Fig. 11.21, Videos 11.1–11.7).[188,226–231] However, specialized training is necessary, and a recent multicenter study has shown complication rates, including AVN, to be in the 20% range. The authors conclude that this procedure should be performed in large centers that have expertise in the procedure.[232] Some centers, however, have shown superior results managing the unstable SCFE via surgical hip dislocation and modified Dunn procedure.[233]

For a type II or III fracture, the reduction maneuver is similar to closed treatment and internal fixation. Similarly, the Watson-Jones approach can be used to assess the quality

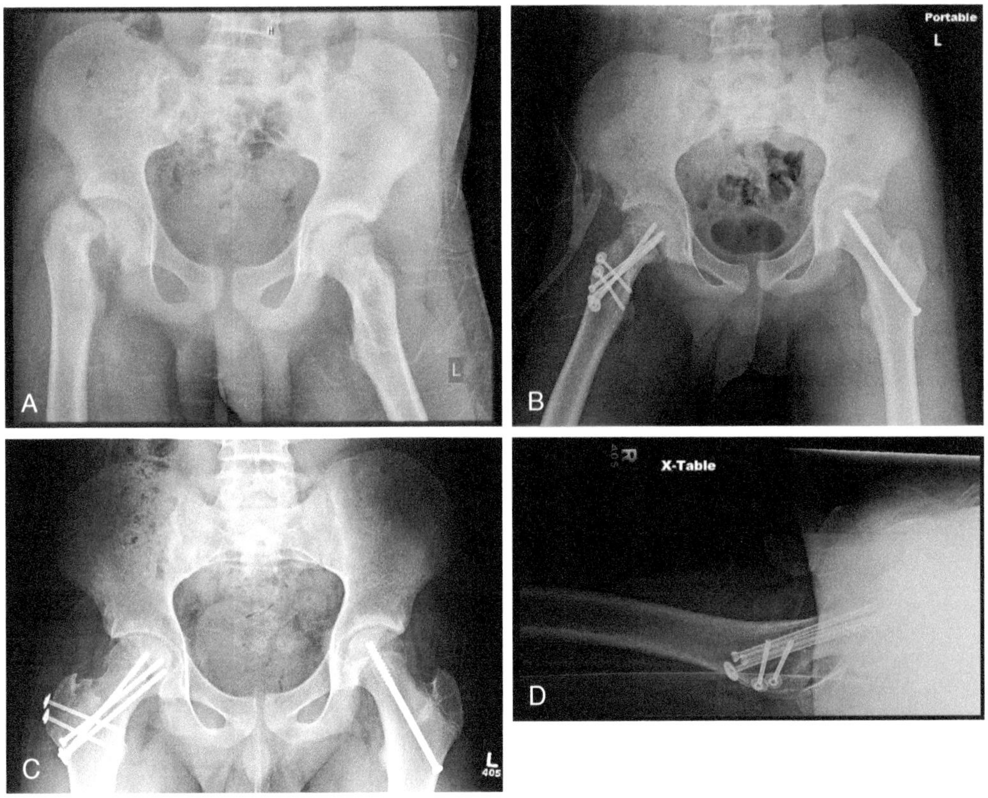

Fig. 11.21 Modified Dunn osteotomy for immediate repair of a slipped capital femoral epiphysis. A 14-year-old boy sustained a mechanical fall while playing hockey and was noted to have an acute slipped capital femoral epiphysis. (A) Anteroposterior pelvic radiograph on initial presentation reveals acute displacement of the femoral epiphysis and deformity of the femoral neck. (B) Postoperative anteroposterior pelvic radiograph after a modified Dunn osteotomy through surgical hip dislocation shows anatomic alignment of the right femoral epiphysis. (C and D) Four months' postoperative anteroposterior pelvic and lateral hip radiographs demonstrate the healed fracture with no avascular necrosis.

of the reduction, or can be performed initially. Internal fixation can then be performed similarly with screws or pins and cerclage wire as needed (Fig. 11.22). If the fracture is not anatomically reduced with simple traction and external rotation, a bone hook or curved retractor can be placed under the medial aspect of the neck to help with the reduction. Additionally, a 2.5-mm half-pin can be placed in the proximal neck fragment, and a 5.0-mm Schanz pin can be inserted percutaneously distal to the lesser trochanter to assist with traction and reduction. The reduction can then be maintained with pointed reduction forceps or K-wires until more permanent fixation is performed (Figs. 11.23 and 11.24). As with closed reduction and internal fixation, the implants can be advanced into the femoral head if there is concern about stability or implant purchase in the proximal fragment. Recent advancements, such as the surgical hip dislocation approach, may also be used for formal open reduction of femoral neck fractures in children. If the patient is under 8 years, a modified approach can be used without osteotomy of the greater trochanteric apophyseal region and provide an adequate view of reduction.

In the rare setting of a Salter-Harris II fracture of the femoral neck in which the Thurston-Holland fragment is anterior, a standard Watson-Jones approach will not adequately expose the fracture; an alternative approach must be considered. A preoperative CT scan with or without three-dimensional reconstructions can help in the evaluation and planning of this fracture pattern. In this setting, a posterior Kocher-Langenbeck approach or surgical hip dislocation approach should be considered. The entrapped soft tissue at the fracture site can be removed, and the superior

retinacular artery can be protected (if not disrupted from the injury) (Fig. 11.25). The outcome is fair to poor if the retinacular artery is noted to be disrupted.

For a type IV fracture, the anesthesia and patient positioning is similar to closed reduction and internal fixation. A standard lateral approach to the proximal femur is used, and the fracture is reduced under direct visualization with the aid of fluoroscopy. In children younger than 6 years of age, two to three pins or screws can be used for fixation. In children 6 to 12 years of age, use of two to three cannulated screws typically gives better fixation and compression than pin constructs. As with most pin/screw constructs in the proximal femur, supplementation with a single leg or one and one-half spica cast can be used. In patients 12 years of age or older, treatment with an intermediate hip screw with or without a derotation screw gives excellent fixation and compression across the fracture site. Proximal femoral locking plates have been developed and can also be used in these fracture patterns, although there is not yet as much clinical experience and literature on these implants. In this setting, a spica cast is typically not necessary, but if there is concern about fracture stability, a hip abduction brace can be used.

POSTOPERATIVE MANAGEMENT

Postoperative management is similar for all fracture types. Toe-touch weight-bearing can be difficult for younger children to comprehend. In this setting, a spica cast with the affected hip flexed to 90 degrees and a period of non-weight-bearing can be used. Alternatively, less flexion at the affected hip can allow toe-touch to partial weight-bearing

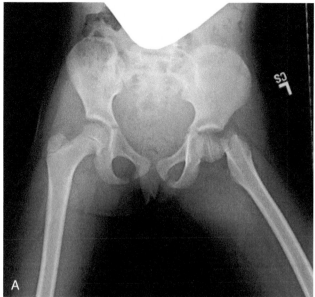

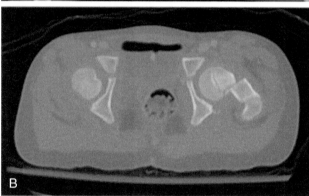

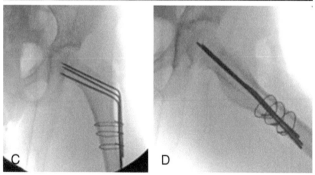

Fig. 11.22 A 4-year-old female was injured in a motor vehicle accident. Left, displaced vertical fracture (A). Preoperative computed tomography scan (B) performed as trauma evaluation revealed left acetabular "fleck" sign suggesting posterior labral injury. Intraoperative fluoroscopy images (C and D) status post–open reduction and internal fixation utilizing Wagner fixation technique and open repair of posterior labrum via modified surgical hip dislocation approach.

but still protect the internal fixation. The period for protection/immobilization is typically 6 weeks. Patients should be followed closely with radiographic evaluation, as cases of late epiphyseal separation have been described.[234]

PHYSICAL THERAPY

Formal physical therapy, other than what is required in the immediate postoperative period for walker or crutch ambulation, is typically not necessary. Adolescents (≥15 years)

may benefit from a gait training or muscle-strengthening program beginning 12 weeks after the injury.

IMPLANT REMOVAL

Implant removal is typically recommended for patients under 6 years of age. If pins or screws were used, they can be removed 6 months after the injury. Lag screws and plate/screw constructs in older children are typically removed between 6 and 12 months postsurgery. Postoperatively, the children should refrain from running or jumping activities for 3 to 4 weeks after implant removal.

PATHOLOGIC FRACTURES

NONOPERATIVE

Nonoperative treatment of pathologic fractures of the femur remains controversial. Typically, the fracture is treated based on the location and the fracture pattern, with special attention to the size of the lesion.[235] Nondisplaced fractures caused by small, benign lesions of the proximal femur in young patients may be treated with hip spica casting. However, the muscle forces about the proximal femur tend to promote varus angulation, even following spica casting. If a biopsy for characterization of the lesion is necessary, the authors will typically stabilize the fracture based on the fracture principles used for traumatic injuries.

OPERATIVE

Operative treatment of pathologic fractures is largely dependent on the underlying pathology and the type of fracture pattern. In the case of a fracture related to an underlying bone condition or benign lesion, the fracture is addressed similarly to traumatic fractures.

TECHNIQUE

The techniques of fixation of pathologic fractures of the proximal femur are similar to those used for traumatic fractures. However, in circumstances in which the lesion comprises a large portion of the femoral neck, fixation can be tenuous. If possible, fixation into the femoral neck that spares the physis is preferred. However, fixation into the femoral head should be performed when stopping short of the physis would result in inadequate fixation. If crossing the physis with fixation, it is recommended that smooth wires be used, similar to the technique described by Wagner.

WAGNER TECHNIQUE

The use of multiple K-wires into the proximal femoral epiphysis has been likened to a "high-angle blade plate equivalent."[236] The technique originated in 1978 by Wagner and has been used to correct coxa vara with low risk to both the proximal femur growth plate and the greater trochanteric apophysis. This technique has been used at the author's institution to treat pathologic femoral neck fractures in which fixation into the proximal femoral physis is necessary to achieve construct stability (Fig. 11.26).

POSTOPERATIVE MANAGEMENT

Postoperative management of pathologic fractures are similar to that of traumatic injuries. If stable fixation is accomplished, postoperative protocols typically include limited

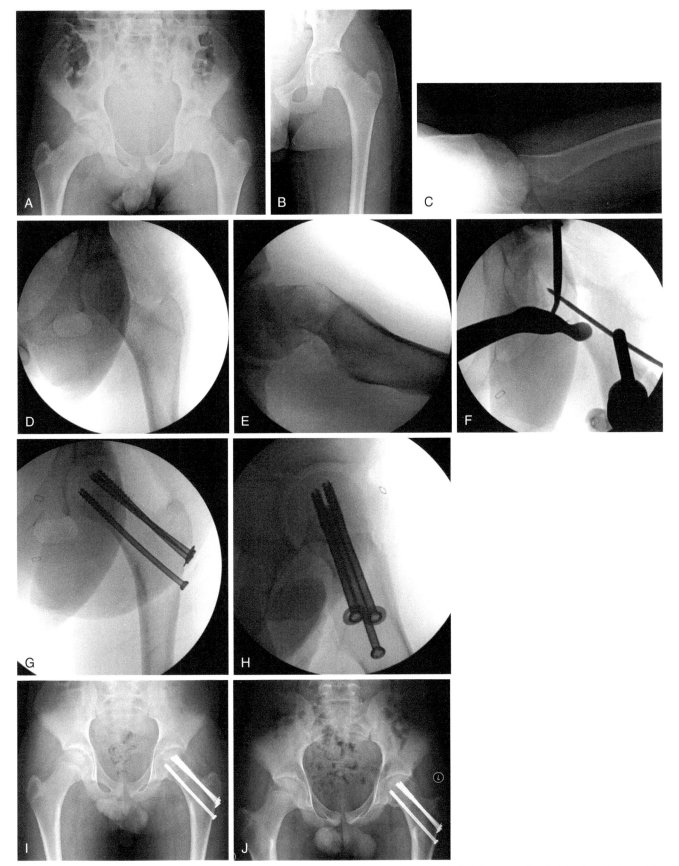

Fig. 11.23 A 12-year-old boy was seen with a left Delbet II femoral neck fracture after a mechanical fall from standing height when his leg got tangled in a chair. (A-C) Preoperative pelvic, anteroposterior, and cross-table lateral hip radiographs show displaced transcervical femoral neck fracture (Delbet II) with comminution. (D-H) Intraoperative fluoroscopic images demonstrate the open reduction and internal fixation with intracapsular hematoma decompression. (I and J) At a 3-month and a 2-year follow-up, radiographic images show the healed fracture with no avascular necrosis. The patient had mild femoroacetabular impingement and underwent an arthroscopic procedure at a later stage.

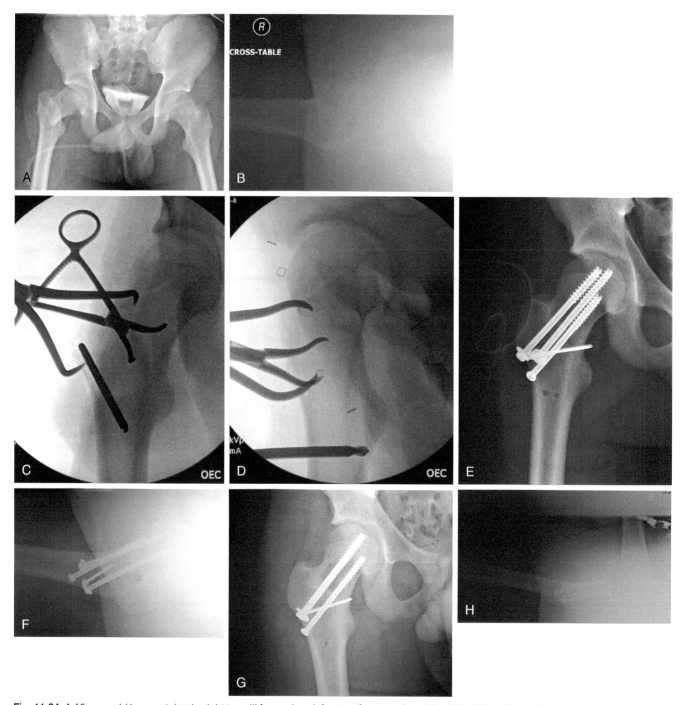

Fig. 11.24 A 15-year-old boy sustained a right type III femoral neck fracture from an all-terrain vehicle injury. (A and B) Anteroposterior pelvic and lateral hip radiographs. (C and D) Intraoperative reduction was achieved with open reduction and a 5.0-mm Schanz pin and pointed reduction forceps. (E and F) Postoperative hip radiographs show adequate alignment. (G and H) Four months' postoperative hip radiographs demonstrate the healed fracture.

weight-bearing until signs of healing are seen on radiographs. In children, supplementation with spica casting is always an option to provide additional protection to the method of fixation.

COMPLICATIONS

Complications after treatment of femoral neck fractures can be divided into early and late complications. Early complications include infection, loss of reduction/fixation, chondrolysis, and AVN, whereas complications such as nonunion,

premature physeal closure, and coxa vara occur in the later postoperative period.[237,238]

INFECTION

Infection is a relatively rare complication after surgical treatment of femoral neck fractures.[239] The risk of septic arthritis has been described in up to 11% of cases seen at a tertiary referral center but is typically quoted at approximately 1%. Outcomes after septic arthritis are poor, as this complication typically results in AVN, collapse, and the subsequent need for future hip arthroplasty.[152]

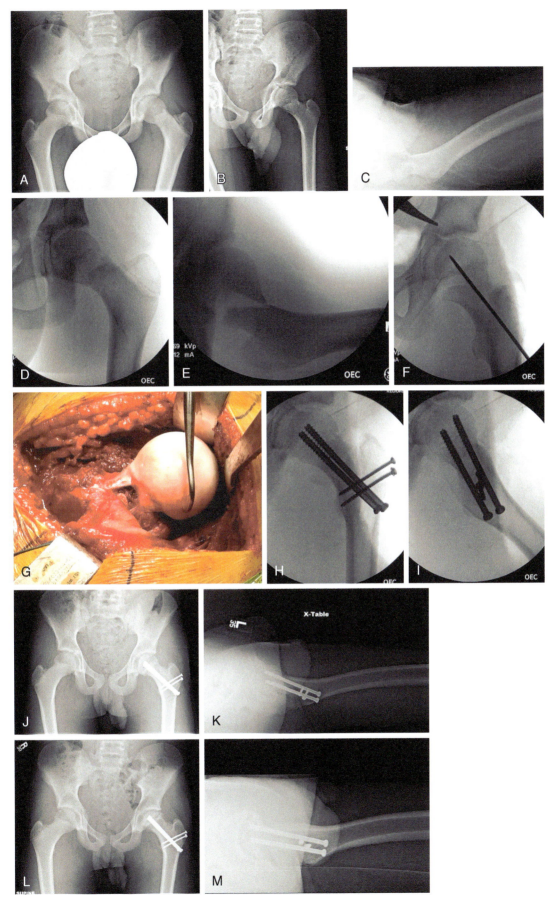

Fig. 11.25 A 13-year-old boy was seen with severe left hip pain from a ski injury. The left hip was in a hyperflexed position with a rare Salter-Harris II femoral neck fracture. (A-C) Preoperative pelvic and hip radiographs. (D-F) Intraoperative fluoroscopic images show a persistent gap at the posterior neck area. The fracture line was in a coronal plane that was not accessible through a traditional Watson-Jones approach. (G) A surgical hip dislocation approach was elected and shows the ruptured retinacular tissue blocking the reduction. (H and I) Anatomic reduction was achieved after the entrapped soft tissue block was gently moved out of the way. (J and K) At a 6-month follow-up, radiographs show the fully healed fracture with no avascular necrosis. (L and M) Avascular necrosis is evident on 12-month follow-up radiographs.

LOSS OF REDUCTION/FIXATION

Complications secondary to loss of reduction are more common in fractures treated with closed reduction and spica casting.[240] Forster et al reported on a case series of three Delbet type III fractures in older children that were initially nondisplaced. These fractures subsequently displaced and were treated with internal fixation with good reported outcomes. Loss of fixation can be seen in instances where fixation stops short of the physis.

CHONDROLYSIS

First described as a complication of femoral neck fracture treatment by Forlin et al in 1992, chondrolysis has not been described as a common complication.[241] Diagnosed by narrowing of the joint space associated with severe limitation of motion, this complication led to poor results in this series of patients.

AVASCULAR NECROSIS

AVN of the femoral head is the most common and devastating complication related to femoral neck fractures.[242–246] Based on the literature, there are three proposed mechanisms that predispose the patient to AVN. The first, which is disruption of the blood vessels that supply the femoral head, is a complication that likely occurs at the time of injury and at this time has no effective treatment. The second, increased intracapsular pressure that causes a local compartment syndrome and decreased perfusion, could conceptually be treated by urgent capsulotomy and decompression of the hip joint. The third mechanism, kinking of the vessels, should be treated by anatomic reduction of the fracture and subsequent unkinking of the vasculature.

The Ratliff classification has been used to describe three subtypes of AVN. Type I involves the entire head, type II is segmental involvement, and type III AVN involves the femoral neck region between the physis and the fracture. Canale and Bourland in 1977 described the end result of 61 cases with an average follow-up of 17 years. The risk of AVN and other complications were directly related to the Delbet type. There was a 100% rate of AVN with type I fractures, 52% with type II fractures, 27% with type III fractures, and 14% with type IV fractures.[171]

NONUNION

The rate of nonunion/delayed union has been reported in up to 21% of cases. This complication is thought to represent inadequate fixation across the fracture, or interposition of tissue in the fracture site seen with closed reduction. Valgus (Pauwels') intertrochanteric osteotomy as described by Magu et al[247] can be used successfully to treat neglected femoral neck fractures. Alternatively, fibular strut autograft to treat delayed Delbet type II and III fractures, as described by Nagi et al, can result in excellent outcomes with a low rate of AVN.[248]

PREMATURE PHYSEAL CLOSURE

PPC of the proximal femur has been reported in up to 65% of all studies.[171,249–251] The proximal femoral physis contributes 13% to 15% of the entire length of the lower extremity and 30% of the growth of the femur. Because of this, the age of the patient at the time of injury plays a significant role in the development of leg-length discrepancy after this complication. The risk of PPC increases when fixation is carried through the physis, and most instances of PPC

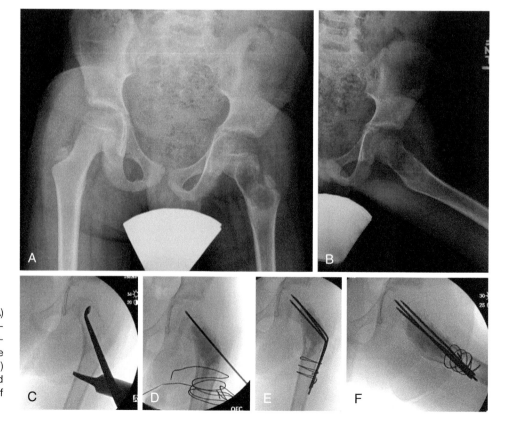

Fig. 11.26 Anteroposterior pelvis (A) and lateral (B) hip radiographs revealing left pathologic femoral neck fracture secondary to unicameral bone cyst. Intraoperative fluoroscopy (C-F) showing curettage, bone grafting, and Wagner osteosynthesis technique of fixation.

are seen in conjunction with AVN. Although common, PPC rarely results in an overall limb-length discrepancy (LLD) greater than 1.5 cm, owing to the relatively slow growth of this physis. However, if the projected LLD at skeletal maturity exceeds 1.5 to 2 cm, contralateral epiphysiodesis can be performed at the appropriate timing to level out the discrepancy.

MISSED ASSOCIATED INJURIES

Missed associated injuries typically occur because of missed or poor visualization of the affected extremity. Concomitant fractures of the femoral shaft, acetabulum, tibia-fibula, and pelvis have all been reported with high-energy pediatric femoral neck fractures.[252] A high index of suspicion, as well as secondary and tertiary surveys of the patient, should be routinely performed to prevent missed injuries.

IATROGENIC SUBTROCHANTERIC FEMUR FRACTURE

Iatrogenic subtrochanteric femur fracture is a well-described complication following cannulated screw fixation for adult femoral neck fractures.[253] It has also been described by Canale et al after treatment for SCFE in which multiple drill holes are used into the femoral neck.[254] Avoiding multiple drill holes in the intertrochanteric or subtrochanteric region and screw placement at or above the lesser trochanteric level should lower the risk of this potentially devastating complication.

FEMOROACETABULAR IMPINGEMENT

Femoroacetabular impingement is thought to be caused by retroversion of a type I femoral neck fracture with a resultant cam deformity and is well described after in situ screw fixation of mild to moderate SCFE.[255,256] The patient will present with groin pain, especially after physical activities. The pain can typically be reproduced with flexion, adduction, and internal rotation of the affected hip. If conservative treatment fails to alleviate the symptoms, osteochondroplasty via hip arthroscopy or open surgical dislocation can be used. Long-standing deformity can be associated with labral tears, which should be addressed concomitantly.

OUTCOMES

Outcomes after treatment for proximal femur fractures are directly related to the number/type of complications encountered.[257–264] The most common and devastating of these complications, AVN, tends to portend a poorer prognosis.

Type I: The results after type I injuries are generally poor, owing to the high rate of AVN. Urgent open reduction and anatomic fixation may reduce the risk of AVN, but a 50% incidence of AVN after this type of injury should be expected.[173,251,265,266] The functional results are poor with type I injuries; however, younger children under 22 months of age may have better outcomes after these injuries. Recent advancements in the modified Dunn procedure may improve these results.

Type II: Results of type II, similar to type I injuries, are generally poor. AVN occurs in a large number of patients.

Because of the need for fixation into the femoral head for stability, PPC develops in approximately 50% to 60% of patients.[171,249–251] Timing of surgery is thought to affect outcomes, and emergent capsulotomy and stable internal fixation with anatomic reduction has been shown to decrease subsequent complications.[124,220,221,267]

Type III: Results of these injuries are generally better than those of the type I and II injuries. The rate of AVN is lower (30%–40%), and because the fracture is at the base of the femoral neck, surgical fixation and the amount of proximal bone available for fixation are increased. The risk of nonunion (10%) can be lessened by compression across the fracture site.[221,268,269]

Type IV: The better results seen with type IV injuries are secondary to the lower rate of AVN seen in these injuries. Coxa vara can result if anatomic reduction is not achieved and is typically seen when traction or casting is used in lieu of internal fixation.[270,271]

HIP DISLOCATIONS

INTRODUCTION/PATHOLOGY

RELEVANT ANATOMY

The relevant osseous and vascular anatomy of the acetabulum and proximal end of the femur have been described earlier in this chapter. Other important structures to the hip joint include the surrounding ligaments, capsule, and muscular attachments. The primary ligamentous support of the hip joint is provided by the iliofemoral ligament (Y ligament of Bigelow). This ligament originates on the anterior-inferior iliac spine and proceeds distally across the anterior aspect of the hip joint and attaches to the anterior intertrochanteric line of the femur. It limits excessive external rotation and hyperextension of the hip. Posteriorly, the ischiofemoral ligament runs deep to the short external rotators and provides additional support to the posterior capsule. Additional ligamentous support is provided by the ligamentum teres connecting the femoral epiphysis and the acetabulum. The external rotators of the hip include the piriformis, obturator internus, obturator externus, superior gemellus, inferior gemellus, and quadratus femoris muscles. An understanding of these structures is key to the treatment of pediatric hip dislocations (Fig. 11.27).

INCIDENCE

Traumatic dislocation of the hip is a rare injury in the pediatric and adolescent population, representing less than 5% of all pediatric dislocations.[272–276] These injuries are not associated with any significant peak age of incidence; however, there is a male predominance with a male:female ratio as high as 4:1.[272,277,278] Although up to 90% of hip dislocations are posterior, anterior dislocations have been reported in children.[279–282] Bilateral hip dislocation is an extremely rare injury, but the treatment principles remain the same.

MECHANISM OF INJURY/BIOMECHANICS

In contrast to pelvic and acetabular fractures, hip dislocation can occur as a result of rather low-energy injury.[283] Younger children (<5 years) require relatively less force to dislocate

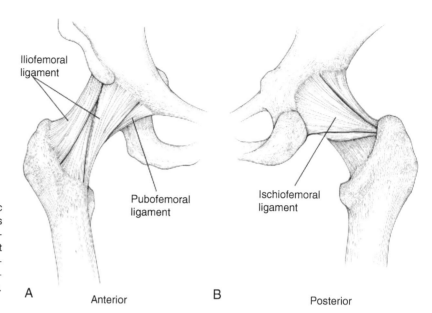

Fig. 11.27 Illustrations demonstrating the anatomic constraints of the hip. (A) The anterior ligamentous constraints of the hip include the iliofemoral and pubofemoral ligaments. (B) The ischiofemoral ligament is the primary posterior restraint. (From Kelly BT, Williams RJ 3rd, Philippon MJ. Hip arthroscopy: current indications, treatment options, and management issues. *Am J Sports Med.* 2003;31(6):1020-1037.)

the hip, which can result from a simple slip or fall.[284] This is because of the overall generalized joint laxity and primarily cartilaginous acetabulum present in very young children. In older children and adolescents, higher-energy mechanisms, including motor vehicle collisions and high-energy sports injuries, are the cause of most hip dislocations.[285,286]

The direction of hip dislocation (anterior vs. posterior) is the result of the position of the femur and direction of force at the time of injury. Posterior hip dislocations result from an axial force along the femur with the hip in a flexed and adducted position. This is commonly seen in head-on motor vehicle collisions when the flexed knee impacts the dashboard or other structure and forces the femoral head posteriorly out of the acetabulum. Additional injuries associated with this mechanism include fractures of the proximal tibia, patella and distal femur, ligamentous knee injuries, femoral shaft fractures, and femoral neck fractures. Anterior dislocations occur when an anteriorly directed force is applied to the posterior aspect of the femur when in an abducted and externally rotated position.

ASSOCIATED INJURIES

Dislocations that occur after low-level falls or with athletic activities are rarely associated with additional injuries. Hip dislocations resulting from high-energy injuries are associated with additional fractures about the hip and pelvis including pelvic ring injuries, acetabular fractures, femoral head fractures, and proximal femur fractures. Presence of an ipsilateral femoral shaft fracture can lead to a missed or delayed diagnosis of concurrent hip dislocation.[29,287,288] As noted in the previous sections of this chapter, more severely injured patients require careful evaluation for head, chest, abdominal, and vascular injuries, as these may be life-threatening.

EVALUATION

HISTORY

Evaluation should begin with a thorough history obtained from the patient, parent, caregiver, or emergency medical services. An understanding of the mechanism and

timing of the injury are important, as both play a role in the patient's treatment and potential outcome. History of high-energy injury should prompt an appropriate evaluation for additional injuries, including those of the head, thorax, and abdomen.

PHYSICAL EXAMINATION

Patients presenting with a hip dislocation will complain of significant hip and groin pain that is exacerbated with motion of the affected extremity. In patients with posterior hip dislocations the affected limb will typically be held in a shortened, flexed, adducted, and internally rotated position. In anterior dislocations, the limb is generally abducted, flexed, and externally rotated. In some patients, the femoral head may be palpable anterior to the obturator foramen. The skin is inspected anteriorly and posteriorly for contusions, abrasions, and open wounds. The femoral, popliteal, dorsalis pedis, and posterior tibial pulses are palpated as common femoral arterial injuries have been reported.[279] In an alert and cooperative child, motor and sensory function of the extremity is evaluated and documented. This examination should be systematically repeated after attempted closed reduction. Younger children may be unable to cooperate with the motor and sensory examination. Thorough examination of the ipsilateral lower extremity is performed to rule out additional fractures and ligamentous injuries.

IMAGING

Patients presenting with concern for hip dislocation or subluxation should undergo radiographic evaluation, starting with an AP pelvis radiograph. The radiograph is carefully studied for fractures of the femoral head, neck, and acetabulum.[289,290] If an acetabular fracture is present, Judet films and CT scan are obtained. Radiographs of the affected hip should also be obtained before reduction attempts when there is concern for associated femoral head or neck fractures. Additionally, in patients with concern for possible nondisplaced physeal fracture of the proximal femur, dynamic fluoroscopic examination before reduction may

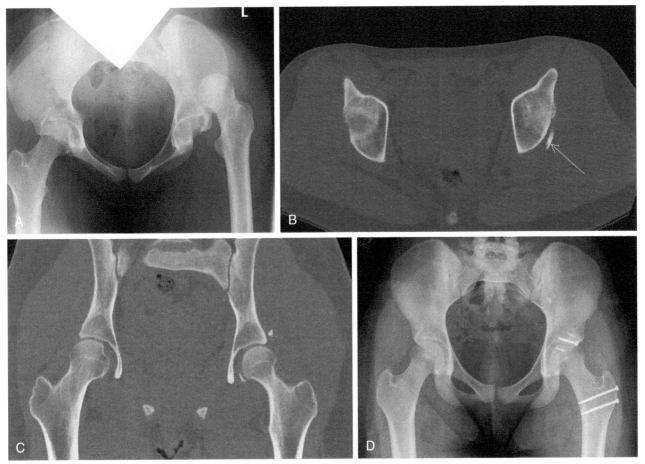

Fig. 11.28 A 16-year-old female injured in a motor vehicle accident. Anteroposterior (AP) pelvis (A) reveals posterior superior left hip dislocation. Postreduction CT scan images (B and C) suggesting large acetabular fleck sign consistent with a posterior labrum osteochondral avulsion. AP pelvis radiograph (D) 6 months' status post left hip surgical dislocation with open reduction and internal fixation posterior labral osteochondral avulsion utilizing two suture anchors and single 3.5 mm cortical screw fixation.

be indicated. It is important to scrutinize all images, as patients with rather benign appearing radiographs can often have much more extensive soft tissue injury present. For example, Blanchard and colleagues reported on a series of pediatric hip dislocations, noting the significance of the acetabular "fleck" sign (Fig. 11.28). In their series, all patients with an acetabular "fleck" sign were found to have a large posterior osteochondral labral avulsion injury requiring fixation.[291] Recognition of these subtle radiographic findings becomes even more important in cases of hip subluxation or dislocation with spontaneous reduction upon presentation.

After closed reduction, the AP pelvis radiograph is repeated to confirm a concentric reduction with symmetric joint space.[292] A postreduction CT scan is typically obtained to ensure concentric reduction and rule out intra-articular loose bodies and fractures of the acetabulum and femoral head.[32,292] In certain settings, when closed reduction has failed, it may be possible to perform CT before open reduction. This study is helpful for delineating loose bodies that need removal, soft tissue interposition that must be addressed, and acetabular fractures that may need stabilization.[32] Recently, a number of studies have demonstrated the superiority of MRI to CT in the diagnosis of soft tissue and cartilaginous injuries associated with hip dislocation in skeletally immature patients.[293–300] The diagnosis of these

injuries is important, as they have significant influence on direction of treatment. However, reduction of the hip should not be delayed for advanced imaging and should be done within the first 6 hours after injury, whenever possible.[280]

SPECIAL STUDIES

In cases where an associated sciatic nerve injury is present, electromyography may be helpful in defining the nature and severity of the injury. However, this is typically delayed until a minimum of 3 weeks after the injury. Arteriography is indicated when physical examination or Doppler studies indicate a major proximal arterial injury.[301] In cases involving infants, ultrasound may be useful to evaluate injury to the hip and other joints.[302,303]

CLASSIFICATION

Although a number of adult hip dislocation classifications exist, no classification has been published specifically for hip dislocation in children. Pediatric hip dislocations have traditionally been grouped according to the age at injury (i.e., 0–5 years, 5–10 years, and 10–15 years), mechanism of injury (high vs low energy), and direction of dislocation (anterior vs posterior). The Stewart-Milford[304] classification of hip dislocations is commonly used in cases with associated acetabular fractures. The Stewart-Milford classification for posterior hip dislocations is as follows:

Grade I: no acetabular fracture or only a minor chip

Grade II: posterior rim fracture; stable after reduction

Grade III: posterior rim fracture with hip instability after reduction

Grade IV: dislocation accompanied by a fracture of the femoral head and neck

TREATMENT

The current standard of care for pediatric hip dislocations begins with urgent closed reduction under conscious sedation or general anesthesia followed by radiographic and CT confirmation of concentric reduction.[198,280,305,306] If a stable, concentric reduction cannot be achieved, open reduction is indicated.[289,292,307,308] Associated acetabular fractures with greater than 2 mm of displacement of the articular surface should undergo open reduction internal fixation, as discussed in the previous section.

EMERGENT TREATMENT

A hip dislocation, like a displaced femoral neck fracture, should be treated in an urgent fashion. Once the patient has been fully evaluated and any life-threatening head, chest, abdominal, and vascular injuries have been addressed, the hip should be reduced. Hip reduction should take precedence over other orthopedic injuries, as time to reduction (> 6 hours) has been directly related to incidence of AVN.[280]

NONOPERATIVE TREATMENT

Nonoperative management of pediatric hip dislocations is rarely indicated, even in missed or delayed presentations.

OPERATIVE TREATMENT

CLOSED REDUCTION

Indications

An anterior or posterior dislocation noted on an AP pelvic radiograph is an indication for closed reduction. In patients with a nondisplaced femoral neck fracture or possible physeal separation, closed reduction must be gentle and be done under fluoroscopic control to ensure that the fracture or the proximal femoral epiphysis does not displace.[309–311] Insertion of percutaneous pins or screws before reduction should be considered in these cases.

Timing

Whenever possible, closed reduction should be performed within 6 hours of injury to minimize the risk of AVN.[193,312]

Preoperative Planning

In cases where an associated acetabular fracture is present, preoperative Judet views and CT/MRI are helpful to plan the appropriate approach and necessary fixation.

Anesthesia and Positioning

Closed reduction performed in the emergency department can typically be performed under conscious sedation. General anesthesia with muscle relaxation is typically used in the operating room. The patient should be positioned supine. In older and larger patients, it is important to have a surgical assistant available to stabilize the pelvis during traction.

Technique

A number of techniques have been described for closed reduction of a posterior hip dislocation.[313–315] Regardless of technique used, adequate sedation and muscle relaxation must be obtained before attempted reduction. This will facilitate ease of reduction while minimizing iatrogenic injury to the proximal femoral physis. The most common and effective method for reduction of a posterior hip dislocation uses the technique described by Allis.[313] The patient is placed in the supine position with an assistant placing direct pressure over the anterior iliac crests. The hip and knee are then flexed to approximately 90 degrees, and the thigh is placed into a position of slight adduction and internal rotation to unlock the femoral head from the posterior lip of the acetabulum. The surgeon places one forearm behind the patient's knee and applies an anteriorly directed force to pull the femoral head over the posterior lip of the acetabulum and reduce the hip joint. If resistance or soft tissue interposition is felt, the surgeon can further adduct and internally rotate the leg to facilitate reduction. It is important not to rotate the thigh forcefully against resistance, as this may cause iatrogenic injury to the proximal femoral physis.

The reduction maneuver for an anterior dislocation requires a more laterally directed force vector. The hip is initially placed into an abducted and slightly flexed position to unlock the femoral head from the anterior acetabulum. Adding knee flexion will allow relaxation of the hamstrings. Traction is then applied directly in line with the long axis of the femur. If this does not result in reduction, the surgeon can use the patient's medial thigh as a lever while slowly adducting the hip until the femoral head is reduced into the acetabulum.

OPEN REDUCTION

Indications

Indications for open reduction include failed closed reduction, nonconcentric closed reduction, dislocation with an associated displaced femoral neck fracture or displaced acetabular fracture, or the presence of an acetabular fleck sign on postreduction CT scan.[277,307,316,317]

Timing

Open reduction should be performed within 6 hours of injury or as soon as possible after failed closed reduction attempts. If surgery is to be delayed for more than a couple of hours, the patient should be placed into traction to help decompress the hip joint and prevent further damage to the articular cartilage. This is of particular importance in the patient with entrapment of an osteochondral fragment within the joint.

Preoperative Planning

The surgical approach for open reduction is typically guided by the direction of the dislocation. Anterior dislocations are typically addressed via the Smith-Peterson approach, and posterior dislocations via the Kocher-Langenbeck approach. Alternatively, the surgical hip dislocation approach

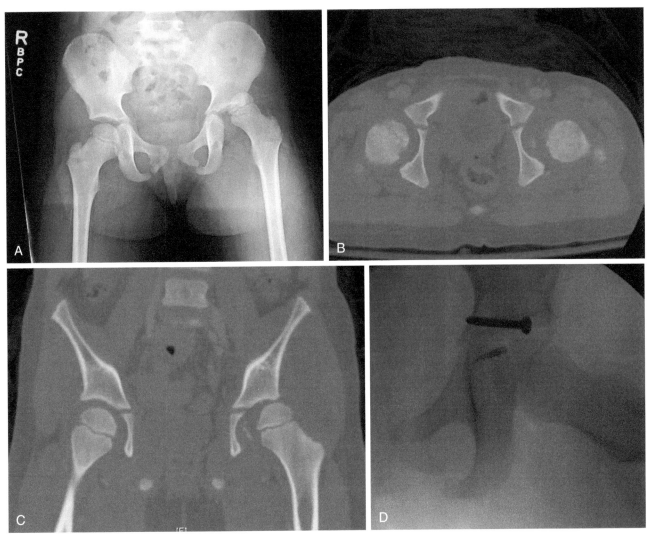

Fig. 11.29 A 4-year old female with left hip pain after falling down stairs. Anteroposterior pelvis (A) shows left posterior superior hip disloca-tion. Postreduction computed tomography (CT) (B and C) suggests acetabular fleck sign with labral interposition and incongruent reduction. Intraoperative fluoroscopy (D) status postmodified surgical hip dislocation approach and open reduction and internal fixation posterior labrum osteochondral avulsion utilizing screw and suture anchor fixation above and below triradiate cartilage.

has been shown to be safe and effective in the treatment of pediatric and adolescent traumatic hip dislocations with nonconcentric reduction, residual instability, or associated intra-articular fractures.[312,318]

Anesthesia and Positioning

The patient is positioned in the lateral decubitus position with the injured hip up when utilizing the Kocher-Langen-beck or surgical hip dislocation approaches. If an anterior Smith-Peterson approach is to be performed, the patient is placed in a supine position. General anesthesia is required.

Technique

For posterior dislocations, a posterior based Kocher-Lan-genbeck approach may be used. Great care must be taken to identify the sciatic nerve, which should be followed prox-imally and distally. This is especially important when neuro-logic deficits have been identified preoperatively. The nerve is carefully inspected in this setting and generally appears contused. The external rotators are evaluated next. In cas-es of failed closed reduction, the piriformis tendon may be found displaced across the acetabulum, blocking reduction of the femoral head.[316,317] The capsule is then inspected and opened to allow visualization and inspection of the labrum. In many cases, the femoral head is buttonholed through the posterior capsule, or the labrum is inverted into the acetab-ulum. Once the soft tissue block is identified, the acetabu-lum must be evaluated for osteocartilaginous loose bodies. A bone hook or external fixator pin in the proximal end of the femur is helpful in laterally displacing the femoral head. Use of a headlamp aids with deep visualization, and small pituitary rongeurs make excellent grasping forceps. In older adolescents, a 5-mm Schanz pin can be inserted dis-tal to the greater trochanteric physis, and a universal chuck can be attached to the pin to provide lateral traction. After the joint is thoroughly irrigated and all blocks to reduction are removed, the femoral head can be reduced into the ac-etabulum. At this point, any associated posterior column or posterior wall fractures can be reduced and internally fixed with smooth K-wires or lag screws in younger children, or with 2.7- or 3.5-mm reconstruction plates in adolescents (Fig. 11.29).

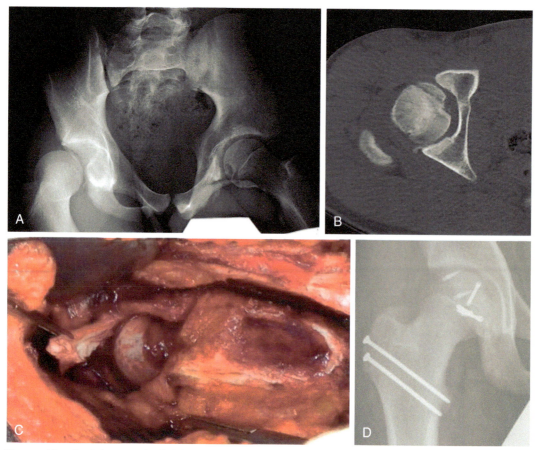

Fig. 11.30 A 14-year-old male status post football injury that occurred while being tackled. Anteroposterior (AP) pelvis (A) reveals right hip posterior dislocation. Postreduction CT scan (B) shows right acetabular "fleck sign" and associated femoral head fracture, small intraarticular loose body. Intraoperative photograph (C) following right hip surgical dislocation approach shows large posterior labral osteochondral avulsion and inferior detachment. Hip radiograph (D) 6 months' status post–open reduction and internal fixation femoral head and posterior labral osteochondral fractures.

In the rare event of an anterior hip dislocation, an anteriorly based approach, such as the direct anterior (Smith-Peterson) or anterolateral (Watson-Jones) approach, is used if closed reduction fails or results in a nonconcentric reduction. Although there is very limited literature on the surgical intervention of anterior hip dislocations, the treatment principles and goals remain the same.

Alternatively, surgical hip dislocation provides excellent exposure for the treatment of pediatric and adolescent hip dislocations.[319,320] This approach is particularly helpful in cases with associated femoral head fractures and large osteochondral labral avulsions. The patient is positioned in the lateral decubitus position on a flat radiolucent table. Verification of full C-arm access and unrestrained hip flexion will ensure adequate exposure. A lateral incision centered over the greater trochanter is used. The fascia lata is incised in line with the skin incision, and the vastus lateralis and gluteus medius muscles are identified. A 1- to 1.5-cm digastric osteotomy of the greater trochanter is performed and retracted anteriorly, as described by Ganz.[321] When performing a surgical hip dislocation approach in the setting of a hip dislocation, it is important to note that there will be an existing traumatic arthrotomy of the hip joint. This arthrotomy can be extended to incorporate a large posterior capsular flap that will protect the piriformis tendon and vascular supply to the femoral head. After dislocation of the femoral head,

the femoral head and acetabulum should be inspected for additional fractures and/or chondral injuries and treated appropriately. The ligamentum teres is often avulsed or attenuated and can be resected to aid in reduction of the hip. If an associated femoral head fracture is present, it can be repaired with the use of either bioabsorbable screws (1.6 mm or 2.0 mm) or cortical screws (2.4 mm, 2.7 mm, or, rarely, 3.5 mm) countersunk below the articular cartilage. Hip dislocations with an associated acetabular fracture can also be treated via this approach. In pediatric and adolescent patients with an associated posterior wall fracture, the fracture typically involves an osteochondral fragment comprised of nonossified cartilage that is avulsed from the posterior acetabular wall along with the posterior labrum. Fixation technique for this injury depends on the size of the fragment. Reattachment of smaller osteochondral labral avulsions can be performed with suture anchors placed along the posterior rim of the acetabulum. Fragments with a large osseous portion can be reduced and fixed with 3.5-mm screws reinforced with additional suture anchor fixation of the posterior labrum (Fig. 11.30).

Large posterior wall fractures are rare in the pediatric and adolescent population. However, if a patient has a large posterior wall fracture that requires direct reduction and plate fixation, a posterior based Kocher-Langenbeck approach may be more appropriate. Use of the surgical hip dislocation approach allows direct visualization of the acetabulum during anchor and screw placement. This allows the surgeon to verify extraarticular placement of any screws or anchors placed.

POSTOPERATIVE CARE AND REHABILITATION

IMMOBILIZATION

Children younger than 6 years are immobilized in a spica cast in slight abduction and neutral extension for 4 to 6 weeks. Older, cooperative children are placed on bed rest or limited activity for 4 weeks and can then be mobilized with crutches for 3 to 4 additional weeks. In cases of fracture-dislocations, immobilization of 6 to 8 weeks is appropriate to allow fracture healing. Hip flexion greater than 60 degrees should be avoided during this period, especially in the presence of posterior wall fractures.

There is no consensus in the literature regarding exact length of immobilization or time to full weight-bearing after pediatric and adolescent hip dislocations. Typically, after the 4 to 8 weeks of immobilization in a cast or with crutches, the patient can be mobilized with progressive weight-bearing, as tolerated. No evidence has been presented that prolonged non-weight-bearing affects the incidence or severity of AVN.[322]

PHYSICAL THERAPY

Physical therapy may be used for initiation of walker or crutch ambulation and hip precautions postoperatively.

IMPLANT REMOVAL

Although not always required, implants in young children should typically be removed within 6 to 12 months after surgery. In adolescents, implants may be safely left in place unless they have migrated to an intra-articular position or there is a possibility of a later reconstructive procedures.

COMPLICATIONS

Complications following traumatic hip dislocation include AVN, sciatic nerve injury, osteoarthritis, and recurrent dislocation.[72,323]

AVASCULAR NECROSIS

AVN is the most common complication following traumatic posterior hip dislocation in children, with a reported incidence of 8% to 18%.[324,325] Although AVN may present as early as 3 months from time of injury, it can develop as late as 2 years after injury.[322] Therefore, patients must be followed with serial radiographs for at least 2 years following a traumatic hip dislocation. Factors associated with an increased risk for development of AVN include high-energy mechanism, older age (>6 years), presence of a femoral head epiphyseal separation, and delay of more than 6 hours from time of injury to reduction.[326,327] Currently, no effective treatment is available; however, acetabular or femoral osteotomy may be considered in certain cases.

SCIATIC NERVE INJURY

Although considered a rare injury, sciatic nerve palsy after traumatic posterior hip dislocation has been reported at rates as high as 24%.[327] Factors associated with sciatic nerve

injury after hip dislocation include older age, high-energy injury, and delayed time to reduction.[327,328] No effective treatment has been published to date. Exploration with neurolysis may have a role if improvement is not demonstrated by 3 to 6 months after injury.

OSTEOARTHRITIS

Osteoarthritis after traumatic hip dislocation in children is rare and is typically the result of AVN of the femoral head. Treatment of posttraumatic osteoarthritis is nonoperative whenever possible and should consist of weight control, modification of activity, walking aids, and antiinflammatory medications. Surgical management should be delayed as long as possible. Options include arthrodesis, femoral and/or periacetabular osteotomy, and arthroplasty.[307]

RECURRENT DISLOCATION

Recurrent dislocation has been reported in children more commonly than adults and generally occurs in those younger than 8 years of age with a posterior dislocation.[29,329] Recurrent anterior dislocation has also been reported, as well as recurrent dislocations after arthroscopic and open hip procedures for various pathologies.[330–335] No clear increase in the incidence has been noted with more severe trauma or an inadequate period of immobilization. Generalized ligamentous laxity, excessive femoral anteversion, an osteocartilaginous defect of the acetabulum, coxa valga, and psychiatric etiology have all been suggested to be associated with recurrent hip dislocations.[336] Evaluation should include a CT or MRI after the first recurrence and subsequent reduction to evaluate for loose bodies in the joint or associated femoral head or acetabular fractures that may have occurred at the time of redislocation. If the reduction is symmetric with no loose bodies, a spica cast should be applied for 6 weeks with the hip abducted 20 to 30 degrees and flexed 45 degrees.[293,337–339] An abduction brace with limitation of hip flexion should be considered for 6 to 12 weeks after removal of the spica cast or as initial treatment. Open surgical exploration with repair of the posterior capsule has also been shown to be an effective treatment. Patients who have more than one recurrence dislocation should undergo posterior capsular reefing.[161,165,340–346]

OUTCOMES

Barring associated sciatic nerve injury or the complications of AVN or heterotopic ossification, one can expect the return of full function in children younger than 10 years by 3 months after injury. Adolescents, especially those who have undergone open reduction and internal fixation of an associated acetabular fracture, may take 6 months to optimize function postoperatively.[346]

Assessment of functional status after hip dislocation includes an evaluation of pain, fatigue, gait, weakness, and motion.[347] Radiographic analysis includes a direct evaluation of the hip for joint space, avascular changes in the femoral head, and osteophytes or sclerosis.[289] A suggested rating scale for outcomes after traumatic hip dislocation is as follows:

Excellent: full motion; no pain, weakness, or fatigue; normal radiograph

Good: no appreciable pain in the hip (except after prolonged work or weight-bearing), no greater than 25% loss of motion, slight osteoarthritic changes on radiographs, normal joint space, no AVN

Fair: mild to moderate pain, moderate limping, moderate osteophytes, moderate narrowing of the joint space

Poor: pain, limping, moderate to extreme limitation of motion, adduction deformity, advanced osteoarthritis, AVN, narrowing of the joint space, or sclerosis of the acetabulum

Few patients reported in the literature have been monitored for more than 5 years. Gartland and Benner followed 50 of 248 children with traumatic hip dislocation to skeletal maturity. Of those patients followed until skeletal maturity, 16 were considered to have a poor outcome. Thirteen of the 16 patients with a poor outcome had either a fracture about the hip or a delay in reduction of greater than 24 hours.[322] Hougaard and Thomsen followed 13 children with traumatic hip dislocation for 5 to 26 years. Twelve of 13 patients underwent reduction within 6 hours of injury and had normal hips. Osteoarthritis developed in one patient who underwent reduction at 37 hours.[347]

CONCLUSION

Traumatic hip dislocation is an uncommon injury in children. Minor trauma tends to be the cause of hip dislocations in young children, whereas greater force is required in adolescents. Urgent reduction should be performed within 6 hours of injury to minimalize the risk of AVN. Muscle relaxation should be obtained for all pediatric hip reduction maneuvers, and femoral neck fractures should be stabilized before hip relocation. Evidence of nonconcentric reduction of the hip should trigger further imaging studies, which may include CT or MRI scans to evaluate for interposed bone and/or soft tissue. A stable, concentric reduction without AVN or complication is the goal of treatment. Delayed presentation or neglected cases of hip dislocation should be openly reduced. Satisfactory outcomes can be seen in the majority of pediatric hip dislocation cases.

REFERENCES

The level of evidence (LOE) is determined according to the criteria provided in the Preface.

1. Amorosa LF, Kloen P, Helfet DL. High-energy pediatric pelvic and acetabular fractures. *Orthop Clin North Am.* 2014;45:483–500. **(LOE IV)**.
2. Karunakar MA, Goulet JA, Mueller KL, Bedi A, Le TT. Operative treatment of unstable pediatric pelvis and acetabular fractures. *J Pediatr Orthop.* 2005;25:34–38. **(LOE IV)**.
3. Bond SJ, Gotschall CS, Eichelberger MR. Predictors of abdominal injury in children with pelvic fracture. *J Trauma.* 1991;31:1169–1173. **(LOE IV)**.
4. DeLuca FN, Keck C. Traumatic coxa vara. A case report of spontaneous correction in a child. *Clin Orthop Relat Res.* 1976;116:125–128. **(LOE V)**.
5. Grisoni N, Connor S, Marsh E, Thompson GH, Cooperman DR, Blakemore LC. Pelvic fractures in a pediatric level I trauma center. *J Orthop Trauma.* 2002;16:458–463. **(LOE IV)**.
6. Habacker TA, Heinrich SD, Dehne R. Fracture of the superior pelvic quadrant in a child. *J Pediatr Orthop.* 1995;15:69–72. **(LOE V)**.
7. Silber JS, Flynn JM. Changing patterns of pediatric pelvic fractures with skeletal maturation: implications for classification and management. *J Pediatr Orthop.* 2002;22:22–26. **(LOE IV)**.
8. Zwingmann J, Aghayev E, Sudkamp NP, et al. Pelvic fractures in children results from the German Pelvic Trauma Registry: a cohort study. *Medicine (Baltimore).* 2015;94:e2325. **(LOE III)**.
9. Silber JS, Flynn JM, Koffler KM, Dormans JP, Drummond DS. Analysis of the cause, classification, and associated injuries of 166 consecutive pediatric pelvic fractures. *J Pediatr Orthop.* 2001;21:446–450. **(LOE IV)**.
10. Gansslen A, Heidari N, Weinberg AM. Fractures of the pelvis in children: a review of the literature. *Eur J Orthop Surg Traumatol.* 2013;23:847–861. **(LOE IV)**.
11. Hart DJ, Wang MY, Griffith P, Gordon McComb J. Pediatric sacral fractures. *Spine (Phila Pa 1976).* 2004;29:667–670. **(LOE IV)**.
12. Bryan WJ, Tullos HS. Pediatric pelvic fractures: review of 52 patients. *J Trauma.* 1979;19:799–805. **(LOE IV)**.
13. Craig CL. Hip injuries in children and adolescents. *Orthop Clin North Am.* 1980;11:743–754. **(LOE IV)**.
14. Heeg M, Klasen HJ, Visser JD. Acetabular fractures in children and adolescents. *J Bone Joint Surg Br.* 1989;71:418–421. **(LOE IV)**.
15. Heeg M, Visser JD, Oostvogel HJ. Injuries of the acetabular triradiate cartilage and sacroiliac joint. *J Bone Joint Surg Br.* 1988;70:34–37. **(LOE IV)**.
16. Schlickewei W, Keck T. Pelvic and acetabular fractures in childhood. *Injury.* 2005;36(suppl 1):A57–A63. **(LOE IV)**.
17. Harrison TJ. The influence of the femoral head on pelvic growth and acetabular form in the rat. *J Anat.* 1961;95:12–24. **(LOE V)**.
18. Ponseti IV. Growth and development of the acetabulum in the normal child. Anatomical, histological, and roentgenographic studies. *J Bone Joint Surg Am.* 1978;60:575–585. **(LOE V)**.
19. Bucholz RW, Ezaki M, Ogden JA. Injury to the acetabular triradiate physeal cartilage. *J Bone Joint Surg Am.* 1982;64:600–609. **(LOE IV)**.
20. Filiberto DM, Fox AD. Preperitoneal pelvic packing: technique and outcomes. *Int J Surg.* 2016;33:222–224. **(LOE IV)**.
21. Hak DJ, Smith WR, Suzuki T. Management of hemorrhage in life-threatening pelvic fracture. *J Am Acad Orthop Surg.* 2009;17:447–457. **(LOE V)**.
22. Pascarella R, Del Torto M, Politano R, Commessatti M, Fantasia R, Maresca A. Critical review of pelvic fractures associated with external iliac artery lesion: a series of six cases. *Injury.* 2014;45:374–378. **(LOE IV)**.
23. Galano GJ, Vitale MA, Kessler MW, Hyman JE, Vitale MG. The most frequent traumatic orthopaedic injuries from a national pediatric inpatient population. *J Pediatr Orthop.* 2005;25:39–44. **(LOE V)**.
24. Godfrey JD. Trauma in children. *J Bone Joint Surg Am.* 1964;46:422–447. **(LOE IV)**.
25. McIntyre Jr RC, Bensard DD, Moore EE, Chambers J, Moore FA. Pelvic fracture geometry predicts risk of life-threatening hemorrhage in children. *J Trauma.* 1993;35:423–429. **(LOE IV)**.
26. Abou-Jaoude WA, Sugarman JM, Fallat ME, Casale AJ. Indicators of genitourinary tract injury or anomaly in cases of pediatric blunt trauma. *J Pediatr Surg.* 1996;31:86–89; discussion 90. **(LOE III)**.
27. Banerjee S, Barry MJ, Paterson JM. Paediatric pelvic fractures: 10 years experience in a trauma centre. *Injury.* 2009;40:410–413. **(LOE IV)**.
28. Beaty JH. Fractures of the hip in children. *Orthop Clin North Am.* 2006;37:223–232, vii. **(LOE IV)**.
29. CDC. Injuries and deaths among children left unattended in or around motor vehicles–United States, July 2000-June 2001. *MMWR Morb Mortal Wkly Rep.* 2002;51:570–572. **(LOE IV)**.
30. Demetriades D, Karaiskakis M, Velmahos GC, Alo K, Murray J, Chan L. Pelvic fractures in pediatric and adult trauma patients: are they different injuries? *J Trauma.* 2003;54:1146–1151; discussion 1151. **(LOE III)**.
31. DeFrancesco CJ, Sankar WN. Traumatic pelvic fractures in children and adolescents. *Semin Pediatr Surg.* 2017;26:27–35. **(LOE V)**.
32. Howard A, Rothman L, McKeag AM, et al. Children in side-impact motor vehicle crashes: seating positions and injury mechanisms. *J Trauma.* 2004;56:1276–1285. **(LOE IV)**.
33. Nabaweesi R, Arnold MA, Chang DC, et al. Prehospital predictors of risk for pelvic fractures in pediatric trauma patients. *Pediatr Surg Int.* 2008;24:1053–1056. **(LOE IV)**.
34. Spiguel L, Glynn L, Liu D, Statter M. Pediatric pelvic fractures: a marker for injury severity. *Am Surg.* 2006;72:481–484. **(LOE IV)**.

35. Hauschild O, Strohm PC, Culemann U, et al. Mortality in patients with pelvic fractures: results from the German pelvic injury register. *J Trauma.* 2008;64:449–455. **(LOE III)**.

36. Ismail N, Bellemare JF, Mollitt DL, DiScala C, Koeppel B, Tepas JJ 3rd. Death from pelvic fracture: children are different. *J Pediatr Surg.* 1996;31:82–85. **(LOE IV)**.

37. Dalal SA, Burgess AR, Siegel JH, et al. Pelvic fracture in multiple trauma: classification by mechanism is key to pattern of organ injury, resuscitative requirements, and outcome. *J Trauma.* 1989;29:981–1000; discussion 1000-1002. **(LOE III)**.

38. Mader TJ. Avulsion of the rectus femoris tendon: an unusual type of pelvic fracture. *Pediatr Emerg Care.* 1990;6:198–199. **(LOE V)**.

39. Mader TJ. Avulsion of the rectus femoris tendon: an unusual type of pelvic fracture. *Pediatr Emerg Care.* 1991;7:126. **(LOE V)**.

40. Martin TA, Pipkin G. Treatment of avulsion of the ischial tuberosity. *Clin Orthop.* 1957;10:108–118. **(LOE IV)**.

41. McKinney BI, Nelson C, Carrion W. Apophyseal avulsion fractures of the hip and pelvis. *Orthopedics.* 2009;32:42. **(LOE IV)**.

42. O'Rourke MR, Weinstein SL. Osteonecrosis following isolated avulsion fracture of the greater trochanter in children. A report of two cases. *J Bone Joint Surg Am.* 2003;85-A:2000–2005. **(LOE IV)**.

43. Resnick JM, Carrasco CH, Edeiken J, Yasko AW, Ro JY, Ayala AG. Avulsion fracture of the anterior inferior iliac spine with abundant reactive ossification in the soft tissue. *Skeletal Radiol.* 1996;25:580–584. **(LOE V)**.

44. Rogge EA, Romano RL. Avulsion of the ischial apophysis. *Clin Orthop.* 1957;9:239–243. **(LOE IV)**.

45. Veselko M, Smrkolj V. Avulsion of the anterior-superior iliac spine in athletes: case reports. *J Trauma.* 1994;36:444–446. **(LOE IV)**.

46. Peterson HA. *Epiphyseal Growth Plate Fractures.* Berlin: Springer; 2007.

47. Rajasekhar C, Kumar KS, Bhamra MS. Avulsion fractures of the anterior inferior iliac spine: the case for surgical intervention. *Int Orthop.* 2001;24:364–365. **(LOE IV)**.

48. Schuett DJ, Bomar JD, Pennock AT. Pelvic apophyseal avulsion fractures: a retrospective review of 228 cases. *J Pediatr Orthop.* 2015;35:617–623. **(LOE IV)**.

49. Wootton JR, Cross MJ, Holt KW. Avulsion of the ischial apophysis. The case for open reduction and internal fixation. *J Bone Joint Surg Br.* 1990;72:625–627. **(LOE V)**.

50. Garvin KL, McCarthy RE, Barnes CL, Dodge BM. Pediatric pelvic ring fractures. *J Pediatr Orthop.* 1990;10:577–582. **(LOE IV)**.

51. Reed MH. Pelvic fractures in children. *J Can Assoc Radiol.* 1976;27:255–261. **(LOE IV)**.

52. Shaath MK, Koury KL, Gibson PD, Adams MR, Sirkin MS, Reilly MC. Associated injuries in skeletally immature children with pelvic fractures. *J Emerg Med.* 2016;51:246–251. **(LOE IV)**.

53. Vazquez WD, Garcia VF. Pediatric pelvic fractures combined with an additional skeletal injury is an indicator of significant injury. *Surg Gynecol Obstet.* 1993;177:468–472. **(LOE III)**.

54. Shaw BA, Holman M. Traumatic lumbosacral nerve root avulsions in a pediatric patient. *Orthopedics.* 2003;26:89–90. **(LOE V)**.

55. Tarman GJ, Kaplan GW, Lerman SL, McAleer IM, Losasso BE. Lower genitourinary injury and pelvic fractures in pediatric patients. *Urology.* 2002;59:123–126; discussion 126. **(LOE IV)**.

56. Torode I, Zieg D. Pelvic fractures in children. *J Pediatr Orthop.* 1985;5:76–84. **(LOE IV)**.

57. Rieger H, Brug E. Fractures of the pelvis in children. *Clin Orthop Relat Res.* 1997;336:226–239. **(LOE IV)**.

58. Holden CP, Holman J, Herman MJ. Pediatric pelvic fractures. *J Am Acad Orthop Surg.* 2007;15:172–177. **(LOE IV)**.

59. Reichard SA, Helikson MA, Shorter N, White RI Jr, Shemeta DW, Haller JA Jr. Pelvic fractures in children—review of 120 patients with a new look at general management. *J Pediatr Surg.* 1980;15:727–734. **(LOE IV)**.

60. Cannada LK, Scovell JF, Bauer B, Podeszwa DA. Open pelvic fracture with vaginal laceration and arterial injury in a pediatric patient. *Am J Orthop (Belle Mead NJ).* 2011;40:415–417. **(LOE V)**.

61. Heinrich SD, Sharps CH, Cardea JA, Gervin AS. Open pelvic fracture with vaginal laceration and diaphragmatic rupture in a child. *J Orthop Trauma.* 1988;2:257–261. **(LOE V)**.

62. Niemi TA, Norton LW. Vaginal injuries in patients with pelvic fractures. *J Trauma.* 1985;25:547–551. **(LOE IV)**.

63. Watts HG. Fractures of the pelvis in children. *Orthop Clin North Am.* 1976;7:615–624. **(LOE IV)**.

64. Ashman CJ, Yu JS, Wolfman D. Satisfaction of search in osteoradiology. *AJR Am J Roentgenol.* 2000;175:541–544. **(LOE V)**.

65. Berbaum KS. Satisfaction of search in osteoradiology. *AJR Am J Roentgenol.* 2001;177:252–253. **(LOE V)**.

66. Slatis P, Huittinen VM. Double vertical fractures of the pelvis. A report on 163 patients. *Acta Chir Scand.* 1972;138:799–807. (LOE.

67. Tile M, Helfet DL, Kellam JF. *Fractures of the Pelvis and Acetabulum.* 3rd ed. Philadelphia: Lippincott Williams & Wilkins; 2003.

68. Young JW, Burgess AR, Brumback RJ, Poka A. Lateral compression fractures of the pelvis: the importance of plain radiographs in the diagnosis and surgical management. *Skeletal Radiol.* 1986;15:103–109. **(LOE II)**.

69. Magid D, Fishman EK, Ney DR, Kuhlman JE, Frantz KM, Sponseller PD. Acetabular and pelvic fractures in the pediatric patient: value of two- and three-dimensional imaging. *J Pediatr Orthop.* 1992;12:621–625. **(LOE IV)**.

70. Kricun ME. Fractures of the pelvis. *Orthop Clin North Am.* 1990;21:573–590. **(LOE V)**.

71. Guillamondegui OD, Mahboubi S, Stafford PW, Nance ML. The utility of the pelvic radiograph in the assessment of pediatric pelvic fractures. *J Trauma.* 2003;55:236–239; discussion 239-240. **(LOE IV)**.

72. Letournel E. *Fractures of the Acetabulum.* Berlin: Springer-Verlag; 1993.

73. Barrett IR, Goldberg JA. Avulsion fracture of the ligamentum teres in a child. A case report. *J Bone Joint Surg Am.* 1989;71:438–439. **(LOE V)**.

74. Ebraheim NA, Coombs R, Jackson WT, Rusin JJ. Percutaneous computed tomography-guided stabilization of posterior pelvic fractures. *Clin Orthop Relat Res.* 1994;307:222–228. **(LOE IV)**.

75. Ruatti S, Courvoisier A, Eid A, Griffet J. Ureteral injury after percutaneous iliosacral fixation: a case report and literature review. *J Pediatr Surg.* 2012;47:e13–e16. **(LOE V)**.

76. Basta AM, Blackmore CC, Wessells H. Predicting urethral injury from pelvic fracture patterns in male patients with blunt trauma. *J Urol.* 2007;177:571–575. **(LOE III)**.

77. Shlamovitz GZ, Mower WR, Bergman J, et al. Lack of evidence to support routine digital rectal examination in pediatric trauma patients. *Pediatr Emerg Care.* 2007;23:537–543. **(LOE IV)**.

78. Sponseller PD. Editorial comment on lower genitourinary injury and pelvic fractures in pediatric patients by Tarman et al. *Urology.* 2002;59:126. **(LOE V)**.

79. Watnik NF, Coburn M, Goldberger M. Urologic injuries in pelvic ring disruptions. *Clin Orthop Relat Res.* 1996;329:37–45. **(LOE IV)**.

80. Alton TB, Gee AO. Classifications in brief: Young and Burgess classification of pelvic ring injuries. *Clin Orthop Relat Res.* 2014;472:2338–2342. **(LOE V)**.

81. Batislam E, Ates Y, Germiyanoglu C, Karabulut A, Gulerkaya B, Erol D. Role of Tile classification in predicting urethral injuries in pediatric pelvic fractures. *J Trauma.* 1997;42:285–287. **(LOE IV)**.

82. Burgess AR, Eastridge BJ, Young JW, et al. Pelvic ring disruptions: effective classification system and treatment protocols. *J Trauma.* 1990;30:848–856. **(LOE IV)**.

83. Shore BJ, Palmer CS, Bevin C, Johnson MB, Torode IP. Pediatric pelvic fracture: a modification of a preexisting classification. *J Pediatr Orthop.* 2012;32:162–168. **(LOE III)**.

84. Ben-Menachem Y, Coldwell DM, Young JW, Burgess AR. Hemorrhage associated with pelvic fractures: causes, diagnosis, and emergent management. *AJR Am J Roentgenol.* 1991;157:1005–1014. **(LOE V)**.

85. Brunette DD, Fifield G, Ruiz E. Use of pneumatic antishock trousers in the management of pediatric pelvic hemorrhage. *Pediatr Emerg Care.* 1987;3:86–90. **(LOE IV)**.

86. Cothren CC, Moore EE, Smith WR, Morgan SJ. Preperitoneal pelvic packing in the child with an unstable pelvis: a novel approach. *J Pediatr Surg.* 2006;41:e17–e19. **(LOE V)**.

87. Osborn PM, Smith WR, Moore EE, et al. Direct retroperitoneal pelvic packing versus pelvic angiography: a comparison of two management protocols for haemodynamically unstable pelvic fractures. *Injury.* 2009;40:54–60. **(LOE III)**.

88. Smith WR, Moore EE, Osborn P, et al. Retroperitoneal packing as a resuscitation technique for hemodynamically unstable patients with pelvic fractures: report of two representative cases and a description of technique. *J Trauma.* 2005;59:1510–1514. **(LOE IV)**.

89. Hornez E, Maurin O, Bourgouin S, et al. Management of exsanguinating pelvic trauma: do we still need the radiologist? *J Visc Surg.* 2011;148:e379–e384. **(LOE IV)**.

90. Aprahamian C, Gessert G, Bandyk DF, Sell L, Stiehl J, Olson DW. MAST-associated compartment syndrome (MACS): a review. *J Trauma.* 1989;29:549–555. **(LOE IV)**.

91. Chia JP, Holland AJ, Little D, Cass DT. Pelvic fractures and associated injuries in children. *J Trauma.* 2004;56:83–88. **(LOE IV)**.

92. Tosounidis TH, Sheikh H, Giannoudis PV. Pelvic fractures in paediatric polytrauma patients: classification, concomitant injuries and early mortality. *Open Orthop J.* 2015;9:303–312. **(LOE IV)**.

93. Cotler HB, LaMont JG, Hansen ST Jr. Immediate spica casting for pelvic fractures. *J Orthop Trauma.* 1988;2:222–228. **(LOE IV)**.

94. Hughes BF, Sponseller PD, Thompson JD. Pediatric femur fractures: effects of spica cast treatment on family and community. *J Pediatr Orthop.* 1995;15:457–460. **(LOE IV)**.

95. Krieg AH, Speth BM, Won HY, Brook PD. Conservative management of bilateral femoral neck fractures in a child with autosomal dominant osteopetrosis. *Arch Orthop Trauma Surg.* 2007;127:967–970. **(LOE V)**.

96. Tolo VT. Orthopaedic treatment of fractures of the long bones and pelvis in children who have multiple injuries. *Instr Course Lect* 2000;49:415–423. **(LOE V)**.

97. Tile M. Pelvic ring fractures: should they be fixed? *J Bone Joint Surg Br.* 1988;70:1–12. **(LOE IV)**.

98. Currey JD, Butler G. The mechanical properties of bone tissue in children. *J Bone Joint Surg Am.* 1975;57:810–814. **(LOE V)**.

99. Hargitai E, Szita J, Doczi J, Renner A. Unstable pelvic fractures in children. *Acta Chir Hung.* 1998;37:77–83. **(LOE IV)**.

100. Junkins EP Jr, Nelson DS, Carroll KL, Hansen K, Furnival RA. A prospective evaluation of the clinical presentation of pediatric pelvic fractures. *J Trauma.* 2001;51:64–68. **(LOE IV)**.

101. Keshishyan RA, Rozinov VM, Malakhov OA, et al. Pelvic polyfractures in children. Radiographic diagnosis and treatment. *Clin Orthop Relat Res.* 1995;320:28–33. **(LOE IV)**.

102. Leonard M, Ibrahim M, McKenna P, Boran S, McCormack D. Paediatric pelvic ring fractures and associated injuries. *Injury.* 2011;42:1027–1030. **(LOE IV)**.

103. Matta JM. Fractures of the acetabulum: accuracy of reduction and clinical results in patients managed operatively within three weeks after the injury. *J Bone Joint Surg Am.* 1996;78:1632–1645. **(LOE IV)**.

104. Musemeche CA, Fischer RP, Cotler HB, Andrassy RJ. Selective management of pediatric pelvic fractures: a conservative approach. *J Pediatr Surg.* 1987;22:538–540. **(LOE IV)**.

105. Quick TJ, Eastwood DM. Pediatric fractures and dislocations of the hip and pelvis. *Clin Orthop Relat Res.* 2005;432:87–96. **(LOE V)**.

106. Rang M. *Children's Fractures.* 2nd ed. Philadelphia: Lippincott; 1983.

107. Rockwood CA, Wilkins KE, King RE, eds. *Fractures in Children.* 3rd ed. New York: Lippincott.

108. Trunkey DD, Chapman MW, Lim RC Jr, Dunphy JE. Management of pelvic fractures in blunt trauma injury. *J Trauma.* 1974;14:912–923. **(LOE IV)**.

109. Schwarz N, Posch E, Mayr J, Fischmeister FM, Schwarz AF, Ohner T. Long-term results of unstable pelvic ring fractures in children. *Injury.* 1998;29:431–433. **(LOE IV)**.

110. Smith W, Shurnas P, Morgan S, et al. Clinical outcomes of unstable pelvic fractures in skeletally immature patients. *J Bone Joint Surg Am.* 2005;87:2423–2431. **(LOE II)**.

111. Alonso JE, Horowitz M. Use of the AO/ASIF external fixator in children. *J Pediatr Orthop.* 1987;7:594–600. **(LOE IV)**.

112. Blasier RD, McAtee J, White R, Mitchell DT. Disruption of the pelvic ring in pediatric patients. *Clin Orthop Relat Res.* 2000;376:87–95. **(LOE III)**.

113. Gansslen A, Hildebrand F, Heidari N, Weinberg AM. Acetabular fractures in children: a review of the literature. *Acta Chir Orthop Traumatol Cech.* 2013;80:10–14. **(LOE IV)**.

114. Holt GE, Mencio GA. Pelvic C-clamp in a pediatric patient. *J Orthop Trauma.* 2003;17:525–527. **(LOE V)**.

115. Koller H, Balogh ZJ. Single training session for first time pelvic C-clamp users: correct pin placement and frame assembly. *Injury.* 2012;43:436–439. **(LOE V)**.

116. Brooks E, Rosman M. Central fracture-dislocation of the hip in a child. *J Trauma.* 1988;28:1590–1592. **(LOE IV)**.

117. Cannada LK, Scovell JF, Bauer B, Podeszwa DA. Open pelvic fracture with vaginal laceration and arterial injury in a pediatric patient. *Am J Orthop (Belle Mead NJ).* 2011;40:415–417. **(LOE V)**.

118. Davidson BS, Simmons GT, Williamson PR, Buerk CA. Pelvic fractures associated with open perineal wounds: a survivable injury. *J Trauma.* 1993;35:36–39. **(LOE IV)**.

119. Maull KI, Sachatello CR, Ernst CB. The deep perineal laceration—an injury frequently associated with open pelvic fractures: a need for aggressive surgical management. A report of 12 cases and review of the literature. *J Trauma.* 1977;17:685–696. **(LOE IV)**.

120. Mosheiff R, Suchar A, Porat S, Shmushkevich A, Segal D, Liebergall M. The "crushed open pelvis" in children. *Injury.* 1999;30(suppl 2):B14–18. **(LOE IV)**.

121. Raffa J, Christensen NM. Compound fractures of the pelvis. *Am J Surg.* 1976;132:282–286. **(LOE IV)**.

122. Rothenberger D, Velasco R, Strate R, Fischer RP, Perry JF Jr. Open pelvic fracture: a lethal injury. *J Trauma.* 1978;18:184–187. **(LOE IV)**.

123. Reff RB. The use of external fixation devices in the management of severe lower-extremity trauma and pelvic injuries in children. *Clin Orthop Relat Res.* 1984;188:21–33. **(LOE IV)**.

124. Carrell B, Carrell WB. Fractures in the neck of the femur in children with particular reference to aseptic necrosis. *J Bone Joint Surg Am.* 1941;23:225–239. **(LOE IV)**.

125. Kim WY, Hearn TC, Seleem O, Mahalingam E, Stephen D, Tile M. Effect of pin location on stability of pelvic external fixation. *Clin Orthop Relat Res.* 1999;361:237–244. **(LOE V)**.

126. Gansslen A, Pohlemann T, Krettek C. [A simple supraacetabular external fixation for pelvic ring fractures]. *Oper Orthop Traumatol.* 2005;17:296–312. **(LOE V)**.

127. Haidukewych GJ, Kumar S, Prpa B. Placement of half-pins for supra-acetabular external fixation: an anatomic study. *Clin Orthop Relat Res.* 2003;411:269–273. **(LOE V)**.

128. Lidder S, Heidari N, Gansslen A, Grechenig W. Radiological landmarks for the safe extra-capsular placement of supra-acetabular half pins for external fixation. *Surg Radiol Anat.* 2013;35:131–135. **(LOE V)**.

129. Poelstra KA, Kahler DM. Supra-acetabular placement of external fixator pins: a safe and expedient method of providing the injured pelvis with stability. *Am J Orthop (Belle Mead NJ).* 2005;34:148–151. **(LOE V)**.

130. Rupp RE, Ebraheim NA, Jackson WT. Anatomic and radiographic considerations in the placement of anterior pelvic external fixator pins. *Clin Orthop Relat Res.* 1994;302:213–218. **(LOE V)**.

131. Solomon LB, Pohl AP, Sukthankar A, Chehade MJ. The subcristal pelvic external fixator: technique, results, and rationale. *J Orthop Trauma.* 2009;23:365–369. **(LOE V)**.

132. Archdeacon MT, Kazemi N, Guy P, Sagi HC. The modified Stoppa approach for acetabular fracture. *J Am Acad Orthop Surg.* 2011;19:170–175. **(LOE V)**.

133. Gansslen A, Hildebrand F, Kretek C. Transverse + posterior wall fractures of the acetabulum: epidemiology, operative management and long-term results. *Acta Chir Orthop Traumatol Cech.* 2013;80:27–33. **(LOE IV)**.

134. Roberts J, Uhl RL, Hospodar PP, MacGloin S. Crescent fracture of the pelvis in a 4-year-old child. *Orthopedics.* 2007;30:666–667, 2007. **(LOE IV)**.

135. Routt Jr ML, Kregor PJ, Simonian PT, Mayo KA. Early results of percutaneous iliosacral screws placed with the patient in the supine position. *J Orthop Trauma.* 1995;9:207–214. **(LOE IV)**.

136. Ziebarth K, Zilkens C, Spencer S, Leunig M, Ganz R, Kim YJ. Capital realignment for moderate and severe SCFE using a modified Dunn procedure. *Clin Orthop Relat Res.* 2009;467:704–716. **(LOE IV)**.

137. Routt Jr ML, Meier MC, Kregor PJ, Mayo KA. Percutaneous iliosacral screws with the patient supine technique. *Oper Tech Orthop.* 1993;3:35–45. **(LOE IV)**.

138. Burn M, Gary JL, Holzman M, et al. Do safe radiographic sacral screw pathways exist in a pediatric patient population and do they change with age? *J Orthop Trauma.* 2016;30:41–47. **(LOE IV)**.

139. Starr AJ, Ortega G, Reinert CM. Management of an unstable pelvic ring disruption in a 20-month-old patient. *J Orthop Trauma.* 2009;23:159–162. **(LOE V)**.

140. Durbin FC. Avascular necrosis complicating undisplaced fractures of the neck of femur in children. *J Bone Joint Surg Br.* 1959;41-B:758–762. **(LOE IV)**.

141. Tonetti J, Carrat L, Blendea S, et al. Clinical results of percutaneous pelvic surgery. Computer assisted surgery using ultrasound compared to standard fluoroscopy. *Comput Aided Surg.* 2001;6:204–211. (**LOE III**).
142. Baskin KM, Cahill AM, Kaye RD, Born CT, Grudziak JS, Towbin RB. Closed reduction with CT-guided screw fixation for unstable sacroiliac joint fracture-dislocation. *Pediatr Radiol.* 2004;34:963–969. (**LOE V**).
143. Takao M, Nishii T, Sakai T, Sugano N. CT-3D-fluoroscopy matching navigation can reduce the malposition rate of iliosacral screw insertion for less-experienced surgeons. *J Orthop Trauma.* 2013;27:716–721. (**LOE IV**).
144. Takeba J, Umakoshi K, Kikuchi S, et al. Accuracy of screw fixation using the O-arm ® and StealthStation ® navigation system for unstable pelvic ring fractures. *Eur J Orthop Surg Traumatol.* 2018;28:431–438. (**LOE IV**).
145. Zwingmann J, Hauschild O, Bode G, Sudkamp NP, Schmal H. Malposition and revision rates of different imaging modalities for percutaneous iliosacral screw fixation following pelvic fractures: a systematic review and meta-analysis. *Arch Orthop Trauma Surg.* 2013;133:1257–1265. (**LOE IV**).
146. Stiletto RJ, Baacke M, Gotzen L. Comminuted pelvic ring disruption in toddlers: management of a rare injury. *J Trauma.* 2000;48:161–164. (**LOE V**).
147. Weber U, Rettig H, Brudet J. [Femoral neck fracture in childhood. II. Results of follow-up]. *Unfallchirurg.* 1985;88:512–517. (**LOE IV**).
148. Metzmaker JN, Pappas AM. Avulsion fractures of the pelvis. *Am J Sports Med.* 1985;13:349–358. (**LOE IV**).
149. Routt ML Jr, Swiontkowski MF. Operative treatment of complex acetabular fractures. Combined anterior and posterior exposures during the same procedure. *J Bone Joint Surg Am.* 1990;72:897–904. (**LOE IV**).
150. Matta JM. Fractures of the acetabulum: accuracy of reduction and clinical results in patients managed operatively within three weeks after the injury. *J Bone Joint Surg Am.* 1996;78:1632–1645. (**LOE IV**).
151. Blair W, Hanson C. Traumatic closure of the triradiate cartilage: report of a case. *J Bone Joint Surg Am.* 1979;61:144–145. (**LOE V**).
152. Davison BL, Weinstein SL. Hip fractures in children: a long-term follow-up study. *J Pediatr Orthop.* 1992;12:355–358. (**LOE IV**).
153. Dente CJ, Feliciano DV, Rozycki GS, et al. The outcome of open pelvic fractures in the modern era. *Am J Surg.* 2005;190:830–835. (**LOE IV**).
154. Scuderi G, Bronson MJ. Triradiate cartilage injury. Report of two cases and review of the literature. *Clin Orthop Relat Res.* 1987;217:179–189. (**LOE IV**).
155. Ganz R, Gerber C. Malunited juvenile fractures in pelvic and hip area. *Orthopade.* 1991;20:346–352. (**LOE IV**).
156. Rangger C, Gabl M, Dolati B, Spiss R, Beck E. [Pediatric pelvic fractures]. *Unfallchirurg.* 1994;97:649–651. (**LOE IV**).
157. Lee DH, Jeong WK, Inna P, Noh W, Lee DK, Lee SH. Bilateral sacroiliac joint dislocation (anterior and posterior) with triradiate cartilage injury: a case report. *J Orthop Trauma.* 2011;25:e111–e114. (**LOE V**).
158. McDonnell M, Schachter AK, Phillips DP, Liporace FA. Acetabular fracture through the triradiate cartilage after low-energy trauma. *J Orthop Trauma.* 2007;21:495–498. (**LOE IV**).
159. Rodrigues KF. Injury of the acetabular epiphysis. *Injury.* 1973;4:258–260.(**LOE V**).
160. Upperman JS, Gardner M, Gaines B, Schall L, Ford HR. Early functional outcome in children with pelvic fractures. *J Pediatr Surg.* 2000;35:1002–1005. (**LOE IV**).
161. Copeland CE, Bosse MJ, McCarthy ML, et al. Effect of trauma and pelvic fracture on female genitourinary, sexual, and reproductive function. *J Orthop Trauma.* 1997;11:73–81. (**LOE III**).
162. Quinby WC Jr. Fractures of the pelvis and associated injuries in children. *J Pediatr Surg.* 1966;1:353–364. (**LOE IV**).
163. Brenneman FD, Katyal D, Boulanger BR, Tile M, Redelmeier DA. Long-term outcomes in open pelvic fractures. *J Trauma.* 1997;42:773–777. (**LOE III**).
164. McDonald GA. Pelvic disruptions in children. *Clin Orthop Relat Res.* 1980;151:130–134. (**LOE IV**).
165. Compere EL, Garrison M, Fahey JJ. Deformities of the femur resulting from arrestment of growth of the capital and greater trochanteric epiphyses. *J Bone Joint Surg Am.* 1940;22:909–1915. (**LOE IV**).
166. Laurent LE. Growth disturbances of the proximal end of the femur in the light of animal experiments. *Acta Orthop Scand.* 1959;28:255–261. (**LOE V**).
167. Allende G, Lezama LG. Fractures of the neck of the femur in children; a clinical study. *J Bone Joint Surg Am.* 1951;33-A:387–395. (**LOE IV**).
168. Bimmel R, Bakker A, Bosma B, Michielsen J. Paediatric hip fractures: a systematic review of incidence, treatment options and complications. *Acta Orthop Belg.* 2010;76:7–13. (**LOE IV**).
169. Boardman MJ, Herman MJ, Buck B, Pizzutillo PD. Hip fractures in children. *J Am Acad Orthop Surg.* 2009;17:162–173. (**LOE IV**).
170. Canale ST. Fractures of the hip in children and adolescents. *Orthop Clin North Am.* 1990;21:341–352. (**LOE IV**).
171. Canale ST, Bourland WL. Fracture of the neck and intertrochanteric region of the femur in children. *J Bone Joint Surg Am.* 1977;59:431–443. (**LOE IV**).
172. Ratliff AH. Fractures of the neck of the femur in children. *J Bone Joint Surg Br.* 1962;44-B:528–542. (**LOE IV**).
173. Swiontkowski MF, Winquist RA. Displaced hip fractures in children and adolescents. *J Trauma.* 1986;26:384–388. (**LOE IV**).
174. Weiner DS, O'Dell HW. Fractures of the hip in children. *J Trauma.* 1969;9:62–76. (**LOE IV**).
175. Winquist RA, Hansen ST Jr, Pearson RE. Closed intramedullary shortening of the femur. *Clin Orthop Relat Res.* 1978;136:54–61. (**LOE IV**).
176. Pritchett JW. *Practical Bone Growth.* Seattle, WA: James W. Pritchett.
177. Gage JR, Cary JM. The effects of trochanteric epiphyseodesis on growth of the proximal end of the femur following necrosis of the capital femoral epiphysis. *J Bone Joint Surg Am.* 1980;62:785–794. (**LOE II**).
178. Boraiah S, Dyke JP, Hettrich C, et al. Assessment of vascularity of the femoral head using gadolinium (Gd-DTPA)-enhanced magnetic resonance imaging: a cadaver study. *J Bone Joint Surg Br.* 2009;91:131–137. (**LOE V**).
179. Maeda S, Kita A, Funayama K, Kokubun S. Vascular supply to slipped capital femoral epiphysis. *J Pediatr Orthop.* 2001;21:664–667. (**LOE IV**).
180. Manninger J, Kazar G, Nagy E, Zolczer L. Phlebography for fracture of the femoral neck in adolescence. *Injury.* 1974;5:244–254. (**LOE IV**).
181. Stromqvist B. Femoral head vitality after intracapsular hip fracture. 490 cases studied by intravital tetracycline labeling and Tc-MDP radionuclide imaging. *Acta Orthop Scand Suppl.* 1983;200:1–71. (**LOE IV**).
182. Swiontkowski MF, Tepic S, Perren SM, Moor R, Ganz R, Rahn BA. Laser Doppler flowmetry for bone blood flow measurement: correlation with microsphere estimates and evaluation of the effect of intracapsular pressure on femoral head blood flow. *J Orthop Res.* 1986;4:362–371. (**LOE V**).
183. Wolcott WE. The evolution of the circulation in the developing femoral head and neck. An anatomic study. *Surg Gynecol Obstet.* 1943;77:61–68. (**LOE V**).
184. Zlotorowicz M, Czubak J, Kozinski P, Boguslawska-Walecka R. Imaging the vascularisation of the femoral head by CT angiography. *J Bone Joint Surg Br.* 2012;94:1176–1179. (**LOE IV**).
185. Chung SM. The arterial supply of the developing proximal end of the human femur. *J Bone Joint Surg Am.* 1976;58:961–970. (**LOE V**).
186. Ogden JA. Changing patterns of proximal femoral vascularity. *J Bone Joint Surg Am.* 1974;56:941–950. (**LOE V**).
187. Trueta J. The normal vascular anatomy of the human femoral head during growth. *J Bone Joint Surg Br.* 1957;39-B:358–394. (**LOE V**).
188. Tucker FR. Arterial supply to the femoral head and its clinical importance. *J Bone Joint Surg Br.* 1949;31B:82–93. (**LOE V**).
189. Mitchell JI. Fracture of the neck of the femur in children. *JAMA.* 1936;107:1603–1606. (**LOE IV**).
190. Morrissy R. Hip fractures in children. *Clin Orthop Relat Res.* 1980;152:202–210. (**LOE V**).
191. Quinlan WR, Brady PG, Regan BF. Fracture of the neck of the femur in childhood. *Injury.* 1980;11:242–247. (**LOE IV**).
192. Chong KC, Chacha PB, Lee BT. Fractures of the neck of the femur in childhood and adolescence. *Injury.* 1975;7:111–119. (**LOE IV**).
193. Honton JL, Bouyala JM. Societe francaise de chirurgie orthopedique et traumatologique. Les fractures transcervicales recentes du femur: symposium. *Rev Chir Orthop.* 1986;72:3–51. (**LOE IV**).

194. Lee DH, Park JW, Lee SH. A transepiphyseal fracture of the femoral neck in a child with 2 widely displaced Salter-Harris III fragments of the capital femoral epiphysis. *J Orthop Trauma.* 2010;24:125–129. **(LOE V)**.

195. Whitman R. Observations on fracture of the neck of the femur in childhood, with especial reference to treatment and differential diagnosis from separation of the epiphysis. *Med Rec.* 1893;8:227–230. **(LOE IV)**.

196. Lindseth RE, Rosene HA Jr. Traumatic separation of the upper femoral epiphysis in a new born infant. *J Bone Joint Surg Am.* 1971;53:1641–1644. **(LOE V)**.

197. Milgram JW, Lyne ED. Epiphysiolysis of the proximal femur in very young children. *Clin Orthop Relat Res.* 1975;110:146–153. **(LOE IV)**.

198. Wojtowycz M, Starshak RJ, Sty JR. Neonatal proximal femoral epiphysiolysis. *Radiology.* 1980;136:647–648. **(LOE IV)**.

199. Letts M, Davidson D, Lapner P. Multiple trauma in children: predicting outcome and long-term results. *Can J Surg.* 2002;45:126–131. **(LOE IV)**.

200. van der Sluis CK, Kingma J, Eisma WH, ten Duis HJ. Pediatric polytrauma: short-term and long-term outcomes. *J Trauma.* 1997;43:501–506. **(LOE IV)**.

201. Colonna PC. Fracture of the neck of the femur in children. *Am J Surg.* 1929;6:793–797. **(LOE IV)**.

202. Gopinathan NR, Chouhan D, Akkina N, Behera P. Case report: bilateral femoral neck fractures in a child and a rare complication of slipped capital epiphysis after internal fixation. *Clin Orthop Relat Res.* 2012;470:2941–2945. **(LOE V)**.

203. Thompson GH, Bachner EJ, Ballock RT. Salter-Harris type II fractures of the capital femoral epiphysis. *J Orthop Trauma.* 2000;14:510–514. **(LOE IV)**.

204. Moon ES, Mehlman CT. Risk factors for avascular necrosis after femoral neck fractures in children: 25 Cincinnati cases and meta-analysis of 360 cases. *J Orthop Trauma.* 2006;20:323–329. **(LOE IV)**.

205. Banskota AK, Spiegel DA, Shrestha S, Shrestha OP, Rajbhandary T. Open reduction for neglected traumatic hip dislocation in children and adolescents. *J Pediatr Orthop.* 2007;27:187–191. **(LOE IV)**.

206. Epstein HC. Traumatic dislocations of the hip. *Clin Orthop Relat Res.* 92:116–142, 1973. **(LOE IV)**.

207. Hamilton CM. Fractures of the neck of the femur in children. *JAMA.* 1961;178:799–801. **(LOE IV)**.

208. Heiser JM, Oppenheim WL. Fractures of the hip in children: a review of forty cases. *Clin Orthop Relat Res.* 1980;149:177–184. **(LOE IV)**.

209. Hughes LO, Beaty JH. Fractures of the head and neck of the femur in children. *J Bone Joint Surg Am.* 1994;76:283–292. **(LOE V)**.

210. Ingram AJ, Bachynski B. Fractures of the hip in children; treatment and results. *J Bone Joint Surg Am.* 1953;35-A:867–887. **(LOE IV)**.

211. Miller WE. Fractures of the hip in children from birth to adolescence. *Clin Orthop Relat Res.* 1973;92:155–188. **(LOE IV)**.

212. Sferopoulos NK, Papavasiliou VA. [Proximal epiphyseal separation of the femur in the newborn: early ultrasonic diagnosis]. *Rev Chir Orthop Reparatrice Appar Mot.* 1994;80:338–341. **(LOE V)**.

213. Niethard FU. Physiopathology and prognosis of femoral neck fractures in childhood. *Hefte Unfallheilkd.* 1982;158:221–232. **(LOE V)**.

214. Pforringer W, Rosemeyer B. Fractures of the hip in children and adolescents. *Acta Orthop Scand.* 1980;51:91–108. **(LOE IV)**.

215. Ratliff AH. Fractures of the neck of the femur in children. *Orthop Clin North Am.* 1974;5:903–924. **(LOE IV)**.

216. Russell RH. A clinical lecture on fracture of the neck of the femur in childhood. *Lancet.* 1898;152:125–126. **(LOE IV)**.

217. Shrader MW, Jacofsky DJ, Stans AA, Shaughnessy WJ, Haidukewych GJ. Femoral neck fractures in pediatric patients: 30 years experience at a level 1 trauma center. *Clin Orthop Relat Res.* 2007;454:169–173. **(LOE IV)**.

218. Hoekstra HJ, Lichtendahl D. Pertrochanteric fractures in children and adolescents. *J Pediatr Orthop.* 1983;3:587–591. **(LOE IV)**.

219. Cheng JC, Tang N. Decompression and stable internal fixation of femoral neck fractures in children can affect the outcome. *J Pediatr Orthop.* 1999;19:338–343. **(LOE III)**.

220. Dora C, Zurbach J, Hersche O, Ganz R. Pathomorphologic characteristics of posttraumatic acetabular dysplasia. *J Orthop Trauma.* 2000;14:483–489. **(LOE IV)**.

221. Gerber C, Lehmann A, Ganz R. Femoral neck fractures in children: a multicenter follow-up study. *Z Orthop.* 1985;123:767. **(LOE IV)**.

222. Lam SF. Treatment of fractures of the neck of the femur in children. *Orthop Clin North Am.* 1976;7:625–632. **(LOE IV)**.

223. Sharma JC, Biyani A, Kalla R, Gupta SP, Arora A, Bhaskar SK. Management of childhood femoral neck fractures. *Injury.* 1992;23:453–457. **(LOE III)**.

224. Song KS, Kim HK. Femoral neck fracture in a child with autosomal-dominant osteopetrosis: failure of spica cast treatment and successful outcome by internal fixation. *J Orthop Trauma.* 2005;19:494–497. **(LOE V)**.

225. Song KS, Kim YS, Sohn SW, Ogden JA. Arthrotomy and open reduction of the displaced fracture of the femoral neck in children. *J Pediatr Orthop B.* 2001;10:205–210. **(LOE IV)**.

226. Gholve PA, Cameron DB, Millis MB. Slipped capital femoral epiphysis update. *Curr Opin Pediatr.* 2009;21:39–45. **(LOE V)**.

227. Gordon JE. It's not as easy as it looks: commentary on an article by Wudhhav N. Sankar, MD, et al. "The modified Dunn procedure for unstable slipped capital femoral epiphysis. A multicenter perspective". *J Bone Joint Surg Am.* 2013;95:e47. **(LOE V)**.

228. Huber H, Dora C, Ramseier LE, Buck F, Dierauer S. Adolescent slipped capital femoral epiphysis treated by a modified Dunn osteotomy with surgical hip dislocation. *J Bone Joint Surg Br.* 2011;93:833–838. **(LOE IV)**.

229. Parsch K, Weller S, Parsch D. Open reduction and smooth Kirschner wire fixation for unstable slipped capital femoral epiphysis. *J Pediatr Orthop.* 2009;29:1–8. **(LOE IV)**.

230. Slongo T, Kakaty D, Krause F, Ziebarth K. Treatment of slipped capital femoral epiphysis with a modified Dunn procedure. *J Bone Joint Surg Am.* 2010;92:2898–2908. **(LOE IV)**.

231. Zhang Q, Chen W, Liu H, Su Y, Pan J, Zhang Y. The anterior dislocation of the sacroiliac joint: a report of four cases and review of the literature and treatment algorism. *Arch Orthop Trauma Surg.* 2009;129:941–947. **(LOE IV)**.

232. Sankar WN, Vanderhave KL, Matheney T, Herrera-Soto JA, Karlen JW. The modified Dunn procedure for unstable slipped capital femoral epiphysis: a multicenter perspective. *J Bone Joint Surg Am.* 2013;95:585–591. **(LOE V)**.

233. Persinger F, Davis RL 2nd, Samora WP, Klingele KE. Treatment of unstable slipped capital epiphysis via the modified Dunn procedure. *J Pediatr Orthop.* 2018;38:3–8. **(LOE III)**.

234. Joseph B, Mulpuri K. Delayed separation of the capital femoral epiphysis after an ipsilateral transcervical fracture of the femoral neck. *J Orthop Trauma.* 2000;14:446–448. **(LOE V)**.

235. Shrader MW, Schwab JH, Shaughnessy WJ, Jacofsky DJ. Pathologic femoral neck fractures in children. *Am J Orthop (Belle Mead NJ).* 2009;38:83–86; discussion 86. **(LOE IV)**.

236. Widmann RF, Hresko MT, Kasser JR, Millis MB. Wagner multiple K-wire osteosynthesis to correct coxa vara in the young child: experience with a versatile 'tailor-made' high angle blade plate equivalent. *J Pediatr Orthop B.* 2001;10:43–50. **(LOE IV)**.

237. Bagatur AE, Zorer G. Complications associated with surgically treated hip fractures in children. *J Pediatr Orthop B.* 2002;11:219–228. **(LOE IV)**.

238. Kay SP, Hall JE. Fracture of the femoral neck in children and its complications. *Clin Orthop Relat Res.* 1971;80:53–71. **(LOE IV)**.

239. Taylor KF, McHale KA. Percutaneous pin fixation of a femoral neck fracture complicated by deep infection in a 12-year-old boy. *Am J Orthop (Belle Mead NJ).* 2002;31:408–412. **(LOE V)**.

240. Forster NA, Ramseier LE, Exner GU. Undisplaced femoral neck fractures in children have a high risk of secondary displacement. *J Pediatr Orthop B.* 2006;15:131–133. **(LOE V)**.

241. Forlin E, Guille JT, Kumar SJ, Rhee KJ. Complications associated with fracture of the neck of the femur in children. *J Pediatr Orthop.* 1992;12:503–509. **(LOE IV)**.

242. Abbas AA, Yoon TR, Lee JH, Hur CI. Posttraumatic avascular necrosis of the femoral head in teenagers treated by a modified transtrochanteric rotational osteotomy: a report of three cases. *J Orthop Trauma.* 2008;22:63–69. **(LOE IV)**.

243. Ng GP, Cole WG. Effect of early hip decompression on the frequency of avascular necrosis in children with fractures of the neck of the femur. *Injury.* 1996;27:419–421. **(LOE III)**.

244. Ramachandran M, Ward K, Brown RR, Munns CF, Cowell CT, Little DG. Intravenous bisphosphonate therapy for traumatic osteonecrosis of the femoral head in adolescents. *J Bone Joint Surg Am.* 2007;89:1727–1734. **(LOE IV).**

245. Seiler JG 3rd, Kregor PJ, Conrad EU 3rd, Swiontkowski MF. Posttraumatic osteonecrosis in a swine model. Correlation of blood cell flux, MRI and histology. *Acta Orthop Scand.* 1996;67:249–254. **(LOE IV).**

246. Tsirikos AI, Shah SA, Riddle E, Stanton RP. Transphyseal fracture-dislocation of the femoral neck: a case report and review of the literature. *J Orthop Trauma.* 2003;17:648–653. **(LOE V).**

247. Magu NK, Singh R, Sharma AK, Ummat V. Modified Pauwels' intertrochanteric osteotomy in neglected femoral neck fractures in children: a report of 10 cases followed for a minimum of 5 years. *J Orthop Trauma.* 2007;21:237–243. **(LOE IV).**

248. Nagi ON, Dhillon MS, Gill SS. Fibular osteosynthesis for delayed type II and type III femoral neck fractures in children. *J Orthop Trauma.* 1992;6:306–313. **(LOE IV).**

249. Lam SF. Fractures of the neck of the femur in children. *J Bone Joint Surg Am.* 1971;53:1165–1179. **(LOE IV).**

250. Ovesen O, Arreskov J, Bellstrom T. Hip fractures in children. A long-term follow up of 17 cases. *Orthopedics.* 1989;12:361–367. **(LOE IV).**

251. Raju KK, Tepler M, Dharapak C, Pearlman HS. Transepiphyseal fracture of the hips in children. *Orthop Rev.* 1984;13:65–77. **(LOE IV).**

252. McDougall A. Fracture of the neck of femur in childhood. *J Bone Joint Surg Br.* 1961;43:16–28. **(LOE IV).**

253. Kloen P, Rubel IF, Lyden JP, Helfet DL. Subtrochanteric fracture after cannulated screw fixation of femoral neck fractures: a report of four cases. *J Orthop Trauma.* 2003;17:225–229. **(LOE V).**

254. Canale ST, Azar F, Young J, Beaty JH, Warner WC, Whitmer G. Subtrochanteric fracture after fixation of slipped capital femoral epiphysis: a complication of unused drill holes. *J Pediatr Orthop.* 1994;14:623–626. **(LOE V).**

255. Ehrensperger J. Fractures of the sacrum and disk herniation: rare lesions in the pediatric surgical patient? *Eur J Pediatr Surg.* 1992;2:173–176. **(LOE IV).**

256. Strehl A, Ganz R. [Anterior femoroacetabular impingement after healed femoral neck fractures]. *Unfallchirurg.* 2005;108:263–273. **(LOE IV).**

257. Jerre R, Karlsson J. Outcome after transphyseal hip fractures. 4 children followed 34-48 years. *Acta Orthop Scand.* 1997;68:235–238. **(LOE IV).**

258. Leung PC, Lam SF. Long-term follow-up of children with femoral neck fractures. *J Bone Joint Surg Br.* 1986;68:537–540. **(LOE IV).**

259. Morsy HA. Complications of fracture of the neck of the femur in children. A long-term follow-up study. *Injury.* 2001;32:45–51. **(LOE IV).**

260. Pape HC, Krettek C, Friedrich A, Pohlemann T, Simon R, Tscherne H. Long-term outcome in children with fractures of the proximal femur after high-energy trauma. *J Trauma.* 1999;46:58–64. **(LOE IV).**

261. Sferopoulos NK, Papavasiliou VA. 'Natural' healing of hip fractures in childhood. *Injury.* 1994;25:493–496. **(LOE IV).**

262. Togrul E, Bayram H, Gulsen M, Kalaci A, Ozbarlas S. Fractures of the femoral neck in children: long-term follow-up in 62 hip fractures. *Injury.* 2005;36:123–130. **(LOE IV).**

263. Yeranosian M, Horneff JG, Baldwin K, Hosalkar HS. Factors affecting the outcome of fractures of the femoral neck in children and adolescents: a systematic review. *Bone Joint J.* 2013;95-B:135–142. **(LOE III).**

264. Young NL, Wright JG. Measuring pediatric physical function. *J Pediatr Orthop.* 1995;15:244–253. **(LOE V).**

265. Gaudinez RF, Heinrich SD. Transphyseal fracture of the capital femoral epiphysis. *Orthopedics.* 1989;12:1599–1602. **(LOE V).**

266. Marsh HO. Intertrochanteric and femoral neck fractures in children. *J Bone Joint Surg Am.* 1967;49:1024. **(LOE IV).**

267. Manninger J, Kazar G, Fekete G, et al. Significance of urgent (within 6h) internal fixation in the management of fractures of the neck of the femur. *Injury.* 1989;20:101–105. **(LOE II).**

268. Flynn JM, Wong KL, Yeh GL, Meyer JS, Davidson RS. Displaced fractures of the hip in children. Management by early operation and immobilisation in a hip spica cast. *J Bone Joint Surg Br.* 2002;84:108–112. **(LOE IV).**

269. Kujat R, Suren EG, Rogge D, Tscherne H. Femoral neck fractures during the growth period. Treatment principles, results, prognosis. *Chirurg.* 1984;55:43–48. **(LOE IV).**

270. Delbet MP. Fractures du col de femur. *Bull Mem Soc Chir.* 1909;35:387–389. **(LOE IV).**

271. Gamble JG, Lettice J, Smith JT, Rinsky LA. Transverse cervicopertrochanteric hip fracture. *J Pediatr Orthop.* 1991;11:779–782. **(LOE V).**

272. Byram G, Wickstrom J. Traumatic dislocation of the hip in children. *South Med J.* 1967;60:805–810. **(LOE IV).**

273. MacFarlane IJA. Survey of traumatic dislocation of the hip in children. Orthopaedic proceedings. *J Bone Joint Surg Br.* 1976;58(suppl 2):267. **(LOE IV).**

274. Mason ML. Traumatic dislocation of the hip in childhood; report of a case. *J Bone Joint Surg Br.* 19554;36-B:630–632. **(LOE V).**

275. Wilson DW. Traumatic dislocation of the hip in children: a report of four cases. *J Trauma.* 1966;6:739–743. **(LOE IV).**

276. Freeman GEJ. Traumatic dislocation of the hip in children, a report of seven cases and review of the literature. *J Bone Joint Surg Am.* 1961;43:401–406. **(LOE IV).**

277. Offierski CM. Traumatic dislocation of the hip in children. *J Bone Joint Surg Br.* 1981;63-B:194–197. **(LOE IV).**

278. Bonnemaison MF, Henderson ED. Traumatic anterior dislocation of the hip with acute common femoral occlusion in a child. *J Bone Joint Surg Am.* 1968;50:753–756. **(LOE V).**

279. Choyce CC. Traumatic dislocation of the hip in childhood, and relation of trauma to pseudocoxalgia: analysis of 59 cases published up to January, 1924. *Br J Surg.* 1924;12:52–59. **(LOE IV).**

280. Elmslie RC. Traumatic dislocation of the hip in a child, aged 7, with subsequent development of coxa plana. *Proc R Soc Med.* 1932;25:1100–1102. **(LOE V).**

281. Glass A, Powell HDW. Traumatic dislocation of the hip in children: an analysis of forty-seven patients. *J Bone Joint Surg Br.* 1961;43:29–37. **(LOE IV).**

282. Jones BG, Kinninmonth AW. Low-energy hip dislocation in the young. *J Trauma.* 2005;58:638–639. **(LOE V).**

283. Sahin V, Karakas ES, Turk CY. Bilateral traumatic hip dislocation in a child: a case report and review of the literature. *J Trauma.* 1999;46:500–504. **(LOE V).**

284. Libri R, Calderon JE, Capelli A, Soncini G. Traumatic dislocation of the hip in children and adolescents. *Ital J Orthop Traumatol.* 1986;12:61–67. **(LOE IV).**

285. Olsson O, Landin LA, Johansson A. Traumatic hip dislocation with spontaneous reduction and capsular interposition. A report of 2 children. *Acta Orthop Scand.* 1994;65:476–479. **(LOE IV).**

286. Barquet A. Traumatic hip dislocation in childhood. A report of 26 cases and review of the literature. *Acta Orthop Scand.* 1979;50:549–553. **(LOE IV).**

287. Ferguson AB Jr, Donaldson WF, Rodriguez EE, et al. Traumatic dislocation of the hip joint in children: a report by the Scientific Research Committee of the Pennsylvania Orthopaedic Society. *J Bone Joint Surg Am.* 1960;42:705–710. **(LOE IV).**

288. Piggot J. Traumatic dislocation of the hip in childhood. *J Bone Joint Surg Br.* 1961;43:38–42. **(LOE IV).**

289. Hoiness P, Roise O. Successful open reduction of a 5-month-old hip dislocation associated with a femoral head fracture. *J Orthop Trauma.* 2003;17:131–134. **(LOE V).**

290. Mohammad S, Port A, Montgomery RJ. Transepiphyseal fracture of the femoral neck with dislocation of the femoral head and fracture of the posterior column of the acetabulum in a child. *J Bone Joint Surg Br.* 2002;84:113–115. **(LOE V).**

291. Blanchard C, Kushare I, Boyles A, Mundy A, Beebe AC, Klingele KE. Traumatic, posterior pediatric hip dislocations with associated posterior labrum osteochondral avulsion: recognizing the acetabular "fleck" sign. *J Pediatr Orthop.* 2016;36:602–607. **(LOE IV).**

292. Price CT, Pyevich MT, Knapp DR, Phillips JH, Hawker JJ. Traumatic hip dislocation with spontaneous incomplete reduction: a diagnostic trap. *J Orthop Trauma.* 2002;16:730–735. **(LOE IV).**

293. Barquet A, Vecsei V. Traumatic dislocation of the hip with separation of the proximal femoral epiphysis. Report of two cases and review of the literature. *Arch Orthop Trauma Surg.* 1984;103:219–223. **(LOE IV).**

294. Godley DR, Williams RA. Traumatic dislocation of the hip in a child: usefulness of MRI. *Orthopedics.* 1993;16:1145–1147. **(LOE V).**

295. Hearty T, Swaroop VT, Gourineni P, Robinson L. Standard radiographs and computed tomographic scan underestimating pediatric acetabular fracture after traumatic hip dislocation: report of 2 cases. *J Orthop Trauma.* 2011;25:e68–e73. (**LOE V**).

296. Mayer SW, Stewart JR, Fadell MF, Kestel L, Novais EN. MRI as a reliable and accurate method for assessment of posterior hip dislocation in children and adolescents without the risk of radiation exposure. *Pediatr Radiol.* 2015;45:1355–1362. (**LOE IV**).

297. Rubel IF, Kloen P, Potter HG, Helfet DL. MRI assessment of the posterior acetabular wall fracture in traumatic dislocation of the hip in children. *Pediatr Radiol.* 2002;32:435–439. (**LOE V**).

298. Speer KP, Spritzer CE, Harrelson JM, Nunley JA. Magnetic resonance imaging of the femoral head after acute intracapsular fracture of the femoral neck. *J Bone Joint Surg Am.* 1990;72:98–103. (**LOE IV**).

299. Thanacharoenpanich S, Bixby S, Breen MA, Kim YJ. MRI is better than CT scan for detection of structural pathologies after traumatic posterior hip dislocations in children and adolescents. *J Pediatr Orthop.* 2018 [epub ahead of print].

300. Vialle R, Pannier S, Odent T, Schmit P, Pauthier F, Glorion C. Imaging of traumatic dislocation of the hip in childhood. *Pediatr Radiol.* 2004;34:970–979. (**LOE IV**).

301. Nerubay J. Traumatic anterior dislocation of hip joint with vascular damage. *Clin Orthop Relat Res.* 1976;116:129–132. (**LOE V**).

302. Keller MS. Musculoskeletal sonography in the neonate and infant. *Pediatr Radiol.* 2005;35:1167–1173; quiz 1293. (**LOE V**).

303. Martinoli C, Valle M, Malattia C, Beatrice Damasio M, Tagliafico A. Paediatric musculoskeletal US beyond the hip joint. *Pediatr Radiol.* 2011;41(suppl 1):S113–S124. (**LOE V**).

304. Stewart MJ, Milford LW. Fracture-dislocation of the hip; an end-result study. *J Bone Joint Surg Am.* 1954;36:315–342. (**LOE IV**).

305. Bunnell WP, Webster DA. Late reduction of bilateral traumatic hip dislocations in a child. *Clin Orthop Relat Res.* 1980;147:160–163. (**LOE V**).

306. Vialle R, Odent T, Pannier S, Pauthier F, Laumonier F, Glorion C. Traumatic hip dislocation in childhood. *J Pediatr Orthop.* 2005;25:138–144. (**LOE IV**).

307. Herrera-Soto JA, Price CT. Traumatic hip dislocations in children and adolescents: pitfalls and complications. *J Am Acad Orthop Surg.* 2009;17:15–21. (**LOE V**).

308. Kutty S, Thornes B, Curtin WA, Gilmore MF. Traumatic posterior dislocation of hip in children. *Pediatr Emerg Care.* 2001;17:32–35. (**LOE V**).

309. Herrera-Soto JA, Price CT, Reuss BL, Riley P, Kasser JR, Beaty JH. Proximal femoral epiphysiolysis during reduction of hip dislocation in adolescents. *J Pediatr Orthop.* 2006;26:371–374. (**LOE IV**).

310. Odent T, Glorion C, Pannier S, Bronfen C, Langlais J, Pouliquen JC. Traumatic dislocation of the hip with separation of the capital epiphysis: 5 adolescent patients with 3-9 years of follow-up. *Acta Orthop Scand.* 2003;74:49–52, 2003. (**LOE IV**).

311. Ratliff AH. Traumatic separation of the upper femoral epiphysis in young children. *J Bone Joint Surg Br.* 1968;50:757–770. (**LOE IV**).

312. Novais EN, Heare TC, Hill MK, Mayer SW. Surgical hip dislocation for the treatment of intra-articular injuries and hip instability following traumatic posterior dislocation in children and adolescents. *J Pediatr Orthop.* 2016;36:673–679. (**LOE IV**).

313. Allis O. *Inquiry into the Difficulties Encountered in the Reduction of Dislocation of the Hip.* Philadelphia: Dornan; 1986.

314. Bigelow H. *The Mechanics of Dislocation and Fracture of the Hip with the Reduction of the Dislocations by the Flexion Method.* Philadelphia: Henry C. Lea; 1869.

315. Stimson L. *Treatise on Dislocation.* Philadelphia: Lea Brothers; 1888.

316. Canale ST, Manugian AH. Irreducible traumatic dislocations of the hip. *J Bone Joint Surg Am.* 1979;61:7–14. (**LOE IV**).

317. Nelson MC, Lauerman WC, Brower AC, Wells JR. Avulsion of the acetabular labrum with intraarticular displacement. *Orthopedics.* 1990;13:889–891. (**LOE V**).

318. Podeszwa DA, De La Rocha A, Larson AN, Sucato DJ. Surgical hip dislocation is safe and effective following acute traumatic hip instability in the adolescent. *J Pediatr Orthop.* 2015;35:435–442. (**LOE IV**).

319. Ganz R, Gill TJ, Gautier E, Ganz K, Krugel N, Berlemann U. Surgical dislocation of the adult hip a technique with full access to the femoral head and acetabulum without the risk of avascular necrosis. *J Bone Joint Surg Br.* 2001;83:1119–1124. (**LOE IV**).

320. Madan SS, Cooper AP, Davies AG, Fernandes JA. The treatment of severe slipped capital femoral epiphysis via the Ganz surgical dislocation and anatomical reduction: a prospective study. *Bone Joint J.* 2013;95-B:424–429. (**LOE IV**).

321. Ganz R, Krushell RJ, Jakob RP, Kuffer J. The antishock pelvic clamp. *Clin Orthop Relat Res.* 1991;267:71–78. (**LOE IV**).

322. Gartland JJ, Benner JH. Traumatic dislocations in the lower extremity in children. *Orthop Clin North Am.* 1976;7:687–700. (**LOE V**).

323. Swiontkowski MF. Complications of hip fractures in children. *Compl Orthop.* 1989;4:58–64. (**LOE V**).

324. Eijer H, Myers SR, Ganz R. Anterior femoroacetabular impingement after femoral neck fractures. *J Orthop Trauma.* 2001;15:475–481. (**LOE IV**).

325. Haliburton RA, Brockenshire FA, Barber JF. Avascular necrosis of the femoral capital epiphysis after traumatic dislocation of the hip in children. *J Bone Joint Surg Br.* 1961;43:43–46. (**LOE IV**).

326. Mehlman CT, Hubbard GW, Crawford AH, Roy DR, Wall EJ. Traumatic hip dislocation in children. Long-term followup of 42 patients. *Clin Orthop Relat Res.* 2000;376:68–79. (**LOE IV**).

327. Pearson DE, Mann RJ. Traumatic hip dislocation in children. *Clin Orthop Relat Res.* 1973;92:189–194. (**LOE IV**).

328. Hillyard RF, Fox J. Sciatic nerve injuries associated with traumatic posterior hip dislocations. *Am J Emerg Med.* 2003;21:545–548. (**LOE IV**).

329. Aufranc OE, Jones WN, Harris WH. Recurrent traumatic dislocation of the hip in a child. *Jama.* 1964;190:291–294. (**LOE V**).

330. Dall D, Macnab I, Gross A. Recurrent anterior dislocation of the hip. *J Bone Joint Surg Am.* 1970;52:574–576. (**LOE V**).

331. Benali Y, Katthagen BD. Hip subluxation as a complication of arthroscopic debridement. *Arthroscopy.* 2009;25:405–407. (**LOE V**).

332. Matsuda DK. Acute iatrogenic dislocation following hip impingement arthroscopic surgery. *Arthroscopy.* 2009;25:400–404. (**LOE V**).

333. Mei-Dan O, McConkey MO, Brick M. Catastrophic failure of hip arthroscopy due to iatrogenic instability: can partial division of the ligamentum teres and iliofemoral ligament cause subluxation? *Arthroscopy.* 2012;28:440–445. (**LOE V**).

334. Nepple JJ, Schoenecker PL, Clohisy JC. Iatrogenic hip subluxation after surgical dislocation successfully treated with periacetabular osteotomy: a case report. *JBJS Case Connect.* 2013;3:e1. (**LOE V**).

335. Ranawat AS, McClincy M, Sekiya JK. Anterior dislocation of the hip after arthroscopy in a patient with capsular laxity of the hip. A case report. *J Bone Joint Surg Am.* 2009;91:192–197. (**LOE V**).

336. Song KS, Choi IH, Sohn YJ, Shin HD, Leem HS. Habitual dislocation of the hip in children: report of eight additional cases and literature review. *J Pediatr Orthop.* 2003;23:178–183. (**LOE IV**).

337. Barquet A. Recurrent traumatic dislocation of the hip in childhood. *J Trauma.* 1980;20:1003–1006. (**LOE V**).

338. Graham B, Lapp RA. Recurrent posttraumatic dislocation of the hip. A report of two cases and review of the literature. *Clin Orthop Relat Res.* 1990;256:115–119. (**LOE IV**).

339. Wilchinsky ME, Pappas AM. Unusual complications in traumatic dislocation of the hip in children. *J Pediatr Orthop.* 1985;5:534–539. (**LOE IV**).

340. Carlson BC, Carlson WO, Baumgarten KM. A transphyseal fracture of the nonossified proximal femoral epiphysis as a result of child abuse: a case report. *JBJS Case Connect.* 2012;2:e42. (**LOE V**).

341. Gaul RW. Recurrent traumatic dislocation of the hip in children. *Clin Orthop Relat Res.* 1973;90:107–109. (**LOE V**).

342. Lieberman JR, Altchek DW, Salvati EA. Recurrent dislocation of a hip with a labral lesion: treatment with a modified Bankart-type repair. Case report. *J Bone Joint Surg Am.* 1993;75:1524–1527. (**LOE V**).

343. Schwartz DL, Haller JA Jr. Open anterior hip dislocation with femoral vessel transection in a child. *J Trauma.* 1974;14:1054–1059. (**LOE V**).

344. Simmons RL, Elder JD. Recurrent posttraumatic dislocation of the hip in children. *South Med J.* 1972;65:1463–1466. (**LOE V**).

345. Weber M, Ganz R. Recurrent traumatic dislocation of the hip: report of a case and review of the literature. *J Orthop Trauma.* 1997;11:382–385. (**LOE V**).

346. Upadhyay SS, Moulton A, Srikrishnamurthy K. An analysis of the late effects of traumatic posterior dislocation of the hip without fractures. *J Bone Joint Surg Br.* 1983;65:150–152. (**LOE IV**).

347. Hougaard K, Thomsen PB. Traumatic hip dislocation in children. Follow up of 13 cases. *Orthopedics.* 1989;12:375–378. (**LOE IV**).

Fractures of the Femoral Shaft   12

Ying Li | Kevin M. Dale | Jeffrey Shilt

INTRODUCTION: SCOPE AND PURPOSE

The treatment of pediatric femur fractures continues to evolve similarly to other pediatric fracture management trends, highlighted by utilization of more invasive methods and the rising percentage of surgical implant fixation. One exception is the use of external fixation, which appears to be on the decline and is not mentioned in the latest American Academy of Orthopaedic Surgeons (AAOS) guidelines.[1,2] This increase in invasive surgical techniques is likely the result of societal expectations that desire rapid return to patient preinjury activity levels with little disruption of caregiver routines. Whether or not it is causal, there is a concomitant decrease in length of hospital stay.[3,4] It is unlikely that this trend will reverse.

ANATOMY AND DEVELOPMENT

As the longest, most voluminous, and strongest bone of the human body, the femur consists of a tubular shaft, hemispheric head, and bicondylar distal end. The femur constitutes approximately 25% of the total adult height. The contribution of femoral growth by the proximal and distal femoral growth plates is approximately 30% and 70%, respectively.[5]

The femur forms from the mesoderm at approximately 4 weeks of embryonic life. Eight weeks after fertilization of the ovum, during the transition from embryonic to fetal life, the primary ossification center of the diaphysis begins transforming from a cartilage anlage into bone. Typically, by 16 weeks, the entire femoral shaft is ossified.[6]

The proximal secondary ossification centers are rarely present at birth. Proximally, the cartilaginous mass develops in three distinct stages: (1) femoral head at 6 months of age, (2) greater trochanter at 3 to 4 years of age, and (3) lesser trochanter at 7 to 9 years of age.[7] The distal secondary ossification centers are present at birth, typically appearing in the third trimester.[8] The use of dual-energy x-ray absorptiometry to evaluate femoral development has introduced some controversy about the actual dates of appearance of these ossification centers in the prenatal period, but does not impact clinical decision making.[9]

The femoral shaft blood supply consists of endosteal and periosteal contributions. An equal proportion of individuals have either one or two nutrient arteries that supply the femoral diaphysis as branches of the deep femoral artery, with the rare contribution of three or more nutrient arteries.[10] The vessels typically enter the shaft posteromedially at the

proximal and distal third junctions, respectively. These nutrient arteries give rise to the endosteal or intramedullary blood supply to the inner two-thirds of the cortex. Generally, there are also two periosteal vessels that supply the outer third of the cortex. One vessel each arises from the femoral and deep femoral arteries.[11] This dual blood supply from both endosteal and periosteal contributions is important because methods of treatment that involve reaming of the intramedullary canal destroy the endosteal blood supply. Fortunately, the intact periosteum and its blood supply remain, allowing adequate blood flow for fracture healing via periosteal remodeling.

Knowledge of the blood supply to the femoral head is imperative in the treatment of femoral shaft fractures. The blood supply to the femoral head is provided primarily from the ascending branches of the medial femoral circumflex artery,[12] the most notable of which is the lateral ascending cervical artery (Fig. 12.1). This branch crosses through the piriformis fossa on its way to the femoral head. This fact precludes utilization of the piriformis entry for rigid nails in immature patients for fear of avascular necrosis.

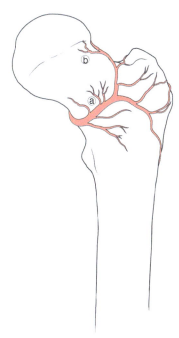

Fig. 12.1 Diagram showing the deep branch of the medial femoral circumflex artery (A) and its ascending branches. The terminal subsynovial branches of the medial femoral circumflex artery (B) are located on the posterosuperior aspect of the neck of the femur and are at risk of injury from intramedullary nailing with a start site in the piriformis fossa.

Femoral osteology is unique. Many of the features are dynamic and evolve from childhood to adulthood. For instance, the orientation of the femoral shaft in relation to the femoral head and neck changes during childhood. The neck-shaft angle and amount of anteversion present in the femoral neck decrease with growth, beginning at 150 degrees and 40 degrees, respectively, and finally resting at 130 degrees and 10 degrees. An anterior bow exists in the upper third of the femoral shaft and is maintained throughout life. This curvature has altered the development of rigid intramedullary nails when used as a treatment option. The anatomy of the greater trochanter deserves attention because it serves as an important landmark in the treatment of femoral shaft fractures when performing antegrade rigid femoral nail fixation using a greater trochanteric approach. In the sagittal plane, the tip of the trochanter is located eccentrically at the junction of the anterior first and middle thirds of the greater trochanter. This point is posterior to the femoral head, as noted on a lateral radiograph. The role of the greater trochanteric apophysis in proximal femoral development is important in treating femoral shaft fractures. Historically, it was believed this ossification center influenced angulation of the femoral neck until approximately 8 years of age, thereby providing an age threshold for which one should not embark on violating with rigid nail entrance without expectation of growth disturbance.[13] More recent studies[14] have confirmed the lack of significant changes in the femoral neck shaft angle or femoral neck diameter when performing trochanteric nailing after this time.

DEMOGRAPHICS AND MECHANISM OF INJURY

The incidence of femur fractures has stabilized since the last edition, and this trend is noted both in the United States and Sweden.[3,4] However, femur fractures continue to represent the most common reason for hospitalization for traumatic pediatric orthopedic injuries in the United States, accounting for 20% of admissions in an updated review of the 2006 Kids' Inpatient Database, a subset of the Healthcare Cost and Utilization Project, which is the largest collection of longitudinal hospital care data in the United States.[4] Femur fractures are costly and seem to correlate with the length of stay. Femur fractures fall only behind spine and pelvic fractures in both categories. Although these are most commonly isolated injuries, femoral fractures can be associated with additional injuries.

Femoral shaft fractures occur twice as often in boys as in girls.[3,4] The incidence of femoral fractures is bimodal, with the initial peak at 2 to 3 years of age and a second peak at 17 to 18 years.

Children experience isolated femoral fractures more often than adults. Fatalities from femoral fractures are rare in children: usually 1 in 600, or 0.17%. Although the mortality rate exceeds that of any other extremity injury, it is one-half the rate of spine and pelvic injuries.[15] Death associated with femoral fractures is generally caused by the presence of multiple associated injuries, particularly in association with significant closed head injuries.

Pediatric femoral fractures most commonly result from motor vehicle accidents (38%) and falls (32%), although they also result from nonaccidental trauma, pathologic causes, and stress syndromes.[4] Fractures associated with nonaccidental trauma more often occur in the distal femur or in combination with the distal femur.[16] Up to 30% of femoral shaft fractures in children younger than 4 years may be the result of inflicted physical abuse, and the most common cause of femoral fractures in nonambulatory infants is child physical abuse. Factors suggestive of child physical abuse include bruises, burns, multiple fractures in various stages of healing, and late presentation.

The femur is a very common location for pathologic fractures in children. These fractures occur through weak bone that lacks normal biomechanical properties as a result of intrinsic processes, such as metabolic bone disease or tumors. Extrinsic processes, such as implant removal or radiation, can also weaken the bone and result in a fracture. Although one-third of pathologic fractures occur in the proximal and distal ends of the femur, the diaphysis remains a relatively common location for fractures resulting from fibrous dysplasia and osteosarcoma.[17,18]

Stress or fatigue fractures occur when an exceptional repetitive force, such as with athletic training, is exerted on bone that fails to remodel. A precipitating event or increase in activity is rarely identified in the history, although the diagnosis is characterized by pain and a limp. This vague presentation is common to many pediatric conditions and creates a diagnostic challenge.

EVALUATION

HISTORY AND PHYSICAL EXAMINATION

The history is important, as treatment varies depending on the mechanism of injury and its associated level of energy. The treatment of a fracture resulting from a high-energy motor vehicle accident is approached differently than a pathologic or stress fracture. High-energy fractures are more likely to have associated soft tissue injury. The presence of significant soft tissue injury or periosteal stripping should influence the treatment options because these injuries are less amenable to closed treatment.

A suspicious history may lead one to investigate nonaccidental trauma as a cause of the fracture. Differentiating between nonaccidental and accidental trauma is anxiety provoking for both the physician and the caregiver. The well-being of the child is paramount, yet preserving a working relationship with the caregivers can be done with care and time. Understanding the demographics and different disease processes responsible for nonaccidental trauma can assist in narrowing the differential diagnosis. That said, the current AAOS clinical practice guideline recommends that children younger than 36 months of age with a diaphyseal femur fracture be evaluated for child abuse.[1,2] The injury plausibility method helps tabulate historical data into the likelihood of injury from falling from stairs, a common occurrence, yet also a common false reason given to explain child abuse.[19]

History can assist with the identification of accompanying injuries. For instance, identifying the occurrence of a pedestrian versus motor vehicle accident alerts one to the possibility of the Waddell triad, which describes the associated head injury, intrathoracic or abdominal injury, and femoral fracture that can occur from such trauma.[16] The Waddell triad is actually less common than originally thought, and the more common ipsilateral upper extremity and pelvic injuries should be closely evaluated.[20]

The physical examination of an injured, conscious child always begins by gaining the patient's trust and reassuring the family. A reliable examination of the injured extremity can begin only after a nonthreatening relationship is established. Careful inspection for obvious deformities or swelling is performed, and any soft tissue defects are measured and recorded. Careful palpation of the nontraumatized areas is done to identify secondary injuries. A motor and sensory examination is performed, and peripheral pulses are documented. The examination of the injured extremity is compared with the status of the uninvolved extremity. Any difference warrants further evaluation.

In patients with ipsilateral fractures proximal and distal to the knee (floating knee), it is imperative to evaluate the vascular status of the extremity more carefully. Hard signs of vascular injury are obvious and include pulsatile hemorrhaging, an expanding hematoma, a palpable thrill or audible bruit, or a pulseless limb. More subtle physical clues include unequal pulses, decreased two-point discrimination distal to the fracture, or a nonpulsatile hematoma. However, physical examination alone is not reliable enough to preclude further workup in high-risk injuries. An arterial pressure index (API) or an ankle-brachial index (ABI) can be used in the emergency department as a screening test. The API is calculated by placing one blood pressure cuff distal to the lower extremity injury, and another is placed on an uninjured upper extremity. A Doppler probe is used to determine the systolic pressure of both extremities. The systolic arterial pressure in the injured extremity is divided by the systolic pressure in the unaffected upper extremity to calculate the API. A value less than 0.9 warrants additional radiographic imaging.[21]

Assessment of the injured portion of the thigh is reserved for last and should be performed gently. Traction, reduction, or wound probing should be minimized in patients likely to undergo surgery. These maneuvers should be conducted in the operating room when possible. The exception is in patients whose deformity and pain can be relieved by manipulation and splinting. If manipulation is performed, serial neurovascular checks should be conducted.

It is imperative during the initial assessment of femoral fractures to search for accompanying injuries. In patients with isolated femoral shaft fractures, hemodynamic insufficiency is rare, and volume support is not customarily required. If a patient is seen with hypotension, hypovolemia, or anemia, further investigation must be performed to identify another cause for the bleeding, other than the femoral fracture. Typically, only patients with additional trauma have significant decreases in both hemoglobin concentrations and hematocrit levels compared with patients with isolated femoral fractures.[22] An obvious decrease in hematocrit or hemoglobin concentration in a child with a femoral fracture nearly always indicates additional injury.[23]

In high-energy trauma, examination is dictated by the Advanced Trauma Life Support protocol. The initial assessment is directed to the airway, breathing, and circulation, and attention to any limb injury is focused on circulatory

(hemorrhage) control from open injuries. All limbs are stripped of clothing during the initial examination. Once the patient is stabilized, a secondary survey can be conducted. The limbs are evaluated for further injury by examination for bruising or deformity and palpation for tenderness, crepitus, diminished pulses, and limited joint range of motion. If the patient is stable, further radiographic imaging can then be performed if additional fractures are a concern.

Ipsilateral intraarticular knee injuries are a very common (16%–70%) associated injury with diaphyseal femoral fractures in the adult population.[24-26] The pediatric incidence is unknown, but one should have increased suspicion for these injuries in older children and adolescents. Cruciate and collateral ligament tears and meniscal and osteochondral injuries can occur. Examination for intraarticular injuries is difficult in the acute care setting. A complete ligamentous examination is most easily obtained intraoperatively after stabilization of the femoral fracture and postoperatively by serial evaluation. Magnetic resonance imaging (MRI) or arthroscopy may be warranted.

IMAGING

High-quality anteroposterior (AP) and lateral plain films that include both the hip and knee joints are generally the only radiographic studies required to diagnose and treat pediatric femoral shaft fractures. The advent of the Picture Archiving and Communication System has greatly facilitated measurement of intramedullary canal size and femoral length.

Many practitioners advocate traction films for evaluating stability and predicting treatment outcomes after femoral fractures. The "telescope test" described by Thompson and colleagues predicts that unacceptable final shortening of 25 mm is 20 times more likely if 30 mm of initial shortening or more was identified during the test. The telescope test is a gentle compressive force applied manually across the fracture site. Radiographs are made on standard cassettes with the x-ray beam perpendicular to the fracture site so that maximum overriding of the fracture fragments can be documented. Interestingly, a resting radiographic overlap was not predictive of the final outcome in this study.[27]

Excessive shortening is the result of associated soft tissue injury. Often, history and physical examination can predict the likelihood of excessive shortening. Documentation of excessive shortening may indicate the use of more invasive treatment methods.

Computed tomography is helpful in the evaluation of physeal or periarticular fractures but is not required in isolated femoral shaft fractures. A bone scan may be useful for the detection of suspected stress or pathologic fractures but is unlikely to yield helpful information in a traumatic fracture. Bone scans have been described as an adjuvant modality for diagnosis of orthopedic injuries missed in the initial screening of multiply injured patients with head injuries.[28]

MRI is valuable for assessment of intraarticular pathology, stress fractures, and pathologic lesions. Ipsilateral epiphyseal, ligamentous, meniscal, and osteochondral pathology are relatively common.[24,26] In particular, one should be concerned about osteochondral injury or bone bruises in patients with persistent knee pain after a healed diaphyseal femoral fracture.

Diaphyseal fractures femur (32-D)

Simple fractures			Wedge/multifragmentary fractures		
Code	Figure	Description	Code	Figure	Description
32 - D/4.1	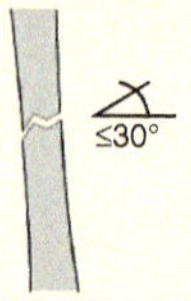	Simple complete transverse (≤30°)	32 - D/4.2	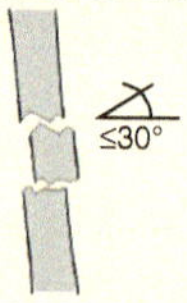	Multifragmentary transverse (≤30°)
32 - D/5.1	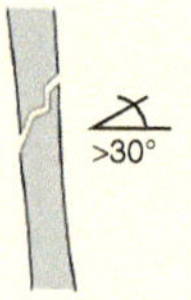	Simple complete oblique or spiral (>30°)	32 - D/5.2	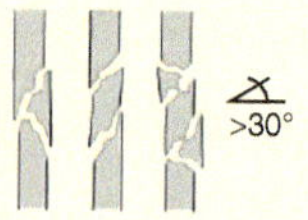	Multifragmentary oblique or spiral (>30°)

Fig. 12.2 Arbeitsgemeinschaft für Osteosynthesefragen (AO) pediatric classification of femoral shaft fractures. (From Slongo TF, Audigé L, AO Pediatric Classification Group, Fracture and dislocation classification compendium for children: the AO pediatric comprehensive classification of long bone fractures (PCCF). *J Orthop Trauma.* 2007;21(Suppl):S135–S160.)

Vascular compromise should be evaluated in an expeditious manner. Arteriograms are the historical gold standard for investigating vascular insufficiency. Assessment with duplex ultrasound, ABI, or both may be useful for determining the need for an arteriogram in equivocal cases. Identification of an arterial injury is more likely to occur when the physician suspects and evaluates for a vascular injury. Physical examination alone has proved inadequate for diagnosing vascular compromise.

CLASSIFICATION

Classification systems provide descriptive information and serve as a basis for selecting optimal treatment, predicting the outcome, and comparing results of various treatment modalities.[29] Maurice E. Müller believed this general theorem and stated that "a classification is useful only if it considers the severity of the bone lesion, and serves as a basis for treatment and for evaluation of the results." He subsequently developed the Arbeitsgemeinschaft für Osteosynthesefragen (AO) classification, which is commonly used in describing adult fractures as combined in the Orthopaedic Trauma Association-AO classification system. In 2007, the AO Pediatric Comprehensive Classification of Long Bone Fractures was developed[30] and the lower extremity component validated in 2017.[31] The femoral shaft fractures are classified as category 32-D, with subcategories 4.1, 4.2, 5.1, and 5.2 (Fig. 12.2).[32]

Though validated, the AO classification system is not commonly used to describe pediatric femoral shaft fractures clinically. Rather, fractures are more commonly classified according to (1) cause, (2) soft tissue integrity, (3) anatomy, and (4) fracture pattern.

The mechanism, chronicity, and other contributing causal factors responsible for fracture contribute to nomenclature. Most fractures can be relegated to high- or low-energy mechanism. Pathologic fractures are considered low energy and are the result of tumors, metabolic disorders, or other processes resulting in abnormal bone biomechanics. Stress fractures occur secondary to repetitive and chronic overuse syndromes. Nonaccidental fractures are caused by intentional harm. Accidental trauma is typically associated with a high-energy mechanism, such as from a motor vehicle accident.

The status of the soft tissue envelope plays an important role in the treatment of femoral fractures and likewise contributes to classifying these fractures. Fractures are considered open if the bone communicates with a wound in the skin and closed if the skin is intact. Ballistic open wounds warrant close attention. In particular, "wadding," which is the barrier between the pellets and gunpowder in shotgun shells, must be accounted for. It is important to note that injuries with intact skin can also have compromised soft tissues. The soft tissue envelope and thick periosteum play a significant role in pediatric fracture stability, and this is inversely proportional to the age of the child. Excessive soft tissue injury and periosteal stripping result in increasing instability and typically require more invasive fixation methods. Bicycle spoke injuries, wringer injuries, and other high-energy mangled extremities are examples where there is extensive soft tissue envelope injury.

Classification by anatomic location of the femoral fracture has important implications for treatment. Femoral shaft fractures are considered to be subtrochanteric, diaphyseal, or supracondylar. Subtrochanteric femoral fractures present unique problems in fracture management. Fractures in this region have limited capacity to compensate for malalignment, and the strong deforming muscle forces place the proximal fragment in a flexed, abducted, and externally rotated position. This malalignment makes maintenance of fracture reduction difficult. The definition of a pediatric subtrochanteric femoral fracture is controversial. Pombo and Shilt[33] advocated that a fracture that occurs within 10% of the total length of the femur below the lesser trochanter should be classified as subtrochanteric. There are other published definitions that do not accommodate the great variability in pediatric femoral length.[34,35] However, a definition that takes into account the wide range of femoral lengths in the pediatric population may be the most accurate and has been found to be useful.[36] Supracondylar femoral fractures historically presented similar problems with definition and management. Butcher and Hoffman[37] defined a supracondylar femoral fracture as one in which

Table 12.1   Recommended Treatment Options for Pediatric Femoral Shaft Fractures

	≤6 Months	6 Months to 5 Years	5 to 11 Years	≥11 Years
Stable fracture	Pavlik	Spica cast	Flexible intramedullary nailing	Rigid trochanteric entry intramedullary nailing
	Spica cast			
Unstable fracture	Pavlik	Spica cast	Flexible intramedullary nailing	Rigid trochanteric entry intramedullary nailing
	Spica cast	Plating	Plating	Plating
		External fixation	External fixation	

the distance from the fracture to the knee joint center was equal to or less than the width of the femoral condyles. Hyperextension of the distal fragment is common secondary to forces from the gastrocnemius muscle. Although less common, a residual flexion deformity at the fracture site can result in interference with patellar tracking.[38] Recognition of these difficult fractures from the more easily treated diaphyseal fractures is critical.

Finally, nomenclature detailing the fracture pattern provides further understanding of its inherent stability. Commonly described fracture patterns include simple transverse, short oblique, long oblique, long spiral, or comminuted. Simple and short oblique fracture patterns are considered "length-stable." Long oblique, long spiral, and comminuted fracture patterns are considered "length-unstable." Specifically, long oblique and comminuted fractures are defined as follows:

Long oblique: The length of the obliquity is twice the diameter of the femur at the level of the fracture.
Comminuted or multifragmentary: More than one continuous fracture is present, of which there are two types:
Butterfly or wedge: The two main fragments maintain some contact.
Complex: No contact is present between the two main fracture fragments.

This differentiation is critical because the method of treatment may need to be modified so that adequate stability is ensured for the specific fracture pattern.

MANAGEMENT

As indicated earlier, patients and their families are increasingly well informed and expect optimal outcomes with the least disruption in their lives. This approach is reasonable but must be tempered by the physician's knowledge of available options, his or her technical ability, and potential complications. The management trend of pediatric femoral shaft fractures has trended toward increased operative treatment and operating more often in younger patients.[39,40] Evidence-based reviews demonstrate fair to good evidence that operative treatment reduces the rate of malunion and total adverse events.[41] This trend, cited in multiple sources in the literature, has reduced inpatient length of stay by nearly 75% and has decreased the overall cost of treatment by more than 60% in comparison with traction alone, and

by almost 30% in comparison with traction followed by casting in certain series.[42,43]

Vascular injuries should always be considered in patients with femoral shaft fractures. Direct arterial repair with or without end-to-end anastomosis, interposition of an autogenous reversed saphenous vein graft, and, in rare cases, ligation are all potential treatment options in patients with direct vessel injury. In blunt trauma, however, endovascular stenting of the involved vessel has been described and may be an acceptable treatment alternative.[44]

EMERGENT TREATMENT

Early surgical stabilization of femoral shaft fractures in children has been shown to decrease hospital stay and intensive care unit stay without increased risk of pulmonary complications.[45,46] Patients who are medically stable should undergo definitive treatment on their initial presentation. Polytrauma patients who are not medically stable enough to undergo definitive fixation can be treated with temporary external fixation or traction with conversion to intramedullary nailing within 2 weeks if their medical condition improves.[47] Although the exact timing of operative management of open fractures is controversial, open fractures should be treated with early antibiotics, urgent irrigation and débridement, and temporary or definitive fracture fixation.[48]

INDICATIONS FOR DEFINITIVE CARE

The treatment of femoral shaft fractures has traditionally been based on chronological age (Table 12.1). Although age may serve as one reasonable guideline, the large variance in patient morphometry and skeletal age precludes this demographic as the sole guide to treatment. Using age alone fails to address problems in children who are extremely large or small for their chronologic age. Hence, many treatment failures occur as a result of mismatching between the biomechanical demands of the fracture and the stability provided by a chosen treatment (Fig. 12.3). For consistency purposes, the authors use an age-based approach, realizing that there is acceptable variability at each end of the age limits proposed to accommodate the aforementioned variance in patient morphometry.

Infants 6 months or younger with femoral shaft fractures can be treated in a Pavlik harness or spica cast. Neonatal fractures heal quickly in 2 to 3 weeks and remodel significantly. Pavlik harness treatment may be preferable secondary to the many reported disadvantages of spica casting.[49–51]

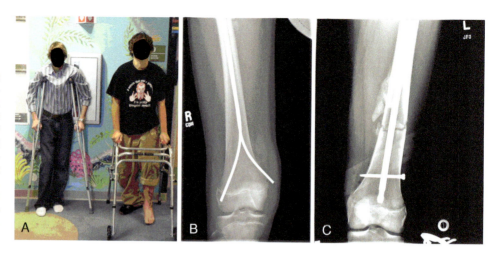

Fig. 12.3 (A) These two adolescent males were seen in the emergency department within an hour of each other. They were both 14 years of age. (B) The patient on the left had a smaller intramedullary canal. He was treated successfully with flexible intramedullary nailing. (C) The patient on the right had physes that were nearly closed, and he weighed 80 kg. He was treated with rigid intramedullary nailing. Age alone is a poor determinant of treatment options.

Children 6 months to 5 years of age with fractures demonstrating less than 2 cm of shortening can be treated with early spica casting or traction with delayed spica casting.[52,53] However, fractures with greater than 2 cm of shortening are unstable and may require an alternative treatment method, such as flexible intramedullary nailing, plating, or external fixation. Fractures are generally considered unstable because of the significant shortening or angulation at initial presentation. Either parameter can occur secondary to excessive soft tissue stripping or the nature of the bony injury, as both are indicative of high-energy injury. Typically, overriding of the fracture segments by 2 cm is an indirect measure of disruption of the periosteal sleeve. The telescope test (described in the "Imaging" section) can be used to determine fracture stability. Long oblique, long spiral, and comminuted fracture patterns are generally length-unstable. In unstable fractures, the authors prefer to use a submuscular plating technique because of the well-reported complications of external fixation.[54–57]

Length-stable fractures of the femur in children 5 to 11 years of age can be treated with flexible intramedullary nailing. Children with femoral shaft fractures treated with flexible intramedullary nailing have been found to have less residual angular deformity, less leg length discrepancy, shorter hospitalization, earlier ambulation, earlier return to school, lower overall cost, better scar acceptance, and higher overall parent satisfaction than children treated with traction and spica casting.[58–60] Earlier advancement to full weight-bearing, shorter time to regain full range of motion, earlier return to school, lower complication rate, and less residual malalignment have also been reported with flexible intramedullary nailing compared with external fixation.[61,62] This technically simple, economic, safe modality of treatment can be used when the intramedullary canal size allows and should be used until it is no longer biomechanically sound to do so.[63] Children who weigh more than 49 kg who are treated with titanium elastic nails are at increased risk of a poor outcome.[64,65] Therefore, an alternative treatment option, such as plating or rigid trochanteric entry intramedullary nailing, should be used. Unstable fractures in this age group can be treated with stainless steel flexible intramedullary nails,[66–68] plating,[69–73] or external fixation.

Finally, children age 11 years to skeletal maturity can be treated with rigid trochanteric entry intramedullary nailing if the femoral canal is large enough to accommodate the

nail. Rigid nailing has been used safely in the treatment of adult femoral shaft fractures for decades. This modality has also been shown to be successful in the pediatric population.[74–77] One notable difference between rigid nailing in adult and pediatric patients is the risk of avascular necrosis of the femoral head. This complication results from injury to the posteriorly based blood supply to the femoral head in patients with open proximal femoral physes. A 2% risk of avascular necrosis of the femoral head has been associated with a rigid nail inserted at the piriformis fossa.[78] The risk of avascular necrosis can be decreased with the use of a lateral trochanteric entry point.[77] Modern pediatric rigid nails are inserted at the lateral aspect of the greater trochanter. Thorough knowledge of the technique is required before use of a rigid trochanteric entry nail in a skeletally immature patient is advised.[76]

These guidelines based on chronological age are general recommendations. The specific characteristics of the fracture and patient's body habitus must be considered. Individual circumstances always dictate fracture management.

NONOPERATIVE TREATMENT

SKIN TRACTION

Skin traction with a Thomas splint or modified Bryant traction has fallen out of favor because of the success of the Pavlik harness at decreasing skin complications, days in the hospital, and cost.[79]

PAVLIK HARNESS

The Pavlik harness makes care of femoral fractures in infants very easy. The ease of application and adjustability, reduced hospital stay and cost, and significant improvement in perineal care all contribute to the attractiveness of this treatment modality.[51] The short-term results are equal to those of hip spica casting.[51] The long-term results show that overgrowth does occur with Pavlik harness treatment and there is significant ability to remodel angular deformity.[80,81]

Technique

Placement of the Pavlik harness does not require anesthesia, and oral pain medication usually suffices during application and subsequent care. Gentle traction is applied to the affected limb while an assistant places the shoulder straps, chest band, and the normal limb in the stirrup. The affected limb

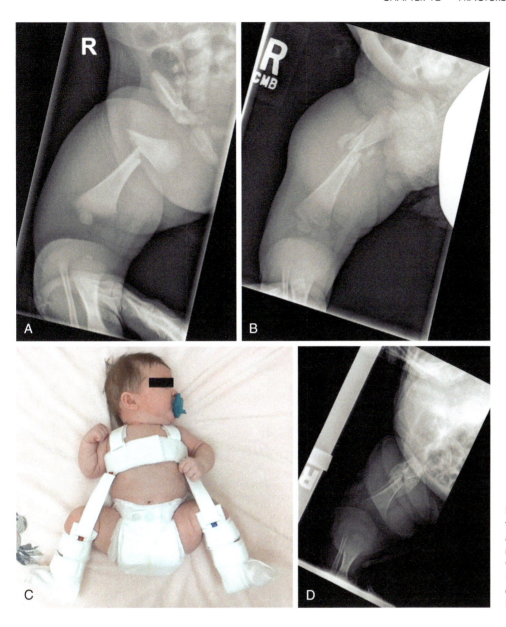

Fig. 12.4 (A) Femur fracture in an infant at time of injury. (B) Follow-up imaging at 2 weeks shows stable alignment and abundant callus formation with Pavlik harness treatment. (C) Infant in a Pavlik harness. (D) Mature callus at 1 month, at which time the Pavlik harness was discontinued.

is then placed in the stirrup with the hip flexed approximately 80 degrees and abducted 45 degrees. Blankets or towels can be placed to support the lateral aspect of the affected leg as needed for patient comfort. The patient is then seen weekly in the clinic until the fracture is healed. This usually takes 3 to 4 weeks in the young infant (Fig. 12.4). Adjustments to the Pavlik harness are made during the first clinic visit based on standard AP and lateral radiographs.

HIP SPICA CASTING

Safe and proper application of a hip spica cast requires thorough training. Careful attention to detail and experienced assistance are critical, which is why the authors prefer spica cast application in the operating room with general anesthesia. However, spica cast application in the emergency room under conscious sedation has been found to be safe and effective for the treatment of pediatric femoral shaft fractures.[82,83] Mansour et al reported that although spica cast application in the emergency room versus the operating room had similar results in terms of fracture reduction and

complications, the children who underwent spica cast application in the operating room had a significantly delayed time from presentation to cast placement, longer hospital length of stay, and higher hospital charges.[83]

Multiple different methods to apply a spica cast have been described. These techniques vary in the type of liner over which the cast is applied, degree of hip and knee flexion, sequence of body parts casted, incorporation of the foot or contralateral limb, casting material, use of a cross bar, and creation of an abdominal window.[84–89] A waterproof cast liner may be preferred over stockinette secondary to the reported benefit of decreased skin excoriation and unplanned cast changes.[90] A single-leg spica cast has been shown to be as effective as a double-leg spica cast for the treatment of pediatric femoral shaft fractures with regard to duration of treatment, femoral shortening, and femoral alignment.[86,88] However, Leu et al found that children treated with a single-leg spica cast were significantly more likely to fit into car seats and fit more comfortably into chairs.[88] In addition, the caregivers of these children took less time off work.

Table 12.2   Summary of Recommendations of the American Academy of Orthopaedic Surgeons Clinical Practice Guideline on the Treatment of Pediatric Diaphyseal Femur Fractures[1,2]

Recommendation	LOE	Strength of Recommendation
We recommend that children <36 months with diaphyseal femoral fractures be evaluated for child abuse.	II	Strong
Treatment with a Pavlik harness or a spica cast are options for infants ≤6 months with diaphyseal femoral fractures.	IV	Limited
We suggest early spica casting or traction with delayed spica casting for children age 6 months to 5 years with diaphyseal femoral fractures with <2 cm of shortening.	II	Strong
When the spica cast is used in children 6 months to 5 years of age, altering the treatment plan is an option if the fracture shortens >2 cm.	V	Limited
It is an option for physicians to use flexible intramedullary nailing to treat children 5 to 11 years of age diagnosed with diaphyseal femoral fractures.	III	Limited
Rigid trochanteric entry nailing, submuscular plating, and flexible intramedullary nailing are treatment options for children 11 years to skeletal maturity diagnosed with diaphyseal femoral fractures, but neither piriformis nor near piriformis entry rigid nailing is a treatment option.	IV	Limited
Regional pain management is an option for patient comfort perioperatively.	IV	Limited
Waterproof cast liners for spica casts are an option for use in children diagnosed with pediatric diaphyseal femoral fractures.	III	Limited

LOE, Level of evidence.

Table 12.3   Acceptable Radiographic Criteria Based on Patient Age[91]

Age (years)	Coronal Angulation (degree)	Sagittal Angulation (degree)	Shortening (cm)
<2	30	30	1.5
2–5	15	20	2
6–10	10	15	1.5
≥11	5	10	1

Jaafar et al reported that a single-leg spica cast allowed patients to walk and resulted in significantly fewer skin problems compared with a double-leg spica cast.[86]

Femoral shaft fractures in young children have great remodeling potential, which is why the AAOS Clinical Practice Guideline for the treatment of pediatric diaphyseal femur fractures suggests spica casting for children age 6 months to 5 years with less than 2 cm of shortening (Table 12.2).[1,2] Acceptable radiographic criteria based on patient age are shown in Table 12.3.[91] Although any residual angular deformity remodels significantly in children younger than 5 years, excessive rotational malunion will not likely correct. Little remodeling is expected in children older than 10 years. Younger children may experience overgrowth of 1 cm to 1.5 cm, and this must be taken into consideration when the spica cast is applied.

Technique

The authors prefer spica cast application in the operating room with general anesthesia. A waterproof pantaloon liner is placed on the patient, and the patient is positioned on the spica table. Radiolucent spica tables are now commercially available, which facilitate verification of fracture alignment with fluoroscopy while the patient is on the spica table. Towels are placed between the waterproof pantaloon liner and the chest and abdomen to provide space for chest and abdominal expansion after the cast is set. A long leg cast with the foot left out is applied first with the knee in 45 degrees to 60 degrees of flexion. Cast padding is rolled onto the extremity with careful attention to keep the knee in stable flexion at all times to prevent bunching of the padding behind the knee. Fiberglass is soaked in room temperature water and then applied using the stretch-relax technique[92] to limit skin surface pressure. A gentle mold is applied at the fracture site. Assistants should use the flats of their hands to support the limb to avoid causing an indentation in the cast that may result in a pressure point and subsequent sore.

The hip is then flexed to 45 degrees, and cast padding is rolled onto the torso to the nipple line. Flexion of the hip to 60 to 75 degrees can be considered for a single-leg spica cast to facilitate positioning in a car seat.[88] The 90-90 position of hip and knee flexion previously recommended should be avoided because of risks of compartment syndrome. The contralateral lower extremity is left out for a single-leg spica

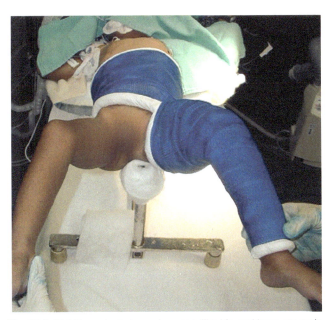

Fig. 12.5 Child in a single-leg spica cast. The hip and knee are maintained in 45 degrees of flexion, and the contralateral lower extremity is left out of the cast. (Courtesy of Steven Frick, MD. Lucille Packard Children's Hospital Stanford, Palo Alto, CA.)

cast (Fig. 12.5). Cast padding is applied to just above the contralateral knee for a double-leg spica cast. The authors prefer a double-leg spica cast in children younger than 2 years for better control of the fracture in smaller children. Adhesive-backed foam or felt can be applied over bony prominences and at the edges of the cast to reduce skin irritation. Fiberglass is then rolled around the torso. Fiberglass is also applied to the contralateral lower extremity for a double-leg spica cast. A strut consisting of four to eight layers of fiberglass can be applied across the hip joint on the side of the fracture to strengthen the cast. The edges of the waterproof pantaloon liner are wrapped down and secured with a final layer of fiberglass.

Finally, the cast is trimmed. The perineal area of a double-leg spica cast must be adequately trimmed so that caregivers have sufficient room for double diapering. The posterior aspect of the cast should be trimmed to just above the intergluteal fold. The edges of the cast are pedaled with waterproof tape. A smaller diaper is then tucked underneath the edges of the cast, and a larger diaper is placed on top of the cast.

A window can be cut over the abdomen to allow abdominal expansion. A connecting bar between the lower extremities may also be added to reinforce the cast. This has been shown to reduce mechanical failure of the spica cast following surgery for developmental dysplasia of the hip.[93] The authors do not find that creation of an abdominal window or addition of a connecting bar is routinely necessary.

A good rule of thumb regarding duration of cast treatment is the patient's age in years plus 2 weeks, resulting in a total treatment time of 4 to 8 weeks. The patient is first seen 1 to 2 weeks after cast application to verify fracture alignment and wedge the cast if necessary. The patient is then followed every 2 to 3 weeks until cast removal.

SKELETAL TRACTION

Skeletal traction is a temporizing measure for older children with isolated fractures until definitive treatment can occur. Pins are usually placed in the distal femur or proximal tibia. Location of pin insertion depends on the status of the knee ligaments and local soft tissues, level of the femoral shaft fracture, ipsilateral extremity trauma, and the child's age.

Proximal tibial pins can result in a growth arrest of the tibial tubercle apophysis and subsequent recurvatum deformity, and should be avoided in children younger than 10 years.[91] Ipsilateral knee instability, meniscal injury, and tibial fracture are other contraindications to placement of a proximal tibial traction pin. A distal femoral traction pin provides better control of a femoral shaft fracture.

Technique

The pin is inserted using aseptic technique. Injection of a local anesthetic in combination with adequate sedation in younger and less cooperative patients is usually sufficient. Local anesthetic should be injected at the skin entry and exit sites, as well as the periosteum. Pin size depends on the type of traction bow. A smaller-diameter pin that is adequately tensioned (Kirschner bow) is more effective than a larger-diameter pin placed in a neutral bow (Böhler bow). A smooth or threaded pin can be used. Threaded pins have more secure fixation in bone but may be at slightly higher risk of pin site complications.

A distal femoral pin is inserted one fingerbreadth above the patella in a medial-to-lateral direction to avoid damage to the femoral artery in Hunter's canal. Conversely, a proximal tibial pin is inserted in a lateral-to-medial direction to prevent injury to the peroneal nerve. Care should be taken to avoid the distal femoral and proximal tibial physes. The proximal tibial apophysis can be injured by errant pin placement. The pin is placed parallel to the joint surface to help maintain fracture alignment. Fluoroscopy is used to guide proper pin insertion, and biplanar radiographs can confirm the pin's location. Pin sites are cleaned daily to try to prevent infection.

The initial traction weight should be enough to slightly elevate the ipsilateral buttock from the mattress. Serial lateral radiographs are obtained every 3 to 4 days to monitor fracture shortening. Lateral radiographs are preferred because the anterior bow of the femur makes AP radiographs less accurate in assessing length. A true AP image can also be difficult to obtain when the child is in traction. The weight is adjusted according to the findings on the serial radiographs. Distraction of the fracture site should be avoided, as this can cause pain and neurovascular injury. Definitive fracture fixation occurs when the child is stable enough to undergo surgery. If the child's condition necessitates that skeletal traction be the definitive treatment, radiographs can be obtained less frequently once fracture callus is noted.

SURGICAL TREATMENT

EXTERNAL FIXATION

Historically, external fixation was recommended for operative management of pediatric femoral shaft fractures. With the advent of flexible nails, the enthusiasm for external fixation has waned. Studies comparing the two methods have demonstrated improved outcomes with flexible nailing.[61,62] Despite these limitations, external fixation can be used in patients with open fractures and fractures associated with neurovascular injury, and in polytrauma patients.[94] Most authors report good results with a variety of external frame constructs, although there is some evidence that dynamic external fixation is superior to static external fixation.[62] Some authors recommend combining external fixation and flexible intramedullary nailing in length-unstable fractures with early frame removal when callus formation is seen, usually around 4 to 6 weeks.[95,96]

Anatomic concerns of frame placement must be addressed. The quadriceps muscle mass is minimally violated when the frame is applied laterally as opposed to when multiplanar constructs are used. Lateral half-pin frames allow for control of the fracture and mobilization of both the hip and knee joints.

An advantage to external fixation is the ability to perform serial adjustments if an adequate initial reduction was not obtained. Serial biplanar radiographs evaluate changes in the fracture, especially in a combative or restless patient, and remanipulation is preferably performed early. The connecting nuts should be tightened at intervals, which will prevent frame loosening.

Technique

The patient is positioned supine on a radiolucent table. If the fracture is open, débridement of the open wound should be performed first. Nonviable skin edges must be sharply excised, all debris removed, and the nonbleeding crushed or contaminated subcutaneous tissue and muscle débrided. The fractured bone ends are inspected and débrided, followed by lavage with copious amounts of normal saline irrigant.

Fluoroscopy directs safe and strategic pin insertion, as well as manipulative reduction. The initial lateral pin is placed farthest from the fracture site in the longer of either the distal or proximal shaft fragments. The pin can be either a 5-mm standard adult pin or a 4-mm pin for smaller children. The pin is placed through a 1-cm stab wound with the use of a sleeve system that allows for saline-cooled predrilling of the bone. The length of connecting bar is then selected to span the comminution or hold the proximal and distal fragments out to length. A carbon fiber rod is preferred for its radiolucency. Two bars are appropriate for length-unstable fracture patterns.

Two pin-bar clamps are placed on each bar. One of the end clamps is attached to the already inserted pin, and manual traction is applied. The second far pin is then placed through another end clamp into the shorter fracture fragment. The reduction is perfected, and the two end pin clamps are tightened to the connecting bars. The bar is positioned in line with the femoral shaft laterally and at least two fingerbreadths from the skin to allow for any thigh swelling. The near pins can then be placed through the remaining clamps.

The soft tissues adjacent to the pins may need to be incised so that hip and knee range of motion is not restricted. The surgeon should passively range the hip and knee and ensure that the skin and deep tissues are adequately released so the most distal pin in the supracondylar region does not entrap the iliotibial band restricting knee motion.

After surgery, pin site care is instituted. Sterile, saline-moistened, cotton-tipped applicators are used to clean the skin of crusted serous fluid and blood around the pins two or three times daily. Gait training and range-of-motion exercises are instituted under the direction of a physical therapist. Patients can be allowed toe-touch weight-bearing ambulation using crutches or a walker. Active and active-assisted range-of-motion exercises of the hip and knee should be performed.

After 6 weeks, radiographic signs of callus formation direct the progression of weight-bearing and activity. When fracture callus is present, spanning all four cortices on biplanar radiographs, the external fixation device and pins can be removed (Fig. 12.6). If minimal radiographic signs of healing are present, the frame is maintained, and the parent and therapist supervise increased weight-bearing. A double-bar external frame can allow dynamization by removal of the most peripheral bar to stimulate fracture healing by further loading of the fracture. Before frame removal, clinical union can be checked by having the patient walk after loosening the frame clamps or completely removing the bar.

Pin removal is painful and causes anxiety in most children and their parents, so it typically requires a return trip to the operating room. After the frame is removed, manual and/or radiographic testing of fracture stability should be performed before pin removal. If the fracture is stable, the pins can be removed, and the pin sites can be débrided with curettes. Manipulation of a stiff knee after frame removal should not be performed because of the risk of iatrogenic refracture. Patients should continue with protected weight-bearing precautions with no torsional or pivoting activities initially and are advanced to full unprotected weight-bearing over the next 3 to 6 weeks. Early, unprotected weight-bearing increases the risk of refracture or a new fracture at the previous pin sites.

FLEXIBLE INTRAMEDULLARY NAILING

Flexible intramedullary nailing is currently the most popular technique for management of length-stable femoral shaft fractures in children 5 to 11 years of age. Flexible nailing has supplanted external fixation by reducing the malunion rate, refracture rate, rate of total adverse events, time to full weight-bearing, time to regain full range of motion, and time to return to school.[41,61,62] Flexible nailing is also preferred to submuscular plating in length-stable fractures because of increased value with shorter operative time, less estimated blood loss, and lower surgical costs.[97]

Titanium elastic nails and stainless steel flexible nails are most commonly used. Several studies have demonstrated that titanium elastic nails produce the best results when used in the management of length-stable fractures involving the middle 60% of the femoral shaft in children 5 to 11 years of age. Because flexible nailing is relatively safe and technically easy to perform, physicians are starting to trend toward surgical treatment in preschool-age children.[39] When compared with spica casting in preschool-age children, those treated with flexible nails show shorter time to ambulation, shorter time to return to school, shorter time to return to full activities, less shortening, less sagittal and coronal angulation, and less malrotation, but more return trips to the operating room, primarily for nail removal.[98–100]

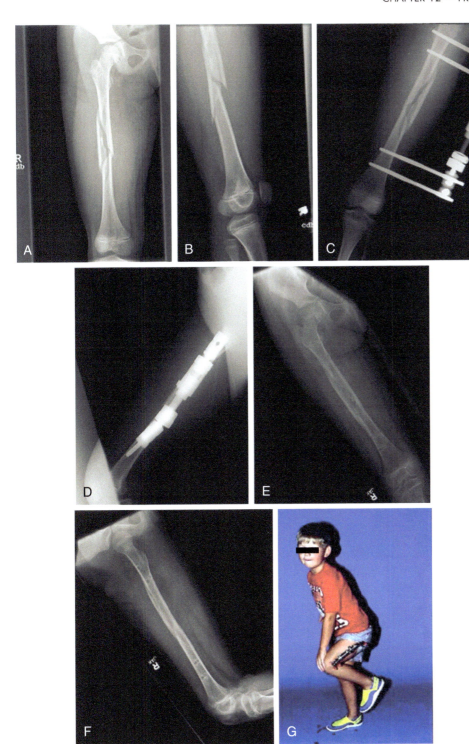

Fig. 12.6 A 7-year-old boy fell off a horse, sustaining this comminuted femoral shaft fracture. (A and B) Anteroposterior (AP) and lateral injury films with traction applied. (C and D) Postoperative AP and lateral films. (E and F) Three months after surgery. (G) Child in a typical external fixator.

Technique

The nail size is determined by the following equation: determine the smallest femoral canal diameter measured on preoperative AP and lateral radiographs and subtract 1 mm with the result divided by 2. This value correlates with the size of each nail (Fig. 12.7). Alternatively, prior studies have used 40% of the narrowest canal diameter to determine nail size.[101,102] Two nails of equal diameter are used in all cases so that the forces are balanced across the fracture site and angular deformity is prevented.[103]

The patient is placed supine on a radiolucent table. Fluoroscopy is used to locate the nail insertion site, which is 2.5 cm proximal to the distal femoral physis. An incision is made on the lateral aspect of the distal thigh from the level of proposed nail insertion and is carried 2 cm distally. This facilitates nail insertion while minimizing the size of the required incision. The subcutaneous tissues and iliotibial band are opened in line with the skin incision to expose the lateral aspect of the distal femoral metaphysis. The lateral cortex is opened with a drill or a sharp awl. The latter

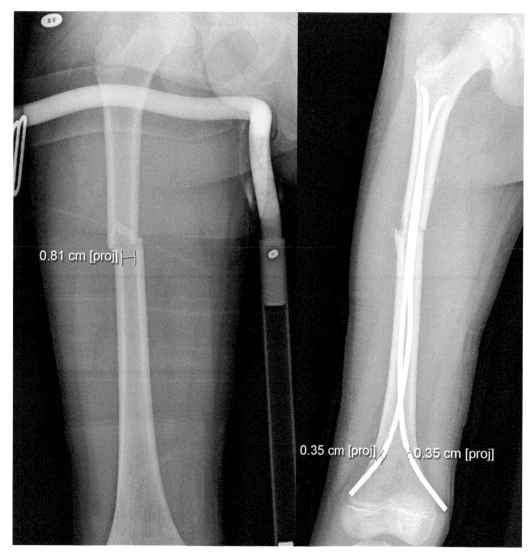

Fig. 12.7 Determination of nail size requires measurement of the smallest diameter of the intramedullary canal. In the case shown here, the canal measured 8 mm. One should subtract 1 mm from the canal diameter, divide that number by 2, and the result is the size of nail required. In this case, two 3.5-mm nails were placed.

method eliminates the need for a power drill and minimizes thermal energy production near the distal femoral physis. The drill or awl is then redirected cephalad so that it makes a 10-degree angle with the lateral cortex. This will allow the nail to glance off the far cortex as it is advanced and will facilitate passage of the nail.

A slight bend is placed at the tip of the nail to facilitate advancement of the nail beyond the far cortex and to assist with fracture reduction. Some surgeons advocate making a gentle C-shaped bend in the nail, with the apex approximating the level of the fracture, to augment stability of the construct.[104,105] This is not always necessary and can make nail passage more difficult. The nail is then inserted in the starting hole, and the intramedullary position is verified with the use of fluoroscopy. The fracture is reduced, and the lateral nail is advanced across the fracture site. If there is an issue passing the lateral nail, the medial nail may be placed before the lateral nail is advanced across the fracture site.

Next, a medial incision is made, and a nail of equal diameter is placed and advanced into the proximal fragment. The final position of the tip of the lateral nail should be just distal to the greater trochanteric apophysis. The tip of the medial nail should lie at the same level but point toward the calcar region of the femoral neck. When the nails are approximately 1 cm from their final position, the nails are trimmed outside the skin. Final impaction is then performed with a tamp, and 1 cm of nail is left outside the bone to facilitate nail remove in the future. The nail tip should not be bent away from the cortex because soft tissue irritation will occur. The stability of the fracture is checked intraoperatively under fluoroscopic guidance. Supplemental external immobilization, such as a knee immobilizer, may be used for length-stable fractures or a cast for length-unstable fractures (Fig. 12.8). As the quadriceps muscle frequently does not function normally in the first 1 to 2 weeks after femoral shaft fracture, a knee immobilizer can facilitate mobilization.

A slight modification in technique may be useful for treatment of subtrochanteric femoral fractures because of the deforming forces from the iliopsoas, hip abductor, and short external rotator muscles. The proximal fracture fragment is in flexion, abduction, and varus, which leads to difficulty obtaining and maintaining fracture reduction.

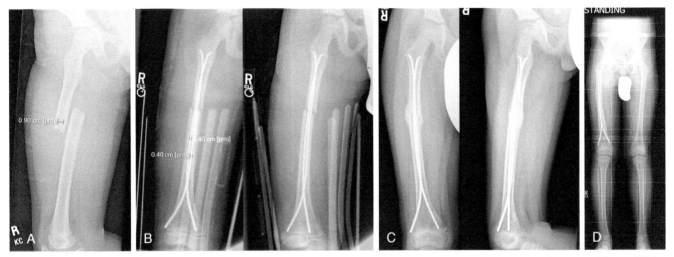

Fig. 12.8 (A) A 8-year-old boy sustained this injury in a motor vehicle crash. The diameter of his intramedullary canal measured 9 mm. (B) Anteroposterior (AP) (*left*) and lateral (*right*) radiographs after nail placement with 4.0-mm nails. The patient was placed in a knee immobilizer postoperatively for added support. (C) AP (*left*) and lateral (*right*) films showing mature fracture callus at 3 months. (D) Alignment films at 9 months showing equal leg lengths.

Traumatic subtrochanteric femoral fractures are also frequently high-energy injuries, resulting in length-unstable fracture patterns. If titanium elastic nails are used, advancement of the tip of the lateral nail into or just distal to the greater trochanteric apophysis and advancement of the medial nail into the femoral neck just short of the proximal femoral physis may increase the stability of the construct.[33]

Patients undergo gait training and hip and knee range-of-motion exercises with a physical therapist on postoperative day 1. Toe-touch weight-bearing restrictions are maintained until radiographs demonstrate clinical evidence of fracture healing, which usually occurs at 4 to 6 weeks postoperatively. Nails are removed after clinical and radiographic evidence of union, usually 6 to 12 months after the index procedure. The timing of nail removal is dependent on soft tissue irritation from the nail tips preventing additional progression in knee function; pain from the nail tips; and convenience for the patient and family. Controversy exists regarding the need for nail removal.[43,59,106,107]

PLATE FIXATION

Open and submuscular plate fixation are alternative treatment options for length-unstable femoral shaft fractures, fractures in the subtrochanteric and supracondylar regions, children 5 to 11 years who weigh more than 49 kg, and children 11 years and older who have a femoral canal that is too narrow for rigid trochanteric entry intramedullary nailing. Some surgeons select plate fixation for both length-stable and length-unstable fractures. Good results have been shown with traditional open compression plating of femoral shaft fractures in children and adolescents.[69,108–113] Although open plating restores length and alignment and provides excellent stability, disadvantages of this technique include extensive soft tissue dissection, which can lead to delayed union or nonunion, greater blood loss, a higher infection rate, pain, and scarring.[109,111]

Submuscular plating has gained increased popularity over the past 15 years because of the minimally invasive technique and reported efficacy for the treatment of length-unstable pediatric femoral shaft fractures and fractures in the subtrochanteric region and distal femoral metaphysis.[70–73,114–118] A biomechanical study comparing titanium elastic nails with locked plating in an oblique and comminuted pediatric femur fracture model showed that locked plating provided a more stable construct.[119] Submuscular plates function as internal "external fixators." Indirect fracture reduction and insertion of longer plates and fewer screws through a minimally invasive approach produce maximum biologic healing.[120] The long plates have an increased working length, which results in decreased strain and less pullout force on the screws, and leads to increased biomechanical stability of the construct. Standard external fixation principles are followed during screw placement; two screws are placed adjacent to the fracture, and the remaining screws are placed widely apart to maximize construct stability.

Technique

Compression Plating. The patient is placed in the supine position on a radiolucent table. A lateral incision is made over the fracture site. The iliotibial band is split longitudinally, and the vastus lateralis is retracted anteriorly. The perforating arteries and veins should be identified and ligated. The proximal and distal fragments are exposed. The fracture is reduced under direct visualization and held with a bone clamp. A femoral distractor can help hold the fracture out to length. Lag screws are inserted across the fracture either independently or through the plate. A 3.5-mm or 4.5-mm narrow stainless steel low-contact dynamic compression plate is used, depending on the size of the femur. The fracture pattern and extent of comminution determine the length of the plate, which should have eight or more holes.

Submuscular Plating. A 3.5-mm or 4.5-mm narrow stainless steel low-contact dynamic compression plate is selected based on the size of the femur. A locking plate may be used for patients with poor bone quality or proximal or distal fractures. The authors prefer using a straight plate, but femur locking plates with an anterior bow are commercially available. The patient is placed in the supine position on a radiolucent table or fracture table. The fracture is provisionally reduced

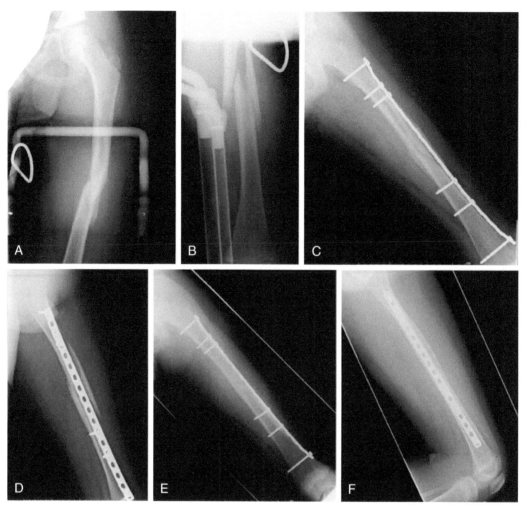

Fig. 12.9 (A and B) Anteroposterior (AP) and lateral radiographs demonstrating a comminuted femoral shaft fracture in a 9-year-old boy. (C and D) AP and lateral radiographs of the femur after submuscular plating. (E and F) AP and lateral radiographs demonstrating fracture union. (From Li Y, Hedequist DJ. Submuscular plating of pediatric femur fractures. *J Am Acad Orthop Surg.* 2012;20:596–603.)

using inline traction, and fluoroscopy is used to determine the length of the plate, which is usually 12 to 16 holes. A plate bender is used to contour the proximal and distal aspects of the plate to match the proximal and distal metaphyseal flares. A small lateral incision is made over the distal femoral metaphysis. The iliotibial band is opened, and the vastus lateralis is elevated anteriorly. A tunnel is made for the plate by passing a Cobb elevator deep to the vastus lateralis in a retrograde manner. This dissection should be extraperiosteal. The plate is then inserted into the submuscular interval and advanced proximally under fluoroscopic guidance while the extremity is held in traction to maintain fracture length. Plate position and reestablishment of fracture length are confirmed with fluoroscopy. Kirschner wires are placed in the proximal and distal ends of the plate for provisional fixation. Persistent recurvatum at the fracture site can be addressed by placing a bolster under the thigh or inserting an additional Kirschner wire through the middle of the plate.

The first screw is placed through the open incision. All other screws are inserted percutaneously using the perfect circle technique with lateral fluoroscopy views. The second screw can be used to achieve indirect fracture reduction by placing it through the plate just proximal or distal to the fracture in the fragment that is farthest from the plate. The

length of the screws that are inserted percutaneously can be more easily and safely determined by placing the depth gauge over the thigh and assessing the length using fluoroscopy rather than placing the depth gauge through the small percutaneous incisions. Tying a suture over the screw head also helps prevent the screw from disengaging from the screwdriver during insertion and facilitates screw exchange if necessary. The authors apply the principles of external fixation and spread the screws wide apart. Three screws proximal and distal to the fracture usually provide enough stability. Lag screws are not necessary (Fig. 12.9). Supplemental external immobilization is not required, although a knee immobilizer may provide comfort and facilitate mobilization. Placement of a cluster of two to three cortical and locking screws through the proximal and distal ends of the plate is another described technique, but these patients are placed in a knee immobilizer postoperatively.[117]

The postoperative course after plate fixation is similar to that after flexible intramedullary nailing. Patients are instructed to remain toe-touch weight bearing for approximately 6 weeks after surgery. Weight-bearing is advanced when healing is noted on radiographs.

Although implant removal in children remains controversial, the authors routinely remove submuscular plates after

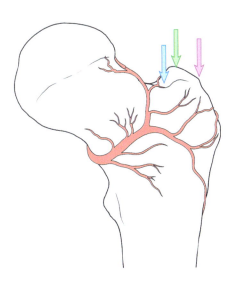
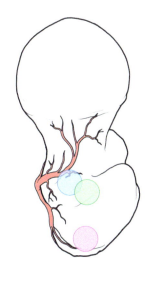

Fig. 12.10 Proximal femoral anatomy showing the piriformis fossa (*blue arrow and circle*), the tip of the greater trochanter (*green arrow and circle*), and the lateral aspect of the greater trochanter (*purple arrow and circle*) with its entry points identified.

complete fracture healing in children with significant growth remaining. Children treated with a distally contoured submuscular plate have been found to develop stress shielding, leg length discrepancy, valgus deformity, bony overgrowth over the plate, and screw tip prominence in the medial thigh as a result of plate migration secondary to growth of the femur.[121] Plates can usually be removed 6 months after the index procedure. Bony overgrowth at the tip of the plate has been noted at the time of removal, and more extensive exposure may be necessary to remove the ingrown bone.[122] Patients can be full weight bearing after plate removal but are restricted from sporting activities to avoid fracture through a screw hole.

RIGID INTRAMEDULLARY NAILING

Rigid intramedullary nailing is a treatment option for children 11 years and older with a femoral shaft fracture and a femoral canal that is large enough to accommodate a rigid nail. Some surgeons use lateral trochanteric entry nailing with small-diameter nails in patients 8 years and older, as trochanteric growth after age 8 is believed to be primarily appositional rather than from the trochanteric apophysis. The safest starting point is at the lateral aspect of the greater trochanter, as this avoids the blood supply to the proximal femur (Fig. 12.10). Avascular necrosis and clinically important proximal femoral deformity have not been reported with the lateral trochanteric nail entry site.[77,78]

Technique

The patient is placed in the supine position on a fracture table or in the lateral position on a radiolucent table. Nerve palsies, particularly of the peroneal nerve in the operative leg, have been reported in pediatric patients who underwent femur fracture fixation on the fracture table.[123] Kelly et al found that increased patient weight was the only significant independent risk factor for development of a nerve palsy in their multivariate analysis.[123] Compartment syndrome in the well leg related to the hemilithotomy position[124,125] and internal rotation malalignment of the fracture[126] have been demonstrated in the adult population when femur fracture fixation is performed on the fracture table. However, the fracture table facilitates the use of inline traction to achieve fracture reduction, keeps the lower extremity in position

and the thigh exposed for the surgical procedure, facilitates fluoroscopic imaging, and requires fewer surgical assistants. Surgeons who prefer the lateral position feel that proper identification of the starting point and insertion of the proximal instrumentation is more easily achieved in the lateral position, particularly in obese patients. When the authors use the fracture table, the well leg is scissored, and every effort is made to minimize the amount of time in traction.

The starting point is just lateral to the tip of the greater trochanter in the AP plane and at the junction of the middle and posterior thirds of the femoral neck in the lateral plane (Fig. 12.10). Rigid nails that are specifically designed for the pediatric population have a greater valgus angulation proximally to accommodate the lateral trochanteric entry site.

The lower extremity is internally rotated to obtain a true AP radiograph of the proximal femur to facilitate proper guide pin placement. A small incision is made approximately 4 fingerbreadths proximal to and in line with the tip of the greater trochanter. Guide pin insertion can be initiated with a mallet to prevent inadvertent plunging into the piriformis fossa. The guide pin starting position should be lateral to the tip of the greater trochanter, with most pediatric orthopedic experts advocating a "far-lateral" insertion, at or lateral to the midpoint of the medial and lateral cortical margins of the greater trochanter on an AP view. After acceptable placement of the guide pin is verified with fluoroscopy, the guide pin is advanced to the lesser trochanter. An entry reamer is advanced over the guide pin, and the ball-tip guide rod is inserted into the intramedullary canal. Fracture reduction is confirmed with fluoroscopy, and the ball-tip guide rod is advanced across the fracture site into the distal femoral metaphysis. Reduction of the fracture is facilitated by judicious placement of bumps or closed fracture reduction tools (mallet, F-tool). If the fracture is very unstable and reduction difficult, passage of the guidewire can be rapidly facilitated by placement of a single 5-mm half-pin in the distal fragment and use of a T-hand chuck to control the distal fragment. The guide wire is positioned fluoroscopically in the center of the medullary canal just proximal to the distal physis. The femoral canal is sequentially reamed. In most cases, reaming to 1.5 mm greater than the diameter of the nail allows passage of the nail. A guide is used to place the proximal interlocking screw.

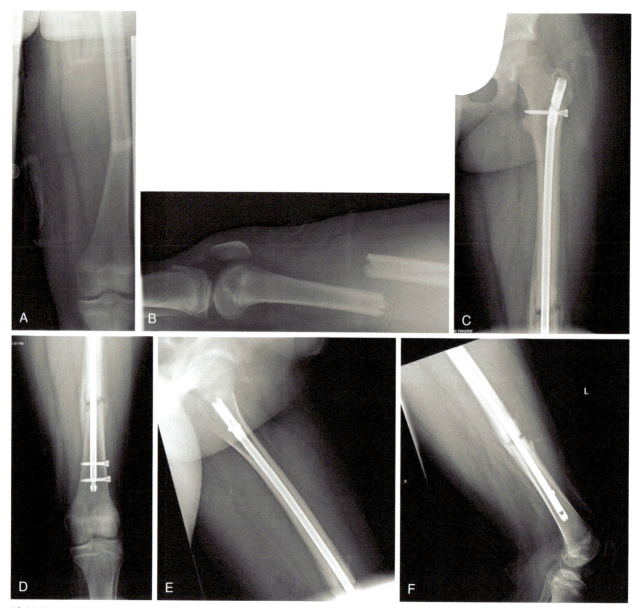

Fig. 12.11 (A and B) Anteroposterior (AP) and lateral radiographs demonstrating a femoral shaft fracture in an 11-year-old girl. This was a grade 1 open fracture that was sustained in a motorcycle accident. (C, D, E and F) AP and lateral radiographs of the femur after rigid trochanteric entry nailing.

Before placement of the distal interlocking screws, the fracture can be compressed manually or by releasing the traction on the fracture table, and proper rotation of the distal fragment should be verified. One to two distal interlocking screws are inserted using the perfect circle technique. Two distal interlocking screws should be placed for unstable and distal fractures, as this has been shown to increase rotational stability (Fig. 12.11).[127] No external immobilization is required.

Patients can advance to weight bearing as tolerated. Patients are followed until clinical and radiographic evidence of fracture healing is noted. The authors do not routinely remove the implants, although some surgeons do remove locked nails in patients with more than 2 years of growth remaining. Survey studies of adult reconstruction surgeons suggest that removal of intramedullary nails can make later reconstructive hip surgery less complicated.

COMPLICATIONS

The risk of different complications is relative to the technique used for fracture management. Table 12.4 lists the risk of complications as reported in the literature.

Nonunion remains a relatively rare complication in pediatric fractures. Despite the low incidence, this is a significant complication, and the femur is the most common bone in which this complication occurs in the pediatric population.[128] Factors that increase this risk include the use of internal fixation, age older than 6 years, infection, open fractures, and high-energy mechanism of injury (Fig. 12.12).

Rotational malalignment and angular malalignment are also notable complications. Although internal fixation has reduced the incidence of malalignment in comparison with nonoperative management and external fixation, malunion

Table 12.4   Risk of Complications by Type of Treatment

	LLD	Skin Necrosis	Prominent Implants	Infection	Malunion	Malrotation	Nonunion	Nerve Injury
Skeletal traction	+	+		+	++	++		+
Hip spica cast	+	+			++	++		+
External fixation				+++	+	+	+	+
Flexible nails	+		+	+	+	+	+	
Compression plating			+	+	+	+	+	
Submuscular plating	+		+		+	+		
Rigid nails	+		+	+	+	+	+	

LLD, Limb length discrepancy; +, mild risk; ++, moderate risk; +++, high risk.

and malrotation still occur with all treatment options. Fortunately, the magnitude of malalignment reported with surgical stabilization is often of little clinical significance and does not result in functional impairment.

LIMB LENGTH DISCREPANCY

Femoral overgrowth reportedly related to increased vascular perfusion to the femoral physes during fracture healing is a well-documented phenomenon after a femoral fracture.[129–132] The overgrowth rarely exceeds 2 cm and typically measures 1 cm. This overgrowth occurs primarily in the first 2 years after the fracture. Overgrowth has been reported with all treatment methods and can occur in the setting of intentional fracture shortening with casting or after anatomic open reduction (Fig. 12.13). When a hip spica cast is applied, 1 cm of overlap of the fracture fragments is recommended in anticipation of future overgrowth (Fig. 12.14).

COMPLICATIONS SPECIFIC TO TREATMENTS

HIP SPICA CASTING
Skin breakdown is the most common complication of spica casting. Use of a waterproof cast liner has been shown to decrease the rate of skin excoriation and unplanned cast changes.[90] However, skin complications can still occur in over 25% of children.[133] DiFazio et al reported that child abuse as a mechanism of injury, younger age, and duration of casting greater than 40 days were predictors for skin complications.[133] The cast should have adequate space to allow for chest and abdominal expansion. This can be accomplished by placing towels between the chest and abdomen and the cast liner before cast application. An anterior window can also be cut in the cast for additional abdominal decompression. Appropriate padding and molding of the cast is important. The 90/90 spica casts should be avoided, as they have been associated with the development of compartment syndrome and Volkmann contracture.[89] These complications can occur when a short leg cast is placed first, and

then traction is applied with the hip and knee flexed at 90 degrees. After the remainder of the cast is applied and traction is released, the fracture shortens and produces pressure on the posterior aspect of the knee (Fig. 12.15). Mubarak et al found that the superficial and deep posterior compartments were most severely affected.[89] Wedging of 90/90 spica casts can cause a peroneal nerve palsy.[134] Immediate cast removal usually leads to resolution of the nerve palsy.

SKELETAL TRACTION
Traction pins should be inserted under fluoroscopic guidance when possible to avoid physeal injury to the distal femur, proximal tibia, and tibial tubercle. Injury to the tibial tubercle apophysis can result in a significant recurvatum deformity, so proximal tibial pins should be avoided in children younger than 10 years. A distal femoral pin is inserted one fingerbreadth above the patella in a medial-to-lateral direction to prevent injury to the femoral artery. A proximal tibial pin is inserted in a lateral-to-medial direction to avoid damage to the peroneal nerve.

EXTERNAL FIXATION
Recurrent fractures at the original fracture site or fractures through pin sites after removal of the external fixator are major complications reported with the use of external fixation. A metaanalysis revealed a correlation of refractures with open fractures, bilateral fractures, and a longer time in the fixator. Factors that may be contributory but were inconclusive included the fracture pattern, dynamization status, fixator type, pin size, and number of pins.[38] Transverse or short oblique fractures and fracture patterns with a small surface area may be at higher risk of refracture because of limited callus formation.

Pin site infections previously occurred in nearly all patients with external fixators and appeared to be closely related to pin loosening. Bone-pin fixation improved with the use of hydroxyapatite pins, and pin-related complications significantly reduced.[135] Pin site care and antibiotic prophylaxis vary by surgeon preference but are important

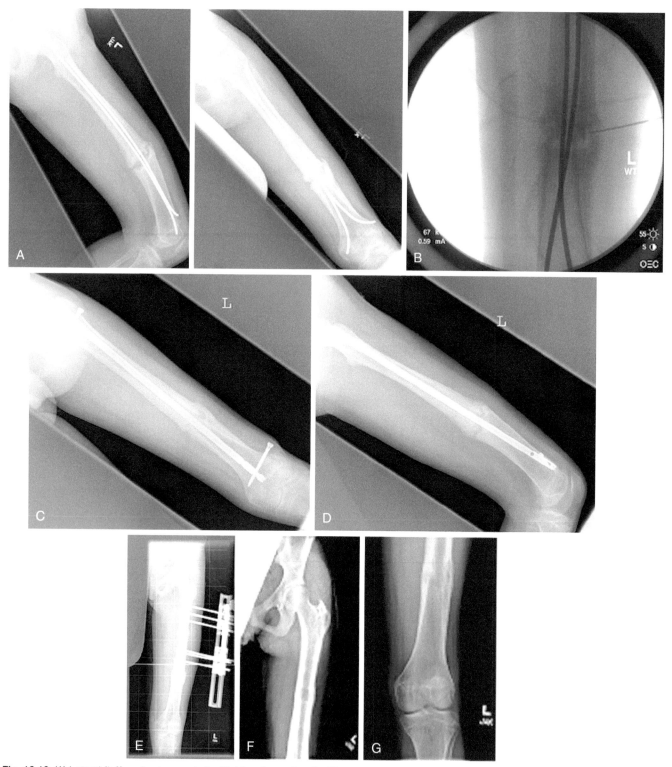

Fig. 12.12 (A) Lateral (*left*) and anteroposterior (*right*) radiographs of a 10-year-old girl seen after initial treatment at an outside facility. She was the victim of a pedestrian versus motor vehicle accident and was treated with flexible intramedullary nails. Eight months later, she was ambulating with a minimal limp but had a limb length discrepancy. (B) After a negative aspiration of the nonunion site, the flexible nails were removed. (C and D) The deformity was reduced, and a rigid nail was placed. (E) The fracture healed uneventfully, and the nail was removed. She then underwent limb lengthening with an external fixator. The distraction site healed proximally (F), and the nonunion healed distally (G).

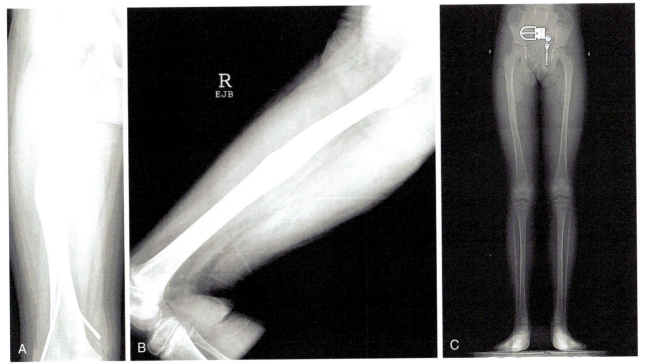

Fig. 12.13 (A and B) Anteroposterior and lateral radiographs demonstrating anatomic reduction after flexible intramedullary nailing in an 8-year-old patient. (C) One year after flexible nail removal, a 1.2-cm limb length discrepancy exists in which the right hemipelvis is higher than the left.

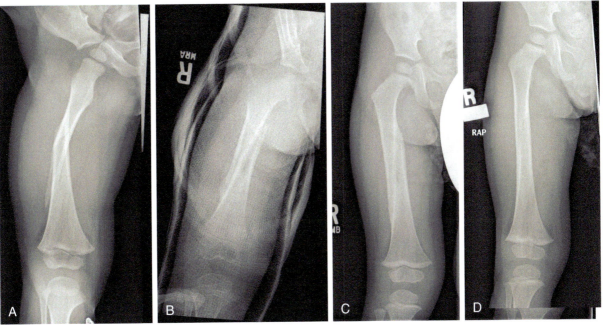

Fig. 12.14 Overgrowth of 1 to 1.5 cm is likely to occur in young children treated with hip spica casting. This must be considered when applying the cast. (A) Represents the initial shortening. (B) Represents the amount of shortening after cast application. (C) Represents the final shortening after cast removal. Commonly, the shortening present on initial x-rays predicts final shortening as depicted here. (D) Overgrowth and remodeling seen at 6 months postinjury.

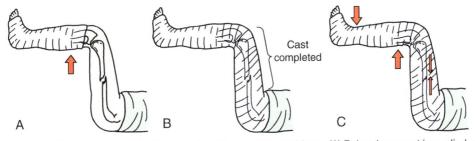

Fig. 12.15 Application of the 90/90 spica cast and pathogenesis of the resulting problems. (A) Below-knee cast is applied while the patient is on the spica frame. (B) Next, traction is applied to the below-knee cast to produce distraction at the fracture site. The remainder of the cast is applied, which fixes the relative distance between the leg and the torso. (C) After the child awakens from general anesthesia, the femur is shortened from muscular contraction, which causes the thigh and leg to slip somewhat back into the spica. This causes pressure to occur at the corners of the cast (see *arrows* at the proximal posterior calf and anterior ankle). (Modified from Mubarak SJ, Frick S, Sink E, et al. Volkmann contracture and compartment syndromes after femur fractures in children treated with 90/90 spica casts. *J Pediatr Orthop.* 2006;26:567.)

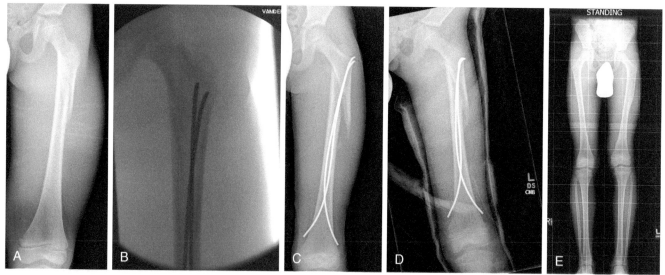

Fig. 12.16 (A) A 6-year-old boy with a spiral subtrochanteric femoral fracture. (B) The patient underwent flexible nailing with titanium elastic nails that stopped short of the femoral neck. (C) At 2 weeks postoperatively, the fracture has angulated and shortened with prominent nail tips proximally. (D) The patient was taken back to the operating room for closed reduction and spica cast placement for additional stabilization. (E) At 9 months, the nails were removed, and the patient has remodeled the fracture with only a 0.5-cm leg length difference.

to prevent serious or chronic infection. The authors recommend daily oral cephalexin and mechanical débridement of the pin sites with sterile saline-soaked swabs. Care to eliminate skin adherence to the pin is emphasized. Acute infections that do not respond to this regimen are given a trial of intravenous antibiotics along with removal of the affected pin.

FLEXIBLE INTRAMEDULLARY NAILING

Children 5 to 11 years of age who weigh less than 49 kg, with a length-stable fracture that involves the middle 60% of the femoral shaft, are the best candidates for titanium elastic nailing. A multicenter retrospective study of pediatric femoral shaft fractures treated with titanium elastic nails found that children 11 years or older were nearly four times more likely to have a poor outcome. The same study reported that children who weighed more than 49 kg had a fivefold increased risk of a poor outcome.[65] Biomechanical evidence supports this weight limit.[64] Increased body mass index under the 49-kg cutoff does appear to affect shortening or malunion.[136] Stainless steel flexible intramedullary nails have increased stiffness and have been shown to have good results in patients over 49 kg.[137]

Length-unstable fractures and fractures that involve the proximal or distal third of the femur are also at higher risk of complications.[72,101,104,138,139] Fracture shortening and angulation leading to prominent or exposed nails, pain at the nail insertion site, limb length discrepancy, and malunion have all been reported in the literature.[101,138,139] An increased rate of unplanned surgery to treat complications has been demonstrated with length-unstable femoral fractures treated with titanium elastic nails.[139] Postoperative immobilization with a single-leg walking spica cast, hip-knee-ankle-foot orthosis, or knee immobilizer may be necessary if stability is a concern. Alternatively, stainless steel flexible nails with or without distal locking may provide improved fixation of length-unstable fractures.[66–68] Although the stiffer material properties of stainless steel produce greater

fracture stability, the concern is that use of these implants could lead to straightening of the normal bow of the pediatric femur.[105]

Subtrochanteric femoral fractures treated with titanium elastic nails have been found to be associated with lower outcome scores and a higher overall complication rate when compared with plating. Complications include fracture malalignment, limb length discrepancy, and pain from prominent implants (Fig. 12.16).[116] A slight modification in nail insertion technique (described in the "Surgical Treatment" section) may improve the stability of the construct and decrease the risk of complications.[33]

PLATING

The extensive soft tissue dissection that is necessary for traditional compression plating can lead to delayed union or nonunion, greater blood loss, a higher infection rate, pain, and scarring.[109,111] The minimally invasive insertion technique used for submuscular plating can avoid many of these complications. Distal femoral shaft fractures treated with open or submuscular plating and fractures in which the plate is placed 20 mm or less from the distal femoral physis may develop a valgus deformity.[140,141] These children should undergo plate removal after fracture healing or undergo long-term follow-up to monitor for development of a deformity. In addition, stress shielding, leg length discrepancy, valgus deformity, bony overgrowth over the plate, and screw tip prominence in the medial thigh have been demonstrated in femur fractures treated with a distally contoured submuscular plate.[121,141] These findings occur as a result of plate migration secondary to growth of the femur and can be avoided by plate removal after fracture healing. More extensive exposure may be necessary to remove the bony overgrowth at the tip of the plate.[122] Refracture through a screw hole after implant removal has been reported.[109]

RIGID INTRAMEDULLARY NAILING

Avascular necrosis of the femoral head has been associated with nail insertion through the piriformis fossa and tip of the greater trochanter. A systematic review found no cases of avascular necrosis with the lateral trochanteric nail entry site, whereas the rate of avascular necrosis was 2% for the piriformis fossa entry site and 1.4% for the tip of the greater trochanter entry site.[78] Nevertheless, the patient and family should be counseled preoperatively about the risk of avascular necrosis with the antegrade rigid intramedullary nailing technique.

Injury to the greater trochanteric physis can occur in skeletally immature patients who undergo rigid intramedullary nailing, resulting in coxa valga, thinning of the femoral neck, and premature closure of the greater trochanteric physis.[142,143] These changes are less likely after 8 years of age because epiphysiodesis of the greater trochanter does not affect the neck-shaft angle.[13] Clinically important proximal femoral deformity has not been noted with rigid intramedullary nailing in older children and adolescents, particularly when the lateral trochanteric entry site is used.[77,144]

GUIDELINES

The AAOS published a Clinical Practice Guideline on the treatment of pediatric diaphyseal femur fractures in 2009.[1] The guideline was reissued in 2015 after a new literature search did not find any additional literature that would alter the original recommendations.[2] A summary of the recommendations is listed in Table 12.2.

CONCLUSION

Pediatric femoral shaft fractures can occur as a result of trauma, nonaccidental trauma, a pathologic disease process, or a stress reaction. Chronological age can be used as a guideline for treatment, although other factors, such as patient weight and fracture pattern, should be taken into consideration. In general, children 6 months or younger can be treated with a Pavlik harness. Children 6 months to 5 years can be treated with a hip spica cast. Length-stable fractures in children 5 to 11 years can be treated with flexible intramedullary nailing, and unstable fractures can be managed with open or submuscular plating. Finally, children 11 years to skeletal maturity can be treated with rigid trochanteric entry intramedullary nailing. Complications exist for all treatment options, and patients and families must be informed of the risks.

REFERENCES

The level of evidence (LOE) is determined according to the criteria provided in the Preface.

1. Kocher MS, Sink EL, Blasier RD, et al. Treatment of pediatric diaphyseal femur fractures. *J Am Acad Orthop Surg.* 2009;17(11):718–725. (**LOE N/A**).
2. Jevsevar DS, Shea KG, Murray JN, Sevarino KS. AAOS Clinical Practice Guideline on the treatment of pediatric diaphyseal femur fractures. *J Am Acad Orthop Surg.* 2015;23(12):e101. (**LOE N/A**).
3. Heideken J, Svensson T, Blomqvist P, Haglund-Akerlind Y, Janarv PM. Incidence and trends in femur shaft fractures in Swedish children between 1987 and 2005. *J Pediatr Orthop.* 2011;31(5):512–519. (**LOE III**).
4. Nakaniida A, Sakuraba K, Hurwitz EL. Pediatric orthopaedic injuries requiring hospitalization: epidemiology and economics. *J Orthop Trauma.* 2014;28(3):167–172. (**LOE IV**).
5. Anderson M, Green WT, Messner MB. The classic. Growth and predictions of growth in the lower extremities by Margaret Anderson, M.S., William T. Green, M.D. and Marie Blail Messner, A.B. from the Journal of Bone and Joint Surgery, 45A:1, 1963. *Clin Orthop Relat Res.* 1978(136):7–21. (**LOE II**).
6. Lee MC, Eberson CP. Growth and development of the child's hip. *Orthop Clin North Am.* 2006;37(2):119–132. (**LOE N/A**).
7. Gardner E, Gray DJ. The prenatal development of the human femur. *Am J Anat.* 1970;129(2):121–140. (**LOE V**).
8. Mahony BS, Callen PW, Filly RA. The distal femoral epiphyseal ossification center in the assessment of third-trimester menstrual age: sonographic identification and measurement. *Radiology.* 1985;155(1):201–204. (**LOE II**).
9. Panattoni GL, D'Amelio P, Di Stefano M, Isaia GC. Ossification centers of human femur. *Calcif Tissue Int.* 2000;66(4):255–258. (**LOE V**).
10. Gupta RK, Gupta AK. A study of diaphyseal nutrient foramina in human femur. *Int J Res Med Sci.* 2016;4(3):706–712. (**LOE V**).
11. Al-Motabagani MAH. The arterial architecture of the human femoral diaphysis. *J Anat Soc India.* 2002;1:27–31. (**LOE V**).
12. Chung SM. The arterial supply of the developing proximal end of the human femur. *J Bone Joint Surg Am.* 1976;58(7):961–970. (**LOE V**).
13. Gage JR, Cary JM. The effects of trochanteric epiphyseodesis on growth of the proximal end of the femur following necrosis of the capital femoral epiphysis. *J Bone Joint Surg Am.* 1980;62(5):785–794. (**LOE III**).
14. Stevens PM, Anderson LA, Gililland JM, Novais E. Guided growth of the trochanteric apophysis combined with soft tissue release for Legg-Calve-Perthes disease. *Strategies Trauma Limb Reconstr.* 2014;9(1):37–43. (**LOE IV**).
15. Galano GJ, Vitale MA, Kessler MW, Hyman JE, Vitale MG. The most frequent traumatic orthopaedic injuries from a national pediatric inpatient population. *J Pediatr Orthop.* 2005;25(1):39–44. (**LOE N/A**).
16. Rewers A, Hedegaard H, Lezotte D, et al. Childhood femur fractures, associated injuries, and sociodemographic risk factors: a population-based study. *Pediatrics.* 2005;115(5):e543–552. (**LOE II**).
17. Ortiz EJ, Isler MH, Navia JE, Canosa R. Pathologic fractures in children. *Clin Orthop Relat Res.* 2005;432:116–126. (**LOE II**).
18. De Mattos CB, Binitie O, Dormans JP. Pathological fractures in children. *Bone Joint Res.* 2012;1(10):272–280. (**LOE N/A**).
19. Pierce MC, Bertocci GE, Janosky JE, et al. Femur fractures resulting from stair falls among children: an injury plausibility model. *Pediatrics.* 2005;115(6):1712–1722. (**LOE II**).
20. Brainard BJ, Slauterbeck J, Benjamin JB. Fracture patterns and mechanisms in pedestrian motor-vehicle trauma: the ipsilateral dyad. *J Orthop Trauma.* 1992;6(3):279–282. (**LOE IV**).
21. Halvorson JJ, Anz A, Langfitt M, et al. Vascular injury associated with extremity trauma: initial diagnosis and management. *J Am Acad Orthop Surg.* 2011;19(8):495–504. (**LOE N/A**).
22. Lynch JM, Gardner MJ, Gains B. Hemodynamic significance of pediatric femur fractures. *J Pediatr Surg.* 1996;31(10):1358–1361. (**LOE IV**).
23. Unal VS, Gulcek M, Unveren Z, Karakuyu A, Ucaner A. Blood loss evaluation in children under the age of 11 with femoral shaft fractures patients with isolated versus multiple injuries. *J Trauma.* 2006;60(1):224–226; discussion 226. (**LOE II**).
24. Kumar B, Borgohain B, Balasubramanian S, Sathyanarayana V, Muthusamy M. Risks of concomitant trauma to the knee in lower limb long bone shaft fractures: a retrospective analysis from a prospective study population. *Adv Biomed Res.* 2014;3:49. (**LOE II**).
25. Dickson KF, Galland MW, Barrack RL, et al. Magnetic resonance imaging of the knee after ipsilateral femur fracture. *J Orthop Trauma.* 2002;16(8):567–571. (**LOE I**).
26. Emami Meybodi MK, Ladani MJ, Emami Meybodi T, et al. Concomitant ligamentous and meniscal knee injuries in femoral shaft fracture. *J Orthop Traumatol.* 2014;15(1):35–39. (**LOE I**).
27. Thompson JD, Buehler KC, Sponseller PD, et al. Shortening in femoral shaft fractures in children treated with spica cast. *Clin Orthop Relat Res.* 1997;338:74–78. (**LOE III**).

28. Heinrich SD, Gallagher D, Harris M, Nadell JM. Undiagnosed fractures in severely injured children and young adults. Identification with technetium imaging. *J Bone Joint Surg Am*. 1994;76(4):561–572. **(LOE IV)**.

29. Burstein AH. Fracture classification systems: do they work and are they useful? *J Bone Joint Surg Am*. 1993;75(12):1743–1744. **(LOE II)**.

30. Slongo T, Audigé L, Schlickewei W, Clavert JM, Hunter J, International Association for Pediatric Traumatology. Development and validation of the AO pediatric comprehensive classification of long bone fractures by the Pediatric Expert Group of the AO Foundation in collaboration with AO Clinical Investigation and Documentation and the International Association for Pediatric Traumatology. *J Pediatr Orthop*. 2006;26(1):43–49. **(LOE II)**.

31. Joeris A, Lutz N, Blumenthal A, Slongo T, Audigé L. The AO Pediatric Comprehensive Classification of Long Bone Fractures (PCCF). *Acta Orthop*. 2017;88(2):129–132. **(LOE IV)**.

32. Slongo TF, Audigé L, AO Pediatric Classification Group. Fracture and dislocation classification compendium for children: the AO Pediatric Comprehensive Classification of Long Bone Fractures (PCCF). *J Orthop Trauma*. 2007;21(suppl 10):S135–S160. **(LOE N/A)**.

33. Pombo MW, Shilt JS. The definition and treatment of pediatric subtrochanteric femur fractures with titanium elastic nails. *J Pediatr Orthop*. 2006;26(3):364–370. **(LOE III)**.

34. Ireland DC, Fisher RL. Subtrochanteric fractures of the femur in children. *Clin Orthop Relat Res*. 1975;(110):157–166. **(LOE IV)**.

35. Jeng C, Sponseller PD, Yates A, Paletta G. Subtrochanteric femoral fractures in children. Alignment after 90 degrees-90 degrees traction and cast application. *Clin Orthop Relat Res*. 1997;(341):170–174. **(LOE IV)**.

36. Parikh SN, Nathan ST, Priola MJ, Eismann EA. Elastic nailing for pediatric subtrochanteric and supracondylar femur fractures. *Clin Orthop Relat Res*. 2014;472(9):2735–2744. **(LOE IV)**.

37. Butcher CC, Hoffman EB. Supracondylar fractures of the femur in children: closed reduction and percutaneous pinning of displaced fractures. *J Pediatr Orthop*. 2005;25(2):145–148. **(LOE IV)**.

38. Carmichael KD, Bynum J, Goucher N. Rates of refracture associated with external fixation in pediatric femur fractures. *Am J Orthop (Belle Mead NJ)*. 2005;34(9):439–444; discussion 444. **(LOE III)**.

39. Roaten JD, Kelly DM, Yellin JL, et al. Pediatric femoral shaft fractures: a multicenter review of the AAOS Clinical Practice Guidelines before and after 2009. *J Pediatr Orthop*. 2017. **(LOE III)**.

40. Naranje SM, Stewart MG, Kelly DM, et al. Changes in the treatment of pediatric femoral fractures: 15-year trends from United States Kids' Inpatient Database (KID) 1997 to 2012. *J Pediatr Orthop*. 2016;36(7):e81–e85. **(LOE III)**.

41. Poolman RW, Kocher MS, Bhandari M. Pediatric femoral fractures: a systematic review of 2422 cases. *J Orthop Trauma*. 2006;20(9):648–654. **(LOE III)**.

42. Gaid M, Jeer P. Cost analysis of managing paediatric femoral shaft fractures: flexible intramedullary nailing versus non-operative management. *Acta Orthop Belg*. 2006;72(2):170–175. **(LOE II)**.

43. Wright JG, Wang EE, Owen JL, et al. Treatments for paediatric femoral fractures: a randomised trial. *Lancet*. 2005;365(9465):1153–1158. **(LOE I)**.

44. Angiletta D, Impedovo G, Pestrichella F, Marotta V, Perilli F, Regina G. Blunt femoropopliteal trauma in a child: is stenting a good option? *J Vasc Surg*. 2006;44(1):201–204; discussion 205. **(LOE IV)**.

45. Hedequist D, Starr AJ, Wilson P, Walker J. Early versus delayed stabilization of pediatric femur fractures: analysis of 387 patients. *J Orthop Trauma*. 1999;13(7):490–493. **(LOE III)**.

46. Loder RT. Pediatric polytrauma: orthopaedic care and hospital course. *J Orthop Trauma*. 1987;1(1):48–54. **(LOE III)**.

47. Della Rocca GJ, Crist BD. External fixation versus conversion to intramedullary nailing for definitive management of closed fractures of the femoral and tibial shaft. *J Am Acad Orthop Surg*. 2006;14(10 Spec No.):S131–S135. **(LOE N/A)**.

48. Skaggs DL, Friend L, Alman B, et al. The effect of surgical delay on acute infection following 554 open fractures in children. *J Bone Joint Surg Am*. 2005;87(1):8–12. **(LOE III)**.

49. Ali M, Raza A. Union and complications after Thomas splint and early hip spica for femoral shaft fractures in children. *J Coll Physicians Surg Pak*. 2005;15(12):799–801. **(LOE III)**.

50. Podeszwa DA, Mooney JF 3rd, Cramer KE, Mendelow MJ. Comparison of Pavlik harness application and immediate spica casting for femur fractures in infants. *J Pediatr Orthop*. 2004;24(5):460–462. **(LOE III)**.

51. Stannard JP, Christensen KP, Wilkins KE. Femur fractures in infants: a new therapeutic approach. *J Pediatr Orthop*. 1995;15(4):461–466. **(LOE IV)**.

52. Burton VW, Fordyce AJ. Immobilization of femoral shaft fractures in children aged 2-10 years. *Injury*. 1972;4(1):47–53. **(LOE III)**.

53. Rasool MN, Govender S, Naidoo KS. Treatment of femoral shaft fractures in children by early spica casting. *S Afr Med J*. 1989;76(3):96–99. **(LOE II)**.

54. Blasier RD, Aronson J, Tursky EA. External fixation of pediatric femur fractures. *J Pediatr Orthop*. 1997;17(3):342–346. **(LOE IV)**.

55. Gregory P, Pevny T, Teague D. Early complications with external fixation of pediatric femoral shaft fractures. *J Orthop Trauma*. 1996;10(3):191–198. **(LOE III)**.

56. Miner T, Carroll KL. Outcomes of external fixation of pediatric femoral shaft fractures. *J Pediatr Orthop*. 2000;20(3):405–410. **(LOE IV)**.

57. Skaggs DL, Leet AI, Money MD, Shaw BA, Hale JM, Tolo VT. Secondary fractures associated with external fixation in pediatric femur fractures. *J Pediatr Orthop*. 1999;19(5):582–586. **(LOE III)**.

58. Buechsenschuetz KE, Mehlman CT, Shaw KJ, Crawford AH, Immerman EB. Femoral shaft fractures in children: traction and casting versus elastic stable intramedullary nailing. *J Trauma*. 2002;53(5):914–921. **(LOE III)**.

59. Flynn JM, Luedtke LM, Ganley TJ, et al. Comparison of titanium elastic nails with traction and a spica cast to treat femoral fractures in children. *J Bone Joint Surg Am*. 2004;86-A(4):770–777. **(LOE II)**.

60. Song HR, Oh CW, Shin HD, et al. Treatment of femoral shaft fractures in young children: comparison between conservative treatment and retrograde flexible nailing. *J Pediatr Orthop B*. 2004;13(4):275–280. **(LOE III)**.

61. Barlas K, Beg H. Flexible intramedullary nailing versus external fixation of paediatric femoral fractures. *Acta Orthop Belg*. 2006;72(2):159–163. **(LOE III)**.

62. Bar-On E, Sagiv S, Porat S. External fixation or flexible intramedullary nailing for femoral shaft fractures in children. A prospective, randomised study. *J Bone Joint Surg Br*. 1997;79(6):975–978. **(LOE II)**.

63. Hunter JB. Femoral shaft fractures in children. *Injury*. 2005;36(suppl 1):A86–A93. **(LOE N/A)**.

64. Li Y, Stabile KJ, Shilt JS. Biomechanical analysis of titanium elastic nail fixation in a pediatric femur fracture model. *J Pediatr Orthop*. 2008;28(8):874–878. **(LOE V)**.

65. Moroz LA, Launay F, Kocher MS, et al. Titanium elastic nailing of fractures of the femur in children. Predictors of complications and poor outcome. *J Bone Joint Surg Br*. 2006;88(10):1361–1366. **(LOE IV)**.

66. Ellis HB, Ho CA, Podeszwa DA, Wilson PL. A comparison of locked versus nonlocked Enders rods for length unstable pediatric femoral shaft fractures. *J Pediatr Orthop*. 2011;31(8):825–833. **(LOE III)**.

67. Rathjen KE, Riccio AI, De La Garza D. Stainless steel flexible intramedullary fixation of unstable femoral shaft fractures in children. *J Pediatr Orthop*. 2007;27(4):432–441. **(LOE III)**.

68. Wall EJ, Jain V, Vora V, Mehlman CT, Crawford AH. Complications of titanium and stainless steel elastic nail fixation of pediatric femoral fractures. *J Bone Joint Surg Am*. 2008;90(6):1305–1313. **(LOE III)**.

69. Caird MS, Mueller KA, Puryear A, Farley FA. Compression plating of pediatric femoral shaft fractures. *J Pediatr Orthop*. 2003;23(4):448–452. **(LOE III)**.

70. Hedequist DJ, Sink E. Technical aspects of bridge plating for pediatric femur fractures. *J Orthop Trauma*. 2005;19(4):276–279. **(LOE N/A)**.

71. Kanlic EM, Anglen JO, Smith DG, Morgan SJ, Pesantez RF. Advantages of submuscular bridge plating for complex pediatric femur fractures. *Clin Orthop Relat Res*. 2004;426:244–251. **(LOE III)**.

72. Sink EL, Faro F, Polousky J, Flynn K, Gralla J. Decreased complications of pediatric femur fractures with a change in management. *J Pediatr Orthop*. 2010;30(7):633–637. **(LOE III)**.

73. Sink EL, Hedequist D, Morgan SJ, Hresko T. Results and technique of unstable pediatric femoral fractures treated with submuscular bridge plating. *J Pediatr Orthop*. 2006;26(2):177–181. **(LOE IV)**.

74. Buford Jr D, Christensen K, Weatherall P. Intramedullary nailing of femoral fractures in adolescents. *Clin Orthop Relat Res.* 1998;(350):85–89. **(LOE II)**.

75. Herndon WA, Mahnken RF, Yngve DA, Sullivan JA. Management of femoral shaft fractures in the adolescent. *J Pediatr Orthop.* 1989;9(1):29–32. **(LOE III)**.

76. Kanellopoulos AD, Yiannakopoulos CK, Soucacos PN. Closed, locked intramedullary nailing of pediatric femoral shaft fractures through the tip of the greater trochanter. *J Trauma.* 2006;60(1):217–222; discussion 222–213. **(LOE IV)**.

77. Keeler KA, Dart B, Luhmann SJ, et al. Antegrade intramedullary nailing of pediatric femoral fractures using an interlocking pediatric femoral nail and a lateral trochanteric entry point. *J Pediatr Orthop.* 2009;29(4):345–351. **(LOE IV)**.

78. MacNeil JA, Francis A, El-Hawary R. A systematic review of rigid, locked, intramedullary nail insertion sites and avascular necrosis of the femoral head in the skeletally immature. *J Pediatr Orthop.* 2011;31(4):377–380. **(LOE III)**.

79. Wang CN, Chen JJ, Zhou JF, Tang HB, Feng YB, Yi X. Femoral fractures in infants: a comparison of Bryant traction and modified Pavlik harness. *Acta Orthop Belg.* 2014;80(1):63–68. **(LOE III)**.

80. Mahajan J, Hennrikus W, Piazza B. Overgrowth after femoral shaft fractures in infants treated with a Pavlik harness. *J Pediatr Orthop B.* 2016;25(1):7–10. **(LOE IV)**.

81. Rush JK, Kelly DM, Sawyer JR, Beaty JH, Warner Jr WC. Treatment of pediatric femur fractures with the Pavlik harness: multiyear clinical and radiographic outcomes. *J Pediatr Orthop.* 2013;33(6):614–617. **(LOE IV)**.

82. Cassinelli EH, Young B, Vogt M, Pierce MC, Deeney VF. Spica cast application in the emergency room for select pediatric femur fractures. *J Orthop Trauma.* 2005;19(10):709–716. **(LOE IV)**.

83. Mansour AA 3rd, Wilmoth JC, Mansour AS, Lovejoy SA, Mencio GA, Martus JE. Immediate spica casting of pediatric femoral fractures in the operating room versus the emergency department: comparison of reduction, complications, and hospital charges. *J Pediatr Orthop.* 2010;30(8):813–817. **(LOE III)**.

84. Epps HR, Molenaar E, O'Connor DP. Immediate single-leg spica cast for pediatric femoral diaphysis fractures. *J Pediatr Orthop.* 2006;26(4):491–496. **(LOE IV)**.

85. Illgen 2nd R, Rodgers WB, Hresko MT, Waters PM, Zurakowski D, Kasser JR. Femur fractures in children: treatment with early sitting spica casting. *J Pediatr Orthop.* 1998;18(4):481–487. **(LOE IV)**.

86. Jaafar S, Sobh A, Legakis JE, Thomas R, Buhler K, Jones ET. Four weeks in a single-leg weight-bearing hip spica cast is sufficient treatment for isolated femoral shaft fractures in children aged 1 to 3 years. *J Pediatr Orthop.* 2016;36(7):680–684. **(LOE III)**.

87. Kiter E, Demirkan F, Kilic BA, Erkula G. A new technique for creating an abdominal window in a hip spica cast. *J Orthop Trauma.* 2003;17(6):442–443. **(LOE V)**.

88. Leu D, Sargent MC, Ain MC, Leet AI, Tis JE, Sponseller PD. Spica casting for pediatric femoral fractures: a prospective, randomized controlled study of single-leg versus double-leg spica casts. *J Bone Joint Surg Am.* 2012;94(14):1259–1264. **(LOE I)**.

89. Mubarak SJ, Frick S, Sink E, Rathjen K, Noonan KJ. Volkmann contracture and compartment syndromes after femur fractures in children treated with 90/90 spica casts. *J Pediatr Orthop.* 2006;26(5):567–572. **(LOE IV)**.

90. Wolff CR, James P. The prevention of skin excoriation under children's hip spica casts using the goretex pantaloon. *J Pediatr Orthop.* 1995;15(3):386–388. **(LOE II)**.

91. Flynn JM, Skaggs DL. *Fractures in Children.* 7th ed. Philadelphia: Lippincott Williams & Wilkins; 2010. **(LOE N/A)**.

92. Davids JR, Frick SL, Skewes E, Blackhurst DW. Skin surface pressure beneath an above-the-knee cast: plaster casts compared with fiberglass casts. *J Bone Joint Surg Am.* 1997;79(4):565–569. **(LOE IV)**.

93. Hosalkar HS, Jones S, Chowdhury M, Chatoo M, Hill RA. Connecting bar for hip spica reinforcement: does it help? *J Pediatr Orthop B.* 2003;12(2):100–102. **(LOE II)**.

94. Quintin J, Evrard H, Gouat P, Cornil C, Burny F. External fixation in child traumatology. *Orthopedics.* 1984;7(3):463–467. **(LOE V)**.

95. Anderson SR, Nelson SC, Morrison MJ. Unstable pediatric femur fractures: combined intramedullary flexible nails and external fixation. *J Orthop Case Rep.* 2017;7(4):32–35. **(LOE V)**.

96. El-Alfy B, Ali AM, Fawzy SI. Comminuted long bone fractures in children. Could combined fixation improve the results? *J Pediatr Orthop B.* 2016;25(5):478–483. **(LOE IV)**.

97. Allen JD, Murr K, Albitar F, Jacobs C, Moghadamian ES, Muchow R. Titanium elastic nailing has superior value to plate fixation of midshaft femur fractures in children 5 to 11 years. *J Pediatr Orthop.* 2018;38(3):e111–e117. **(LOE III)**.

98. Assaghir Y. The safety of titanium elastic nailing in preschool femur fractures: a retrospective comparative study with spica cast. *J Pediatr Orthop B.* 2013;22(4):289–295. **(LOE III)**.

99. Heffernan MJ, Gordon JE, Sabatini CS, et al. Treatment of femur fractures in young children: a multicenter comparison of flexible intramedullary nails to spica casting in young children aged 2 to 6 years. *J Pediatr Orthop.* 2015;35(2):126–129. **(LOE III)**.

100. Ramo BA, Martus JE, Tareen N, Hooe BS, Snoddy MC, Jo CH. Intramedullary nailing compared with spica casts for isolated femoral fractures in four and five-year-old children. *J Bone Joint Surg Am.* 2016;98(4):267–275. **(LOE III)**.

101. Flynn JM, Hresko T, Reynolds RA, Blasier RD, Davidson R, Kasser J. Titanium elastic nails for pediatric femur fractures: a multicenter study of early results with analysis of complications. *J Pediatr Orthop.* 2001;21(1):4–8. **(LOE IV)**.

102. Luhmann SJ, Schootman M, Schoenecker PL, Dobbs MB, Gordon JE. Complications of titanium elastic nails for pediatric femoral shaft fractures. *J Pediatr Orthop.* 2003;23(4):443–447. **(LOE IV)**.

103. Green JK, Werner FW, Dhawan R, Evans PJ, Kelley S, Webster DA. A biomechanical study on flexible intramedullary nails used to treat pediatric femoral fractures. *J Orthop Res.* 2005;23(6):1315–1320. **(LOE V)**.

104. Flynn JM, Luedtke L, Ganley TJ, Pill SG. Titanium elastic nails for pediatric femur fractures: lessons from the learning curve. *Am J Orthop (Belle Mead NJ).* 2002;31(2):71–74. **(LOE IV)**.

105. Ligier JN, Metaizeau JP, Prevot J, Lascombes P. Elastic stable intramedullary nailing of femoral shaft fractures in children. *J Bone Joint Surg Br.* 1988;70(1):74–77. **(LOE IV)**.

106. Cramer KE, Tornetta P 3rd, Spero CR, Alter S, Miraliakbar H, Teefey J. Ender rod fixation of femoral shaft fractures in children. *Clin Orthop Relat Res.* 2000;376:119–123. **(LOE II)**.

107. Mazda K, Khairouni A, Pennecot GF, Bensahel H. Closed flexible intramedullary nailing of the femoral shaft fractures in children. *J Pediatr Orthop B.* 1997;6(3):198–202. **(LOE IV)**.

108. Abbott MD, Loder RT, Anglen JO. Comparison of submuscular and open plating of pediatric femur fractures: a retrospective review. *J Pediatr Orthop.* 2013;33(5):519–523. **(LOE III)**.

109. Eren OT, Kucukkaya M, Kockesen C, Kabukcuoglu Y, Kuzgun U. Open reduction and plate fixation of femoral shaft fractures in children aged 4 to 10. *J Pediatr Orthop.* 2003;23(2):190–193. **(LOE III)**.

110. Fyodorov I, Sturm PF, Robertson Jr WW. Compression-plate fixation of femoral shaft fractures in children aged 8 to 12 years. *J Pediatr Orthop.* 1999;19(5):578–581. **(LOE III)**.

111. Kregor PJ, Song KM, Routt Jr ML, Sangeorzan BJ, Liddell RM, Hansen Jr ST. Plate fixation of femoral shaft fractures in multiply injured children. *J Bone Joint Surg Am.* 1993;75(12):1774–1780. **(LOE IV)**.

112. Ward WT, Levy J, Kaye A. Compression plating for child and adolescent femur fractures. *J Pediatr Orthop.* 1992;12(5):626–632. **(LOE IV)**.

113. Ziv I, Rang M. Treatment of femoral fracture in the child with head injury. *J Bone Joint Surg Br.* 1983;65(3):276–278. **(LOE III)**.

114. Abdelgawad AA, Sieg RN, Laughlin MD, Shunia J, Kanlic EM. Submuscular bridge plating for complex pediatric femur fractures is reliable. *Clin Orthop Relat Res.* 2013;471(9):2797–2807. **(LOE IV)**.

115. Kuremsky MA, Frick SL. Advances in the surgical management of pediatric femoral shaft fractures. *Curr Opin Pediatr.* 2007;19(1):51–57. **(LOE N/A)**.

116. Li Y, Heyworth BE, Glotzbecker M, et al. Comparison of titanium elastic nail and plate fixation of pediatric subtrochanteric femur fractures. *J Pediatr Orthop.* 2013;33(3):232–238. **(LOE III)**.

117. Samora WP, Guerriero M, Willis L, Klingele KE. Submuscular bridge plating for length-unstable, pediatric femur fractures. *J Pediatr Orthop.* 2013;33(8):797–802. **(LOE IV)**.

118. Stoneback JW, Carry PM, Flynn K, Pan Z, Sink EL, Miller NH. Clinical and radiographic outcomes after submuscular plating (SMP) of pediatric femoral shaft fractures. *J Pediatr Orthop.* 2018;38(3):138–143. **(LOE IV)**.

119. Porter SE, Booker GR, Parsell DE, et al. Biomechanical analysis comparing titanium elastic nails with locked plating in two simulated pediatric femur fracture models. *J Pediatr Orthop.* 2012;32(6):587–593. **(LOE V)**.

120. Rozbruch SR, Müller U, Gautier E, Ganz R. The evolution of femoral shaft plating technique. *Clin Orthop Relat Res.* 1998;(354):195–208. **(LOE III)**.

121. Kelly B, Heyworth B, Yen YM, Hedequist D. Adverse sequelae due to plate retention following submuscular plating for pediatric femur fractures. *J Orthop Trauma.* 2013;27(12):726–729. **(LOE IV)**.

122. Pate O, Hedequist D, Leong N, Hresko T. Implant removal after submuscular plating for pediatric femur fractures. *J Pediatr Orthop.* 2009;29(7):709–712. **(LOE IV)**.

123. Kelly BA, Naqvi M, Rademacher ES, et al. Fracture table application for pediatric femur fractures: incidence and risk factors associated with adverse outcomes. *J Pediatr Orthop.* 2017;37(6):e353–e356. **(LOE III)**.

124. Anglen J, Banovetz J. Compartment syndrome in the well leg resulting from fracture-table positioning. *Clin Orthop Relat Res.* 1994;(301):239–242. **(LOE V)**.

125. Meldrum R, Lipscomb P. Compartment syndrome of the leg after less than 4 hours of elevation on a fracture table. *South Med J.* 2002;95(2):269–271. **(LOE V)**.

126. Stephen DJ, Kreder HJ, Schemitsch EH, Conlan LB, Wild L, McKee MD. Femoral intramedullary nailing: comparison of fracture-table and manual traction. A prospective, randomized study. *J Bone Joint Surg Am.* 2002;84-A(9):1514–1521. **(LOE I)**.

127. Hajek PD, Bicknell Jr HR, Bronson WE, Albright JA, Saha S. The use of one compared with two distal screws in the treatment of femoral shaft fractures with interlocking intramedullary nailing. A clinical and biomechanical analysis. *J Bone Joint Surg Am.* 1993;75(4):519–525. **(LOE V)**.

128. Arslan H, Subasy M, Kesemenli C, Ersuz H. Occurrence and treatment of nonunion in long bone fractures in children. *Arch Orthop Trauma Surg.* 2002;122(9-10):494–498. **(LOE IV)**.

129. Corry IS, Nicol RO. Limb length after fracture of the femoral shaft in children. *J Pediatr Orthop.* 1995;15(2):217–219. **(LOE IV)**.

130. Griffin PP, Green WT. Fractures of the shaft of the femur in children: treatment and results. *Orthop Clin North Am.* 1972;3(1):213–224. **(LOE N/A)**.

131. Stephens MM, Hsu LC, Leong JC. Leg length discrepancy after femoral shaft fractures in children. Review after skeletal maturity. *J Bone Joint Surg Br.* 1989;71(4):615–618. **(LOE IV)**.

132. Sulaiman AR, Joehaimy J, Iskandar MA, Anwar Hau M, Ezane AM, Faisham WI. Femoral overgrowth following plate fixation of the fractured femur in children. *Singapore Med J.* 2006;47(8):684–687. **(LOE IV)**.

133. DiFazio R, Vessey J, Zurakowski D, Hresko MT, Matheney T. Incidence of skin complications and associated charges in children treated with hip spica casts for femur fractures. *J Pediatr Orthop.* 2011;31(1):17–22. **(LOE III)**.

134. Weiss AP, Schenck Jr RC, Sponseller PD, Thompson JD. Peroneal nerve palsy after early cast application for femoral fractures in children. *J Pediatr Orthop.* 1992;12(1):25–28. **(LOE IV)**.

135. Moroni A, Vannini F, Mosca M, Giannini S. State of the art review: techniques to avoid pin loosening and infection in external fixation. *J Orthop Trauma.* 2002;16(3):189–195. **(LOE N/A)**.

136. Nielsen E, Andras LM, Bonsu N, Goldstein RY. The effects of body mass index on treatment of paediatric femur fractures managed with flexible intramedullary nails. *J Child Orthop.* 2017;11(5):393–397. **(LOE III)**.

137. Shaha J, Cage JM, Black S, Wimberly RL, Shaha SH, Riccio AI. Flexible intramedullary nails for femur fractures in pediatric patients heavier than 100 pounds. *J Pediatr Orthop.* 2018;38(2):88–93. **(LOE III)**.

138. Narayanan UG, Hyman JE, Wainwright AM, Rang M, Alman BA. Complications of elastic stable intramedullary nail fixation of pediatric femoral fractures, and how to avoid them. *J Pediatr Orthop.* 2004;24(4):363–369. **(LOE IV)**.

139. Sink EL, Gralla J, Repine M. Complications of pediatric femur fractures treated with titanium elastic nails: a comparison of fracture types. *J Pediatr Orthop.* 2005;25(5):577–580. **(LOE III)**.

140. Heyworth BE, Hedequist DJ, Nasreddine AY, Stamoulis C, Hresko MT, Yen YM. Distal femoral valgus deformity following plate fixation of pediatric femoral shaft fractures. *J Bone Joint Surg Am.* 2013;95(6):526–533. **(LOE IV)**.

141. May C, Yen YM, Nasreddine AY, Hedequist D, Hresko MT, Heyworth BE. Complications of plate fixation of femoral shaft fractures in children and adolescents. *J Child Orthop.* 2013;7(3):235–243. **(LOE IV)**.

142. Gonzalez-Herranz P, Burgos-Flores J, Rapariz JM, Lopez-Mondejar JA, Ocete JG, Amaya S. Intramedullary nailing of the femur in children. Effects on its proximal end. *J Bone Joint Surg Br.* 1995;77(2):262–266. **(LOE IV)**.

143. Raney EM, Ogden JA, Grogan DP. Premature greater trochanteric epiphysiodesis secondary to intramedullary femoral rodding. *J Pediatr Orthop.* 1993;13(4):516–520. **(LOE IV)**.

144. Gordon JE, Swenning TA, Burd TA, Szymanski DA, Schoenecker PL. Proximal femoral radiographic changes after lateral transtrochanteric intramedullary nail placement in children. *J Bone Joint Surg Am.* 2003;85-A(7):1295–1301. **(LOE IV)**.

Fractures Around the Knee in Children

13

Mauricio Silva | Richard E. Bowen | Rachel M. Thompson

INTRODUCTION

Traumatic forces applied to an immature knee result in fracture patterns that differ from those seen in adults. As in other anatomic regions in a growing child, the cartilaginous structures around the knee are weaker than the ligaments and tendons that insert onto them, making them more vulnerable to injury. Fractures involving the epiphyses require accurate reduction to minimize the risk of growth disturbances that could lead to significant angular deformity or leg length discrepancy. As in adults, fractures involving the articular surfaces require meticulous reduction to restore joint congruity to best assure long-term functionality. As the knee matures into adolescence, adult-type cartilaginous and ligamentous injuries become more prevalent and should be considered when evaluating injuries in this population.

FRACTURES OF THE DISTAL FEMORAL METAPHYSIS

Although the total reported incidence of supracondylar femur fractures account for 12% of all femoral fractures in children,[1] the incidence of displaced fractures in otherwise healthy children is significantly smaller. These fractures only account for 3% of all pediatric femur fractures.[2]

PERTINENT ANATOMY

In managing distal femoral metaphyseal fractures, it is important to remain cognizant of a few key neurovascular structures positioned in close proximity to the distal end of the femur, namely the femoral/popliteal artery and the peroneal and tibial nerves. This anatomy becomes more important when considering percutaneous fixation in this region. The femoral artery runs through the adductor canal, where it is in close proximity to the medial cortex of the distal femur as it descends and enters the posterior compartment. It becomes the popliteal artery as it emerges from the adductor hiatus and enters the popliteal fossa more distally. As the popliteal artery enters the popliteal fossa (sometimes referred to as the popliteal space), only a thin layer of fat separates the artery from the posterior surface of the femoral metaphysis. As the artery is relatively tethered proximally to the femur at the adductor hiatus and distally to the fibrous arch over the soleus muscle, it

is vulnerable to injury from the metaphyseal spike that occurs with a supracondylar femur fracture. Within the popliteal fossa, five geniculate arteries originate from the popliteal artery: paired superior and inferior branches and an unpaired middle geniculate. Although these arteries anastomose with the anterior tibial recurrent artery, they are diminutive and cannot provide sufficient blood supply to the lower part of the leg if the popliteal artery is occluded or disrupted.[3]

The tibial nerve lies adjacent to the popliteal artery in the popliteal fossa, descending into the posterior compartment of the leg. The common peroneal nerve branches from the sciatic nerve, more proximally, above the popliteal fossa and descends along the lateral border of the fossa adjacent to the medial border of the biceps femoris muscle. The nerve descends distally between the biceps femoris muscle and the lateral head of the gastrocnemius, becoming subcutaneous behind the fibular head. It then wraps around the neck of the fibula, deep to the peroneus longus muscle. Because of its location and proximal and distal tethering, the common peroneal nerve can be injured by a displaced distal femoral fracture, much like the popliteal artery, especially when the injury results from hyperextension and/or varus stress. This structure is also specifically at risk with proximal tibial traction pin insertion.

MECHANISM OF INJURY

Distal femoral metaphyseal fractures most often result from a direct blow to the anterior or lateral aspect of the thigh or a fall from height, resulting, most commonly, in a transverse fracture pattern. In children younger than 4 years of age, especially in nonambulatory children, nonaccidental trauma should be considered. The lack of a reasonable explanation, an unreasonable delay in seeking medical care, and/or the presence of concomitant injuries should raise the level of suspicion for a nonaccidental cause. Specifically, corner fractures, or bucket-handle lesions, at the level of the distal metaphysis are pathognomonic for nonaccidental trauma—these occur almost always in children less than 12 months of age.[4] However, other fracture patterns have been associated with child abuse as well. In fact, Arkader[5] published a series of complete transverse distal femoral metaphyseal fractures, in which 20 of 29 fractures were in children less than 1 year of age. Of those 20, 75% were associated with or were highly suspicious for child abuse.

In older children, nondisplaced fractures and stress fractures may occur as an overuse injury. These patients present with local pain and tenderness, and radiographs typically reveal robust periosteal bone reaction. Pathologic fracture should be considered in these patients.[6] Distal femoral metaphyseal fractures have also been reported in association with certain musculoskeletal conditions, including osteogenesis imperfecta, spina bifida, spinal muscular atrophy, and hemophilia.[1]

EVALUATION

EXAMINATION

Patients with a fracture of the distal femoral metaphysis present with local soft tissue swelling, tenderness, and deformity at the distal thigh and knee. The skin must be inspected for a possible open fracture. Because of the neurovascular anatomy previously described, a careful neurovascular examination is mandatory.

The presence and strength of a pedal pulse should be documented. The use of a Doppler ultrasound may aid in assessing the circulation to the limb if pulses are not palpable. An assessment of the ankle-brachial index (ABI) should be considered in any patients with a clinical examination concerning for vascular injury. If the limb is ischemic, a gentle reduction maneuver may restore circulation. Absent or diminished pulses may warrant vascular imaging. However, if the limb is frankly ischemic and the location of the vascular injury is clear, vascular exploration and early restoration of perfusion should not be delayed for imaging.

The function of the common peroneal and tibial nerves should additionally be tested and documented at initial evaluation. The peroneal nerve is tested with ankle dorsiflexion and great toe extension; the tibial nerve is tested with plantar flexion. The peroneal nerve is specifically at risk with either a direct blow to the posterolateral corner of the knee (e.g., from a car bumper) or from a stretch injury at the time of greatest displacement.

Ongoing serial evaluation of the lower extremity is important during the first few days after presentation so that a developing compartment syndrome may be detected promptly. This examination includes a neurological and a vascular examination. Compartment pressures should be measured if clinical signs and symptoms of a compartment syndrome are noted.

IMAGING

Anteroposterior (AP) and lateral radiographs of the distal end of the femur should be ordered and evaluated. As with any long bone fracture, radiographs of the entire bone should be taken, necessarily including the joint above and below the injury. Accordingly, radiographs of the entire femur, including the hip and knee, should be obtained at initial evaluation. These fractures, in general, do not require advanced imaging modalities, with the exception of vascular imaging for ischemic limbs.

CLASSIFICATION

Fractures of the distal femoral metaphysis in children are classified descriptively by the fracture pattern (transverse, oblique), the degree of displacement, and the presence or absence of comminution.

EMERGENT TREATMENT

If the limb is ischemic, a gentle reduction may restore circulation, as was mentioned in "Evaluation." The injured extremity should be splinted in a position of comfort after initial evaluation. Traction, either skin or skeletal, may be useful in multiply injured patients or medically compromised patients when definitive management will be delayed. The neurovascular status should be serially monitored pending definitive management of the fracture. This may include serial ABIs if vascular injury is suspected.

NONOPERATIVE TREATMENT

Given the nature of the deforming forces on this fracture, the significant risk for displacement, and the burden of nonoperative treatment in these fractures, nonoperative treatment is rarely recommended. Nonoperative treatment may be appropriate for truly nondisplaced fractures. Although a single-leg spica cast provides the most secure immobilization, especially in more obese children, a long leg cast may suffice for very distal fractures. This decision should be made by the treating physician, based on his/her judgement of fracture location and stability. Fractures treated in this manner must be closely followed, as the risk of subsequent displacement is present.

TRACTION AND CAST APPLICATION

Traction and cast application is less commonly used as definitive treatment currently as compared with previous generations. This technique has been largely replaced by operative management, given the overall burden that both traction and casting introduce to the hospital system, the patient, and the patient's family. However, the technique of balanced traction described below may be useful for temporary immobilization in the polytraumatized patient to maintain length and alignment of the fracture while definitive management is provided. Casting following traction may be used in patients who cannot tolerate surgical management for any reason.

In this technique, traction is applied to the lower extremity, maintaining proper reduction of the fracture until enough callus has formed to be safely maintained in a spica cast or long leg cast. In a young child, skin traction can be applied to the lower part of the leg, but skeletal traction is preferable in children older than 3 years of age.

Skeletal traction with the use of a Steinmann pin may be applied through the distal end of the femur or the proximal tibia. Regardless of site chosen, the pin is applied aseptically under local or general anesthesia. For distal femoral traction, the pin should be inserted medial to lateral so that the risk of injury to the femoral artery in the region of the adductor canal is minimized. For proximal tibial traction, the pin should be inserted in a lateral-to-medial direction so that the risk of injury to the peroneal nerve is minimized. Care should also be taken to avoid the proximal tibial physis and tibial tubercle apophysis.

Because of the muscle forces that act on the fracture fragments in this fracture pattern, the use of a single-traction pin may not maintain adequate alignment. Double-pin traction is often required. A proximal tibial pin provides longitudinal traction, but an additional distal femoral pin inserted into the distal femoral fragment may be required to provide an anteriorly directed force to achieve satisfactory sagittal alignment.[7] Similarly, if the distal femoral fragment is long enough, two pins may be inserted into the femoral fragment proximal to the physis to achieve the same desired result. Staheli[8] described a double-pin traction technique in which one pin is placed through the metaphysis and a second pin is placed through the epiphysis. The two pins are attached to an external fixation apparatus through which traction is applied. The patient is then placed in 90/90 traction. Once early callus forms and sagittal plane alignment is satisfactory, the knee is straightened gradually, and traction can be removed if the sagittal alignment is maintained on radiographs. Any residual coronal malalignment can be corrected with cast placement while the callus is still relatively soft.

The duration of immobilization varies with the age of the patient—3 to 4 weeks in the very young and 6 to 8 weeks in older children, which is determined by radiographic signs of adequate healing. After removal of the cast, rehabilitation is required to strengthen the quadriceps and hamstring. Weight-bearing is as tolerated, but assistive devices—crutches or a walker—are used for mobilization until knee motion and thigh strength are adequate to allow for independent ambulation. Return to regular activities is permitted after the quadriceps has regained normal strength and full range of motion of the knee joint has been achieved.

This technique may be complicated by pressure ulcers from prolonged immobilization, varus malalignment, and premature closure of the anterior part of the proximal tibial physis with proximal tibial traction, which will result in a recurvatum deformity. Careful cast application and management can prevent coronal malalignment. Meticulous proximal tibial pin placement will help avoid injuring the physis and tibial tubercle apophysis, although there are reported cases of premature tibial tubercle arrest occurring in association with femoral fractures, in the absence of tibial traction.[9] Malalignment in the sagittal plane may result in an apparent hyperextension or flexion deformity of the knee with associated limitations in range of motion. In a young child, this deformity largely remodels with time, as it is in the plane of motion of the knee.

SURGICAL TREATMENT

Surgical treatment has largely replaced nonoperative management in these fractures and is indicated for essentially all displaced fractures of the distal metaphysis of the femur, as the muscle forces acting on the distal fragment make obtaining and maintaining proper alignment of displaced fractures difficult without internal or external fixation. Generally, the distal fragment displaces posteriorly, into recurvatum, because of the pull of the gastrocnemius. If the fracture line is just proximal to the distal insertion of the adductor magnus, the distal fragment may also angulate into a varus position. To counteract these muscular forces, surgical options include external fixation, closed or open reduction with percutaneous pin fixation followed by the application of a long leg cast, open reduction with internal fixation, and submuscular bridge plating.

EXTERNAL FIXATION

External fixation is an effective tool used to reduce and stabilize distal femoral metaphyseal fractures (Fig. 13.1). The best situations for the use of external fixation for this injury are in polytraumatized patients and those with an open fracture, an associated vascular injury, and/or a floating knee.

In cases of polytrauma with multiple fractures, abdominal injury, or head injury, stabilizing the fracture with an external fixator is quick and safe, allowing for other diagnostic studies and/or operative procedures. In persistently comatose children, external fixation provides stability of the fracture while introducing minimal surgical risks. Given the high rate (>90%) of neurologic recovery in children following traumatic brain injury,[10] it is important to treat all fractures in children with head injuries with the assumption that full neurologic recovery will occur.

In addition to polytrauma stabilization, external fixation greatly facilitates wound care in open fractures. Further, stabilization of the distal part of the femur with an external fixator allows for easier care of concomitant injuries—vascular injury and/or an associated tibial fracture. Further, external fixation may limit the cost of prolonged hospitalization that occurs with the use of traction while providing more mechanical stability and decreasing the burden of care placed on the family.

In utilizing an external fixator to manage a distal femoral metaphyseal fracture, several technical points should be kept in mind.[10] Pins should be inserted from lateral to medial under image intensifier control through uninjured skin, whenever possible. The distal pin(s) should be placed at least 1 cm (preferably 2 cm) proximal to the physis to avoid potential thermal injury during insertion, as well as injury from a possible pin tract infection. Once the pins are placed and the external fixator bar is connected, a reduction can be achieved with manual traction and knee flexion to counteract the forces of the gastrocnemius on the distal fragment. In transverse fractures, an end-to-end reduction is attempted; in oblique fractures, bayonet apposition with approximately 5 mm of overlap should be considered in children younger than 10 years to minimize the effect of limb overgrowth. After preliminary placement of the frame, final adjustments to coronal and axial alignment can be made under fluoroscopic guidance.

Pin care is taught to the caregiver while in the hospital, and the authors recommend that it should be continued daily. Typical pin care consists of daily cleaning with either normal saline– or hydrogen peroxide–soaked Q-tip or gauze. Some experts recommend only daily bathing and soap and water cleaning of external fixation pin sites. Partial weight-bearing with crutches can be initiated early. Once radiographs reveal callus formation, weight-bearing is progressed to full.

Once the fracture is healed clinically and radiographically (at least three cortices with bridging callus on AP and lateral views),[11] typically occurring between 6 and 12 weeks from the time of the injury (depending on the age of the patient), the device may be removed in the outpatient setting. In most older children and all adolescents, it is best to leave the external fixator on for the full 12 weeks to minimize the risk of refracture after frame removal.

Potential complications include pin tract infection, malunion, refracture through either a pin tract or the original fracture site, and growth disturbances. Although not entirely

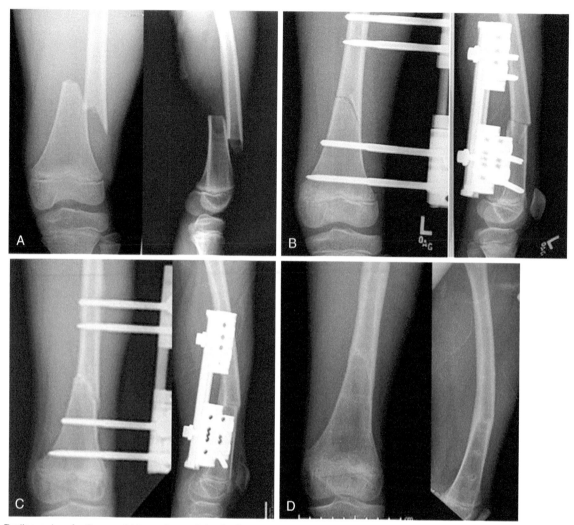

Fig. 13.1 Radiographs of a 9-year-old boy who sustained a fracture of the distal end of the femur. (A) Anteroposterior and lateral radiographs of the distal part of the femur and knee showing a distal femoral fracture, with significant displacement and shortening. (B) The fracture was reduced in the operating room, and the reduction was held with an external fixator. (C) Anteroposterior radiograph of the knee and distal end of the femur showing healing of the fracture 3 months after the injury. (D) Radiograph obtained 1 year after the injury demonstrating good distal femoral alignment and advanced remodeling.

preventable, the risk of pin tract infections is reduced with diligent pin care. If they do occur, pin tract infections should be treated with a short course (7–14 days) of oral antibiotics. However, if drainage persists or if erosion around the pin is apparent on radiographs, the pin should be exchanged and the original tract should be surgically débrided. Alternatively, if there is sufficient stability at the fracture site, the entire fixator can be removed and replaced with a cast until the fracture is fully healed.

Malunion can be prevented with placement of the fixator, paying specific attention to rotational and coronal reduction at the time of placement. Injury to the distal femoral physis is avoidable if the pins are placed at least 1 cm proximal to the physis. The pins should always be inserted under image intensifier control to avoid direct injury to the physis.

Refracture occurs more often with fractures treated with external fixation than with other methods. A fracture may occur through the initial fracture site if the frame is removed prematurely.[11] A fracture may also occur through a pin site, particularly in young children in whom large 5-mm fixator pins have been used.

CLOSED REDUCTION AND PERCUTANEOUS PIN FIXATION

Closed reduction and percutaneous pin fixation supplemented by the application of a long leg cast is a commonly used treatment modality for supracondylar femur fractures. This technique is particularly useful in younger patients in whom the metaphyseal fracture is quite distal (Fig. 13.2).

Under general anesthesia, the fracture is reduced typically with knee flexion and traction, and smooth pins are inserted in a retrograde crossed fashion under image intensifier control. It is preferable to insert the pins through the distal metaphysis, provided that sufficient metaphyseal length is available for placement. If there is not sufficient metaphysis distal to the fracture site for stable fixation, the pins may be inserted through the distal femoral epiphysis, crossing the physis, as described in detail for distal femoral physeal fractures. If so, smooth pins should be used. The pins are left percutaneously for ease of removal and bent at the skin to avoid proximal migration. A long leg cast is applied with the knee immobilized in 20 to 30 degrees of flexion. The pins can usually be removed after 4 weeks to decrease the

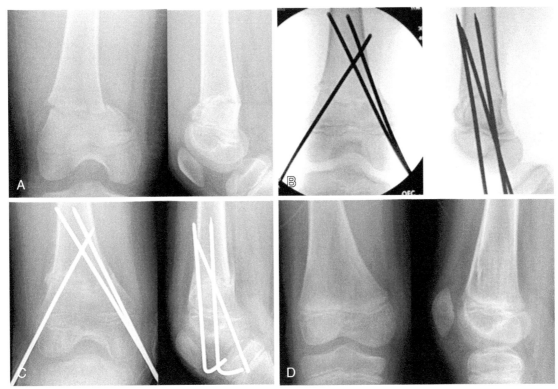

Fig. 13.2 A 10-year-old boy sustained an injury to his right knee. (A) Anteroposterior and lateral radiographs of the distal end of the femur show a complete supracondylar femoral fracture with medial displacement and extension of the distal fragment. (B) Because of the proximity of the injury to the physis, the fracture was reduced and pinned percutaneously. (C) Three weeks after surgery, early signs of healing are noted, and the pins are removed. (D) Six months after surgery, the fracture has healed in an anatomic position, and the distal femoral physis appears to be viable.

risk of pin-site infection. The cast is then replaced, and after 6 to 8 weeks, immobilization is discontinued. Damage to the femoral vessels on the medial side has been suggested as a potential complication of this method.[1] Butcher and Hoffman[2] have recommended that the lateral pin(s) should be placed posteriorly and directed anteriorly so that damage to the femoral vessels near the adductor hiatus is avoided. Although smooth pins that transgress the growth plate carry a theoretical risk of potential growth disturbance, the small diameter of the pins relative to the physeal area makes this complication unlikely.[2]

Alternatively, Parikh et al[12] published a small series of supracondylar femur fractures that were fixated with elastic nails, which resulted in radiographic healing in all seven patients with adequate alignment and no major complications. When there is adequate metaphyseal bone stock for placement of elastic nails, this is a reasonable option, avoiding the need for obligatory supplemental casting.

OPEN REDUCTION AND INTERNAL FIXATION

Open reduction and internal fixation is also appropriate for fractures that are irreducible by closed means and/or in the setting of vascular injury. The most common reason for failure to obtain adequate closed reduction is the presence of interposed muscle between fracture fragments. If repair of an arterial injury is required, internal fixation prevents excessive motion at the fracture site and protects the repair.

The surgical approach depends on the indication for open surgery. If interposed muscle is blocking reduction, a direct lateral approach allows the quadriceps muscle to be reflected anteriorly and provides adequate access to the

distal end of the femur for manual reduction. If arterial repair is required, the incision should be placed posteromedial to allow access to the femoral and popliteal arteries, as well as the saphenous vein, if vein grafting is necessary.

Rigid internal fixation, as is commonly used in adults, is not usually necessary in children. Percutaneous fixation can be successfully combined with open reduction.[13] This technique allows for the required access for reduction or vascular exploration and is associated with excellent radiographic and clinical results in a small series of widely displaced pulseless fractures, drawing parallels to pulseless supracondylar humerus fracture management. As in closed reduction and percutaneous fixation, fixation should be supplemented with a long leg cast. Of note, in the setting of a vascular injury, an external fixator may be more appropriate stabilization. The fixation choice should be agreed upon in conjunction with the surgeon who is treating the vascular injury, if not the same surgeon treating the fracture.

Compression plate fixation is rarely indicated to treat distal femoral metaphyseal fractures in a growing child, except perhaps in older/larger children and in the polytrauma setting. In this situation, compression plating may be a useful alternative and does not cause excessive femoral overgrowth.[14] The plate is generally removed 6 to 9 months following placement. Lateral plate fixation has been associated with the development of distal femoral valgus deformity in distal femoral shaft fractures. The etiology is not fully understood, and there is not a defined association between removal of hardware or retaining hardware and propensity to develop this deformity.[15]

More recently, Lin and colleagues[16] described open reduction and internal fixation utilizing a pediatric physeal slide traction plate for fixation of comminuted distal femur fractures in children. They reported excellent outcomes in 16 children treated with this device after a mean follow-up of 36 months. They recommended this device as a safe and effective treatment option for children with comminuted distal femur fractures. Other authors have advocated the use of proximal humerus plates for the fixation of these fractures, as they are appropriately sized for the distal femur in the pediatric population and provide locking fixation options.[17] A number of plate design options are now available to maximize the possible number of screws in the distal metaphyseal segment.

SUBMUSCULAR BRIDGE PLATING

Submuscular bridge plating is an alternative option for treating these fractures.[18–21] This technique is especially advantageous for managing comminuted and unstable fracture patterns (Fig. 13.3). The procedure is performed with the use of an image intensifier. A precontoured plate is tunneled proximally through a small distal incision deep to the vastus lateralis muscle. Reduction of the fracture is achieved manually, and the plate is secured to the femur with percutaneously placed screws proximal and distal to the fracture site. A plate with locking options should be used in fractures with limited bone stock available for fixation distally.[21]

No immobilization is required postoperatively, and the patients are encouraged to begin immediate knee range of motion. Toe-touch weight-bearing is maintained until early callus is evident radiographically. The plate may be removed 6 to 9 months after fixation, as is the case with compression plating. Minimized soft tissue dissection used in this technique is believed to result in rapid fracture healing and faster return of function as compared with traditional open reduction and plate fixation.

OUTCOME

In the absence of neurovascular complications, the outcome of fractures of the distal femoral metaphysis is excellent. Fractures in this region heal rapidly, and early return to full activities is the rule.

COMPLICATIONS

Malunion is a potential complication after the treatment of a distal femoral metaphyseal fracture. Sagittal plane deformity has a good capacity for remodeling, depending on the age of the patient. Coronal plane malunion has limited remodeling potential. Significant residual varus or valgus deformity may be addressed by guided growth or osteotomy, as can distal femoral valgus deformity associated with lateral plating.

Avoiding malunion requires knowledge of lower extremity anatomy and bony anatomic morphology. The anatomic axis of the shaft of the femur differs from the mechanical (weight-bearing) axis. The mechanical axis passes through the head of the femur and the middle of the knee joint and generally subtends an angle of 3 degrees from the vertical. The anatomic axis that runs through the shaft of the femur has an average valgus angulation of 6 degrees relative to the vertical axis. The knee joint line is typically parallel to the ground, and the anatomic femoral axis subtends an 81-degree lateral distal femoral angle relative to the knee joint. For each patient, it is important to confirm this angle by comparing it to the contralateral femur because individual variations do occur.

FRACTURES OF THE DISTAL FEMORAL PHYSIS

Fractures of the distal femoral physis account for 1.4% to 5.5% of all physeal injuries[22–24] and slightly more than 1% of all pediatric fractures.[22]

PERTINENT ANATOMY

The distal femoral epiphyseal ossification center is present in a full-term newborn infant. With subsequent growth, this ossification center rapidly expands to fill both condylar regions. The distal femoral physis is the largest and most rapidly growing physis in the body. It contributes almost 70% of the growth of the femur and 40% of the longitudinal growth of the entire leg, averaging approximately 1 cm of growth

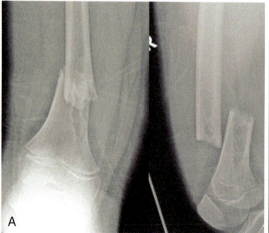
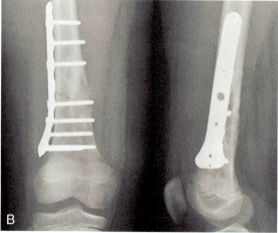

Fig. 13.3 An 8-year-old boy sustained a twisting injury to his leg while running. (A) Anteroposterior (AP) and lateral radiographs of the distal femur demonstrating a pathologic fracture of the distal femur through a nonossifying fibroma. (B) AP and lateral radiographs after application of a submuscular bridge plate showing excellent alignment of the fracture.

yearly until maturity.[25,26] Closure of this growth plate usually occurs between 14 and 16 years of age in girls and between 16 and 18 years in boys.[27] Any injury that partially or completely disrupts growth of the distal end of the femur may lead to significant angular deformity or foreshortening of the extremity. The younger the patient is at the time of injury, the greater the potential for these sequelae.

The distal epiphysis includes the entire articular surface of the lower end of the femur and serves as the origin for part of the gastrocnemius muscle.[28] Both the medial and lateral collateral ligaments originate from the distal femoral epiphysis. When a varus or valgus force is exerted on the knee, ligamentous injury is uncommon. Rather, the force most commonly dissipates through the distal femoral physis, resulting in a physeal fracture.

The configuration of the distal femoral physis is unique and has been well described by Roberts.[29] The distal surface of the metaphysis consists of four gentle mounds, one in each quadrant of the cross-sectional area. These mounds fit into four shallow depressions on the proximal surface of the epiphysis. This complex anatomy has been well-demonstrated by three-dimensional magnetic resonance imaging (MRI) modeling.[30] Although this undulating contour probably provides resistance to shear and torsional forces, it may also predispose regions of the epiphysis to grind against the metaphyseal projections when a separation occurs, resulting in germinal layer injury. This complex anatomy may help explain the frequency of growth disturbances following distal femoral physeal injury.

The relevant vascular anatomy has been outlined in the preceding section.

MECHANISM OF INJURY

The majority of these fractures are sustained in pedestrian versus automobile accidents or are sports related.[31–34] Riseborough and colleagues[33] observed that fractures in the juvenile group—ages 2 to 11 years—were invariably caused by severe trauma (i.e., motor vehicle accident), whereas fractures in the adolescent age group were most often sports related.

Because the physis provides less resistance to traumatic forces than the attached ligaments, a varus or valgus stress applied to an immature knee more often results in physeal separation than in collateral ligament injury. If hyperextension of the knee occurs, the epiphysis may displace anteriorly.[35] This mechanism of injury is similar to the mechanism that results in adult knee dislocations. It is important to recognize this pattern of injury as the potential for associated neurovascular injury is high. Posterior displacement of the epiphysis is relatively uncommon and results from a posteriorly directed force applied to the anterior aspect of a flexed knee.

As noted in the preceding section, children who are seen with injuries to the distal femur who are younger than 4 years, especially those younger than 1 year or who are nonambulatory, should be evaluated for nonaccidental trauma. The lack of a reasonable explanation for the injury, an unreasonable delay in seeking medical care, or the presence of additional injuries should raise the level of suspicion. A corner fracture, or bucket-handle lesion, at the level of the distal metaphysis is correlated with nonaccidental trauma.[4]

Distal femoral physeal separation can also occur at birth. These injuries are rare and have been associated with breech presentation, macrosomia, and difficult delivery.[33,36–38] Although the clinical appearance of these injuries may be confused with septic arthritis of the knee, clinical suspicion for physeal separation and close evaluation of the radiographs will usually reveal the diagnosis.[37,38]

EVALUATION

EXAMINATION

A patient with a distal femoral physeal fracture will present with a painful knee effusion, local soft tissue swelling, and tenderness over the physis. Symptoms vary depending on the displacement of the fracture. With displaced fractures, the patient is unable to bear weight on the injured limb, and deformity—most commonly varus or valgus—may be readily evident. In these cases, it is the metaphyseal fragment that is visually and palpably prominent medially or laterally. In an anteriorly displaced hyperextension injury, the patella is prominent, and dimpling of the anterior skin is often evident. With posterior displacement of the epiphysis, the distal metaphyseal fragment is prominent proximal to the patella.

IMAGING

Orthogonal radiographs should be obtained upon presentation. Oblique radiographs may reveal minimally displaced fractures (Fig. 13.4). Plain radiographs underestimate the displacement of Salter-Harris type III fractures by 100% on average (3 mm vs. 6 mm), which can result in missed diagnoses at initial evaluation in nearly 40% of patients with these fracture.[39] As such, Lippert et al[40] recommend advanced imaging for all suspected Salter-Harris type III distal femoral fractures. Advanced imaging is further useful in detecting the presence of a coronal shear injury.[38,41,42] Type III fractures, additionally, have a 12% reported incidence of concomitant soft tissue injuries, the majority of which are anterior cruciate ligament (ACL) injuries as reported by Pennock et al[39] most recently, and consistent with previous publications.[43–45] Accordingly, MRI may provide useful information in these patients.

If plain radiographs are inconsistent with obvious fracture but knee instability has been noted on clinical examination, stress radiographs have been historically advocated. However, stress radiographs are painful and risk further damage to the physis.[46] Alternatively, Stanitski[46] suggests immobilizing the extremity and obtaining a follow-up radiograph in 10 to 14 days to document the presence of a healing physeal fracture. Likewise, multiple authors advocate for MRI, ultrasound, and even computed tomography (CT) evaluation to identify nondisplaced physeal fractures in the pediatric population given correlating physical examination.[47–53]

CLASSIFICATION

The most commonly used classification system for distal femoral epiphyseal fractures is that of Salter and Harris (Fig. 13.5).[54] Type I fractures are characterized by complete separation through the physis without any involvement of the adjacent metaphysis or epiphysis. In type II fractures—the most common type as reported by Basener et al[55]—the

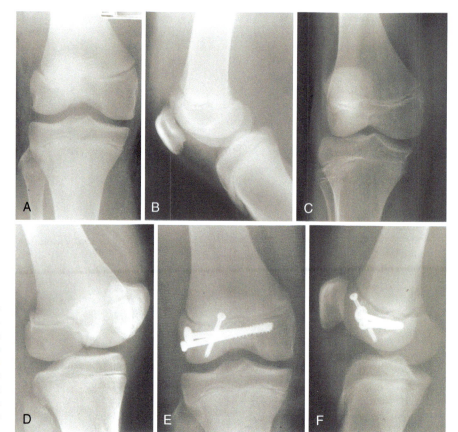

Fig. 13.4 (A and B) Anteroposterior and lateral radiographs of a 15-year-old boy who sustained an injury to his knee. Radiographs do not reveal an obvious fracture. (C) An oblique radiograph shows a Salter-Harris type III fracture of the physis of the distal femur. (D through F) The fracture was treated with open reduction and internal fixation. Radiographs show that excellent alignment of the fracture was achieved.

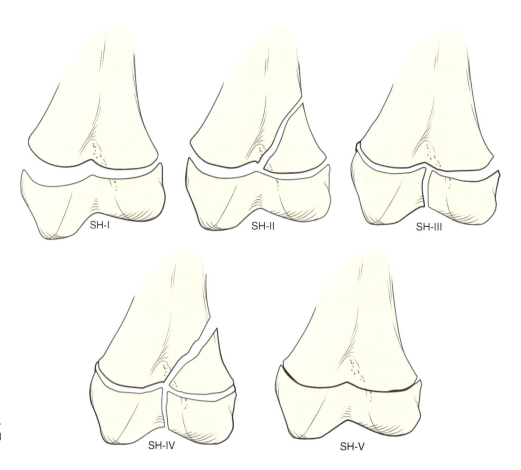

Fig. 13.5 Salter-Harris classification system for distal femoral epiphyseal injuries.

fracture line traverses the physis before exiting obliquely across one corner of the metaphysis, which results in a roughly triangular-shaped Thurston-Holland metaphyseal fragment. Displacement is usually toward the side of the metaphyseal fragment. The periosteum is generally intact on the side of the metaphyseal fragment and may aid in maintaining reduction of the fracture. Interposed soft tissue that may impede reduction is most likely found on the side opposite to the metaphyseal fragment. A type III injury consists of a fracture through the physis exiting through the epiphysis into the joint. A type IV injury describes a vertical, intraarticular fracture that traverses the epiphysis, physis, and metaphysis. Type V fractures are crush injuries to the physeal cartilage. These rare injuries are usually diagnosed late.

Coronal fractures of the femoral condyles—Hoffa fractures—have been described in children.[41,42,56–58] Depending on the location of the fracture line, these injuries may be classified as type III Salter-Harris fractures, or they may be entirely intraepiphyseal (Fig. 13.6).

EMERGENT TREATMENT

A careful neurovascular examination is required in all distal femoral physeal fractures but especially in hyperextension injuries. The presence and strength of the pedal pulses and the function of the common peroneal and posterior tibial nerves should be documented. An assessment of the ABI should be considered in any patients with a clinical examination concerning for vascular injury. If the clinical findings of acute ischemia are present—pallor, coolness, cyanosis, or delayed capillary refilling—reduction of the fracture should be attempted as soon as possible, as in ischemic distal femoral metaphyseal fracture. If vascularity is not restored after reduction, immediate vascular exploration is indicated. In the absence of an obviously ischemic limb, patients with any findings concerning for decreased perfusion or vascular injury should be carefully monitored for signs of late ischemia or compartment syndrome and may warrant advanced vascular imaging.[59–61] As described for fractures of the distal femoral metaphysis, serial neurovascular examinations should be performed during the first few days following fracture so as not to miss a developing compartment syndrome or intimal tear with thrombosis.

After initial examination and providing any necessary emergent treatment, the injured extremity should be splinted in a position of comfort and elevated to the level of the heart.

NONOPERATIVE TREATMENT

Nonoperative treatment with a long leg cast is appropriate for nondisplaced Salter-Harris type I and II injuries. The duration of immobilization varies with the age of the patient. Spica cast immobilization can be considered for short, obese children or unreliable patients.[31,33,62] Patients treated nonoperatively should be observed closely and have follow-up radiographs taken 5 to 7 days after initial treatment to identify and address any interval displacement.

Although nondisplaced type III and IV injuries can be treated with cast immobilization and close clinical follow-up, percutaneous fixation with pins or screws supplemented by

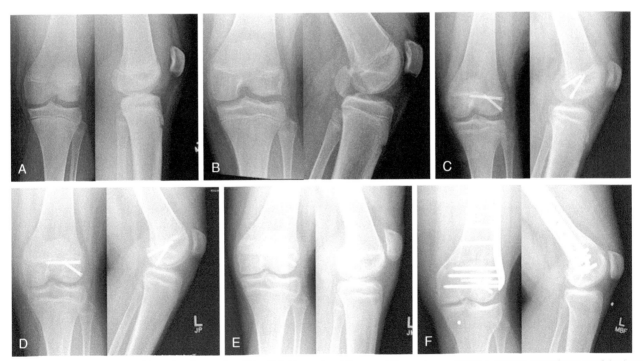

Fig. 13.6 (A) Anteroposterior and lateral radiographs of the distal femur in a 12-year-old boy who sustained a coronal shear fracture of the lateral femoral condyle. The fracture line is barely visible on the lateral radiograph and was not diagnosed. (B) The patient was next seen 2 weeks later. Radiographs clearly show the fracture. (C) The fracture was treated by open reduction and internal fixation. (D) Six months later, the fracture is healed, and the patient has fully recovered the function of his knee. (E) The patient is lost to follow-up and returns 4 years later with a valgus deformity caused by premature physeal closure of the lateral aspect of the distal femoral physis. (F) A corrective osteotomy is performed, obtaining restoration of the anatomic alignment.

cast immobilization is typically preferable to prevent physeal or articular incongruity. In fact, some authors advocate for operative fixation of all type III and IV fractures, as imaging modalities may underestimate intra-articular displacement.[62] As such, Wall and May[62] recommend a 3-cm medial or lateral parapatellar incision when treating these fractures, allowing direct palpation of the joint surface during reduction and fixation.

SURGICAL TREATMENT

Surgical treatment is indicated for all displaced fractures of the distal femoral physis. Treatment options for this injury include closed reduction and percutaneous pin fixation followed by application of a long leg cast and open reduction and internal fixation.

CLOSED REDUCTION AND PERCUTANEOUS FIXATION

Closed reduction and percutaneous fixation is recommended for displaced type I and II fractures and for nondisplaced type III and IV fractures.

The reduction technique varies depending on the displacement of the fracture. In general, the surgical assistant secures the proximal thigh while the surgeon accentuates the deformity, applies longitudinal traction, and ultimately reduces the distal fragment into the appropriate position. General anesthesia and muscle paralysis will help ensure that this reduction maneuver is performed with attention not to further damage the physis through forceful reduction. In instances in which the distal fragment is displaced anteriorly, the reduction maneuver may be performed with the patient placed in either the supine or prone position.

Internal fixation makes subsequent displacement less likely, allows the use of a long leg cast with a greater margin of safety, and avoids having to place the knee in an extreme position of flexion or extension to maintain the reduction.[33,63–66] After the fracture is reduced under image intensifier control, smooth transphyseal pins are inserted retrograde in a crossed fashion for type I injuries and type II injuries with small metaphyseal fragments (Fig. 13.7). The pins should cross above (not at) the physis and engage the metaphyseal cortices. The pins are bent to avoid migration. They may be bent and cut beneath the skin or percutaneously. They can alternatively be advanced to exit the skin proximally, proximal to the knee joint, where they can be bent and left percutaneously. Type II fractures with an adequately sized metaphyseal fragment on both AP and lateral views are best stabilized with all-metaphyseal cannulated screws (Fig. 13.8). Type III fractures are best stabilized with all-epiphyseal pins or cannulated screws (Fig. 13.9). Type IV fractures are stabilized with all-metaphyseal smooth pins or screws with supplementary all-epiphyseal fixation, if necessary (Figs. 13.10 and 13.11).

After fixation is achieved, the knee is brought through a full range of motion under fluoroscopy to confirm the stability of the construct. A long leg cast is applied with the knee immobilized in 20 to 30 degrees of flexion. Percutaneous pins should be removed at 4 weeks so that the risk of infection is reduced. Cast immobilization should continue for a total of 6 weeks but may require longer in older children.

OPEN REDUCTION AND INTERNAL FIXATION

Open reduction is indicated for all type I and II fractures that cannot be accurately reduced by closed methods or if an arterial injury has occurred at the time of fracture. If the epiphysis is displaced laterally, a medial approach provides visualization of any obstacles to reduction and avoids disruption of the intact lateral periosteal hinge. If the epiphysis is displaced medially, a lateral approach is recommended for similar reasons. A posterior approach should be used if arterial exploration is indicated. Once the fracture is reduced, fixation is achieved as described above.

Open reduction with internal fixation is further recommended for all displaced type III and IV fractures to restore congruity of the articular surface. Because type III and IV fractures are intra-articular, an approach that provides adequate visualization to both the articular surface and the physis or metaphysis is required.

Type III fractures are approached through an anteromedial or anterolateral arthrotomy, depending on the location of the vertical component of the fracture through the epiphysis. Alternatively, arthroscopically assisted reduction is a viable alternative to those surgeons with that skillset.[39] Once accurate reduction is achieved, the fracture is stabilized with all-epiphyseal partially threaded cancellous screws placed across the fracture under image intensifier control (Fig. 13.9).

For type IV fractures, the chosen approach should allow for visualization of the epiphyseal and metaphyseal fracture line. Once accurate reduction is achieved, the fracture is stabilized with one or two all-metaphyseal cancellous partially threaded screws. An all-epiphyseal screw is added only if adequate stability of the fracture cannot be achieved by fixation of the metaphyseal fragment alone.

Postoperative immobilization can be achieved with a long leg cast or knee immobilizer based on surgeon preference in addition to the patient's age and perceived reliability. If secure fixation is achieved and a knee immobilizer is used for supplemental immobilization, early range of motion of the knee may be encouraged. Supplemental immobilization can be discontinued 6 weeks postoperatively, beginning a rehabilitation protocol focused on recovering knee range of motion. Weight-bearing should be avoided until radiographs confirm that the fracture is fully healed.

Open reduction and internal fixation is further indicated for coronal shear fractures. The fracture is exposed through a medial or lateral parapatellar approach, depending on which condyle is affected. After anatomic reduction, interfragmentary lag screws are placed through and buried beneath the articular cartilage without crossing the physis. Postoperatively, a long leg cast or brace is used. As with type III and type IV fractures, early range of motion of the knee may be encouraged, but weight-bearing should be avoided until radiographs confirm fracture healing.

OUTCOME

Outcomes associated with fractures of the distal femoral physis are generally good. The patient should continue to be followed clinically and radiographically after fracture union to allow for early identification of growth disturbances.

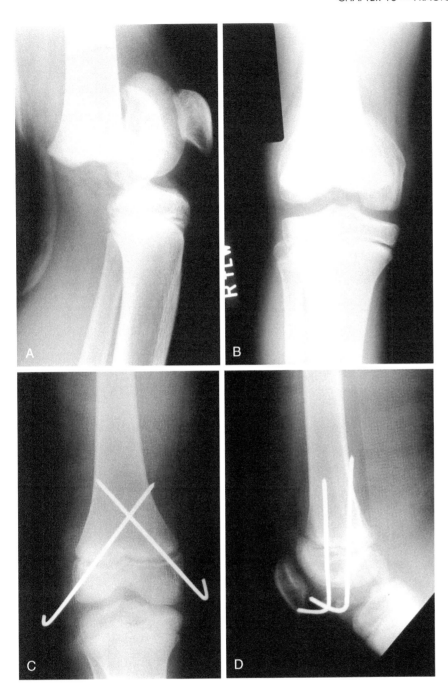

Fig. 13.7 Salter-Harris type I fracture of the distal femoral physis in a 13-year-old boy. The patient sustained a hyperextension injury of the knee without any neurovascular injury. (A) Lateral radiograph of the knee showing a completely displaced Salter-Harris type I physeal injury of the distal end of the femur along with anterior displacement of the femoral condyles. (B) Anteroposterior (AP) radiograph of the same knee demonstrating displacement of the condyles. (C) AP radiograph after closed reduction and percutaneous pinning showing anatomic restoration of the fracture. Note that the pins are smooth and have crossed the physis. (D) Lateral radiograph of the knee showing anatomic reduction of the fracture. (Courtesy of Dr. Vernon T. Tolo, Children's Hospital Los Angeles, Los Angeles, CA.)

COMPLICATIONS

LATE DISPLACEMENT

Loss of initial reduction may occur in fractures treated by closed reduction and cast immobilization. Close clinical and radiological follow-up is essential in such cases to ensure early identification of any loss of reduction, allowing for surgical correction of the displacement. In addition, some patients may initially present with a displaced fracture several days after injury. Although evidence is generally lacking, the consensus of most authorities is that displaced type I and II fractures should not undergo manipulative reduction after 7 to 10 days for fear of causing further physeal injury.[67] It is probably better to accept a malunion after this period of time and to allow the fracture to heal and remodel rather than performing a late open reduction. Depending on patient age and outcome, residual deformity can be addressed with an osteotomy or with guided growth. Unlike type I and II fractures, type III and IV fractures with late displacement should undergo open reduction and internal fixation to restore articular congruity.

NEUROVASCULAR INJURY

The incidence of an associated compartment syndrome has been estimated to be approximately 1%. Volkmann ischemic contracture has been reported in two patients in a series of 151 distal femoral physeal fractures.[31] Although the reported incidence of this complication is low, the consequences are often devastating. The importance of early recognition and prompt intervention in children who demonstrate the signs and symptoms of compartment syndrome cannot be overemphasized.

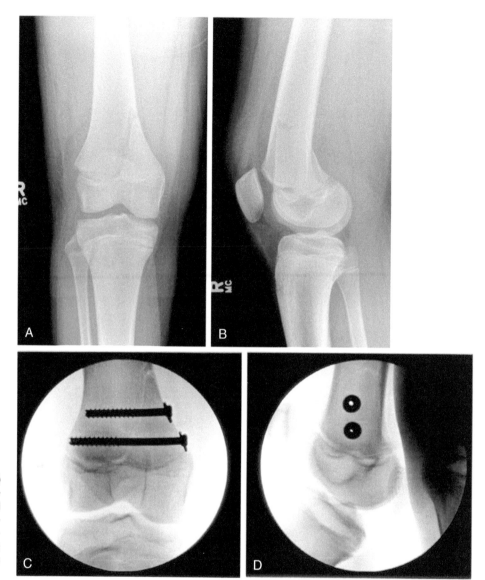

Fig. 13.8 (A and B) Anteroposterior (AP) and lateral radiographs of the distal femur in a 15-year-old boy who sustained a Salter-Harris type II fracture of the distal femoral physis. (C and D) AP and lateral radiographs after closed reduction and stabilization of the fracture with two cannulated screws.

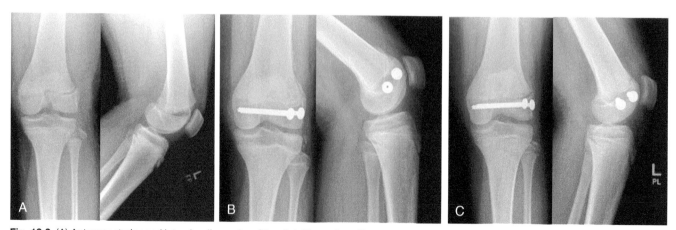

Fig. 13.9 (A) Anteroposterior and lateral radiographs of the distal femur in a 12-year-old boy who sustained a Salter-Harris type III fracture of the distal femoral physis. (B) Radiographs obtained 1 month after an open reduction and internal fixation with all-epiphyseal screws was performed. (C) Four months after the original injury, the fracture is healed in an anatomic position.

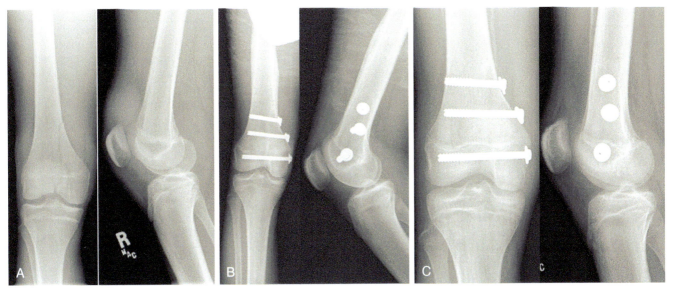

Fig. 13.10 (A) Anteroposterior and lateral radiographs of the distal femur in a 16-year-old boy who sustained a Salter-Harris type IV fracture of the distal femoral physis. (B) Radiographs obtained 1 month after an open reduction and internal fixation achieved with a combination of metaphyseal and epiphyseal screws. (C) Ten months after the original injury, the fracture is healed in an anatomic position.

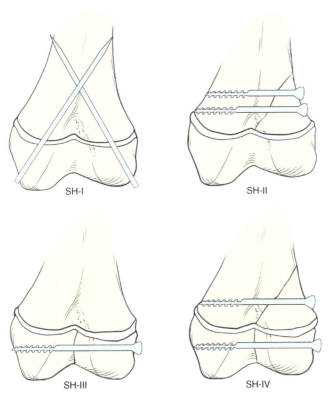

Fig. 13.11 Stabilization techniques for distal femoral epiphyseal fractures using smooth pins or partially threaded cancellous lag screws.

Associated peroneal nerve palsy has also been reported by Eid et al[31] to be as high as 7.3%, resolving in all cases within 3 months of injury without the need for routine surgical exploration. However, in cases in which the neurologic deficit persists beyond 3 months, electromyographic testing should be considered, and further intervention may be warranted.

LIGAMENT AND MENISCAL INJURY

A number of authors have reported concomitant distal femoral physeal fractures and ligamentous injuries.[31,43–45,68,69] Most often, the ligamentous injuries are not appreciated at the time the physeal injuries are treated. In these instances, laxity of the knee joint is discovered after the fracture has healed. Anterior laxity has been reported most frequently, followed by lateral and medial laxity. These reports emphasize the need for continued follow-up after fracture union as well as consideration of advanced imaging at the time of presentation.

GROWTH DISTURBANCE

Although the prognosis for a fracture of the distal femoral physis is generally good, growth arrest and angular deformity are more common than one might expect according to the Salter-Harris classification.[31–34,55,69–71] A meta-analysis by Basener and colleagues[55] reviewed 564 fractures involving the distal femoral physis. Overall, 52% of patients developed a growth disturbance. This complication occurred in 36% of type I fractures, 58% of type II fractures, 49% of type III fractures, and 64% of type IV fractures. Unexpectedly high rates of physeal disturbances following distal femoral physeal fractures may be associated with the large forces required to cause physeal separation at this site, especially in younger patients whose thicker periosteal and perichondrial sheaths typically provide greater stability.[33]

Growth disturbances are more likely to occur in fractures that are initially displaced,[32,55,66,70,71] in younger patients,[31,33] and in those in which anatomic reduction is not achieved.[32] Riseborough[33] observed that fractures occurring in children with ages between 2 and 11 years were more likely to result in growth disturbances than similar fractures in adolescents, as they were typically a result of higher-energy trauma. The association between high-energy mechanism and growth disturbances has been corroborated by more recent series.[64] Further, transphyseal fixation increases risk for growth disturbance. Although we advocate for transphyseal smooth cross-pin fixation in type I and some type II fractures, there is animal evidence that physeal bars may result from even small-diameter smooth pin fixation that crosses the physis.[72]

Careful clinical evaluation is recommended at 6-month intervals after the injury to assess lower extremity alignment and leg length. Serial long leg alignment films should be obtained every 6 months as well. In addition to angular deformities and complete growth disturbances, partial inhibition of growth, or growth deceleration, can occur after distal femoral physeal injuries and can be identified with serial radiographic examinations.[33] Isolated instances of growth stimulation after these fractures have also been reported.[66] Therefore, these patients should be monitored until skeletal maturity. Multiple authors have reported following the configuration of Harris-Park growth lines to detect a growth disturbance early after fracture treatment. If these lines extend across the entire metaphysis in both planes and remained parallel to it, a growth arrest is unlikely.[64,73]

Leg length inequalities estimated to result in less than a 2-cm differential at skeletal maturity require no treatment. If the estimated discrepancy at maturity is between 2 and 5 cm, an appropriately timed epiphysiodesis of the contralateral extremity may be indicated. For inequalities estimated at maturity to be more than 5 cm, lengthening should be considered.

Angular deformities may result from either malunion or partial growth arrest. Significant angular deformity caused by malunion may be managed by osteotomy or, when appropriate, by guided growth through hemiepiphysiodesis. Treatment options for a progressive angular deformity caused by a partial growth disturbance include osseous bridge resection, osteotomy, or completing the epiphysiodesis in the remaining portion of the physis. Osseous bridge resection may be considered for lesions involving less than 50% of the physis in children who have at least 2 years of growth remaining.[29,74,75] Results are best if the osseous bar is located peripherally. The surgical incision is made either laterally or medially, depending on the location of the bar. The area of resection is determined preoperatively based on advanced imaging with either an MRI or CT scan. A high-speed burr is employed to resect the osseous bridge until normal physeal cartilage is visualized circumferentially within the defect. The defect is then packed with either autogenous fat or methyl methacrylate (Cranioplast) to prevent reformation of the osseous bridge. Small metal markers placed in the metaphysis and the epiphysis aid follow-up evaluation of growth resumption. If varus or valgus deformity of the distal end of the femur is greater than 20 degrees at the time of bridge resection, a distal femoral osteotomy should also be performed to realign the knee joint.[75] Guided growth with hemiepiphysiodesis of the preserved half of the physis may be considered as an adjunct in lesser degrees of deformity in children with sufficient skeletal growth remaining.

An osteotomy with complete epiphysiodesis may be necessary when the bridge is too large to excise or in children who are approaching skeletal maturity.

NONUNION

Nonunion has been reported in coronal shear fractures involving the femoral epiphysis.[42,58] These reports highlight the importance of early diagnosis and treatment of these uncommon injuries by open reduction and internal fixation.

OSTEOCHONDRAL FRACTURES

An osteochondral fracture of the knee is most commonly seen in adolescent patients. It is often associated with patellar dislocation, being present in up to 75% of acute patellar dislocations in children and adolescents.[76–78]

PERTINENT ANATOMY

The etiology of these fractures is likely related to the unique structure of the cartilage-bone interface in the developing knee. Multiple authors have postulated that the pediatric population is most susceptible to these fractures because the calcified cartilage layer is immature. This results in a weakened cartilaginous-bone interface.[79,80] One relatively recent histopathologic study concluded that adolescents were particularly susceptible to osteochondral fractures because of structural changes that occur in the anchoring region of the osteochondral junction during skeletal maturation.[80] They demonstrated that fingers of compliant cartilage penetrate deep into the subchondral bone in immature tissue, providing a strong cartilaginous anchor. In mature tissue, articular cartilage is secured to the subchondral bone by a well-defined layer of calcified cartilage. During adolescence, the interdigitating fingers are replaced with a calcified matrix before the mature calcified cartilage layer is fully developed. This makes the adolescent more susceptible to failure in the osteochondral region.

MECHANISM OF INJURY

Osteochondral fractures of the knee most often result from either a direct force exerted on a flexed knee or, more commonly, shearing forces associated with acute patellar dislocation.[81–84] These injuries most commonly occur in adolescents. When associated with patellar dislocation, these fractures occur when the dislocated patella slides tangentially over the surface of the lateral femoral condyle.[77] The fracture may occur during either the dislocation or relocation. Rorabeck and Bobechko[84] estimated that osteochondral fractures occur in approximately 5% of all acute patellar dislocations occurring in children. Nietosvaara and colleagues[77] found associated osteochondral fractures, either capsular avulsions or intra-articular loose bodies, in 28 of 72 children (39%) after an acute patellar dislocation. Stanitski and Paletta[85] reported articular injuries in 34 of 48 older children and adolescents (71%) following acute patellar dislocation. More recently, Seeley and colleagues[78] noted 46 osteochondral injuries in 122 children (38%) with acute patellar dislocation.

EVALUATION

EXAMINATION

Most patients with an osteochondral fracture report a twisting injury on a flexed knee. Usually, a painful "snap" is heard or felt. The child may report a sensation of "giving way" or that the knee "went out of joint." Hemarthrosis occurs rapidly, and weight-bearing is difficult or impossible.

A child with an osteochondral fracture presents with a painful, swollen joint. The child may hold the knee in 10 degrees to 15 degrees of flexion, and any attempts at range of motion are resisted. Tenderness may be elicited over the injured portion of the articular surface. The patient may also have a positive patellar apprehension sign and exhibit tenderness over the medial patellar retinaculum. One should ascertain the presence of hypermobility in other joints, as adolescents without generalized joint laxity have a twofold increased incidence of articular lesions after acute patellar dislocation.[86]

IMAGING

Radiographic evaluation should include orthogonal views of the knee, as well as tunnel and patellar skyline views. Osteochondral fractures may be difficult to diagnose with plain radiographs alone, especially if the ossified portion of the fragment is small.[85–88] Although CT imaging[89] was previously the gold standard in evaluating these injuries, MRI is the current gold standard for visualizing the size and location of osteochondral fragments.[78,90,91] In fact, MRI confirmed an osteochondral injury that was not seen on plain radiographs in 21 of 46 children (44%) in one series.[78] These injuries have been reportedly identified through diagnostic arthroscopy as well.[77,85,86,88,89,92–94]

CLASSIFICATION

Rorabeck and Bobechko[84] described three fracture patterns following acute patellar dislocations: inferomedial fracture of the patella, fracture of the lateral femoral condyle, and a combination of the two (Fig. 13.12). Fractures involving the medial femoral condyle are less common and usually result from a direct blow to the knee.

EMERGENT TREATMENT

After examination, the affected extremity should be splinted in a position of comfort and elevated. If a tense hemarthrosis is present, it may be aspirated to relieve pain. Neurovascular function should be monitored pending definitive treatment.

NONOPERATIVE TREATMENT

Nonoperative management with a short period of knee immobilization may be elected for very small osteochondral or chondral-only fragments. Arthroscopic evaluation and treatment is reserved in these cases for persistent mechanical symptoms or effusion.[92] Once the swelling has subsided, rehabilitation of the knee can be initiated.

SURGICAL TREATMENT

Most authorities recommend early operative management of acute osteochondral fractures of the knee.[27,81–84,93] Whether the fragment is excised or replaced depends on the size and origin of the fragment. However, authors do not agree on the size of the fragment that mandates reduction and fixation. In general, if the fragment is small and from a non–weight-bearing surface, it may be excised arthroscopically. Larger fragments originating from weight-bearing areas should be replaced.

Osteochondral fractures can be fixated with the use of several techniques approached through an arthrotomy or arthroscopically (Fig. 13.13). Countersunk mini-fragment screws (Fig. 13.14)[82,93]; headless variable-pitch compression screws[95–97]; small, threaded Steinmann pins inserted in a retrograde fashion[27]; fibrin sealant or other adhesives[93,98,99]; and bioabsorbable pegs (Fig. 13.15)[100–102] have all been used with similar results. Of note, aseptic synovitis has been reported in patients treated with intraarticular biodegradable internal fixation.[103]

Postoperative protocols vary depending on the degree of stability achieved at the time of surgery. If adequate stability of the fracture is achieved, a postoperative knee immobilizer can be applied, and early range of motion of the joint and quadriceps muscle-strengthening exercises can be initiated. Full weight-bearing is restricted until there is radiographic evidence of fracture healing.

When an acute patellar dislocation requires excision or reattachment of an osteochondral fragment, several authors have recommended concomitant procedures to realign the extensor apparatus of the knee to prevent redislocation, especially when factors associated with patellofemoral malalignment are present.[81–84,92–94]

OUTCOME

Although outcomes following fixation or arthroscopic removal of osteochondral fractures of the knee are generally good, treatment is guided only on retrospective case series. Several studies have described satisfactory short- and intermediate-term outcomes following fixation of osteochondral fractures in children and adolescents.[100,102,104,105] One study suggested that patients with fractures involving the

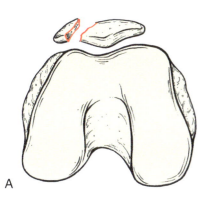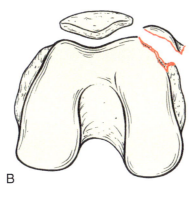

A   B

Fig. 13.12 Diagrammatic representation of the medial pole of the patella (A) and an osteochondral fracture of the lateral femoral condyle (B), both secondary to patellar dislocation. Radiographs may appear normal, but the hemarthrosis aspirate will contain fat droplets. Arthroscopy is indicated when these chondral or osteochondral fractures are suspected.

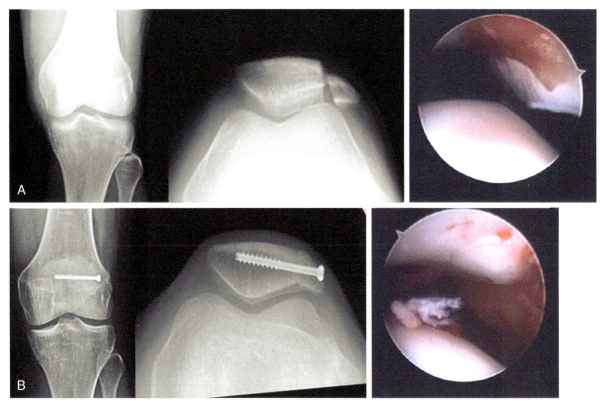

Fig. 13.13 Radiographs of a 17-year-old female who had a fall on her knee. (A) Anteroposterior and lateral radiographs of her knee showing a lateral osteochondral fracture. The patient undergoes arthroscopic repair of the fracture. Intraoperative image demonstrates significant intra-articular step-off on the patellar articular surface. (B) Anteroposterior and lateral radiographs obtained postoperatively demonstrating an anatomic reduction and hardware in good position. Intra-operative image demonstrating complete restoration of the articular surface of the patella.

weight-bearing of the lateral femoral condyle may have a poorer outcome than those with fractures that lie outside of the weight-bearing surface.[78] Further research is needed to determine whether surgical repair of these injuries will prevent the development of osteoarthritis in the long term.

COMPLICATIONS

Complications of surgical treatment include quadriceps atrophy and loss of motion. Kramer and Pace[92] observed that partially threaded cannulated screws may leave an indentation on the articular surface and, if not countersunk, may abrade the tibial surface, requiring later removal. They also noted that headless screws, despite being placed deep to the articular surface, may back out over time, requiring removal.

FRACTURES OF THE PATELLA

The patella is the largest sesamoid bone in the body. It lies within the tendon of the quadriceps, and functions to increase the efficiency of the quadriceps as a knee extensor. In general, patellar fractures in children are uncommon, representing about 1% of all pediatric fractures.[106–110] Most fractures of the body of the patella are seen in adolescents, whereas sleeve-type avulsion fractures are seen more commonly in children.

PERTINENT ANATOMY

The patella begins to ossify between 3 and 5 years of age. Ossification often begins as multiple foci that gradually coalesce. As the patellar ossification center expands, the peripheral margins may appear irregular and may be associated with accessory ossification centers.[111] Incomplete coalescence of a superolaterally located accessory center of ossification results in a bipartite patella, which may be confused with a fracture. When present, a bipartite patella is usually evident by 12 years of age and may persist into adult years.[112] Ossification of the patella is generally complete by late adolescence.

MECHANISM OF INJURY

Transverse or comminuted fractures of the main body of the patella rarely occur in children because the patella is largely cartilaginous and has greater mobility than in adults. Most of these injuries occur in adolescence when ossification is nearly complete[113] (Fig. 13.16). As in adults, fractures of the patella in children may result from either direct or indirect forces.[114] An avulsion fracture of the inferior or superior[108,115] pole of the patella, the so-called sleeve fracture, is an indirect injury caused by a powerful contraction of the quadriceps muscle applied to a flexed knee. These fractures usually occur in individuals involved in explosive acceleration activities, such as jumping.

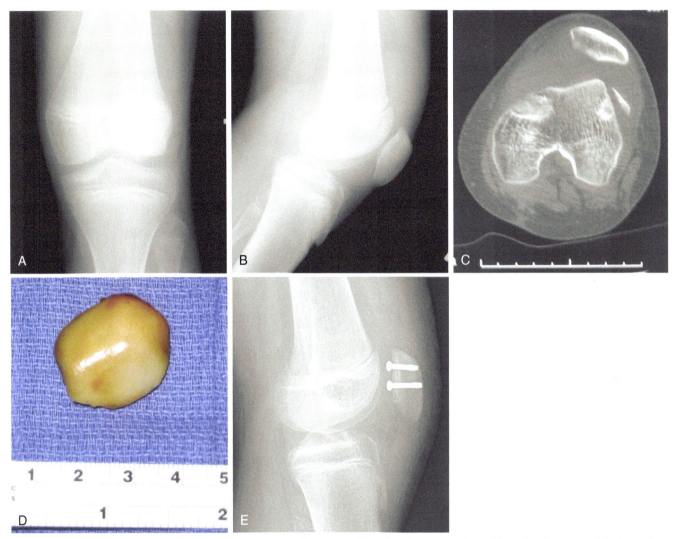

Fig. 13.14 An 11-year-old girl dislocated her patella while playing soccer. (A and B) Anteroposterior and lateral radiographs of the knee show no obvious fracture. (C) Computed tomography shows a large osteochondral fracture off the medial facet of the patella. (D) Appearance of the fragment at operation. (E) Her fracture was stabilized with the use of two cannulated screws whose heads were countersunk below the articular surface. A lateral retinacular release and a medial retinacular imbrication were performed to provide optimal tracking of the patella.

Fractures of the patella have also been attributed to repetitive stress. Hensal and colleagues[116] reported bilateral simultaneous fractures of the patella that resulted from indirect trauma in a 17-year-old boy. At surgery, sclerosis of the fracture edges was thought to be indicative of underlying areas of stress reaction. Iwaya and Takatori[117] described lateral longitudinal fractures of the patella occurring in three children ages 10 to 12 years. The authors attributed these to repetitive activities. Ogden and colleagues[112] suggested that instances of painful bipartite patella may be because of a chronic stress fracture.

EVALUATION

EXAMINATION

A patient with a fracture of the main body of the patella usually has local tenderness and soft tissue swelling. Hemarthrosis of the knee joint is often present. Active extension of the knee, especially against resistance, is usually difficult. If the disruption is minimal, the child might be able to lift the leg by internally rotating the affected limb using tension of the fascia lata. A palpable gap at either the upper or the lower end of the patella, in association with swelling, pain, and functional limitation, indicates the presence of a sleeve fracture. A high-riding patella (patella alta) suggests that the extensor mechanism has been disrupted.

With marginal fractures, local tenderness and swelling over the affected region of the patella may be the only findings present. In these injuries, straight leg raising may often be possible. The presence of an avulsion fracture of the medial margin suggests the diagnosis of acute patellar dislocation that may have reduced spontaneously.[118] With an associated dislocation, other findings such as medial retinacular tenderness and a positive apprehension sign may also be present.

IMAGING

Orthogonal radiographs of the affected patella are needed to evaluate fractures of the main body of the patella. Transverse fractures are best visualized on the lateral view. A lateral radiograph taken with the knee in 30 degrees of flexion may better define the soft tissue stability and true extent of displacement that is present.[27,118]

Small flecks of bone adjacent to the superior or inferior pole in a patient who has sustained an acute injury may indicate the presence of a sleeve fracture. Lateral radiographs of both the injured and unaffected knee in 30 degrees of flexion are usually sufficient to confirm the presence of patella alta on the injured side when a sleeve fracture is suspected. MRI may be helpful for detecting a sleeve fracture when the diagnosis is not clear from the clinical and plain radiographic findings. Marginal fractures that are oriented longitudinally may be best seen on a skyline view of the patella.

CLASSIFICATION

Fractures of the patella in children are generally classified according to the location, pattern, and degree of displacement. One fracture unique to children is the so-called sleeve fracture that traditionally was described as occurring through the cartilage on the inferior pole of the patella (Fig. 13.17). This fracture is most commonly seen in children 8 to 12 years of age. With this injury, a large sleeve of cartilage is pulled off the main body of the patella along with a small piece of bone from the distal pole. Grogan and colleagues[118] observed that avulsion fractures may involve any region of the periphery of the patella. They described four patterns of injury: superior, inferior, medial (which often accompanies an acute dislocation of the patella), and lateral (which they attributed to chronic stress caused by repetitive pulling from the vastus lateralis muscle). Other authors have further described the occurrence and treatment of the less common superior sleeve fracture.[108]

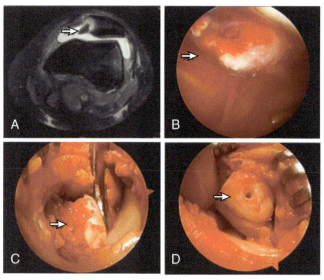

Fig. 13.15 A 16-year-old male sustained a patellar dislocation. (A) Axial magnetic resonance image demonstrates a 2 × 2-cm osteochondral fracture *(arrow)* of the medial patella. (B) Arthroscopic appearance of fragment *(arrow)*. (C) Fragment after arthrotomy *(arrow)*. (D) Fragment after open reduction and internal fixation with a bioabsorbable screw.

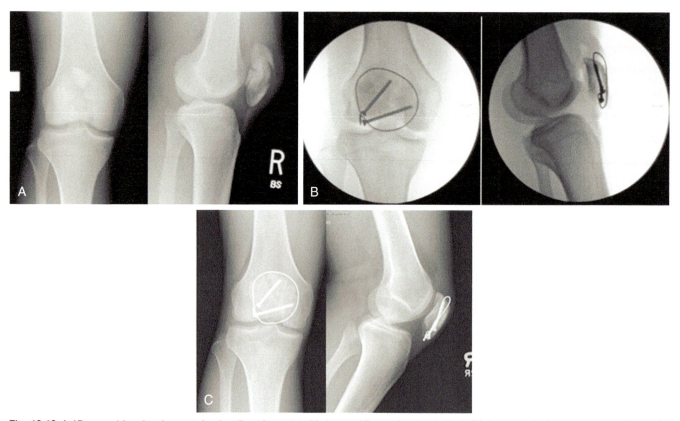

Fig. 13.16 A 17-year-old male who sustained a direct impact to his knee while playing basketball. (A) Anteroposterior and lateral radiographs demonstrating a severely comminuted patellar fracture. (B) Intraoperative fluoroscopic images obtained after open reduction and internal fixation using cerclage wires and cannulated screws. Note the restoration of the articular surface. (C) Anteroposterior and lateral radiographs obtained 8 months after the original injury, demonstrating healing of the fracture.

EMERGENT TREATMENT

After examination, the patient with a patellar fracture should have the injured extremity elevated and splinted in a position of comfort, and ice should be applied to control swelling. If a tense hemarthrosis is present, it may be aspirated to relieve pain. The neurovascular function of the affected extremity should be monitored pending definitive treatment.

NONOPERATIVE TREATMENT

Closed treatment in a cylinder cast or knee immobilizer with the knee in full extension is recommended for nondisplaced transverse fractures and small marginal fractures,

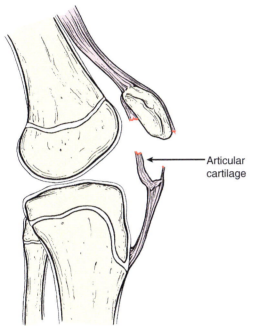

Fig. 13.17 Sleeve fracture of the patella. A small segment of the distal pole of the patella is avulsed with a relatively large portion of the articular surface.

Articular cartilage

particularly if active extension of the knee is present. The patient may be permitted to bear weight as tolerated with crutches. The immobilization can be removed in 4 to 6 weeks when healing is complete, and gradual range-of-motion exercises can be initiated.

SURGICAL TREATMENT

The treatment guidelines for transverse patellar fractures in children are generally the same as those for adults.[109,113] Operative treatment is necessary for transverse fractures that show more than 3 mm of diastasis or step-off at the articular surface, and for sleeve fractures.[27,109] Fixation may be achieved with the use of the modified tension band technique with a wire loop around two longitudinally placed K-wires (Fig. 13.18). The use of an absorbable suture, as an alternative to the more traditional stainless steel wire, or as a fixation method, either through bone tunnels or in association with bone anchors, has also been described.[119–124] Other fixation options include a circumferential wire loop (Fig. 13.16), interfragmentary screws, or cannulated screws in combination with a tension band wire[125,126] The retinaculum should be repaired at the time of osseous fixation. Comminuted fractures of the distal pole are best managed by partial patellectomy.[119] Total patellectomy is reserved for injuries in which the comminution is widespread and not amenable for fixation.

OUTCOME

Although the outcome following treatment of a fracture of the patella is generally good, there is no evidence stronger than retrospective case series to guide treatment of these injuries in children.[110] Reported results are poorer after fractures that show greater displacement and comminution.[113] The long-term outcome may also be influenced by accompanying cartilage damage.[110] Further research is needed to determine whether surgical repair of these injuries will provide satisfactory function and prevent the development of osteoarthritis in the long term.

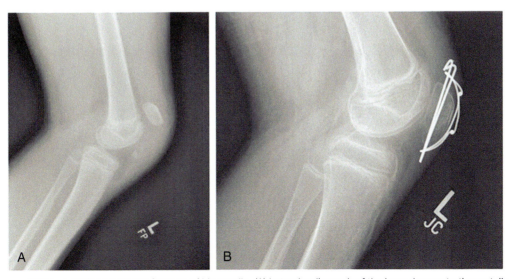

Fig. 13.18 A 10-year-old boy sustained a sleeve fracture of his patella. (A) Lateral radiograph of the knee demonstrating patella alta and a small, visible fragment of bone avulsed off the inferior pole. (B) Lateral radiograph 2 months postoperatively showing a healed fracture.

COMPLICATIONS

Complications that may occur after displaced patellar fractures that are not adequately reduced include patella alta, extensor lag, and quadriceps atrophy.[27,121]

TIBIAL EMINENCE FRACTURE

The anterior tibial eminence, or anterior tibial spine, is the distal site of attachment of the ACL. Fractures of the tibial eminence are rare, occurring in about 3 per 100,000 children every year, but represent about 2 % to 5% of pediatric knee injuries in which an effusion is present.[127] These fractures are seen most commonly in children between 8 and 14 years of age.

PERTINENT ANATOMY

Before complete ossification of the proximal end of the tibia is achieved, the surface of the anterior tibial spine is cartilaginous.[128] The ACL arises from the medial side of the lateral femoral condyle and attaches distally in the anterior intercondylar region of the tibia. The anterior horn of the lateral meniscus is attached in close proximity. The femoral attachment of the posterior cruciate ligament is to the lateral surface of the medial femoral condyle. Distally, this ligament attaches to the posterior intercondylar area of the proximal tibia.

MECHANISM OF INJURY

When excessive tension is applied to the ACL, the incompletely ossified tibial spine offers less resistance than the ligament, and the tensile stress thus leads to failure through the cancellous bone beneath the tibial spine.

Tibial spine fractures are most likely to be caused by hyperextension or valgus and external rotation of the knee. Traumatic forces that would normally rupture the ACL in an adult may instead lead to a tibial spine fracture in a child, usually involving the anterior spine and rarely the posterior spine.[129,130] Posterior tibial spine fractures are more likely to occur in skeletally mature individuals (Fig. 13.19).[101]

Historically, the most common event associated with fracture of the tibial spine is a fall from a bicycle. Some authors have gone as far as saying that a child who has a painful, swollen knee after falling from a bicycle must be assumed to have a tibial spine fracture until it is proved otherwise.[29,128] More recently, these fractures have commonly been reported to occur in children participating in sports activities or in children involved in motor vehicle accidents.[131]

EVALUATION

EXAMINATION

A patient with a fracture of the tibial spine usually presents with knee pain and an effusion and is reluctant to bear weight. The knee is usually held in a slightly flexed position because of hamstring spasm.

IMAGING

Early recognition of the degree of injury to the knee in children, including a complete radiologic assessment, is of cornerstone importance to minimize the risk of misdiagnosis, delayed surgical treatment, and long-term sequelae.[132] AP and lateral radiographs demonstrate a tibial spine fracture. The degree of displacement is best evaluated on the lateral view. The base of the tibial spine must be carefully inspected on the lateral view for discontinuity of the bony margin. When routine radiographs show only small flecks of bone in the intercondylar notch, CT or MRI may be useful for further evaluating the injury. MRI is also useful in evaluating concomitant injuries such as meniscal or cartilaginous injuries to the knee. Recently, Mitchell et al[131] found, either by preoperative MRI or at the time of surgery, that 33% and 12% of patients with type II and III tibial spine fractures, respectively, had a concomitant meniscal tear.

CLASSIFICATION

Meyers and McKeever[128,133] classified tibial spine fractures into three main types (Fig. 13.20). In type I fractures, the fragment is minimally displaced and shows only slight elevation of the anterior margin. In type II fractures, the avulsed fragment has a posterior hinge, and the anterior portion is

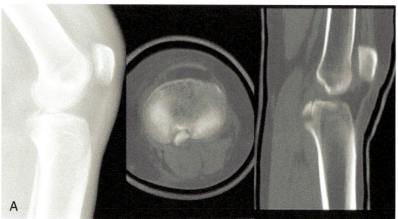
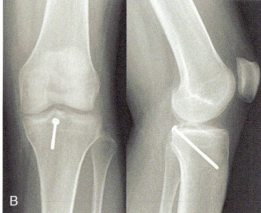

Fig. 13.19 (A) Lateral radiograph and axial and sagittal computed tomography images of the knee of a 16-year-old boy who sustained an avulsion of the posterior tibial spine. (B) Anteroposterior and lateral radiograph of the knee after open reduction and internal fixation of the fracture of the posterior tibial spine through a posterior approach.

elevated from its bone bed. In type III fractures, the avulsed fragment is completely displaced and may be rotated. Later, Zaricznyj[134] described a fourth type of tibial spine fracture involving excessive comminution of the fracture fragment.

EMERGENT TREATMENT

After examination, the patient with a tibial eminence fracture should have the injured extremity elevated and splinted in a position of comfort. To relieve pain, knee aspiration should be considered if a tense hemarthrosis is present. Injection of local anesthesia may facilitate a subsequent attempt at reduction and immobilization of the fracture. The neurovascular function of the affected extremity should be monitored pending definitive treatment.

NONOPERATIVE TREATMENT

The type of fracture and the amount of displacement guide treatment of a tibial eminence fracture. Type I fractures and type II fractures that are minimally displaced may be treated by closed means. If a tense hemarthrosis is present, it should be aspirated under sterile conditions, and a long leg cast should be applied. There is no general agreement as to the ideal amount of knee flexion needed to maintain reduction of a tibial spine fracture in a cast. Bakalim and Wilppula[135] described 10 patients treated by closed reduction and immobilization in hyperextension, noting good results in seven of eight patients with adequate follow-up. Beaty and Kumar[27] recommended immobilizing the knee in 10 degrees to 15 degrees of flexion. Similarly, Meyers and McKeever[133] recommended immobilizing the knee in 20 degrees of flexion. Fyfe and Jackson,[136] noting that the ACL is taut in extension, recommended that the knee be immobilized in 30 to 40 degrees of flexion to relax the ligament. After the cast is applied, radiographs should be taken to confirm reduction of the tibial spine fragment. Radiographs should be repeated in 1 to 2 weeks to ensure that displacement has not occurred. The cast is usually removed 4 weeks after the original injury, in 6 weeks, when gentle range-of-motion exercises can begin.

SURGICAL TREATMENT

Operative reduction, either through a limited anteromedial or anterolateral arthrotomy[137,138] or arthroscopically assisted,[139,140] is indicated for irreducible type II fractures and all type III fractures. Failure to accurately reduce displaced fractures is often because of interposed meniscus, ligament, or soft tissue. Kocher and associates[141] noted entrapment of the anterior horn of the medial meniscus, the intermeniscal ligament, or the anterior horn of the lateral meniscus in 26% of type II fractures and 65% of type III fractures. Mitchell et al[131] reported similar findings. The choice of surgical technique is still a matter of controversy. When comparing open and arthroscopically assisted techniques with regard to quality of reduction, arthrofibrosis rate, and final postoperative clinical and functional scores, Edmonds et al[142] reported no statistical differences. Greater range-of-motion deficits and more laxity with anterior drawer and Lachman tests have been reported for pediatric tibial spine fractures treated through an arthroscopically assisted technique when compared with those treated using an arthrotomy.[127,131] However, significantly lower rates of laxity based on pivot-shift testing have been reported in patients treated using an arthroscopically assisted technique.[127,131]

When reduction is obtained through an anteromedial arthrotomy, the fragment may be secured by passing an absorbable suture through the cartilaginous portion of the fracture fragment and either the anterior lip of the tibial epiphysis or the edge of the anterior portion of the meniscus. Alternatively, the fragment can be secured with smooth K-wires.[134] In an adolescent patient with a small fragment, fixation may be achieved by weaving a suture (either nonabsorbable or absorbable) through the ACL with the ends passed through drill holes in the anterior portion of the tibia.[27,143] Screw fixation, with either metallic or absorbable screws, can be achieved if the bone fragment is large enough to hold secure purchase of a screw (Figs. 13.21 and 13.22).[137–140]

Arthroscopic-assisted reduction and fixation may be preferred based on the experience of the surgeon and is indicated for displaced type II fractures, type III fractures, and

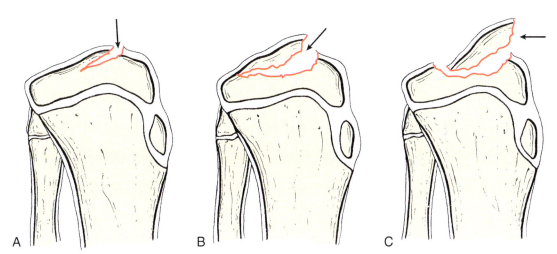

Fig. 13.20 Meyers and McKeever classification of fractures of the anterior tibial spine. (A) Type I fracture with no displacement of the fracture. (B) Type II fracture with elevation of the anterior portion of the anterior tibial spine but with the fracture posteriorly reduced. (C) Type III fracture that is totally displaced.

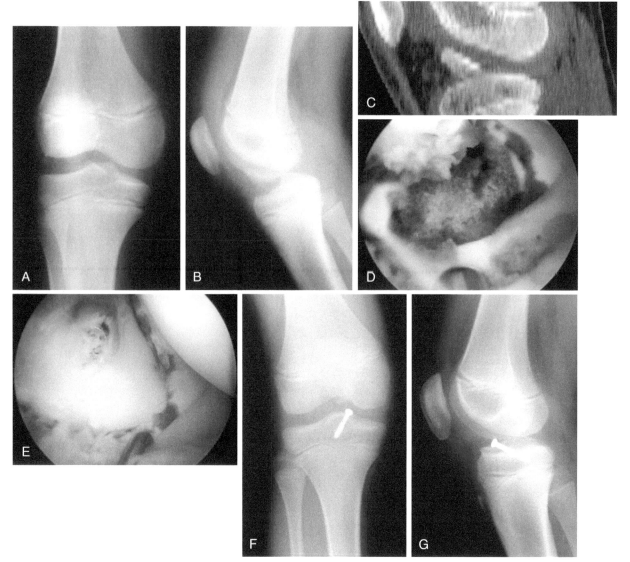

Fig. 13.21 Ten-year-old boy who sustained a type III fracture of the anterior tibial spine as a result of a dirt bike accident. On arrival at the emergency department, he had a large, painful effusion of his knee. (A) Anteroposterior (AP) radiograph of the patient's knee. A displaced fracture of the anterior tibial spine is noted to be elevated from its normal position. (B) On a lateral radiograph of the knee, the completely displaced fracture of the anterior tibial spine is seen to be displaced superiorly. (C) A sagittal reconstruction computed tomographic scan easily demonstrates the fracture fragment displaced from its normal position. (D) Arthroscopic view of the fracture. The bed of the fracture is seen in the middle of the photograph, and the anterior horn of the meniscus is located in the lower portion of the photograph. The fractured fragment is seen superiorly and partially overlying the superolateral portion of the fracture bed. (E) The fragment has been replaced and internally fixed with a screw. One can see the fragment anatomically reduced into its bed. The screw has been partially countersunk into the fracture fragment. A small hook is seen retracting the anterior horn of the meniscus. (F) Postoperative AP radiograph demonstrating that the fragment has been reinserted into its normal position and is well secured with a single cancellous screw. The screw remains entirely within the epiphysis. (G) On this lateral radiograph, the fragment has been reduced anatomically and is internally fixed with a cancellous screw that is directed posteriorly so that the screw has adequate bone surface contact yet remains within the epiphysis and does not risk injuring the physis. (Courtesy of Dr. Neil E. Green, Vanderbilt Children's Hospital, Nashville, TN.)

type IV fractures. Suture fixation[144,145] through the ACL and smaller bone fragments can be performed with the use of basic arthroscopic suture-passing techniques. Sutures can be tied through bone tunnels on the anterior tibial cortex. Several recent studies have compared the efficacy of different methods of suture fixation and types of sutures.[146–148] For a more detailed description of arthroscopic reduction techniques, including suture and screw fixation, the reader is directed to the recent review article by Anderson and Anderson.[149]

At the time of surgery, if a meniscal tear is found, meniscal repair is undertaken. A preoperative MRI is of value if surgical exposure is via arthrotomy, which makes visualization of posterior meniscal tears difficult. Meniscal repair technique will depend on the surgical exposure used to treat the tibial spine fracture and the meniscal tear characteristics.

Depending on the stability of the fixation, a cast or brace is applied with the knee immobilized in 10 degrees to 20 degrees of flexion for 3 to 4 weeks. Once healing is evident on radiographs, range of motion of the knee is initiated. After

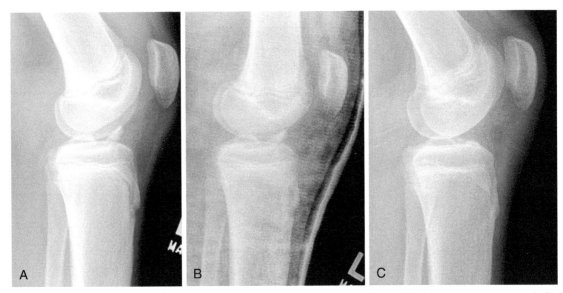

Fig. 13.22 Lateral radiographs of the knee of an 11-year old boy. (A) A type II fracture of the tibial intercondylar eminence is found. (B) After attempted closed reduction (by knee extension), there is no change from the initial radiograph. This is usually the result of a meniscus blocking fracture reduction. (C) Four months postoperatively showing excellent reduction and fracture healing after open reduction and fixation of the fracture using an absorbable screw.

immobilization is discontinued, most patients will benefit from physical therapy consisting of knee range-of-motion and quadriceps-strengthening exercises. A standard ACL reconstruction rehabilitation program can be used, and return to sports activities is allowed when the injured knee has comparable strength and motion to the unaffected knee, usually 4 to 6 months after injury.

OUTCOME

In general, the outcome treatment of tibial eminence fractures in children is good. Some residual knee laxity may be present but does not appear to adversely affect outcome.[150] One study noted poorer outcomes in patients treated for type IV fractures.[151]

Malunion, nonunion, and knee stiffness should be minimized by good surgical technique and appropriate rehabilitation.

COMPLICATIONS

NONUNION AND MALUNION

Nonunion of properly treated fractures is rare, but malunion of type III injuries has been reported. These patients may be seen with clinical instability and a mechanical block to full extension of the knee. For symptomatic patients, mobilization of the tibial spine, excision of excess bone, and reattachment of the tibial fragment in the reduced position may be used to treat the malunion.[136,152]

RESIDUAL KNEE LAXITY

Several authors have documented anterior cruciate laxity and some loss of full knee extension after tibial spine fractures, even those that have healed in an anatomic position.[138,153–157] Laxity has been attributed to the interstitial tearing of the ACL that probably occurs before the fragment is avulsed.[150,153,156–158] During arthroscopic reduction of tibial spine fractures, Kocher and coworkers[155] observed

that, although grossly intact, the ACL often appeared hemorrhagic within its sheath. Late laxity varies according to the severity of the initial injury. When compared with type I injuries, greater laxity has been noted after types II and III fracture.[154,157] Despite the laxity, relatively few patients complain of pain or instability.

Few long-term outcome studies of this injury have been reported. Janarv and colleagues[150] monitored 61 children with anterior tibial spine fractures for an average of 16 years. Although most of their patients had a good clinical outcome at latest follow-up, these authors found no evidence to suggest that the anterior knee laxity that resulted from the injury diminished over time. Because of the persistent anterior knee laxity that has been documented in several articles, the long-term prognosis for this injury remains uncertain, and families of patients with this injury should be counseled accordingly.

STIFFNESS

Stiffness may occasionally occur after either closed or operative treatment of tibial spine fractures and can be a difficult problem to manage. Physical therapy consisting of active and active-assisted range-of-motion exercises and the use of dropout casts may be helpful. If persistent stiffness remains, consideration should be given to manipulation under general anesthesia and arthroscopic lysis of adhesions. Overzealous manipulation has led to fractures of the distal femur and proximal tibia and should be avoided.[159]

Patel and associates[160] found that patients who began range of motion within 4 weeks after treatment of a tibial eminence fracture experienced an earlier return to full activity and a decreased likelihood of eventual arthrofibrosis compared with a group of patients who were immobilized for longer than 4 weeks. Vander Have and colleagues[161] reported a series of 32 patients with arthrofibrosis after treatment of a tibial eminence fracture. Some 29 patients eventually regained full range of motion, but three patients had physeal fractures with manipulation under anesthesia. The authors emphasized the importance of rigid fixation and starting early range of motion in treatment of these fractures. Similarly, May and coworkers[151] reviewed the results of surgery in 22 patients with displaced type II, III, or IV fractures treated by a variety of surgical fixation methods. One factor that predicted return to previous activity level was instituting early range of motion. A recent systematic review showed that knee stiffness was also more likely to occur with type III and IV fractures.[162] Other factors that have been identified as possibly associated with the development of stiffness include performing the surgery in a delayed fashion (≥7 days from injury) and having prolonged operative times (≥120 minutes).[163]

TIBIAL TUBERCLE FRACTURE

Tibial tubercle fractures are relatively uncommon injuries, have a reported incidence of 0.4% to 2.7% of all pediatric fractures,[164–166] and occur most often in boys between 12 and 17 years of age. Sports activities, especially basketball and competitive jumping events, are most commonly associated with this injury.[167–173]

PERTINENT ANATOMY

The proximal tibial physis contributes not only to longitudinal growth of the tibia but also to development of the tibial tubercle. The tibial tubercle, or tibial tuberosity, initially develops as an anterior extension of the proximal tibial physis at around 12 to 15 weeks of gestation.[111] At birth, the tubercle is located approximately near the level of the proximal tibial epiphysis; distal migration occurs after birth.

The epiphyseal ossification center of the proximal part of the tibia appears between the first and third months of life. The ossification center of the tibial tubercle begins in its distal region between the ages of 7 and 9 years and then gradually extends toward the proximal end of the tibia. During adolescence, a small, cartilaginous bridge that eventually dissipates separates these two ossification centers. The physis of the tibial tubercle closes between the ages of 13 and 15 years in girls and 15 and 19 years in boys.[111]

Ogden[111] has observed that the physis underlying the tibial tubercle is initially composed almost exclusively of fibrocartilage rather than the columnar physeal cartilage that is usually present in a region of growth. He suggested that this unusual cytoarchitecture allows the tubercle to better resist the normal tensile stresses applied to it by the quadriceps muscle through the patellar tendon. As the tubercle undergoes progressive ossification, the growth plate underlying the tubercle changes from fibrocartilage to columnar physeal cartilage. Because the tensile strength of columnar cartilage is less than that of fibrocartilage, these changes render the tubercle less able to resist violent tensile stresses, thus making it potentially more vulnerable to separation.

The anterior tibial recurrent artery contributes to the blood supply of the tibial tubercle and has potential clinical implications. Wall[174] demonstrated, by anatomic dissection, numerous leash-like branches of the anterior tibial recurrent artery that terminate along the lateral border of the tibial tubercle. When these vessels were sectioned in a cadaver, he observed that they tended to retract laterally and distally under the fascia and into the muscles of the anterior compartment. The author concluded that continued bleeding from these vessels into the anterior compartment could lead to a compartment syndrome. Pape and colleagues[175] reported two adolescent boys in whom a compartment syndrome developed after an avulsion fracture of the tibial tubercle. They cited bleeding from branches of the anterior tibial recurrent artery as a predisposing factor for this complication.

MECHANISM OF INJURY

This injury usually is the result of active extension of the knee with violent contraction of the quadriceps muscle, as occurs with jumping, or an abrupt passive flexion against a contracted quadriceps muscle, as occurs when a football player is tackled.[167,170,173,176] Sleeve fractures of the tibial tubercle, representing an avulsion of thick periosteum, cartilage, and small bone fragments, have been described in adolescents.[177,178]

Several authors have suggested that Osgood-Schlatter disease may predispose an individual to abrupt disruption of the tibial tubercle.[170,172,173,176] Osgood-Schlatter disease is a common cause of knee pain in active children between the ages of 10 and 14 years. These patients usually present with tenderness directly over the tibial tubercle. Although this condition is self-limited and resolves when the physis of the tibial tubercle closes, affected children may require activity restrictions to allow resolution of symptoms during the early stages. Rosenberg and colleagues[79] concluded, on the basis of imaging studies, that this condition was caused by inflammation of the patellar tendon at its insertion into the tubercle rather than involvement of the bone. According to Ogden and colleagues,[172] Osgood-Schlatter disease appears to involve only the anterior portion of the ossification center of the tubercle; the physis is not involved. They postulated that this condition might somehow alter the physis of the tubercle by increasing the amount of columnar cartilage relative to fibrocartilage, thus predisposing the patient to acute avulsion of the entire tubercle. In a recent systematic review, 23% of patients with a tibial tubercle fracture had concomitant Osgood-Schlatter disease.[179]

EVALUATION

EXAMINATION

Patients with a fracture of the tibial tubercle are seen with local soft tissue swelling and tenderness directly over the fracture site. Patients with nondisplaced type I injuries are usually able to extend the knee against gravity, and knee effusion is not generally present. In type II and type III injuries, active knee extension is not possible. Most of these patients have hemarthrosis of the knee joint. Patella alta may be clinically evident and proportional to the displacement of the fracture fragment.

IMAGING

Accurate lateral radiographs of the tubercle are essential for evaluating this injury. Because the tubercle is just lateral to the midline of the tibia, the best profile is obtained with the tibia in slight internal rotation. Oblique radiographs of the proximal end of the tibia are helpful to fully visualize the extension of the fracture into the knee joint.[172] Small flecks of bone anterior to the distal apophysis accompanied by a patella alta may suggest the presence of a displaced type I injury (Fig. 13.23). Davidson and Letts[180] described three patients with these radiographic findings that were associated with small subchondral fragments of bone along with an extensive avulsion of periosteum from the proximal tibia. Other authors reported similar cases.[181,182] Pandya and colleagues[183] reported that the presence of intra-articular involvement is largely underestimated by plain radiography. They suggested that a CT scan or an MRI should be obtained in selected patients to assess the amount of intra-articular involvement and the presence of accompanying meniscal tears, coronary ligament injuries, and osteochondral defects.

Kramer and colleagues[184] observed that the presence of multiple calcified fragments below the patella in a patient with radiographs showing a tibial tubercle fracture may indicate the presence of a simultaneous avulsion of the tibial tubercle and patellar ligament.

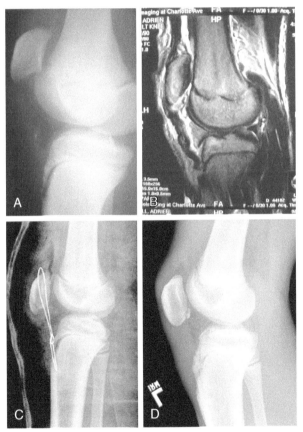

Fig. 13.23 Lateral radiograph of a 13-year-old male who sustained a tear of his patellar tendon both from the patella and the tibial tubercle from high jumping. (A) Lateral radiograph demonstrating the high-riding patella and the small fragments of bone seen just above the tibial tubercle. (B) Magnetic resonance imaging showing avulsion of the patellar tendon from both the tibial tubercle and the inferior pole of the patella. The tendon was repaired at both ends. (C) Postoperative lateral radiograph demonstrating that the patella is back in its normal position. A wire was passed around the superior pole of the patella and through a drill hole in the tibia to reinforce the tendon repair. (D) Radiograph at a 9-month follow-up demonstrates maintenance of the normal patellar position. Clinically, the patient's knee examination results were normal, and he has returned to high jumping. (Courtesy of Dr. Neil E. Green, Vanderbilt Children's Hospital, Nashville, TN.)

CLASSIFICATION

Watson-Jones[185] classified fractures of the tibial tubercle into three types. In the first type, a small fragment of the distal portion of the tubercle is avulsed. In the second type, the entire secondary center of the tubercle is hinged upward, and the apex of the angulation is at the level of the proximal tibial physis. In the third type, the fracture line propagates through the proximal tibial physis into the knee joint.

Ogden and colleagues[172] modified this classification to place greater emphasis on intra-articular extension of the fracture and comminution of the tubercle (Figs. 13.24 and 13.25). In type 1, only the most distal portions of the tubercle are involved. Subtype A is a fracture through the ossification center of the tubercle with little displacement. In subtype B, the fragment is separated from the metaphysis. Type II injuries involve separation of the entire ossification center of the tubercle. The fracture occurs through the area bridging the main tibial and tubercle ossification centers. In subtype B, the ossification center of the tubercle is comminuted, and the more distal fragment may be proximally displaced. Type III fractures extend into the joint surface. In subtype B, the fracture fragment is comminuted.

Other authors have proposed additions to the classification scheme of Ogden and colleagues. Frankl and coauthors[181] proposed adding a type IC to describe an avulsion fracture of the tibial tubercle with accompanying avulsion of the patellar ligament. Both Ryu and Debenham[186] and others[187,188] proposed adding a type IV injury in which the separation of the physis beneath the tubercle extends posteriorly, leading to a separation of the entire proximal tibial epiphysis. This injury is identical to a flexion-type Salter-Harris type I or II fracture of the proximal tibial physis as described by other authors.[189–191] McKoy and Stanitski[192,193] proposed adding a type V injury, which combines types III and IV, producing an inverted "Y"–shaped fracture line. More recently, Pandya and coauthors[183] proposed an entirely new classification scheme to emphasize the importance of intra-articular extension of these injuries.

EMERGENT TREATMENT

After examination, the patient with a fracture of the tibial tubercle should have the injured extremity elevated and splinted in a position of comfort, and ice should be applied to control swelling. Because this injury has been associated with the development of a compartment syndrome,[164,165,173,175,183,194] a careful evaluation of the circulation, sensation, and motor function of the limb should be performed. The presence or absence of pain with passive extension of the toes and the frequency of pain medication required by the patient should be documented and monitored pending definitive treatment of the injury.

NONOPERATIVE TREATMENT

Nondisplaced type I fractures can be treated successfully by immobilization in a cylinder or long leg cast with the knee in full extension for 4 to 6 weeks, followed by progressive rehabilitation of the quadriceps.

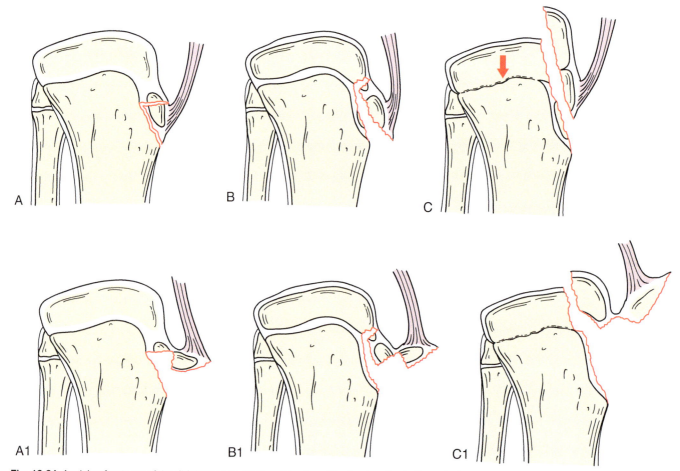

Fig. 13.24 Avulsion fractures of the tibial tubercle. (A) Type I fracture. The fracture line is through the secondary ossification center. In subtype A, the displacement is minimal. (A1) In subtype B, the fragment is hinged anteriorly and proximally. (B) Type II fracture. The fracture occurs through the junction of the ossification centers of the proximal end of the tibia and the tuberosity. In subtype A, the fragment is not comminuted. (B1) In subtype B, the fragment is comminuted and may be more proximally displaced. (C) A type III fracture is a true Salter-Harris type III injury that is intra-articular. In subtype A, the tubercle and anterior part of the proximal tibial epiphysis form a single unit. (C1) In subtype B, the fragment is comminuted, and the site of fragmentation is at the junction of the ossification centers of the proximal end of the tibia and the tuberosity.

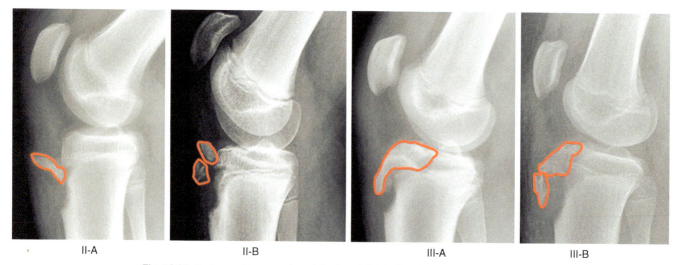

Fig. 13.25 Radiographic examples of displaced tibial tubercle fractures, by subtypes.

SURGICAL TREATMENT

Type IB and nearly all type II and type III injuries require operative treatment.[172] Osseous fixation may be achieved with cancellous screws placed from anterior to posterior.

The surgical approach is anterior, parallel with the patellar tendon, either medially or laterally. Hematoma and any interposed soft tissue, such as a flap of periosteum, are removed to facilitate accurate reduction. The menisci should be inspected for tears or peripheral detachments in all type III injuries.[172]

With the knee in full extension, the fracture is reduced and provisionally held in position with a Steinmann pin through the fracture fragment into the metaphysis. Under image intensifier control, a cancellous screw is placed in an anterior-to-posterior direction through the proximal tibial metaphysis. Wiss and colleagues[173] recommended that 4.0-mm cancellous screws be used rather than larger implants, such as 6.5-mm screws, to lessen the incidence of bursitis that may develop over prominent screwheads. Washers may be helpful in preventing the screwhead from sinking below the cortical surface. If solid fixation is not achieved with a single screw, a second screw can be added (Fig. 13.26). The continuity of the patellar ligament and avulsed periosteum is also repaired. If severe comminution is present, a tension-holding suture may be necessary to secure the repair. The insertion of the quadriceps should be assessed and repaired if found to be disrupted.[166,184] A prophylactic fasciotomy of the anterior compartment may be considered at the time of open reduction, especially if swelling of the anterior compartment is present.

After operative reduction, a cylinder or long leg cast with the knee immobilized in complete extension is worn for 4 to 6 weeks, followed by progressive rehabilitation of the quadriceps. Return to regular activities is permitted after the quadriceps has regained normal strength and after full range of motion of the knee joint has been achieved. Mirbey and coworkers[171] permitted their patients to resume sports activities at an average of 3 months after injury. After type II and type III fractures, Ogden and colleagues[172] observed that patients took between 16 and 18 weeks after cast removal to return to their preinjury activity levels.

OUTCOME

The reported outcome of treatment of tibial tubercle fractures is generally favorable in the short term. Growth disturbances and residual stiffness do not appear to be a common problem. Long-term outcome studies pertaining to the treatment of this injury are lacking. Recently, Riccio et al[195] reported on 19 pediatric patients who were evaluated clinically and functionally at an average of 3 years after surgical fixation of a tibial tubercle fracture. Although the operated side has a similar knee range of motion of that of the normal, contralateral side, it had a smaller thigh circumference and significant quadriceps extension strength deficits on 26% of the extremities. Validated, self-reported functional outcome scores (Tegner-Lysholm Scale and Pediatric International Knee Documentation Committee Scale) revealed fair and poor results in up to 35% of the operated extremities. The authors concluded that despite promising objective results, clinical outcomes measured by subjective validated self-reported surveys are not all excellent in patients undergoing surgical treatment of tibial tubercle fractures.[195]

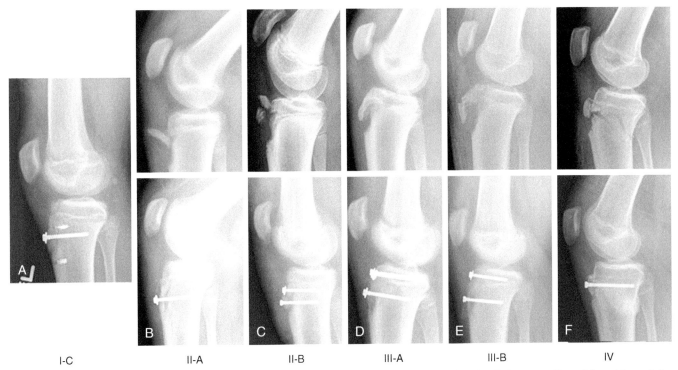

| I-C | II-A | II-B | III-A | III-B | IV |

Fig. 13.26 Pre- and postoperative radiographs of patients with tibial tubercle fractures. (A) A tibial tubercle fracture with avulsion of the patellar ligament (type I–C), requiring screw fixation of the fracture fragment and reattachment of the patellar tendon with sutures. (B and C) Type II-A and B fractures fixed with all metaphyseal screws. (D and E) Type III-A and B fractures, fixed with a combination of metaphyseal and epiphyseal screws. (F) A tibial tubercle fracture extending posteriorly with separation of the entire proximal tibial epiphysis (type IV).

COMPLICATIONS

GROWTH DISTURBANCE

A significant growth disturbance is uncommon after tibial tubercle fractures because most of these injuries occur when the physis is nearing normal closure. However, the potential for genu recurvatum exists in younger patients who sustain these fractures. Brey and colleagues[164] recently reported three patients who developed a recurvatum deformity after tibial tubercle fractures. In addition, minor (<2 cm) limb length discrepancies have infrequently been reported.[179]

COMPARTMENT SYNDROME

Compartment syndrome, presumably caused by tearing of nearby branches of the anterior tibial recurrent artery, has been reported after tibial tubercle fractures.[164,165,173,175,183,194] Patients who are treated by closed methods should be carefully monitored.

The presence of a posterior metaphyseal fracture accompanying a type II tibial tubercle injury may indicate a greater risk of development of a compartment syndrome.[164,183] These comminuted fractures likely represent higher-energy injuries that could potentially lead to greater vascular disruption. Because these fractures require operative treatment, a prophylactic anterior compartment fasciotomy at the time of surgery should be carefully considered in these patients; however, serial examination to detect a compartment syndrome is also a reasonable alternative.

PROMINENT HARDWARE

Bursitis over prominent screwheads necessitates removal of the implant, which is the most common complication in surgical treatment of these fractures.[179] Avoiding the use of larger screws may minimize the risk of this problem.[173]

FRACTURES OF THE PROXIMAL TIBIAL PHYSIS

Although trauma to the region of the knee is quite common in children, fractures of the proximal tibial epiphysis are rare and account for less than 2% of all physeal injuries.[22–24] Several anatomic structures appear to protect the proximal tibial physis from injury.[196,197]

PERTINENT ANATOMY

The epiphyseal ossification center of the proximal part of the tibia usually appears between the first and third months of life.[28] The proximal tibial physis contributes approximately 55% of the length of the tibia and 25% of the length of the entire leg and averages approximately 6 mm of growth each year until maturity.[25,26] Closure of this growth plate is usually complete by 13 to 15 years in girls and 15 to 18 years in boys. Blanks and colleagues[189] showed that the closure of the growth plate proceeds from posterior to anterior. Any injury that partially or completely disrupts growth of the proximal end of the tibia may lead to angular deformity and/or shortening of the extremity. The younger the child at the time of such injury, the greater the potential for these sequelae.

As noted, several anatomic structures appear to protect the proximal tibial physis from injury.[196,197] Laterally, the upper end of the fibula buttresses the physis. Anteriorly, the distal projection of the tibial tubercle over the metaphysis provides stability. Posteromedially, the insertion of the semimembranosus muscle spans the physis. Several authors have suggested that the proximal tibial physis may also be protected from traumatic stress because insertion of the collateral ligaments directly into the epiphysis is limited.[29,197–200] They noted that the lateral collateral ligament inserts into the head of the fibula and has no tibial attachment, whereas the medial collateral ligament has only a minor attachment to the epiphysis, and most of the ligament inserts distally into the metaphysis. In contrast, Ogden[28] has described dense attachments of the collateral ligaments and joint capsule into the epiphyseal perichondrium, both medially and laterally. He believes that the protection afforded to the proximal tibial physis is more likely as a result of anatomic factors other than the insertion of the collateral ligaments.

Of all physeal fractures, those of the proximal physis of the tibia have the greatest potential for disastrous vascular compromise.[199–201] The local vascular anatomy primarily accounts for this high risk of associated injury.

As the popliteal artery passes distally beneath the soleal arch, it divides into three branches: the anterior tibial, peroneal, and posterior tibial arteries. The vessels of this trifurcation pass distally; the peroneal artery usually terminates in the lower part of the leg, and the anterior tibial (dorsalis pedis) and posterior tibial arteries provide circulation to the foot. Just below the level of the trifurcation, the anterior tibial artery pierces the interosseous membrane as it courses into the anterior compartment of the leg and causes the arteries to be relatively tethered and immobile at this location. Because this trifurcation occurs just distal to the proximal tibial physis, any posterior displacement of the proximal end of the metaphysis may stretch or tear the popliteal artery (Fig. 13.27). Most reported cases of proximal tibial fractures associated with vascular damage are hyperextension injuries.

MECHANISM OF INJURY

Most proximal tibial physeal fractures are caused by either a hyperextension or abduction force applied to a fixed knee. The majority of these injuries occur in adolescents either during sports activities or as the result of a motor vehicle accident.[199,200] An unusual avulsion injury involving the proximal tibial physis may occur during sports activities that involve jumping.[167,186,189,191] In this flexion-type injury, the fracture begins as a tibial tubercle avulsion before propagating through the entire proximal tibial physis and exiting to include a portion of the posterior tibial metaphysis (Fig. 13.28). Blanks and colleagues[189] suggested that this fracture pattern occurs in older adolescents because, by that age, the posterior portion of the physis has already begun to close. A recent report of bilateral simultaneous nondisplaced proximal tibial Salter-Harris type II fractures in an otherwise healthy 14-year-old athlete with vitamin D deficiency highlights the need for a careful evaluation, including a metabolic workup, when facing any unusual presentation of these fractures.[202]

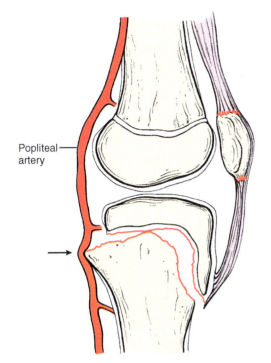

Fig. 13.27 Lateral drawing of a knee showing a displaced proximal tibial physeal injury that also demonstrates the risk of arterial injury because of the close proximity of the popliteal artery to the proximal end of the tibia.

Popliteal artery

As described for the distal femoral physis, a metaphyseal corner lesion involving the proximal tibial physis in infants is a strong indicator of child abuse. These lesions usually involve the medial aspect of the metaphysis and should be sought in any case of suspected abuse.[203]

EVALUATION

EXAMINATION

A description of the accident should be elicited to determine the direction of the force that caused the injury.

A patient with a fracture of the proximal tibial physis usually presents with pain, local soft tissue swelling, and tenderness directly over the physis. Often, hemarthrosis is present. In displaced fractures, deformity is evident, and the patient is unable to bear weight on the injured limb.

Because displaced fractures of the proximal tibial epiphysis may have partially or completely reduced before the patient is evaluated, an arterial injury must be considered in every patient with this injury (Fig. 13.29).[199,204] A careful neurovascular examination must be performed, with documentation of the presence of the dorsalis pedis and posterior tibial pulses and the function of the posterior tibial and peroneal nerves. Doppler ultrasound may be useful in assessing the distal pulses. Absent or diminished pulses may warrant appropriate vascular imaging or ABI assessment.

If clinical findings of acute ischemia are present—extremity pallor, coolness, cyanosis, or delayed capillary refilling—reduction of the displacement should be performed as soon as possible. If these findings are still present after the

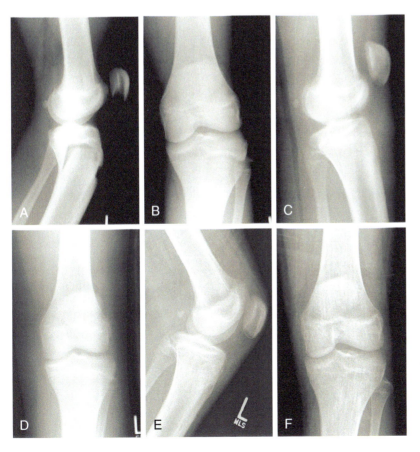

Fig. 13.28 A 15-year-old boy sustained an injury to his knee while playing basketball. (A and B) Anteroposterior (AP) and lateral radiographs of the knee showing a flexion-type Salter-Harris type II fracture of the proximal tibia. (C and D) The fracture was reduced with the use of traction followed by extension of the knee. A long leg cast was applied. (E and F) AP radiographs of the knee made after healing show that excellent alignment of the fracture has been maintained.

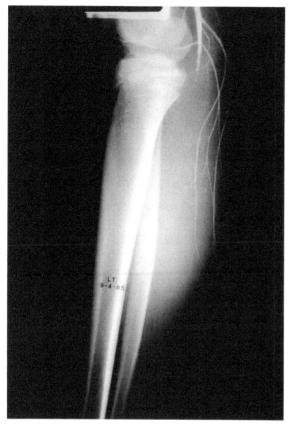

Fig. 13.29 Arteriogram of the knee and proximal end of the tibia of a 13-year-old patient who sustained a complete popliteal artery injury as a result of a displaced proximal tibial type I physeal injury that reduced spontaneously. (Courtesy of Dr. Neil E. Green, Vanderbilt Children's Hospital, Nashville, TN.)

reduction maneuver and the location of the vascular injury is clear, immediate vascular exploration is indicated and should not be delayed for imaging studies. In the absence of an obviously ischemic limb, patients with an abnormal pulse or those who recover pulses and perfusion after reduction of the fracture should be carefully monitored at appropriate intervals and may warrant arteriography[59–61] or ABI assessment. The presence or absence of pain on hyperextension of the toes should be recorded as a baseline measure to detect the possible development of an anterior compartment syndrome. Patients with proximal tibial physeal fractures can develop a slow, progressive popliteal artery insufficiency, even in the presence of foot pulses.[205] As described for fractures of the distal femoral metaphysis and physis, ongoing evaluation of the lower extremity is important during the first few days after the fracture so that a developing arterial insufficiency or compartment syndrome may be detected promptly.[206]

IMAGING

Orthogonal radiographs of the proximal part of the tibia and knee usually reveal the fracture. When there is clinical suspicion of a fracture through the proximal tibial physis but no radiographic evidence of it, one might consider to immobilize the knee and take a follow-up radiograph in 10 days to confirm the presence of a healing fracture.[46] MRI may be useful for revealing a fracture in a patient thought to have an occult injury to the growth plate (Fig. 13.30),[47,49,51,52] or a purely intraepiphyseal stress injury of the incompletely ossified proximal tibial epiphysis.[207] CT may be helpful for diagnosis and planning treatment of a type III or IV fracture.

CLASSIFICATION

The most commonly used classification system for fractures of the proximal epiphysis of the tibia is that of Salter and Harris,[54] as described earlier for the distal part of the femur. It is also useful to classify these injuries according to the direction of displacement so that associated complications can be anticipated and treatment can be guided (Fig. 13.31). Hyperextension injuries carry a high risk of vascular injury. In valgus injuries, which are probably the most common type, there is often an associated lateral metaphyseal fragment and fracture of the proximal fibula. Varus injuries are less common. Flexion injuries are seen in late adolescence. Understanding the direction and displacement of these fractures is often helpful in reducing and stabilizing them. Several authors have reported triplane fractures of the proximal tibia.[208–211] Like the triplane fracture that commonly occurs at the distal physis of the tibia, these rare injuries are likely caused by the asymmetric manner in which the proximal tibial physis undergoes closure.

Avulsion fractures of the lateral tibial condyle may occur in children. Sferopoulos and colleagues[212] described two types. The first—the Segond fracture—is a small, vertical intraepiphyseal avulsion involving the midportion of the lateral tibial condyle, distal to the plateau but proximal to the physis. The appearance of this fracture was associated with tibial spine fractures in two of five patients. The second was an avulsion fracture of the Gerdy tubercle. In this type of fracture, the detached fragment was larger, more anterior, and involved a part of the articular surface in addition to the physeal plate.[212] In addition, Dietz and colleagues[213] observed that a Segond fracture represents substantial evidence of major injury to the lateral joint capsule. This fracture also has a strong association with rupture of the ACL.

EMERGENT TREATMENT

If extremity pallor, coolness, cyanosis, or delayed capillary refilling (the clinical findings of acute ischemia) are present, reduction of the displacement should be performed as soon as possible. If these findings are still present after the reduction maneuver and the location of the vascular injury is clear, immediate vascular exploration is indicated and should not be delayed for imaging studies.

After examination and providing any emergent treatment that is warranted, the patient should have the injured extremity elevated and splinted in a position of comfort, and ice should be applied to control swelling. The neurovascular status of the limb should be monitored pending definitive treatment of the injury. Measuring the ABI should be considered if pulses are diminished.

NONOPERATIVE TREATMENT

The goals of treatment are to obtain and maintain anatomic reduction and avoid further damage to the growth plate.

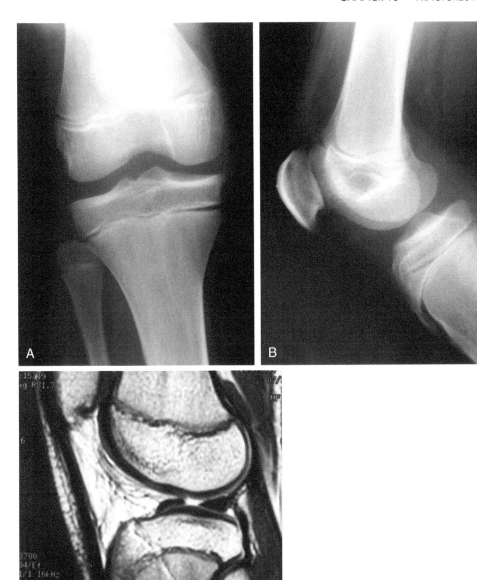

Fig. 13.30 A 13-year-old boy sustained an injury to his right knee. (A and B) Anteroposterior and lateral radiographs failed to reveal a fracture. (C) Magnetic resonance imaging revealed a nondisplaced Salter-Harris type IV fracture of the proximal end of the tibia.

Both the fracture type and the degree of displacement determine the form of treatment. Closed reduction and long leg cast immobilization is best reserved for nondisplaced Salter-Harris type I and type II fractures. Weight bearing is not recommended for 2 to 3 weeks so that the risk of further damage to the physis and possible displacement of the fracture is minimized. Follow-up radiographs are obtained in 5 to 7 days so that any displacement can be identified promptly and addressed.

Although nondisplaced and minimally displaced Salter-Harris type III and type IV injuries may be managed by cast immobilization alone, it may be preferable to stabilize these fractures with the use of percutaneous wires or cannulated screws to maintain alignment of the physis and assure congruity of the articular surface.

Closed reduction and cast immobilization may also be used to treat displaced type I and type II fractures if the reduction appears stable and the limb does not need to be immobilized in an extreme position to maintain reduction. The type II flexion epiphyseal injury is reduced with the use of traction and extension of the knee. These fractures tend to be stable with the knee extended. Usually, the reduction can be maintained by immobilization of the extremity in a long leg cast with the knee in extension.[186,189,191]

The advantage of closed reduction and cast immobilization is that it may be done with the use of analgesia or sedation, thus avoiding the need to place the child under general anesthesia. The disadvantage is the risk of a loss of reduction. If this option is selected, it is important to obtain follow-up radiographs in 5 to 7 days so that any loss of alignment can be addressed. With the possible exception of the flexion-type injury, stabilization of the reduced fracture with percutaneous placement of pins and screws followed by cast immobilization is often preferable to cast immobilization alone for most reducible proximal tibial physeal separations when there is any question as to the stability of the reduction. Before opting for closed treatment of a flexion type fracture, the surgeon should obtain a CT scan to exclude an intraarticular component that may not be visible on plain radiographs.[183]

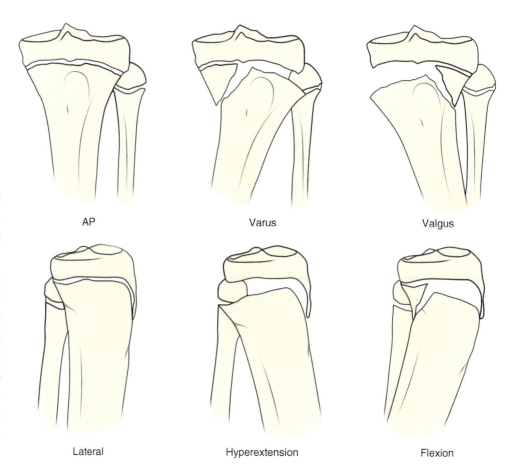

AP   Varus   Valgus

Lateral   Hyperextension   Flexion

Fig. 13.31 Classifying fractures of the proximal tibial physis according to the direction of displacement may be helpful in anticipating associated complications and in guiding treatment. *Varus fractures* are treated by reduction and application of a long leg cast with the knee in extension and valgus molding. *Valgus fractures* are treated by reduction and application of a long leg cast with the knee in extension and varus molding. *Hyperextension fractures* have a higher risk of vascular complications. *Flexion fractures* tend to be stable with the knee extended and can usually be treated by cast immobilization with the knee extended. *AP,* Anteroposterior.

SURGICAL TREATMENT

Surgical treatment is indicated for most displaced fractures of the proximal tibial physis to control the alignment during the healing process. Treatment options for this injury include closed reduction and percutaneous pin fixation followed by application of a long leg cast, as well as open reduction and internal fixation.

CLOSED REDUCTION AND PERCUTANEOUS FIXATION

Closed reduction and percutaneous fixation is recommended for most displaced type I and II fractures to avoid loss of reduction and for most nondisplaced type III and IV fractures to assure congruity of the articular surface. Displaced fractures should be gently reduced under general anesthesia so that further damage to the growth plate is minimized.

The technique of reduction will vary depending on the direction of the displacement of the proximal fracture fragment. Reduction of the fracture is best done under image intensifier control. The surgeon applies longitudinal traction to the leg while the thigh is stabilized by an assistant. For hyperextension injuries, traction followed by flexion of the distal fragment usually achieves reduction. These fractures tend to be unstable. Often, the reduction is most stable with the knee immobilized in marked flexion, a position that may increase the risk of vascular compromise and should be avoided. Transphyseal smooth pins are useful for stabilizing the reduction[201,214] and avoiding the need to immobilize the knee in extreme flexion (Fig. 13.32). The use of internal fixation allows the knee to be immobilized in 20 to 30 degrees of flexion in a long leg cast, a position that poses less risk to the circulation and makes subsequent displacement less likely. The cast may be bivalved to accommodate swelling. Bed rest with the leg slightly elevated is maintained for 24 to 48 hours, and the neurovascular status of the child is carefully monitored at appropriate intervals.

Salter-Harris types I and II valgus injuries are reduced by longitudinal traction followed by application of a gentle varus stress. If the fracture is deemed stable, a long leg cast is applied with the knee in extension, and varus molding is used. If the fracture is unstable, smooth, crossed transphyseal pins can be used to stabilize the reduction. In type II fractures with a large lateral fragment, the fracture may be stabilized with the use of pins or screws across the metaphyseal portion of the fracture (Fig. 13.33). After reduction and stabilization of the fracture, a long leg cast is applied with the knee in extension. Types I and II varus injuries are managed in a similar manner except that after closed reduction, valgus molding is applied to the long leg cast.

OPEN REDUCTION AND INTERNAL FIXATION

If satisfactory closed reduction cannot be achieved by closed means, open reduction is required. It is more often needed in type II than type I fractures. The most common reason that closed reduction of these fractures may fail is the interposition of soft tissue in the fracture site.[196] If arterial repair is required, open reduction and internal fixation is

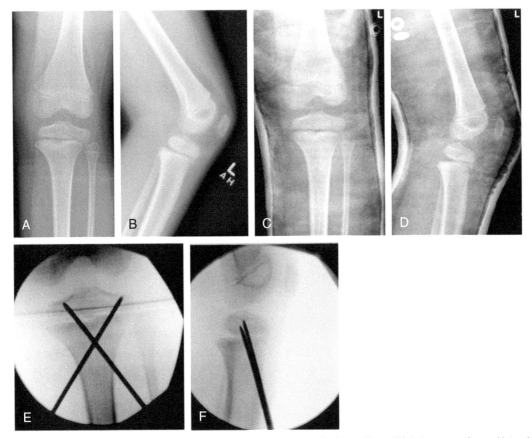

Fig. 13.32 An 8-year-old boy sustained an injury to his left knee without neurovascular injury. (A and B) Anteroposterior and lateral radiographs of the knee showing a hyperextension-type Salter-Harris type I fracture of the proximal tibia. (C and D) Radiographs obtained in a cast show some displacement of the fracture. (E and F) The fracture was reduced, closed, and stabilized with two smooth pins.

first performed through a posterior approach. Stabilization of the injury prevents excessive motion at the fracture site, thus affording protection to the vascular repair.

In patients not undergoing vascular exploration, open reduction of type I fractures may be done through an anterior approach, lateral to the tibial tubercle. In type II fractures, the incision is made over the metaphyseal fragment. Hematoma and any interposed soft tissue are removed to facilitate anatomic reduction. Smooth Steinmann pins may be used to stabilize the fracture. Postoperative management is similar to that described for fractures treated by closed reduction.

Displaced type III and type IV fractures are treated by open reduction and internal fixation to align the physis and restore congruity of the joint surface. After reduction, stabilization of the fracture may be achieved with the use of either smooth pins or screws inserted horizontally to avoid crossing the physis. Type III fractures may have associated injuries to the meniscus or collateral ligaments.[68,197,200,215,216] However, there does not appear to be sufficient information in the literature to suggest that early operative repair of the ligament is superior to simple immobilization that accompanies the treatment of the fracture.

Postoperative care is similar to that described earlier for displaced type I and type II injuries. Because these are intraarticular fractures, weight-bearing after a type III or type IV injury should not be started until radiographs confirm that the fracture is fully healed.

COMPLICATIONS

LATE DISPLACEMENT

The approach to a child who is seen several days after injury with a displaced fracture of the proximal tibial physis is similar to that described earlier in the section on fractures of the distal femoral physis.

NEUROVASCULAR INJURY

The incidence of arterial injury and compartment syndrome after fracture of the proximal tibial physis is difficult to accurately determine because of the relative rarity of these injuries. Burkhart and Peterson[199] reported two patients with arterial injury in a series of 28 children with a fracture of the proximal tibial physis. In their series of 34 patients with this injury, Shelton and associates[200] observed two patients with an arterial injury and a third who developed a compartment syndrome. Wozasek and colleagues[201] reported four patients with vascular complications seen among 30 children with proximal tibial physeal injuries. Tjoumakaris and Wells[204] described a popliteal artery transection in an adolescent following a minimally displaced type III fracture. Although the reported number of children who developed these complications is small, many of them required amputation. The importance of early recognition and prompt intervention in children who demonstrate the signs and symptoms of arterial insufficiency cannot be overemphasized. Peroneal nerve injuries have also been reported to accompany these fractures.[199–201]

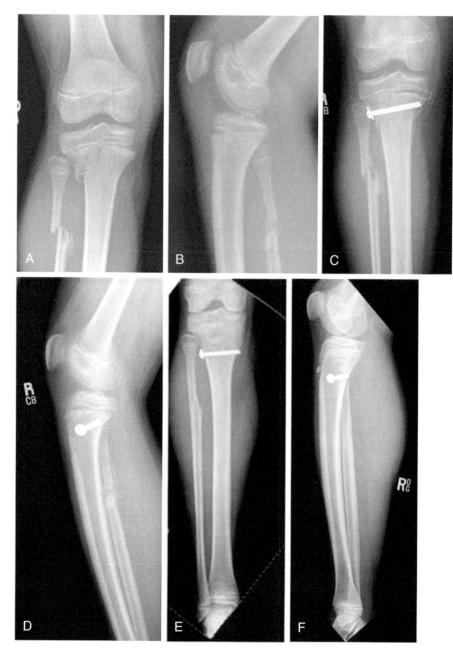

Fig. 13.33 An 11-year-old boy sustained an injury to his left knee. (A and B) Anteroposterior and lateral radiographs of the knee showing a valgus-type Salter-Harris type II fracture of the proximal tibia. The fracture was treated by closed reduction and stabilization with a cannulated screw. (C and D) Radiographs obtained 1 month after the fracture showing evidence of healing. (E and F) Radiographs obtained 1 year later. The patient is fully active without symptoms.

GROWTH DISTURBANCE

In general, the prognosis for a fracture of the proximal tibial epiphysis is good. Although shortening and angular deformity can be seen after these fractures,[217] it is less common than after fractures of the distal femoral physis because injuries to the proximal tibial physis tend to occur in older children and adolescents, and the proximal tibial physis contributes less to overall growth of the limb than does the distal femoral physis. The younger the child is at the time of a proximal tibial physeal injury, the greater the likelihood of the development of shortening and angular deformity.

Open injuries to the proximal tibial physis have a much poorer prognosis. These fractures are often the result of a lawn mower injury.[199] Angular deformities, either occurring alone or in combination with limb shortening, are frequently seen after these injuries.

Careful clinical evaluation is recommended at 6-month intervals after an injury to the proximal tibial physis to assess lower extremity alignment and leg length. Comparative radiographs of both lower extremities should be taken in both the AP and lateral planes.[218]

Angular deformities may be caused by either malunion or a partial growth disturbance. Significant angular deformity resulting from malunion may be managed by osteotomy or, when appropriate, by hemiepiphysiodesis. Treatment options for progressive angular deformity caused by a partial growth disturbance include osseous bridge resection, osteotomy, or epiphysiodesis of the remaining portion of the physis. Osseous bridge resection and interpositional free fat may be considered for lesions involving less than 50% of the physis.[74,75] Because the proximal tibial epiphysis averages approximately 6 mm of growth each year until maturity, children should have at least 3 years of growth remaining before osseous bridge resection is considered. A recurrent bar formation has been reported in up to one-third of patients undergoing resection, usually because of graft dislocation out of the resection cavity.[219] The use of poly(lactic-co-glycolic acid) scaffolds, as compared with the traditional fat graft, has been shown to increase the amount of cartilage and reduce the amount of bony bar reformation in a pilot animal study of simulated proximal tibial physeal injuries.[220]

An osteotomy with epiphysiodesis of the remaining portion of the physis may be necessary when the bridge is too large to excise or in children who are nearing completion of growth. Lengthening may be combined with angular correction in children who have both an angular deformity and significant shortening.[221,222]

Patients may occasionally be seen with physeal arrest of the anterior portion of the proximal tibial physis in association with a nonphyseal fracture of the lower extremity.[221,223,224] Pappas and colleagues[224] suggested that in these patients, an injury to the proximal tibial physis may have been overlooked because attention was directed to a more obvious injury. Patients who have fractures of the lower extremities that do not appear to involve the growth plate should be carefully assessed and monitored for a possible physeal injury.

PROXIMAL TIBIAL METAPHYSEAL FRACTURES

Fractures of the proximal metaphysis of the tibia are uncommon injuries in children. Two types of these fractures deserve special mention: a minimally displaced valgus greenstick fracture and a more displaced injury that results from higher-energy trauma. Valgus greenstick fractures are commonly referred to as *Cozen fractures,* named for the orthopedic surgeon who first described the propensity for these injuries to develop a progressive valgus deformity.[225] The displaced proximal tibial fracture has been called the *arterial hazard fracture* by Rang[226] because of the association of this fracture with vascular injury.

VALGUS GREENSTICK FRACTURE

MECHANISM OF INJURY
The more common type of fracture in this region is a minimally displaced, transversely oriented greenstick fracture. These injuries most commonly occur in children younger than 10 years and are usually the result of low-energy trauma such as playground falls or bicycle or trampoline accidents.[227–230]

EVALUATION
On clinical evaluation, the patient with a greenstick fracture of the proximal metaphysis of the tibia is seen with local pain, swelling, and tenderness at the fracture site. Patients with more displaced fractures are unable to bear weight. Associated neurovascular problems are uncommon. AP and lateral radiographs of the proximal end of the tibia, including the knee, will reveal the fracture. Radiographs show the fracture line usually extends two-thirds of the way across the tibial metaphysis, although, in some instances, the fracture

line may continue completely across the metaphysis. An associated fracture of the proximal end of the fibula is infrequent. Even though the fracture is relatively nondisplaced, a fracture gap on the medial side is often present.

EMERGENT TREATMENT
The patient with a greenstick fracture of the proximal tibial metaphysis should have the injured extremity elevated and splinted in a position of comfort pending definitive treatment.

NONOPERATIVE TREATMENT
Initial management of these fractures is nonoperative. Treatment should be directed at closing the medial metaphyseal gap at the fracture site. Reduction is best accomplished with the use of image intensifier control while the patient is under general anesthesia, although many centers perform the reduction under conscious sedation. The knee is straightened, and varus stress is applied across the fracture site. If reduction of the fracture has been obtained, a long leg cast is applied with the knee in nearly full extension; varus molding is used at the fracture site. Healing of these fractures is usually complete by 4 to 6 weeks.

SURGICAL TREATMENT
If the fracture gap cannot be reduced by closed means, the pes anserinus or periosteum may be interposed in the fracture site.[231] In this rare instance, it may be necessary to remove the impediments to reduction through a small medial incision over the fracture site. After operative reduction, internal fixation is unnecessary.

COMPLICATIONS
Despite their innocuous appearance, these fractures often tend toward progressive valgus angulation during the period of fracture healing, as well as after union of the fracture (Fig. 13.34). The most common problem associated with a greenstick fracture of the proximal tibial metaphysis is progressive valgus angulation. The angulation occurs most rapidly during the first 12 months after the injury and continues at a slower rate for as long as 18 to 24 months.[227,232,233] It is important to emphasize to parents the possibility of subsequent deformity, despite adequate and appropriate treatment of the fracture.

Although the exact cause of the deformity is unknown, relative overgrowth of the proximal tibial physis, presumably caused by fracture-induced hyperemia, probably plays a key role.[227,234] Increased radionuclide activity at the proximal tibial growth plate, with proportionally greater uptake on the medial side, has been reported after a fracture of the proximal tibial metaphysis.[234] In a series of children with posttraumatic tibia valga, Ogden and colleagues[227] found both a generalized increase in longitudinal growth of the injured tibia that occurred both proximally and distally and eccentric proximal medial overgrowth in every patient.

Although the valgus deformity resulting from the proximal tibial metaphyseal fracture is unsightly to parents, several authors have reported spontaneous improvement of the deformity with time.[232,233,235–237] Therefore, a period of observation before considering any surgical options is recommended. There is no evidence to suggest that bracing has any influence on this particular deformity. In addition,

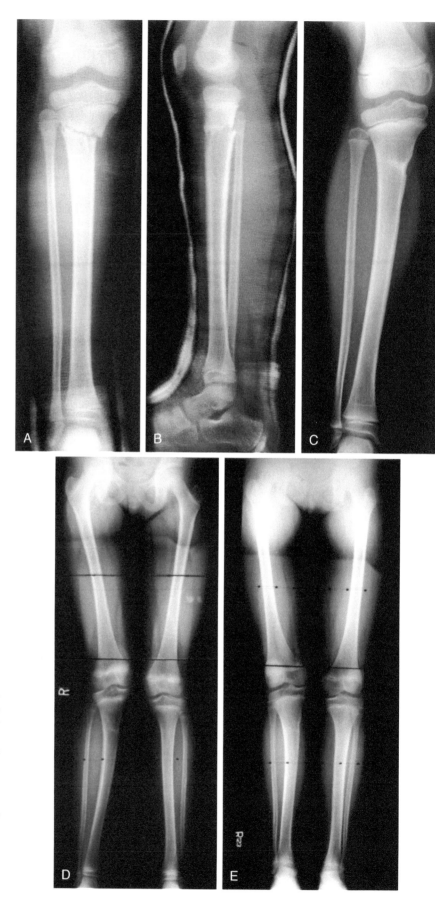

Fig. 13.34 A 5-year-old girl sustained a fracture of the proximal metaphysis of the tibia. (A) An anteroposterior (AP) radiograph made after closed reduction of the fracture and application of a long leg cast shows that the fracture is properly aligned. (B) A lateral radiograph shows excellent reduction in the sagittal plane. (C) An AP radiograph made 1 year after the fracture shows that a valgus deformity has developed. (D) An AP radiograph taken 2.5 years after the injury reveals that the deformity is still evident. (E) An AP radiograph taken 3 years and 2 months after the injury shows that the overall alignment of the lower extremities has improved.

both recurrence of deformity and compartment syndrome have been reported after corrective tibial osteotomy for this problem.[235,238]

McCarthy and colleagues[236] compared the results of operative versus nonoperative treatment in a series of children with posttraumatic tibia valga. These authors found no significant difference in lower extremity alignment between the operative and nonoperative groups at the time of injury, at maximal deformity, or at latest follow-up. Tuten and colleagues[237] monitored seven patients with acquired valgus deformity after a proximal metaphyseal fracture for an average of 15 years postinjury and found that spontaneous improvement of the angulation occurred in all patients and resulted in a clinically well-aligned limb in most. They concluded that patients with this deformity should be monitored through skeletal maturity and that operative intervention should be reserved for patients who have symptoms from malalignment. Alternatively, Morin et al[239] recommended early temporary hemiepiphysiodesis using a two-hole plate to correct posttraumatic tibia valgus deformity in young children. They advised waiting at least 1 year after the original fracture to offer the surgical intervention. They reported 19 patients who underwent hemiepiphysiodesis of the proximal medial physis of the tibia, obtaining correction of the mechanical axis and the proximal medial tibial angle in all but one patient. Seven patients required repeated procedures as a result of either under- or overcorrection of the deformity. Permanent growth arrest did not occur in their series but remains a potential complication of this procedure.[239]

DISPLACED FRACTURE OF THE PROXIMAL TIBIAL METAPHYSIS

The other type of fracture of the proximal tibial metaphysis is produced by higher-energy trauma. These displaced fractures often injure the anterior tibial artery and may lead to a compartment syndrome in the lower part of the leg. The fibula is generally fractured and displaced with the proximal end of the tibia and may be associated with an injury to the peroneal nerve. Because this fracture is prone to neurovascular problems, Rang[226] has labeled this injury the *arterial hazard fracture*.

MECHANISM OF INJURY

As noted earlier, these injuries are usually the result of higher-energy trauma such as an automobile versus pedestrian accident or a fall from a height.

EVALUATION

The evaluation of this injury is similar to that described earlier for fractures of the proximal tibial physis. A patient with a fracture of the proximal tibial metaphysis usually presents with pain, deformity, local soft tissue swelling, and tenderness directly over the physis. If the clinical findings of acute ischemia are present, reduction of the displacement should be performed as soon as possible. The presence or absence of pain on hyperextension of the toes should be recorded as a baseline and monitored to detect the possible development of an anterior compartment syndrome. After evaluation and necessary emergent treatment are concluded, the injured extremity should be elevated and splinted in a position of comfort, and ice should be applied.

NONOPERATIVE TREATMENT

If adequate closed reduction can be obtained and no signs of compartment syndrome are apparent, a long leg cast may be applied with the knee immobilized in slight flexion. After reduction, the cast is bivalved, the leg is slightly elevated, and the patient is closely monitored for compartment syndrome over the next 24 to 48 hours.

OPERATIVE TREATMENT

Open reduction is indicated if a satisfactory closed reduction cannot be obtained. This may be as a result of interposition of soft tissue. The fracture may be stabilized with smooth Steinmann pins. Postoperatively, a splint is applied for monitoring of the extremity. A cast is applied after an appropriate period of observation. If a fasciotomy is required to treat a compartment syndrome, either external or internal fixation is needed to stabilize the fracture until wound healing is sufficient to apply a long leg cast.

PROXIMAL FIBULAR METAPHYSEAL AND PHYSEAL FRACTURES

Most proximal fibular fractures accompany proximal tibial physeal or metaphyseal fractures. Although these fractures do not require anatomic reduction, careful evaluation of peroneal nerve function is needed whenever this injury is seen on radiographs.

Physeal fractures of the proximal portion of the fibula are among the rarest of physeal injuries.[240,241] These fractures typically occur during adolescence, so growth disturbance is not generally a problem. If instability of the knee ligaments is not present, a long leg or cylinder cast for 3 to 4 weeks is sufficient for management. Normal function and return to athletic activities can be expected.

OPEN INJURIES IN THE KNEE REGION

Open fractures near the knee joint require thorough evaluation for determination of whether the joint was entered at the time of injury. Sometimes, the examiner can look into the knee joint through the wound, and the diagnosis is easy. Radiographs showing air within the knee joint can be used as presumptive evidence that the wound communicates with the joint. A CT scan of the knee can sometimes be useful for excluding intraarticular penetration. If the diagnosis is less clear, a saline loading test may be performed.[242] Under sterile conditions, 30 mL to 50 mL of saline or other physiologic fluid is injected into the knee through intact skin. If the wound communicates with the knee joint, the injected fluid will leak out through the wound. Once penetration of the knee joint has been confirmed, sterile dressings are applied to the wound, tetanus prophylaxis is given, if indicated, and broad-spectrum antibiotics are started intravenously. Thorough wound débridement and irrigation of the joint are performed through a formal arthrotomy.[243] If possible, the knee joint is closed over a suction drain. Similarly, the open fracture is irrigated and débrided. The type of closure selected will depend on the size and extent of the fracture. Although no general consensus exists in the literature, as with other open fractures, antibiotics are generally continued for 2 to 5 days after the operation.

In open fractures caused by penetrating trauma such as a bullet, fracture management is somewhat different. If the bullet is a low-velocity missile causing little adjacent soft tissue injury, an open fracture of the femoral or tibial shaft does not usually require formal irrigation and débridement. However, if the bullet has lodged in the knee joint or has passed through it, arthrotomy is recommended for removal of osseous and cartilaginous fragments and for extraction of the bullet. Even if a bullet is not mechanically causing a problem with knee motion, a retained bullet within the knee joint may lead to elevated serum lead levels.[244]

With gunshot wounds to the knee, vascular injury should be considered, especially when the path of the bullet is in close proximity to the popliteal vessels. Arteriography or exploration may be necessary if the bullet trajectory is in the posterior region of the knee and clinical evidence of vascular disruption is apparent. Once the wound and soft tissue injuries have been addressed, the fracture may require external fixation to allow for dressing changes; however, management has to be individualized for each open fracture in this region.

REFERENCES

The level of evidence (LOE) is determined according to the criteria provided in the Preface.

1. Smith NC, Parker D, McNicol D. Supracondylar fractures of the femur in children. *J Pediatr Orthop.* 2001;21(5):600–603. (**LOE IV**).
2. Butcher CC, Hoffman EB. Supracondylar fractures of the femur in children: closed reduction and percutaneous pinning of displaced fractures. *J Pediatr Orthop.* 2005;25(2):145–148. (**LOE IV**).
3. Green NE, Allen BL. Vascular injuries associated with dislocation of the rk. *J Bone Joint Surg Am.* 1977;59(2):236–239. (**LOE III**).
4. Beals RK, Tufts E. Fractured femur in infancy: the role of child abuse. *J Pediatr Orthop.* 1983;3(5):583–586. (**LOE IV**).
5. Arkader A, Friedman JE, Warner WC Jr, Wells L. Complete distal femoral metaphyseal fractures: a harbinger of child abuse before walking age. *J Pediatr Orthop.* 2007;27(7):751–753. (**LOE IV**).
6. Davies AM, Carter SR, Grimer RJ, Sneath RS. Fatigue fractures of the femoral diaphysis in the skeletally immature simulating malignancy. *Br J Radiol.* 1989;62(742):893–896. (**LOE IV**).
7. Griffin PP. Fractures of the femoral diaphysis in children. *Orthop Clin North Am.* 1976;7(3):633–638. (**LOE V**).
8. Staheli LT. Fractures of the shaft of the femur. In: Rockwood CA, Wilkins KE, King RE, eds. *Fractures in Children.* Philadelphia: J.B. Lippincott Company; 1984:1121–1163. (**LOE IV**).
9. Bowler JR, Mubarak SJ, Wenger DR. Tibial physeal closure and genu recurvatum after femoral fracture: occurrence without a tibial traction pin. *J Pediatr Orthop.* 1990;10(5):653–657. (**LOE IV**).
10. Tolo VT. External fixation in multiply injured children. *Orthop Clin North Am.* 1990;21(2):393–400. (**LOE V**).
11. Skaggs DL, Leet AI, Money MD, Shaw BA, Hale JM, Tolo VT. Secondary fractures associated with external fixation in pediatric femur fractures. *J Pediatr Orthop.* 1999;19(5):582–586. (**LOE IV**).
12. Parikh SN, Nathan ST, Priola MJ, Eismann EA. Elastic nailing for pediatric subtrochanteric and supracondylar femur fractures. *Clin Orthop Relat Res.* 2014;472(9):2735–2744. (**LOE IV**).
13. Su Y, Nan G. ORIF with percutaneous cross pinning via the posterior approach for paediatric widely displaced supracondylar femoral fractures. *Injury.* 2016;47(6):1242–1247. (**LOE IV**).
14. Kregor PJ, Song KM, Routt Jr ML, Sangeorzan BJ, Liddell RM, Hansen ST Jr. Plate fixation of femoral shaft fractures in multiply injured children. *J Bone Joint Surg Am.* 1993;75(12):1774–1780. (**LOE IV**).
15. Heyworth BE, Hedequist DJ, Nasreddine AY, Stamoulis C, Hresko MT, Yen YM. Distal femoral valgus deformity following plate fixation of pediatric femoral shaft fractures. *J Bone Joint Surg Am.* 2013;95(6):526–533. (**LOE IV**).
16. Lin D, Lian K, Hong J, Ding Z, Zhai W. Pediatric physeal slide-traction plate fixation for comminuted distal femur fractures in children. *J Pediatr Orthop.* 2012;32(7):682–686. (**LOE IV**).
17. Abdelgawad AA, Kanlic EM. Pediatric distal femur fixation by proximal humeral plate. *J Knee Surg.* 2013;26(suppl 1): S45–S49. (**LOE V**).
18. Abdelgawad AA, Sieg RN, Laughlin MD, Shunia J, Kanlic EM. Submuscular bridge plating for complex pediatric femur fractures is reliable. *Clin Orthop Relat Res.* 2013;471(9):2797–2807. (**LOE IV**).
19. Baker P, McMurtry I, Port A. The treatment of distal femoral fractures in children using the LISS plate: a report of two cases. *Ann R Coll Surg Engl.* 2008;90(4):4–6. (**LOE IV**).
20. Kanlic EM, Anglen JO, Smith DG, Morgan SJ, Pesantez RF. Advantages of submuscular bridge plating for complex pediatric femur fractures. *Clin Orthop Relat Res.* 2004;(426):244–251. (**LOE IV**).
21. Sink EL, Hedequist D, Morgan SJ, Hresko T. Results and technique of unstable pediatric femoral fractures treated with submuscular bridge plating. *J Pediatr Orthop.* 2006;26(2):177–181. (**LOE IV**).
22. Mann DC, Rajmaira S. Distribution of physeal and nonphyseal fractures in 2,650 long-bone fractures in children aged 0-16 years. *J Pediatr Orthop.* 1990;10(6):713–716. (**LOE IV**).
23. Peterson CA, Peterson HA. Analysis of the incidence of injuries to the epiphyseal growth plate. *J Trauma.* 1972;12(4):275–281. (**LOE N/A**).
24. Peterson HA, Madhok R, Benson JT, Ilstrup DM, Melton LJ 3rd. Physeal fractures: Part 1. Epidemiology in Olmsted County, Minnesota, 1979-1988. *J Pediatr Orthop.* 1994;14(4):423–430. (**LOE IV**).
25. Anderson M, Geen WT, Messner MB. Growth and predictions of growth in the lower extremities. *J Bone Joint Surg Am.* 1963;45-A:1–14. (**LOE IV**).
26. Pritchett JW. Longitudinal growth and growth-plate activity in the lower extremity. *Clin Orthop Relat Res.* 1992;(275):274–279. (**LOE IV**).
27. Beaty JH, Kumar A. Fractures about the knee in children. *J Bone Joint Surg Am.* 1994;76(12):1870–1880. (**LOE V**).
28. Ogden JA. *Skeletal Injury in the Child.* 2nd ed. Lea & Febiger; 1990.
29. Roberts JM. Operative treatment of fractures about the knee. *Orthop Clin North Am.* 1990;21(2):365–379. (**LOE V**).
30. Craig JG, Cramer KE, Cody DD, Hearshen DO, Ceulemans RY, van Holsbeeck MT, et al. Premature partial closure and other deformities of the growth plate: MR imaging and three-dimensional modeling. *Radiology.* 1999;210(3):835–843. (**LOE IV**).
31. Eid AM, Hafez MA. Traumatic injuries of the distal femoral physis. Retrospective study on 151 cases. *Injury.* 2002;33(3):251–255. (**LOE IV**).
32. Lombardo SJ, Harvey Jr JP. Fractures of the distal femoral epiphyses. Factors influencing prognosis: a review of thirty-four cases. *J Bone Joint Surg Am.* 1977;59(6):742–751. (**LOE IV**).
33. Riseborough EJ, Barrett IR, Shapiro F. Growth disturbances following distal femoral physeal fracture-separations. *J Bone Joint Surg Am.* 1983;65(7):885–893. (**LOE IV**).
34. Stephens DC, Louis E, Louis DS. Traumatic separation of the distal femoral epiphyseal cartilage plate. *J Bone Joint Surg Am.* 1974;56(7):1383–1390. (**LOE IV**).
35. Grogan DP, Bobechko WP. Pathogenesis of a fracture of the distal femoral epiphysis. A case report. *J Bone Joint Surg Am.* 1984;66(4):621–622. (**LOE V**).
36. Banagale RC, Kuhns LR. Traumatic separation of the distal femoral epiphysis in the newborn. *J Pediatr Orthop.* 1983;3(3). 396–368. (**LOE V**).
37. Krosin MT, Lincoln TL. Traumatic distal femoral physeal fracture in a neonate treated with open reduction and pinning. *J Pediatr Orthop.* 2009;29(5):445–448. (**LOE V**).
38. Mangurten HH, Puppala B, Knuth A. Neonatal distal femoral physeal fracture requiring closed reduction and pinning. *J Perinatol.* 2005;25(3):216–219. (**LOE V**).
39. Pennock AT, Ellis HB, Willimon SC, Wyatt C, Broida SE, Dennis MM, et al. Intra-articular physeal fractures of the distal femur: a frequently missed diagnosis in adolescent athletes. *Orthop J Sports Med.* 2017;5(10):2325967117731567. (**LOE IV**).
40. Lippert WC, Owens RF, Wall EJ. Salter-Harris type III fractures of the distal femur: plain radiographs can be deceptive. *J Pediatr Orthop.* 2010;30(6):598–605. (**LOE IV**).
41. Flanagin BA, Cruz AI, Medvecky MJ. Hoffa fracture in a 14-year-old. *Orthopedics.* 2011;34(2):138–130. (**LOE V**).

42. Tripathy SK, Aggarwal A, Patel S, Goyal T, Priya N. Neglected Hoffa fracture in a child. *J Pediatr Orthop. B.* 2013;22(4):339–343. **(LOE V)**.

43. Brone LA, Wroble RR. Salter-Harris type III fracture of the medial femoral condyle associated with an anterior cruciate ligament tear. Report of three cases and review of the literature. *Am J Sports Med.* 1998;26(4):581–586. **(LOE IV)**.

44. Rafee A, Kumar A, Shah SV. Salter-Harris type III fracture of the lateral femoral condyle with a ruptured posterior cruciate ligament: an uncommon injury pattern. *Arch Orthop Trauma Surg.* 2007;127(1):29–31. **(LOE V)**.

45. Torg JS, Pavlov H, Morris VB. Salter-Harris type-III fracture of the medial femoral condyle occurring in the adolescent athlete. *J Bone Joint Surg Am.* 1981;63(4):586–591. **(LOE IV)**.

46. Stanitski CL. Stress view radiographs of the skeletally immature knee: a different view. *J Pediatr Orthop.* 2004;24(3):342. **(LOE IV)**.

47. Carey J, Spence L, Blickman H, Eustace S. MRI of pediatric growth plate injury: correlation with plain film radiographs and clinical outcome. *Skeletal Radiol.* 1998;27(5):250–255. **(LOE IV)**.

48. Chauvin N, Jaramillo D. Occult distal femoral physeal injury with disruption of the perichondrium. *J Comput Assist Tomogr.* 2012;36(3):310–312. **(LOE V)**.

49. Gufler H, Schulze CG, Wagner S, Baumbach L. MRI for occult physeal fracture detection in children and adolescents. *Acta Radiol.* 2013;54(4):467–472. **(LOE IV)**.

50. Kritsaneepaiboon S, Shah R, Murray MM, Kleinman PK. Posterior periosteal disruption in Salter-Harris Type II fractures of the distal femur: evidence for a hyperextension mechanism. *AJR Am J Roentgenol.* 2009;193(6):W540–W545. **(LOE IV)**.

51. Naranja Jr RJ, Gregg JR, Dormans JP, Drummond DS, Davidson RS, Hahn M. Pediatric fracture without radiographic abnormality. Description and significance. *Clin Orthop Relat Res.* 1997;(342):141–146. **(LOE IV)**.

52. White PG, Mah JY, Friedman L. Magnetic resonance imaging in acute physeal injuries. *Skeletal Radiol.* 1994;23(8):627–631. **(LOE IV)**.

53. Little RM, Milewski MD. Physeal fractures about the knee. *Curr Rev Musculoskelet Med.* 2016;9(4):478–486. **(LOE V)**.

54. Salter RB, Harris R. Injuries involving the epiphyseal plate. *J Bone Joint Surg Am.* 1963;45:587–622. **(LOE V)**.

55. Basener CJ, Mehlman CT, DiPasquale TG. Growth disturbance after distal femoral growth plate fractures in children: a meta-analysis. *J Orthop Trauma.* 2009;23(9):663–667. **(LOE IV)**.

56. Bali K, Mootha AK, Prabhakar S, Dhillon MS. Isolated Hoffa fracture of the medial femoral condyle in a skeletally immature patient. *Bull NYU Hosp Jt Dis.* 2011;69(4):335–338. **(LOE V)**.

57. Lal H, Bansal P, Khare R, Mittal D. Conjoint bicondylar Hoffa fracture in a child: a rare variant treated by minimally invasive approach. *J Orthop Traumatol.* 2011;12(2):111–114. **(LOE V)**.

58. McDonough PW, Bernstein RM. Nonunion of a Hoffa fracture in a child. *J Orthop Trauma.* 2000;14(7):519–521. **(LOE V)**.

59. Applebaum R, Yellin AE, Weaver FA, Oberg J, Pentecost M. Role of routine arteriography in blunt lower-extremity trauma. *Am J Surg.* 1990;160(2):221–224. **(LOE III)**.

60. Kendall RW, Taylor DC, Salvian AJ, O'Brien PJ. The role of arteriography in assessing vascular injuries associated with dislocations of the knee. *J Trauma.* 1993;35(6):875–878. **(LOE IV)**.

61. Treiman GS, Yellin AE, Weaver FA, Wang S, Ghalambor N, Barlow W, et al. Examination of the patient with a knee dislocation. The case for selective arteriography. *Arch Surg.* 1992;127(9):1056–1062. **(LOE IV)**.

62. Wall EJ, May MM. Growth plate fractures of the distal femur. *J Pediatr Orthop.* 2012;32(suppl 1):S40–46. **(LOE IV)**.

63. Edmunds I, Nade S. Injuries of the distal femoral growth plate and epiphysis: should open reduction be performed? *Aust N Z J Surg.* 1993;63(3):195–199. **(LOE III)**.

64. Garrett BR, Hoffman EB, Carrara H. The effect of percutaneous pin fixation in the treatment of distal femoral physeal fractures. *J Bone Joint Surg Br.* 2011;93(5):689–694. **(LOE IV)**.

65. Graham JM, Gross RH. Distal femoral physeal problem fractures. *Clin Orthop Relat Res.* 1990;(255):51–53. **(LOE V)**.

66. Thomson JD, Stricker SJ, Williams MM. Fractures of the distal femoral epiphyseal plate. *J Pediatr Orthop.* 1995;15(4):474–478. **(LOE IV)**.

67. Egol KA, Karunakar M, Phieffer L, Meyer R, Wattenbarger JM. Early versus late reduction of a physeal fracture in an animal model. *J Pediatr Orthop.* 2002;22(2):208–211. **(LOE III)**.

68. Bertin KC, Goble EM. Ligament injuries associated with physeal fractures about the knee. *Clin Orthop Relat Res.* 1983;(177):188–195. **(LOE IV)**.

69. Buess-Watson E, Exner GU, Illi OE. Fractures about the knee: growth disturbances and problems of stability at long-term follow-up. *Eur J Pediatr Surg.* 1994;4(4):218–224. **(LOE IV)**.

70. Arkader A, Warner Jr WC, Horn BD, Shaw RN, Wells L. Predicting the outcome of physeal fractures of the distal femur. *J Pediatr Orthop.* 2007;27(6):703–708. **(LOE IV)**.

71. Ilharreborde B, Raquillet C, Morel E, et al. Long-term prognosis of Salter-Harris type 2 injuries of the distal femoral physis. *J Pediatr Orthop B.* 2006;15(6):433–438. **(LOE IV)**.

72. Dahl WJ, Silva S, Vanderhave KL. Distal femoral physeal fixation: are smooth pins really safe? *J Pediatr Orthop.* 2014;34(2):134–138. **(LOE III)**.

73. Ogden JA. Growth slowdown and arrest lines. *J Pediatr Orthop.* 1984;4(4):409–415. **(LOE V)**.

74. Kasser JR. Physeal bar resections after growth arrest about the knee. *Clin Orthop Relat Res.* 1990;(255):68–74. **(LOE V)**.

75. Peterson HA. Partial growth plate arrest and its treatment. *J Pediatr Orthop.* 1984;4(2):246–258. **(LOE V)**.

76. Matelic TM, Aronsson DD, Boyd DW Jr, LaMont RL. Acute hemarthrosis of the knee in children. *Am J Sports Med.* 1995;23(6):668–671. **(LOE V)**.

77. Nietosvaara Y, Aalto K, Kallio PE. Acute patellar dislocation in children: incidence and associated osteochondral fractures. *J Pediatr Orthop.* 1994;14(4):513–515. **(LOE IV)**.

78. Seeley MA, Knesek M, Vanderhave KL. Osteochondral injury after acute patellar dislocation in children and adolescents. *J Pediatr Orthop.* 2013;33(5):511–518. **(LOE IV)**.

79. Rosenberg ZS, Kawelblum M, Cheung YY, Beltran J, Lehman WB, Grant AD. Osgood-Schlatter lesion: fracture or tendinitis? Scintigraphic, CT, and MR imaging features. *Radiology.* 1992;185(3):853–858. **(LOE IV)**.

80. Flachsmann R, Broom ND, Hardy AE, Moltschaniwskyj G. Why is the adolescent joint particularly susceptible to osteochondral shear fracture? *Clin Orthop Relat Res.* 2000;(381):212–221. **(LOE III)**.

81. Ahstrom JP Jr. Osteochondral fracture in the knee joint associated with hypermobility and dislocation of the patella. Report of eighteen cases. *J Bone Joint Surg Am.* 1965;47(8):1491–1502. **(LOE IV)**.

82. Hammerle CP, Jacob RP. Chondral and osteochondral fractures after luxation of the patella and their treatment. *Arch Orthop Trauma Surg.* 1980;97(3):207–211. **(LOE V)**.

83. Mayer G, Seidlein H. Chondral and osteochondral fractures of the knee joint—treatment and results. *Arch Orthop Trauma Surg.* 1988;107(3):154–157. **(LOE IV)**.

84. Rorabeck CH, Bobechko WP. Acute dislocation of the patella with osteochondral fracture: a review of eighteen cases. *J Bone Joint Surg Br.* 1976;58(2):237–240. **(LOE IV)**.

85. Stanitski CL, Paletta GA Jr. Articular cartilage injury with acute patellar dislocation in adolescents. Arthroscopic and radiographic correlation. *Am J Sports Med.* 1998;26(1):52–55. **(LOE IV)**.

86. Stanitski CL. Articular hypermobility and chondral injury in patients with acute patellar dislocation. *Am J Sports Med.* 1995;23(2):146–150. **(LOE III)**.

87. Rosenberg NJ. Osteochondral fractures of the lateral femoral condyle. *J Bone Joint Surg Am.* 1964;46:1013–1026. **(LOE IV)**.

88. Vahasarja V, Kinnunen P, Serlo W. Arthroscopy in the diagnostics and treatment of non-acute knee disorders in children. *Eur J Pediatr Surg.* 1996;6(1):25–28. **(LOE IV)**.

89. Gilley JS, Gelman MI, Edson DM, Metcalf RW. Chondral fractures of the knee. Arthrographic, arthroscopic, and clinical manifestations. *Radiology.* 1981;138(1):51–54. **(LOE IV)**.

90. Mink JH, Deutsch AL. Occult cartilage and bone injuries of the knee: detection, classification, and assessment with MR imaging. *Radiology.* 1989;170(3 Pt 1):823–829. **(LOE IV)**.

91. Wessel LM, Scholz S, Rusch M, Kopke J, Loff S, Duchene W, et al. Hemarthrosis after trauma to the pediatric knee joint: what is the value of magnetic resonance imaging in the diagnostic algorithm? *J Pediatr Orthop.* 2001;21(3):338–342. **(LOE IV)**.

92. Kramer DE, Pace JL. Acute traumatic and sports-related osteochondral injury of the pediatric knee. *Orthop Clin North Am.* 2012;43(2):227–236, vi. **(LOE V)**.

93. Ten Thije JH, Frima AJ. Patellar dislocation and osteochondral fractures. *Neth J Surg.* 1986;38(5):150–154.

94. Ure BM, Tiling T, Roddecker K, Klein J, Rixen D. Arthroscopy of the knee in children and adolescents. *Eur J Pediatr Surg.* 1992;2(2):102–105. **(LOE IV)**.

95. Lewis PL, Foster BK. Herbert screw fixation of osteochondral fractures about the knee. *Aust N Z J Surg.* 1990;60(7):511–513. **(LOE IV)**.

96. Rae PS, Khasawneh ZM. Herbert screw fixation of osteochondral fractures of the patella. *Injury.* 1988;19(2):116–119. **(LOE V)**.

97. Wombwell JH, Nunley JA. Compressive fixation of osteochondritis dissecans fragments with Herbert screws. *J Orthop Trauma.* 1987;1(1):74–77. **(LOE IV)**.

98. Gaudernak T, Zifko B, Skorpik G. Osteochondral fractures of the knee and the ankle joint. Clinical experiences using fibrin sealant. *Acta Orthop Belg.* 1986;52(4):465–478. **(LOE V)**.

99. Harper MC, Ralston M. Isobutyl 2-cyanoacrylate as an osseous adhesive in the repair of osteochondral fractures. *J Biomed Mater Res.* 1983;17(1):167–177. **(LOE III)**.

100. Gkiokas A, Morassi LG, Kohl S, Zampakides C, Megremis P, Evangelopoulos DS. Bioabsorbable pins for treatment of osteochondral fractures of the knee after acute patella dislocation in children and young adolescents. *Adv Orthop.* 2012;2012:249687. **(LOE IV)**.

101. Matsusue Y, Nakamura T, Suzuki S, Iwasaki R. Biodegradable pin fixation of osteochondral fragments of the knee. *Clin Orthop Relat Res.* 1996;(322):166–173. **(LOE IV)**.

102. Walsh SJ, Boyle MJ, Morganti V. Large osteochondral fractures of the lateral femoral condyle in the adolescent: outcome of bioabsorbable pin fixation. *J Bone Joint Surg Am.* 2008;90(7):1473–1478. **(LOE IV)**.

103. Barfod G, Svendsen RN. Synovitis of the knee after intraarticular fracture fixation with Biofix. Report of two cases. *Acta Orthop Scand.* 1992;63(6):680–681. **(LOE V)**.

104. Chotel F, Knorr G, Simian E, Dubrana F, Versier G. Knee osteochondral fractures in skeletally immature patients: French multicenter study. *Orthop Traumatol Surg Res.* 2011;97(suppl 8):S154–S159. **(LOE IV)**.

105. Lee BJ, Christino MA, Daniels AH, Hulstyn MJ, Eberson CP. Adolescent patellar osteochondral fracture following patellar dislocation. *Knee Surg Sports Traumatol Arthrosc.* 2013;21(8):1856–1861. **(LOE IV)**.

106. Bates DG, Hresko MT, Jaramillo D. Patellar sleeve fracture: demonstration with MR imaging. *Radiology.* 1994;193(3):825–827. **(LOE V)**.

107. Hunt DM, Somashekar N. A review of sleeve fractures of the patella in children. *Knee.* 2005;12(1):3–7. **(LOE V)**.

108. Maripuri SN, Mehta H, Mohanty K. Sleeve fracture of the superior pole of the patella with an intra-articular dislocation. A case report. *J Bone Joint Surg Am.* 2008;90(2):385–389. **(LOE V)**.

109. Ray JM, Hendrix J. Incidence, mechanism of injury, and treatment of fractures of the patella in children. *J Trauma.* 1992;32(4):464–467. **(LOE IV)**.

110. Schmal H, Strohm PC, Niemeyer P, Reising K, Kuminack K, Sudkamp NP. Fractures of the patella in children and adolescents. *Acta Orthop Belg.* 2010;76(5):644–650. **(LOE IV)**.

111. Ogden JA. Radiology of postnatal skeletal development. X. Patella and tibial tuberosity. *Skeletal Radiol.* 1984;11(4):246–257. **(LOE V)**.

112. Ogden JA, McCarthy SM, Jokl P. The painful bipartite patella. *J Pediatr Orthop.* 1982;2(3):263–269. **(LOE IV)**.

113. Maguire JK, Canale ST. Fractures of the patella in children and adolescents. *J Pediatr Orthop.* 1993;13(5):567–571. **(LOE IV)**.

114. Makhdoomi KR, Doyle J, Moloney M. Transverse fracture of the patella in children. *Arch Orthop Trauma Surg.* 1993;112(6):302–303. **(LOE IV)**.

115. Gettys FK, Morgan RJ, Fleischli JE. Superior pole sleeve fracture of the patella: a case report and review of the literature. *Am J Sports Med.* 2010;38(11):2331–2336. **(LOE V)**.

116. Hensal F, Nelson T, Pavlov H, Torg JS. Bilateral patellar fractures from indirect trauma. A case report. *Clin Orthop Relat Res.* 1983;(178):207–209. **(LOE V)**.

117. Iwaya T, Takatori Y. Lateral longitudinal stress fracture of the patella: report of three cases. *J Pediatr Orthop.* 1985;5(1):73–75. **(LOE IV)**.

118. Grogan DP, Carey TP, Leffers D, Ogden JA. Avulsion fractures of the patella. *J Pediatr Orthop.* 1990;10(6):721–730. **(LOE IV)**.

119. Bostman O, Kiviluoto O, Santavirta S, Nirhamo J, Wilppula E. Fractures of the patella treated by operation. *Arch Orthop Trauma Surg.* 1983;102(2):78–81. **(LOE IV)**.

120. Weber MJ, Janecki CJ, McLeod P, Nelson CL, Thompson JA. Efficacy of various forms of fixation of transverse fractures of the patella. *J Bone Joint Surg Am.* 1980;62(2):215–220. **(LOE III)**.

121. Bruijn JD, Sanders RJ, Jansen BR. Ossification in the patellar tendon and patella alta following sports injuries in children. Complications of sleeve fractures after conservative treatment. *Arch Orthop Trauma Surg.* 1993;112(3):157–158. **(LOE V)**.

122. Houghton GR, Ackroyd CE. Sleeve fractures of the patella in children: a report of three cases. *J Bone Joint Surg Br.* 1979;61-B(2):165–168. **(LOE IV)**.

123. Wu CD, Huang SC, Liu TK. Sleeve fracture of the patella in children. A report of five cases. *Am J Sports Med.* 1991;19(5):525–528. **(LOE IV)**.

124. Sturdee SW, Templeton PA, Oxborrow NJ. Internal fixation of a patella fracture using an absorbable suture. *J Orthop Trauma.* 2002;16(4):272–273. **(LOE V)**.

125. Berg EE. Bipolar infrapatellar tendon rupture. *J Pediatr Orthop.* 1995;15(3):302–303. **(LOE V)**.

126. Carpenter JE, Kasman RA, Patel N, Lee ML, Goldstein SA. Biomechanical evaluation of current patella fracture fixation techniques. *J Orthop Trauma.* 1997;11(5):351–356. **(LOE III)**.

127. Adams AJ, Talathi NS, Gandhi JS, Patel NM, Ganley TJ. Tibial spine fractures in children: evaluation, management, and future directions. *J Knee Surg.* 2018;31(5):374–381. **(LOE V)**.

128. Meyers MH, McKeever FM. Fracture of the intercondylar eminence of the tibia. *J Bone Joint Surg Am.* 1959;41-A(2):209–220. **(LOE IV)**.

129. Pandya NK, Janik L, Chan G, Wells L. Case reports: pediatric PCL insufficiency from tibial insertion osteochondral avulsions. *Clin Orthop Relat Res.* 2008;466(11):2878–2883. **(LOE V)**.

130. Ross AC, Chesterman PJ. Isolated avulsion of the tibial attachment of the posterior cruciate ligament in childhood. *J Bone Joint Surg Br.* 1986;68(5):747. **(LOE V)**.

131. Mitchell JJ, Sjostrom R, Mansour AA, Irion B, Hotchkiss M, Terhune EB, et al. Incidence of meniscal injury and chondral pathology in anterior tibial spine fractures of children. *J Pediatr Orthop.* 2015;35(2):130–135. **(LOE IV)**.

132. Leeberg V, Sonne-Holm S, Krogh CJ, Wong C. Fractures of the knee in children—what can go wrong? A case file study of closed claims in The Patient Compensation Association covering 16 years. *J Child Orthop.* 2015;9(5):391–396. **(LOE IV)**.

133. Meyers MH, McKeever FM. Fracture of the intercondylar eminence of the tibia. *J Bone Joint Surg Am.* 1970;52(8):1677–1684. **(LOE IV)**.

134. Zaricznyj B. Avulsion fracture of the tibial eminence: treatment by open reduction and pinning. *J Bone Joint Surg Am.* 1977;59(8):1111–1114. **(LOE IV)**.

135. Bakalim G, Wilppula E. Closed treatment of fracture of the tibial spines. *Injury.* 1974;5(3):210–212. **(LOE IV)**.

136. Fyfe IS, Jackson JP. Tibial intercondylar fractures in children: a review of the classification and the treatment of mal-union. *Injury.* 1981;13(2):165–169. **(LOE V)**.

137. Kendall NS, Hsu SY, Chan KM. Fracture of the tibial spine in adults and children. A review of 31 cases. *J Bone Joint Surg Br.* 1992;74(6):848–852. **(LOE IV)**.

138. Wiley JJ, Baxter MP. Tibial spine fractures in children. *Clin Orthop Relat Res.* 1990;(255):54–60. **(LOE V)**.

139. Mah JY, Adili A, Otsuka NY, Ogilvie R. Follow-up study of arthroscopic reduction and fixation of type III tibial-eminence fractures. *J Pediatr Orthop.* 1998;18(4):475–477. **(LOE IV)**.

140. Medler RG, Jansson KA. Arthroscopic treatment of fractures of the tibial spine. *Arthroscopy.* 1994;10(3):292–295. **(LOE IV)**.

141. Kocher MS, Micheli LJ, Gerbino P, Hresko MT. Tibial eminence fractures in children: prevalence of meniscal entrapment. *Am J Sports Med.* 2003;31(3):404–407. **(LOE IV)**.

142. Edmonds EW, Fornari ED, Dashe J, Roocroft JH, King MM, Pennock AT. Results of displaced pediatric tibial spine fractures: a comparison between open, arthroscopic, and closed management. *J Pediatr Orthop.* 2015;35(7):651–656. **(LOE III)**.

143. Brunner S, Vavken P, Kilger R, Vavken J, Rutz E, Brunner R, et al. Absorbable and non-absorbable suture fixation results in similar outcomes for tibial eminence fractures in children and adolescents. *Knee Surg Sports Traumatol Arthrosc.* 2016;24(3):723–729. **(LOE III)**.

144. Lehman RA Jr, Murphy KP, Machen MS, Kuklo TR. Modified arthroscopic suture fixation of a displaced tibial eminence fracture. *Arthroscopy.* 2003;19(2):E6. (**LOE IV**).

145. Matthews DE, Geissler WB. Arthroscopic suture fixation of displaced tibial eminence fractures. *Arthroscopy.* 1994;10(4):418–423. (**LOE IV**).

146. Anderson CN, Nyman JS, McCullough KA, et al. Biomechanical evaluation of physeal-sparing fixation methods in tibial eminence fractures. *Am J Sports Med.* 2013;41(7):1586–1594. (**LOE II**).

147. Hapa O, Barber FA, Suner G, et al. Biomechanical comparison of tibial eminence fracture fixation with high-strength suture, EndoButton, and suture anchor. *Arthroscopy.* 2012;28(5):681–687. (**LOE III**).

148. Schneppendahl J, Thelen S, Twehues S, et al. The use of biodegradable sutures for the fixation of tibial eminence fractures in children: a comparison using PDS II, Vicryl and FiberWire. *J Pediatr Orthop.* 2013;33(4):409–414. (**LOE II**).

149. Anderson CN, Anderson AF. Tibial eminence fractures. *Clin Sports Med.* 2011;30(4):727–742. (**LOE V**).

150. Janarv PM, Westblad P, Johansson C, Hirsch G. Long-term follow-up of anterior tibial spine fractures in children. *J Pediatr Orthop.* 1995;15(1):63–68. (**LOE IV**).

151. May JH, Levy BA, Guse D, Shah J, Stuart MJ, Dahm DL. ACL tibial spine avulsion: mid-term outcomes and rehabilitation. *Orthopedics.* 2011;34(2). 89–10. (**LOE IV**).

152. Lipscomb AB, Anderson AF. Open reduction of a malunited tibial spine fracture in a 12-year-old male. A case report. *Am J Sports Med.* 1985;13(6):419–422. (**LOE IV**).

153. Bachelin P, Bugmann P. Active subluxation in extension, radiological control in intercondylar eminence fractures in childhood. *Z Kinderchir.* 1988;43(3):180–182. (**LOE IV**).

154. Baxter MP, Wiley JJ. Fractures of the tibial spine in children. An evaluation of knee stability. *J Bone Joint Surg Br.* 1988;70(2):228–230. (**LOE IV**).

155. Kocher MS, Foreman ES, Micheli LJ. Laxity and functional outcome after arthroscopic reduction and internal fixation of displaced tibial spine fractures in children. *Arthroscopy.* 2003;19(10):1085–1090. (**LOE IV**).

156. Smith JB. Knee instability after fractures of the intercondylar eminence of the tibia. *J Pediatr Orthop.* 1984;4(4):462–464. (**LOE IV**).

157. Willis RB, Blokker C, Stoll TM, Paterson DC, Galpin RD. Long-term follow-up of anterior tibial eminence fractures. *J Pediatr Orthop.* 1993;13(3):361–364. (**LOE IV**).

158. Gronkvist H, Hirsch G, Johansson L. Fracture of the anterior tibial spine in children. *J Pediatr Orthop.* 1984;4(4):465–468. (**LOE IV**).

159. Simonian PT, Staheli LT. Periarticular fractures after manipulation for knee contractures in children. *J Pediatr Orthop.* 1995;15(3):288–291. (**LOE IV**).

160. Patel NM, Park MJ, Sampson NR, Ganley TJ. Tibial eminence fractures in children: earlier posttreatment mobilization results in improved outcomes. *J Pediatr Orthop.* 2012;32(2):139–144. (**LOE III**).

161. Vander Have KL, Ganley TJ, Kocher MS, Price CT, Herrera-Soto JA. Arthrofibrosis after surgical fixation of tibial eminence fractures in children and adolescents. *Am J Sports Med.* 2010;38(2):298–301. (**LOE IV**).

162. Gans I, Baldwin KD, Ganley TJ. Treatment and management outcomes of tibial eminence fractures in pediatric patients: a systematic review. *Am J Sports Med.* 2014;42(7):1743–1750. (**LOE IV**).

163. Watts CD, Larson AN, Milbrandt TA. Open versus arthroscopic reduction for tibial eminence fracture fixation in children. *J Pediatr Orthop.* 2016;36(5):437–439. (**LOE III**).

164. Brey JM, Conoley J, Canale ST, et al. Tibial tuberosity fractures in adolescents: is a posterior metaphyseal fracture component a predictor of complications? *J Pediatr Orthop.* 2012;32(6):561–566. (**LOE IV**).

165. Frey S, Hosalkar H, Cameron DB, Heath A, David HB, Ganley TJ. Tibial tuberosity fractures in adolescents. *J Child Orthop.* 2008;2(6):469–474. (**LOE IV**).

166. Mosier SM, Stanitski CL. Acute tibial tubercle avulsion fractures. *J Pediatr Orthop.* 2004;24(2):181–184. (**LOE IV**).

167. Balmat P, Vichard P, Pem R. The treatment of avulsion fractures of the tibial tuberosity in adolescent athletes. *Sports Med.* 1990;9(5):311–316. (**LOE V**).

168. Chow SP, Lam JJ, Leong JC. Fracture of the tibial tubercle in the adolescent. *J Bone Joint Surg Br.* 1990;72(2):231–234. (**LOE IV**).

169. Christie MJ, Dvonch VM. Tibial tuberosity avulsion fracture in adolescents. *J Pediatr Orthop.* 1981;1(4):391–394. (**LOE IV**).

170. Levi JH, Coleman CR. Fracture of the tibial tubercle. *Am J Sports Med.* 1976;4(6):254–263. (**LOE IV**).

171. Mirbey J, Besancenot J, Chambers RT, Durey A, Vichard P. Avulsion fractures of the tibial tuberosity in the adolescent athlete. Risk factors, mechanism of injury, and treatment. *Am J Sports Med.* 1988;16(4):336–340. (**LOE IV**).

172. Ogden JA, Tross RB, Murphy MJ. Fractures of the tibial tuberosity in adolescents. *J Bone Joint Surg Am.* 1980;62(2):205–215. (**LOE IV**).

173. Wiss DA, Schilz JL, Zionts L. Type III fractures of the tibial tubercle in adolescents. *J Orthop Trauma.* 1991;5(4):475–479. (**LOE IV**).

174. Wall JJ. Compartment syndrome as a complication of the Hauser procedure. *J Bone Joint Surg Am.* 1979;61(2):185–191. (**LOE V**).

175. Pape JM, Goulet JA, Hensinger RN. Compartment syndrome complicating tibial tubercle avulsion. *Clin Orthop Relat Res.* 1993;(295):201–204. (**LOE IV**).

176. Bowers KD Jr. Patellar tendon avulsion as a complication of Osgood-Schlatter's disease. *Am J Sports Med.* 1981;9(6):356–359. (**LOE V**).

177. Williams D, Kahane S, Chou D, Vemulapalli K. Bilateral proximal tibial sleeve fractures in a child: a case report. *Arch Trauma Res.* 2015;4(3):e27898. (**LOE IV**).

178. Desai RR, Parikh SN. Bilateral tibial tubercle sleeve fractures in a skeletally immature patient. *Case Rep Orthop.* 2013;2013:969405. (**LOE IV**).

179. Pretell-Mazzini J, Kelly DM, Sawyer JR, Esteban EM, Spence DD, Warner WC Jr, et al. Outcomes and complications of tibial tubercle fractures in pediatric patients: a systematic review of the literature. *J Pediatr Orthop.* 2016;36(5):440–446. (**LOE III**).

180. Davidson D, Letts M. Partial sleeve fractures of the tibia in children: an unusual fracture pattern. *J Pediatr Orthop.* 2002;22(1):36–40. (**LOE IV**).

181. Frankl U, Wasilewski SA, Healy WL. Avulsion fracture of the tibial tubercle with avulsion of the patellar ligament. Report of two cases. *J Bone Joint Surg Am.* 1990;72(9):1411–1413. (**LOE V**).

182. Mayba II. Avulsion fracture of the tibial tubercle apophysis with avulsion of patellar ligament. *J Pediatr Orthop.* 1982;2(3):303–305. (**LOE V**).

183. Pandya NK, Edmonds EW, Roocroft JH, Mubarak SJ. Tibial tubercle fractures: complications, classification, and the need for intra-articular assessment. *J Pediatr Orthop.* 2012;32(8):749–759. (**LOE III**).

184. Kramer DE, Chang TL, Miller NH, Sponseller PD. Tibial tubercle fragmentation: a clue to simultaneous patellar ligament avulsion in pediatric tibial tubercle fractures. *Orthopedics.* 2008;31(5):501. (**LOE V**).

185. Watson-Jones R. Injuries of the knee. In: E.& S. Livingstone, ed. *Fractures and Joint Injuries.* 3rd ed. Edinburgh and London: E. & S. Livingstone; 1956: 751–800. (**LOE IV**).

186. Ryu RK, Debenham JO. An unusual avulsion fracture of the proximal tibial epiphysis. Case report and proposed addition to the Watson-Jones classification. *Clin Orthop Relat Res.* 1985;(194):181–184. (**LOE V**).

187. Donahue JP, Brennan JF, Barron OA. Combined physeal/apophyseal fracture of the proximal tibia with anterior angulation from an indirect force: report of 2 cases. *Am J Orthop (Belle Mead NJ).* 2003;32(12):604–607. (**LOE V**).

188. Inoue G, Kuboyama K, Shido T. Avulsion fractures of the proximal tibial epiphysis. *Br J Sports Med.* 1991;25(1):52–56. (**LOE IV**).

189. Blanks RH, Lester DK, Shaw BA. Flexion-type Salter II fracture of the proximal tibia. Proposed mechanism of injury and two case studies. *Clin Orthop Relat Res.* 1994;(301):256–259. (**LOE V**).

190. Merloz P, de CC, Butel J, Robb JE. Bilateral Salter-Harris type II upper tibial epiphyseal fractures. *J Pediatr Orthop.* 1987;7(4):466–467. (**LOE V**).

191. Vyas S, Ebramzadeh E, Behrend C, Silva M, Zionts LE. Flexion-type fractures of the proximal tibial physis: a report of five cases and review of the literature. *J Pediatr Orthop B.* 2010;19(6):492–496. (**LOE IV**).

192. McKoy BE, Stanitski CL. Acute tibial tubercle avulsion fractures. *Orthop Clin North Am.* 2003;34(3):397–403. (**LOE IV**).

193. Aerts BR, Ten BB, Jakma TS, Punt BJ. Classification of proximal tibial epiphysis fractures in children: four clinical cases. *Injury.* 2015;46(8):1680–1683. (**LOE IV**).

194. Curtis JF. Type IV tibial tubercle fracture revisited: a case report. *Clin Orthop Relat Res.* 2001;(389):191–195. **(LOE V)**.

195. Riccio AI, Tulchin-Francis K, Hogue GD, Wimberly RL, Gill CS, Collins D, et al. Functional outcomes following operative treatment of tibial tubercle fractures. *J Pediatr Orthop.* 2017:10. **(LOE IV)**.

196. Ciszewski WA, Buschmann WR, Rudolph CN. Irreducible fracture of the proximal tibial physis in an adolescent. *Orthop Rev.* 1989;18(8):891–893. **(LOE V)**.

197. Gill JG, Chakrabarti HP, Becker SJ. Fractures of the proximal tibial epiphysis. *Injury.* 1983;14(4):324–331. **(LOE IV)**.

198. Aitken AP, Ingersoll RE. Fractures of the proximal tibial epiphyseal cartilage. *J Bone Joint Surg Am.* 1956;38-A(4):787–796. **(LOE V)**.

199. Burkhart SS, Peterson HA. Fractures of the proximal tibial epiphysis. *J Bone Joint Surg Am.* 1979;61(7):996–1002. **(LOE IV)**.

200. Shelton WR, Canale ST. Fractures of the tibia through the proximal tibial epiphyseal cartilage. *J Bone Joint Surg Am.* 1979;61(2):167–173. **(LOE IV)**.

201. Wozasek GE, Moser KD, Haller H, Capousek M. Trauma involving the proximal tibial epiphysis. *Arch Orthop Trauma Surg.* 1991;110(6):301–306. **(LOE IV)**.

202. Harb Z, Malhi A. Bilateral simultaneous avulsion fractures of the proximal tibia in a 14-year-old athlete with vitamin-D deficiency. *Case Rep Orthop.* 2015;2015:783046. **(LOE IV)**.

203. Kleinman PK, Marks SC Jr. A regional approach to the classic metaphyseal lesion in abused infants: the proximal tibia. *AJR Am J Roentgenol.* 1996;166(2):421–426. **(LOE IV)**.

204. Tjoumakaris FP, Wells L. Popliteal artery transection complicating a non-displaced proximal tibial epiphysis fracture. *Orthopedics.* 2007;30(10):876–877. **(LOE V)**.

205. Shinomiya R, Sunagawa T, Nakashima Y, Nakabayashi A, Makitsubo M, Adachi N. Slow progressive popliteal artery insufficiency after neglected proximal tibial physeal fracture: a case report. *J Pediatr Orthop B.* 2018;27(1):35–39. **(LOE V)**.

206. Tileston K, Frick S. Proximal tibial fractures in the pediatric population. *J Knee Surg.* 2018;31(6):498–503. **(LOE V)**.

207. Tony G, Charran A, Tins B, Lalam R, Tyrrell PN, Singh J, et al. Intra-epiphyseal stress injury of the proximal tibial epiphysis: preliminary experience of magnetic resonance imaging findings. *Eur J Radiol.* 2014;83(11):2051–2057. **(LOE IV)**.

208. Conroy J, Cohen A, Smith RM, Matthews S. Triplane fracture of the proximal tibia. *Injury.* 2000;31(7):546–548. **(LOE V)**.

209. Hermus JP, Driessen MJ, Mulder H, Bos CF. The triplane variant of the tibial apophyseal fracture: a case report and a review of the literature. *J Pediatr Orthop B.* 2003;12(6):406–408. **(LOE V)**.

210. Kanellopoulos AD, Yiannakopoulos CK, Badras LS. Triplane fracture of the proximal tibia. *Am J Orthop (Belle Mead NJ).* 2003;32(9):452–454. **(LOE V)**.

211. Patari SK, Lee FY, Behrens FF. Coronal split fracture of the proximal tibia epiphysis through a partially closed physis: a new fracture pattern. *J Pediatr Orthop.* 2001;21(4):451–455. **(LOE V)**.

212. Sferopoulos NK, Rafailidis D, Traios S, Christoforides J. Avulsion fractures of the lateral tibial condyle in children. *Injury.* 2006;37(1):57–60. **(LOE IV)**.

213. Dietz GW, Wilcox DM, Montgomery JB. Segond tibial condyle fracture: lateral capsular ligament avulsion. *Radiology.* 1986;159(2):467–469. **(LOE IV)**.

214. Robert M, Khouri N, Carlioz H, Alain JL. Fractures of the proximal tibial metaphysis in children: review of a series of 25 cases. *J Pediatr Orthop.* 1987;7(4):444–449. **(LOE IV)**.

215. Poulsen TD, Skak SV, Jensen TT. Epiphyseal fractures of the proximal tibia. *Injury.* 1989;20(2):111–113. **(LOE IV)**.

216. Hill BW, Rizkala AR, Li M. Clinical and functional outcomes after operative management of Salter-Harris III and IV fractures of the proximal tibial epiphysis. *J Pediatr Orthop B.* 2014;23(5):411–418. **(LOE IV)**.

217. Vrettakos AN, Evaggelidis DC, Kyrkos MJ, Tsatsos AV, Nenopoulos A, Beslikas T. Lower limb deformity following proximal tibia physeal injury: long-term follow-up. *J Orthop Traumatol.* 2012;13(1):7–11. **(LOE IV)**.

218. Gautier E, Ziran BH, Egger B, Slongo T, Jakob RP. Growth disturbances after injuries of the proximal tibial epiphysis. *Arch Orthop Trauma Surg.* 1998;118(1-2):37–41. **(LOE V)**.

219. Hasler CC, Foster BK. Secondary tethers after physeal bar resection: a common source of failure? *Clin Orthop Relat Res.* 2002;(405):242–249. **(LOE IV)**.

220. Clark A, Hilt JZ, Milbrandt TA, Puleo DA. Treating proximal tibial growth plate injuries using poly(lactic-co-glycolic acid) scaffolds. *Biores Open Access.* 2015;4(1):65–74. **(LOE III)**.

221. Olerud C, Danckwardt-Lilliestrom G, Olerud S. Genu recurvatum caused by partial growth arrest of the proximal tibial physis: simultaneous correction and lengthening with physeal distraction. A report of two cases. *Arch Orthop Trauma Surg.* 1986;106(1):64–68. **(LOE V)**.

222. Pennig D, Baranowski D. Genu recurvatum due to partial growth arrest of the proximal tibial physis: correction by callus distraction. Case report. *Arch Orthop Trauma Surg.* 1989;108(2):119–121. **(LOE V)**.

223. Hresko MT, Kasser JR. Physeal arrest about the knee associated with non-physeal fractures in the lower extremity. *J Bone Joint Surg Am.* 1989;71(5):698–703. **(LOE IV)**.

224. Pappas AM, Anas P, Toczylowski Jr HM. Asymmetrical arrest of the proximal tibial physis and genu recurvatum deformity. *J Bone Joint Surg Am.* 1984;66(4):575–581. **(LOE IV)**.

225. Cozen L. Fracture of the proximal portion of the tibia in children followed by valgus deformity. *Surg Gynecol Obstet.* 1953;97(2):183–188. **(LOE IV)**.

226. Rang M. Tibia. In: *Children's Fractures.* 2nd ed. Philadelphia: J.B. Lippincott Company; 1983:297–307.

227. Ogden JA, Ogden DA, Pugh L, Raney EM, Guidera KJ. Tibia valga after proximal metaphyseal fractures in childhood: a normal biologic response. *J Pediatr Orthop.* 1995;15(4):489–494. **(LOE IV)**.

228. Choi ES, Hong JH, Sim JA. Distinct features of trampoline-related orthopedic injuries in children aged under 6 years. *Injury.* 2018;49(2):443–446. **(LOE IV)**.

229. Kakel R. Trampoline fracture of the proximal tibial metaphysis in children may not progress into valgus: a report of seven cases and a brief review. *Orthop Traumatol Surg Res.* 2012;98(4):446–449. **(LOE IV)**.

230. Arkink EB, van der Plas A, Sneep RW, Reijnierse M. Bilateral trampoline fracture of the proximal tibia in a child. *Radiol Case Rep.* 2017;12(4):798–800. **(LOE IV)**.

231. Weber BG. Fibrous interposition causing valgus deformity after fracture of the upper tibial metaphysis in children. *J Bone Joint Surg Br.* 1977;59(3):290–292. **(LOE V)**.

232. Skak SV. Valgus deformity following proximal tibial metaphyseal fracture in children. *Acta Orthop Scand.* 1982;53(1):141–147. **(LOE IV)**.

233. Zionts LE, MacEwen GD. Spontaneous improvement of post-traumatic tibia valga. *J Bone Joint Surg Am.* 1986;68(5):680–687. **(LOE IV)**.

234. Zionts LE, Harcke HT, Brooks KM, MacEwen GD. Posttraumatic tibia valga: a case demonstrating asymmetric activity at the proximal growth plate on technetium bone scan. *J Pediatr Orthop.* 1987;7(4):458–462. **(LOE V)**.

235. Balthazar DA, Pappas AM. Acquired valgus deformity of the tibia in children. *J Pediatr Orthop.* 1984;4(5):538–541. **(LOE IV)**.

236. McCarthy JJ, Kim DH, Eilert RE. Posttraumatic genu valgum: operative versus nonoperative treatment. *J Pediatr Orthop.* 1998;18(4):518–521. **(LOE IV)**.

237. Tuten HR, Keeler KA, Gabos PG, Zionts LE, MacKenzie WG. Posttraumatic tibia valga in children. A long-term follow-up note. *J Bone Joint Surg Am.* 1999;81(6):799–810. **(LOE IV)**.

238. Dal MA, Manes E, Cammarota V. Post-traumatic genu valgum in children. *Ital J Orthop Traumatol.* 1983;9(1):5–11. **(LOE IV)**.

239. Morin M, Klatt J, Stevens PM. Cozen's deformity: resolved by guided growth. *Strategies Trauma Limb Reconstr.* 2018;13(2):87–93. **(LOE IV)**.

240. Abrams J, Bennett E, Kumar SJ, Pizzutillo PD. Salter-Harris type III fracture of the proximal fibula. A case report. *Am J Sports Med.* 1986;14(6):514–516. **(LOE V)**.

241. Brenkel IJ, Prosser AJ, Pearse M. Salter type 2 fracture separation of the proximal epiphysis of the fibula. *Injury.* 1987;18(6):421–422. **(LOE V)**.

242. Voit GA, Irvine G, Beals RK. Saline load test for penetration of periarticular lacerations. *J Bone Joint Surg Br.* 1996;78(5):732–733. **(LOE IV)**.

243. Patzakis MJ, Dorr LD, Ivler D, Moore TM, Harvey JP Jr. The early management of open joint injuries. A prospective study of one hundred and forty patients. *J Bone Joint Surg Am.* 1975;57(8):1065–1070. **(LOE IV)**.

244. Linden MA, Manton WI, Stewart RM, Thal ER, Feit H. Lead poisoning from retained bullets. Pathogenesis, diagnosis, and management. *Ann Surg.* 1982;195(3):305–313. **(LOE IV)**.

Fractures of the Tibia and Fibula

14

George H. Thompson

INTRODUCTION

Nonphyseal fractures of the tibia and fibula are among the most common injuries involving the lower extremities in children and adolescents.[1–6] They are second only to fractures of the femur as a cause for hospital admissions for pediatric trauma.[2] Most can be treated nonoperatively with satisfactory long-term results and minimal complications. However, certain tibial fractures pose unique problems that must be carefully evaluated and treated to avoid complications.

PATHOLOGY

RELEVANT ANATOMY

The shafts of the tibia and fibula are composed of a proximal metaphysis, central diaphysis, and distal metaphysis. The blood supply to the tibia is from (1) a nutrient artery, which is a branch of the posterior tibial artery that enters at the junction of the distal and middle thirds of the tibia and is responsible for the endosteal or medullary blood supply; (2) periosteal vessels, which are segmented and enter from muscular attachments; and (3) epiphyseal vessels. The inner two-thirds of the cortex is supplied by the endosteal vessels, and the outer third is supplied by the periosteal vessels. Proximally, the epiphyseal and periosteal vessels are branches of the medial and lateral inferior geniculate arteries from the popliteal artery. The collateral circulation is rich proximally, especially on the medial aspect.[7] Tibia fractures distal to the nutrient artery may deprive the distal fragment of its medullary blood supply, and, in such cases, the distal end of the tibia must rely on its periosteal and metaphyseal blood supply for healing. This supply is limited because of a lack of muscle attachment, and a slower rate of healing generally results. Periosteal and soft tissue stripping of the distal fracture from the injury or surgical intervention further slows the healing process.

The blood supply to the fibula is from the peroneal artery, which gives off a nutrient artery that enters the diaphysis just proximal to its midpoint. The rest of the artery supplies multiple segmental musculoperiosteal vessels that pass circumferentially around the fibula and supply both the fibula and the adjacent muscles.

From a surgical perspective, remember that the popliteal artery descends between the posterior aspects of the medial and lateral femoral condyles. It passes between the medial and lateral heads of the gastrocnemius muscle and along the distal border of the popliteus muscle before dividing into the anterior and posterior tibial arteries. The anterior tibial artery passes anteriorly between the two heads of the tibialis posterior muscle and enters the anterior compartment of the leg by passing through the proximal aspect of the interosseous membrane at the flare of the proximal tibial and fibular metaphyses.[7] Displaced fractures in this region may damage the anterior tibial artery.[8] Fortunately, such injuries rarely occur. The foramen in the interosseous membrane is long and narrow; it affords some protection inasmuch as the anterior tibial artery is allowed to move both proximally and distally. Corrective varus or valgus osteotomies of the proximal portion of the tibia can also damage the anterior tibial artery. Subperiosteal dissection in the region below the tibial tubercle helps protect this vessel.

FRACTURE PATTERNS

Fracture patterns involving the tibial and fibular diaphyses include compression (torus), incomplete tension-compression (greenstick), and complete fractures. Plastic deformities can also occur but predominantly involve the fibula. Complete fractures are further classified according to the direction of the fracture (i.e., spiral, oblique, or transverse) and as comminuted or segmental. Approximately 37% of tibial fractures are comminuted.[6] Tibial and fibular fractures may also be open or closed, depending on the integrity of the overlying skin and soft tissues.

PREVALENCE

Fractures of the tibial and fibular shafts are the most common long bone fractures of the lower extremity[2,3,5,6] and represent approximately 15% of all pediatric fractures.[1] They occur more frequently in boys than in girls. Parrini and colleagues[5] reported on 1027 long bone fractures in children between 1 and 11 years of age, including 326 tibial fractures (32%); 157 were isolated fractures of the tibia, and 169 fractures were of both the tibia and fibula. Cheng and Shen[1] studied 3350 children with 3413 limb fractures and also found tibial shaft fractures to be the most common lower extremity fracture, with a relatively static prevalence of 9% to 12% throughout various pediatric age groups.

An epidemiologic study by Karrholm and associates[3] in Sweden in 1981 showed an annual incidence of 190 tibial fractures per 10,000 boys between infancy and 18 years of age and 110 tibial fractures per 10,000 girls in the same age range. In boys, the incidence peaked between 3 and 4 years of age and again between 15 and 16 years of age. The first peak involved predominantly spiral or oblique fractures, and the second peak involved primarily transverse fractures. In girls, the incidence was relatively even up to 11 to 12 years of age, and the tendency was toward a declining incidence with advancing age.

MECHANISMS OF INJURY

Fractures of the tibia and fibula may be the result of direct or indirect forces. Direct trauma frequently produces a transverse fracture or segmental fracture pattern, whereas indirect forces are typically rotational and produce an oblique or spiral fracture.

In a 1982 study by Karrholm and associates,[3] motor vehicle accidents involving children as passengers, as bicycle riders, or as pedestrians were the most common mechanism of tibial fractures. The age range of children in motor vehicle accidents was 8 to 14 years. Of interest, injuries from winter sports activities had almost the same incidence as motor vehicle accidents in girls. Falls were the most common mechanism of injury in young children. In a 1988 study by Shannak[6] of 142 tibial shaft fractures, motor vehicle accidents caused 63% of the fractures; falls, 18%; direct violence, 15%; and sports, only 4%. A 2007 study by Kute and associates[9] evaluated the trauma database of a pediatric level I trauma center and found that, of 238 patients admitted after all-terrain vehicle accidents, 63% of patients had fractures; of those, 14% occurred in the tibia and fibula.

CONSEQUENCES OF INJURY

Despite the frequency of pediatric tibial and fibular fractures, the consequences for most children are minimal. These fractures heal readily with minimal complications. Children typically have a rapid return to normal activities, including sports, and minimal disability. However, in a small percentage of cases, especially those involving open fractures or severe soft tissue injury, residual disability may occur.

ASSOCIATED INJURIES

It is not uncommon for children who sustain tibial and fibular fractures to have associated injuries, especially children who are victims of high-energy trauma, such as from motor vehicle–related accidents. In the study by Karrholm and associates,[3] 27 of 480 children (6%) with tibial and fibular fractures sustained associated injuries, of which the most common were head injuries, fractures of the femur, and injury to an upper extremity. Other body areas (i.e., face and neck, chest, and abdomen) may also be injured, depending on the severity of the trauma. Children with open tibial fractures have the highest incidence of associated injuries.[10–15]

CLASSIFICATION

A classification of nonphyseal fractures of the tibia and fibula is presented in Box 14.1. A modification of the classification of Dias,[16] this classification divides the tibial and fibular shafts into their three major anatomic areas: proximal metaphysis, diaphyses, and distal metaphysis. Fractures of the tibial and fibular diaphyses are subdivided according to the location (proximal third, middle third, and distal third) and

---

> ### Box 14.1   Classification of Tibial and Fibular Fractures
>
> Fractures of the proximal tibial metaphysis
> Fractures of the tibial and fibular shafts
> Isolated fractures of the tibial shaft
> Isolated fractures of the fibular shaft
> Fractures of the distal tibial metaphysis
>
> Modified from Dias LS. Fractures of the tibia and fibula. In: Rockwood CA Jr, Wilkins KE, King RE, eds. *Fractures in Children*. Philadelphia: J.B. Lippincott; 1984:983-1041.[16]

---

the combination of bones fractured. This classification is useful for determining treatment methods and understanding potential long-term results and possible complications.

The recently proposed AO Pediatric Comprehensive Classification of Long Bone Fractures has recently been shown to be clinically relevant with regard to growth and recovery.[17,18] However, further studies for confirmation are necessary.

DIAGNOSIS

HISTORY

The typical symptom of a tibial or fibular fracture is pain. However, the severity of the pain varies with the magnitude of the injury, the mechanism, and the age of the child. Frequently, a history is unavailable because the injury was not observed and the child is unable to verbalize symptoms or the mechanism of injury. In these cases, child abuse or battered child syndrome must also be considered (see Chapter 20). In young children, an inability to walk may be the only sign or symptom. If the child is able to speak, it is important to ascertain the mechanism of injury, if possible.

PHYSICAL EXAMINATION

Because pain is the major symptom in a tibial or fibular shaft fracture, it is important to have the child point to the most painful area. Palpation in this area may reproduce or increase the child's discomfort. Deformity is not a common finding in young children because many tibial fractures are nondisplaced. Swelling or edema of the lower part of the leg also varies according to the mechanism of injury, the extent of soft tissue injury, and the presence of displacement. Usually, the soft tissue swelling is maximal at the fracture site. Stress examination may reveal instability or crepitation but invariably increases pain. A stress examination is usually unnecessary when a fracture is suspected. Injured extremities with a suspected tibial fracture are best splinted before radiographic evaluation, usually with a long leg posterior plaster splint. This relieves pain, prevents additional injury to the soft tissues, and allows for more accurate positioning of the extremity for radiographs.

Nerve damage in association with closed tibial and fibular fractures is very uncommon (see "Neurologic Injury" section). However, in all fractures, it is important to check dorsiflexion and plantar flexion of the foot and toes, as well as sensation, especially to touch. Nerve damage, if present, is most likely the result of a direct injury to the peroneal nerve at the proximal fibular metaphysis.

Arterial injuries associated with a closed tibial shaft fracture are also very uncommon (see "Vascular Injury" section). The peripheral pulses of the dorsalis pedis and posterior tibial arteries must be evaluated and recorded at the initial physical examination. Arterial injuries are most likely to be associated with a displaced proximal tibial metaphyseal fracture or an open fracture. Capillary circulation, sensation to the toes, pain on passive stretching, and pain out of proportion to the injury must be monitored carefully because compartment syndromes can occur in children after tibial fractures (see "Compartment Syndrome" section).

The soft tissues of the lower part of the leg must also be evaluated. It is important to assess the integrity of the skin at the fracture site. Fractures related to bicycle spoke injuries may ultimately result in full-thickness skin loss requiring delayed skin grafting. Any evidence of skin penetration at the fracture site is an indication that the fracture is open and contaminated (see "Open Tibial and Fibular Fractures" section).

RADIOGRAPHIC EVALUATION

When a tibial or fibular shaft fracture is suspected, radiographs must be taken. After splinting of the injured extremity, anteroposterior (AP) and lateral radiographs are obtained. They must include the knee and ankle joints to rule out an associated epiphyseal fracture. Comparison radiographs of the opposite extremity may be indicated in complicated injuries, but this situation is unusual. Occasionally, incomplete fractures, such as a torus fracture, may be difficult to visualize. A spiral fracture of the tibial shaft with an intact fibula may be visible on only one view. It is therefore imperative that orthogonal radiographs always be obtained. Oblique radiographs may be beneficial if the initial radiographic appearance is normal but a fracture is suspected.

SPECIAL DIAGNOSTIC STUDIES

Special diagnostic imaging studies of the tibia and fibula may include ultrasonography, technetium bone scans, computed tomography (CT), and magnetic resonance imaging (MRI).

Ultrasonography[19] was recently shown to be at least as successful as radiography in diagnosing tibia fractures in both children and adults. Although not commonly used, it can be considered in difficult cases or when radiography may not be readily available.

Technetium bone scans may be useful in identifying occult fractures, especially in infants. Park and colleagues[20] found that bone scans could be used to differentiate occult fractures of the femur or tibia from early acute osteomyelitis in infants. Images obtained early (1–4 days after the onset of symptoms) demonstrated a subtle increase in uptake along the entire length of the injured bone when an occult fracture was present. The distribution of uptake was similar regardless of the fracture pattern. In early acute osteomyelitis, focal uptake was observed at the site of infection. Technetium bone scan can also be useful in toddler's and stress fractures.

CT of the tibia can be used to assess torsional alignment after complex unilateral fractures. It can also be used in the assessment of pathologic fractures of the tibia to determine the presence, size, and intralesional contours of the lesion. MRI can be used to detect early stress fractures accurately. This procedure, although expensive, avoids the high doses of radiation incurred with bone scans and CT.

MANAGEMENT

FRACTURES OF THE PROXIMAL TIBIAL METAPHYSIS

Proximal tibial metaphyseal fractures are relatively uncommon injuries that generally occur in children between 3 and 6 years of age (range, 1–12 years).[7,21–27] The male-to-female ratio of approximately 3:1 closely parallels the incidence of tibial fractures by gender in children. These fractures are typically the result of a direct injury to the lateral aspect of the extended knee. Most of these fractures have minimal or no displacement and appear benign radiographically; however, they may, in fact, be followed by a posttraumatic valgus deformity. Greenstick and complete fractures are most commonly associated with a valgus deformity.[26,28] Such deformities are unusual after a torus fracture. In a greenstick fracture, the medial cortex (tension side) fractures while the lateral cortex (compression side) remains intact or hinges slightly. If the lateral cortex hinges, a valgus deformity occurs. However, displacement is not usually seen, and apposition remains normal. The fibula is typically intact but may occasionally sustain either a fracture or plastic deformation. Radiographically, the degree of angulation can be difficult to ascertain unless radiographs are obtained of both lower extremities symmetrically positioned on a long cassette and the true angulation is measured. Oblique views and, occasionally, fluoroscopy may be beneficial in defining the fracture and any angulation.

There have been numerous reports of posttraumatic genu valgum after proximal tibial fractures.[7,22,23,25,26,28–37] Interestingly, similar valgus deformities may occur in association with other conditions affecting the proximal tibial metaphysis, such as acute and chronic osteomyelitis, harvesting of a bone graft, excision of an osteochondroma, and osteotomy.

The incidence of a valgus deformity after a proximal tibial metaphyseal fracture varies greatly, ranging from 0% to 62%.[25,26,28] Theories regarding the cause of valgus deformity have included injury to the lateral aspect of the proximal tibial physis, inadequate reduction,[26] premature weight bearing, hypertrophic callus formation, dynamic muscle action, soft tissue interposition (periosteum, pes anserinus, medial collateral ligament),[34,35,38] tethering from an intact fibula, and asymmetric growth stimulation. However, valgus deformity has been reported after complete fractures of the proximal ends of the tibia and fibula.[28,29]

Currently, most authors attribute valgus deformity to asymmetric growth of the proximal part of the tibia.[7,24,29,31–33,36,39,40] Houghton and Rooker,[40] in experimental studies with immature rabbits, found that medial hemicircumferential division of the periosteum resulted in valgus overgrowth. They believed that if the medial periosteum is torn during a proximal tibial metaphyseal fracture, asymmetric overgrowth occurs and produces a valgus deformity. Spontaneous correction with growth has also been observed.[24,32,33,37]

Aronson and colleagues[39] in 1990 reported on an experimental model with immature rabbits that confirmed asymmetric growth as the cause of posttraumatic valgus deformity. Twenty-two 8-week-old rabbits were divided into two equal groups. In one group, the periosteum on the medial aspect of the proximal tibial metaphysis was excised, and a partial osteotomy involving the medial half of the metaphysis was performed. In the other group, the same procedure was performed on the lateral side. Parallel K-wires were inserted above and below the partial osteotomy. A valgus deformity (mean of 12 degrees) occurred in the first group, and a varus deformity (mean of 10 degrees) developed in the second. In each animal, the K-wires remained parallel, thus indicating that the deformity occurred at the physis. Despite the asymmetric growth, the light microscopic appearance of the physes was normal. The deformities were therefore attributed to asymmetric physeal growth, which was not demonstrable histologically. Ogden[7] reported that the normal circulation to the knee has a more extensive medial geniculate blood supply, especially in the proximal tibial region, than a lateral geniculate supply, which may be responsible for transient eccentric growth. Zionts and colleagues[36] supported the concept of eccentric growth by demonstrating, in quantitative scintigraphic studies, proportionally greater uptake on the medial side than the lateral side and overall increased uptake on the injured as compared with the uninjured side. In 1995, Ogden and colleagues[24] performed detailed measurements of the metaphyseal-diaphyseal-metaphyseal distances medially and laterally of the injured and noninjured tibias of 17 children with 19 proximal tibial metaphyseal fractures (2 children had bilateral fractures) monitored for a mean of 3.7 years (range, 2–7 years). The difference between the medial and lateral sides of the injured tibias was 7.4 mm, which was an indication of eccentric medial growth. Interestingly, the 3.3-mm difference noted between the injured and uninjured lateral sides was a reflection of overall growth stimulation on the injured side. These observations occurred with or without an intact fibula.

It is clear from these studies that a valgus deformity is not usually a complication of the initial reduction but, instead, is secondary to differential growth between the medial and lateral aspects of the proximal tibial epiphysis.

EVOLUTION OF TREATMENT

It is now accepted that a valgus deformity stabilizes and then improves with growth and development. The deformity usually develops within 5 months of injury, reaches its maximum within 18 to 24 months, stabilizes, and then begins to improve by a combination of longitudinal growth and physeal (proximal and distal) realignment.[24,32,33,37] Unfortunately, no data indicate how much improvement can be anticipated. Ippolito and Pentimalli[23] observed that deformities of 15 degrees or less usually remodeled completely, especially in young children. More severe deformities did not completely remodel.

Zionts and MacEwen[37] monitored seven children with posttraumatic tibia valga for a mean of 39 months after injury. These children ranged in age from 11 months to 6 years. It was found that the valgus deformity progressed most rapidly during the first year after injury and then continued at a slower rate for as long as 17 months; overgrowth of the tibia accompanied the valgus deformity. The mean overgrowth was 1 cm (range, 0.2–1.7 cm). Clinical correction with subsequent growth occurred in six of the seven patients. These authors recommended a conservative approach to management of both the acute fracture and the subsequent valgus deformity. If the valgus deformity fails to correct satisfactorily by early adolescence, growth modulation of the proximal tibial physis is preferred over a tibial osteotomy when there is substantial growth remaining. They also recommended that the mechanical tibiofemoral angle, as described by Visser and Veldhuizen,[34] be used to measure the alignment of the lower extremity rather than Drennan's metaphyseal-diaphyseal angle. The latter measures only the alignment of the proximal end of the tibia. This angle is useful in the immediate postinjury stage but not in the follow-up period because considerable correction of the deformity is a result of distal realignment.[24,26,34,37] The distal tibial epiphysis tends to reorient itself perpendicular to the pressure forces, thereby resulting in eccentric growth and an S-shaped appearance of the tibia radiographically.

In an experimental study in dogs, Karaharju and associates[41] observed that the tibial physes changed their direction of growth after an osteotomy and residual valgus angulation. In the study by Ogden and colleagues,[24] no true correction of the proximal tibia valga was observed, but eccentric growth was present distally and led to realignment of the ankle joint toward its normal parallel alignment with the floor and knee.

McCarthy and associates[32] in 1998 made similar observations in their study of 15 children with posttraumatic genu valgum, of whom 10 were treated nonoperatively and 5 operatively. At approximately 4 years of follow-up, they found essentially no difference in the complementary physeal shaft and tibiofemoral angles and maximal valgus deformity of the two groups. They recommended nonoperative treatment and observation, especially for children aged 4 years or younger when injured.

Tuten and associates[33] in 1999 reevaluated the seven children of Zionts and MacEwen[37] at a mean follow-up of 15.3 years (range, 10.4–19.9 years). Every patient had spontaneous improvement of the metaphyseal-diaphyseal and mechanical tibiofemoral angles. However, most of the correction was thought to have occurred in the proximal end of the tibia. The mechanical axis of the limb remained lateral to the center of the knee joint in every patient, and the mean deviation was 15 mm (range, 3–24 mm). The affected tibia was slightly longer. The affected knee score was excellent in five patients and fair in two. One patient required a tibial osteotomy because of knee pain secondary to malalignment. The authors concluded that posttraumatic tibia valga should be observed throughout growth and that operative intervention should be reserved for patients with symptoms from malalignment.

CURRENT ALGORITHM

Most proximal tibial metaphyseal fractures can be treated nonoperatively with closed reduction techniques. Treatment consists of correction of any valgus angulation of greenstick fractures and immobilization in a long leg cast with the knee in extension for 4 to 6 weeks or until the fracture is well united. Slight overcorrection, if possible, may be desirable.[7] Displaced fractures require reduction as well as correction of any residual valgus angulation. However, normal apposition is not always necessary. Currently, indications for operative management of these fractures are limited. An inability to correct a significant valgus deformity under general anesthesia rather than failure to close the medial fracture gap is probably the major indication. The latter is usually indicative of soft tissue entrapment, but this complication does not contribute to subsequent overgrowth.

After satisfactory fracture reduction and cast application, fracture alignment should be assessed radiographically at least weekly for the first 1 to 2 weeks after injury. Any loss of alignment should be corrected.

SPECIAL CONSIDERATIONS FOR MULTIPLE TRAUMATIC INJURIES

Children who are victims of multiple traumatic injuries may sustain an unrecognized proximal tibial metaphyseal fracture, especially if an ipsilateral femoral shaft fracture is present. Bohn and Durbin[42] reported three males with proximal tibial metaphyseal fractures and ipsilateral femoral fractures in whom posttraumatic genu valgum and lower extremity overgrowth of 1.8 to 2.2 cm developed. In one, a 20-degree deformity resolved over a 5-year period. It is important that during the secondary survey, the lower part of the legs be carefully evaluated for occult injuries and that radiographs be obtained in cases of suspected fractures. The presence of a proximal tibial metaphyseal fracture may necessitate a change in treatment plan for the other musculoskeletal injuries. If an associated femoral shaft fracture is present, stabilization by either internal or external fixation may be necessary so that adequate closed reduction of the proximal tibial metaphyseal fracture can be achieved and maintained.

TREATMENT OPTIONS

Nonoperative Management

The vast majority of angulated or displaced proximal tibial metaphyseal fractures are amenable to closed reduction and immobilization in a long leg plaster cast. Such management is almost always performed under general anesthesia to ensure adequate relaxation and pain relief. In some instances, the intact lateral cortex of a greenstick fracture must be fractured to achieve correct alignment. Once satisfactory alignment is obtained, the lower extremity is immobilized in a long leg cast with the knee in extension. An AP radiograph of both lower extremities on a long cassette should document correction of the valgus deformity and symmetric alignment with the opposite uninvolved extremity. Slight overcorrection (5 degrees, if possible) is desirable to counter any valgus overgrowth. A lateral radiograph of the fractured tibia should also be obtained. Burton and Hennrikus[43], in 2016, felt that a varus mold in the cast minimized the potential for valgus deformity.

After a satisfactory closed reduction, repeated radiographs are obtained weekly for the first 3 weeks to assess maintenance of alignment. These radiographs consist of a non-weight-bearing AP view of both lower extremities on a long cassette and a lateral view of the fractured extremity. Subtle changes in alignment may not be appreciated unless both extremities are included on the radiograph. Any loss of alignment should be corrected by cast wedging techniques or a repeated attempt at closed reduction. Repeated closed reduction may require general anesthesia, depending on the age of the child, the amount of correction necessary,

and the degree of healing. Immobilization is continued until the fracture is well healed radiographically.

Surgical Management

Surgery is rarely indicated. Usually, the best alignment by closed reduction is accepted. Only if significant residual valgus deformity is present, with or without closure of the medial fracture gap (entrapped soft tissue), is open reduction considered. At surgery, after any entrapped soft tissue has been removed, the fracture can typically be reduced anatomically and the periosteum repaired. Internal fixation is not generally necessary, and fracture alignment is maintained by a long leg plaster cast with the knee in extension. The child is then monitored as described for nonoperative management.

Open proximal tibial metaphyseal fractures are rare but can occur in children who are victims of polytrauma. They are managed in the same manner as other open tibial shaft fractures (see "Open Tibial and Fibular Fractures" section). An external fixator may be necessary for stabilization, especially in children with segmental bone loss, instability, or other significant fractures or body area injuries. Epiphyseal pins may be necessary in these fractures to achieve adequate stability.

The final step in either management method is to advise the family that even though satisfactory or anatomic alignment of the fracture has been obtained, valgus deformity and tibial overgrowth are possible as a natural consequence of this fracture. Such counseling prepares the family for this complication, should it occur. The necessity of long-term follow-up must be emphasized.

Valgus Deformities

Treatment of valgus deformities after proximal tibial metaphyseal fractures is controversial. Conservative management with an orthosis has been suggested, but there is no evidence to substantiate the efficacy of this method.[16,23] Surgical correction was initially believed to be necessary. Salter and Best[25] reported that 10 of 13 patients with valgus deformity required tibial osteotomy for correction. Balthazar and Pappas[29] pointed out that, even with osteotomies, the valgus deformity can recur. Such recurrence has been attributed to the same asymmetric overgrowth phenomenon that led to the valgus deformity initially. In their six patients who had osteotomies, the valgus deformity recurred, although to a lesser degree. Similar results were reported by DalMonte and colleagues,[22] who observed recurrent valgus deformities in 7 of 16 patients (44%) after proximal tibial osteotomies. No significant difference was seen in the prevalence of recurrence in children younger than 5 years (60%) and those between 5 and 10 years of age (36%), except that the younger children experienced a greater recurrent deformity. These authors concluded that the osteotomy is essentially a second fracture and therefore has the same pathologic factors. Recurrent valgus deformity after corrective osteotomy has been observed by others.[28,31]

Zionts and MacEwen[37] and Tuten and associates[33] recommend that most valgus deformities be observed until early adolescence. If spontaneous improvement fails to provide sufficient clinical correction or if the malalignment is causing pain, a proximal tibial varus shortening osteotomy and fibular diaphyseal osteotomy may be necessary. Zionts and

MacEwen[37] also suggested medial epiphysiodesis as another method for simultaneous correction of both the angular deformity and any remaining lower extremity length inequality. Medial epiphysiodesis has also been recommended by Robert and associates.[28] Although tibial overgrowth is not usually excessive, it may be important for both the valgus and the overgrowth to be corrected simultaneously if surgery is performed.

Currently guided growth by temporary tethering of the proximal medial tibial physis using small plate or screws is favored. These are removed following deformity correction with growth. Morin et al[44] recently reported on 19 patients with posttraumatic tibia valgus who were satisfactorily treated with this technique. The rationale was twofold: correction of the proximal tibial valgus and reduce the tibial length discrepancy.

FOLLOW-UP CARE AND REHABILITATION

Once fracture healing is complete, the long leg cast can be removed. Initially, the child is allowed full weight-bearing, and knee range-of-motion exercises are encouraged. Failure to achieve satisfactory knee motion within 2 to 4 weeks of cast removal is an indication for supervised physical therapy, but such therapy is rarely necessary. Radiographic follow-up at 3-month intervals is usually performed during the first year and should consist of a standing AP view of both lower extremities on a long cassette for assessment of alignment. Orthogonal radiographs or scanograms may be necessary if significant tibial overgrowth has occurred. It is important that all children be monitored for at least 2 years after a fracture. Longer follow-up is necessary if a valgus deformity or significant lower extremity length inequality occurs.

RESULTS

It appears that in approximately 50% of children who sustain proximal tibial metaphyseal fractures, a clinically apparent valgus deformity, tibial overgrowth, or both will develop. Zionts and MacEwen[37] showed that the maximal deformity induced by overgrowth is present by approximately 18 months after the injury. Improvement begins thereafter, and maximal improvement has usually been achieved by 4 years after the injury. Minor residual deformities may continue to correct with subsequent growth and physeal alignment. Significant deformities persisting after 12 years of age may require surgical correction.

AUTHORS' PREFERRED METHOD OF TREATMENT

In the initial management of an acute fracture, any angular or valgus deformity may be corrected, or even slightly overcorrected, by nonoperative closed reduction techniques under general anesthesia. The parents must be warned of possible valgus deformity and tibial overgrowth. To evaluate alignment after closed reduction, adequate radiographs must be obtained. Alignment of the lower extremities should be assessed on an AP view of both lower extremities symmetrically positioned on a long cassette. With this method, the true alignment of the tibia can be measured directly and compared with the opposite side. If correction of a valgus deformity cannot be achieved by closing the medial fracture gap or fracturing the lateral cortex, open reduction is indicated. Failure to close the medial fracture site is typically indicative of soft tissue interposition from the periosteum,

pes anserinus, medial collateral ligament, or a combination thereof. After satisfactory reduction is achieved, a long leg cast is applied with the knee in extension. Only by having the knee in extension is it possible to radiographically assess alignment of the tibia. The child is reevaluated radiographically at weekly intervals for the first 3 weeks after the injury. Any change in position of the alignment in the cast is an indication for cast wedging or repeated closed reduction.

Treatment of valgus deformities is not usually considered for 2 to 3 years after injury, depending on the age of the patient and the degree of valgus. The authors do not believe that the use of orthoses or night splints corrects or alters the growth abnormality. Families are advised that approximately 50% correction of any valgus deformity will occur during the first 3 to 4 years after injury (Fig. 14.1). Only after this time is it possible to determine whether further treatment is necessary. If the maximal valgus deformity exceeds 20 degrees, the residual deformity may be too severe to accept, and growth modulation or an osteotomy may be necessary. Valgus deformities are not generally clinically significant until they are 5% to 10% greater than on the normal side.

If a corrective osteotomy is performed, it is usually a closing wedge proximal tibial and oblique diaphyseal fibular osteotomy. It is important that a fasciotomy of the anterior compartment be performed to minimize the risk of compartment syndrome. The deformity should be slightly overcorrected at the time of surgery because of the tendency for recurrence. Internal fixation with staples or crossed Steinmann pins can be used. Compression plates can also be considered, but they require a second, more extensive operative procedure for removal. The authors recommend stabilization after the osteotomy to maintain alignment and prefer percutaneous crossed Steinmann pins or a simple external fixation system consisting of a single threaded Steinmann pin placed above and below the osteotomy and secured with an external fixation clamp. This simple technique maintains apposition and prevents rotation and angulation. The leg is then immobilized in a long leg cast with the knee in extension. The child is closely monitored radiographically to assess alignment and healing. Once the osteotomy site has healed (usually in 6 weeks), the Steinmann pins are removed, typically in an outpatient clinic.

Temporary stapling or growth modulation of the medial aspect of the proximal tibial epiphysis is the most attractive treatment option because it allows correction with growth and does not provide the same magnitude of stimulation as a corrective osteotomy, which can contribute to recurrence.[45]

After satisfactory healing, the child is allowed full weight-bearing, and knee range-of-motion exercises are encouraged. If satisfactory motion of the knee has not been obtained after 2 weeks, supervised physical therapy is instituted. The child should be monitored for at least 2 years to observe for recurrent valgus deformity, tibial overgrowth, or both. Standing radiographs are obtained at 3- to 6-month intervals, and scanograms are obtained annually.

FRACTURES OF THE TIBIAL AND FIBULAR SHAFTS

Fractures involving both the tibial and the fibular diaphyses are more common than isolated fractures of the tibia.[5,6] In Shannak's 1988 review[6] of 117 children with tibial shaft fractures, 85 (73%) had an associated fracture of the fibula.

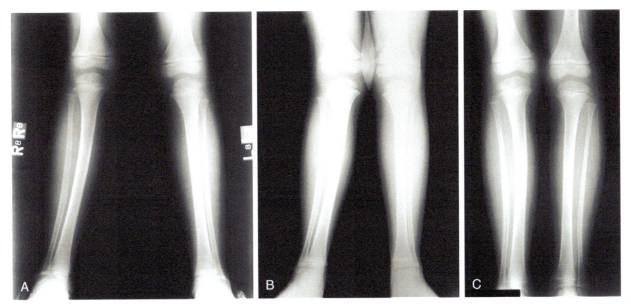

Fig. 14.1 (A) Anteroposterior standing radiograph of the lower extremities of a 5-year-old boy who sustained a nondisplaced fracture of the right proximal tibial metaphysis 15 months previously. The fracture healed uneventfully. The valgus deformity occurred shortly after cast removal. In terms of the mechanical axis, the right knee has a 22-degree valgus alignment versus 5 degrees on the left. (B) A repeated radiograph 1 year later demonstrates improvement in the right genu valgum to approximately 18 degrees. Overgrowth of the tibia is also occurring. Observe the increased width between the distal tibial physis and the physeal growth arrest line on the right compared with the left. (C) Repeated radiograph 40 months after injury showing further improvement in alignment of the right tibia. Although the tibia is longer, the genu valgum measures only 12 degrees. A significant proportion of the realignment has occurred in the distal end of the tibia. The articular surface of the right ankle joint is now parallel to the ground and perpendicular to the weight-bearing axis.

The mean age at fracture was 8 years (range, 1–15 years). Boys were involved three times more frequently than girls. The middle or lower third of the tibial shaft was involved in 104 fractures (90%). Oblique (35%) and comminuted (32%) were the most common fracture patterns. Only four fractures (3%) were open. Parrini and colleagues[5] also found that tibial and fibular fractures were more common than isolated tibial shaft fractures in children between 1 and 11 years of age. Similar findings were reported by Yang and Letts in 1997.[45] Typically, fractures of both the tibia and the fibula require greater energy than an isolated tibial shaft fracture does. They generally result from direct injury rather than from rotation, as occurs in the latter. This mechanism accounts for the increased incidence of oblique, transverse, and comminuted fracture patterns.

EVOLUTION OF TREATMENT

The major problems with fractures of the tibial and fibular shafts are shortening, angulation, and malrotation. Valgus deformities are common because of the action of the long flexor muscles of the lower leg. However, these problems are not usually severe, and almost all fractures are amenable to nonoperative or closed methods of treatment. In the study by Shannak,[6] the 117 pediatric tibial shaft fractures were followed for a mean of 3.9 years (range, 3–10 years); it was determined that satisfactory results can almost always be expected with conservative treatment and that surgery is usually not indicated or justified. Shortening of 5 mm or less is compensated for by growth acceleration, and mild varus angulations undergo spontaneous correction. Unfortunately, valgus malalignment and rotational deformities persist and must be corrected. However, in certain situations, surgical management with either internal or external fixation may

be advantageous. These select indications are presented in Box 14.2.

CURRENT ALGORITHM

Nearly all closed tibial and fibular shaft fractures in children can be managed by nonoperative techniques. Nondisplaced fractures are immobilized in a long leg cast with the knee flexed 20 to 60 degrees.[6] Depending on the fracture pattern,

---

Box 14.2 Indications for Internal or External Fixation of Pediatric Tibial and Fibular Fractures

Open fractures
Type III and some type II
Segmental bone loss
Unstable closed fractures
Segmental
Neurovascular injuries
Multiple traumatic injuries
Severe body area injuries
Head injuries with spasticity or combativeness
Ipsilateral femoral fractures
Multiple fractures
Soft tissue abnormalities
Burns
Skin loss
Compartment syndromes (fasciotomies)

Modified from Thompson GH, Wilber JH, Marcus RE. Internal fixation of fractures in children and adolescents. A comparative analysis. *Clin Orthop Relat Res.* 1984;188:10-20.

the child is not allowed to bear weight for 3 to 4 weeks or until early radiographic healing is evident. A long leg cast with the knee extended may then be applied; full weight-bearing is allowed until complete healing has occurred. In distal third fractures, a patellar tendon-bearing (PTB) cast or short leg cast may, instead, be applied.

Displaced closed fractures require closed reduction, and strict attention must be paid to maintenance of tibial length and correct angulation and rotation alignment. This procedure can usually be accomplished with manipulation and application of a long leg cast with the knee flexed 20 degrees to 60 degrees. If the tibial fracture is oblique or comminuted, maintenance of length may be difficult, and surgical treatment may need to be considered. After application of the long leg cast, the patient must be monitored closely, usually weekly for 2 to 3 weeks, so that maintenance of fracture alignment can be assessed. Minor alterations in angulation can be corrected by cast wedging techniques. When the fracture is stable both clinically and radiographically, usually 4 to 6 weeks after the injury, a long leg weight-bearing cast with the knee in extension, or possibly a PTB or short leg cast, depending on the fracture type and location, may be applied for an additional 2 to 3 weeks until the fracture is well healed.

Unstable closed fractures (oblique or comminuted) in a child who is a victim of polytrauma may benefit from the more aggressive operative methods of management, particularly external fixation or elastic stable intramedullary rods. The latter are currently being used with greater frequency.

SPECIAL CONSIDERATIONS FOR MULTIPLE TRAUMATIC INJURIES

Children who have multiple traumatic injuries and additional long bone fractures or significant injuries to other body areas may benefit from having their fractures stabilized surgically (see Box 14.2). Surgical stabilization enhances their overall care by improving both stability and mobility. The child is more easily cared for, and other diagnostic studies such as CT and MRI are facilitated because the child can be transported and properly positioned in the gantry. A common method of surgical stabilization of pediatric tibial and fibular fractures is external fixation. A variety of half-pin cantilever systems and small-pin transfixation rings have been used for external fixation of tibial fractures in children.[46-48] The former is the preferred method because of the ease and speed of application and the decreased risk of neurovascular injury; in addition, this system does not block surgical exposure to any associated wounds. The Taylor spatial frame can also be considered as another method of external fixation.[49] Wires, pins, and screws are occasionally used as surgical adjuncts. Compression plates and screws are not generally recommended because of the dissection necessary for application, the increased risk of infection, and the need for a second procedure for hardware removal. Flexible intramedullary rods, which avoid injuries to the proximal and distal tibial epiphyses, are becoming a popular newer alternative.[50-52]

TREATMENT OPTIONS

Closed fractures of the tibial and fibular diaphyses in children are usually uncomplicated, and their healing is typically rapid compared with similar fractures in adults. Current treatment methods consist of nonoperative and surgical management.

Nonoperative Management

Most closed fractures of the tibial and fibular shafts can be managed by closed reduction and immobilization in a long leg cast.[6] Displaced fractures usually require reduction under general anesthesia, whereas nondisplaced fractures can frequently be managed with a cast after sedation. This first cast usually has the knee flexed 20 degrees to 60 degrees to discourage weight-bearing. Once satisfactory alignment has been achieved, the fracture is assessed radiographically at weekly intervals for the first 3 weeks. Minor changes in alignment can be corrected with cast wedging techniques. Significant loss of alignment may require repeated closed reduction under general anesthesia. After 1 to 4 weeks, depending on the type of fracture and degree of radiographic healing, a weight-bearing long leg cast with the knee in extension may be applied.[6] The cast is worn until fracture healing is complete. In patients with fractures in the lower third of the tibia and fibula, a PTB cast, or possibly a short leg cast, may be used instead. A functional brace, as described by Sarmiento and Latta,[53] can also be considered for older adolescents. Sarmiento's group applied the functional brace approximately 2 weeks after the injury and initial treatment with a long leg plaster cast. They reported minimal problems with shortening, angulation, malrotation, and delayed union or nonunion.

The major problem when both the tibial and the fibular shafts are fractured is shortening.[6] Angulation can also develop inasmuch as the long flexor muscles tend to produce a valgus rather than a varus deformity at the fracture. Recurvatum may also occur, especially in children with considerable soft tissue swelling at the time of initial reduction and cast application. Wedging of the cast by opening or closing techniques may be required to correct the angulation.[6] Often, it is best to wait 1 to 2 weeks for the soft tissue swelling to resolve and for the fracture to develop some stability. If considerable swelling is observed initially, it may be better to apply a posterior splint and then perform the definitive manipulative reduction 4 to 7 days later when the swelling has subsided, the risk of compartment syndrome has passed, and a more appropriate, well-fitting cast can be applied.

For unstable fractures of the tibial and fibular diaphyses, especially those that are displaced, comminuted, and with appreciable shortening, other methods of closed management have been proposed. A long leg cast with the knee flexed and the foot in mild plantar flexion can be effective. After 3 weeks, the cast is changed, and the foot is brought to the neutral position. Shannak[6] recommended skeletal traction with a Steinmann pin through the os calcis of the heel. After 10 to 14 days, sufficient healing has usually occurred to allow application of a long leg cast with the knee in extension. These methods are rarely used today. Most authors prefer surgical stabilization with some type of external or internal fixation.

Surgical Management

Acceptable parameters for alignment for nonoperative management include up to 5 degrees of varus or valgus angulation, less than 5 degrees of sagittal angulation, and 1.0 cm or less of shortening.[4] Translation of the entire shaft is acceptable in a child 8 years of age or younger, and up to 50% translation is acceptable in older children and adolescents.

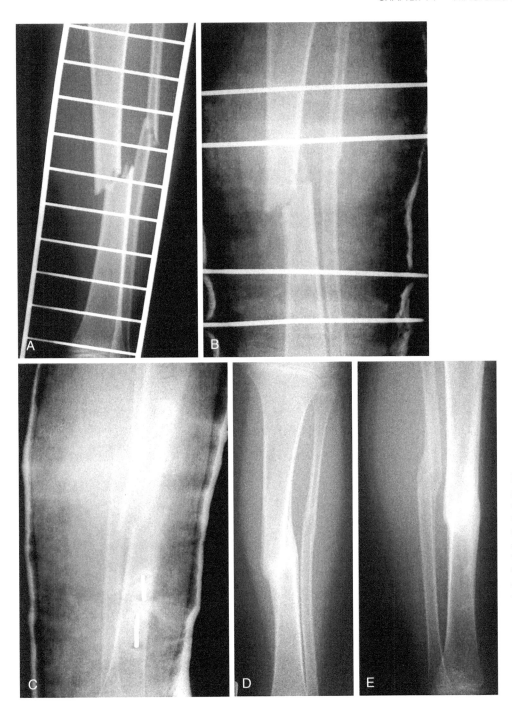

Fig. 14.2 (A) Anteroposterior radiograph of the lower part of the left leg of a 6-year-old girl with a closed fracture of the tibia and fibula. This injury was sustained in an automobile-pedestrian accident in Israel. (B) The fractures were unstable, and stable closed reduction could not be obtained. As a consequence, pins in plaster, closed reduction, and a long leg non-weight-bearing cast were used to achieve and maintain satisfactory alignment. (C) Lateral view demonstrating satisfactory alignment. (D) AP radiograph 4 months postinjury and after returning to the United States. Good healing and satisfactory alignment are evident. (E) Lateral view.

The principles of surgical management of pediatric fractures are distinctly different from those used in skeletally mature adults. When surgical management is indicated for a pediatric fracture, the general principles of Spiegal and Mast[54] must be considered. These principles are applicable both in polytrauma patients and in those with specific tibial fractures. The principles applicable to tibial shaft fractures include: (1) satisfactory, possibly anatomic, alignment should be achieved, with particular attention to rotation and angular orientation; (2) internal fixation devices, if used, should be easy to remove; (3) rigid fixation to maintain fracture alignment rather than to allow for immediate mobilization of the lower leg is usually the goal; therefore, a supplemental plaster cast may be required; and (4) external fixators, when used, should be removed as soon as any soft tissue wounds have healed or the fracture is stable and will not become displaced. Cast immobilization is continued until complete healing has occurred. The choice of surgical treatment of pediatric fractures should be guided by analyzing the extent of soft tissue injury, the location of the fracture, the fracture pattern, and the extent of other associated injuries.

External Fixation. External skeletal fixation has been a common surgical treatment for pediatric tibial and fibular fractures, particularly those that are very comminuted and unstable or associated with severe overlying soft tissue injury[7,10,11,14,46–48,55–58] (see Box 14.2). Techniques include pins above and below the fractures that are incorporated into a plaster cast (Fig. 14.2) or a variety of commercial half-pin and ring fixator systems. External fixation is usually maintained until adequate callus formation has been achieved and the fracture is stable. At that time, the fixator is removed and replaced by a long leg cast with the knee in extension. Tolo[48] reported that the use of external fixators increased the healing time and was associated with a significant prevalence (50%) of superficial pin tract infections and a high rate of refracture. Three of 13 tibial fractures (23%) refractured 5 to 10 months after injury. Whether the refractures were caused by stress shielding, premature frame removal, or relative ischemia from the local trauma was unknown. All three refractures healed with immobilization in long leg casts. In 2007, Myers and colleagues,[57] in a study of 31 consecutive high-energy tibial fractures, reported a significant incidence of complications with external fixation. These included malunion, delayed union, wound infection, osteomyelitis, and lower extremity length discrepancy. There were no refractures.

The advantages of external fixation of pediatric tibial shaft fractures include rigid immobilization, direct surveillance of the lower part of the leg and any associated wounds, facilitation of wound dressing and management, patient mobilization for other diagnostic studies and management of other body area injuries, and possible application under local anesthesia in severely injured children. The use of the Taylor spatial frame has recently been shown to be a newer method of external fixation, particularly in unstable fractures in older children and adolescents.[49]

Internal Fixation. Closed or open reduction with internal fixation of pediatric tibial and fibular diaphyseal fractures are not commonly indicated, but their frequency is increasing.[59,60] Operative techniques include limited internal fixation with K-wires, Steinmann pins, and cortical lag screws; compression plates and screws (Fig. 14.3); and elastic stable intramedullary rods.

Compression plates and screws require extensive dissection and periosteal stripping, which can increase the risk of infection or delayed union or nonunion because of further disruption of the blood supply to the bone. Nevertheless, they are an acceptable technique in closed, comminuted fractures when satisfactory alignment by nonoperative techniques cannot be achieved. Newer percutaneous techniques for plate application have been described, and this modification will likely decrease the rate of these complications. Reamed intramedullary nails can be considered for older adolescents approaching skeletal maturity.[50]

Elastic stable intramedullary rods are gaining popularity in pediatric fractures, including tibial shaft fractures. In 1985, Ligier and colleagues[61] from France reported on the results of using two flexible intramedullary rods in 19 pediatric tibial fractures. Such treatment produced elastic stability at the fracture site, which enhanced the formation of bridging external callus by eliminating shear forces and allowing compression forces across the fracture site. One rod was inserted through the medial and the other through the lateral proximal tibial metaphysis, distal to the physis and posterior to the apophysis of the tibial tubercle, and then passed distally across the fracture site to terminate proximal to the distal tibial physis. They reported that no cast immobilization was necessary, and all fractures healed within 3 months. The major indications

for intramedullary fixation were predominantly for unstable fractures that failed nonoperative management. In 1988, Verstreken and associates[62] from Belgium also used the technique of elastic stable rodding in children. They recommended its use for tibial fractures with contralateral lower limb injuries in children 6 years and older, especially those who had sustained multiple injuries from trauma. In 2001, Qidwai[63] reported on 84 tibial fractures, including 30 open fractures treated with a similar technique of intramedullary K-wires (2.5–3.5 mm in diameter). The mean age at fracture was 10.2 years (range, 4–15 years), and 54 had an associated fibular fracture. The fractures healed at a mean of 9.5 weeks (range, 8–14 weeks), and the implants were removed at a mean of 5.6 months postoperatively. The mean follow-up was 18 months (range, 13–16 months). No delayed unions, nonunions, or lower extremity length discrepancies greater than 1.0 cm were observed. No postoperative infections occurred in the 54 closed fractures. However, in the 30 open fractures, five postoperative infections (four superficial and one deep) were reported. The author concluded that the technique was simple and produced good clinical, radiographic, and functional results. In another study, O'Brien and colleagues[64] followed 16 unstable tibial fractures treated by flexible nailing (three of which were open), and all healed uneventfully. In a comparison study of 31 consecutive tibial fractures, including 16 patients managed with flexible intramedullary nails and 15 patients managed with external fixation, Kubiak and colleagues[65] demonstrated improved functional results with the former. This included eight open fractures in the intramedullary nailing group and five open fractures in the external fixator group. Gicquel and colleagues[55] noted that insufficient bending of the medial nail may lead to valgus malunion when both the tibia and fibula are fractured. Other authors have recently reported satisfactory results with low complication rates using elastic stable intramedullary nails.[50–52,66–68] Other options include percutaneous pin fixation.[1]

FOLLOW-UP CARE AND REHABILITATION

Most children with tibial and fibular fractures do not require physical therapy for rehabilitation. They usually regain full knee and ankle motion within the expected time and return to full activities much sooner than their parents and orthopedic surgeons would like. An inability to regain full knee and ankle motion within 2 to 3 weeks after the cast is removed is a common indication for physical therapy. Normal activities, including sports, can be allowed once motion is regained, muscle strength returns to normal, and radiographs show solid union, usually 4 to 6 weeks after the last cast is removed. The child is then monitored at 3- to 6-month intervals for approximately 2 years to assess function, leg length, and resolution of any residual problems such as mild angulation.

RESULTS

The results after nonoperative management of uncomplicated closed tibial and fibular shaft fractures are uniformly satisfactory. The fractures heal rapidly, depending on age, and minor discrepancies in length and angulation may correct spontaneously with subsequent growth.[6]

Approximately 25% of children with tibial and fibular shaft fractures have minor tibial length inequalities and

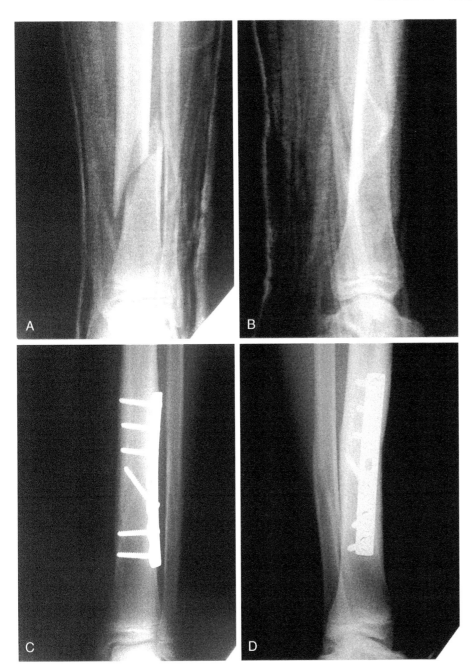

Fig. 14.3 (A) Anteroposterior (AP) radiograph of the lower part of the left leg of a 13-year-old boy with an unstable oblique fracture of the distal ends of the tibia and fibula. (B) A lateral radiograph more clearly demonstrates the fibular fracture. (C) AP radiograph 18 months after open reduction and internal fixation of the fibular fracture. The fractures are well healed. (D) Lateral view.

angulatory changes at initial healing.[6] Significant rotational problems are fortunately uncommon. Because the amount of overgrowth of the tibia and fibula secondary to fracture stimulation is small, it is important to maintain adequate length during healing. In tibial fractures in boys older than 12 years and in girls older than 10 years, an attempt must be made to achieve full length. The amount of shortening that can be accepted after closed reduction of these fractures is 5 to 10 mm in girls 3 to 10 years of age and in boys 3 to 12 years of age.[6,69] Older children and adolescents require alignment that is as close to anatomic as possible. Younger children may have overgrowth in both the tibia and femur, whereas older children and young adolescents may actually experience growth retardation. The type of fracture and the presence of residual angulation do not appear to affect the amount of overgrowth. The growth stimulation process is usually complete 2 years after injury. Reynolds[69]

demonstrated that, within 3 months of injury, the rate of growth was at its maximum and was 38% in excess of normal. The growth rate then decreased but remained significantly elevated for 2 years; it returned to normal in the tibia approximately 40 months after injury.

It is also important to correct any coexistent angular or rotational deformity. Angular deformities may improve with growth, but rotational malalignment does not.[6] Varus deformities of up to 15 degrees in young children can undergo spontaneous correction.[6] However, valgus and posterior angulation tend to persist, as do rotational deformities, particularly medial or internal rotation. In uncomplicated fractures, function can be expected to return to normal.

Gordon and associates[70] reviewed 51 tibial shaft fractures in 50 patients treated with elastic stable intramedullary nailing. The cohort included 25 closed fractures and 26 open fractures. Of the fractures, 21 were treated with closed nailing and 30 required open reduction. Only one patient (2%) developed an infection; the patient had a grade II open tibial fracture and developed osteomyelitis after fracture union. Fifty of the 51 fractures healed in acceptable alignment. A 13.6-year-old patient required an osteotomy 23 weeks postoperatively to correct a valgus-procurvatum deformity. Some 44 of the 50 fractures healed without appreciable limb length discrepancy. Three patients had asymptomatic lengthening, and four had asymptomatic shortening. Five fractures had delayed healing (range, 31–55 weeks): three healed with repeated casting, and two went on to nonunion and required repeated surgical intervention to achieve healing. Of note, three of the five fractures that had delayed healing were closed injuries.

Recently, Kinney and colleagues[71] studied 74 adolescents with closed displaced tibial shaft fractures: 57 managed by closed technique and 17 operatively. The results were similar except those treated nonoperatively were more likely to experience displacement and require surgery.

AUTHORS' PREFERRED METHOD OF TREATMENT

Because closed tibial and fibular fractures in children usually heal rapidly and with satisfactory long-term results, the authors recommend closed reduction and immobilization in a long leg cast for the majority of cases. Only a small percentage of closed fractures require operative management with either external or internal fixation.

Most nondisplaced fractures are managed by a long leg cast applied with the knee in 20 degrees to 60 degrees of flexion. Weight-bearing is avoided for 2 to 3 weeks; a long leg cast is then applied with the knee in extension, and toe-touch weight-bearing is allowed. Once callus formation is visible, the cast may be changed to either a PTB or a short leg cast, depending on the fracture location and the degree of radiographic healing.

Displaced fractures of the tibia and fibula are reduced under general anesthesia. When displacement is present, extensive injury to the surrounding soft tissues has usually occurred. These children have an increased risk of compartment syndrome and are admitted to the hospital for observation after reduction and immobilization in either a posterior splint or a long leg cast, depending on the degree of soft tissue swelling. If a splint is used initially, the long leg cast should be applied 4 to 7 days later to allow resolution of the soft tissue swelling; the procedure is usually performed under general anesthesia. After immobilization, the patient is evaluated radiographically at weekly intervals for the first 3 weeks. If alignment is lost, the need for cast wedging or repeated closed reduction must be considered. In most cases, the displacement is minor and can be managed by cast wedging.

For an unstable fracture with unacceptable alignment after closed reduction, an external fixator may be necessary. The authors prefer half-pin systems. They are easy to apply, but care must be taken to avoid injury to the proximal and distal tibial physes. The use of fluoroscopy ensures safe application of these devices. These systems control length, angulation, and rotation. They are typically supplemented with a posterior splint for the first several weeks to immobilize both the knee and the ankle for comfort. Depending on the age and reliability of the child, partial weight-bearing may be allowed 2 to 4 weeks after injury. Transverse

fractures that heal with small areas of callus may require longer periods with the frame in place to prevent recurrent deformity. Once callus is confirmed radiographically and any associated wounds have healed, the external fixation device is removed and replaced with a long leg or PTB cast until fracture healing is complete.

Elastic stable intramedullary nailing has become a common method of treatment (Fig. 14.4). The nail size should be selected so that approximately 80% of the tibial canal is filled by the nails. Care must be taken to avoid injury to the proximal tibial epiphysis and tibial tubercle during rod insertion. However, burying the pins beneath the skin obviates the need for pin care and enables access to the overlying soft tissues. Some patients do develop reactive bursae over the ends of the nails if they protrude from the bone too much.

In summary, the general indications for operative management include comminuted fractures, displaced fractures with an intact fibula, and displaced fractures in adolescents.[72] Open fractures may also benefit by external and internal fixation.

ISOLATED FRACTURES OF THE TIBIAL DIAPHYSIS

Fractures of the tibial shaft with an intact fibula are common in children.[5,6,30,45,73] They can be either incomplete tension-compression (greenstick) or complete fractures. Shannak[6] and Parrini and colleagues[5] found fractures involving both the tibia and fibula to be the most common. Shannak[6] reported that only 32 (27%) of 117 children with tibial fractures had isolated tibial diaphyseal fractures.

Teitz and colleagues[73] reported that falls were the most common mechanism of injury, followed by skiing and motor vehicle accidents. Most fractures were spiral and involved the middle or distal third of the shaft. In 1997, a study by Yang and Letts[45] found that the mean age at injury was 8.1 years (range, 0.3–17 years); 77 (81%) were because of indirect trauma, and 69 (73%) occurred in the distal third of the tibia. It therefore appears that fractures involving both the tibia and the fibula are more commonly the result of severe, high-energy accidents, such as motor vehicle accidents, whereas isolated tibial shaft fractures result from less severe types of trauma, such as falls or sporting accidents.

Isolated tibial fractures are caused predominantly by torsional forces, and most are localized in the distal third or at the junction of the middle and distal thirds of the tibia.[45] The most common mechanism of torsion was lateral rotation of the body while the foot was in a fixed position on the ground. The fracture line began distally on the anteromedial surface of the tibia and progressed proximally to the posterolateral aspect. The intact fibula and periosteum prevent significant displacement or shortening. However, angulation can occur, especially varus angulation. When the fibula is intact, the tendency toward shortening is converted to a torsional deformity at the fracture site, and a varus deformity is produced. This abnormality is caused predominantly by the effect of the long flexor muscles across the fracture site inducing a rotational force. Yang and Letts[45] found that secondary varus angulation was most likely to develop in oblique and spiral fractures. Transverse fractures tended not to angulate.

Teitz and colleagues[73] corroborated clinical observations with biomechanical studies on tibial fractures with an intact

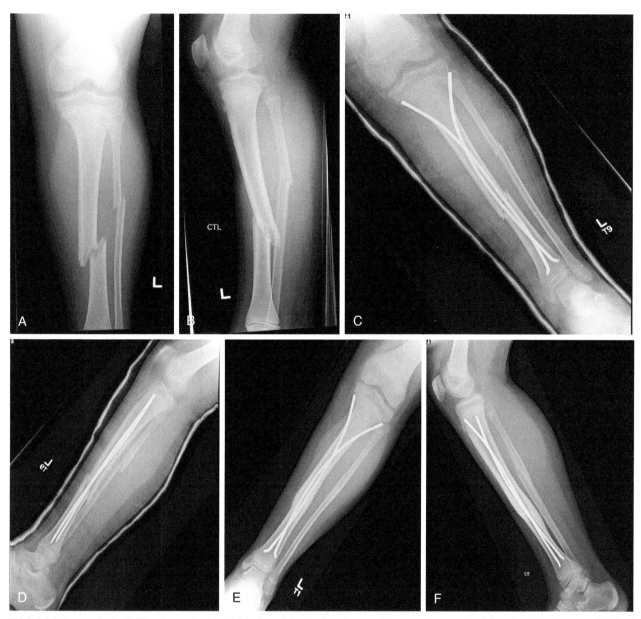

Fig. 14.4 (A) Anteroposterior (AP) radiograph of the left tibia and fibula of a 10-year-old male who was struck by a truck that ran a red light. There is an oblique, displaced fracture of the tibial diaphysis and a more proximal fracture at the fibula. (B) Lateral radiograph demonstrates the displacement and angulation. (C) AP radiograph following closed reduction and internal fixation with elastic stable intramedullary rods of the tibia. (D) Lateral postoperative radiograph. (E) AP radiograph 6 months postoperatively demonstrating that the tibial alignment is well maintained and both fractures are well healed. The rods were subsequently removed. (F) Lateral radiograph confirms maintenance of alignment and satisfactory healing.

fibula. They found that when the fibula remains intact, a tibiofibular length discrepancy develops and causes altered strain patterns in the tibia and fibula. These strain patterns may lead to delayed union, nonunion, or malunion of the tibia. They found a lower incidence of these complications in children and adolescents and attributed it to greater compliance of their fibulas and soft tissues.

Treatment of an isolated tibial shaft fracture is predominantly nonoperative and consists of immobilization in a long leg cast alone (Fig. 14.5).[5,6,30,45,73] Closed reduction may be necessary, especially if a varus deformity greater than 15 degrees is present along with coexistent plastic deformation of the fibula. Flexing the knee 30 degrees to 90 degrees and placing the foot in some degree of plantar flexion during

the first 2 or 3 weeks may negate some of the deforming force from the long toe flexors. Children should be monitored radiographically at weekly intervals for the first 3 weeks because secondary varus angulation can occur, especially in those with oblique and spiral fractures. A repeated attempt at closed reduction may be necessary if the angulation exceeds 15 degrees. After fracture stability is achieved, a long leg weight-bearing cast with the knee in extension is applied. The cast is usually maintained until healing is complete. A PTB cast, fracture brace, or short leg cast can be used for distal fractures. Indications for surgical intervention in children with isolated tibial shaft fractures are limited. Even in children with multiple traumatic injuries, these fractures can be treated by simple immobilization with

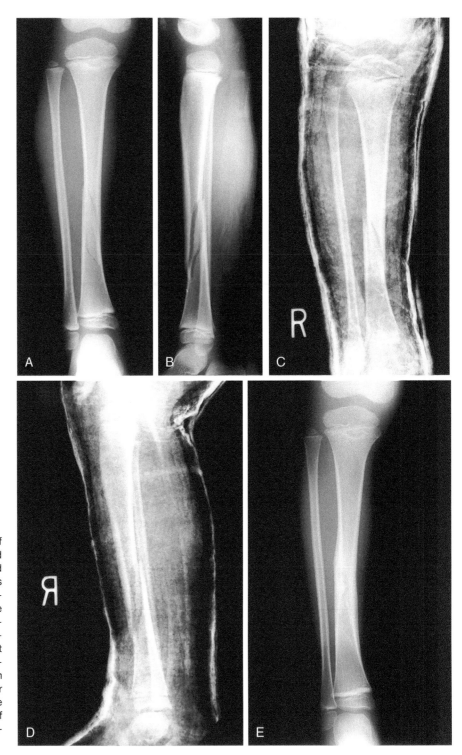

Fig. 14.5 (A) Anteroposterior radiograph of the lower part of the right leg of a 4-year-old boy who fell through a boat hatch. An isolated spiral fracture of the distal third of the tibia is apparent. The fibula is intact. (B) A lateral radiograph demonstrates that the spiral fracture is minimally displaced. (C) Slight varus angulation of 5 degrees occurred during immobilization in a long leg plaster cast. Shortening at the fracture site was minimal. (D) A lateral radiograph shows no change in alignment from the initial radiographs. (E) Three months after injury, the fracture is well healed. Despite the slight varus angulation, the articular surface of the ankle is parallel to the floor and perpendicular to the weight-bearing axis.

a long leg cast. Severe soft tissue damage, such as with burns or open fractures, or a diaphyseal fracture with significant residual angulation may be better managed by open reduction and internal fixation or an external fixator. Qidwai[63] recently reported on 30 isolated tibial shaft fractures treated by intramedullary fixation with 2.5- to 3.5-mm K-wires. The fractures healed quickly, and no postoperative infections occurred in the closed fractures. Others have reported on successful use of flexible intramedullary nails.[30,50–52,65,66,70] Canavase and colleagues[30] recently studied 80 patients with displaced closed tibial shaft fractures with an intact fibula.

Some 54 patients were treated nonoperatively and 26 patients surgically. The results at 2 years follow-up were essentially the same functional and radiographic outcomes.

SPECIAL TIBIAL SHAFT FRACTURES

TODDLER'S FRACTURE
In children between 9 months and perhaps 6 years of age, torsion of the foot may produce an oblique fracture of the distal aspect of the tibial shaft without a fibular fracture.[74–79] The term *toddler's fracture* was first used by Dunbar and

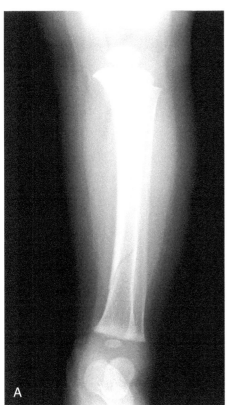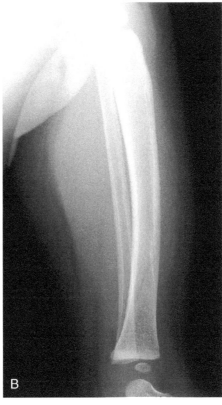

Fig. 14.6 (A) Toddler's fracture in a 9-month-old girl. She fell while taking her first independent steps. A faint oblique fracture is seen crossing the distal tibial diaphysis and terminating medially and distally. This fracture healed with 2 weeks of immobilization in a long leg plaster cast. (B) A lateral radiograph shows that the fracture is barely visible and has no displacement.

colleagues[75] in 1964. These fractures are usually the result of a trivial or seemingly innocuous event, such as tripping while walking or running, stepping on a ball or toy, or falling from a modest height. It is most common in younger children, hence the name.[75,79]

The physical findings and radiographic appearance are often subtle. These children are typically seen because of failure to bear weight, a limp, or pain when forced to stand on the involved extremity. Usually, the child does not have any soft tissue swelling, ecchymoses, or deformity. Localized tenderness is the most common physical finding. Local warmth may be noted during palpation at the fracture site.[79] The traumatic episode may not have been witnessed.[78]

AP and lateral radiographs of the entire tibia and fibula may demonstrate a spiral fracture of the distal third of the tibia. However, the radiographic results may also be normal.[75,76,79,80] The characteristic finding is a faint oblique fracture line crossing the distal tibial diaphysis and terminating medially. When routine radiographic results are normal but a fracture is suspected, oblique views may be beneficial.[75] The fracture line may be visualized on only one film. If a fracture is suspected but not visualized, immobilization is still indicated. A technetium bone scan may reveal increased uptake, thereby confirming the fracture. However, such scanning is rarely indicated unless the child is febrile and osteomyelitis is a concern. Repeated radiographs 7 to 10 days after injury usually demonstrate subperiosteal new bone formation, thereby substantiating the fracture. Halsey and associates[76] recently reported that of 39 children with a suspected toddler's fracture and negative results on initial radiographs, 16 (41%) had a toddler's fracture confirmed on follow-up radiographs. They believed that children with conclusive physical findings and negative radiographs had a

"preoperative diagnosis" of a toddler's fracture and should be treated. Lewis and Logan[81] performed sonograms on three cases of suspected toddler's fracture and found a layer of low reflectivity superficial to the tibial cortex and an elevated periosteum. The diagnosis was later confirmed by radiographic periosteal reaction.

Treatment of a toddler's fracture is usually by immobilization in a long leg cast for 2 to 4 weeks, depending on the age of the child (Fig. 14.6). When the fracture is discovered 2 weeks or more after injury, immobilization may not be necessary, provided that callus formation is adequate and the child has no tenderness on stress examination. Bauer and Lovejoy[80] recommended only a short leg walking boot or cast. Return to weight-bearing was the same for both.

Tenenbien and colleagues[79] differentiated the radiographic features of a typical toddler's fracture from those of child abuse or the battered child syndrome. In the latter, the fracture is usually midshaft and less oblique. It is important to distinguish between these two entities. In a review by Oudjhane and associates[78] of 500 consecutive radiographic evaluations of children younger than 5 years with an acute limp, excluding cases of child abuse, occult fracture of the tibia or fibula was the most common cause (56 cases). These fractures occurred predominantly in the distal metaphysis, occasionally in the proximal metaphysis, and only rarely in the diaphysis. Similar findings were reported by Mellick and Reesor.[77]

BATTERED CHILD SYNDROME

Fractures are second only to soft tissue injuries as the most common finding in battered child syndrome. Approximately 25% to 50% of abused children have fractures.[82] The humerus, femur, and tibia are the most commonly fractured long bones in published series, in various order. In some series, the metaphyseal bucket-handle or corner fracture pattern is the most frequent type, but in recent publications, the transverse pattern was more common. In 1986, Kleinman and colleagues,[83] in a combined histologic and radiographic study, demonstrated that a corner fracture is not an avulsion of the metaphyses at the site of attachment of the periosteum or ligaments but, instead, is a subepiphyseal fracture through the most immature portion of the metaphysis. Depending on the size of the injury, the degree of involvement of the metaphysis, and the radiographic projection, the lesion may appear as a bucket-handle fracture, a corner fracture, or metaphyseal radiolucency. Thus, these fractures are complete rather than avulsion types.

King and colleagues,[82] in a review of 750 children seen at the Children's Hospital of Los Angeles between 1971 and 1981 who were considered to be victims of battered child syndrome, found that 189 children (25%) sustained 429 total fractures. The median age was 7 months, with the range being 1 month to 13 years. Most were 2 years or younger. In this series, the most commonly fractured bones were the humerus, tibia, and femur. However, the most commonly fractured bones per patient were the humerus, femur, and tibia. Of all the long bone fractures, 48% were transverse, 26% were spiral, 16% were avulsion, 10% were oblique, and only 1.5% were comminuted fractures. When fracture combinations were analyzed, avulsion or metaphyseal corner fractures were the fourth most common pattern involving the proximal third of the tibia. Twenty-eight percent of the patients had a history of previous fractures. Ultimately, 10 of the children (5%) died.

The diagnosis of battered child syndrome requires a high index of suspicion. Typically, the injuries are unobserved, and the parents' descriptions are vague. Physical examination may reveal soft tissue injuries in various stages of healing, failure to thrive, and emotional abnormalities resulting from deprivation and fear. Another potential problem is distinguishing between nonaccidental injuries and osteogenesis imperfecta. Usually, diagnosis of the latter is not difficult because of the existence of a family history and the presence of fractures at birth, blue sclerae, dentinogenesis imperfecta, and other characteristic findings. However, these factors may not always be present. In a comparison of fracture patterns in these two disorders, Dent and Paterson[84] found that in osteogenesis imperfecta the peak incidence for fractures was between 2 and 4 years of age; lower limb fractures, especially the distal portion of the femur and the tibial diaphysis, were more frequent than upper extremity fractures, and severe displacement of the fracture fragments was more common. Metaphyseal, spiral, and transverse fractures were common, whereas greenstick and torus fractures were not. However, even when the diagnosis of osteogenesis imperfecta is clear, the possibility of nonaccidental injury must be considered because the two conditions can coexist. In addition, most children with osteogenesis imperfecta and fractures do not have associated bruising or soft tissue injuries. When soft tissue injuries are present, the possibility of child abuse must be considered.

Care must also be taken in distinguishing a toddler's fracture from fracture in an abused child. Mellick and Reesor[77] recognized another accidental spiral tibial fracture that occurs in children between 2 and 6 years of age. It is similar to a toddler's fracture and overlaps the same age range, although it requires more energy and is more visible radiographically. The fracture begins more proximally at the middle rather than the distal third of the tibia. The fibula is not involved. This fracture is usually the result of a fall with a torque or rotational component. Most tibial fractures in abused children are diaphyseal and transverse rather than distal and spiral. In addition, a concomitant fracture of the fibular shaft is suggestive of an abused child because the energy necessary to fracture both bones is much greater than that causing a toddler's fracture or an isolated spiral fracture in an older child. Skeletal surveys are necessary in suspected cases to assess for previous healing fractures and evidence of subperiosteal new bone formation secondary to blunt trauma. If a truly accidental origin cannot be confirmed immediately, the child requires admission to the hospital and evaluation by the child abuse team.

Management of tibial fractures in battered children is similar to that described for isolated tibial and combined tibial and fibular shaft fractures. Closed reduction with simple cast immobilization is usually sufficient in these young children. The most important aspect is the diagnosis and appropriate intervention to prevent further injuries and possible death.

BICYCLE SPOKE INJURIES

Bicycle spoke injuries of the lower extremity, especially over the medial malleoli, are relatively common in children.[3,24,85–87] They may be caused by the lower part of the leg becoming trapped between the spokes of the wheel and the frame of the bicycle when the child is being transported as a passenger. They may also result from motorcycle wheel spoke injuries.[87] Despite the mechanism, these injuries can produce severe compression or crushing of the soft tissues over the foot and ankle. A fracture may also result (Fig. 14.7).[78] Karrholm and associates[3] reported that 39 of 462 pediatric tibial and fibular shaft fractures (8%) were caused by spoke injuries. Izant and colleagues[86] reviewed 60 cases of bicycle spoke injuries and found that most of the children were between 2 and 8 years old (mean, 5 years). In almost every instance, the injury occurred while two children were on a bicycle built for one.

The initial appearance of the extremity can be deceiving. The skin may appear to only be abraded, but over the next 2 to 3 days, an area of full-thickness skin loss may develop. These injuries bear a striking similarity to wringer injuries of the upper extremity. Izant and colleagues[86] recognized three aspects of this injury: (1) laceration of the tissues from the knifelike action of the spokes, (2) crushing from impingement between the wheel and the bicycle frame, and (3) shearing injuries from the coefficient of these two forces. Lacerations usually involve the area over the medial malleoli or the Achilles tendon. Simple suture closure may result in dehiscence of the wound, which may prolong secondary healing. The decision to perform a skin graft must await adequate demarcation of the area of necrosis and wide débridement. The most common site of skin necrosis is over the malleoli, where the skin and subcutaneous tissues are thin. All children with spoke injuries should be admitted to the hospital for observation. Treatment recommendations after fracture management, if necessary, include well-padded splints over dressings, mild elevation, and frequent

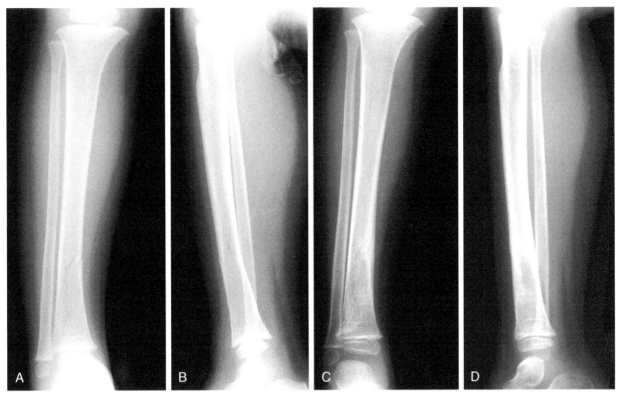

Fig. 14.7 (A) Anteroposterior radiograph of the lower portion of the right leg of a 3-year-old girl demonstrating an oblique fracture of the distal end of the right tibia and an intact fibula. This injury occurred when her leg was trapped between bicycle spokes and a rear fender support while sitting in an unprotected rear passenger seat. The skin and subcutaneous tissues were contused and abraded, but no lacerations occurred. (B) A lateral radiograph demonstrates mild anterior angulation of the fracture. (C) Two months after the injury, the fracture is well healed. (D) Lateral radiograph demonstrating no change in alignment.

wound inspection. Débridement is performed as necrosis becomes apparent, followed by early split-thickness skin grafting. Closure of initial lacerations is done only after careful débridement, and special attention should be paid to defatting the thick skin flaps when the laceration involves the heel.

SLIDE INJURIES

Gaffney,[88] in 2009, found that of 58 tibial fractures treated over an 11-month period, eight (13.8%) occurred while on a playground slide. In all eight cases, the child was sitting on an adult's lap; the child's leg became stuck between the adult and the slide or fixed against the slide while the child and adult continued downwards. All of these fractures were nondisplaced and had an intact fibula. The average patient age was 20.6 months. Parents and caretakers should be educated not to allow their children to sit in their lap while going down a slide.

TRAMPOLINE FRACTURES

Fractures from trampolines are on the rise, especially those involving the upper and lower extremities. Loder and associates[89] reported from a national database that tibia/fibula and ankle fractures were the most common lower extremity fractures. These are treated based on fracture patterns and displacement.

STRESS FRACTURES

Pediatric stress fractures are uncommon and frequently lead to misdiagnosis, especially in young children.[90] The pattern of stress fractures in children is different from that in adults. The tibia and fibula are the most common pediatric bones to sustain stress fractures, and boys are affected more frequently than girls. Stress fractures are more common in adolescents and are similar to those in adults. A stress fracture incurred by a young child may resemble osteomyelitis or a malignant process.

Children typically are seen with mild pain and a limp that was gradual in onset. Although no history of a specific injury may be elicited, frequently, an older child has participated in vigorous physical activities, such as sports, to which the child is unaccustomed or not properly conditioned. In a review of pediatric stress fractures, Walker and colleagues[91] found the proximal third of the tibia to be the most common site, and these fractures usually occurred after 10 years of age. The pain is typically relieved by rest and exacerbated by returning to activities. The most common positive physical finding is local tenderness to palpation or percussion over the fracture site. Typically, no soft tissue swelling, erythema, or ecchymoses are present.

The radiographic diagnosis of a stress fracture of the tibia and fibula is frequently difficult, especially in young children.[92] Radiographic changes may even be absent. Pediatric tibial stress fractures most commonly involve the posteromedial or posterolateral aspect of the proximal third of the tibia. They do not occur in the anterior aspect. Engh and colleagues[92] recognized that the typical radiographic changes occur in three phases. Initially, a small area of radiolucency is seen in the cortex in the posterior wall of the tibia. This abnormality is associated with some metaphyseal and endosteal increase in bone density and a fine haze of periosteal reaction. These findings are usually present 2 to 3 weeks after the onset of symptoms, but this phase is often missed in children. No linear fracture is seen radiographically, and follow-up radiographs show a gradual increase in periosteal and endosteal new bone formation. The second phase is sometimes associated with the appearance of a definite incomplete defect in the posterior cortex. If a complete fracture does not occur, the third phase involves maturation and partial resorption of the periosteal and endosteal new bone formation. If a fracture line becomes apparent, it is typically that of a nondisplaced fracture, and the characteristic radiographic sequence then follows.

In difficult cases, technetium bone scans may be of benefit. Bone scans are a highly sensitive technique for the early diagnosis of stress fractures, and the findings on bone scans can be identified long before radiographic changes. The typical bone scan appearance of a stress fracture of the tibia consists of a sharply marginated oval or fusiform area of increased radiodensity located posteromedially. It occasionally extends the width of the bone at the area of involvement. The medial aspect of the tibial cortex is more commonly involved. Currently, MRI is also beneficial in recognizing stress fractures while avoiding the use of ionizing radiation. Findings include intraosseous bands of very low signal intensity that are continuous with the cortex, as well as juxtacortical or periosteal findings of high signal intensity.

Stress fractures of the fibula can also occur. The process may still be seen in children who participate in vigorous athletic activities, although the fibula may sustain a stress fracture at a younger age than other bones.

Clinical examination usually shows an area of tenderness proximal to the lateral malleolus. The involved area is generally tender to palpation, and mild soft tissue swelling may be present. Plain radiographs may be diagnostic, but in difficult cases, a technetium bone scan or MRI may be indicated.

Treatment of tibial or fibular stress fractures is usually conservative. In most cases, restriction of physical activities relieves the discomfort and allows the fracture to heal. Occasionally, immobilization in a long or short leg plaster cast, depending on the involved bone, may be necessary for 2 to 4 weeks in children with significant discomfort. A stress fracture of the distal end of the fibula may also be treated with a removable air stirrup splint.

IPSILATERAL TIBIAL AND FEMORAL FRACTURES

Ipsilateral tibial and femoral shaft fractures in children are severe injuries, usually the result of high-velocity accidents such as motor vehicle collisions.[70,42,93,94] As a consequence, these fractures are commonly open and associated with other body area injuries. These fractures produce the so-called floating knee.

Bohn and Durbin[42] in 1991 reviewed 44 consecutive ipsilateral femoral and tibial fractures in 42 children and skeletally immature adolescents. Thirty patients (32 limbs) had a mean follow-up of 5.1 years (range, 1–14 years), and 19 were available for personal examination and radiographs. The 24 boys and 6 girls had a mean age of 10.5 years (range, 3.6–16.6 years). Twenty-seven of the children sustained their fractures in automobile-related accidents, including 17 automobile-pedestrian accidents. Twelve of the 30 children had one or both fractures open, 17 children had at least one additional fracture, and 15 had another body area injury, especially cranial.

Closed methods of treatment of both fractures were used in 18 patients. Ten patients had operative stabilization of one fracture, and 10 had operative stabilization of both fractures. Eight patients had operative fixation of their femoral fractures (i.e., closed intramedullary rod, open intramedullary rod, or compression plate and screws), including one of the three open fractures. Twenty-three patients (24 limbs) had their tibial fractures treated by closed reduction and cast immobilization. External fixation was used in five open fractures, and pins in plaster were used in four unstable fractures. One fracture was treated by open reduction and internal fixation.

Bohn and Durbin[42] also found age to be the most important variable related to the clinical course. Of the 15 patients who were younger than 10 years, the mean time to unsupported weight-bearing was 13 weeks, and the mean combined femoral and tibial overgrowth was 1.8 cm. Three children had early complications. Of the 15 patients who were older than 10 years, 8 had early complications, the mean time to unsupported weight-bearing was 20 weeks, and femoral and tibial growth varied. The younger children were treated successfully with closed techniques for both fractures, whereas the older children were more successfully treated with reduction and surgical stabilization of the femoral fracture. The older group had the highest incidence of complications, including four with unrecognized ipsilateral knee ligament injuries. These injuries included four anterior cruciate ligament tears and two medial collateral ligament injuries. Careful examination of the knee was recommended at the time of initial evaluation. Of the 19 patients who were personally evaluated by the authors, only seven had normal function. The remainder had compromised results consisting of lower extremity length inequality, angular deformity, or knee instability.

In 2000, Yue and associates[94] studied 29 children (30 extremities) with ipsilateral femoral and tibial fractures treated nonoperatively (group 1) and operatively with rigid stabilization of one or both fractures (group 2). The mean follow-up was 8.6 years (range, 1.1–18.6 years). The nonoperative group consisted of 16 patients (16 extremities) treated by skeletal traction of the femoral fracture, closed reduction and splinting or casting of the tibial fracture, and an eventual hip spica cast. The operative group of 13 patients (14 extremities) had one or both fractures treated by open reduction and internal fixation (Fig. 14.8). The same criteria of Bohn and Durbin[42] were used in the evaluation of these patients to make the studies comparable. Despite higher modified injury scores and skeletal injury scores, the children and adolescents treated operatively had significantly reduced hospital stays (20.1 vs. 34.9 days, respectively), decreased time to unsupported weight-bearing (16.8 vs. 22.3 weeks), and fewer complications. Operative stabilization of the femur had a significant effect on decreasing the length of the hospital stay and the time to unassisted weight-bearing. The patients were also analyzed according to their age at injury: 9 years or younger and 10 years and older. The younger children treated nonoperatively had an increased rate of lower extremity length inequality, angular malunion, and need for a secondary surgical procedure when compared with younger children treated operatively with rigid fixation. On the basis of the results of this study, the authors recommended operative stabilization of at least the femur and preferably both fractures in a child with a floating knee, even for younger children.

TIBIAL FRACTURES IN CHILDREN WITH NEUROMUSCULAR DISORDERS

Children with neuromuscular disorders such as myelomeningocele, paraplegia from spinal cord injury or tumor, head injury, spinal muscular atrophy, muscular dystrophy, cerebral palsy, and arthrogryposis multiplex congenita, especially those who are nonambulatory, are at risk of fractures and epiphyseal displacement of the tibia and fibula.[95,96] These fractures must be treated in accordance with the underlying diagnosis and the degree of functional impairment. Although comprehensive care programs, including aggressive orthotic management and appropriately timed surgery, may prevent fractures by increasing the exposure of bone to weight-bearing, maximal function may expose the patient to an increased risk of fractures.

The major pathophysiologic change in the bones of children with neuromuscular disorders is osteopenia. Abnormal mechanical properties secondary to lack of weight-bearing and normal joint motion result in osteoporosis and inherent fragility and predispose to fractures even after minimal trauma. Osteoporotic bone has been demonstrated to have less strength and stiffness than normal bone. Developing bone deprived of neuromuscular activity has diminished cross-sectional area, cortical thickness, and bone circumference, and qualitatively and quantitatively inferior bone results. Proper muscle activity is crucial for normal growth

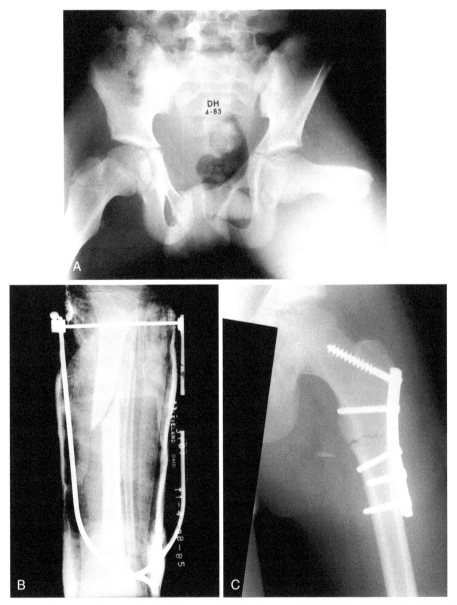

Fig. 14.8 (A) Anteroposterior radiograph of the pelvis of an 11-year-old boy who was struck by an automobile. A closed, displaced left subtrochanteric femoral fracture can be seen. Minimally displaced fractures of the right superior and inferior pubic rami have occurred. This child also sustained an ipsilateral closed, displaced tibial and fibular shaft fracture. The subtrochanteric fracture was initially treated with skeletal traction via a threaded Steinmann pin through the proximal part of the tibia. (B) The tibial fracture was reduced and immobilized in a long leg plaster cast incorporating the proximal tibial traction pin. Unfortunately, alignment of both the femoral and tibial fractures was unsatisfactory. (C) The left subtrochanteric femoral fracture was subsequently managed by open reduction and internal fixation with a compression plate and screws.

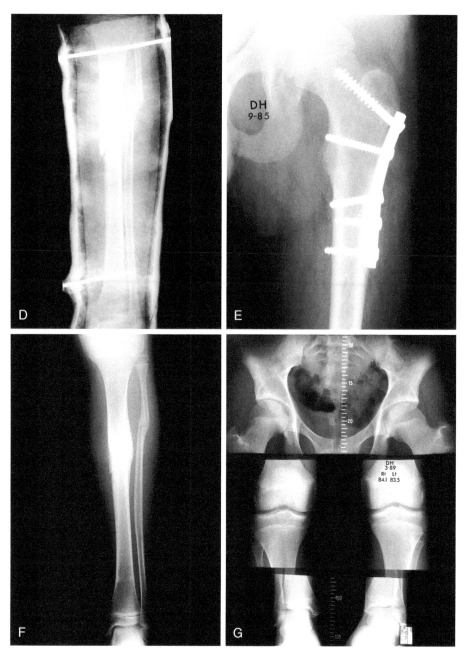

Fig. 14.8, cont'd (D) The left tibial and fibular fractures were treated by a repeated attempt at closed reduction and immobilization in a long leg cast after the addition of a second threaded Steinmann pin distal to the tibial fracture. Satisfactory alignment was achieved and maintained. This radiograph was obtained 2 months after injury. (E) A radiograph taken 5 months after injury demonstrates that the subtrochanteric fracture is well healed. (F) The tibial and fibular fractures also healed satisfactorily. (G) A scanogram obtained 47 months after injury demonstrates only 6 mm of shortening in the left lower extremity. The patient is almost skeletally mature and is asymptomatic.

and development of bone. Although decreased bone mass may result from loss of motor function, when sensory loss is also present, the bone effects are increased. In these cases, epiphyseal separation can occur, including that of the proximal and distal tibial epiphyses or the distal fibular epiphysis. This can occur with minimal or no injury and may resemble osteomyelitis both clinically and radiographically.

Neuromuscular disorders in children disturb the normal pattern of bone growth and development in a variety of ways and result in bone with thin cortices and decreased mass. Loss of muscle and weight-bearing forces produces abnormal bone and joint shape. Associated soft tissue contractures

resulting from muscle imbalance and weakness may also predispose to fractures by placing excessive stress on the adjacent metaphyseal regions, especially about the knee.

The clinical features of fractures of the tibia and fibula in a child with a neuromuscular disease are commonly modified. Fractures may occur with no history of trauma or after a trivial injury. Even gentle physical therapy and passive exercise may unintentionally cause a fracture. Boytim and colleagues[95] recognized that infants with myelodysplasia, thoracic and upper lumbar neurologic levels, and soft tissue contractures were prone to fractures during physical therapy. Common physical signs include warmth, erythema, and swelling. If sensation is normal, pain is obviously present. However, in the absence of sensation, as occurs in myelomeningocele and spinal cord injury, a fever may also be present. The erythrocyte sedimentation rate may also be elevated, but serum calcium, phosphorus, and alkaline phosphatase values are usually normal.

Whatever the underlying neuromuscular disorder, the goals of treatment are to achieve satisfactory alignment of the extremity and return the patient to the preinjury level of function. The major principle is to provide minimal immobilization of the patient and the limb compatible with union in a satisfactory position. What constitutes an acceptable position is based on the ambulatory abilities of the individual. Functional alignment, including rotation, must be achieved so that standing, walking, use of an orthosis, or wheelchair sitting will not be compromised. In displaced fractures in patients who cannot ambulate, less than perfect alignment may be adequate. The specific method of treatment is individualized for the child, the underlying diagnosis, and the functional level.

Fractures of the tibia and fibula in children with neuromuscular diseases are characterized by rapid healing and the absence of serious displacement. As a consequence, nonoperative methods are usually sufficient, as well as desirable. In nonambulatory children, bulky cotton roll dressings or pillow splints may be all that is necessary to maintain satisfactory alignment of the fractured tibia. Plaster or thermoplastic splints may also be used. Once the acute swelling subsides, the patient's orthosis may be used to support the fracture. If a child is able to stand, standing should be allowed as soon as possible after injury. If the fracture displacement, angulation, or rotation is too severe, a short or long leg plaster cast may be required.

Matejczyk and Rang[96] reviewed the distribution of fractures in children with neuromuscular disorders at the Hospital for Sick Children in Toronto. They found that most fractures occurred in the region of the knee joint. The femur, followed by the tibia, was most commonly fractured, especially the distal femoral and proximal tibial metaphyses. In children with myelodysplasia, fractures tended to occur predominantly in areas with no functioning muscles. Fractures occurred most often after falls and removal of postoperative hip spica casts or after immobilization for other reasons. In children with cerebral palsy, only severely involved patients had an increased risk of extremity fracture. This is probably related to severe, preexisting diffuse osteoporosis. Internal fixation may be necessary when spasticity precludes nonoperative management.

PATHOLOGIC FRACTURES

Fractures through preexisting osseous tumors, benign or malignant, may be the first indication of a pathologic process (see Chapter 4). These fractures are usually realigned and temporarily immobilized in a long leg posterior splint while a thorough evaluation of the pathologic lesion is performed. Pathologic fractures in the proximal metaphysis may result in an acquired valgus deformity. Jordan and associates[31] reported a 14-degree valgus deformity over a 2-year period in a 4-year-old boy after fracture through a large simple bone cyst in the proximal end of the tibia. The deformity spontaneously corrected to 4 degrees over the next 7 years. Definitive management is based on the diagnosis and natural history of the lesion.

ISOLATED FRACTURES OF THE FIBULAR DIAPHYSIS

Isolated fracture of the fibular shaft is rare and usually the result of a direct blow to the lateral aspect of the leg. These fractures may be compression (torus), incomplete tension-compression (greenstick), complete, or plastic deformation (bend) fractures. Such fractures typically heal with only simple immobilization (Fig. 14.9). A peroneal nerve palsy may accompany a proximal fibular fracture in direct injuries to the nerve itself. Complications in healing and subsequent growth are rare; however, it is important to exclude the presence of an associated physeal injury of the distal end of the tibia because a high fracture of the fibula can be seen in pronation-eversion/external rotation injuries to the ankle.[96]

FRACTURES OF THE DISTAL TIBIAL METAPHYSIS

Fractures of the distal tibial metaphysis are uncommon. Domzalski and colleagues[97] found only 26 distal tibial metaphyseal fractures in a series of 1068 tibial fractures. Falls were the most common cause. The fractures were primarily transverse and oblique. Most were displaced. Valgus angulation was associated with recurvatum, whereas varus angulation was associated with procurvatum. The fractures tended to occur in younger children. The mean age at injury was 6 years (range, 2–14 years). Nondisplaced fractures were treated with a long leg cast until initial healing allowed a change to a short leg cast. Displaced fractures were treated by closed reduction under conscious sedation or general anesthesia and then a long leg cast. Only one fracture required transcutaneous pin stabilization. All fractures healed within 6 weeks. No vascular complications or compartment syndromes occurred. Minor residual angular deformities were present but were not significant. However, Jung and colleagues[98] recently reported that 20 of 606 distal tibia fractures developed a posttraumatic tibiofibular synostosis. Twelve were focal, whereas 8 were extensive. Twelve patients were asymptomatic. In addition to symptoms, 5 patients needed 10 degrees or more of ankle valgus and distal fibular shortening. The most common fracture pattern leading to a synostosis was an oblique distal tibia fracture and commented fibula fracture. Overall operative intervention is rarely necessary, although displaced unstable fractures are now more frequently treated by closed or open reduction followed by internal fixation. Elastic stable intramedullary nails,[68,99] percutaneous plating,[100] and percutaneous pinning[101] have recently been reported as possible with excellent results and a very low complication.

Fractures of the distal tibial metaphysis generally heal quickly and without significant deformity (Fig. 14.10). They are not associated with the problems of asymmetric overgrowth and progressive angular deformity that occur in fractures of the proximal metaphysis.

OPEN TIBIAL AND FIBULAR FRACTURES

Open fractures of the tibia and fibula in children are serious injuries with a high complication rate.[10–15,63,102–108] They are invariably the result of high-velocity trauma. Motor vehicle–related accidents account for more than 80% of open fractures, and most occur in children older than 2 years. Even

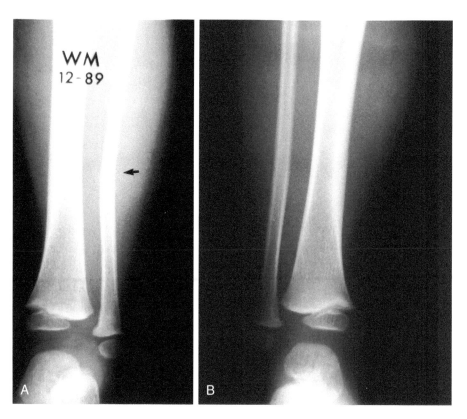

WM
12-89

Fig. 14.9 (A) Anteroposterior radiograph of the lower part of the left leg of a 2-year-old child who was observed to be limping. No history of injury was elicited. Plastic deformation of the distal third of the fibula has produced a slight valgus deformity *(arrow)*. (B) Comparison view of the lower portion of the right leg. The fibula is normal.

in adolescents, athletic activities account for less than 5% of open fractures. Although some open tibial fractures may involve the proximal or distal tibial metaphyses, most occur in the diaphyses or shafts. Approximately 20% of gunshot associated fractures in children and adolescents involve the tibia.[109]

The prevalence of open tibial and fibular shaft fractures in children varies between 2% and 14%.[6,13,15] It has been estimated that 1% of open tibial fractures occur before the age of 2 years, 15% to 20% from 2 to 6 years of age, and about 40% each in those aged 6 to 10 years and 10 to 14 years. The rarity of open fractures in children younger than school age is related to their small body mass and large amount of protective subcutaneous fat. In addition, young children in this age group are rarely exposed to high-velocity injuries that threaten life rather than limb.

Because most open tibial and fibular fractures are caused by severe trauma, the incidence of other body area injuries is high. These injuries include other fractures, closed head injuries, and blunt abdominal and chest trauma[6,10–15,102,104–106,108] (see Chapter 5). The prevalence of associated injuries in children with open tibial fractures has varied between 15% and 74% in recent studies.[10–15,106,108] In closed fractures, both the tibia and the fibula are fractured in about 33% of cases, whereas in open fractures, both bones are fractured approximately 85% of the time.[13] Comminution is also more common in open fractures. It occurs in approximately 33% of open fractures as opposed to only 5% to 10% of closed fractures.

ASSESSMENT AND INJURY CLASSIFICATION

Recent studies indicate that these fractures are best managed similarly to open fractures in adults. The type and incidence of complications are similar, but children appear to have better long-term results.[103,108] The Gustilo classification system of open tibial fractures, which was based on adult injuries, is also used to classify pediatric open tibial and fibular fractures and to guide subsequent management.

Despite advances in prehospital resuscitation and the development of free flaps and microvascular reconstruction, many limbs with severe open fractures, including those with vascular compromise or partial amputation, cannot be salvaged. Some of the most severe open tibial fractures may be better managed with a below-knee amputation than with extensive reconstructive procedures that may leave the patient with a poor cosmetic result and only marginal functionality. Severity indices provide some guidance when the decision is between limb salvage and amputation. For example, the Mangled Extremity Severity Score is a rating scale for lower extremity trauma based on skeletal and soft tissue damage, limb ischemia, shock, and age of the patient. However, reproducibility of the score has been questioned. Furthermore, to what extent this score is useful for the assessment of pediatric lower extremity injury is not known at this time. Minimal requirements for a functional restorable limb include (1) an intact or restorable blood supply, and (2) a sufficient sleeve of viable muscle to provide for stable soft tissue coverage and limb function that is superior to a below-knee amputation. When amputation is inevitable, early intervention enhances patient survival, reduces pain and disability, and shortens the length of hospitalization.

TREATMENT

The goals of treatment of open tibial fractures in children are the same as for adults: (1) preventing wound sepsis, (2) ensuring healing of soft tissues, (3) achieving bone union, and (4) returning the patient to optimal function.[110] Measures to achieve these goals include emergency resuscitation

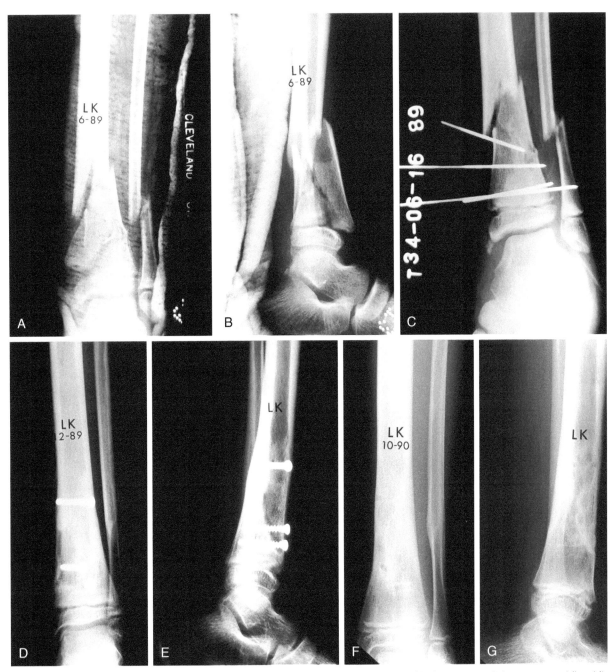

Fig. 14.10 (A) Anteroposterior radiograph of the lower portion of the left leg of a 9-year-old girl who was struck by an automobile while riding her bicycle. A very comminuted fracture involving the left distal tibial metaphysis is evident. In addition, she has a Salter-Harris type II distal tibial epiphyseal fracture. (B) A lateral radiograph demonstrates displacement of the anteromedial portion of the metaphysis of the Salter-Harris type II epiphyseal fracture. (C) Limited internal fixation was performed because the fracture was unstable, and satisfactory alignment could not be achieved by closed reduction. Initial alignment was obtained with multiple K-wires followed by cortical screws. (D) Nine months after surgery, the fractures have healed, and the distal tibial physis remains open. (E) Lateral radiograph confirming no evidence of premature physeal closure. (F) Fourteen months after surgery, the screws have been removed. The distal tibial physis is open, and normal growth and development are occurring. (G) Lateral radiograph 14 months after surgery.

and a thorough initial evaluation focusing in sequence on vital functions, limb-threatening injuries, and then the extremity fracture that is compromising the soft tissues. Other important measures include appropriate antimicrobial therapy, extensive and possibly repeated wound débridement, fracture stabilization, measures that facilitate wound closure, early autogenous cancellous bone grafting, and vigorous rehabilitation (Fig. 14.11). These measures are discussed in more detail in Chapters 5 and 6.

After initial resuscitation and careful assessment of the whole patient, priorities and plans for the treatment of all injuries are established with participation of the key medical services while the patient is still in the emergency department. There, the patient receives tetanus prophylaxis and the appropriate antibiotic or antibiotics.

More extensive evaluation of the wound, the initial débridement, and stabilization of the principal fracture fragments occur in the operating room. Fracture stabilization reduces pain, prevents additional injuries to surrounding soft tissues, decreases the spread of bacteria, and allows for early soft tissue and bone repair. For fractures with more extensive soft tissue injury, the method of stabilization must allow for free limb access to assess limb viability and to carry out repeated débridement. It must also be sufficiently rigid to permit early range-of-motion exercises of adjacent joints and possibly partial weight-bearing.

Iobst and colleagues[111] conducted a retrospective review of 41 patients with type I open fractures treated nonoperatively; eight of these fractures were of the tibia. No open wounds were closed primarily, and patients received an average of 6.97 doses of intravenous antibiotics. Of the 41 patients included in the review, only a 15-year-old male with a tibial fracture had a complication—a deep infection. The authors concluded that pediatric type I open fractures could be treated nonoperatively with acceptable outcomes. However, they recommend careful consideration of traditional irrigation and débridement in patients older than 12 years with open lower extremity fractures.

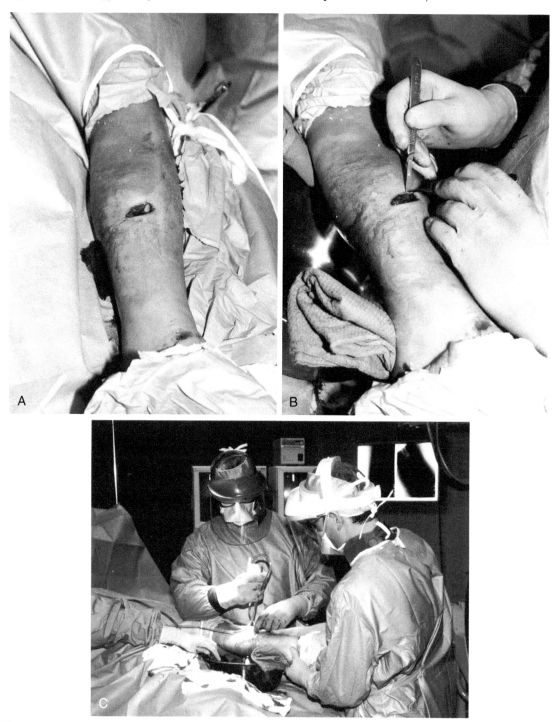

Fig. 14.11 (A) Intraoperative clinical photograph of a type IIIB open tibial and fibular shaft fracture in an 11-year-old girl who was struck by an automobile. (B) Débridement of the skin margins, subcutaneous tissues, and muscle and direct visualization of the fracture and inspection of the bone ends. (C) Pulsed irrigation with 10 L of normal saline.

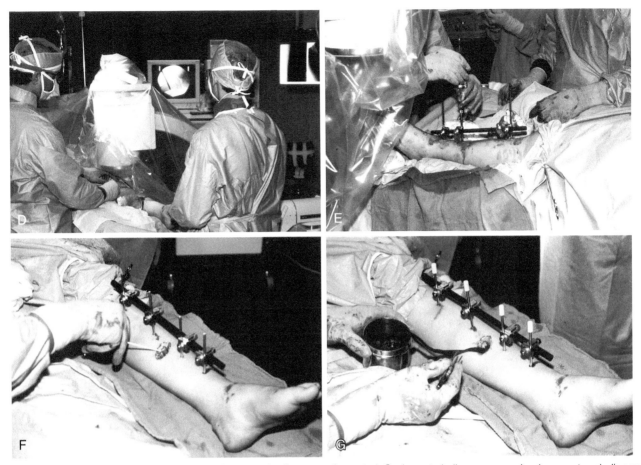

Fig. 14.11,cont'd (D) Application of an external fixator under fluoroscopic control. Such control allows proper pin placement and alignment, avoids possible physeal injury, and facilitates final reduction. (E) Final adjustments of the half-frame external fixator. (F) Tissue for culture is obtained intraoperatively after débridement, irrigation, and application of the external fixator. (G) Packing of the wound. In this case, povidone-iodine (Betadine)–soaked gauze was used, followed by the application of sterile dressings and a long leg posterior plaster splint.

Splints and Casts

Plaster splints and plaster-reinforced cotton-wool dressings (Robert Jones dressings) can be used for the early care of some stable type I and type II open fractures.[6] Once the soft tissue swelling has subsided and the wounds are closed, better fracture stabilization is needed. In many children, such stabilization can be achieved with a well-padded long leg cast with the knee in approximately 10 degrees of flexion.[13,108] Younger children, up to 8 years of age, can be immobilized in a long leg cast until their fractures are healed, usually 6 to 10 weeks after injury. In older children, the long leg cast is exchanged for a well-molded short leg cast after 4 to 5 weeks, when early callus formation is evident radiographically. The short leg cast remains in place for another 1 to 2 months, when most open tibial fractures have healed.

External Fixation

Splints and casts cannot prevent shortening of unstable fractures. Such lesions, including most type II and type III open fractures, which may require prolonged observation, repeated débridement, secondary flap procedures, or bone grafts, are best managed with external fixators.[57,106,108,112] When properly applied, external fixators allow free access to the wound for repeated débridement. The fixator frames should be of sufficient rigidity to prevent further injuries to the soft tissues, preserve length, and allow progressive weight-bearing with dynamization.[13,46,102,106,112]

In older children and adolescents, external fixators designed for adults are ideal. However, for smaller children, fixators used for adult wrist fractures or a combination of smaller pins with adult clamps and connecting rods is more appropriate (Fig. 14.12). The diameter of the fixator pins should not exceed a quarter of the diameter of the tibia; thus, pins with diameters ranging from 2.5 to 4 mm are most appropriate for children younger than 12 years.

To construct fixator frames of sufficient rigidity, many surgeons use such optimizing methods as a wide pin spread, dual longitudinal bars, and two-plane unilateral or two-plane bilateral designs. Nevertheless, with the exception of athletic or obese teenagers, simple one-plane unilateral frames routinely achieve sufficient rigidity for early weight-bearing. Ring fixators using wires under tension are useful for treating tibial fractures with extensive comminution and fractures extending close to the epiphyseal plates. These devices, which are generally more versatile than unilateral frames, are also preferred for correction of length discrepancy, malalignment, and soft tissue contracture. Ring fixators and Taylor spatial frames, however, tend to obstruct the wound.

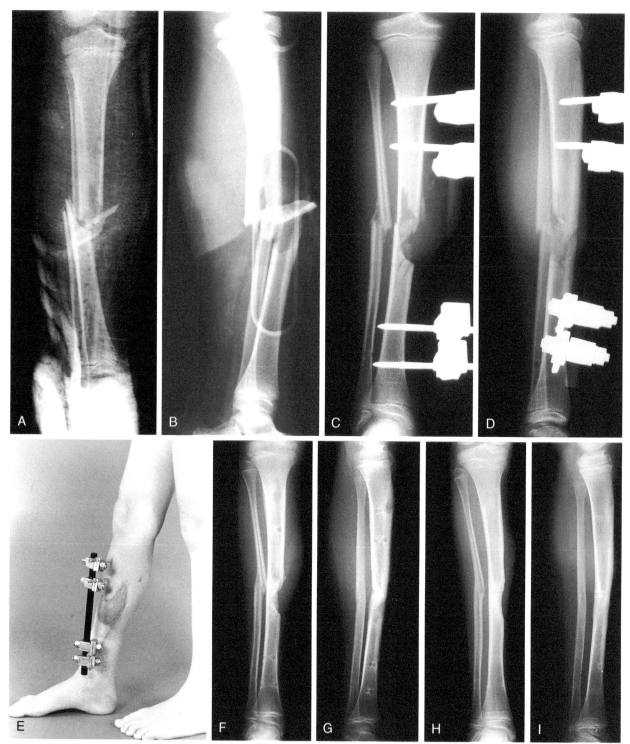

Fig. 14.12 (A) Anteroposterior (AP) radiograph of the lower part of the right leg of a 6-year-old girl with a comminuted, displaced type IIIB open fracture of the tibial and fibular diaphyses. These fractures were sustained when she was struck by an automobile. (B) A lateral radiograph demonstrates malrotation and a large, transversely oriented tibial fracture segment. (C) Radiograph obtained 1 month after débridement, removal of the devascularized tibial fracture fragment, irrigation, stabilization with an external fixator, and a soleus muscle rotation flap covered with a meshed, split-thickness skin graft. A large residual defect is present in the tibia. Limb length was maintained because of reduction of the lateral cortices of the tibia. (D) Lateral radiograph demonstrating satisfactory alignment. (E) Clinical photograph 2 months after injury. The wounds are well healed, and the patient is allowed partial weight-bearing with crutches. Cancellous bone grafting of the tibial defect was performed at this time. (F) AP radiograph 3 months after injury and 1 month after cancellous bone grafting and removal of the external fixator. The tibial defect is healing satisfactorily. The patient then had 2 months of additional immobilization in a short leg weight-bearing fiberglass cast. (G) Lateral radiograph showing maintenance of satisfactory alignment. (H) Six months after injury, excellent reconstitution of the tibial defect has occurred. At this time, the patient was allowed unprotected weight-bearing. (I) Lateral radiograph demonstrating excellent healing and alignment.

Optimal stabilization with minimal complications requires that three basic criteria be followed when external fixators are applied: (1) they should not damage vital anatomy, (2) they should provide sufficient wound access for débridement and secondary procedures, and (3) the frame should be appropriate to the mechanical demands of the patient.[112] Occasionally, pins may be inserted into the epiphysis. Great care must be taken when pins are placed periarticularly because the undulating shape of the physis creates an unsafe zone that varies in width from 1 to 2 cm.[46] Pins injuring the physis can cause growth disturbances. Epiphyseal pins also demand meticulous pin care to prevent osteomyelitis and septic arthritis. With careful technique and the use of an image intensifier, epiphyseal pins can be placed safely and can be highly effective in the management of fractures, especially those with a comminuted metaphyseal component.

Internal Fixation

Although the use of screws, plates, and intramedullary nails has revolutionized the treatment of open tibial fractures in adults, they have had less influence on the care of these injuries in children. Screws alone may have a place in the fixation of simple metaphyseal fractures but lack the axial and bending stability needed to hold tibial shaft fractures. In both adults and children, plating of tibial fractures has been accompanied by a higher infection rate. As long as the proximal tibial physis is open, standard intramedullary nails are contraindicated. Flexible intramedullary rods have become an alternative to external fixation.[63,108] In 2001, Qidwai[63] reported intramedullary fixation in 30 open tibia fractures, including 9 type I, 10 type II, and 11 type III (8 type IIIA and 3 type IIIB) fractures. Eighteen patients underwent primary wound closure, whereas 12 had delayed wound closure. Five patients (17%) had a postoperative infection—four superficial and one deep. The latter occurred in a type IIIB fracture that underwent delayed wound closure. All infections were successfully treated by débridement and intravenous antibiotics. All fractures healed rapidly with good functional outcomes. Kubiak and colleagues,[65] in 2005, in their comparative study of flexible intramedullary nailing and external fixation for tibial fractures, including open fractures, recommended the former for open tibial fractures without segmental bone loss and limited comminution. The complication rate was low, and improved functional results were seen. Access to open wounds is facilitated because the ends of the rods are buried beneath the skin and do not obstruct access for dressing changes and other procedures.

FOLLOW-UP CARE AND REHABILITATION

Once the soft tissues have healed and bone union progresses, rehabilitation is accelerated. Typically, range-of-motion exercises of the knee and ankle are followed by muscle strengthening and gait training. It is important that children undergo long-term follow-up for assessment of their ultimate outcomes with respect to function, alignment, and lower extremity length equality.

RESULTS

As external fixation of fractures gained popularity in adults, it began to be used in children, especially in those with open tibial fractures. The initial results were controversial because of a high incidence of infection and refracture after removal of the devices.[42,46,48]

Between 1989 and 1995, numerous large, relatively standardized studies investigating open tibial fractures in children were conducted.[10–12,14,15] The studies used the Gustilo classification and followed the associated treatment recommendations. These studies have demonstrated the true spectrum of pediatric open tibial fractures. Uncomplicated healing typically occurs in type I fractures, whereas delayed union, infection, nonunion, and other complications increase progressively in type II and type III fractures (Fig. 14.13).

In 1995, Kreder and Armstrong[14] reviewed 56 open tibial fractures in 55 children. The mean age at injury was 10 years (range, 3–17 years); most injuries occurred in boys and were related to motor vehicle accidents. These children had 14 type I, 16 type II, and 26 type III injuries (12 type IIIA, 8 type IIIB, and 6 type IIIC). Most of their patients had other body area injuries. Four patients died in the first 48 hours after injury. Four patients with five injured extremities (7%) required amputation, including four of the six type IIIC injuries. Infections occurred in eight patients and eight extremities (four superficial and four deep infections), which yielded a prevalence of 14%. Twenty-three fractures were treated by external fixation. Fourteen children experienced delayed union or nonunion. The 10 children with delayed union required prolonged immobilization and subsequently healed. The four patients with nonunion each underwent bone grafting and internal fixation before union was obtained. At follow-up, two extremities required treatment for lower extremity length discrepancy, and three required treatment for malunion. Important factors leading to complications were older age, severity of the injury, neurovascular injury, and a delay in getting the patient to the operating room.

Since 1995, most studies have focused on specific fixation methods, more severe injuries, and the factors that most clearly affect prognosis.[11,102–107] Buckley and colleagues,[104] in 1996, reviewed 20 children with type III open tibial fractures. There were 7 type IIIA, 10 type IIIB, and 3 type IIIC fractures. Some 90% of these patients required repeated débridement, and most had their fractures initially stabilized with an external fixator. To cover the wounds, 25% required split-thickness skin grafts, 15% needed local muscle flaps, and 30% underwent free muscle transfers. Three patients with segmental bone loss were treated with autologous bone grafts after the soft tissue injuries had healed. The limbs in three patients who had interpositional vein grafts for injuries to one or both tibial arteries survived, although the grafts failed. In one of these patients, a deep infection and delayed union with 3.5 cm of shortening developed. Osteomyelitis developed in three patients (30%) with type IIIB fractures. The average healing time was 29 weeks (range, 8–104 weeks) for all type III tibial fractures, 16 weeks for type IIIA fractures, 35 weeks for type IIIB fractures, and 36 weeks for type IIIC fractures. Simple fractures healed in 16 weeks, and comminuted fractures healed in 33 weeks. Fractures without bone loss healed in 24 weeks, and those with a segmental bone defect healed at an average of 59 weeks. The average healing time for uninfected fractures was 29 weeks, whereas those with osteomyelitis required 33 weeks for union. Only two patients had a leg length discrepancy in excess of 1 cm. All patients with osteomyelitis were successfully treated, and no amputations were necessary. The

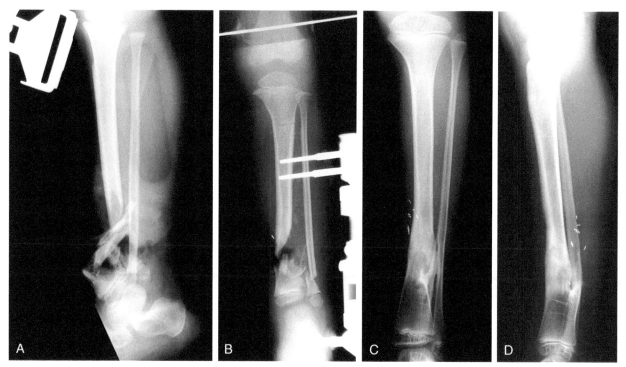

Fig. 14.13 (A) Anteroposterior radiograph of the lower portion of the left leg of a 3-year-old boy who sustained an open, comminuted, type IIIC fracture of the distal ends of the tibia and fibula when he was struck by an automobile. The closed ipsilateral femoral shaft fracture compromised circulation to the left foot. An arteriogram demonstrated occlusion of both the anterior tibial and the peroneal arteries. Blood flow through the posterior tibial artery was intact. (B) Radiograph 1 month after extensive débridement, irrigation, application of an external fixator, vascular repair, wound coverage with a rotational skin flap, and cancellous bone grafting. The femoral shaft fracture was treated with skeletal traction through the distal part of the femur. (C) Radiograph 28 months after injury. The child experienced delayed union and required two additional bone grafts. He ultimately underwent a free microvascular muscle transfer and split-thickness skin grafting to obtain vascularized soft tissue coverage over the fracture. Union ultimately occurred. The patient has equal leg length and normal function. (D) Lateral radiograph confirming satisfactory alignment, although slight posterior angulation is present.

authors concluded that with proactive wound care and fracture management, children with severe open fractures of the tibia have a good prognosis for limb salvage.

Cullen and colleagues[105] also in 1996 reported satisfactory results in 40 children with open fractures treated by stabilization with two or more large transcutaneous threaded Steinmann pins. Although the pins were left long, they were removed in the operating room, and a long leg cast was placed when there was evidence of early callus formation. This occurred at a mean of 7 weeks (range, 2–15 weeks) after injury. They reported a low incidence of complications using this technique.

Blasier and Barnes,[103] in 1996, also reviewed 33 consecutive open fractures of the tibia prospectively and focused, in particular, on the relationship of age to various treatment parameters. They separated their patient population into children younger than 12 years (group A) and those 12 years or older (group B). Both groups were similar regarding mechanism, severity of soft tissue injury, and method of immobilization. The authors found that patients in group A had significantly fewer complications, a lower rate of osteomyelitis, a diminished need for bone grafts, and faster healing times. These results confirmed the previous observations of Cramer and associates,[11] who reported average healing times of 3 months for type I fractures, 4.6 months for type II fractures, 6.8 months for type IIIA fractures, 17.8 months for type IIIB fractures, and 11.6 months in the only type IIIC fracture in the study.

Bartlett and colleagues[102] in 1997 reported that the type II and type III fractures of 19 of 23 patients were stabilized with external fixators. Fracture union occurred at a mean of 13.1 weeks: 11.5 weeks in type II fractures and 13.8 weeks in type III fractures. Seven patients had pin tract drainage but no chronic infection. There was one compartment syndrome and six patients with lower extremity length discrepancy, including three with overgrowth. No patient had greater than a 1-cm discrepancy. No nonunions, malunions, or refractures occurred.

Myers and colleagues,[57] in 2007, reported on 31 consecutive high-energy tibial fractures, of which 19 were open. There were three grade I, nine grade II, and seven grade III fractures. They reported a significant rate of complications secondary to both the injury and the external fixation system. These included malunion, delayed union, nonunion, wound infection, osteomyelitis, pin tract infection, and lower extremity length inequality. Complications were increased in open fractures and in older children and young adolescents.

A retrospective review comparing 14 patients with open tibial shaft fractures with 16 patients with closed fractures who underwent flexible intramedullary nailing by Pandya and Edmonds[113] in 2012 concluded that this was an acceptable intervention for open tibial shaft fractures. The study included 2 grade I fractures, 10 grade II fractures, and 2 grade IIIA fractures. They found that the risk of infection and wound complications was not significantly greater than that seen in patients with closed injuries. However, they also found a significantly increased incidence of bone healing complications in grade II and IIIA fractures treated with flexible intramedullary nailing, including nonunion, delayed union, malunion, leg length discrepancy, and growth arrest. Patients with open fractures also had a higher rate of secondary procedures (e.g., wound débridement, cast wedging/remanipulation, and secondary surgical procedures for malunion or nonunion). Some 79% of the patients in the open fracture group returned to the operating room to have the hardware removed compared with more than 90% of the closed fracture group. The authors also noted two systemic complications encountered in the open fracture group. Both patients had closed head injuries (one with an epidural hematoma and one with an intraventricular hemorrhage) and developed increased intracranial pressures perioperatively; both ultimately resolved postoperatively.

Summary of Recent Studies

In reviewing recently published articles, it appears that between 5% and 15% of all fractures of the tibia and fibula are open. The vast majority of these fractures are caused by collisions of motor vehicles with pedestrians or bicycles and falls from heights. About 30% of these injuries are type I, 40% are type II, and another 30% are type III in severity. The severity of the soft tissue injury directly correlates with the number and severity of associated injuries, which occur in about 25% of those with type I, 50% with type II, and 80% with type III open fractures. About 3% of patients sustain a compartment syndrome. Amputation rates are difficult to estimate because primary amputations are not usually reported. Many open tibial fractures, particularly those of lesser severity, are managed with primary wound closure and immobilization in a long leg cast, whereas repeated débridement and external fixation have become the accepted standard of care for the most severe injuries. Expected complication rates are 30% for infection, 40% for delayed union, 5% for nonunion, 6% for malunion, and about 2% for lower extremity length discrepancy in excess of 1 cm. According to recent studies, children younger than 12 years fare significantly better than those who are older.[105,108] They have fewer complications, and healing times are faster than in older children and adolescents. This difference may relate to the energy of the trauma involved in older children. These studies show that expert care of even type IIIB and type IIIC fractures may still result in overall outcomes superior to below-knee amputation.[63,104–106]

For children with large traumatic tibial defects, an ipsilateral fibular transfer can be considered. Keenan and colleagues[114] reported on two such cases with satisfactory outcomes. The defects were 10 and 11 cm in length and placed in an intercalary position and secured with screws. Other options include Ilizarov bone transport.[115]

AUTHORS' PREFERRED METHOD OF TREATMENT

Tetanus prophylaxis, parenteral antibiotics, and thorough wound débridement remain key for the optimal care of open tibial fractures. Wound débridement should take place within 24 hours of injury. Skaggs and colleagues,[116] in a multicenter study of 554 open pediatric fractures, showed no difference in infection rates between débridement performed within 6 hours and that performed 7 to 24 hours

after injury. Administration of early antibiotics is the prerequisite in preventing acute infections. There is good evidence that primary loose wound closure is well tolerated in lower grade injuries,[12,105] but, in most type III lesions, repeated débridement is usually required. Stable fractures with minimal soft tissue injury can be successfully managed with a long leg cast. However, most children with multiple injuries, those with second- and third-degree burns or other skin conditions, those with unstable fracture patterns, and children with higher-grade open wounds are best treated with external fixation.[104] Simple unilateral frames are ideal for most diaphyseal fractures, but ring fixators are more effective in highly comminuted lesions, in some metaphyseal fractures close to the growth plate, and in fractures with bone loss that may eventually require bone transport. The authors do not normally use plates and screws because of their higher complication rates[104] but do consider use of flexible intramedullary nails in older children with unstable fracture patterns.

COMPLICATIONS

DELAYED UNION

Delayed union (≥6 months) in closed pediatric tibial fractures is uncommon. The total time to satisfactory healing depends on the child's age and the type of fracture.

Typically, younger children heal faster than older children.[117] In addition, comminuted, displaced fractures take longer to heal than simple nondisplaced fractures in which the periosteum is intact. A delay in healing usually represents inadequate vascularization of the fracture site. This problem may be caused by an injury to the nutrient artery, the overlying musculature or periosteum, or a combination thereof. Additional time for revascularization and healing is therefore necessary. Moreover, inadequate immobilization that allows motion at the fracture site may contribute to delayed union or possibly to nonunion.

Delayed union after closed tibial fractures is usually managed by autogenous bone grafting from the iliac crest and proper immobilization until healing occurs. Internal or external fixation may be beneficial, especially in children with instability or malalignment.

In open fractures, delayed union is more common.[117] The reported prevalence has been between 5% and 36%.[10–15,63,104,105,108] This increase is predominantly the result of compromised vascularity, as discussed previously.

NONUNION

Nonunion of closed pediatric tibial fractures is very uncommon. Lewallen and Peterson,[118] in a study of 30 nonunions of long bone fractures, including 15 tibial fractures, found that they tend to occur in older children and adolescents, in high-energy fractures, and in open fractures (13 cases), especially those with soft tissue loss and infection. The association of nonunion with open fractures is clearly evident in recent publications on this subject, although Buckley and colleagues[104] reported two nonunions (20%) in their series of type III fractures. Other studies involving open tibial fractures have shown a low occurrence of nonunion, usually 10% or less.[14,105]

An autogenous bone graft from the iliac crest and appropriate fracture stabilization form the basis of treatment of pediatric tibial nonunion. In patients with inadequate vascularization of the fracture site, delayed muscle or myocutaneous flap reconstruction with microvascular techniques and cancellous bone grafting may be beneficial in achieving union. Immobilization can be accomplished with external fixation, flexible intramedullary rods, or plates and screws. Ring fixators (Ilizarov) and callotasis have been used successfully for tibial nonunion associated with bone loss.[117] The authors prefer external fixation because it does not require a second procedure for metal removal, and the soft tissue damage at the time of the initial bone grafting is less severe. Flexible intramedullary rods can be considered for nonunion.[11]

ANGULAR DEFORMITY

Angular deformities after closed or open tibial fractures are primarily caused by inadequate alignment before union and occasionally by transient asymmetric overgrowth. The latter is typically associated with a proximal tibial metaphyseal fracture, which has already been discussed.

Fractures of long bones, including the tibia, in children with angular deformities may undergo spontaneous correction with subsequent skeletal growth.[6,10,108,119] Certain generalities can be stated regarding remodeling: (1) the younger the child, the greater the capacity for correction; (2) the closer the fracture to the physis, the more the remodeling potential; (3) the smaller the angular deformity, the more complete the correction should be; and (4) residual angulation in the same plane as the movement of the adjacent joints has a greater capacity for correction. Correction of residual angular deformities results from a combination of asymmetric epiphyseal growth, both proximally and distally, and remodeling of the fracture site according to Wolff's law. However, the amount of correction is not predictable and varies with each long bone.

Shannak[6] identified several factors associated with spontaneous correction of angulated tibial malunions. These factors included varus and anterior angulation, spiral fractures, and younger age at injury (more remaining skeletal growth). He reported that 43 (37%) of 117 children had residual varus or valgus angulation. In 25 children, it was mild and varied from 1 degree to 10 degrees, and in 18 children it was moderate, being greater than 10 degrees but less than 22 degrees. At a mean follow-up of 3.9 years (range, 1–10 years), 91 children had no residual angulation, 20 had 1 degree to 10 degrees, and only 6 had more than 10 degrees. Thus, one-third of the children with greater than 10 degrees of angulation had persistent deformity, which was typically valgus or anterior angulation, or both. Even when remodeling is incomplete at the diaphyseal level, epiphyseal realignment, both proximally and distally, compensates for some of the residual deformity. Such compensation occurs with varus more than with valgus deformities and with posterior more than with anterior deformities.

Management of angular deformities is prevention. It is important that tibial fractures be monitored closely radiographically and that any residual angulation in the frontal and sagittal planes be corrected before fracture healing. Angulations up to 10 degrees can be accepted in young children (≤8 years of age) because many will improve with growth. Deformities greater than 10 degrees need to be corrected before healing, especially in older children and adolescents, because corrective procedures (osteotomy or hemiepiphysiodesis) may be required at a later time. After 12 years of age, remodeling will be less than 25%.[6]

MALROTATION

Pediatric tibial fractures that are allowed to heal in a malrotated position will not correct or remodel with subsequent skeletal growth. External rotation of the distal fracture fragment results in an out-toed gait, as well as increased stress along the medial aspect of the knee and pronation of the ankle and foot. Internal rotation of the distal fracture fragment results in an in-toed gait. It may also produce internal rotation at the knee joint level and supination of the foot.

Fortunately, the incidence of functionally significant rotational malunion is low. In Shannak's series,[6] three of 117 children (3%) had rotational deformities: two internal and one external. These deformities persisted after 3.9 years of follow-up. All three children were 12 years or older at injury. Bohn and Durbin[80] reported no rotational malalignment in 30 children (32 limbs) with ipsilateral femoral and tibial fractures monitored for a mean of 5.1 years. Yue and associates[94] reported one malrotation in 16 patients with ipsilateral femoral and tibial fractures treated nonoperatively and none in the 13 patients (14 extremities) treated by operative stabilization.

It is important that accurate rotational alignment be achieved during reduction of a tibial fracture with the use of either nonoperative or operative techniques. Any degree of malrotation should be avoided. If adequate radiographic assessment cannot be made by matching cortical widths of the proximal and distal fragments, CT, including views of the opposite intact tibia, can be helpful. If the fracture is allowed to heal in excessive rotational malalignment, surgical correction may be necessary.

ASYMMETRIC PROXIMAL TIBIAL PHYSEAL CLOSURE

Asymmetric closure of the proximal tibial physis with subsequent genu recurvatum is a rare complication after a nonphyseal tibial fracture.[120] It has also been described after femoral shaft fractures, Osgood-Schlatter disease, avulsion fractures of the tibial tubercle, tibial tubercle transfer, prolonged immobilization for congenital (developmental) dislocation of the hip, excessive pressure on the tibial tubercle from a cast or brace, skeletal traction, and minor trauma.

Cases of premature cessation of epiphyseal growth about the knee joint have been described after both femoral and tibial shaft fractures.[120–122] Genu recurvatum deformity secondary to anterior closure of the proximal tibial physis has also been seen, despite K-wires, clearly distal to the tibial tubercle.[120,122] The mean age at injury for children who seem to be at increased risk of this complication is between 10 and 12 years. The clinical deformity is usually noticed 1 to 3 years later.

The cause of closure of the anterior aspect of the proximal tibial physis is unknown. Hresko and Kasser[120] speculated on two possible mechanisms: (1) direct blunt trauma to the subcutaneous tibial tubercle resulting in anterior growth arrest and recurvatum, or (2) a compression injury to the anterior part of the proximal tibial physis generated by hyperextension of the knee. These mechanisms may damage the perichondral ring of the tibial tubercle or the periosteum at the edge of the tubercle, which, during healing, results in the formation of an osseous bridge. The initial injury is not recognizable radiographically.

Genu recurvatum deformities are best managed by an opening wedge osteotomy of the proximal end of the tibia with triangular iliac crest bone grafts. Epiphysiodesis of the remainder of the proximal tibial physis is necessary to prevent recurrence. It is important that the osteotomy restore the normal posterior slope of the articular surface of the proximal part of the tibia. Care must be taken to not excessively stretch the skin anteriorly because such stretching may predispose to wound dehiscence and skin necrosis. Osteotomy followed by lengthening (callotasis) can also be used. Fasciotomy of the anterior compartment and closed suction drainage should be performed to minimize the risk of compartment syndrome. Epiphysiodesis of either or both the distal femoral and proximal tibial epiphyses of the contralateral extremity may be required in children with significant tibial shortening to achieve equal lower extremity length at skeletal maturity.

In a young child with an angular deformity less than 20 degrees, resection of the osseous bridge and interposition with fat or other inert material may restore growth and allow spontaneous correction.[123] When the deformity exceeds 20 degrees, a corrective osteotomy combined with osseous bridge resection is recommended.

Recently, Navascues and associates[121] reported on seven patients with premature central closure of the distal femoral or proximal tibial physis or both after tibial diaphyseal fractures. All patients were 12 to 15 years of age at injury, and mild lower extremity length discrepancies (8 to 30 mm) subsequently developed. No children had angular deformities. The exact cause of the premature closure was unknown, but a vascular component was suspected.

LOWER EXTREMITY LENGTH INEQUALITY

As with other long bone fractures in children, the periosteal stripping, callus formation, and increased blood flow to the involved bone result in stimulation of the adjacent physes and a transient acceleration in growth. However, it does not occur with the same magnitude as in femoral shaft fractures, with the possible exception of children with open tibial fractures. Tibial overgrowth of approximately 5 mm can be expected in girls 3 to 10 years of age and in boys 3 to 12 years of age. Older children and young adolescents may actually have growth retardation induced by the fracture. Additional overgrowth of 1 to 3 mm can occur in the ipsilateral femur. The overgrowth is not usually affected by the fracture pattern or any residual angulation and lasts for 1 to 2 years after injury. Shannak,[6] however, found that comminuted fractures, proximal and distal fractures, and fractures with significant shortening had the greatest overgrowth. Similar results were reported in the Italian literature in 1985.[5]

Open fractures, especially those treated by external fixation, also seem to have a greater propensity for overgrowth than would normally be anticipated.[10,42,46,48,105] Tolo[48] reported overgrowth of 1 to 1.4 cm in three of 13 open tibial fractures. He recommended slight overriding of the fracture fragments in children between 2 and 12 years of age to compensate for this expected overgrowth. Cullen and colleagues[105] reported overgrowth of 1 cm or more in five of 40 patients (13%) treated by transcutaneous Steinmann pin fixation. All had grade I injuries and were 12 years of age or younger at injury.

Overgrowth and the resultant length inequality of the lower extremities also appear to be a problem in younger children whose fractures are reduced end on or anatomically.[10,104,105] Open reduction and the use of intramedullary rods in open and closed fractures may cause overgrowth, if it is assumed that the proximal physis is not injured. Qidwai[63] reported no cases of overgrowth of 1.0 cm or greater in 84 tibial fractures, including 30 open fractures treated by intramedullary fixation.

It has been demonstrated that a mean of 5 mm (range, 5–12 mm) of length discrepancy occurs normally in the lower extremities of healthy children. Therefore, some degree of luck is involved in obtaining equal leg lengths, especially if the fractured extremity was originally the longer one.

Thus it is important that accurate restoration of length be achieved in the management of pediatric tibial shaft fractures. Fortunately, most instances of shortening are not clinically significant. Discrepancies of 2 cm or less as an adult do not usually produce a limp or predispose to other problems. If overgrowth or shortening should occur, the child must be monitored with periodic radiographic measurements (scanograms) and bone age determinations to assess the behavior of the discrepancy and determine whether epiphysiodesis will be necessary to achieve relatively equal lower extremity lengths at skeletal maturity.

VASCULAR INJURY

Vascular injuries in association with closed tibial shaft fractures are very uncommon in children.[8,42] When vascular injuries secondary to tibial fractures are present, they are usually the result of high-velocity injuries and open fractures, such as occur in motor vehicle accidents.[10,12,15,42,121] Males are more commonly involved than females. Between 1% and 18% of open tibial fractures in the most recent studies had associated vascular injuries (type IIIC).[10–15,104] These injuries frequently lead to amputation.

Vascular injuries in association with closed tibial fractures are most often seen with displaced fractures of the proximal metaphysis or diaphysis.[8,42,121] Fractures in the proximal tibial metaphysis may damage the anterior tibial artery as it passes in a posterior-to-anterior direction through the interosseous membrane. Proximal tibial diaphyseal fractures may also damage the popliteal artery or its trifurcation of the posterior tibial, anterior tibial, and peroneal arteries.[42] Injuries involving the popliteal and posterior tibial arteries are associated with poorer outcomes than those involving the anterior tibial and peroneal arteries.[124] Isolated injuries to the posterior tibial artery as a consequence of a tibial shaft fracture are very rare.

Prompt recognition, evaluation, and vascular reconstruction are critical for initial limb salvage and avoidance of late complications. The cardinal signs of an arterial injury are known as the five Ps: pulselessness, pain, pallor, paresthesias, and paralysis.[123] However, the presence of audible pulses on Doppler flowmetry does not exclude an arterial injury. If such an injury is suspected, an arteriogram should be obtained. Compartment syndromes can have many of the same features as an arterial injury and may also occur after vascular repair (see "Compartment Syndrome" section). Fasciotomies at the time of vascular repair have been recommended.[42] If a fasciotomy is not performed, sequential or continuous compartment pressure assessments need to be taken.

Another potential vascular complication after tibial fractures is a traumatic arterial spasm. A diffuse arterial spasm without a specific arterial injury can occur and result in gangrene. Children appear to be more susceptible to this condition than adults. Russo[125] reported a 9-year-old boy who sustained a type IIIC open tibial, fibular, and calcaneus fracture; a traumatic arterial spasm developed and resulted in gangrene of the lower part of the leg and foot that required below-knee amputation. Arteriography showed only a diffuse arterial spasm. The spasm was not relieved by vasodilating agents. Treatment options for this rare condition, as discussed by Russo,[125] include intraarterial injection of vasodilating agents such as papaverine, sodium nitroprusside, reserpine, tolazoline, and prostaglandin E. Surgical measures may include external irrigation with warm lactated Ringer solution, application of local anesthetics or 32% papaverine, and adventitial stripping. If these measures fail, dilatation of the artery with mechanical dilators or catheters may be beneficial.

Treatment of fractures associated with arterial injury in children is controversial. Generally, the fracture is stabilized by external or internal fixation before arterial repair. However, Friedman and Jupiter[8] demonstrated satisfactory results with conservative management. Each case must be individualized, and the vascularity to the lower portion of the leg should be restored as rapidly as possible. Some fracture patterns may prevent initial vascular repair and necessitate reduction and stabilization before repair. If limb viability is in question, the arterial repair should be performed first, or an intraluminal shunt should be used. When limb viability is not in question, the fracture should be stabilized first to allow for more normal anatomic restoration of the bone and soft tissue.

NEUROLOGIC INJURY

Neurologic injuries associated with pediatric tibial fractures are uncommon, even in open fractures. The most common neurologic injury involves the peroneal nerve as it passes around the lateral aspect of the proximal end of the fibula. The nerve is more likely to be damaged by a direct blow than by a fracture fragment. It is important when fractures occur in this area that the function of the muscles innervated by the peroneal nerve be well documented. Bohn and Durbin[42] reported two transient, partial peroneal nerve palsies in children with ipsilateral femoral and tibial fractures. One occurred during skeletal traction, and the other occurred at the time of injury or during fracture reduction and application of a hip spica cast. In studies on open tibial fractures in children, the prevalence has varied widely. Some studies have reported no neurologic injuries,[11,12,15] whereas others have reported a prevalence between 2% and 14%.[10,14,104,105] The peroneal and posterior tibial nerves are the most frequently injured nerves.

COMPARTMENT SYNDROME

A compartment syndrome caused by bleeding and extravasation of tissue fluid into one or more of the four compartments of the lower part of the leg can and does occur in children.[126–129] Increased tissue pressure results in an increased net force per unit area exerted on the vessels within one or more compartments. This force increases local venous pressure, which decreases the local arteriovenous gradient and reduces local blood flow and oxygenation; as a consequence, local tissue function (muscle and nerve) and viability are compromised. The tolerance for increased compartment pressure varies with the local arterial pressure, the duration of the pressure, and, possibly, the local metabolic needs of the tissues. Prompt diagnosis and surgical decompression are essential for preserving the viability and function of tissues within the compartment. Failure to diagnose and treat compartment syndrome may result in irreversible ischemia of the extrinsic muscles of the lower part of the leg and, possibly, amputation.[128,130] Mubarak and Carroll,[128] in 1979, presented a review of 55 children with compartment syndromes that included 11 children with lower leg compartment syndromes, 5 of whom experienced complications of tibial shaft fractures. All but one patient had a delay in diagnosis of greater than 3 days. As a result, one below-knee amputation and 10 cases of residual functional deficit (5 severe, 4 moderate, and 1 mild) occurred.

Although most compartment syndromes occur in closed fractures, the presence of an open fracture with supposed compartment disruption does not preclude the possibility.[10–13,105,126,127] It is more likely to occur in type I or type II injuries, in which compartment disruption may be limited.[10–12,102] The incidence varies between 2% and 18% in these series. However, other authors have reported no cases of compartment syndrome in their studies on open tibial fractures.[14,15,104]

The clinical findings of compartment syndrome are subjective, and detection depends heavily on patient cooperation. In children, such cooperation can be difficult because of pain, fear, and anxiety. The classic five Ps (pain, pallor, paresthesias, paralysis, and pulselessness) may not be present, requiring the physician a high index of suspicion during evaluation. Intracompartmental pressure measurements by a variety of techniques allow a more objective method of evaluating and monitoring compartment pressure (see Chapter 5 for more detail). The first and most important symptom of an impending acute compartment syndrome is pain out of proportion to that expected from the fracture. Bae and colleagues,[126] in a study of acute compartment syndromes in children, observed that an increasing requirement for pain medication was a sensitive indicator of a developing compartment syndrome. Other potential signs include restlessness, agitation, and increasing anxiety.

The earliest clinical finding is a swollen and tense compartment caused by the increased intracompartmental pressure. Pain with passive stretching of the muscles in the involved compartment is a common finding but is subjective.[128,131] Unfortunately, children with sensory deficits resulting from a proximal nerve injury may not exhibit stretching pain, even in the presence of elevated intracompartmental pressure.

The most reliable physical finding of a compartment syndrome is sensory deficit.[132] Most compartments of the lower part of the leg are traversed by nerves with distal sensory distribution. Decreased sensation to light touch, pinprick, or two-point discrimination in the distal sensory distribution is an important finding. However, differentiating between paresthesias from a proximal nerve injury and a compartment syndrome can be difficult, especially in children.

Except in the presence of major arterial injury, peripheral pulses and capillary filling are usually intact in children with compartment syndrome.[132] As a consequence, the presence of palpable distal pulses and good capillary filling is no assurance that a compartment syndrome does not exist.

The most complex problem after a tibial shaft fracture is distinguishing among compartment syndrome, arterial occlusion, and proximal nerve injury (neurapraxia).[132,133] These conditions frequently coexist, and their clinical findings can overlap. Mubarak and Hargens[133] developed an algorithm to assist in differentiating them and in choosing appropriate treatment. Arterial injuries normally have absent peripheral pulses but no increased compartment pressure. Children with neurapraxia have no pain with passive stretching of muscles within a given compartment, no increased compartment pressure, and normal peripheral pulses. These characteristics are generalities, and each child must be carefully evaluated for these possibilities.

Mubarak and colleagues[134] identified three groups of patients in whom it is difficult to elicit and interpret the physical findings of compartment syndrome and in whom measurement of intracompartmental pressure may be extremely helpful: (1) patients who are unresponsive; (2) those who are uncooperative or unreliable, as commonly occurs in young children; and (3) those with peripheral nerve deficits attributable to other causes, such as peroneal nerve palsy.

Several methods have been developed for the measurement of compartment pressure, including needle, continuous infusion, wick catheter, and slit catheter techniques. The last technique affords an accurate method for continuous monitoring of intracompartmental pressure.[132] The pressure threshold for diagnosis of compartment syndrome varies for each of these techniques. The orthopedic surgeon must be familiar with the advantages, disadvantages, and pressure thresholds for each technique. However, common thresholds include pressures 30 mm Hg of the diastolic blood pressure.[126] Whitesides and associates[135] suggest that tissue perfusion depends not on the absolute compartment pressure but on the difference between the patient's blood pressure and the compartment pressure, known as ΔP. A ΔP of greater than 30 mm Hg is considered suggestive of compartment syndrome and is an indication for fasciotomy when the appropriate clinical picture is present. The use of ΔP has been shown in several studies to be more reliable than absolute compartment pressures for identifying compartment syndrome. It is also more useful in patients with abnormal physiology, such as those who are hypotensive or in shock.[136] It is important that pressure measurements be taken at the level of the fracture because pressure declines at increasing distances proximal and distal to the fracture. Incorrect technique could result in a serious underestimation of maximal compartment pressure.

The anterior compartment syndrome occurs most often after a fracture of the tibial shaft and is characterized by pain referred to the anterior compartment on passive flexion of the toes and mild weakness of the extensor hallucis longus followed by the extensor digitorum longus. The last sign to appear is hypoesthesia in the first web space.[130] Although the anterior compartment syndrome is the most common, other compartments may be involved concomitantly or individually. A deep posterior compartment syndrome can occur in children and is characterized by pain, plantar hyperesthesia, weakness of toe flexion, pain on passive toe and ankle extension, and tenseness of the fascia between the tibia and the triceps surae in the distal medial part of the leg. Bohn and Durbin[42] have reported on the sequelae of unrecognized deep posterior compartment syndrome. These patients are seen with clawed toes, intrinsic muscle wasting, and limited ankle and subtalar motion secondary to fibrous contractures of the muscles of the deep posterior compartment.

Because involvement of multiple compartments is common, it is now recommended that during the initial evaluation, pressure measurements be made in all four compartments and, if a fasciotomy is required, all compartments be released simultaneously.[102,126,130]

Incipient compartment syndromes can also exist and should be suspected in children who complain of inordinate pain under the cast but in whom no frank signs of compartment syndrome are present. The first step in the management of incipient compartment syndrome involves bivalving the cast and splitting the underlying padding. Rorabeck[131] stated that bivalving a long leg cast in a patient with a fracture of the tibial shaft and cutting the underlying padding may reduce compartment pressure by as much as 50%. Elevation of an extremity with incipient compartment syndrome is not recommended. It was noted both experimentally and clinically that elevation of the limb above the level of the heart reduced the mean arterial pressure and therefore reduced blood flow to the compartment.[128] In addition, elevation reduces the arteriovenous gradient and hence increases the susceptibility of the limb to compartment syndrome by reducing oxygen perfusion to the muscles. An extremity with an incipient compartment syndrome should be positioned at the level of the heart to promote arterial inflow.

In an established compartment syndrome, the patient has the clinical signs and symptoms of a compartment syndrome along with elevation of intracompartmental pressure. Rorabeck[131] identified the indications for surgical decompression in patients with established compartment syndrome. These indications include (1) clinical signs of an acute compartment syndrome with demonstrable motor or sensory loss, (2) elevated compartment pressure above 35 mm Hg when either the slit or the wick catheter technique is used or above 40 mm Hg when the needle technique is used in a conscious or unconscious patient, and (3) interrupted arterial circulation to an extremity for more than 4 hours. The most common methods for decompression of all four compartments of the lower part of the leg in an established compartment syndrome include partial fibulectomy, perifibular fasciotomy, and double-incision fasciotomy.

Partial fibulectomy is a historical method of decompression in adults. It is particularly useful for a deep posterior compartment syndrome. However, it is usually contraindicated in children because of the risk of residual pseudarthrosis of the fibula, which may result in fibular shortening from asymmetric growth and a valgus deformity of the ankle, as well as external tibial torsion.[137] This risk is especially high when fibulectomy is performed in children 10 years or younger. Friedman and Jupiter[8] used either a fibulectomy, which leaves the periosteum intact, or multiple-incision fasciotomies for their pediatric patients who had fractures associated with vascular injuries. The former allowed reformation of the fibula. Bone grafting is an alternative for fibular pseudarthrosis after partial fibulectomy. Perifibular fasciotomy has the advantage of allowing access to all four compartments through a single lateral incision. This technique is useful, provided that the anatomy of the extremity has not been distorted. The double-incision technique has been used by Mubarak and colleagues[134] and was studied extensively by Rorabeck.[131] The procedure is easy to perform, and no structures are likely to be damaged, with the exception of the saphenous vein medially. This technique allows easy access to all four compartments. It is important to perform generous skin incisions because the skin envelope can also contribute to increased compartment pressure.

Fracture management after fasciotomies in children is controversial. Mubarak and Carroll[128] recommended either internal or external fixation of pediatric tibial fractures associated with compartment syndrome to allow for easier management of the fasciotomy wounds. One of the major reasons for stabilization is that fasciotomies convert a closed fracture into an open fracture that, in most cases, must be left open and later closed secondarily. In a child, such stabilization may not always be necessary. The decision regarding fracture stabilization must be made on the basis of associated injuries and fracture stability. If rigid stabilization is necessary, it usually involves the use of an external fixator. In certain cases, however, young children may be treated conservatively with a long leg posterior splint followed by a long leg plaster cast for 4 to 8 weeks.

OSTEOPENIA

Essentially all pediatric patients with a tibial fracture (with or without a fibular fracture) will undergo a period of cast immobilization and non-weight-bearing. Although it is well documented in the adult population that this immobilization and non-weight-bearing results in a decrease in bone mineral content and density, little has been written on this phenomenon in otherwise healthy pediatric patients with lower extremity fractures. Ceroni and associates[138] performed a longitudinal matched case-control study comparing the bone mineral density and content in otherwise healthy adolescents. They found significantly decreased bone mineral density and bone mineral content in the injured extremity at the fracture site and adjacent sites in the same extremity but no significant difference in bone mineral density/bone mineral content Z-scores of L2–L4 or total body. This decrease was not as profound as that seen in adults but does raise the questions of how long patients should be kept from participating in sports and vigorous activity and whether the affected side ever regains the lost bone mineral density and content.

REFERENCES

The level of evidence (LOE) is determined according to the criteria provided in the Preface.

1. Cheng JCY, Shen WY. Limb fracture pattern in different pediatric age groups: a study of 3,350 children. *J Orthop Trauma.* 1993;7:15–22. (**LOE IV**).
2. Galano GJ, Vitale MA, Kessler MW, et al. The most frequent traumatic orthopaedic injuries from a national pediatric inpatient population. *J Pediatr Orthop.* 2005;25:39–44. (**LOE V**).
3. Karrholm J, Hansson LI, Svensonn K. Incidence of tibio-fibular shaft and ankle fractures in children. *J Pediatr Orthop.* 1982;2:386–396. (**LOE IV**).
4. Mashru RP, Herman MJ, Pizzutillo PD. Tibial shaft fractures in children and adolescents. *J Am Acad Orthop Surg.* 2005;13:345–352. (**LOE V**).
5. Parrini L, Paleari M, Biggi F. Growth disturbances following fractures of the femur and tibia in children. *Ital J Orthop Traumatol.* 1985;11:139–145. (**LOE IV**).
6. Shannak AO. Tibial fractures in children: follow-up study. *J Pediatr Orthop.* 1988;8:306–310. (**LOE IV**).
7. Ogden JA. Tibia and fibula. In: Ogden JA, ed. *Skeletal Injury in the Child.* 2nd ed. Philadelphia: W.B. Saunders; 1991:587–591.
8. Friedman RJ, Jupiter JB. Vascular injuries and closed extremity fractures in children. *Clin Orthop Relat Res.* 1984;188:112–119. (**LOE IV**).
9. Kute B, Nyland JA, Roberts CS, et al. Recreational all-terrain vehicle injuries among children. *J Pediatr Orthop.* 2007;27:851–855. (**LOE IV**).
10. Buckley SL, Smith G, Sponseller PD, et al. Open fractures of the tibia in children. *J Bone Joint Surg Am.* 1990;72:1462–1469. (**LOE IV**).
11. Cramer KA, Limbird TJ, Green NE. Open fractures of the diaphysis of the lower extremity in children. Treatment, results, and complications. *J Bone Joint Surg Am.* 1992;74:218–232. (**LOE IV**).
12. Hope PG, Cole WG. Open fractures of the tibia in children. *J Bone Joint Surg Br.* 1992;74:546–553. (**LOE IV**).
13. Irwin A, Gibson P, Ashcroft P. Open fractures of the tibia in children. *Injury.* 1995;26:21–24. (**LOE IV**).
14. Kreder HJ, Armstrong P. A review of open tibia fractures in children. *J Pediatr Orthop.* 1995;15:482–488. (**LOE IV**).
15. Yasko A, Wilber JH. Open tibial fractures in children. *Orthop Trans.* 1989;13:547–548. (**LOE IV**).
16. Dias LS. Fractures of the tibia and fibula. In: Rockwood CA Jr, Wilkins KE, King RE, eds. *Fractures in Children.* Philadelphia: J.B. Lippincott; 1984:983–1041.
17. Audigé L, Slongo T, Lutz N, Blumenthal A, Joeris A. The AO pediatric comprehensive classification of long bone fractures (PCCF). *Acta Orthop.* 2017;88:133–139. (**LOE IV**).
18. Joeris A, Lutz N, Blumenthal A, Slongo T, Audigé L. The AO pediatric comprehensive classification of long bone fractures (PCCF). *Acta Orthop.* 2017;88:129–132. (**LOE IV**).
19. Kozaci N, Ay MD, Avci M, et al. The comparison of point-of-care ultrasonography and radiography in the diagnosis of tibia and fibula fractures. *Injury.* 2017;48:1628–1635. (**LOE III**).
20. Park H-M, Kernek CB, Robb JA. Early scintigraphic findings of occult femoral and tibia fractures in infants. *Clin Nucl Med.* 1988;13:271–275. (**LOE III**).
21. Brammer TJ, Rooker GD. Remodeling of valgus deformity secondary to proximal metaphyseal fracture of the tibia. *Injury.* 1998;29:558–560. (**LOE IV**).
22. DalMonte A, Manes E, Cammarota V. Posttraumatic genu valgum in children. *Ital J Orthop Traumatol.* 1985;11:5–11. (**LOE IV**).
23. Ippolito E, Pentimalli S. Post-traumatic valgus deformity of the knee in proximal tibial metaphyseal fractures in children. *Ital J Orthop Traumatol.* 1984;10:103–108. (**LOE IV**).
24. Ogden JA, Ogden DA, Pugh L, et al. Tibia valga after proximal metaphyseal fractures in childhood: a normal biologic process. *J Pediatr Orthop.* 1995;15:489–494. (**LOE IV**).
25. Salter RB, Best T. The pathogenesis and prevention of valgus deformity following fractures of the proximal metaphyseal region of the tibia in children. *J Bone Joint Surg Am.* 1973;55:1324. (**LOE V**).
26. Skak SV, Toftgard T, Torben DP. Fractures of the proximal metaphysis of the tibia in children. *Injury.* 1987;18:149–156. (**LOE IV**).
27. Stevens PM, Pease F. Hemiepiphysiodesis for post-traumatic tibial valgus. *J Pediatr Orthop.* 2006;26:385–392. (**LOE IV**).

28. Robert M, Khouri N, Carlioz H, et al. Fractures of the proximal tibial metaphysis in children: review of a series of 25 cases. *J Pediatr Orthop.* 1987;7:444–449. (**LOE IV**).

29. Balthazar DA, Pappas AM. Acquired valgus deformity of the tibia in children. *J Pediatr Orthop.* 1984;4:538–541. (**LOE IV**).

30. Canavese F, Botnari A, Andreacchio A, et al. Displaced tibial shaft fractures with intact fibula in children: nonoperative management versus operative treatment with elastic stable intramedullary nailing. *J Pediatr Orthop.* 2016;36:67–672. (**LOE III**).

31. Jordan SE, Alonso JE, Cook FF. The etiology of valgus angulation after metaphyseal fractures of the tibia in children. *J Pediatr Orthop.* 1987;7:450–457. (**LOE IV**).

32. McCarthy JJ, Kim DH, Eilert RE. Posttraumatic genu valgum: operative versus nonoperative treatment. *J Pediatr Orthop.* 1998;18:518–521. (**LOE IV**).

33. Tuten HR, Keeler KA, Gabos PG, et al. Posttraumatic tibia valga in children: a long-term follow-up note. *J Bone Joint Surg Am.* 1999;81:799–810. (**LOE IV**).

34. Visser JD, Veldhuizen AG. Valgus deformity after fracture of the proximal tibial metaphysis in childhood. *Acta Orthop Scand.* 1982;53:663–667. (**LOE IV**).

35. Weber BG. Fibrous interposition causing valgus deformity after fracture of the upper tibial metaphysis in children. *J Bone Joint Surg Br.* 1977;59:290–292. (**LOE IV**).

36. Zionts L, Harcke TH, Brooks KM, et al. Posttraumatic tibia valga: a case demonstrating asymmetric activity of the proximal growth plate on technetium bone scan. *J Pediatr Orthop.* 1987;7:458–462. (**LOE IV**).

37. Zionts LE, MacEwen GD. Spontaneous improvement of posttraumatic tibia valga. *J Bone Joint Surg Am.* 1986;68:680–687. (**LOE IV**).

38. Coates R. Knock-knee deformity following upper tibial "greenstick" fractures. *J Bone Joint Surg Br.* 1977;59:516. (**LOE IV**).

39. Aronson DD, Stewart MC, Crissman JD. Experimental tibial fractures in rabbits simulating proximal tibial metaphyseal fractures in children. *Clin Orthop Relat Res.* 1990;255:61–67. (**LOE N/A**).

40. Houghton GR, Rooker GD. The role of the periosteum in the growth of long bones: an experimental study in the rabbit. *J Bone Joint Surg Br.* 1979;61:218–220. (**LOE N/A**).

41. Karaharju EO, Ryoppy SA, Makinen RJ. Remodeling by asymmetrical epiphyseal growth. *J Bone Joint Surg Br.* 1976:58 122–126. (**LOE N/A**).

42. Bohn WW, Durbin RA. Ipsilateral fractures of the femur and tibia in children and adolescents. *J Bone Joint Surg Am.* 1991;73:429–439. (LOE IV).

43. Burton A, Hennrikus W. Cozen's phenomena revisited. *J Pediatr Orthop B.* 2016;6:551–555. (**LOE IV**).

44. Morin M, Klatt J, Stevens PM. Cozen's deformity: resolved by guided growth. *Strategies Trauma Limb Reconstr.* 2018;13:87–93. (**LOE IV**).

45. Yang J-P, Letts RM. Isolated fractures of the tibia with intact fibula in children: a review of 95 patients. *J Pediatr Orthop.* 1997;17:347–351. (**LOE IV**).

46. Alonso JE, Horowitz M. Use of the AO/ASIF external fixator in children. *J Pediatr Orthop.* 1987;7:594–600. (**LOE IV**).

47. Gregory RJH, Cubison TCS, Pinder IM, et al. External fixation of lower limb fractures of children. *J Trauma.* 1992;33:691–693. (**LOE IV**).

48. Tolo VT. External skeletal fixation in children's fractures. *J Pediatr Orthop.* 1983;3:435–442. (**LOE IV**).

49. Al-Sayyad MJ. Taylor spatial frame in the treatment of pediatric and adolescent tibial shaft fractures. *J Pediatr Orthop.* 2006;26:164–170. (**LOE IV**).

50. Court-Brown CM, Byrnes T, McLaughlin G. Intramedullary nailing of tibial diaphyseal fractures in adolescents with open physes. *Injury.* 2003;34:781–785. (**LOE IV**).

51. Goodwin RC, Gaynor T, Mahar A, et al. Intramedullary flexible nail fixation of unstable pediatric tibial diaphyseal fractures. *J Pediatr Orthop.* 2005;25:570–576. (**LOE IV**).

52. Salem KH, Lindemann I, Keppler P. Flexible intramedullary nailing in pediatric lower limb fractures. *J Pediatr Orthop.* 2006;26:505–509. (**LOE IV**).

53. Sarmiento A, Latta LL. 450 closed fractures of the distal third of the tibia treated with a functional brace. *Clin Orthop Relat Res.* 2004;428:261–271. (**LOE IV**).

54. Spiegal PG, Mast JW. Internal and external fixation of fractures in children. *Orthop Clin North Am.* 1980;11:405–421. (**LOE IV**).

55. Gicquel P, Giacomelli MC, Basic B, et al. Problems of operative and non-operative treatment and healing in tibial fractures. *Injury.* 2005;36(suppl 1):A44–A50. (**LOE IV**).

56. Grimard G, Naudie D, Laberge LC, et al. Open fractures of the tibia in children. *Clin Orthop Relat Res.* 1996;332:62–70. (**LOE IV**).

57. Myers SH, Spiegel D, Flynn JM. External fixation of high-energy tibia fractures. *J Pediatr Orthop.* 2007;27:537–539. (**LOE IV**).

58. Norman D, Peskin B, Ehrenraich A, et al. The use of external fixators in the immobilization of pediatric fractures. *Arch Orthop Trauma Surg.* 2002;122:379–382. (**LOE IV**).

59. Stenroos A, Laaksonen T, Nietosvaara N, Jalkanen J, Nietosvaara Y. One in three of pediatric tibia shaft fractures is currently treated operatively: a 6-year epidemiological study in two university hospitals in Finland treatment of pediatric tibia shaft fractures. *Scand J Surg.* 2018;107(3):269-274. (**LOE III**).

60. Stenroos A, Jalkanen J, Sinkumpu JJ, et al. Treatment of unstable pediatric tibia shaft fractures in Finland. *Eur J Pediatr Surg.* 2018;29(3):247-252. (**LOE III**).

61. Ligier JN, Metaizeau JP, Prevot J, et al. Elastic stable intramedullary pinning of long bone shaft fractures in children. *Z Kinderchir.* 1985;40:209–212. (**LOE IV**).

62. Verstreken L, Delronge G, Lamoureux J. Orthopaedic treatment of paediatric multiple trauma patients. *Int Surg.* 1988;73:177–179. (**LOE IV**).

63. Qidwai SA. Intramedullary Kirschner wiring for tibia fractures in children. *J Pediatr Orthop.* 2001;21:294–297. (**LOE IV**).

64. O'Brien T, Weisman DS, Ronchetti P, et al. Flexible titanium nailing for the treatment of the unstable pediatric tibial fracture. *J Pediatr Orthop.* 2004;24:601–609. (**LOE IV**).

65. Kubiak EN, Egol KA, Scher D, et al. Operative treatment of tibial fractures in children: are elastic stable intramedullary nails an improvement over external fixation? *J Bone Joint Surg Am.* 2005;87:1761–1768. (**LOE IV**).

66. Berger P, DeGraaf JS, Leemans R. The use of elastic intramedullary nailing in the stabilization of paediatric fractures. *Injury.* 2005;36:1217–1220. (**LOE IV**).

67. Heo J, Oh CW, Park KH, et al. Elastic nailing of tibia shaft fractures in young children up to 10 years of age. *Injury.* 2016;47:832–836. (**LOE III**).

68. Shen K, Cai H, Wang Z, Xu Y. Elastic stable intramedullary nailing for severely displaced distal tibial fractures in children. *Medicine (Baltim).* 2016;95:e4980. (**LOE III**).

69. Reynolds DA. Growth changes in fractured long-bones: a study of 126 children. *J Bone Joint Surg Br.* 1981;63-B:83–88. (**LOE IV**).

70. Gordon JE, Gregush RV, Schoenecker PL, et al. Complications after titanium elastic nailing of pediatric tibial fractures. *J Pediatr Orthop.* 2007;27:442–446. (**LOE IV**).

71. Kinney MC, Nagle D, Bastrom T, Linn MS, Schwartz AK, Pennock AT. Operative versus conservative management of displaced tibial shaft fractures in adolescents. *J Pediatr Orthop.* 2016;36:661–666. (**LOE III**).

72. Gordon JE, O'Donnell JC. Tibia fractures: what should be fixed? *J Pediatr Orthop.* 2012;32(SUAAI I):S52–S61. (**LOE V**).

73. Teitz CC, Carter DR, Frankel VH. The problems associated with tibial fractures with intact fibulae. *J Bone Joint Surg Am.* 1980;62:770–776. (**LOE IV**).

74. Donnelly F. Toddler's fracture of the fibula. *Am J Roentgenol.* 2000;175:922. (**LOE III**).

75. Dunbar JS, Owen HF, Nogrady MD, et al. Obscure tibial fracture of infants—the toddler's fracture. *J Can Assoc Radiol.* 1964;25:136–144. (**LOE IV**).

76. Halsey MF, Finzel KC, Carrion WV, et al. Toddler's fracture: presumptive diagnosis and treatment. *J Pediatr Orthop.* 2001;21:152–156. (**LOE IV**).

77. Mellick LB, Reesor K. Spiral tibial fractures of children: a commonly accidental spiral long bone fracture. *Am J Emerg Med.* 1990;8:234–237. (**LOE IV**).

78. Oudjhane K, Newman B, Oh KS, et al. Occult fractures in preschool children. *J Trauma.* 1988;28:858–860. (**LOE V**).

79. Tenenbien M, Reed MH, Black GB. The toddler's fracture revisited. *Am J Emerg Med.* 1990;8:208–211. (**LOE IV**).

80. Bauer JM, Lovejoy SA. Toddler's fracture: time to weight-bear with regard to immobilization type and radiographic monitoring. *J Pediatr Orthop.* 2019; 39(6):314-317. **(LOE III).**

81. Lewis D, Logan P. Sonographic diagnosis of toddler's fracture in the emergency department. *J Clin Ultrasound.* 2006:34:190-194. **(LOE III).**

82. King J, Diefendorf D, Apthorp J, et al. Analysis of 429 fractures in 189 battered children. *J Pediatr Orthop.* 1988; 8(5):585-589. **(LOE IV).**

83. Kleinman PK, Marks SC, Blackbourne B. The metaphyseal lesion in abused infants: a radiologic-histopathologic study. *AJR Am J Roentgenol.* 1986;146:895–905. **(LOE IV).**

84. Dent JA, Paterson CR. Fractures in early childhood: osteogenesis imperfecta or child abuse? *J Pediatr Orthop.* 1990;10:542–544. **(LOE IV).**

85. Agarwal A, Pruthi M. Bicycle-spoke injuries of the foot in children. *J Orthop Surg (Hong Kong).* 2010;18:338–341. **(LOE IV).**

86. Izant RJ, Rothman BF, Frankel V. Bicycle spoke injuries of the foot and ankle in children: an underestimated "minor" injury. *J Pediatr Surg.* 1969;4:654–656. **(LOE IV).**

87. Mak CY, Chang JH, Lui TH, Ngai WK. Bicycle and motorcycle wheel spoke injury in children. *J Orthop Surg (Hong Kong).* 2015;23:56–58. **(LOE III).**

88. Gaffney JT. Tibia fractures in children sustained on a playground slide. *J Pediatr Orthop.* 2009;29:606–608. **(LOE IV).**

89. Loder RT, Schultz W, Sabatino M. Fractures from trampolines: results from a national database, 2002-2011. *J Pediatr Orthop.* 2014;34:683–690. **(LOE III).**

90. Niemeyer P, Weinberg A, Schmitt H, et al. Stress fractures in the juvenile skeletal system. *Int J Sports Med.* 2006;27:242–249. **(LOE IV).**

91. Walker RN, Green NE, Spindler KP. Stress fractures in skeletally mature patients. *J Pediatr Orthop.* 1996;16:578–584. **(LOE IV).**

92. Engh CA, Robinson RA, Milgram J. Stress fractures in children. *J Trauma.* 1970;10:532–541. **(LOE IV).**

93. Letts M, Vincent N, Gouw G. The "floating knee" in children. *J Bone Joint Surg Br.* 1986;68:442–446. **(LOE IV).**

94. Yue JJ, Churchill RS, Cooperman DR, et al. The floating knee in the pediatric patient. Nonoperative versus operative stabilization. *Clin Orthop Relat Res.* 2000;376:124–136. **(LOE IV).**

95. Boytim MJ, Davidson RS, Charney E, et al. Neonatal fractures in myelomeningocele patients. *J Pediatr Orthop.* 1991;11:28–30. **(LOE IV).**

96. Matejczyk MB, Rang M. Fractures in children with neuromuscular disorders. In: Houghton GR, Thompson GH, eds. *Problematic Musculoskeletal Injuries in Children.* London: Butterworths; 1983:178–192.

97. Domzalski ME, Lipton GE, Lee D, et al. Fractures of the distal tibial metaphysis in children: patterns of injury and results of treatment. *J Pediatr Orthop.* 2006;26:171–176. **(LOE IV).**

98. Jung ST, Wang SI, Moon YJ, Mubarak SJ, Kim JR. Posttraumatic tibiofibular synostosis after treatment of distal tibiofibular fractures in children. *J Pediatr Orthop.* 2017;37:532–536. **(LOE IV).**

99. Cravino M, Canavese F, DeRosa V, et al. Outcome of displaced distal tibial metaphyseal fractures in children between 6 and 15 years of age treated by elastic stable intramedullary nails. *Eur J Orthop Surg Traumatol.* 2014;24:1603–1608. **(LOE IV).**

100. Masquijo JJ. Percutaneous plating of distal tibial fractures in children and adolescents. *J Pediatr Orthop B.* 2014;23:207–211. **(LOE IV).**

101. Brantley J, Majumdar A, Jobe JT, Kallur A, Salas C. A biomechanical comparison of pin configurations used for percutaneous pinning of distal tibia fractures in children. *Iowa Orthop J.* 2016;36:133–137. **(LOE III).**

102. Bartlett CS 3rd, Weiner LS, Yang EC. Treatment of type II and type III open tibia fractures in children. *J Orthop Trauma.* 1997;11:357–362. **(LOE III).**

103. Blasier RD, Barnes CL. Age as a prognostic factor in open tibial fractures in children. *Clin Orthop Relat Res.* 1996;331:261–264. **(LOE IV).**

104. Buckley SL, Smith GR, Sponseller PD, et al. Severe (type III) open fractures of the tibia in children. *J Pediatr Orthop.* 1996;16:627–634. **(LOE IV).**

105. Cullen MC, Roy DR, Crawford AH, et al. Open fracture of the tibia in children. *J Bone Joint Surg Am.* 1996;78:1039–1046. **(LOE IV).**

106. Jones BG, Duncan RD. Open tibial fractures in children under 13 years of age—10 years experience. *Injury.* 2003;34:776–780. **(LOE IV).**

107. Levy AS, Wetzler M, Lewars M, et al. The orthopaedic and social outcome of open tibia fractures in childhood. *Orthopaedics.* 1997;20:593–598. **(LOE IV).**

108. Robertson P, Karol LA, Rab GT. Open fractures of the tibia and femur in children. *J Pediatr Orthop.* 1996;16:621–626. **(LOE IV).**

109. Naranje SM, Gilbert SR, Stewart MG, et al. Gunshot-associated fractures in children and adolescents treated at two level 1 pediatric trauma centers. *J Pediatr Orthop.* 2016;36:1–5. **(LOE IV).**

110. Stewart DG, Kay RM, Skaggs DL. Open fractures in children. Principles of evaluation and management. *J Bone Joint Surg Am.* 2005;87:2784–2798. **(LOE V).**

111. Iobst CA, Tidwell MA, King WF. Nonoperative management of pediatric type I open fractures. *J Pediatr Orthop.* 2005;25:513–517. **(LOE IV).**

112. Behrens F, Searls K. External fixation of the tibia. Basic concepts and prospective evaluation. *J Bone Joint Surg Br.* 1986;68:246–254. **(LOE III).**

113. Pandya NK, Edmonds EW. Immediate intramedullary flexible nailing of open pediatric tibial shaft fractures. *J Pediatr Orthop.* 2012;32:770–776. **(LOE IV).**

114. Keenan AJ, Keenan OJ, Tubb C, Wood AM, Rowlands T, Christensen SE. Ipsilateral fibular transfer as a salvage procedure for large traumatic tibial defects in children in an austere environment. *J R Army Med Corps.* 2016;162:476–478. **(LOE IV).**

115. Abdelkhalek M, El-Alfy B, Ali AM. Ilizarov bone transport versus fibular graft for reconstruction of tibial defects in children. *J Pediatr Orthop B.* 2016;25:556–560. **(LOE III).**

116. Skaggs DL, Friend L, Alman B, et al. The effect of surgical delay on acute infection following 554 open fractures in children. *J Bone Joint Surg Am.* 2005;87:8–12. **(LOE IV).**

117. Liow RYL, Montgomery RJ. Treatment of established and anticipated nonunion of the tibia in childhood. *J Pediatr Orthop.* 2002;22:754–760. **(LOE IV).**

118. Lewallen RP, Peterson HA. Nonunion of long bone fractures in children: a review of 30 cases. *J Pediatr Orthop.* 1985;5:135–142. **(LOE IV).**

119. Friberg S. Remodeling after fractures healed with residual angulation. In: Houghton GR, Thompson GH, eds. *Problematic Musculoskeletal Injuries in Children.* London: Butterworths; 1983:77–100.

120. Hresko MT, Kasser JR. Physeal arrest about the knee associated with non-physeal fractures in the lower extremity. *J Bone Joint Surg Am.* 1989;71:698–703. **(LOE IV).**

121. Navascues JA, Gonzalez-Lopez JL, Lopez-Valverde S, et al. Premature physeal closure after tibial diaphyseal fractures in adolescents. *J Pediatr Orthop.* 2000;20:193–196. **(LOE IV).**

122. Pappas AM, Anas P, Toczylowski HM Jr. Asymmetrical arrest of the proximal tibial physis and genu recurvatum deformity. *J Bone Joint Surg Am.* 1984;66:575–581. **(LOE IV).**

123. Peterson HA. Partial growth plate arrest and its treatment. *J Pediatr Orthop.* 1984;4:246–258. **(LOE IV).**

124. Waikakul S, Sakkarnkosol S, Vanadurongwan V. Vascular injuries in compound fractures of the leg with initially adequate circulation. *J Bone Joint Surg Br.* 1998;80:254–258. **(LOE II).**

125. Russo VJ. Traumatic arterial spasm resulting in gangrene. *J Pediatr Orthop.* 1985;5:486–488. **(LOE IV).**

126. Bae DS, Kadiyala RK, Waters PM. Acute compartment syndrome in children: contemporary diagnosis, treatment, and outcome. *J Pediatr Orthop.* 2001;21:680–688. **(LOE IV).**

127. Grottkau BE, Epps HR, DiScala C. Compartment syndrome in children and adolescents. *J Pediatr Surg.* 2005;40:678–682. **(LOE IV).**

128. Mubarak SJ, Carroll NC. Volkmann's contracture in children: aetiology and prevention. *J Bone Joint Surg Br.* 1979;61-B:285–293. **(LOE IV).**

129. Willis RH, Rorabeck CH. Treatment of compartment syndromes in children. *Orthop Clin North Am.* 1990;21:401–412. **(LOE V).**

130. Rorabeck CH, MacNab I. Anterior tibial compartment syndrome complicating fractures of the shaft of the tibia. *J Bone Joint Surg Am.* 1976;58:549–550. **(LOE IV).**

131. Rorabeck CH. The treatment of compartment syndromes of the leg. *J Bone Joint Surg Br.* 1984;66-B:93–97. **(LOE IV).**

132. Mubarak SJ. A practical approach to compartmental syndromes. Part II. Diagnosis. *Instr Course Lect.* **(LOE V).**

133. Mubarak SJ, Hargens AR. Diagnosis and management of compartmental syndromes. In: *American Academy of Orthopaedic Surgeons: Symposium on Trauma to the Leg and its Sequelae.* St. Louis: C.V. Mosby; 1981.

134. Mubarak SJ, Owens CA, Hargens AR, et al. Acute compartment syndromes: diagnosis and treatment with the aid of the wick catheter. *J Bone Joint Surg Am.* 1978;60:1091–1095. **(LOE III)**.

135. Whitesides TEJ, Haney TC, Morimoto K, et al. Tissue pressure measurements as a determinant for the need of fasciotomy. *Clin Orthop Relat Res.* 1975;113:43–51. **(LOE III)**.

136. Shadgan B, Menon M, O'Brien P, et al. Diagnostic techniques in acute compartment syndrome of the leg. *J Orthop Trauma.* 2008;22:581–587. **(LOE V)**.

137. Gonzalez-Herranz P, del Rio A, Burgos J, et al. Valgus deformity after fibular resection in children. *J Pediatr Orthop.* 2003;24:55–59. **(LOE IV)**.

138. Ceroni D, Martin X, Delhumeau C, et al. Effects of cast-mediated immobilization on bone mineral mass at various sites in adolescents with lower extremity fracture. *J Bone Joint Surg Am.* 2012;94:208–216. **(LOE IV)**.

15 Fractures and Dislocations of the Foot and Ankle

Shital N. Parikh | Jaime R. Denning

INTRODUCTION

Fractures and injuries about the foot and ankle in children are common and can have an important functional impact. Foot and toe fractures are among the top 10 pediatric orthopedic injuries,[1] and physeal injuries about the ankle are the second most common growth plate fracture.[2] A pain-free and deformity-free foot and ankle after injury allows a child the freedom to run, play, and explore the environment. If a residual deformity lingers after injury, the child limps, which causes distress for the parents, who may feel that they did not do enough to prevent their child's problem. The child might be teased by peers and may have an arthritic problem that causes pain and leads to limitations later in life.

With increased and more competitive sports participation and activities, possible decreasing age for puberty, and increased functional demands, many older children and adolescents sustain adult-type injuries. Pilon fractures, syndesmotic injuries, Lisfranc fracture-dislocations, and comminuted fractures of calcaneus or talus are uncommon fracture patterns in children. For complex injury patterns that are not typical for pediatric patients, it would be beneficial to team up with adult orthopedic trauma specialists for optimal patient care. Our collected thoughts and those of our referenced colleagues are intended to guide the reader to a safe resolution of foot and ankle injuries in children.

THE ANKLE

RELEVANT ANATOMY

The ankle joint is a true mortise joint, or a modified hinge joint, that consists of three bones: the tibia, fibula, and talus. The joint essentially moves in only one plane, from plantar flexion to dorsiflexion. The lateral malleolus allows minimal rotation to accommodate the changing width of the talar dome. The talar dome is broader anteriorly than posteriorly and, as a result, allows less rotation when the foot is in dorsiflexion than when it is in plantar flexion. The anatomic relationships and limited joint motion render the distal fibular epiphysis particularly vulnerable to crushing and twisting injuries (Fig. 15.1).

The ligaments about the ankle are attached to the epiphyses (Fig. 15.2). The deltoid ligament arises from the tip of the medial malleolus distal to the growth plate; it consists of two sets of fibers—superficial and deep. The superficial fibers originate from the anterior portion of the medial malleolus (anterior colliculus) and span out to attach to the calcaneus, navicular, and talus. The deep portion of the deltoid ligament originates from the posterior portion of the medial malleolus (posterior colliculus and intercollicular groove) and inserts into the medial surface of the talus. On the lateral aspect of the ankle, support is provided by three separate ligaments. Their tension and spatial orientation change according to the position of the ankle joint: plantar flexion, neutral, or dorsiflexion. These ligaments have their origin on the fibula distal to the physis. The anterior talofibular ligament runs anteriorly and medially from the anterior margin of the lateral malleolus to the talus anteriorly. The posterior talofibular ligament runs horizontally from the sulcus on the back of the lateral malleolus to the posterior aspect of the talus. The calcaneofibular ligament extends downward and slightly posterior from the tip of the lateral malleolus to a tubercle on the lateral aspect of the calcaneus; it is in close relationship to the peroneal tendons and their sheath. In general, the growth plate is more likely than the ligaments to fail during the years of skeletal development because of tensile weakness in the growth plate.

The tibiofibular syndesmosis consists of four ligaments—the anterior and posterior inferior tibiofibular ligaments, the interosseous ligament, and the anterior transverse ligament—in addition to the interosseous membrane. The anterior tibiofibular ligament runs downward between the anterior margin of the tibia and fibula; its origin in the fibula is also distal to the growth plate. The tibiofibular syndesmosis is rarely injured in children because the ligament is stronger than the growth plates, which tend to give more easily. In an adolescent in whom the growth plate has closed, disruption of the tibiofibular syndesmosis can occur.

The distal tibial physis begins to close about 18 months before complete cessation of tibial growth, first closing in its midportion, then medially, and finally laterally.[3] Longitudinal growth of the distal tibial epiphysis ceases at about 12 years of age in girls and 13 years in boys.[4] The fusion process does not occur uniformly but is instead asymmetric (Fig. 15.3). Fusion begins in the area of the tibial "hump," which is located centrally and is seen on the anteroposterior (AP) view as a small bump over the area of the medial edge of the talus. As fusion progresses, the medial part of the plate closes and then progresses posteriorly; finally, the anterolateral part of the plate fuses. The average time to fusion is 18 months. The fused part of the epiphyseal plate is no longer weak and prone to fracture but becomes an area of relative strength.[4] The irregular fusion pattern and the resulting

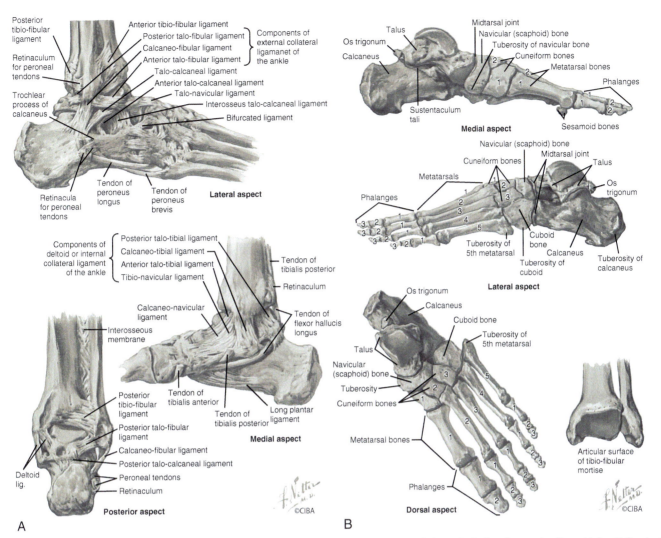

Fig. 15.1 (A and B) The anatomic bones of the foot and ankle; anteroposterior and lateral views, including ligaments. (From Netter F. Surgical anatomy of the foot and ankle. *Clin Symp.* 1965;17:1.)

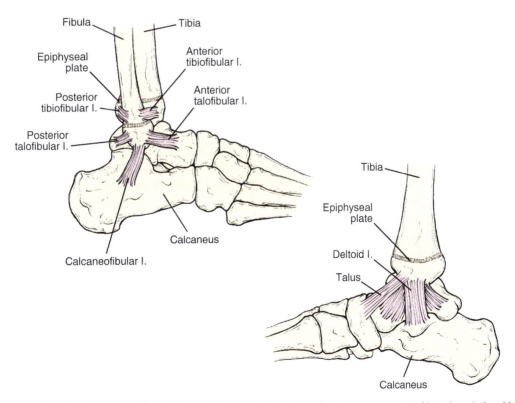

Fig. 15.2 The ligaments of the foot. Medial and lateral views of the ankle showing the ligamentous anatomy. Note the relationship of the physes to the ligaments. (From MacNealy GA, Rogers LF, Hernandez R, et al. Injuries of the distal tibial epiphysis: systematic radiographic evaluation. *AJR Am J Roentgenol.* 1982;138:683. Copyright 1982, American Roentgen Ray Society.)

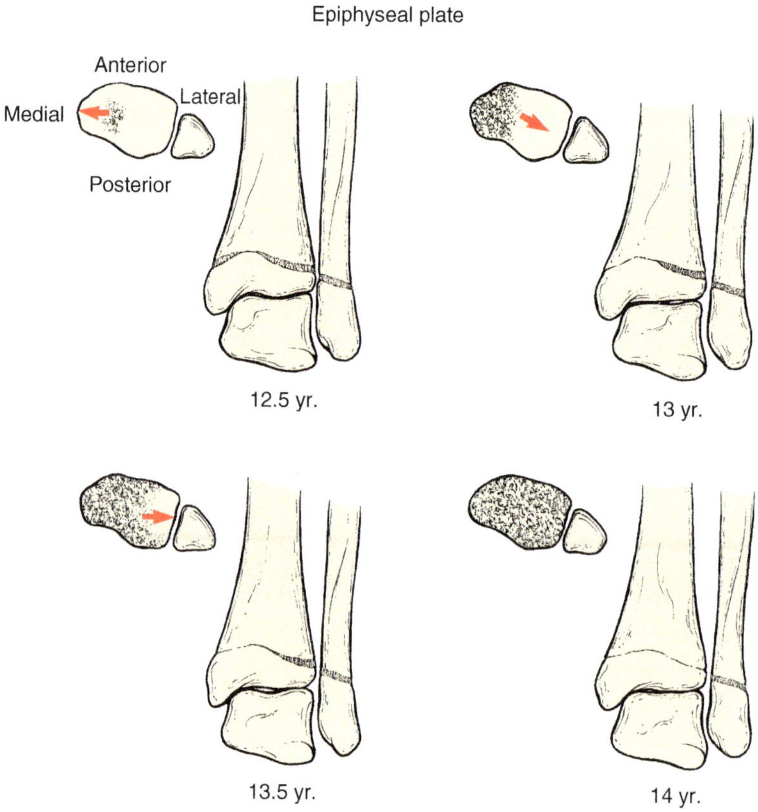

Epiphyseal plate

Anterior

Medial   Lateral

Posterior

12.5 yr.

13 yr.

13.5 yr.

14 yr.

Fig. 15.3 Average age of onset and normal fusion pattern in the distal tibial epiphysis. (From MacNealy GA, Rogers LF, Hernandez R, et al. Injuries of the distal tibial epiphysis: systematic radiographic evaluation. *AJR Am J Roentgenol.* 1982;138:683. Copyright 1982, American Roentgen Ray Society.)

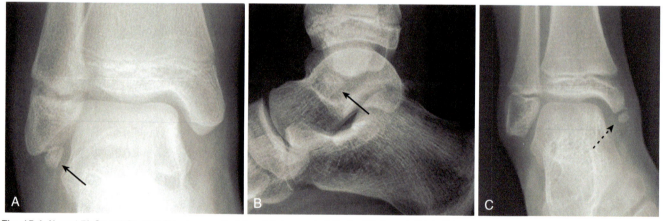

Fig. 15.4 (A and B) Os subfibulare (*black arrows*) at the distal aspect of fibula. (C) Os subtibiale (*black dashed arrow*) distal to medial malleolus. These well-rounded and well-corticated ossicles represent ossification variants or remote injuries and may be confused as acute fractures.

areas of relative strength and weakness are responsible for the unusual transitional fracture patterns; specifically, juvenile Tillaux and triplane fractures.

Accessory ossicles of the malleoli are common in skeletally immature individuals. They usually appear between the ages of 7 and 10 years and eventually fuse with the secondary ossification center of the malleolus at skeletal maturity.[5] The lateral ossicle has been termed the *os subfibulare*, and the medial ossicle is termed the *os subtibiale* (Fig. 15.4). Most of these ossification variations are identified only fortuitously, when radiographs are taken to evaluate an injury to the ankle or foot. They may represent remote injury or

may be confused with a sleeve fracture-avulsion of the lateral or medial malleolus. If the patient is symptomatic and the presence of a lesion is uncertain, a contralateral ankle radiograph can help differentiate ossification variant from an avulsion fracture. A positive magnetic resonance image (MRI) after failure of nonoperative treatment may support a diagnosis of injury.

INCIDENCE AND MECHANISM OF INJURY

Ankle fractures account for 5% of childhood fractures.[6] Injuries are commonly caused by indirect violence in which the fixed foot is forced into eversion-inversion, plantar flexion, external rotation, or dorsiflexion. Fractures may also be sustained by direct violence: the history is then usually an automobile accident, a fall from a height, or participation in contact sports. Injuries to the lower part of the leg and foot are more common in boys and usually occur between the ages of 10 and 15 years.[7–10] Those about the ankle constitute 10% to 25% of all physeal injuries. The distal tibial epiphysis is the second most common site of epiphyseal fracture in children, after the distal end of the radius.[9] The bone of a child is more capable of elastic and plastic deformation than is an adult bone.[11] Ligamentous injuries have traditionally been considered to be rare because the ligaments are stronger than the physes, but a recent prospective cohort study has shown that a combination of lateral ligament and bony injury coexists in 90% of suspected Salter-Harris type I fractures of the distal fibula.[12] The forces are transmitted to the medial part of the tibia by the ligamentous pull of the deltoid ligaments. Laterally, forces are transmitted by the anterior and posterior tibiofibular ligaments, the anterior and posterior talofibular ligaments, and the calcaneofibular ligaments.[13] The tendency for physeal compression during adduction injury is also greater. With an adduction injury, medial migration of the talus is usually blocked by the medial malleolus, and the medial malleolus is subsequently fractured.

CONSEQUENCES OF INJURY

The prognosis for injuries to the foot and ankle involves several criteria. The skeletal maturity of the patient determines the resulting bone, ligament, and/or growth plate injury. At different skeletal ages, the same mechanical twisting, torsional force, or related trauma to the foot and leg causes different injuries. Children are more prone to epiphyseal injuries, which, of course, are subject to more complications than are shaft or metaphyseal injuries. The more severe the injury (e.g., open fracture, grossly contaminated, or comminuted with or without soft tissue crushing), the greater the possibility of secondary devitalization with consequent delayed union, nonunion, pseudarthrosis, or osteomyelitis. The adequacy of reduction directly influences the rate of union; less healing time is required when bone contact is more. In addition, anatomic reduction is especially important for growth plate fractures because anatomic alignment reduces the incidence of angular deformity and shortening secondary to growth arrest, as well as degenerative arthritis secondary to persistent joint incongruity and instability. The prognosis after fractures involving the distal end of the tibia in children depends on the skeletal maturity of the patient, the severity of the injury, the fracture type, the degrees of comminution and displacement of the fracture, and the adequacy of reduction.[10]

RADIOLOGIC EVALUATION

In recent years, clinical prediction rules that focus on eliciting bony tenderness have led to refinement in the use of plain film radiography of the pediatric ankle; that is, the need for radiography has been reduced by approximately 25% without missing any fractures.[14] Although some institutional variation has been reported,[15] multiple studies have now shown that both doctors and nurses can effectively apply such decision rules (also referred to as ankle rules) in ambulatory care settings.[14] As per "low-risk ankle rules" in children, if tenderness or swelling is only confined to the distal fibula or adjacent lateral ligaments, then ankle radiographs are not required.[16] As per "Ottawa ankle rules," ankle radiographs are required if there is pain near the malleoli and one or more of: inability to bear weight; bony tenderness at the posterior edge; or bony tenderness at the tip of either malleolus. In a prospective comparative study, there was 63% reduction in requirement of ankle radiographs using low-risk ankle rules, compared with only a 12% reduction using the Ottawa ankle rules.[16] Despite these ankle rules, most institutions in North America would recommend standard three-view (i.e., AP, lateral, and mortise) radiographs for evaluation of ankle injuries. Consideration may be given to more selective use of radiographs during follow-up of known injuries.[17]

Besides evaluation of bones and joints on radiographs, one should assess the soft tissue very carefully. The normal fat stripe surrounding a bone may be thickened after a nondisplaced fracture. In addition, joint effusion after nondisplaced articular fractures may result in a positive fat pad, or synovial sign, especially in the anterior aspect of the ankle over the talar neck or posteriorly, with displacement of the Achilles tendon fat stripe (Fig. 15.5).

Computed tomography (CT) is recommended for imaging intraarticular fractures. CT scan can better define the fracture geometry and help measure articular gap, step-off, or displacement. It can also help in surgical planning for size, number, and trajectory of implant placement, especially when percutaneous approach is planned. In a study focused on triplane fractures, compared with radiographs, raters changed the definition of the fracture pattern in 46% of cases, degree of displacement in 39%, treatment plan in 27%, and either the number or orientation of screws in 41% of cases after reviewing the CT.[18] Paradoxically, a European survey of surgeons revealed that 50% used CT selectively and only 38% used CT routinely in their management of triplane fractures.[19] This may simply reflect a high level of confidence in allowing orthopedic plain-film interpretation to drive surgical decision-making. In an adult cadaver Tillaux fracture setting, plain radiographs were shown to be accurate to within 1 mm 75% of the time, whereas CT achieved this goal only 50% of the time.[20] However, CT was more sensitive than plain radiographs in detecting fractures with greater than 2 mm of displacement. It must be remembered that, in contrast to plain radiography, CT exposes the child to substantial amounts of radiation.[21] Newer CT imaging protocols have tried to minimize radiation. The newer cone-beam CT (CBCT) radiation dose is similar to that of an adult extremity radiograph, and its application has been studied in pediatric foot and ankle injuries.[22] Other advantages of CBCTs are their dynamic capabilities to scan the extremity in weightbearing position and possible installation in the clinic for easy access.

MRI utility in acute pediatric foot and ankle injuries is conflicted in the literature. Intraarticular bone fragments of unknown origin on radiographs could be further evaluated by MRI. After treatment, if the patient has any stiffness or ankle instability, MRI is indicated to exclude any intraarticular cartilaginous (silent) fragments or severe ligamentous injury, respectively.

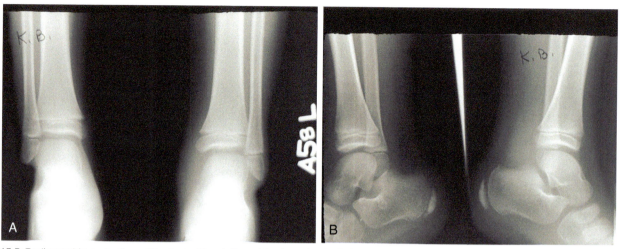

Fig. 15.5 Radiographic evaluation of the foot with notation of the fat stripe (soft tissue shadows). (A) The right side is normal. Note the increase in soft tissue density adjacent to and below the medial malleolus on the left side. (B) The left lateral ankle view *(right side)* shows an increase in the soft tissue posterior to the ankle joint. The soft tissue density is limited by the fat stripe just anterior to the Achilles tendon shadow.

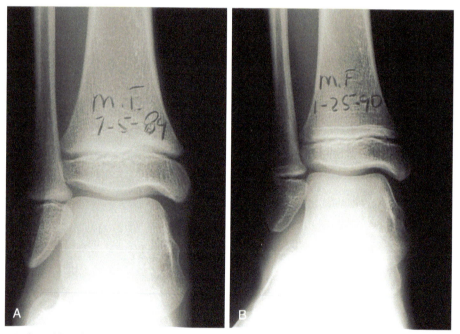

Fig. 15.6 "Sprain" injury to the ankle, with the subsequent development of Park-Harris lines. (A) A radiograph taken at the time of injury demonstrates soft tissue swelling below the malleoli. (B) Six months later, a horizontal line is seen just superior to the physis of both the tibia and fibula—the Park-Harris growth arrest line. The line should always be horizontal and parallel to the physis when growth is normal.

When fractures about the ankle in children are monitored, it is extremely important to observe the Park-Harris growth arrest lines.[23] These lines represent transient calcification of physeal cartilage during injury repair and are an excellent marker for observing growth after injury. The lines are parallel to the physis if growth is occurring normally (Fig. 15.6). In children with physeal damage, the line may be tented or angular.

CLASSIFICATION

In 1978, Dias and Tachdjian[7] introduced a classification of children's fractures that incorporated the concepts of Lauge-Hansen adult classification. To classify the fracture properly, radiographs are necessary; AP, lateral, and mortise views must be taken. In their classification (Table 15.1), the first part of the type name describes the position of the foot at the moment of trauma, and the second notes the abnormal force applied to the ankle joint: supination-inversion, pronation-eversion/external rotation, supination-plantar flexion, or supination-external rotation (Fig. 15.7).

The Salter-Harris classification has been used for fractures of the distal end of the tibia. It is familiar and easier to use compared with Dias-Tachdjian classification. Spiegel and colleagues[10] (Fig. 15.8) monitored 184 of a series of 237 fractures of the distal end of the tibia, fibula, or both for an average of 28 months after injury. Using the Salter-Harris classification, they differentiated three groups according to their risk of shortening of the leg, angular deformity of the bone, or incongruity of the joint. The low-risk group consisted of

TABLE 15.1   Classification of Physeal Injuries of the Ankle in Children

Type	Grade	Position of Foot	Injuring Force	Pattern of Fracture	Comment
Supination-inversion	1	Supinated	Inversion	Usually Salter-Harris type I or II fracture-separation of the distal fibular physis Occasionally rupture of the lateral ligament or fracture of the tip of the lateral malleolus	Displacement minimal and almost always medial
	2	Supinated	Inversion	Usually Salter-Harris type III or IV fracture of the medial part of the tibial epiphysis Rarely Salter-Harris type I or II fracture with medial displacement of the entire tibial epiphysis	Caution: Risk of up to 50% growth arrest without surgery, 2% with surgery
Supination-plantar flexion	1	Supinated	Plantar flexion	Commonly Salter-Harris type II fracture of the tibial epiphysis Rarely Salter-Harris type I fracture of the tibial physis No associated fracture of the fibula Metaphyseal fragment and displacement posterior Fracture line is best seen on a lateral radiograph	Prognosis good Caution: Do not damage growth plate by forced manipulation Posterior displacement will remodel
Supination-external rotation	1	Supinated	External rotation	Salter-Harris type II fracture of the distal tibial epiphysis with long spiral fracture of the distal tibia starting laterally at distal tibial growth plate	Up to 35% risk of distal tibial growth arrest
	2	Supinated	External rotation	Grade 1 plus spiral fracture of the distal fibular shaft	
Pronation-eversion/lateral rotation	1	Pronated	Eversion-lateral rotation	Salter-Harris type II fracture of the distal tibial epiphysis Metaphyseal fragment lateral or posterolateral Displacement lateral or posterolateral	Greater than 50% risk of distal tibial growth arrest
	2			Fibular fracture short, oblique, 4–7 cm from tip of the lateral malleolus	
Miscellaneous					
Adolescent Tillaux	—	Neutral?	Lateral rotation	Salter-Harris type III fracture of the lateral part of the distal tibial epiphysis Should not be any metaphyseal fragment Displacement anterolateral	Medial part of the distal tibial physis closed
Triplane, three fragments	—	?	Lateral rotation	Fracture in three planes—coronal, sagittal, and transverse Combination of Salter-Harris types II and III Fracture produces three fragments	Medial part of the distal tibial physis open
Triplane, two fragments	—	?	Lateral rotation	Fracture in three planes—coronal, sagittal, and transverse Combination of Salter-Harris types II and III	Medial part of the distal tibial physis usually closed
Comminuted fracture of the distal end of the tibia	—	?	Crushing injuries Direct violence	Comminuted fracture involving the distal tibial epiphysis Physis often damaged Fibula fracture at various levels	Poor prognosis

(From Tachdjian MO. *Pediatric Orthopedics*. 2nd ed. Philadelphia: W.B. Saunders; 1990.)

89 patients, 6.7% of whom had complications; this group included all type I and type II fibular fractures, all type I tibial fractures, type III and type IV tibial fractures with less than 2 mm of displacement, and epiphyseal avulsion injuries. The high-risk group consisted of 28 patients, 32% of whom had complications; this group included type III and type IV tibial fractures with 2 mm or more of displacement, juvenile Tillaux fractures, triplane fractures, and comminuted tibial epiphyseal fractures (type V). The unpredictable group consisted of 66 patients, 16.7% of whom had complications; only type II tibial fractures were included. The incidence and types of complications were correlated with the type of fracture (Carothers and Crenshaw classification), the severity of displacement or comminution, and the adequacy of reduction.[10]

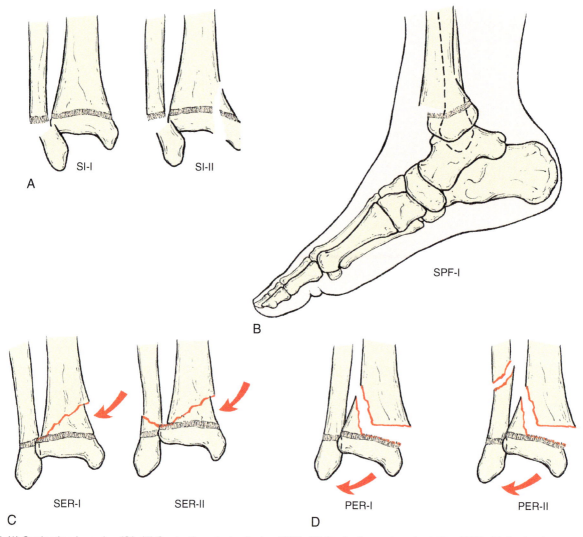

Fig. 15.7 (A) Supination-inversion (*SI*). (B) Supination-plantar flexion (*SPF*). (C) Supination-external rotation (*SER*). (D) Supination-external rotation (*PER*). (From Dias LS, Tachdjian MO. Physeal injuries of the ankle in children. *Clin Orthop Relat Res.* 1978;136:230.)

Despite their complexity, ankle fractures in children can be roughly divided into avulsion and epiphyseal fractures.[24] Adequately reduced avulsion fractures can be expected to heal well; epiphyseal fractures, however, may give rise to late complications. Vahvanen and Alto[24] proposed that classification of ankle fractures in children be based on radiographic findings, primarily with respect to epiphyseal lesions, and on a simple grouping with regard to risk for clinical purposes: group I, low-risk avulsion fractures and epiphyseal separations; and group II, high-risk fractures through the epiphyseal plate. The authors agree with this simplistic concept. Most avulsion fractures in children heal very well and have few complications; those that involve the epiphyseal plate tend to lead to either failure of continued growth because of damage to the endochondral ossification sequence or the potential for arthritis from intraarticular gaps or step-offs greater than 2 mm.

INDICATIONS FOR SURGICAL TREATMENT

Primary indications for surgical treatment include open fractures, inability to obtain or maintain adequate closed reduction, displaced articular fractures, displaced physeal fractures, or massive soft tissue injury.

SURGICAL TECHNIQUE

Every effort should be made to reduce the fracture anatomically and obtain accurate alignment of the physis and articular surface. It is strongly recommended that most displaced injuries be treated under general anesthesia with adequate muscle relaxation. During reduction maneuvers, more traction and less manipulation would help to minimize further injury to the physis.

If anatomic reduction can be achieved by closed manipulation, consideration should be given to stabilizing the fracture with percutaneously placed cannulated screws or Kirschner wires. The goals are quite clearly anatomic reduction and stable internal fixation. Indirect reduction as an adjunct to closed manipulation is extremely effective in treating children's ankle fractures. It is most effective when the fracture is fresh or before an interfragmentary clot has formed. Indirect reduction of medial malleolar and Tillaux fractures can be performed by using a guide pin through the distal fragment as a levering device, or "joystick," to anatomically align the fragment; direct manual compression is then applied, and the pin is advanced across the fracture site. Percutaneous placement of pointed reduction forceps can help to achieve reduction and compression if required (Fig. 15.9). Once anatomic reduction is achieved, partially threaded cannulated screw can be placed over the pin and across the fracture to achieve compression and maintain stability. Depending on the size of the fracture fragment, K-wires may be used for definitive fixation. Ankle arthroscopy can be used as an adjunct for assessment and treatment of articular surface injuries involving the distal tibia or the

talar dome, or to address intraarticular osteochondral fragments (Fig. 15.10).

If one has to perform open reduction for intraarticular fracture, adequate exposure of the physis and the articular surface would help. Every effort should be made to diminish the amount of soft tissue dissection by placing the incision over the area of the fracture gap. One can usually encounter tear of the periosteum at the level of the fracture, and little additional dissection is necessary. Surgery should be performed in a physeal-respecting manner, and one should avoid putting instruments in the physis or forcefully manipulating the physis. By irrigating the wound, removing any clots, and extracting any bony debris by gentle curettage, it is usually possible to realign the fracture anatomically. If anatomic reduction is prevented by a small metaphyseal fragment, such as that found with a Salter-Harris type IV fracture, it is possible to remove the metaphyseal fragment and obtain anatomic alignment of the epiphysis without damaging the physeal line. On occasion, a periosteal flap may prevent adequate reduction and may need to be extracted from the fracture site. Once anatomic alignment has been achieved, one could temporarily pin the epiphysis to the intact portion of the epiphysis and, if the metaphyseal fragment is large enough, then metaphysis to the metaphysis. Definitive fixation using cannulated screw can then be performed across the epiphysis and the metaphyseal fragment. The authors strongly recommend *against* placing a screw obliquely across the physis in a growing child. Unless evidence of closure of the middle of the physis is seen, the authors would not place an oblique screw across the fracture site as placed in adults for medial malleolar fractures. If the fracture geometry requires placement of hardware across the physis, then smooth K-wires could be used instead of a screw. Transarticular pins or multiple passes across the physis should be avoided (Fig. 15.11).

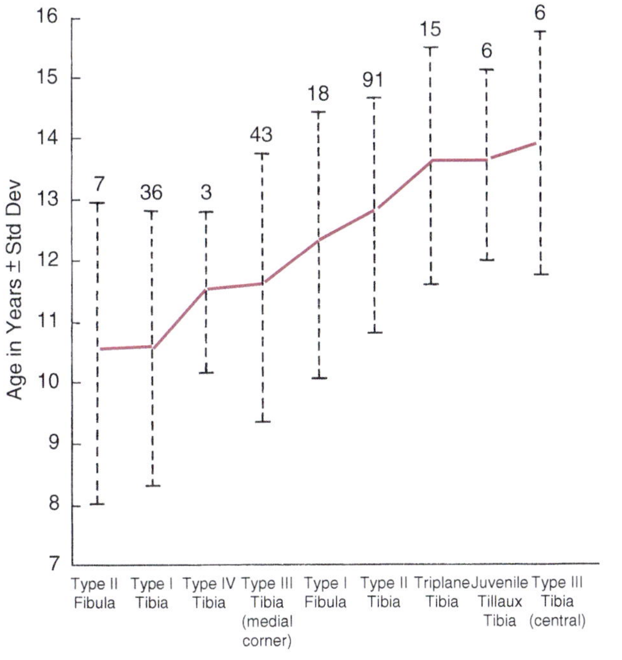

COMMENTS ON SPECIFIC FRACTURE PATTERNS

INTRODUCTION

The Dias-Tachdjian pediatric ankle fracture classification has stood the test of time as a useful tool for categorizing and understanding these injuries. The authors would estimate that this classification system easily accounts for more than

Fig. 15.8 Type of fracture based on age (age vs. type of fracture). (From Spiegel PG, Cooperman DR, Laros GS. Epiphyseal fractures of the distal ends of the tibia and fibula. A retrospective study of two hundred and thirty-seven cases in children. *J Bone Joint Surg Am.* 1978;60:1046-1050.)

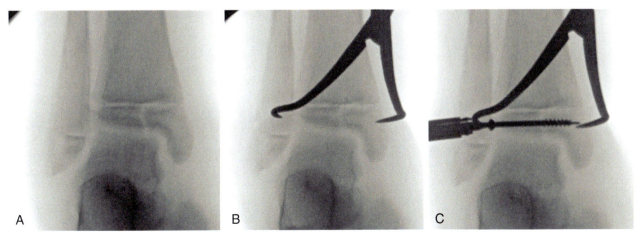

Fig. 15.9 (A) Tillaux fracture. (B) Indirect reduction using pointed reduction clamp placed percutaneously on medial malleolus and just anterior to the fibula. (C) Partially threaded cancellous screw with threads across the fracture site would allow for further fracture compression.

90% of the nontransitional ankle fractures encountered in children. Outcome studies have also indicated prognostic differences among the various categories and the ability of surgical intervention to improve treatment results. Universal agreement does not exist because some authors have emphasized that the risk of growth arrest may simply be linked to higher-energy injuries.[25] Other authors have also voiced skepticism about the ability of surgery to reduce the overall risk of growth arrest.[26]

SUPINATION-INVERSION

The supination-inversion mechanism is considered to be the most common of the pediatric ankle fracture patterns. This makes immediate sense because the first stage of this injury pattern is a Salter-Harris I or II fracture of the distal fibula (usually nondisplaced), a ubiquitous fracture in pediatric orthopedic trauma clinics. At times this injury may amount to a *physis-opathy* or *physis-itis* (which amounts to a stress fracture) of the distal fibular growth plate. More commonly, the radiographic appearance of the osseous distal fibula is normal, and pain, tenderness, and swelling ("goose egg") on clinical examination make the diagnosis.

For distal fibular physeal fracture, recent literature has challenged the previous notion that physis, being weaker than ligament, is more prone to injury in children and adolescents. There is now some evidence that Salter-Harris type I fracture of the distal fibula is not as common as was previously reported.[12] In a prospective study of 135 children with lateral ankle injury, normal radiographs, and MRI, only 4 patients had true physeal fracture of the distal fibula; 108 (80%) had ligament injuries (ankle sprain), and 27 (22%) had bone contusions. Some 35% of those with ligamentous injury were found to have an associated occult fibular avulsion fracture. There was no difference in outcomes when all patients were treated with a removable ankle brace for a

month.[27] These findings can decrease the overtreatment of these injuries.

The second stage of this injury, after bony or ligamentous injury on the lateral side, involves a Salter-Harris type III or IV injury of the medial malleolus. This typically attracts much attention, but it must be remembered that the distal fibula fractures first and the medial malleolus fractures second. After separation of the distal fibular epiphysis, the inversion-adduction force of the talus striking the medial malleolus produces the resultant fracture pattern. Radiographs typically show the fracture to involve less than one-third of the mediolateral distance across the epiphysis because the fracture line extends vertically to the physis and exits medially through the physis (Fig. 15.12). Determining the precise extent of displacement in these fractures is crucial because a significant gap may lead to nonunion, delayed union, or growth arrest. As the fracture unites, the ossification process above and below the physis may span the growth plate and form a bony bridge anchored in the metaphyseal and epiphyseal calluses. The width and, in turn, the strength of that bridge depend on the size of the residual interfragmentary gap. A thin, weak bridge after Salter-Harris III or IV fracture of the medial malleolus in a young patient (<10 years of age) may break spontaneously, and normal growth may continue.[28,29,30]

As mentioned earlier, the medial malleolar fracture fragment (either a Salter-Harris type III or IV) usually attracts the most attention, and most of the following discussion focuses on it. In the past, when these fractures were treated via closed reduction and cast immobilization, the rate of growth arrest (particularly of the medial malleolar growth region) may have often exceeded 50%.[8] However, with current concepts of anatomic reduction and stable internal fixation, these growth-related complications may be seen in as few as 2% of patients.[31] Thus the precedent for surgical treatment is rather strong in this fracture pattern.

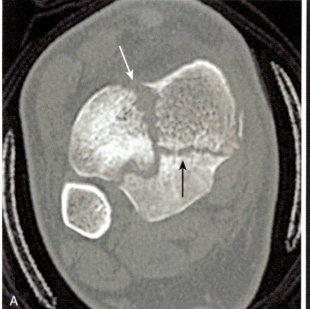
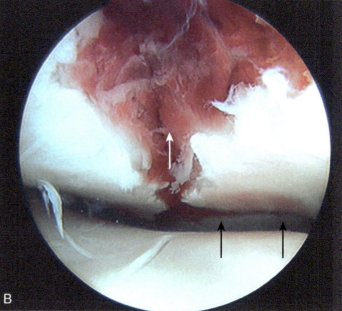

Fig. 15.10 The anterior gap (*white arrow*) on the computed tomography scan (A) and arthroscopic evaluation (B) is correlated. Similarly, the undisplaced posterior fracture line (*black arrows*) can be verified through ankle arthroscopy. During percutaneous fracture fixation for intraarticular fractures, arthroscope or arthrogram can be used to confirm the articular surface reduction.

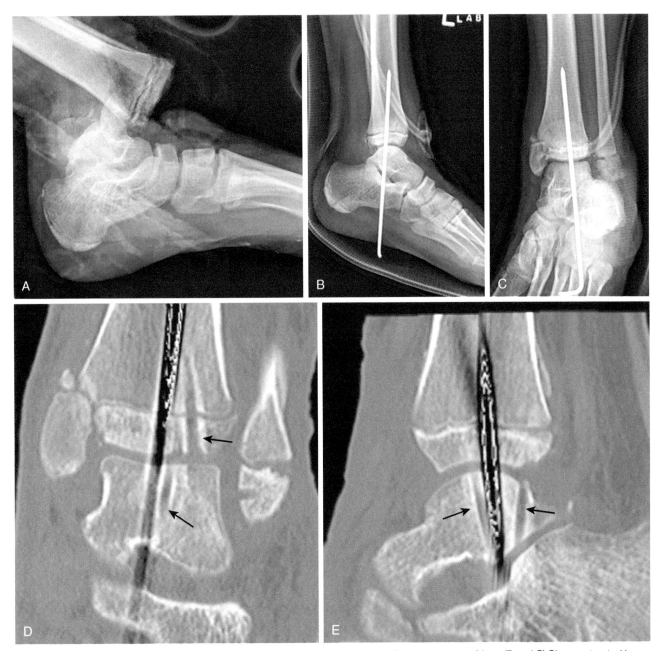

Fig. 15.11 (A) Open ankle fracture-dislocation in an 11-year-old girl following pedestrian versus car accident. (B and C) She was treated by open reduction and transarticular placement of Steinmann pin to maintain joint reduction and stability. (D and E) Computed tomography scan of the ankle. Multiple passes of the pin (*arrows*) through the articular surface and through the distal tibial physis should be avoided; an external fixator should be considered in such cases.

For a displaced medial malleolar fracture, either closed or open reduction and internal fixation is the preferred treatment. A percutaneous cannulated screw can be inserted in the epiphysis quite neatly and allows excellent control if closed reduction to within 2 mm is achieved (Fig. 15.12). In soft bone, a washer can be used as a one-hole plate to distribute forces generated by the screw head, thus allowing the possibility of greater interfragmentary compression. However, a washer can be prominent and may require later hardware removal if it leads to irritation. If logistically possible, percutaneous procedures are less traumatic and result in less operative exposure with less potential for vascular compromise and infection. Most of these fractures have remarkably small Thurston-Holland (metaphyseal spike)

fragments that do not lend themselves to fracture fixation. Rarely, the articular surface may have comminution or marginal impaction (Fig. 15.13). If in doubt, a preoperative CT scan can help to identify this. For such fractures, the articular surface is aligned using open reduction techniques, and the smaller articular fragments can be held by small (0.035 or 0.045 inch) K-wires. These wires can be embedded in bone or pulled out from the lateral side and cut outside the skin for later removal after fracture healing. They can be supported by screws using the raft technique. In a minority of cases, the fibula may merit formal reduction and smooth K-wire fixation.

After reduction and stable internal fixation of the medial malleolar fragment and after appropriate attention to

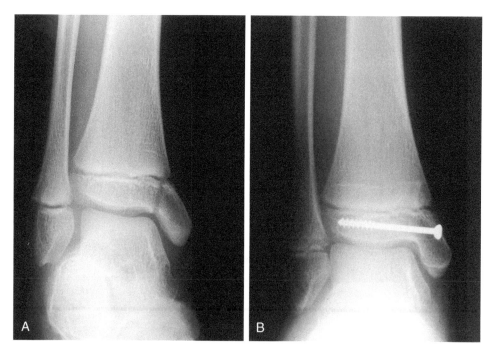

Fig. 15.12 Supination-inversion grade II. Salter-Harris type III fracture treated by a percutaneous interfragmentary screw. (A) In this adduction injury, the fracture occurred just above the super-omedial aspect of the talar dome. The fracture line of the epiphysis ends at the physis. (B) The injury was treated by closed reduction and a percutaneous interfragmentary screw. Note the horizontal Park-Harris line, indicative of normal growth after treatment. The screw should never cross an open growth plate obliquely.

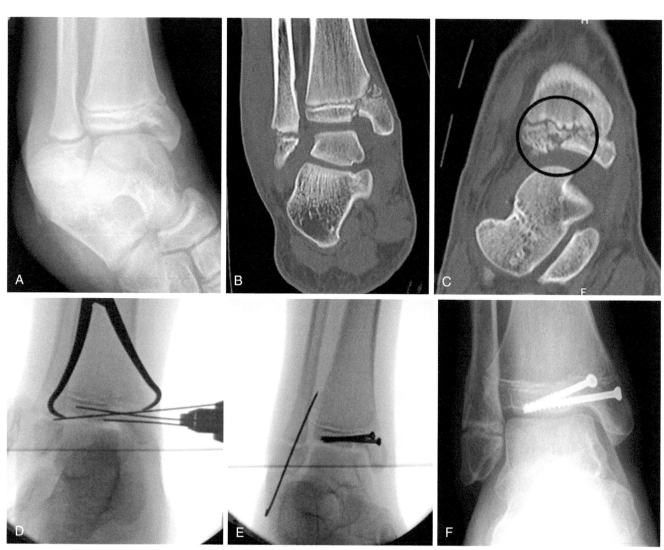

Fig. 15.13 (A) Salter-Harris type IV fracture of medial malleolus fracture in 14-year-old boy following fall off a trampoline. Coronal (B) and sagittal (C) computed tomography scan showing comminution of the fracture (*black circle*). (D) During open reduction and internal fixation, multiple K-wires were used to reconstruct the articular surface. (E) Raft screws were used to maintain the joint surface reduction, besides fixation of the medial malleolus fracture fragment. Fibula fracture fixation is optional but does add stability to fracture fixation. (F) Follow-up radiograph 1 year later shows well-healed fracture and intact articular surface.

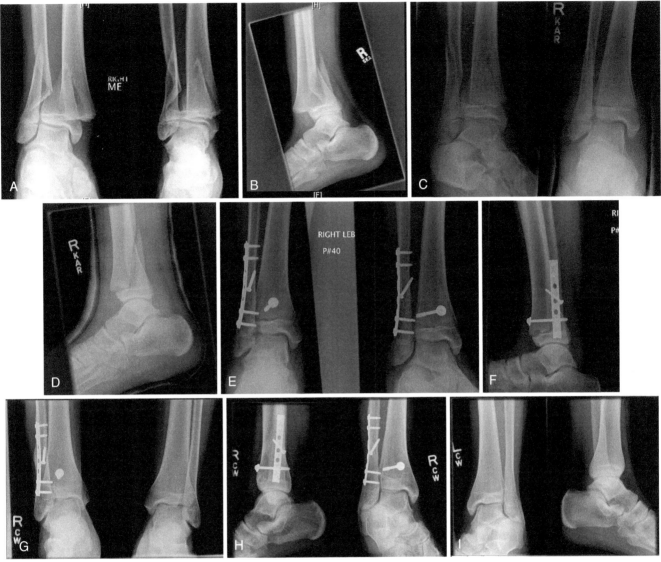

Fig. 15.14 Supination-external rotation fracture of the right ankle in a 14-year, 11-month male patient. (A) Initial mortise and anteroposterior views demonstrating fractures of the distal fibula and distal tibia (with a large medially based Thurston-Holland fragment). (B) Lateral injury radiograph illustrates anterodistal to posteroproximal orientation of the fibula fracture. (C and D) Unacceptable alignment on mortise, anteroposterior, and lateral views after effort at closed reduction. (E and F) Anatomic alignment after open reduction with internal fixation. (G, H, and I) Multiple views of both ankles at 1-year follow-up showing complete healing and fortuitous simultaneous closure of growth plates of both ankles.

the distal fibular fracture, non-weightbearing cast immobilization is added for about 4 weeks. Routine hardware removal is controversial. The recommendation for removing epiphyseal screws is based on a cadaveric study that showed that subchondral distal tibia screws increased peak contact pressure and force across the tibiotalar joint.[32] In clinical practice, however, the authors do not routinely remove the epiphyseal screws and have not encountered any problems by retaining the implants permanently. If a decision is made to remove the screw, it should be performed in the first year. After that, screw removal may be challenging if bony growth covers the screw head. Removing such a screw late may then subject the extremity to more trauma than simply leaving it in place. The authors have no experience with the use of bioabsorbable implants for the management of these fractures, although reported study has not shown any differences in the rate of nonunion, unplanned secondary surgeries, or complications between bioabsorbable and metal screws.[33]

Certainly, in selected cases, closed reduction and cast immobilization of this injury may be successful when the fracture is not displaced and anatomic reduction is maintained.

SUPINATION-EXTERNAL ROTATION

This pediatric ankle injury pattern has been recognized for quite some time.[34,35] The supination-external rotation mechanism is considered to first result in a physeal fracture of the distal tibia that typically has a rather large and medially based (to posteromedially based) Thurston-Holland fragment. Continuation of these injury forces results in a nonphyseal fracture of the distal fibula. This pediatric injury pattern mimics the adult pattern of the same name in that, when the fibula is involved, its distal diaphyseal fracture line extends along an anterodistal-to-posteroproximal line (Fig. 15.14).

The displacement of the supination-external rotation injury is typically not subtle. The ankle is swollen and painful,

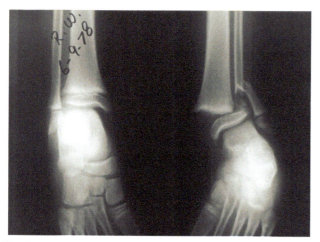

Fig. 15.15 Pronation-external rotation Salter-Harris type II fracture of the distal end of the tibia with a fibular shaft fracture. This Salter-Harris type II fracture is an abduction injury. The Thurston-Holland fragment sign on the distal end of the tibia is on the lateral aspect.

and the deformity is obvious. The apex of the deformity is usually anterolateral, and the previously mentioned oblique-to-spiral-oblique fibular fracture is virtually always present. Interposed periphyseal periosteum is certainly a possibility but has a somewhat lower likelihood simply because of the large size of the associated Thurston-Holland fragment. Anatomic reduction is the goal, with axial forces being applied via manual calcaneal traction and a variable amount of internal rotation followed by dorsiflexion. Postreduction images must be critically evaluated with respect to restoration of overall anatomic ankle alignment, significant residual physeal widening, and persistent fibular displacement.

The treating orthopedic surgeon must decide how much displacement is acceptable in these supination-external rotation injuries. These extraarticular fractures are very different from the displaced intraarticular fractures of the previously discussed supination-inversion category. Nonetheless, concern exists about premature distal tibial growth arrest because of residual physeal displacement and abnormal joint forces secondary to fibular malunion. The amount of displacement that may trigger surgical intervention may be as little as 3 mm of physeal gapping and 2 mm or more of fibular displacement (shortening). Barmada et al reported the rate of premature physeal closure after Salter-Harris type I and II distal tibial fractures to be 60% if there was more than 3 mm residual physeal gap after fracture reduction, and the rate decreased to 17% if there was no residual gap.[36] They recommended open reduction of these fractures to remove interposed periosteum if residual gap after fracture reduction was more than 3 mm. Subsequent study by the same group, however, did not report any significant change in the rate of premature physeal closure based on residual fracture gap or operative intervention.[26] The authors do not recommend routine removal of interposed periosteum unless it is required to obtain satisfactory fracture alignment. Literature documenting the remodeling potential of these Salter-Harris type II fractures is scarce. It has been suggested in the literature that a premature physeal closure rate for this injury pattern could be as high as 35%.[37] Thus, anatomic reduction and stable internal fixation is becoming more common than in the past. The large Thurston-Holland fragment

associated with these injuries lends itself to stable internal fixation with one or even two cannulated screws.

If the fibular fracture remains displaced or if increased stability at the ankle is deemed necessary, especially in adolescents, then the fibular fracture can be treated with open reduction and internal fixation using lag screw and neutralization plate. Adult literature has reported on abnormal tibiotalar joint forces after fibular malunion, but this has not been studied in children.[38,39] The authors do not routinely stabilize the fibula in children.

PRONATION-EVERSION-EXTERNAL ROTATION

The pronation-eversion- external rotation fracture pattern was originally described by Dias and Tachdjian[7] as a single stage injury, almost as if the respective tibial and fibular injuries occurred at the same time. However, it is commonly taught that this pediatric ankle fracture involves fracture of the distal tibial growth plate first (frequently with a rather small but easily seen laterally based Thurston-Holland fragment) followed by a rather transverse and substantially higher fracture of the fibular diaphysis (Fig. 15.15). Once again, this fibular fracture more closely mimics the fibular fracture associated with the adult pronation-external rotation ankle fracture pattern. Displacement of this pediatric ankle fracture is almost never subtle in that the translation (lateral) and angulation (apex medial) of the distal tibial epiphyseal fragment is substantial; angulation (apex medial) of the fibular shaft fracture is equally impressive.

Carothers and Crenshaw[35] expressed their greatest concern for growth arrest after pronation-external rotation injuries. These concerns have been echoed by contemporary authors as premature physeal closure rates that exceed 50% have been reported.[37] As mentioned earlier, removal of interposed periosteum to decrease residual physeal gap after fracture reduction is controversial, unless it is required for satisfactory fracture alignment[26,36] (Fig. 15.16). An impediment to anatomic reduction (besides interposed periosteum) could be interposed tibialis posterior tendon (Fig. 15.17). A high-energy mechanism of injury has also been implicated in growth arrest of such ankle fractures.[25] Such concerns led to Carothers and Crenshaw's reduction of these injuries under anesthesia and their selective use of internal fixation (even in 1955).[35] For the typical fracture pattern of the tibia with small metaphyseal fragment, one or two smooth K-wires across the physis are usually sufficient for fracture stabilization. If the Thurston-Holland fragment is large enough, then screw fixation across the metaphyseal fragment could be performed (Fig. 15.17). Standard plate fixation of the fibular fracture may add to the stability of the construct, if needed.

SUPINATION-PLANTAR FLEXION

This is the only mechanism that is considered to result in a displaced growth plate fracture of the distal tibia without any associated fibular fracture. The tibial Thurston-Holland fragment is variable in size but is predominantly posterior in location. It is clear from multiple published series that this plantar flexion injury is the least common of the pediatric ankle injury patterns.[34,35,37] Displacement is also typically subtle, and the lateral radiograph is the most likely to show mild widening of the tibial physis (Fig. 15.18). It is controversial if removal of interposed periosteum would decrease

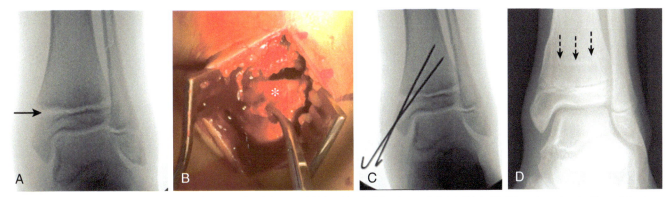

Fig. 15.16 A 13-year-old boy with pronation-eversion injury and Salter-Harris I fracture of distal tibial. (A) After closed reduction of fracture, there is persistent widening of the physis and valgus alignment at the fracture site. The patient underwent open reduction (B), removal of the interposed periosteum (*asterisk*) from the physis, and (C) internal fixation using smooth K-wires across the physis. The K-wires were removed at 4 weeks postoperative in the clinic. At 2 years' follow-up (D), a symmetric Park-Harris line (*dashed arrows*), parallel to the physis, indicates normal growth. (From Parikh SN, Mehlman CT. The community orthopaedic surgeon taking trauma call: pediatric ankle fracture pearls and pitfalls. *J Orthop Trauma.* 2017;31(Suppl 6):S27-S31.)

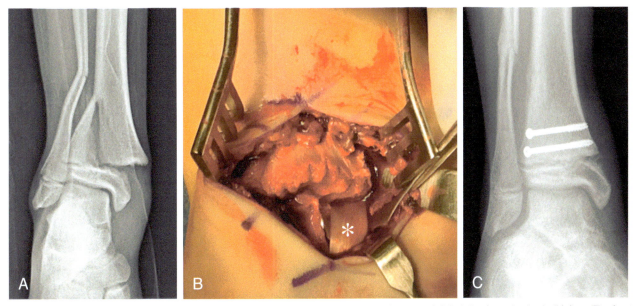

Fig. 15.17 (A) A 14-year-old with pronation-eversion fracture with Salter-Harris type II fracture of tibia following a basketball injury. The fracture was irreducible under general anesthesia. (B) A medial approach was performed and the interposed tibialis posterior tendon (*asterisk*) was removed, allowing for fracture reduction. (C) The large metaphyseal fragment allowed for placement of two cannulated screws for fracture fixation. Once reduced, the guide wires for fracture fixation were placed from medial to lateral through the exposed fracture site, and cannulated screws were then placed percutaneously from lateral to medial direction.

the rate of physeal closure.[26] No special studies are required for this injury because the diagnosis is fairly straightforward.

Growth arrest after the supination-plantar flexion mechanism can occur even after undisplaced fracture. The reported rate of growth disturbance has been 24%.[40] The treating surgeon's decision must be guided by an appreciation of the amount of physeal displacement and estimation of the amount of remaining growth. Clearly, there is little need for reduction of mild residual physeal displacement aimed at decreasing the likelihood of growth arrest in a patient with very little remaining growth. If it is determined that significant growth remains and the surgeon opts for surgical treatment, removal of interposed periosteum could be considered, because it is fairly common in this injury pattern (Fig. 15.18). After anatomic reduction, internal fixation may often be achieved with smooth K-wire across the physis or with

a cannulated screw in the posterior metaphyseal fragment if the fragment is large enough. Non-weightbearing cast immobilization is indicated for several weeks after surgery for purposes of pain control and fostering undisturbed fracture healing.

OTHER FRACTURE PATTERNS

TYPE V FRACTURE

The Salter-Harris type V injuries are extremely rare and appear to result from axial compression. These injuries supposedly cause partial or complete physeal arrest by virtue of a crush injury to the germinal cells of all or a portion of the physis. In such an injury, no obvious fracture of the epiphysis or metaphysis can be found, and the initial radiograph may show no evidence of injury. The diagnosis of a type V

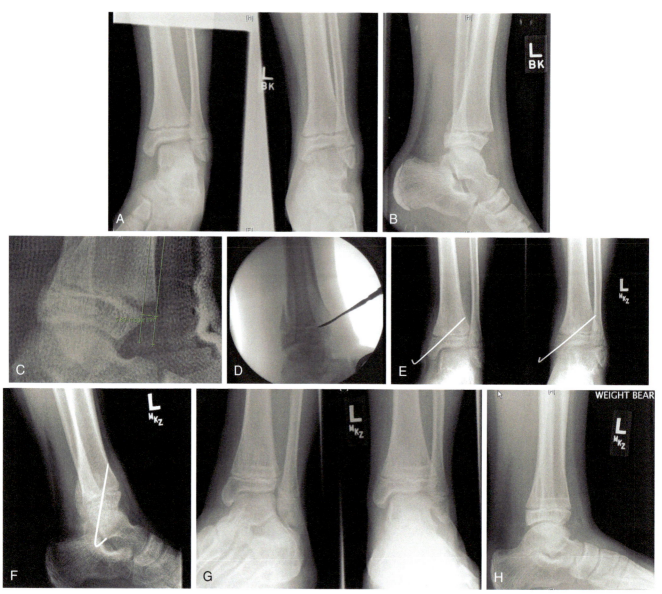

Fig. 15.18 Supination-plantar flexion fracture of the left ankle in a 13-year, 1-month male patient. (A) Initial mortise and anteroposterior views that demonstrate an intact fibula, physeal widening of the distal tibia, and presence of a Thurston-Holland fragment. (B) Lateral radiograph demonstrates posteriorly translated Salter-Harris II fracture with a posteriorly oriented Thurston-Holland fragment. (C) Displacement of almost 6 mm remains after closed reduction. (D) Open reduction included gentle removal of interposed periosteum. (E) Postoperative mortise and anteroposterior radiographs show smooth K-wire fixation just before pin removal at 4 weeks. (F) Postoperative lateral radiograph showing anatomic reduction. (G) One-year follow-up mortise and anteroposterior radiographs showing symmetric Park-Harris line. (H) A 1-year follow-up lateral view also showing a "good" Park-Harris line.

injury is therefore a retrospective one made only after premature closure has been established in a growth plate that was previously considered uninjured (Fig. 15.19). It is believed that this injury causes unrecognized damage to physeal cells either directly or secondary to injury to the blood supply of the germinal cell layer of the physis.

Two cases of tibial fracture have been reported in which symmetric premature closure of the entire proximal tibial physis caused a leg-length discrepancy without any angular deformity. A compression injury to the entire physis would be unlikely unless a uniform longitudinal force were the mechanism of injury, as in a fall from a height. However, the clinical history and the configuration of the associated fractures were not consistent with a purely longitudinal force in their cases. Peterson and Burkhart[41] believed the proposition to be speculative that premature closure of the growth plate results from compression at the time of the accident. Because the two cases cited by Salter and Harris[42] did not have a normal radiographic appearance at the time of injury, another fracture type could have been present. These investigators further concluded that all type V injuries reported in the literature involved the knee.[41] On review of the literature, they concluded that the common factor in all these conditions, including the trauma cases, seemed to be prolonged immobilization. Thus, an intriguing possibility is that posttraumatic physeal fusion is not always caused by direct damage to the growth plate at the time of injury but rather by factors associated with immobilization, like ischemia.

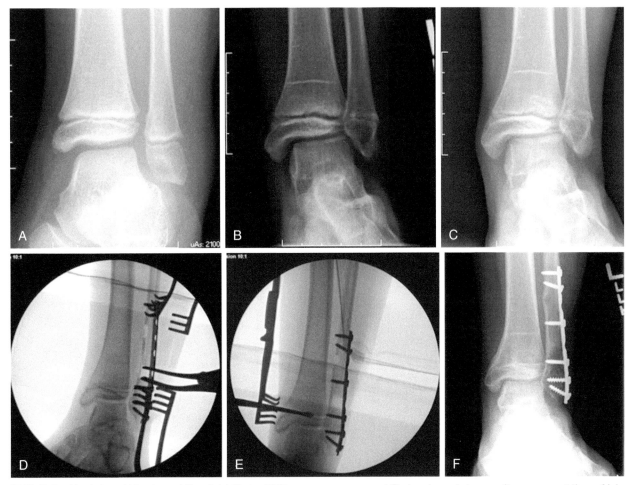

Fig. 15.19 Salter-Harris type V fracture of the distal fibula. (A) There was no apparent fibular physeal abnormality on x-ray at time of injury for this 8-year-old girl. (B) Follow-up x-ray 2 years later (asymptomatic) shows physeal arrest of fibula and normal Park-Harris line of distal tibia. (C) A year later (3 years after injury), she is still asymptomatic, but there is a resulting angular deformity of the ankle from fibular growth arrest from presumed type V physeal injury and continued distal tibial growth. (D and E) Intraoperative fluoroscopy showing fibular lengthening osteotomy with fixation (and correction of ankle angular deformity) and distal tibial epiphysiodesis. (F) One-year follow-up from osteotomy/epiphysiodesis with healed fibular osteotomy and maintenance of angular correction.

TYPE VI FRACTURE

Ablation of the perichondrial ring has been categorized as a type VI injury. Avulsion or compression injury to the periphery of the physis is rarely seen. Lawn mower injuries and degloving injuries, which occur when the leg is dragged across concrete or pavement, may remove the perichondrial ring (Fig. 15.20). The ensuing callus may cause the development of a bridge between the metaphysis and epiphysis as described by Rang.[11] The ankle would drift progressively into varus.

TYPE VII FRACTURE

Transepiphyseal fractures (type VII fracture) are uncommon and have to be differentiated from os subfibulare.[43] In a study comparing 11 patients with type VII distal fibular intraepiphyseal fracture to 12 patients with os subfibulare, the authors provided diagnostic radiographic criteria to differentiate these two injuries. Type VII fractures had long, irregular fracture line through the middle third of the distal fibular epiphysis, and those with symptomatic os subfibulare had a smooth-edged ossicle within the inferior third of the epiphysis. It is important to differentiate between these two entities because it has treatment implications (Fig. 15.21).

Adolescent Pilon Fracture

Letts et al reported on eight pilon fractures in seven adolescents with a mean age of 15 years, 10 months.[44] A pilon fracture was defined as a fracture of tibial plafond with displacement of tibial articular surface greater than 5 mm with variable comminution and variable involvement of the fibula and the talus. All patients were treated with open reduction and internal fixation (Fig. 15.22). There were three poor results as a result of posttraumatic arthrosis in two cases (necessitating ankle arthrodesis) and residual distal tibial articular deformity in one patient. Another patient with a growth arrest did not have any clinical implications because of him being near skeletal maturity. The results demonstrate difficulty in treatment of this subset of patients.

For adolescent pilon fractures, the authors recommend CT scan for detailed evaluation of intraarticular fractures, diligent assessment of the soft tissues, and appropriate timing for definitive fixation. If there is excessive soft tissue swelling, definitive fixation should be delayed for 10 to 14 days until the swelling subsides and the "wrinkle" test is present. Patients need to be counseled preoperatively regarding possible complications like wound healing, infection, nonunion, malunion, growth arrest, stiffness, and osteoarthritis.

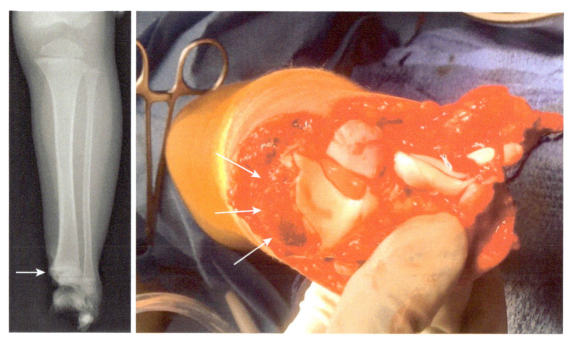

Fig. 15.20 Radiograph of type VI distal tibia fracture resulting from a lawn mower injury in a 3-year-old boy, and the correlating clinical photo showing the axial view of the distal tibia articular surface with the medial malleolus sheared off through the physis (*white arrows*).

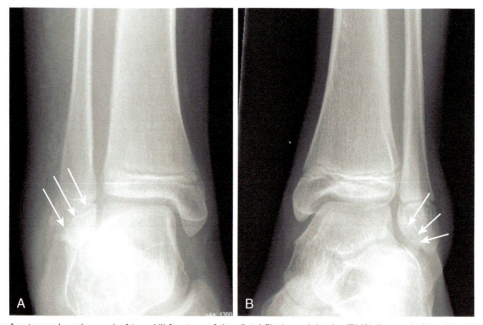

Fig. 15.21 (A) Sharp fracture edges (*arrows*) of type VII fracture of the distal fibular epiphysis. (B) Well-rounded ossicle at the inferior aspect of the distal fibula (*arrows*) indicating os subfibulare.

TRANSITIONAL FRACTURES

The juvenile fracture of Tillaux and triplane fractures are considered to be transitional fractures. These fractures occur in and about the early part of the second decade during the pubescent transition to skeletal maturity. They occur as a result of an external rotational force. The pattern of closure of the distal tibial physis (i.e., middle, medial, and lateral) is responsible for propagation of the fracture after injury.

Juvenile Fracture of Tillaux

The juvenile fracture of Tillaux is an isolated fracture of the lateral portion of the distal tibial epiphysis (Fig. 15.23). With external rotation, the anterior tibiofibular ligament holds firmly to the tibial epiphysis, which separates through the junction of the middle and lateral open physis. When displacement of the fragment is minimal, the vertical and horizontal fracture lines may be difficult to visualize. It is a Salter-Harris type III epiphyseal fracture, and mild or moderate displacement of the fragment may be present. The pattern of the injury is thought to result from the closure sequence of the distal tibial physis.[45]

The distal physis of the tibia closes first on its medial half at the age of 13 or 14 years; the lateral part closes at 14.5 to 16 years. Closure of the distal tibial physis occurs first in the

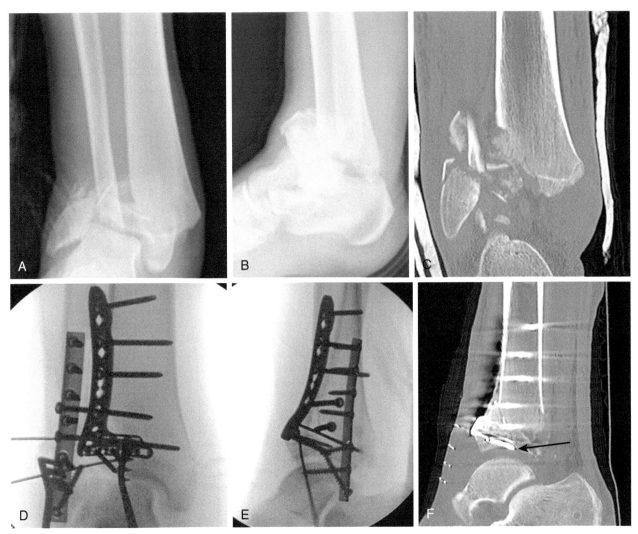

Fig. 15.22 A 17-year-old boy with closing physis, who sustained a pilon fracture of the distal tibia (A and B) when he jumped over a fence and landed on a rock. The computed tomography (CT) scan (C) demonstrates comminution in the epiphysis. (D and E) His initial treatment involved external fixation. Once the swelling subsided, he underwent definitive treatment with open reduction and internal fixation. Postoperative CT scan (F) shows the tip of the screw violating the articular surface (*arrow*). The intraoperative fluoroscopy image (E) can underestimate the position of the hardware.

middle, then in the medial, and finally in the lateral physis (Fig. 15.3). Because the lateral physis is still open, the fracture crosses through it. The fracture line extends from the articular surface proximally; it traverses the epiphysis and then continues along the physis laterally. It is equivalent to the Tillaux lesion in adults. Local tenderness and swelling may be seen over the anterolateral aspect of the distal tibial epiphysis.

For truly nondisplaced fractures, conservative treatment using cast immobilization is preferred. Close follow-up and weekly radiographs should be obtained to make sure that the fracture does not displace once swelling subsides. CT scan can provide an accurate assessment of true displacement, which can help with treatment decisions (Fig. 15.24). CT can also help for surgical planning of size and trajectory of screw. For displaced fractures, closed reduction should be performed in the operating room by gentle internal rotation of the foot. If closed reduction is successful, the authors recommend percutaneous fixation with a 4-mm partially threaded, cannulated screw.[46] K-wires could be used for

definitive fixation if the fragment is small or comminuted. A below-knee non-weightbearing cast is applied for 3 to 4 weeks. If closed reduction is not satisfactory, open reduction with transfixion may be required. The screw can cross the physis in this particular situation because the middle and medial sections of the growth plate are usually closed (Fig. 15.24). If the growth plate is not closed or closing, the implant should not cross the physis. Growth discrepancy is an unusual sequela of this injury because most of the physis has closed. The more significant complication is nonunion or arthritis resulting from either a step-off of the articular surface or a residual gap greater than 2 mm.[47]

Triplane Fracture

A triplane fracture is an injury unique to the closing distal tibial growth plate. The fracture line crosses the articular surface through the epiphysis, the physis, and finally the posterior tibial metaphysis in the sagittal, transverse, and coronal planes, respectively. The multiplanar Salter-Harris type IV injury created is thought to be caused by external

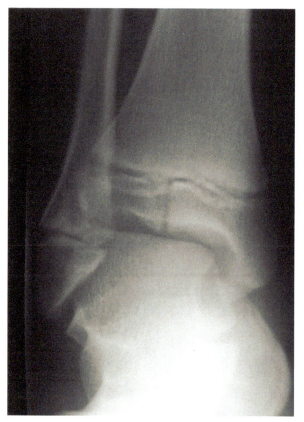

Fig. 15.23 This nondisplaced Salter-Harris type III fracture was treated by cast immobilization with an uneventful outcome.

rotation of a supinated foot. The triplane fracture occurs earlier in adolescence than the juvenile Tillaux fracture because the epiphyseal plate is still completely open in early adolescence, thus allowing the horizontal fracture to run through its entire anterior portion. In the older group, the growth plate's medial area has already closed, so the horizontal break extends only through its anterolateral portion and is met by the vertical fracture near the closed medial epiphyseal line.[48]

Radiographic Evaluation. Triplane fractures of the distal end of the tibia are sometimes quite difficult to identify on plain radiographs. AP, lateral, and mortise views should be taken. The fracture appears to be a Salter-Harris type III injury on the AP view and a Salter-Harris type II injury on the lateral projection (Fig. 15.25). In the AP projection, the fracture can be seen as a vertical line crossing the central area of the epiphysis, with widening of the mortise. The appearance in this projection is remarkably similar to that of a juvenile Tillaux fracture, and care must be taken not to confuse the two. Mortise views may show more displacement than the AP ones.[48] The apparent Salter-Harris type II fracture seen on the lateral view may be minimally displaced and occasionally obscured. It may be misinterpreted as fibula fracture at times. This radiographic fracture pattern in a growing child should always suggest a triplane fracture. An associated fibular fracture has been shown to occur in 37% of triplane cases (40 of 107 cases).[49–51] CT studies have simplified identification of all facets of this injury. Depending on closure of the distal tibial physis, the fracture may consist of one, two, or three fragments in addition to the

tibial shaft (Table 15.2). Thus triplane fractures are said to come in two-part, three-part, and four-part varieties.[50] Data from five published series of triplane fractures reveal that two-part fractures are the most common, representing 60% of cases (85 of 141), three-part fractures comprise 38% (53 of 141), and four-part fractures occur only in 2% of cases (3 of 141).[3,48–51]

Denton and Fischer[52] described a medial triplane fracture caused by adduction and axial loading. Kärrholm[53] stated that such a fracture type occurs at a low peak age and is associated with complications such as medial growth retardation or arrest, and they stressed that it should not be confused with other types of triplane fractures. Lutz Von Laer[54] has quite appropriately stated that a transitional fracture such as the triplane fracture "strains the spatial imagination of the surgeon." Several authors have summarized the major triplane fracture patterns,[51,55,56] and these findings are illustrated in Fig. 15.26.

Intramalleolar triplane fractures have been reported.[57,58] Shin and associates[58] published a classification of intramalleolar triplane fractures and pointed out that three-dimensional CT has great advantages over plain radiographs and two-dimensional CT for evaluating this injury. They described three classes: intraarticular fracture at the junction of the tibial plafond and medial malleolus (type 1), intraarticular fracture of the medial malleolus (type 2), and extraarticular fracture (type 3), which is the most prevalent. Operative reduction is required when intraarticular incongruity exists. The extraarticular triplane fractures that extend through the medial malleolus (instead of tibiotalar joint) can be treated nonoperatively with satisfactory outcomes[57] (Fig. 15.27).

Ertl and associates[48] completed a long-term (3- to 13-year) follow-up of this intraarticular fracture and found that it led to significant arthritis in adults when less than anatomic reduction was achieved. Although symptoms were absent on early follow-up, about half their patients were symptomatic at long-term evaluation. Kärrholm[53] published the results of 21 of his cases with a 4-year follow-up and a review of the literature (209 cases); in total, about 80% displayed excellent results, 16% had minor symptoms, and 4% had more pronounced symptoms combined with degenerative changes. When the epiphyseal fracture extended into the weightbearing arch of the ankle, residual displacement of greater than 2 mm was associated with suboptimal results. In Rapariz and associates' series,[51] of the 35 patients treated for triplane fractures, the only two patients in whom degenerative changes were seen in their ankle radiographs were those with residual intraarticular displacement of 3 mm. Anatomic reduction by either closed or open means is mandatory in the treatment of triplane fractures.

The choice between open and closed reduction depends on the amount of residual displacement after reduction. Impending growth arrest is not usually a consideration because the growth plate is approaching closure. Even though this fracture seems to be intrinsically unstable, it is only at the articular surface; where permanent disruption definitely predisposes to degenerative joint disease, that loss of reduction is crucial. Anatomic reduction of the articular surface is mandatory. Ertl and associates[48] found that none of their patients with initial displacement of greater than 3 mm on AP or mortise radiographs had successful closed reduction.

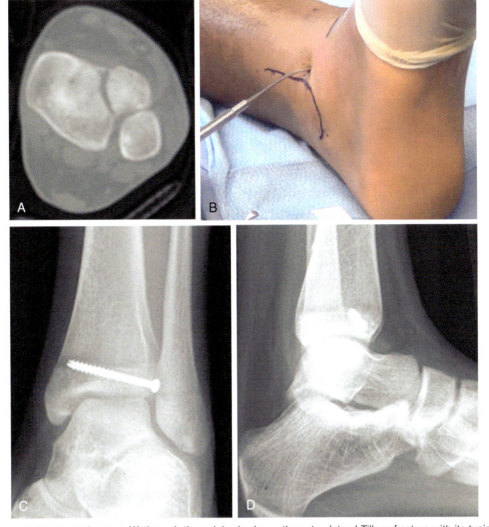

Fig. 15.24 Axial computed tomography scan (A) through the epiphysis shows the anterolateral Tillaux fracture with its typical fracture line. (B) Percutaneous fixation performed by insertion of screw in the epiphysis, starting just anterior to the anterior aspect of fibula. (C and D) The screw can be inserted obliquely through the physis, as the medial aspect of the physis is already closed.

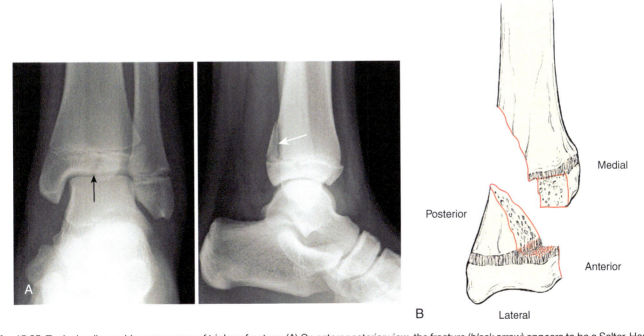

Fig. 15.25 Typical radiographic appearance of triplane fracture. (A) On anteroposterior view, the fracture (*black arrow*) appears to be a Salter-Harris type III fracture, similar to Tillaux fracture. (B) On lateral view, the posterior metaphyseal fracture (*white arrow*) appears to be a Salter-Harris type II fracture of distal tibia. The fracture actually represents a Salter-Harris type IV fracture of distal tibia. (B) Artist's rendition of a two-fragment triplane fracture. (B, From MacNealy GA, Rogers LF, Hernandez R, et al. Injuries of the distal tibial epiphysis: systematic radiographic evaluation. *AJR Am J Roentgenol.* 1982;138:688. Copyright 1982, American Roentgen Ray Society.)

TABLE 15.2   Number of Fracture Fragments Associated With Triplane Fractures

Author	Year	Two-Part	Three-Part	Four-Part	Fibula
McNealy et al[71]	1982	14	5	0	?
Ertl et al[29]	1988	4	11	0	?
Rapariz et al[100]	1996	12	23	0	17
El-Karef et al[28]	2000	12	6	3	5
Brown et al[8]	2004	43	8	0	18
Totals:		85/141	53/141	3/141	40/107
%		60%	38%	2%	37%

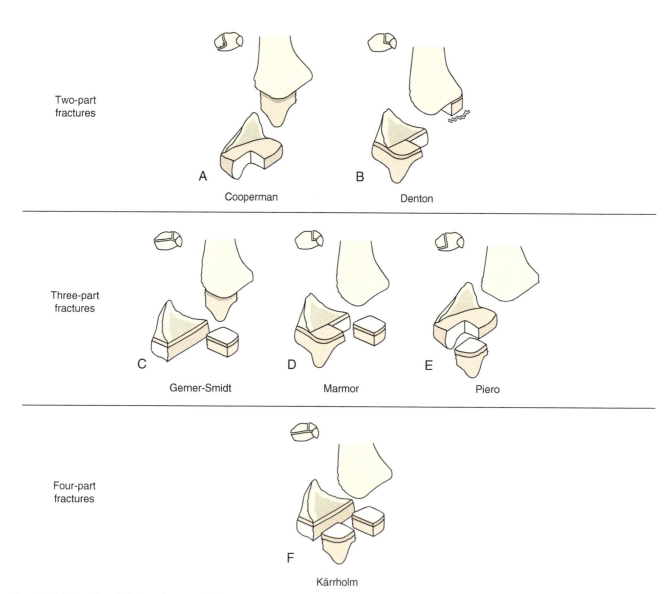

Two-part fractures

A   Cooperman

B   Denton

Three-part fractures

C   Gerner-Smidt

D   Marmor

E   Piero

Four-part fractures

F   Kärrholm

Fig. 15.26 Hierarchy of triplane fractures (with eponyms). (A) Tillaux position contiguous with Salter-Harris IV position and medial malleolus intact. (B) Medial malleolus position contiguous with Salter-Harris IV position and Tillaux segment intact. (C) Medial malleolus intact. (D) Tillaux fragment disrupted, plus Denton-type fragment. (E) Free fragment medial malleolus. (F) Medial malleolus, Salter-Harris IV, and Tillaux fragments are all present. (Modified from Rapariz JM, Ocete G, Gonzalez-Herranz P, et al. Distal tibial triplane fractures: long-term follow-up. *J Pediatr Orthop.* 1996;16:113-118.)

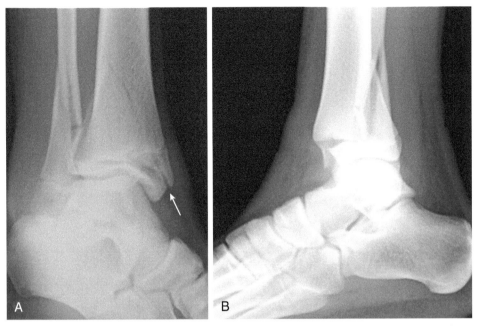

Fig. 15.27 Anteroposterior (A) and lateral (B) radiograph of an extraarticular triplane fracture. On the lateral view, the fracture may appear to be similar to an intraarticular triplane fracture, but on the anteroposterior view, the fracture exits through the medial malleolus (*arrow*) instead of the joint surface.

Interposition of soft tissue at the fracture site was responsible for the failure of closed reduction in six of eight open operations. The soft tissue was identified as periosteum in five patients and was found to be the extensor hallucis longus tendon in one.[48] A diastasis or step-off of more than 2 mm in any plane at the articular surface requires anatomic reduction.[47]

Management. General anesthesia is required for complete relaxation. The knee is flexed to 90 degrees, and the foot is plantar flexed and internally rotated. If anatomic reduction is achieved, percutaneous partially threaded 4-mm cannulated interfragmentary screws are placed (Fig. 15.28). Preoperative CT scan can help in planning for percutaneous placement of screws. The axial cut through the epiphysis helps to plan for the intraarticular fracture reduction and fixation. The axial cut above the physis helps to plan the trajectory of the metaphyseal screw. Pointed reduction clamps could be used to maintain reduction during percutaneous fixation. Usually, a lateral to medial epiphyseal screw is placed first for fixation of the intraarticular Tillaux part of the triplane fracture. Next, a metaphyseal screw is placed from anterior to posterior for stabilization of the posterior metaphyseal fragment that is visualized on lateral view. The trajectory of these two screws are nearly perpendicular to each other. More screws can be placed depending on the size of the fracture fragments. The extremity is placed in a non-weight-bearing below-knee cast for 4 weeks.

If the intraarticular gap after reduction is greater than 2 mm, open reduction is necessary. Open reduction is not easy and may require anterolateral and posteromedial approaches to reduce the fractures under direct visualization. Only after the posteromedial fragment is reduced can the anterolateral (Tillaux) fragment be reduced. Through an anterolateral approach, the anterolateral fragment is identified and displaced. The posteromedial fragment, if displaced, is first reduced under direct visualization by internal rotation

and dorsiflexion of the foot. When reduced, the posteromedial fragment is typically fixed with a cannulated screw. If the posteromedial fragment cannot be reduced by manipulation, it should be reduced under direct visualization through a posteromedial incision. If displaced, the fibular fracture is reduced next. Finally, the displaced anterolateral fragment (Tillaux) is reduced and fixed with a cannulated screw (Fig. 15.29).[59] A non-weightbearing, below-knee cast is placed for 4 weeks. In a recent study comparing percutaneous fixation (17 patients) to open reduction and internal fixation (48 patients) for transitional fractures, there were significantly higher rate of complications from open surgery (19% vs. 0%); these complications included symptomatic hardware, nerve/muscle injury, persistent pain, and infection.[60]

Distal tibial growth is nearly complete when this injury occurs, so shortening from growth arrest is rarely a problem. Ertl and associates' long-term reevaluation[48] showed marked deterioration with time in ankles in which reduction of the articular surface was not accomplished. At an average of more than 6 years after injury, the result was that 15 patients had declined at least one grade. None of these patients improved during follow-up after injury to the articular cartilage. Even in individuals with anatomic reduction, delayed long-term symptoms still occurred. The symptomatic patients monitored for 20 years were only in their third decade and could experience continued deterioration. Residual 2- to 3-mm displacement of the articular cartilage in the weightbearing area may result in late-onset degenerative arthritis.[48]

Choudhry et al evaluated functional outcomes after treatment of 78 transitional fractures (58 triplane and 20 Tillaux fractures). Some 60% of patients had closed reduction and percutaneous fixation, 33% had closed reduction, and 5% had open reduction and internal fixation. They reported good medium-term outcomes when the residual gap or step

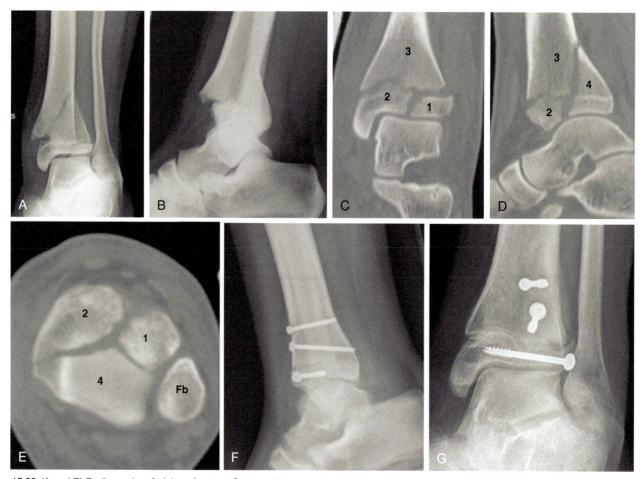

Fig. 15.28 (A and B) Radiographs of triplane fracture. Computed tomography scan imaging in coronal (C), sagittal (D), and epiphyseal axial (E) plane show a four-part triplane fracture. All four fracture parts are numbered. Typical percutaneous fixation of triplane fracture involves lateral to medial epiphyseal screw and anterior to posterior metaphyseal screw, as shown on postoperative lateral (F) and anteroposterior (G) radiographs. *Fb,* Fibula.

off was less than 2.5 mm, and these results did not deteriorate at longer-term follow-up (4–10 years).[61]

Syndesmotic Injuries. Syndesmotic injuries in children are rare, but they do occur. Study of normative radiographic values of syndesmosis in children showed that the medial clear space could not be reliably assessed in children less than 8 years of age because of insufficient ossification of medial malleolus.[62] Similarly, lack of tibiofibular overlap (less than 6 mm is considered abnormal in adults) and increased tibiofibular clear space (more than 6 mm is considered abnormal in adults) could be normal in children because of delayed ossification of incisura fibularis.[63] Sung et al performed radiographic measurements on 590 children and concluded that the criteria for absolute radiographic values used in adults to assess the syndesmosis could not be applied to children, but these values should be compared with the contralateral side. If there was more than 50% difference in the values for tibiofibular overlap, tibiofibular clear space, and medial clear space on comparison radiographs of opposite ankle, then further imaging (MRI or CT) should be performed to confirm the diagnosis.[64]

For management of syndesmotic injuries in children and adolescents, it has been reported that presence of fibular fracture, medial clear space greater than 5 mm, and closed tibial physis had 44 times, 8 times, and 5 times the odds of requiring surgical intervention, respectively.[6] For surgical

fixation, there are lack-of-outcomes studies or comparison studies to recommend suture-button fixation over standard screw fixation of syndesmosis in children.[65]

Triplane Fracture with Ipsilateral Tibial Shaft Fracture. Jarvis and Miyanji[66] reported on six patients with distal tibial triplane fractures in conjunction with completely separate (noncontiguous) fractures of the ipsilateral tibial shaft. The average age at the time of injury was 14 years, which is the typical age for a transitional fracture of the ankle. Contrary to conventional thinking, all injuries were secondary to low-energy falls. All tibial shaft fractures were midshaft spiral or short oblique and were minimally displaced. Similarly, all but one triplane fracture were minimally displaced (gap, <2 mm). Diagnosis of the distal triplane fracture was delayed in two cases. Although all patients in the study were treated satisfactorily with closed reduction and casting with the ankle in internal rotation, the treatment may vary based on patient and fracture characteristics. The authors have treated five patients with this combination and would recommend focused ankle examination in an adolescent with a tibial shaft fracture and dedicated ankle radiographs for suspected injuries (Fig. 15.30). Because of the injury's potential for long-term sequelae, a high index of suspicion should be maintained so that the ankle fracture is not missed.

Extensor Retinaculum Compartment Syndrome. Mubarak[67] described extensor retinaculum syndrome of the ankle after

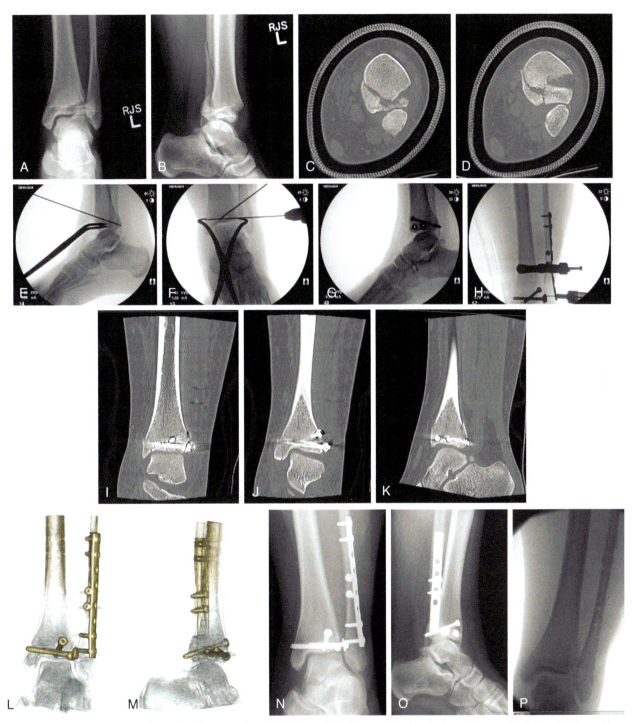

Fig. 15.29 A 13-year, 4-month female patient (approaching skeletal maturity) who sustained a displaced three-part triplane fracture with associated fibular fracture of her left ankle. (A) Mortise view clearly demonstrating displaced anterolateral fragment (Tillaux fragment). (B) Lateral radiograph illustrating comminuted distal tibial epiphysis and associated oblique fibular fracture. (C) A computed tomography (CT) scan cut above the physis illustrating posteriorly located Thurston-Holland fragment. (D) CT scan below the physis demonstrating the so-called Mercedes sign, which confirms the free Tillaux fragment. (E through H) Selected fluoroscopic images illustrating the sequence of fracture fragment fixation and reduction tactics. (I through K) Postoperative two-dimensional CT imaging. (L and M) Postoperative three-dimensional CT imaging. (N and O) Six-month follow-up plain radiographs. (P) All implants removed and growth plates clearly closed at 1-year anniversary.

injury to the distal tibial physis in six children aged 10 to 15 years. All had sustained a Salter-Harris type II or type IV fracture (triplane fracture) with anterior displacement of the tibia into the tunnel of the superior extensor retinaculum. The clinical findings related to compartment syndrome included severe pain and swelling of the ankle, hypoesthesia or anesthesia in the first web space, weakness of extensor halluces longus and extensor digitorum communis, and pain with passive flexion of the great toe. Three patients were seen with a displaced fracture and the clinical finding of extensor retinaculum syndrome, whereas three patients developed symptoms 24 to 48 hours after reduction and

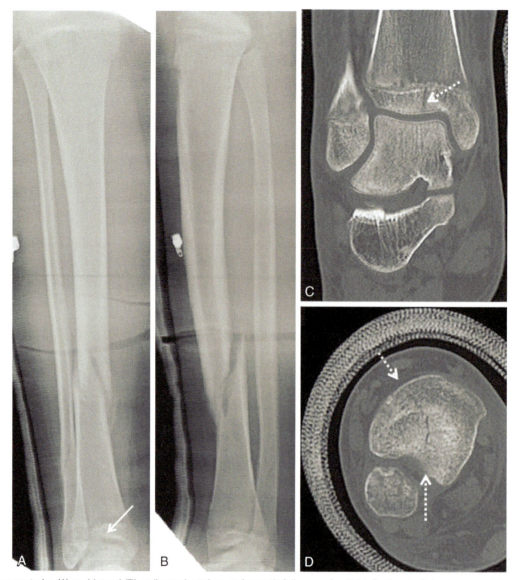

Fig. 15.30 Anteroposterior (A) and lateral (B) radiographs taken at 1-month follow-up for tibial-fibular shaft fracture in a 14-year-old boy. The triplane ankle fracture (*arrow*) is seen; it was initially missed. The coronal (C) and axial (D) computed tomographic scans show that the ankle triplane fracture was not displaced (<2 mm of displacement), and the fracture was healing (*dashed arrows*). Conservative treatment was continued, and the patient had a satisfactory outcome.

internal fixation of the fracture. Compartment syndrome was confirmed by measurement of intracompartmental pressures under general anesthesia after fracture reduction, which was greater than 40 mm Hg beneath the superior extensor retinaculum but less than 20 mm Hg in the anterior compartment. All patients had relief of their symptoms within 24 hours of treatment, which consisted of release of the superior extensor retinaculum with a 10- to 12-cm longitudinal incision over the distal tibia and fracture stabilization. The inferior extensor retinaculum should not be released because bowstringing of the extensor tendons at the ankle may occur (Fig. 15.31). After surgical decompression, one patient developed osteomyelitis, and two patients had persistent weakness of the extensor hallucis longus and hypoesthesia in the first web space. On the basis of a cadaveric study, Haumont and colleagues[68] confirmed the anatomic cause of extensor retinaculum syndrome: they found that the muscle fibers of the extensor hallucis longus extend un-

der the superior extensor retinaculum and that the region is more susceptible to ischemia if the blood supply in this area is tenuous. They recommended ankle immobilization in neutral dorsiflexion to decrease the risk of compartment syndrome because fewer muscle fibers extend under the retinaculum in this position.

DISLOCATION OF THE ANKLE JOINT

Ankle dislocation without a fracture is a rare event that has prompted isolated case reports in the literature.[69] Most dislocations are posteromedial and manifest as open injuries on the anterolateral side of the joint, with gross disruption of the lateral capsular ligamentous complex (Fig. 15.32). The majority of patients are young adults; few ankle dislocations have been reported in children (Fig. 15.11).[69,70] Nusem and associates[70] reported a closed posterior ankle dislocation in a 12-year-old girl that was successfully treated with closed

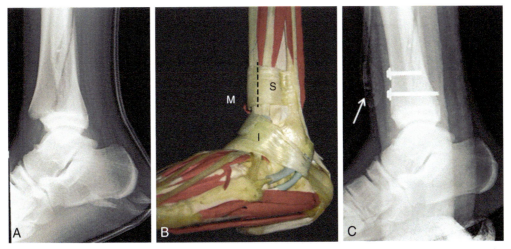

Fig. 15.31 (A) A 14-year-old male patient with a Salter-Harris type II fracture of the distal tibia (as a component of his supination-external rotation injury) with anterior displacement of the metaphysis and resultant extensor retinaculum compartment syndrome. (B) The anatomic model shows the extensor muscle fibers extending under the superior extensor retinaculum *(S)*. At surgery, the superior retinaculum is cut longitudinally *(black dashed line)*. The inferior extensor retinaculum *(I)* is not released. *M,* Medial side. (C) At the time of compartment release, internal fixation of the fracture is performed. The anterior wound is typically left open for later closure. A vacuum-assisted closure *(arrow)* was used for this patient.

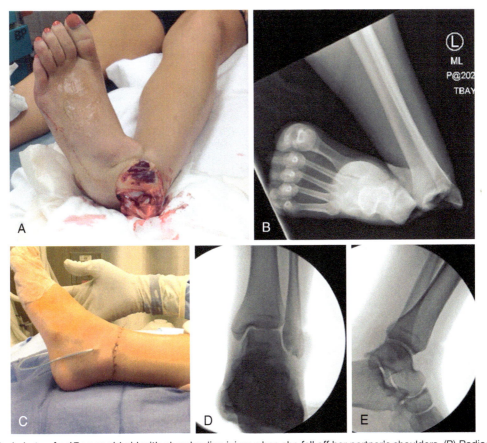

Fig. 15.32 (A) Clinical photo of a 17-year-old girl with cheerleading injury when she fell off her partner's shoulders. (B) Radiograph shows ankle dislocation without any fractures. (C) The open ankle dislocation was treated with immediate surgical débridement, joint reduction, repair of lateral ligaments, and wound closure. At 1 year, patient was back to full activities, and (D) and (E) radiographs appear normal.

reduction and a short leg cast. Most posterior or medial dislocations are stable in neutral or slight dorsiflexion. In this position, the torn lateral ligamentous complex is approximated.

The mechanism of injury is generally marked plantar flexion with inversion. Local distraction occurs anterolaterally, with rapid rupture of the lateral ligamentous complex from front to back or through the fibular physis in children. This injury is akin to a flexion-distraction injury in the spine. In addition to separation of the lateral ligamentous complex, the physis, or both, the skin, extensor tendons, and neurovascular structures frequently rupture in an open dislocation. As the plantar-flexed foot is carried into inversion, varus tilting and rotation of the talus occur, followed by dislocation, usually in the posteromedial position. The deltoid ligament is always injured; however, except in cases of gross displacement, it usually retains a significant amount of integrity and provides a posteromedial hinge that affords stability when the ankle is reduced and held in dorsiflexion. If the ankle remains unstable after reduction or if an open injury precludes repair/fixation, an external fixator should be used to stabilize the ankle. Transarticular pins should be avoided, as they not only violate the articular surface but also violate the physis (Fig. 15.11).

Most of these injuries are open, and débridement and irrigation of the joint are required. In an adult, the lateral ligamentous structures are repaired; however, in a child, in whom the injury is transphyseal through the fibula, the talofibular ligaments appear to be intact, and anatomic reduction and fixation of the fibular physis are normally all that is necessary. The wound may be closed over a drain if the soft tissues will allow it; otherwise, delayed primary closure and possibly skin grafting are required. The ankle is placed in a compressive protective dressing for 7 to 10 days, after which a non-weightbearing cast in the neutral plantigrade position is worn for 4 to 6 weeks. After cast removal, progressive weightbearing is permitted after rehabilitation restores ankle motion, strength, and proprioception.

COMPLICATIONS OF INJURIES TO THE DISTAL TIBIAL AND FIBULAR GROWTH PLATES

ANGULAR DEFORMITY SECONDARY TO ASYMMETRIC ARREST OF THE DISTAL TIBIAL GROWTH PLATE

The deformity is usually varus and is most frequently seen after Salter-Harris type III and IV medial malleolar injuries. An adduction injury most commonly results in a varus deformity. After an adduction injury, a direct compressive force applied to the epiphyseal plate by the talus results in premature closure of that part of the plate and subsequent angular deformity (Fig. 15.33). Anatomic reduction by open or closed means is necessary when the fracture involves the medial malleolus (Salter-Harris type III or IV) because incomplete anatomic reduction results in later deformity.[8] Anatomic reduction and fixation usually prevent this problem.

Premature physeal closure and angular deformity can also be seen after Salter-Harris type I and II fracture of the distal tibia. The rates of physeal arrest and deformity are more dependent on initial mechanism of injury and initial displacement rather than residual displacement after fracture reduction.[25] The reported rate of physeal arrest after pronation-external rotation (28.8%–54%) has been more than supination-external rotation type injury (11.4%–35%).[37,62] Although 6 of 15 patients with physeal arrest after pronation-external rotation type injury had greater than 10-degree angular deformity, none of the patients with physeal arrest after supination-external rotation or supination-plantar flexion type injury had angular deformities.[40]

Opening or closing wedge osteotomies have been used successfully to correct deformity and lessen minimal leg-length

discrepancy caused by partial growth arrest. Epiphysiodesis of the distal ends of the tibia and fibula may be performed to prevent an angular deformity if the child has less than 2 years of growth remaining. Correction by epiphysiolysis (also known as physeal bar resection) may be successful if less than 50% of the cross-sectional area of the physis is involved.[5] If greater than 10 degrees to 20 degrees of angular deformity has occurred, multiple authors recommend also performing a corrective osteotomy at the time of physeal bar resection.[71,72] Epiphysiolysis is an adequate if not excellent procedure when partial growth arrest of the distal part of the tibia has occurred.[73,74] The child should have 2 or more years of growth remaining. Traditionally, CT has been the most common imaging method used to determine the size of the physeal bar. MRI is another modality for imaging physeal bars. The amount of involvement of the growth plate can be documented graphically by the use of anterior and lateral polycycloidal tomography to map the physeal bar.[75] Imaging data can be processed to yield both three-dimensional-rendered and projection physeal maps that are particularly useful in preoperative planning (Fig. 15.34). Careful evaluation of MRI information regarding physeal bar size is recommended, as discrepancy in estimated size can occur (Fig. 15.35).

Even though the physician has made the family aware of the potential for physeal arrest or has discussed the radiographs demonstrating angulation of the Park-Harris growth arrest line, if the child does not complain of pain, that child may not be returned for follow-up. Most often, the child is seen sometime later because of the development of a varus deformity. The technique of placing a proximal window in the metaphysis and approaching the bar from above for central bars and directly for peripheral ones has been successful.[76] For central bars, arthroscopic-assisted bar resection is an alternative.[77] A percutaneous guide-pin is inserted from the metaphysis into the center of the bar. This is followed by reaming with a cannulated reamer from the ACL set. The resection is verified using arthroscope (Fig. 15.36). It is most important that the bar be completely excised and that, after excision, normal-appearing physeal cartilage be identified circumferentially. An interposition substance is necessary to prevent rebridging, and subcutaneous fat[78] or methyl methacrylate (Cranioplast) has been used most often. Methyl methacrylate appears to be a more attractive option because it allows immediate weightbearing. However, if indicated, removal of the interpositional substance may be difficult. Compromised host immunity has been associated with release of the methyl methacrylate monomer.[79,80] If the angular deformity of the ankle exceeds 20 degrees, a corrective osteotomy should be included. Nearly normal longitudinal growth and correction of moderate angular deformities can be expected with bridges that occupy less than 25% of the physis. It is important to place metallic markers (a small K-wire or vascular clip) into the epiphysis and metaphysis to determine whether growth results from the epiphysiolysis. Berson and colleagues[81] suggested a decision-making process that they used to divide their 24 patients into three groups: group 1 consisted of children with less than 2 years of growth remaining, less than 9 degrees of predicted angulation, and less than 2 cm of predicted discrepancy. This group was treated by observation. Group 2 consisted of children with less than 9 degrees of existing angulation, more than 2 cm of predicted

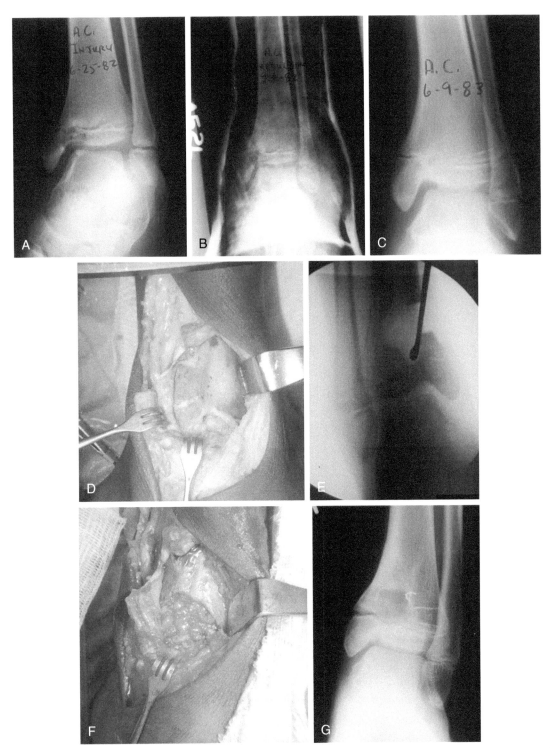

Fig. 15.33 This child sustained a Salter-Harris type IV medial malleolar fracture of the distal end of the tibia that resulted in a growth plate injury. The growth plate injury, in turn, resulted in a physeal bar that caused a varus deformity. The bar was removed, fat was interposed, and growth was reestablished. (A) Initial radiograph of the ankle showing minimal displacement. (B) Radiograph through a plaster cast, consistent with anatomic reduction. (C) Radiograph 1 year later showing a bony bar. Note the Park-Harris line angulated from the bar. (D) Intraoperative photograph showing a bone bridge across the growth plate. (E) Intraoperative Polaroid radiograph showing a curette across the resected physeal bar. (F) Operative photograph showing fat through the bone window. (G) Anteroposterior radiograph after excision of the bar and resumption of growth. The metallic clips are used as markers to monitor future growth.

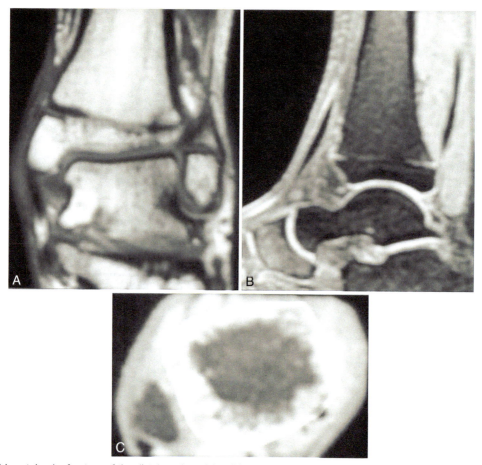

Fig. 15.34 This child sustained a fracture of the distal portion of the tibia that resulted in a growth plate injury. The growth plate injury, in turn, resulted in a large physeal bar. Rarely is there documentation of the circumferential diameter of a physeal bar as illustrated in this figure. (A) Coronal T1-weighted magnetic resonance imaging (MRI) of the ankle showing obliteration of the physis in its middle segment (high signal intensity); the peripheral linear low signal intensity represents the open physis. (B) Sagittal gradient-recalled echo MRI of the ankle showing a large bony bar (low signal intensity); the line of high signal intensity represents the open physis. (C) A gradient-recalled echo maximal intensity projection image in the axial plane outlining the perimeter of the distal tibial physis and showing a large centrally located physeal bar *(represented by the central area of low signal intensity)*. (Case referred by Dr. Tal Laor, Cincinnati, OH.)

leg-length discrepancy, or more than 9 degrees of predicted angulation. This group was treated with bilateral distal tibial and fibular epiphysiodesis. Group 3 consisted of children with more than 9 degrees of existing angulation and greater than 2 cm of predicted leg-length discrepancy. This group was treated by osteotomy to correct the angulation and either lengthening or epiphysiodesis to correct the leg-length discrepancy. They did not include physeal bar excision because they did not have great success with it. This approach resulted in satisfactory correction in 22 of 24 patients.

Takakura and colleagues[82] reported their results after opening wedge osteotomy for the treatment of posttraumatic varus deformity of the ankle. A corrective osteotomy was indicated for children only when they had ankle pain after walking for long distances, had difficulty participating in sports, and had a progressive deformity as well as uneven wear of the sole of the shoe, with more rapid wear on the lateral part. In four of the nine cases discussed, the initial injury was an epiphyseal fracture of the distal end of the tibia. The average age of these patients was 14 years, and the average follow-up was 9 years. The tibial shaft and the tibial joint surface angle (TAS angle) on the

AP radiograph was an average of 73 degrees in this group (this angle is 88 degrees in healthy Japanese). The ankle joint radiographs also showed evidence of subchondral sclerosis and osteophyte formation. The osteotomy was performed 2 to 3 cm proximal to the epiphyseal plate, and an oblique osteotomy of the fibula was performed first (Fig. 15.37). The space created anteromedially was filled with iliac crest bone graft. The average time for osseous union was 6.5 weeks, and the average postoperative TAS angle was 89 degrees. Improvement in leg-length discrepancy was also reported. On latest follow-up, these patients were able to participate in physical education classes at school, and two of them were able to participate in competitive basketball and athletic activities.

Foster and colleagues[83] published a report on the early use of free fat interpositional grafts in severe physeal injuries of the distal end of the tibia, particularly in injuries with complete peripheral detachment of the zone of Ranvier. The physeal, cancellous epiphyseal, and metaphyseal debris were removed, fractures were stabilized, and fat grafting was performed. After an average follow-up of 4 years (for distal tibial injuries), no angular deformity of the leg was present, and the distal tibial growth plate remained open.

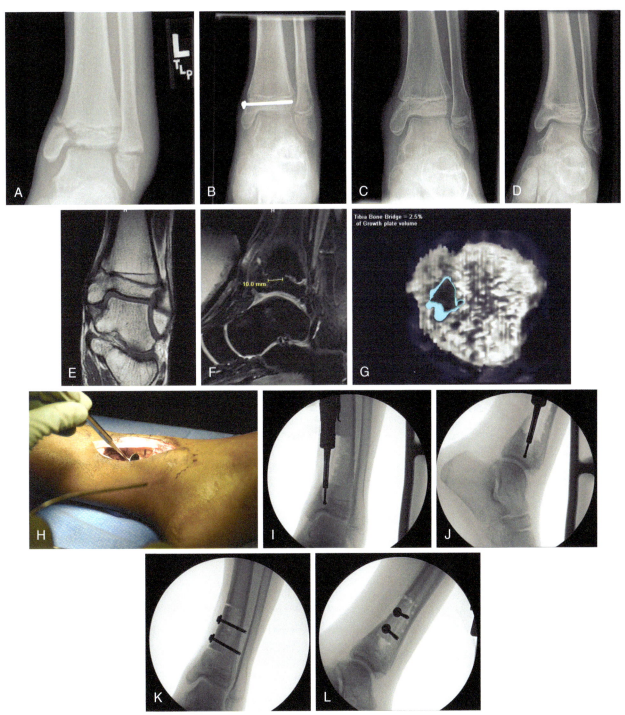

Fig. 15.35 An 11-year, 4-month male patient sustained a supination-inversion grade 2 injury to his left ankle and had partial growth arrest that required alternative treatment. (A) Injury radiograph. (B) An 8-week follow-up radiograph. (C) A 4-month follow-up radiograph showing narrowed medial physis. (D) A 1-year follow-up view demonstrating clear growth arrest with an asymmetric Park-Harris line and varus angular deformity. (E) Coronal magnetic resonance imaging (MRI) illustrating growth arrest. (F) Sagittal MRI showing an anteromedial bar measuring in the 10 mm range (the treating surgeon found a larger bar intraoperatively). (G) Calculated bar size of less than 5% based on MRI data. (H) Clinical photograph showing the use of a metaphyseal window and dental mirror during the procedure. (I and J) Intraoperative fluoroscopic views of the extent of bar resection with the use of a surgical burr. (K and L) Fluoroscopic views of replacement and fixation of the "manhole cover" of the metaphyseal window. (M) Absence of treatment effect 5 months after physeal bar resection. (N) Subsequent corrective osteotomies of distal tibia and fibula. (O and P) Mortise and lateral radiographs of the left ankle at 3 years' follow-up from original injury and 2 years' follow-up after the effort at physeal bar resection. (Courtesy Junichi Tamai, MD, Cincinnati, OH.)

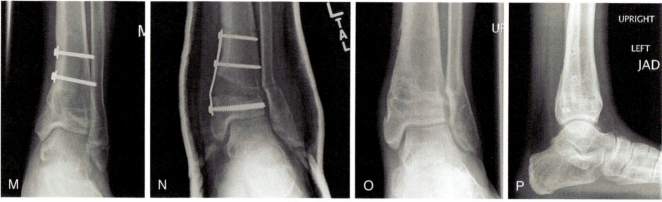

Fig. 15.35, cont'd

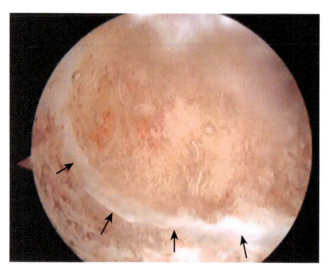

Fig. 15.36 Endoscopic verification of removal of bony bar. The physis (*arrows*) should be seen all the way around without any bone bridging across it, to ascertain complete excision of the bar.

ANGULAR DEFORMITY SECONDARY TO GROWTH ARREST OF THE DISTAL FIBULAR GROWTH PLATE

Growth arrest of the distal fibular physis is a rare complication of distal fibular growth plate fractures. This complication may result in lateral wedging of the distal tibial epiphysis and valgus malalignment of the ankle joint. When the deformity is detected early, screw epiphysiodesis of the distal tibial physis may suffice; otherwise, a corrective osteotomy aimed at leveling the joint surface is necessary (Fig. 15.38; see Fig. 15.19).

ANGULAR DEFORMITY SECONDARY TO MALUNION

This unusual complication is seen more frequently in older adolescents. Angulation of less than 20 degrees can be expected to remodel in children younger than 10 years. The authors tend to give injuries with less than 20 degrees of angulation approximately 2 years to remodel to within 10 degrees or to within limits acceptable to the parents before considering an osteotomy. Angulation of less than 15 degrees rarely causes functional disability. Residual valgus deformities are generally more acceptable than varus deformities. Angular deformities in the plane of motion tend to remodel more readily. A supramalleolar osteotomy is usually considered when the child is too old for epiphysiolysis, as a complement to bar excision in an older child, or when residual varus or valgus angulation is greater than 20 degrees.

LEG-LENGTH DISCREPANCY

Direct bone lengthening is another option in the management of growth problems after fractures. Approximately 10% to 30% of lengthening procedures on the lower extremity are performed for correction of discrepancies after injury to the growth plates. One-stage step-cut procedures or opening or closing wedge osteotomies may be performed for the correction of discrepancies within 1 inch. Greater discrepancies can be addressed by contralateral open or closed epiphysiodesis or by ipsilateral leg lengthening. The axial distraction osteogenesis and callotasis methods used for lengthening the leg by means of periosteal stimulation of bone are currently most popular. They have been found to be quite satisfactory in the management of limb-length inequality. The most popular techniques use the monaxial fixator or the circular frame. The monaxial fixator frame is less bulky than the circular frame lengthener, but it may cause the tibia to go into valgus unless it is applied in an AP direction instead of laterally. The circular frame is preferred when angular and rotational deformity is associated with tibial shortening and length discrepancy.

OSTEOARTHRITIS

Osteoarthritis may occur secondary to persistent residual joint incongruity. The condition usually follows failure to achieve anatomic reduction of intraarticular gaps greater than 2 mm. The use of current radiographic imaging technology may increase awareness of this problem and prevent its occurrence. Prevention may be achieved by open or closed anatomic reduction and stabilization.

Another cause of osteoarthritis may be unappreciated damage to articular cartilage. The impact of the trauma may damage the subchondral plate. Irreversible damage to these cartilage cells causes localized failure of the articular weight-bearing surface, which leads to shearing down to subchondral bone and chondrolysis. In addition, damage may occur to the articular component of the tibia, the talar dome, or both (Fig. 15.39).

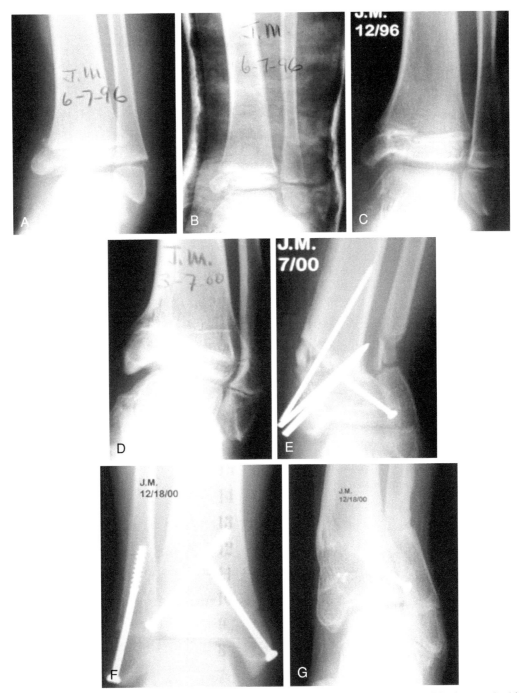

Fig. 15.37 This child sustained a Salter-Harris type IV medial malleolar fracture of the distal end of the tibia that resulted in a growth plate injury, as well as a Salter-Harris type I distal fibular fracture that went on to normal healing. The tibial growth plate injury, in turn, resulted in a physeal bar involving greater than 50% of the physis that produced a significant varus deformity. (A) Initial anteroposterior (AP) radiograph of the ankle showing displacement of the medial malleolar fracture, as well as the fibular physeal fracture. (B) AP radiograph through a plaster cast consistent with anatomic reduction. (C) Radiograph 6 months later illustrating the Park-Harris growth lines of both the fibula and the tibia. Note on the fibula that the Park-Harris growth line is horizontal and shows consistent growth from the physis. The Park-Harris line of the tibia ends in the medial aspect of the tibial metaphysis immediately lateral to the Poland hump (most often associated with physeal injuries). Failure of continuous parallel growth of the Park-Harris line of the tibia in addition to angulation of it into the area of the previous fracture site (Poland hump) is highly indicative of an early physeal bar. Unfortunately, the patient was not referred at that time. (D) An AP radiograph of the ankle at the authors' institution revealed the continued obliquity of the Park-Harris line into the area of physeal arrest. Note that the ankle has gone into significant varus and that the lateral physis is still open. (E) An opening wedge supramalleolar osteotomy was performed in addition to a lateral tibial physeal screw epiphysiodesis and a fibular osteotomy. (F) Postoperative radiograph showing screw epiphysiodesis performed on the distal ends of the contralateral tibia and fibula to minimize future leg-length discrepancy. (G) Final correction obtained after removal of the hardware except for the lateral tibial epiphysiodesis screw.

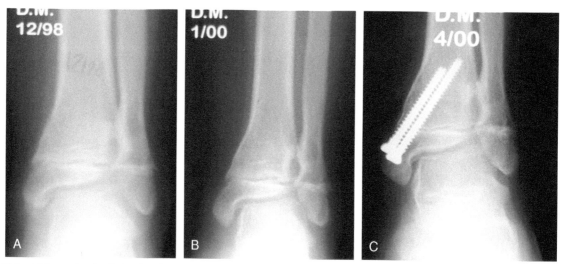

Fig. 15.38 This child sustained a Salter-Harris type I fracture of the distal tibial physis and a Salter-Harris type V fracture of the distal end of the fibula at the age of 8 years. The fractures were treated by closed reduction and casting. The fibular growth plate injury, in turn, resulted in a physeal bar that caused a mild valgus deformity of the ankle joint. The deformity appeared to be progressive and thus warranted treatment. (A) Radiograph of the ankle 1 year after injury showing distal fibular arrest with the fibular physis at the same level as the tibial physis. In normal growth of children without neurologic conditions, the fibular physis should never be above the level of the joint line. Note in this child the symmetric Park-Harris line of the distal end of the tibia. The child did not have any incremental Park-Harris line of the distal fibular physis inferring physeal arrest. (B) Radiographs 1 year after injury showing worsening of the valgus malalignment of the ankle as the distal tibial epiphysis increases in size and incorporates its secondary ossification center. (C) Radiographs 2 months after screw epiphysiodesis of the medial aspect of the distal tibial physis was carried out to prevent further progression of the ankle valgus deformity.

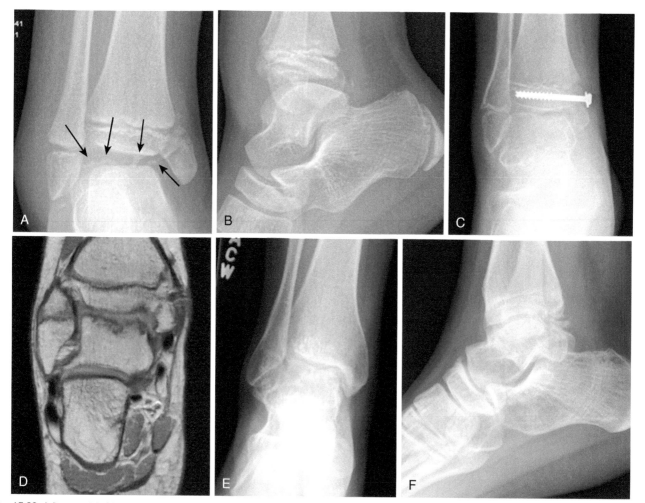

Fig. 15.39 A 9-year-old girl sustained an injury to her ankle after fall from height while rock climbing. Anteroposterior (A) and lateral (B) radiographs show displaced fracture of medial malleolus and intraarticular bony debris (*arrows*). (C) Ankle arthroscopy was performed for joint débridement, and the medial malleolus fracture was treated with an epiphyseal screw, which was later removed once the fracture healed. (D) Magnetic resonance imaging, 1 year after injury, shows the irregular degenerative surface of the talar dome. (E and F) Radiographs taken 4 years after the injury show degenerative changes affecting the tibiotalar joint. Patient does not have pain or swelling but has stiffness with about 20 degrees of ankle motion.

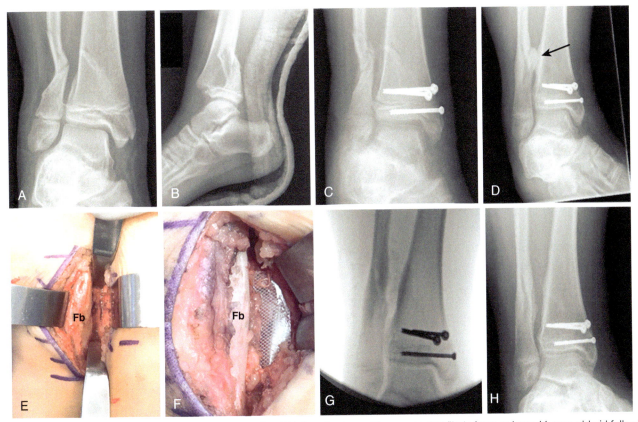

Fig. 15.40 (A and B) Anteroposterior and lateral radiographs of triplane fracture with comminuted fibula fracture in an 11-year-old girl following roller-skating injury. (C) Fracture was treated with closed reduction and internal fixation. (D) At 9 months following injury, patient had increasing pain over the ankle joint. Radiographs show localized tibiofibular synostosis (*arrow*). (E and F) The synostosis was excised, and a silastic sheet with local subcutaneous fat was interposed between the tibia and the fibula (*Fb*). (G) Fluoroscopic image after excision of synostosis. (H) Radiograph 1 year later shows adequate excision of synostosis without recurrence. There was no fibular shortening, but the distal fibular physis has increased angulation.

POSTTRAUMATIC DISTAL TIBIOFIBULAR SYNOSTOSIS

Jung et al reported on 20 patients with synostosis after treatment of distal tibiofibular fractures.[84] The mean age was 8.4 years, and the most common fracture configuration was oblique tibial fracture with comminuted fibular fracture. The synostosis was either focal (*n* = 12) or extensive (*n* = 8). All patients had proximal migration of distal fibular physis, and five patients demonstrated ankle valgus of more than 10 degrees. The patients present either with pain or deformity. The recommended treatment for symptomatic synostosis is surgical excision with interposition of fat or silastic sheet. A concurrent osteotomy may be required to correct deformity. The risk of recurrence should be considered and discussed with the family before surgical treatment (Fig. 15.40).

ROTATIONAL DEFORMITIES

This complication is unusual and, if significant, can be easily corrected by a supramalleolar osteotomy. Both bones may have to undergo osteotomy based on extent of desired rotational correction; however, it may not be necessary to transfix the fibula.

NONUNION OR DELAYED UNION

These complications are uncommon but may occur. Intraarticular fractures that are treated nonoperatively and have persistent gap may fail to unite (Fig. 15.41). Similarly, persistent gap after internal fixation of intraarticular fracture may lead to nonunion (Fig. 15.42). Operative management of nonunion or delayed union would include open reduction and internal fixation with or without bone graft.

AVASCULAR NECROSIS OF THE DISTAL TIBIA AFTER PHYSEAL INJURY

This extremely rare condition was first reported in the English-language literature in 1950.[85] Posttraumatic osteonecrosis (ON) after a distal tibial fracture in a skeletally immature patient is rare. A case of a 10-year-old healthy boy with a missed diagnosis of Salter-Harris type I fracture of the distal tibia was reported.[86] The patient developed ON of the distal tibial metaphysis that was treated conservatively. At 2 years' follow-up, he had mild ankle valgus deformity that could have been secondary to growth arrest. Another 11-year-old boy sustained a seemingly undisplaced Salter-Harris type II fracture of the distal tibia.[87] He developed symptomatic and biopsy-proven ON of distal tibial metaphysis, which resolved over a 2-year period.

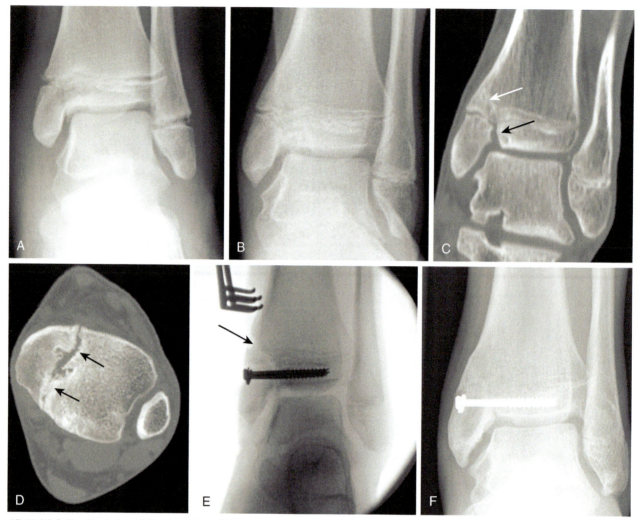

Fig. 15.41 (A) Salter-Harris type IV fracture of medial malleolus treated conservative. (B) At 1 year, patient continued to have ankle pain. (C and D) Computed tomography scan showed healing of the metaphyseal fragment (*white arrow*) and nonunion of the epiphyseal part of the fracture (*black arrows*). (E) A metaphyseal osteotomy was performed (*arrow*), the intraarticular fragment was compressed, and internal fixation was performed. (F) Radiograph taken 9 months after surgery. Patient has remained asymptomatic because of fracture fixation.

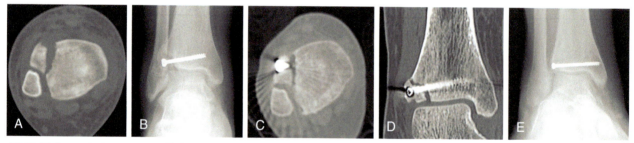

Fig. 15.42 (A) Computed tomography (CT) scan of Tillaux fracture in a 15-year-old boy. (B) The fracture was treated with closed reduction and internal fixation. Patient continued to have pain, and CT scan (C and D) 5 months after initial surgery showed nonunion of the fracture. The screw was placed along the correct trajectory, but fracture site was not sufficiently compressed. (E) Revision surgery was performed with open reduction, bone grafting from metaphyseal tibia, and internal fixation. The fracture went on to heal with a satisfactory outcome.

THE FOOT

ANATOMY

The foot has 26 bones and a variable number of sesamoids and accessory ossicles (Fig. 15.43). All are held together by interconnecting ligaments. The five rays of the foot each contain a metatarsal and its phalanges: two for the first toe and three for the others. The epiphysis of the first metatarsal is located at its proximal end, similar to a phalanx, rather than at the distal end, as it is for the other metatarsals.

The first three rays have a cuneiform bone at the base; the fourth and fifth share the cuboid bone at the base. The tarsal navicular is interposed between the head of the talus

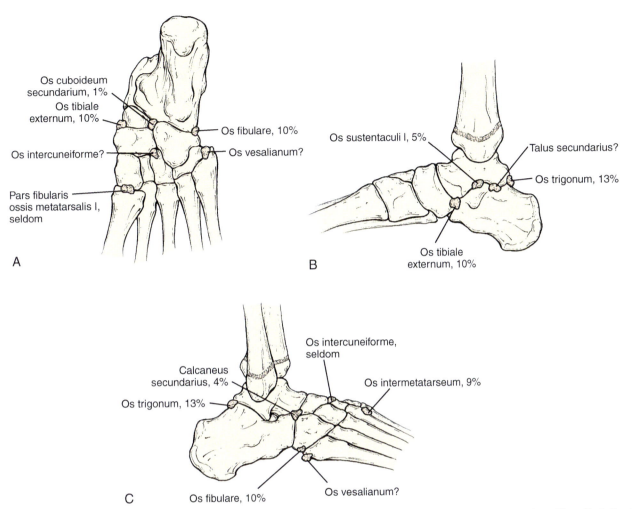

Os cuboideum secundarium, 1%
Os tibiale externum, 10%
Os intercuneiforme?
Pars fibularis ossis metatarsalis I, seldom
Os fibulare, 10%
Os vesalianum?

A

Os sustentaculi I, 5%
Os tibiale externum, 10%
Talus secundarius?
Os trigonum, 13%

B

Calcaneus secundarius, 4%
Os trigonum, 13%
Os intercuneiforme, seldom
Os intermetatarseum, 9%
Os fibulare, 10%
Os vesalianum?

C

Fig. 15.43 The normal bones of the foot and the accessory ossicles. (A) Plantar view. (B) Medial view. (C) Lateral view. (From Tachdjian MO. *Pediatric Orthopedics.* 2nd ed. Philadelphia: W.B. Saunders; 1990.)

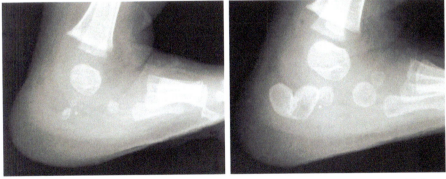

Fig. 15.44 The presence of multiple calcaneal centers usually implies a malformation syndrome. This patient with four calcaneal centers, which eventually fused, had Williams (Beuren) elfin facies syndrome. (From Oestrich AO, Crawford AH. *Atlas of Pediatric Orthopaedic Radiology.* New York: Thieme; 1985.)

and the cuneiform, and the talus sits "sidesaddle" on the calcaneus. Thus, the talus lies roughly in the axis of the first ray, and the calcaneus lies in the axis of the fourth ray.

The foot is customarily divided into the forefoot, midfoot, and hindfoot (i.e., metatarsus, midtarsus, and tarsus). The forefoot contains the five metatarsals and 14 phalanges; it is separated from the midfoot by the tarsometatarsal joint

(of Lisfranc). The midfoot contains the three cuneiforms, the navicular, and the cuboid, and it is separated from the hindfoot by the transverse midtarsal joint (of Chopart). The hindfoot contains two bones: the talus and the calcaneus. The reader is referred to comprehensive articles by Mann[88] and Morris[89] for a thorough description and discussion of foot and ankle biomechanics.

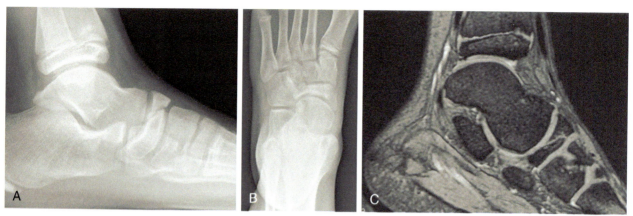

Fig. 15.45 Foot radiographs (A and B) taken for evaluation of occasional foot pain in a 12-year-old boy without any previous history of injury. Radiograph shows a fracture line through the navicular. Magnetic resonance imaging (C) shows bipartite navicular without any increased uptake in the navicular.

The foot presents myriad interesting anatomic features. It is not well ossified at birth, and of the tarsal bones present at birth, only the calcaneus and talus are fully ossified; however, the cuboid ossifies shortly after birth. The calcaneus may be bifid in certain syndromes (e.g., Larsen and Williams syndromes) (Fig. 15.44), and this variation may be interpreted as a fracture. The cartilaginous model is retained for an extended period. Similarly, the talus or navicular could be bipartite and could be confused with fractures (Fig. 15.45).

Reduction of foot deformities after fractures in children is important because remodeling cannot always be predicted with growth. Approximately 50% of the mature length has been achieved in 1-year-old girls and 1.5-year-old boys. In contrast, the femur and tibia do not reach 50% of their length until 3 years before comparable physeal closure in the long bones.[90] Therefore, severe malalignment after foot fractures does not usually have enough time to correct spontaneously.

TYPES OF INJURIES

The previous author (Alvin H. Crawford, MD) undertook a review of foot injuries managed at our institution (Table 15.3).[46] Some 215 patients were identified, and their charts and radiographs were examined; 175 patients with 213 definitive fractures and follow-up to completion of treatment were identified and reviewed. Coexistent unrecognized fractures of the distal ends of the tibia and fibula occurred in 8% of all fractures studied. Conditions initially mistaken as fractures were talofibular ligament tears, tarsal coalition, foreign bodies, and sesamoid fractures, each occurring once. Of the children in this study, 62% were boys, and 38% were girls. The left side was involved in 64% of cases, and the right side was involved in 36%.[46] This study is referred to throughout the discussion of foot fractures.

Most foot fractures result from direct violence, such as being crushed by a falling object, being run over by the wheel of an automobile, falling, or jumping from a height. The foot is so flexible and resilient that force applied to it is usually transmitted higher up and causes ankle and leg injuries. The soft tissue component of a foot injury is most

TABLE 15.3   Distribution of 213 Foot Fractures/Dislocations in 175 Patients

Area of Injury	Number of Fractures	Percentage
Metatarsals	157	74
Lesser (2–4)	104 (66.24)	49
Base of first	14 (8.91)	6.6
Base of fifth	39 (24.84)	18.3
Navicular	9	4.2
Talus	4	1.9
Calcaneus	4	1.9
Cuboid	2	0.9
Cuneiform	1	0.45
Phalanges	31	14.6
Proximal	20 (64.51)	9.4
Distal	9 (29.0)	4
Middle	2 (6.45)	0.9
Sesamoid	1	0.45
Dislocation (MP/IP)	4	1.9

(From Crawford AH. Fractures about the foot in children. A radiographic analysis. Cincinnati Children's Hospital, Cincinnati, OH, 1991 [unpublished data].)

IP, Interphalangeal; *MP,* metaphalangeal.

important, and if the area is swollen and tense, elevation and decompression should be instituted early. Preservation of soft tissues, particularly the ligaments essential to long-term function of the longitudinal and transverse arches, is just as important as actual fracture reduction in restoring complete function to an injured foot. Fractures involving a joint surface carry a worse prognosis than do nonarticular fractures, especially when the tarsal bones are involved.

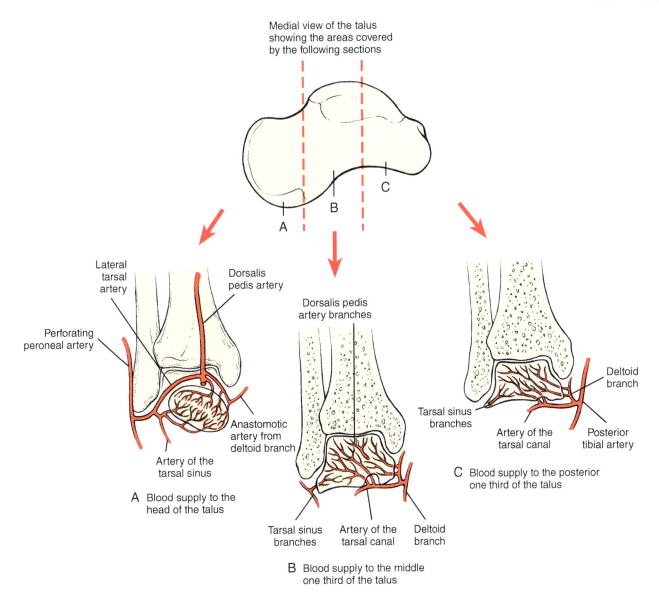

Medial view of the talus
showing the areas covered
by the following sections

A

B

C

Lateral tarsal artery

Dorsalis pedis artery

Perforating peroneal artery

Anastomotic artery from deltoid branch

Artery of the tarsal sinus

A Blood supply to the head of the talus

Dorsalis pedis artery branches

Tarsal sinus branches **Artery of the tarsal canal** **Deltoid branch**

B Blood supply to the middle one third of the talus

Deltoid branch

Tarsal sinus branches **Artery of the tarsal canal** **Posterior tibial artery**

C Blood supply to the posterior one third of the talus

Fig. 15.46 Diagram showing the blood supply to the talus in coronal sections. (A) Tuberosity, (B) dome, and (C) neck. (From Mulfinger GL, Trueta J, Trueta J. Blood supply of the talus. *J Bone Joint Surg Br.* 1970;52:160-167.)

Articular fractures in mobile joints require anatomic reduction so that early degenerative arthritis can be prevented.

TALUS

In a recent study by Thermann and colleagues,[91] the prevalence of talar fractures was found to be 0.08% of all childhood fractures. It takes nearly twice the force to fracture a child's talus than to fracture the ankle or other tarsals.[92] Because talus fractures are most often high-energy injuries (i.e., fall from height with forced ankle dorsiflexion), the treating provider should have a high index of suspicion to look for concomitant injuries.

This infrequent injury in children is a potential problem injury because of the precarious blood supply to the talus.[93] The posterior tibial artery gives off small branches that enter the region of the posterior tubercle to supply a portion of the body of the talus. The anterior tibial artery creates small branches that enter the superior surface of the head and neck of the talus. Formation of the primary talar ossification center depends on a functioning vascular supply

(Fig. 15.46). When compared with adults, children appear to have less dominance of a single system with retrograde flow from the neck into the body, and avascular (ischemic) necrosis is a rare complication after a talar fracture. Much of its surface is covered by articular cartilage, and only the constricted neck is left to accept the majority of nutrient vessels. Unfortunately, the neck is the area where most injuries occur. A displaced fracture of the neck of the talus is consistent with impending avascular necrosis (AVN).[94] Talar neck fractures can be overlooked in children and may become apparent only after the onset of AVN (Fig. 15.47). AVN may not be appreciated for up to 6 months after injury.

TYPES OF FRACTURES
Talar Neck and Body Fractures

The most common talar fracture occurs through the talar neck, followed by talar body. Talar head fractures are rare. The mechanism of injury for talar neck fracture is forced dorsiflexion of the foot, wedging the talar neck against the

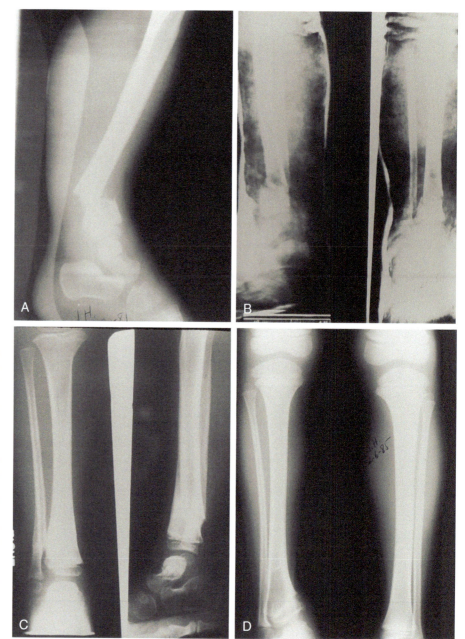

Fig. 15.47 An example of unrecognized injury to the talus resulting in osteonecrosis. This child sustained a tibial fracture that was reduced and healed uneventfully. He was subsequently noted to have avascular necrosis of the talus over the dome. Another unrecognized injury was a Salter-Harris type IV injury to the medial malleolus. The injury resulted in a severe varus deformity that finally caused his return to the hospital. (A) Lateral radiograph of the leg showing a displaced, posteriorly angulated distal tibial fracture. The talar fracture was not recognized. (B) Anteroposterior (AP) and lateral radiographs of the leg showing adequate reduction. (C) AP and lateral radiographs 2 months later showing avascular necrosis of the talar dome that had not been recognized. (D) The patient was seen in consultation 3.5 years after the injury because of an ankle varus deformity secondary to growth arrest of the medial malleolar fracture. The talus was collapsed, and the ankle or subtalar joint had very little motion.

anterior edge of distal tibia. The amount of displacement correlates with the age of the patient; most fractures in children less than 12 years of age are minimally displaced and are significantly displaced in those greater than 12 years of age.[95]

Ankle pain, swelling, and decreased joint motion may be noted. Weightbearing is painful. Radiographs reveal the injury in most cases (Fig. 15.48). A CT scan can help to better define the fracture geometry. Angulation of up to 30 degrees can usually be accepted, particularly in younger children less than 8 years of age. The apex of the angulation is in a plantar direction. Gentle, maximal plantar flexion with image intensification control under general anesthesia should be performed if the angulation is greater than 30 degrees. One has to weigh the risk of further displacement and vascular compromise against acceptance of the angulation. Rarely does the angulation inhibit ankle motion. If plantar flexion is required to maintain

reduction, a non-weightbearing, above-knee cast is worn for 3 to 4 weeks, followed by a walking boot. Treatment otherwise consists of a below-knee, non-weightbearing cast for 3 to 4 weeks. Two-thirds of patients less than 12 years of age were successfully treated nonoperatively in one series without ON.[95] Radiographs should be monitored for evidence of subchondral osteopenia of the proximal fragment. Vascular resorption (Hawkins sign) is an indication that the blood supply is intact.[96]

Displaced talar neck fractures tend to occur in older children.[97] These fractures require anatomic reduction. In one series, 13 of 16 adolescents greater than 12 years of age required surgical treatment for displaced fractures.[95] Early reduction by open or closed means enhances fracture healing but may not influence the occurrence of AVN. The common surgical approaches use anteromedial and anterolateral incisions (Fig. 15.49). Because the distal tibial growth

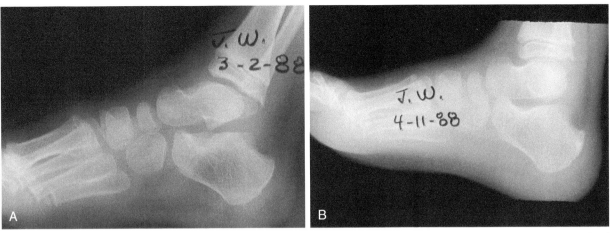

Fig. 15.48 Minimally angulated talar neck fracture in a 6-year-old boy after a dorsiflexion injury to his foot. (A) Lateral radiograph at the time of injury. Minimal plantar angulation is seen. (B) Lateral radiograph at the time of healing. The neck remains slightly angulated.

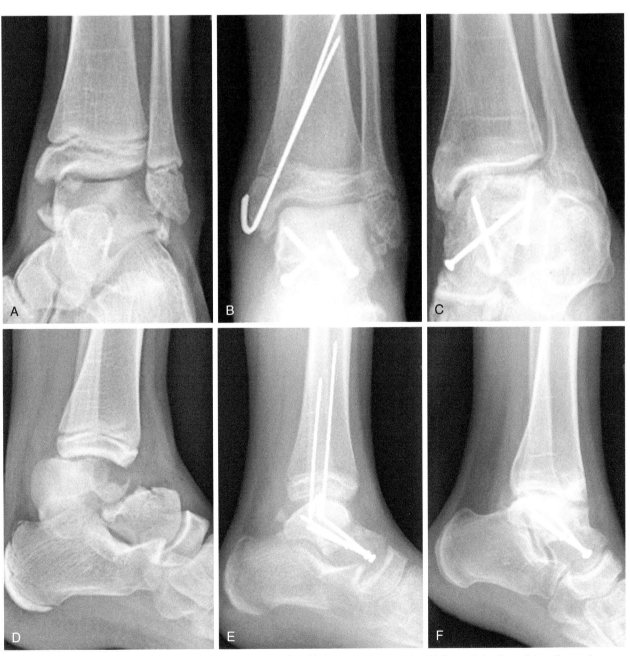

Fig. 15.49 (A and D) An 11-year-old female with a fall from a 10-foot-high rope swing sustained talar neck fracture dislocation and concurrent bimalleolar ankle fracture. (B and E) She underwent immediate open reduction and internal fixation of the talar neck and medial malleolus fracture. Radiographs taken 6 months after fracture fixation show healed fracture but osteonecrosis of talar body. (C and F) Two years after injury, she had pan-talar arthritis that has so far been adequately treated with activity modification only.

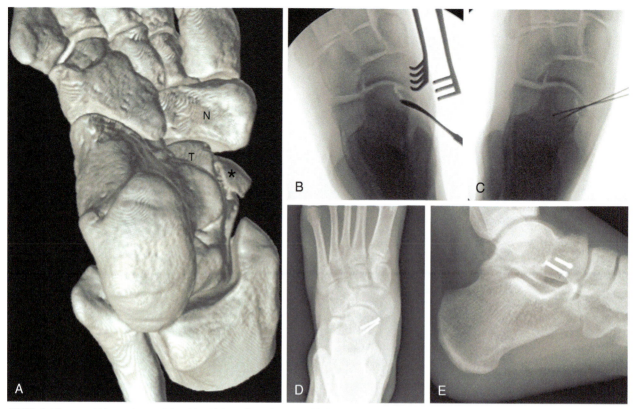

Fig. 15.50 A 14-year-old boy who sustained foot injury after a jump and fall during football. He sustained a talonavicular (*TN*) fracture dislocation along with other midfoot injuries. Computed tomography scan (A) shows talar head fracture (*asterisk*) with joint incongruity. (B and C) Intraoperative fluoroscopic images show open reduction and tentative fixation using K-wires. (D and E) Postoperative radiographs show definitive fixation of talar head fracture using headless screws.

plates are closing, a medial malleolar osteotomy may be performed to allow direct visualization of the fracture. Two screws, one bigger screw or multiple K-wires are placed to achieve interfragmentary compression. The direction of the screw from anterior to posterior or vice versa is controversial. If the screws are placed from posterior to anterior, a posterolateral approach is used. Recently, percutaneous reduction of fracture using intrafocal K-wires and percutaneous stabilization of the fracture using two cannulated screws has been reported.[98] When this technique of percutaneous reduction and fixation in 23 children was compared with open technique in 26 children, there was shorter time to healing (8 vs. 11 weeks), decreased nonunion rates (0 vs. 5), and decreased AVN rates (0 vs. 3). Following reduction and fixation, a below-knee cast is applied with the ankle plantar-flexed 20 degrees for 4 to 6 weeks. The parents should be strongly advised of the possibility of AVN. Radiographs of the talus should be monitored for evidence of subchondral osteopenia of the proximal fragment, indicating adequate blood flow to the talar body (positive Hawkins sign is a good prognostic indicator). If no Hawkins sign is apparent and the proximal fragment becomes sclerotic, a patellar tendon-bearing (PTB) brace is recommended for prevention of talar collapse.[99] The difficulty in predicting AVN in younger pediatric patients is that the Hawkins sign is not reliable in the cartilaginous pediatric talar dome.[100]

Talar Head Fracture

Fracture of the talar head is rare, and only few case reports have been published. Because the fracture is intraarticular

and involves talonavicular articulation, anatomic reduction is desirable (Fig. 15.50). Of seven cases reported in the literature, two were managed operatively: one using interfragmentary screw and one using K-wire. Two cases were managed nonoperatively. Three cases were diagnosed late, and the patients received no initial treatment.[101]

Compression Fracture of the Dome of the Talus

This injury is rare in children. The cartilage-to-bone ratio tends to cushion the impact of the tibial and subtalar joints, and the bone is well protected in the mortise. These compression fractures are most common in older adolescents and young adults; thus, they are not discussed here in detail (Fig. 15.51).

Lateral Process Fracture

The lateral process of talus is a wedge-shaped projection from the lateral wall of the talus with its apex directed laterally. The superolateral surface articulates with the distal fibula, and the inferolateral surface is a part of the posterior facet of the subtalar joint. The lateral talocalcaneal ligament and the anterior talofibular ligament attach to the lateral process.

Kirkpatrick and colleagues[102] showed that lateral process fractures represented 15% of all the ankle injuries related to snowboarding in their study. A common mechanism for this fracture is dorsiflexion of the ankle and inversion of the hindfoot. The patient typically presents with pain and swelling over the anterior talofibular ligament, thus mimicking an ankle sprain. The physician should be very suspicious of

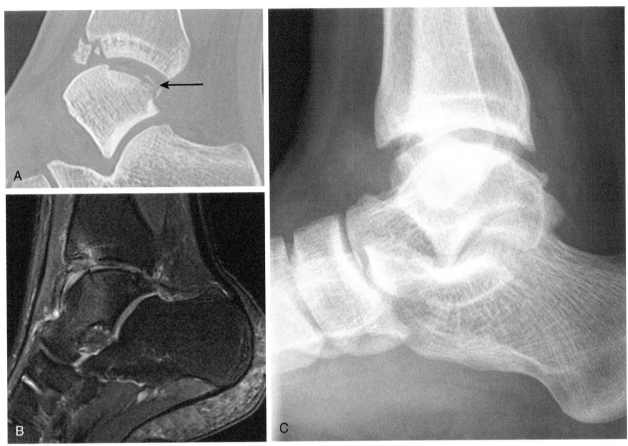

Fig. 15.51 A 16-year-old boy sustained a fall from height. Computed tomography scan (A) shows impaction fracture of the dome of the talus and bone debris in the joint (*arrow*), treated with arthroscopic joint débridement. Magnetic resonance imaging (B) 6 months after injury show the step-off of the talar dome with thinning of articular cartilage. (C) Radiograph 4 years after injury shows early degenerative changes of tibiotalar joint with anterior and posterior osteophytes from distal tibia. Patient is asymptomatic at this time.

anterolateral ankle pain in a snowboarder. Many of these fractures are not visible on plain radiographs and hence are often missed (Fig. 15.52). In one study, the missed diagnosis rate for lateral process talus fractures was 42% (5/12).[103] If missed, the fracture can lead to painful nonunion. If clinical suspicion is high or with delayed presentation, MRI/CT scan would help to diagnose the fracture and plan the treatment.

Treatment of nondisplaced fractures or small, extraarticular avulsion fractures consists of non-weightbearing in a below-knee cast for 4 weeks, followed by a walking cast or brace. If the fracture fragment is intraarticular but small or comminuted, excision and weightbearing as tolerated would be the favored treatment option.[102,104] For larger, displaced fractures, open reduction and internal fixation should be performed.[105]

COMPLICATIONS

Complications of talar fractures depend on the location of the fracture line and the amount of displacement. In a series of 21 talar fractures in children and adolescents, there was persistent pain in 10 fractures (47.6%), 3 cases of nonunion (14.3%) (Fig. 15.53), 3 cases of AVN (14.3%; of which, 1 required ankle and subtalar fusion), and arthrosis developing in 1 or more surrounding joint(s) in 12 fractures (57.1%).[97] Of the 12 fractures in adolescents 16 to 18 years of age, 9 (75%) developed arthrosis, and 2 (16.7%) subsequently

required arthrodesis. Thus the incidence of displaced talar fractures and associated complications increased with age. In another series of 29 talar fractures in children, higher rates of complication corresponded to the amount of displacement, age of the patient, and high-energy mechanism.[106] Posttraumatic arthritis occurred in 25% of pediatric patients, which followed an average of 11 years after talus fracture. One of the most common complication after reduction of fractures with significant displacement is AVN.

Avascular Necrosis

In a study of 24 children and adolescents with talus fractures, none of the patients younger than 12 years of age had ON, whereas 5 out of 15 patients older than 12 years had ON.[95] The patients in the older age group had higher displacement of talar fracture and underwent more surgical treatment compared with the younger group. AVN/ON, however, can happen even in nondisplaced/occult talus fractures in children.[14] The talus is the anatomic keystone for the ankle joint; it is the linchpin between the anatomic foot and ankle. Collapse of the talar dome may occur after AVN of the talus, but this condition is extremely rare in children younger than 10 years of age. Talkhani and colleagues[107] reported a case of AVN of the talus after a minimally displaced talar neck fracture in a 6-year-old child. The authors had a similar case in a 5-year-old child (Fig. 15.47). The anatomy and function of the talus are usually

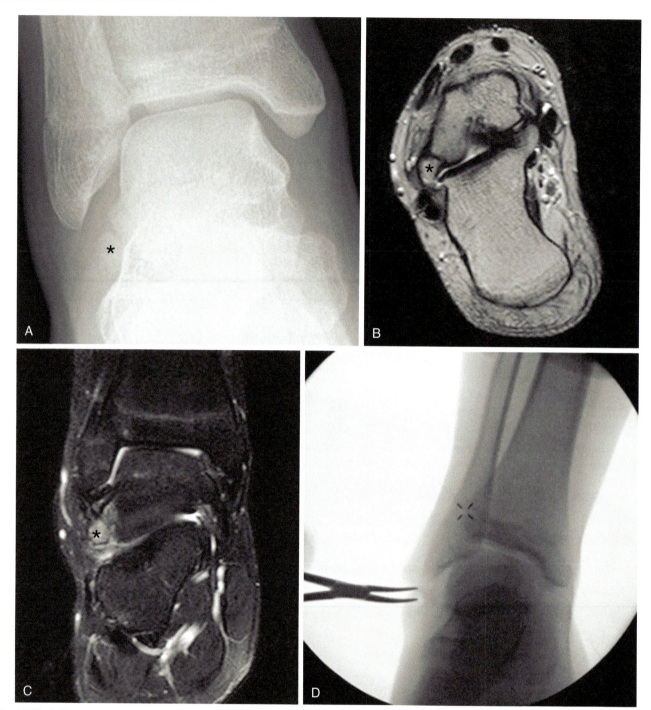

Fig. 15.52 A 16-year-old boy presented with ongoing pain on the lateral aspect of his ankle, about 4 months after an ankle sprain. (A) Radiographs show fracture of the lateral process of the talus (*asterisk*). Magnetic resonance imaging (B and C) shows the fracture with increased uptake. (D) Because of the small size of the fracture fragment, it was excised with satisfactory outcome.

stable until the collapse occurs. The subsequent alteration in its shape leads to ankle joint incongruity, instability, and, later, degenerative joint disease. A bone scan or MRI can be performed early after treatment of all displaced talar fractures to exclude AVN. It has been questioned whether the avoidance of weightbearing has an effect on the outcome of talar AVN. Management is usually similar to that for Legg-Calvé-Perthes disease, with no weightbearing and active motion in a PTB-articulated ankle brace until evidence of revascularization.

AVN developed in 5 of 17 children with nondisplaced fractures of the talus, as reported by Canale and Kelly[94] and by Letts and Gibeault.[108] Consequently, Gross[109] suggested that children may be as much at risk of the development of AVN as adults after nondisplaced fractures. These reports contradict the prevailing philosophy that pediatric AVN is unusual because displacement is uncommon in children.

Hawkins,[96] in 1970, detailed his experience with a series of 57 fractures of the talus in adults and outlined a useful classification. Type I fractures were nondisplaced, and in his

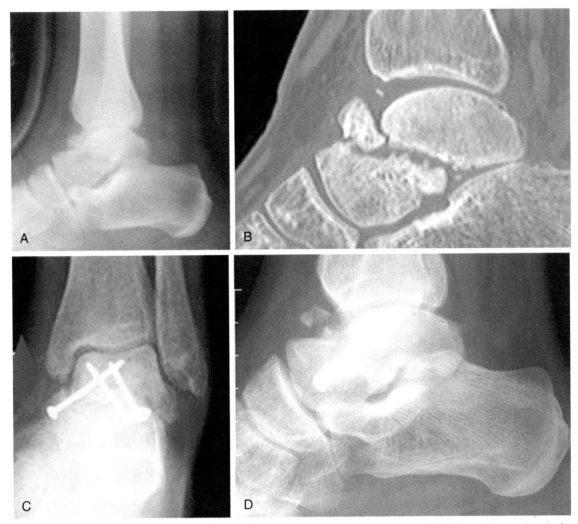

Fig. 15.53 A 17-year-old girl presented 3.5 months after polytrauma (pedestrian struck by motor vehicle) with a talar neck malunion/nonunion. (A) The injury was initially treated in a cast. Subsequently, she was ambulating with mild pain and varus deformity of her ankle. (B) Computed tomography scan showed nonunion of talar neck fracture with comminution. (C) Immediate postoperative radiograph after treatment with open reduction, bone grafting, and internal fixation of the talar neck nonunion using two dorsal incisions. The fracture healed, and she returned to cheerleading. (D) Final 2-year follow-up lateral x-ray show fracture healing and heterotopic bone above the talar neck, but the patient had only intermittent ankle pain, and no additional intervention has been required.

series, AVN did not appear. Type II fractures were displaced, with subtalar dislocation or subluxation. All united, but the rate of AVN was 42%. Type III fractures were accompanied by subluxation or dislocation at the subtalar and ankle joints, and a 91% rate of AVN was found in this group.[96] After injury and reduction, the Hawkins sign, a radiolucent subchondral line, is usually an indication that the blood supply is intact, even though AVN may have occurred. Because this sign accompanies disuse atrophy, it may be absent in children immobilized for only brief periods. A bone scan can demonstrate whether AVN has occurred and has been used by Canale and Kelly[94] to determine when weightbearing can be resumed. The authors have treated talar AVN by PTB bracing in an effort to decrease weightbearing on the hindfoot and prevent collapse. This method has not been completely successful; in one child, the talus underwent flattening, and stiffness of the ankle and shortening of the extremity occurred. Pain has not been a consistent complaint, but 5 years after the injury, the child is only 10 years old, and symptoms may occur as maturity progresses. It is

too early to recommend any of the newer pharmacologic treatments (like statins) or newer methods of injecting bisphosphonates, bone marrow aspirate, or bone morphogenic protein in the area of ON to prevent collapse and allow regeneration; these ideas are borrowed from studies related to femoral head ON.

OS TRIGONUM

The talus has two posterior tubercles; the lateral tubercle is larger than the medial, and the posterior talofibular ligament inserts on the lateral tubercle.[110] The tendon of flexor hallucis longus (FHL) traverses the groove between the two tubercles. The normal ossification process within the body of the talus is characterized by progressive posterior extension toward the posterior tubercles. The secondary centers of ossification of the tubercles appear at age 8 to 10 years in girls and 11 to 13 years in boys, and then fuse in a year. An elongated lateral process of talus is named the Steida process. The os trigonum represents failed fusion of the secondary ossification center of the lateral tubercle or stress

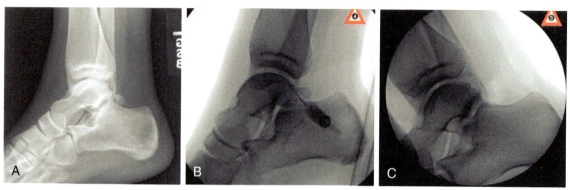

Fig. 15.54 (A) Lateral radiograph showing os trigonum posterior to the talus in a patient with pain in this location with horseback riding. (B) A diagnostic and therapeutic steroid injection was performed with temporary but complete relief of pain. (C) Surgical excision of the os trigonum was performed through a posterolateral approach.

fracture of the Steida process from repeated forced plantar flexion of the foot. Other etiologic factors include symptomatic synchondrosis, painful scar tissue, or posterior tibiotalar impingement. Radiographic studies suggest that the prevalence of os trigonum may be as high as 14% to 25% and that the condition is usually bilateral and asymptomatic.

The prevalence of os trigonum syndrome is high in ballet dancers who perform with the foot in forced plantar flexion and in certain sports like soccer, downhill running, or kicking.[111] Symptoms include stiffness, especially in plantar flexion, chronic pain, swelling behind the ankle, and decreased function. On examination, there is posterolateral tenderness at the ankle, between the Achilles and peroneal tendons. Os trigonum syndrome often coexists with FHL tenosynovitis. Lateral radiographs show evidence of chondro-osseous separation (Fig. 15.54). When the clinical findings are difficult to differentiate from other causes of posterior ankle pain, MRI or a positive response to a fluoroscopically guided injection of local anesthetic into the region of the synchondrosis between the os trigonum and the posterior aspect of the talus can help confirm the diagnosis.[112] Initial treatment consists of rest, activity modifications, antiinflammatory medications, and physical therapy. Although the radiographs may not change, the patient can be asymptomatic and can gradually return to activities. If conservative treatment fails, then surgical excision can be performed using open (posterolateral) or arthroscopic approach.

OSTEOCHONDRAL FRACTURES

Lesion of the osteochondral surface of the talus could be traumatic in origin (osteochondral fracture) or it could be the result of underlying osteochondritis dissecans (OCD). Osteochondral fractures of the talus usually result from eversion-inversion injuries.[113,114] A history of trauma has been reported in 64% to 92% of patients.[113,115,116] The OCD lesions may have been present before the injury; the recent injury may have triggered symptoms. The true etiology of OCD lesion is not known, although repetitive stress, vascular insult, and trauma have been implicated as causative factors. Systemic and genetic factors play a role as well because OCD has been described in siblings and has been associated with dwarfism[117–120] and with endocrine abnormalities. Extreme obesity carries a three times increased risk of OCD compared with normal-weight children.[121] Based on an

epidemiologic study, females had 1.5 times greater risk for ankle OCD compared with males, and the age group of 12 to 19 years had nearly seven times the risk for ankle OCD compared with the 6- to 11-year age group.[122]

Medial OCD is more common; is located more posteriorly; and is a deeper "cup-shaped" lesion, and the clinician is not always able to elicit a history of injury. Lateral OCD is less common; is located more anteriorly; is a shallower, "wafer-shaped" lesion; and is generally caused by a more significant injury. In addition, the lateral fragment has a greater tendency to become displaced into the joint. The patient may be asymptomatic or may complain of ankle pain with an associated limp. Swelling and other mechanical symptoms are typically not present.

Berndt and Harty[113] coined the term *torsional impaction*, which is useful in understanding the mechanism of injury in these lesions. They classified the lesion into four stages: (1) a small area of compression of subchondral bone; (2) a partially detached osteochondral fragment; (3) a completely detached osteochondral fragment remaining in the crater; and (4) a displaced osteochondral fragment (Fig. 15.55). They suggested that the lesion may represent nonunion of an osteochondral fracture or separation of articular cartilage and underlying subchondral bone by means of a localized vascular insult. They produced the posteromedial lesion by inversion and plantar flexion of the foot combined with external rotation of the tibia. Traumatic inversion and ankle dorsiflexion and compression of the talus against the lateral malleolus produce the anterolateral lesion, which may be accompanied by rupture of the lateral ligaments.

The OCD fragment consists of viable hyaline cartilage with underlying necrotic bone. The radiolucent line between the dead bone and the remainder of the talus is formed by a dense layer of fibrous connective tissue that acts as a barrier to capillary ingrowth. The primary objective of any treatment is to obtain bony union between the osteochondrotic fragment and the remainder of the talus. MRI can help if detachment or displacement of the fragment cannot be identified on plain radiographs. MRI findings that have been reported in osteochondral lesions are a low-intensity area on T1-weighted images and signal rims observed between the talar bed and the osteochondral fragment on T2-weighted images; the first suggests the presence of the lesion, and the second evaluates the stability of the lesion. However, MRI does tend to overestimate the stage and stability of OCD. In

Stage I   Stage II   Stage III   Stage IV

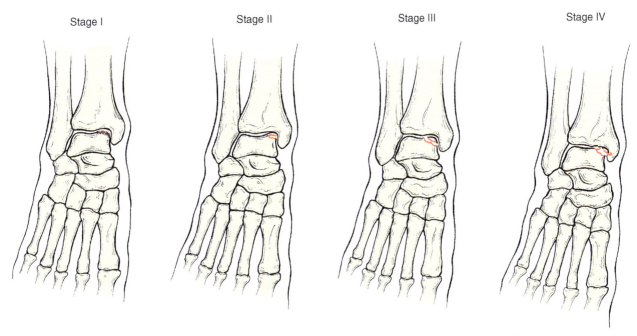

Fig. 15.55 The four stages of an osteochondral lesion of the talus according to the classification of Berndt and Harty: stage I, a small area of subchondral compression; stage II, a partially detached fragment; stage III, a completely detached fragment remaining in the crater; and stage IV, a fragment that is loose in the joint. (From Canale ST, Belding RM. Osteochondral lesions of the talus. *J Bone Joint Surg Am.* 1980;62:97-102.)

a study of 17 patients with juvenile OCD of talus, the preoperative MRI showed stage II OCD in 12 patients and stage III OCD in 5 patients. Arthroscopy revealed stage I OCD in five patients, stage II OCD in eight patients, and stage III OCD in three patients.[123] Postoperative MRI of these lesions is useful in assessing healing of osteochondral lesions. MRI findings that suggest healing are a decreasing size of the low-intensity area on T1-weighted images and disappearance of the signal rims behind the osteochondral fragment on T2-weighted images.[124]

Taranow and colleagues[125] suggested a new classification for talar osteochondral lesions. The classification uses findings from preoperative MRI and arthroscopy. The condition of the cartilage and bone together determines the type of surgical treatment. Cartilage is classified as viable and intact (grade A) or breached and nonviable (grade B). The bone component is described as follows: stage 1 is subchondral compression or a bone bruise, which appears as a high signal on T2-weighted images; stage 2 lesions are subchondral cysts and are not seen immediately; stage 3 lesions are partially separated or detached fragments in situ; and stage 4 represents displaced fragments. When drilling was indicated, retrograde drilling was suggested in patients with grade A cartilage.

Canale and Belding[114] recommended that undisplaced lesions be treated conservatively with casts and that displaced lesions be treated with excision and curettage. The literature is pessimistic about the use of a cast and non-weightbearing to obtain healing of lateral OCD.[113,114] At our institution, after 6 months of nonoperative treatment of talar OCD in 31 skeletally immature patients with a mean age of 11.9 years, 77% continued to have persistent lesions on radiograph, 16% had complete clinical and radiographic healing, and 6% had severe pain after cast removal that required surgery.[126] In those with radiographic persistent lesions and after an extra 6 months of nonoperative treatment, 42% had to undergo

surgery for unhealed lesions and pain, whereas 46% had no symptoms despite persistent lesions on radiographs. Thus, the success rate of nonoperative treatment was limited.

For nondisplaced lesions in children younger than 10 years, nonoperative treatment should be initiated. This would involve the application of a below-knee, non-weightbearing cast for 4 weeks. After an interval of 3 to 4 weeks, another cast could be placed for 4 weeks if progressive healing is noted on radiographs. Displaced lesions and those that do not respond to non-weightbearing warrant surgical intervention. Because arthroscopic treatment of these lesions has yielded outcomes as good as or better than arthrotomy, the authors advocate this method. Advantages of arthroscopic surgery include minimal iatrogenic trauma during surgery and rapid mobilization of patients after surgery. The authors recommend arthroscopically assisted retrograde drilling of the OCD lesion in patients in whom continuity of the cartilaginous surface and stability of the lesion have been confirmed, possibly allowing easier access to posteromedial lesions (Fig. 15.56). For larger lesions, open reduction and fixation of unstable osteochondral fragment is recommended; a transmalleolar osteotomy may be required. The authors prefer arthroscopic débridement of the lesion and pick arthroplasty (microfracture) of the base if the overlying cartilage is breached or not healthy (Fig. 15.57). If the fragment is completely detached and the bed of the defect is forming granulation tissue or fibrocartilage, then simple excision of the fragment may be indicated. Outcomes of surgical treatment are generally acceptable. The reoperation rate after three common procedures performed for OCD in 109 ankles were 31%, 23%, and 19% for transarticular drilling (59 ankles), fixation using bioabsorbable implants (22 ankles), and excision microfracture (27 ankles), respectively.[127] Female sex and elevated body mass index were bad prognostic factors.

In summary, surgery is to be recommended infrequently in the prepubescent age group because children usually do

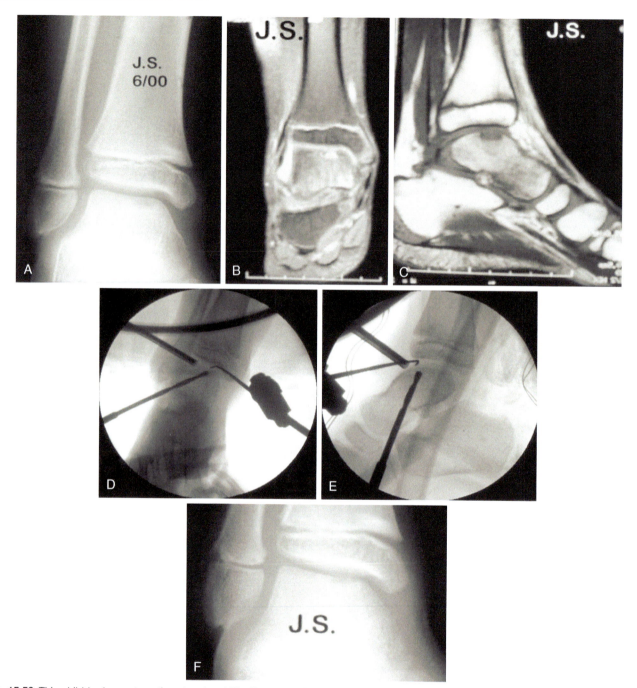

Fig. 15.56 This child had symptomatic osteochondritis dissecans of the talus that failed to respond to 6 months of nonoperative treatment. The child was then treated by arthroscopically guided transtalar retrograde drilling of the lesion. (A) Anteroposterior (AP) radiograph of the ankle showing the medial talar osteochondritic lesion. (B) Coronal T2-weighted magnetic resonance imaging (MRI) revealing a stable lesion. (C) Sagittal spin-echo MRI also shows the lesion to be stable. (D and E) Intraoperative Polaroid radiographs showing transtalar retrograde drilling with the arthroscope in the ankle joint. (F) AP radiograph of the ankle 3 months postoperatively showing no evidence of extension of the lesion. (Courtesy Dr. Eric Wall, Cincinnati, OH.)

well after a period of activity modification, immobilization, or both. In patients aged 6 to 11 years, only 1 of 13 (7.7%) OCD lesions required surgery; in the 12- to 19-years-of-age group, 26 of 72 (36.1%) OCD lesions required surgery.[128] Thus, for postpubescent and adolescent patients, surgical treatment is frequently recommended.

OCD of the talar head is rare. Four children, aged 9, 10, 16, and 16 years, have been reported having it. One patient had a history of trauma. Three patients had nonoperative

symptomatic treatment, and one required surgical excision and drilling because of persistent symptoms and was doing well at the 2-year follow-up.[129,130]

SUBTALAR DISLOCATIONS

Subtalar dislocations are very rare in children and adolescents, and literature regarding pediatric subtalar dislocations is limited to case reports.[131,132] In a metaanalysis of 359 patients with subtalar dislocations, Hoexum et al found the common

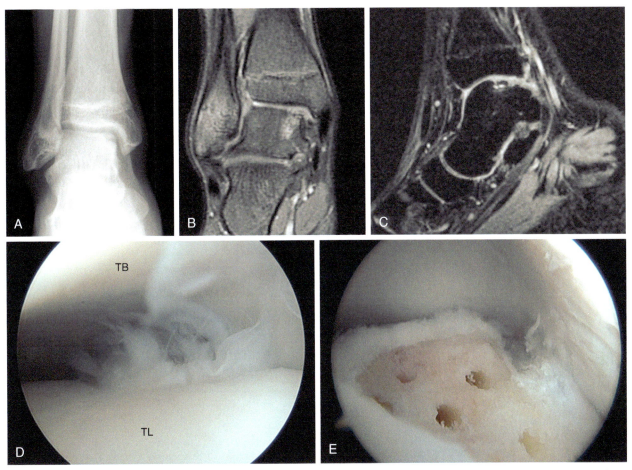

Fig. 15.57 (A) Radiograph of a 16-year-old girl with ankle pain shows osteochondritis dissecans (OCD) of medial talar dome of talus. (B and C) Magnetic resonance imaging shows signs of instability including increased edema, small subchondral cysts, and breach of articular cartilage. (D) At arthroscopy, the fibrillated edges of affected cartilage are seen. (E) Debridement of the OCD lesion up to normal, healthy cartilage edges, and microfracture was performed. *TB,* Tibia; *TL,* talus.

mechanisms of injury to be motor vehicle accident (44%), fall (33%), and sports related (14%). The dislocation is either medial (72%–75%) or lateral (17%–26%), and rarely, posterior or anterior (1%–2%).[133] Some 20% to 25% of subtalar dislocations are open, more lateral than medial.[133] Closed or open reduction should be attempted. If the ankle is stable after reduction, then a splint is applied, followed by a cast for 4 to 6 weeks. The reduction techniques and common impediments to reduction are described in Table 15.4. As a result of the high rate of peritalar fractures associated with subtalar dislocations, postreduction CT scan is recommended.[133] Long-term complications after subtalar dislocations include AVN, arthritis, and soft tissue complications/infection, especially after open dislocations.

CALCANEUS

Essex-Lopresti[134] reported only 12 patients between the ages of 9 and 20 years among 241 with fractures of the calcaneus. Thomas,[135] in 1969, reported five boys age 6 to 12 years who had sustained fractures of the calcaneus. Matteri and Frymoyer[136] reported three fractures of the calcaneus in children. Schmidt and Weiner[137] detected 59 fractures of the calcaneus in patients younger than 20 years, 46 of which were in skeletally immature children. One-third of

their patients had associated injuries; three sustained lumbar vertebral fractures. In adults, 10% of patients with calcaneal fractures have spinal injuries, whereas only 5% of children have such injuries. Despite this lower prevalence, however, children should still be examined for spinal injuries. Calcaneal fractures were initially unrecognized in 16 of the 59 fractures reviewed. Most of these fractures were minimal, which led to the conclusion that the injury has a benign prognosis. Inokuchi and colleagues[138] reported on 20 fractures of the calcaneus in children 14 years or younger, and Brunet[139] reported on 19 fractures in 17 patients 13 years or younger.

CLASSIFICATION

The patterns of fractures modified from Rowe by Ogden[140] include the following: type 1, fracture of the tuberosity, sustentaculum tali, or anterior process; type 2, a beak fracture or avulsion fracture of the tendocalcaneus insertion; type 3, an oblique fracture in the posterior portion of the bone not involving the subtalar joint and similar to a metaphyseal fracture of a longitudinal bone; type 4, involvement of the subtalar region, with or without actual articular involvement; type 5, a central depression fracture with varying degrees of comminution; and type 6, involvement of the secondary ossification center (Table 15.5). Schmidt and Weiner[137]

TABLE 15.4   Subtalar Dislocation

Direction of Dislocation	Frequency	Mechanism of Dislocation	Reduction Technique	Percent Irreducible by Closed Means	Usual Blocks to Reduction
Medial	72%–75%	Forced inversion of a plantarflexed foot	With knee in flexion, plantarflex, invert, and pull foot distally to unlock talar head from navicular. Then dorsiflex and evert the foot with direct pressure on prominent talar head.	10%	Talar head buttonholed through superior extensor retinaculum or EDB. Rarely talonavicular joint capsule, neurovascular bundle, peroneal tendons
Lateral	17.26%	Eversion of a dorsiflexed foot	With knee and hip in flexion, dorsiflex, evert, and pull foot distally. Then plantarflex and invert foot under the talus while applying medial pressure to talar head.	40%	Tibialis posterior or FDL slung around talar head
Posterior or anterior	1%–2%	Posterior: heavy plantarflexion of foot. Anterior: anterior traction of foot with fixed lower leg	With knee flexed, apply axial traction to the foot.	-	-

EDB, Extensor digitorum brevis; *FDL,* flexor digitorum longus.

TABLE 15.5   Calcaneal Fracture Patterns

Type	Description
1	Fracture of the tuberosity Fracture of the sustentaculum tali Fracture of the anterior process
2	"Beak" fracture Avulsion fracture of the tendocalcaneus insertion
3	Oblique fracture in the posterior portion not involving the subtalar joint; corresponds to a metaphyseal fracture of a longitudinal bone
4	Fracture involving the subtalar region with or without actual articular involvement
5	Central depression with varying degrees of comminution
6	Involvement of the secondary ossification center

(From Rowe CR, Sakellarides HT, Freeman PA, Sorbie C. Fractures of the os calcis: a long-term follow-up study of 146 patients. *JAMA* 1963;184:920. Copyright 1963, American Medical Association.)

developed a composite classification to include the compound fractures that are so common with lawn mower injuries in children (Fig. 15.58). The soft tissue injury is usually serious and includes significant bone loss, cartilage loss, and loss of insertion of the Achilles tendon.

For adolescent patients, intraarticular fracture patterns mimic those seen in adults and are better classified using Sanders CT classification.[141] Based on this classification, the posterior facet fracture on a coronal CT image could be nondisplaced (type I), displaced in two parts (type II), displaced in three parts (type III) or displaced and comminuted with more than three parts (type IV). The prognosis is worse with higher grades of fractures.

MANAGEMENT OF CALCANEUS FRACTURES

The calcaneus is largely cartilaginous in young children. Fracture of the calcaneus is a common, disabling injury in adults, yet it is rarely reported in infancy or in early childhood.[136] However, it is probably the most frequent tarsal injury seen in children.[137]

Stress or occult fractures may occur, and clinicians should be concerned about a young child who refuses to bear weight or who limps, especially when no radiographic evidence of a fracture can be found.[119] Schindler and colleagues[119] reported on five children 14 to 33 months of age treated for calcaneal fractures who had a history of trauma followed by limping or refusal to walk. Their initial radiographic results were negative. Four patients were treated with above-knee casts with the presumptive diagnosis of fracture, and one was treated with a bandage. All fractures healed without complications, and although no advanced imaging was performed, radiographs taken 2 to 4 weeks after treatment confirmed the diagnosis. Depending on the degree of primary ossification, a stress fracture is extremely difficult to diagnose early. Later, a sclerotic oblique line may be seen over the trabecular pattern, which is an indication of the reparative process. A below-knee, weightbearing cast for 3 to 4 weeks is usually sufficient treatment.

Heel pain may be a result of overuse or a symptom of systemic disease such as osteomyelitis or leukemia. The appearance of the secondary ossification center of the calcaneus is often fragmented on radiographs and leads to the assumption that an injury is present. This pattern of fragmentation of the apophysis in young children is more the rule than the exception. The clinical condition of pain about the heel with this radiographic finding carries the diagnosis of Sever disease. Sever disease is considered to be an overuse syndrome or the result of repetitive microtrauma (Fig. 15.59).

Most calcaneal fractures result from a significant fall. Radiographs are usually taken in the AP, lateral, and axial planes, although internal and external oblique views of the foot, as well as a CT scan, may be necessary. On the lateral view, the Böhler angle (normal adult values, 25 degrees to 40 degrees) and crucial angle of Gissane (normal adult values, 100 degrees to 130 degrees) can be measured to estimate fracture severity (Fig. 15.60). For pediatric patients (0–14 years), the Böhler angle ranges from 14.3 degrees to 58.1 degrees, and the angle of Gissane ranges from 90.1 degrees to 147 degrees.[142] The increased variability in pediatric age group is secondary to irregular and insufficient ossification of calcaneus, and contralateral radiograph can help to decide the normal values for the child. If the patient sustained a significant fall from a height, AP and lateral views of the thoracolumbar spine should be taken to exclude a

vertebral fracture (Fig. 15.61). Calcaneal injuries may also result from vehicular and lawn mower accidents (Fig. 15.62) or from a heavy object falling onto the foot (Fig. 15.63).

Intraarticular injuries affect the subtalar joint and are most often caused by the inferior protruding lateral process of the talus. The process jams superiorly into the calcaneus during impact, and the calcaneus fractures in a dorsal-to-plantar direction. Most young children with fractures of the calcaneus are assumed to have ankle sprains. The initial radiographs may not show the fracture, and in suspected cases, an MRI is indicated. A nondisplaced fracture of the calcaneus is treated by immobilization. This injury in children produces minimal disability in comparison with fractures of the calcaneus in adults. For a displaced calcaneal fracture, initial treatment should be directed toward the soft tissue swelling, which may be extensive. One should make every effort to achieve anatomic reduction of all articular surfaces to prevent subsequent degenerative joint disease. After reduction, the foot and ankle should be immobilized in a well-padded compression dressing, and the leg should be elevated for 2 to 3 days. A cast should not be applied until the bulk of the swelling has subsided. A below-knee walking cast is

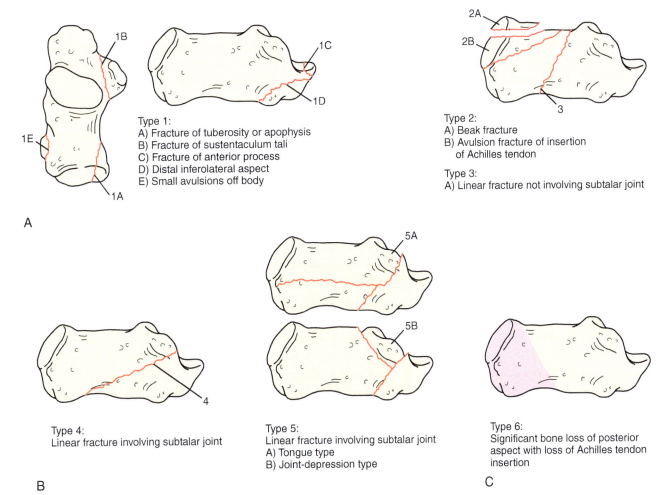

Type 1:
A) Fracture of tuberosity or apophysis
B) Fracture of sustentaculum tali
C) Fracture of anterior process
D) Distal inferolateral aspect
E) Small avulsions off body

Type 2:
A) Beak fracture
B) Avulsion fracture of insertion of Achilles tendon

Type 3:
A) Linear fracture not involving subtalar joint

Type 4:
Linear fracture involving subtalar joint

Type 5:
Linear fracture involving subtalar joint
A) Tongue type
B) Joint-depression type

Type 6:
Significant bone loss of posterior aspect with loss of Achilles tendon insertion

Fig. 15.58 Classification used to evaluate calcaneal fracture patterns in children. (A) Extraarticular fractures. (B) Intraarticular fractures. (C) Type 6 injury, with significant soft tissue injury, bone loss, and loss of insertion of the Achilles tendon. (From Schmidt TL, Weiner DS. Calcaneal fractures in children. An evaluation of the nature of the injury in 56 children. *Clin Orthop Relat Res.* 1982;171:151.)

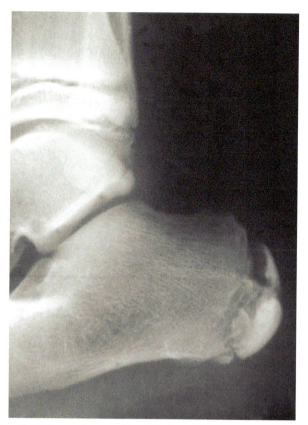

Fig. 15.59 Sever disease. Note the fragmentation of the calcaneal apophysis. Heel pain diagnosed as Sever disease is probably an overuse syndrome.

sufficient for immobilization of most calcaneal fractures not requiring open reduction. After open reduction, a well-padded below-knee cast is indicated for 3 to 4 weeks. Cole and colleagues[143] reported on avulsion fractures of the tuberosity of the calcaneus in children and reviewed the literature. In contrast to the usual recommendation to treat skeletally immature patients with calcaneal fractures by immobilization, they recommend open reduction and internal fixation. Of the four patients in their series (all of whom were older than 12 years), open reduction and internal fixation gave the best results. None of their patients had displaced intraarticular injuries, and the purpose of the open reduction was to prevent any functional loss from a shortened heel cord. The recommendation is to first attempt closed reduction under general anesthesia and to place the child in an above-knee cast with the knee in flexion and the ankle in 30 to 45 degrees of plantar flexion. If closed reduction fails and if the degree of displacement is such that functional disability, nonunion, or breakdown of soft tissue is likely, the fracture should be treated by open reduction and internal stabilization plus avoidance of fixation across the immature calcaneal apophysis.

Intraarticular fractures prevail in adult series (56%–75%). In one series,[137] 37% of children sustained intraarticular fractures, and 63% sustained extraarticular fractures. A review of the association between fracture type and age further illustrated that extraarticular fractures were more characteristic of younger children. In children through the age of 7 years, 92% of the fractures were extraarticular. From ages 8 through 14 years, 61% of the

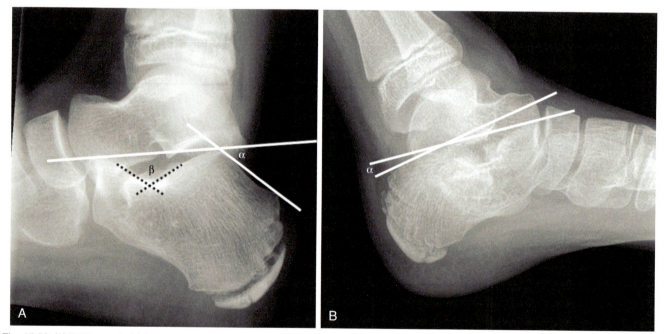

Fig. 15.60 (A) Böhler angle (α) is calculated on the lateral radiograph as the angle between a line from the highest point of tuberosity to highest point of the posterior facet and a line connecting the highest point of anterior process to highest point of posterior facet. The crucial angle of Gissane (β) is calculated as the angle between a line along the posterior facet of calcaneus and line from anterior process of calcaneus to the sulcus calcaneus. (B) The Böhler angle (α) is decreased in this 9-year-old boy who sustained a calcaneus fracture after fall from height, indicating loss of calcaneus height.

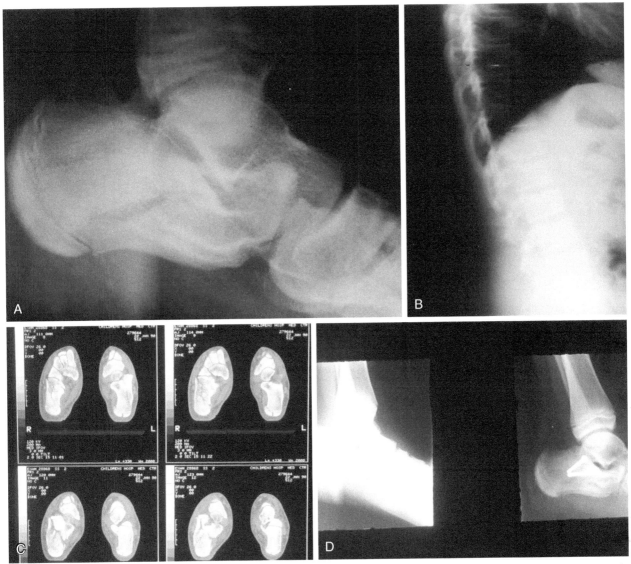

Fig. 15.61 Comminuted calcaneal fracture in association with a thoracolumbar spine injury. This child jumped from a height and sustained a calcaneal fracture; he also had back pain. The lateral thoracolumbar spine film shows a compression injury at the T12-L1 junction. The calcaneal fracture was treated by open reduction and internal fixation. (A) Lateral view of the foot showing a comminuted, dorsally displaced calcaneal fracture. (B) Lateral thoracolumbar spine radiograph showing mild compression fractures of T12, L1, and L2. (C) Multiple coronal-view computed tomographic scans of both feet revealing a comminuted right calcaneal fracture and nondisplaced fractures of the left calcaneus. (D) Preoperative and postoperative lateral views of the right foot show reduction and fixation with two cortical screws.

fractures were extraarticular. In children 15 years and older, the adult pattern was present, in that 38% of the fractures were extraarticular and 62% were intraarticular. The predominance of extraarticular fractures in younger children seems predictable in view of the fact that the mechanism of the vertical compressive load (e.g., a fall) is responsible for most intraarticular fractures and occurs twice as frequently in adults as in children. In addition, the resiliency of the cartilage and adjacent soft tissues tends to act as a resorbing factor in children who sustain vertical compressive loads. It is probable that the ability to absorb the stress from vertical loading results in fewer displaced intraarticular fractures in children than in adults. On the contrary, two series in the literature reported a predominance of intraarticular fractures in children; the first is by de Beer and associates,[144] who reported on

nine fractures in eight patients age 18 months to 12 years (mean, 6 years); they found that six of the nine fractures (66%) were intraarticular. The second report is by Brunet,[139] who reported on 19 fractures in 17 patients age 1.6 to 13 years (mean, 6.2 years); 14 of the 19 fractures (74%) were intraarticular.

Inokuchi and associates[138] reported on 20 calcaneal fractures, and ages at the time of injury ranged from 1 to 14 years (mean, 8.2 years). The fractures were extraarticular in 12 and intraarticular in eight. Four of the intraarticular fractures were associated with displacement. Only two cases required surgical intervention: one was a displaced avulsion fracture of the Achilles tendon insertion, and the other was a displaced intraarticular fracture of the joint depression type. The results were favorable in all patients except one, who sustained an associated

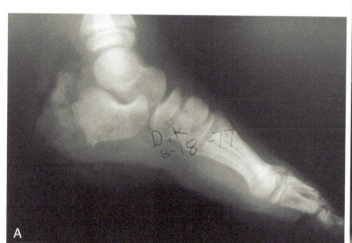

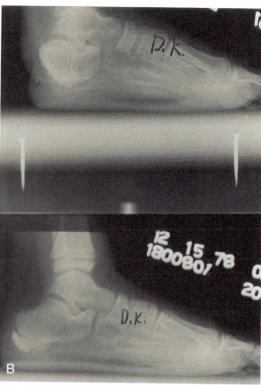

Fig. 15.62 This child sustained a lawn mower injury that clipped away the posterior half of the calcaneus. After injury, the bone had minimal posterior growth. (A) Lateral radiograph of the foot showing extensive soft tissue and bony injury to the posterior of the calcaneus. The wound was débrided, and the Achilles tendon was sutured to bone. Unfortunately, the apophysis was crushed and had to be discarded. (B) Comparison lateral views of both feet 1.5 years later showing loss of the calcaneal apophysis and failure of continued posterior growth of the bone.

neurologic injury after an L5 burst fracture. Inokuchi and colleagues[138] concluded that surgical therapy should be performed on displaced avulsion fractures of the portion of the calcaneus where the Achilles tendon inserts and on intraarticular fractures in which displacement is present (Fig. 15.64).

Brunet[139] reported on the long-term results of the treatment of the 19 calcaneal fractures mentioned previously. Follow-up ranged from 13.2 to 22.7 years (average, 16.8 years). Extraarticular fractures occurred in 6, and intraarticular fractures occurred in 14. The fracture pattern of these 14 intraarticular fractures consisted of two tongue-type, two centrolateral, one involving the sustentaculum tali, six grossly comminuted, and three minimally displaced. All fractures were managed in casts without manipulative reduction, with the exception of one that required open treatment for wound débridement. At follow-up, a few children complained of cramps in the foot with abrupt barometric pressure changes and sensitivity to cold weather. All but two patients had full or slightly reduced range of motion of the subtalar joint, and these two patients sustained an ipsilateral fracture of the neck of the talus. All patients were unaware of any functional restriction resulting from their injury. They could all walk comfortably on uneven ground. Mild to moderately severe osteoarthritic changes were seen in two patients on radiographic assessment: one involved the subtalar joint, and the other involved the calcaneocuboid joint. Many who sustained joint depression and comminution had been and were still involved in high-performance sports

such as long-distance running. It was suggested that children younger than 10 years have sufficient remodeling potential at the damaged articular surfaces of the calcaneum that when the immature talus grows into the defect produced by the depressed calcaneus, the final result is relative anatomic congruity of the subtalar joint.

Petit et al reported their results of open reduction and internal fixation in 14 displaced intraarticular calcaneus fractures in children (mean age, 11.7 years).[145] Thirteen patients received a buttressing lateral plate (Fig. 15.65). There were seven tongue-type and seven joint depression type based on Essex-Lopresti classification. There were nine type II and five type III fractures as per Sanders classification. The average preoperative and postoperative Böhler angles were 11.8 and 28.4 degrees. Functional outcomes were satisfactory. Four minor complications (two wound dehiscence, one hardware irritation, and one peroneal tendon irritation) were reported.

For intraarticular fractures in adolescents, a more aggressive approach of anatomic reduction and internal fixation is favored. The traditional L-shaped lateral incision and internal fixation has been associated with wound problems and infection. Instead, a limited open (sinus tarsi) approach to the posterior facet and K-wire fixation in 25 children with a mean age of 9.8 years has had favorable results in pediatric calcaneus fracture.[146] Feng et al described the technique of closed reduction and percutaneous fixation in 14 displaced intraarticular fractures in children (mean age, 11.2 years).[147] The authors used Schanz pins and K-wires to achieve reduction

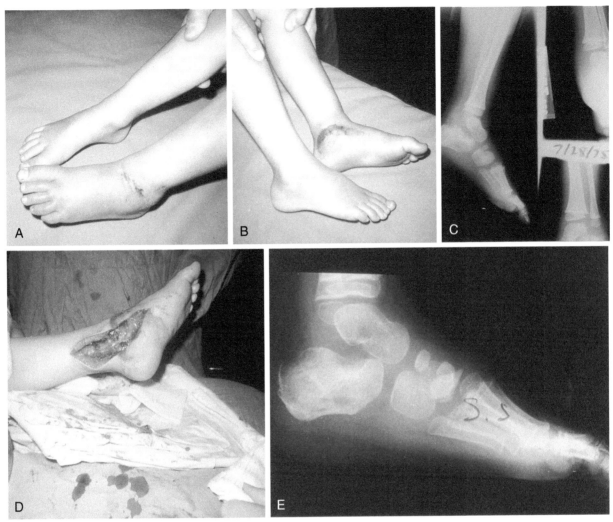

Fig. 15.63 This child was watching her father erect a wall of concrete blocks when one of the blocks fell on her left foot and caused tremendous swelling of the foot and toes. A clinical diagnosis of impending compartment syndrome was made. Immediate decompression was carried out to save the foot. The fracture healed uneventfully. Swelling and congestion of the foot and toes constitute a surgical emergency. (A) Anterior clinical photograph of both feet showing the tension edema of the foot and toes. (B) Side view showing swelling of the medial aspect of the left foot with focal blanching "ischemia" on the plantar portion. (C) Anteroposterior, lateral, and mortise views. (D) Operative photograph at the time of decompression. (E) Follow-up lateral radiograph of the foot. The calcaneus is healed, and the wounds were approximated by delayed primary closure.

and provisional fixation, followed by cannulated screw insertion for definitive fixation.

COMPLICATIONS

Subtalar arthritis may occur with persistent displacement and instability of osteochondral fractures in the subtalar joint. Late surgery to reduce and align the joint surfaces is rarely successful, and subtalar or triple arthrodesis may be required. In Brunet's long-term study,[139] subtalar joint osteoarthritis developed in only one of 14 intraarticular fractures. This patient was 11.8 years old at the time of the injury and had a severely comminuted fracture of his calcaneus. The patient had minimal symptoms and scored 90 out of 100 on the American Orthopaedic Foot and Ankle Society rating score. Injury to the growth plate has been noted after an open fracture caused by a lawn mower injury (Fig. 15.62); otherwise, growth plate injury to the calcaneus is extremely rare.

NAVICULAR BONE

The tarsal navicular bone is injured only occasionally in children, and the fracture is rarely displaced. Nine navicular fractures were seen in 175 fractures reviewed at our institution.[148]

Because of the variability in ossification, a fracture may be confused with Köhler disease. The radiographic picture of a sclerotic, thin, fragmented tarsal navicular bone, commonly called Köhler disease, may represent repetitive microtrauma, an abnormal ossification pattern, or an overuse syndrome (Fig. 15.66). In Waugh's study of 52 boys and 52 girls,[149] on radiographs taken at 6-month intervals from 2 to 5 years, 10 boys and 16 girls showed abnormal ossification. Radiographs of the foot taken for other reasons often show irregularity of tarsal navicular ossification. It is still questioned whether Köhler disease is a normal variant or represents overuse. Treatment of this injury is usually uncomplicated because the bone is minimally displaced, if at all.

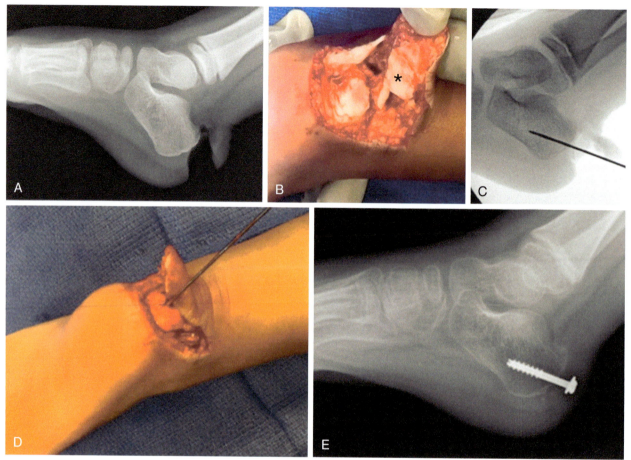

Fig. 15.64 A 5-year-old child with open calcaneal apophysis avulsion fracture with detachment of Achilles tendon insertion. (A) The fracture cannot be seen on initial radiograph, as the apophysis is cartilaginous. (B) Clinical evaluation demonstrates the fractured apophyseal fragment (*asterisk*), and the Achilles tendon attached to the fracture fragment. (C and D) The fracture was irrigated, débrided, and fixed provisionally with a guide pin. (E) Definitive fixation was performed using a cannulated screw, which was removed 7 months later after healing of the soft tissues and after clinically healed calcaneal fracture.

Borges and colleagues[150] found that patients treated without casting had symptoms lasting an average of 10 months. Patients treated with casting were completely asymptomatic within an average of 3 months. Treatment with a below-knee walking cast for about 8 weeks rendered the individual pain free in the shortest period. The average time required for complete restoration of normal bone structure was 1 year and 4 months, with a minimum of 4 months and a maximum of 4 years.

Another variant of navicular ossification is the bipartite navicular (Fig. 15.45). It may be confused with a fracture when the patient presents with midfoot pain after an injury. The absence of high-velocity trauma should alert the physician against the diagnosis of fracture. MRI can help to exclude the diagnosis of fracture, if in doubt. Conservative treatment is recommended. Attempts at surgical fixation have not been successful in achieving union.[151]

The most frequent navicular fracture in children is a dorsal proximal chip fracture, which is best seen on a lateral radiograph of the foot (Fig. 15.67). This injury may represent an avulsion pull-off of an apophyseal fragment from the dorsal tarsal ligament. Treatment of this injury is usually uncomplicated because of the lack of or minimal displacement.

A below-knee walking cast is applied for 3 to 4 weeks. Even though the small chip may not unite to the navicular body, the symptoms subside.

Displaced fractures of the navicular in adolescents are usually associated with severe trauma and other fractures/dislocations. Soft tissue injury and swelling should be monitored. If soft tissues are compromised and there are multiple fractures/dislocations, an external fixator may be placed. CT scan may help to delineate the fracture pattern and help surgical planning. The authors recommend anatomic reduction (usually open reduction) and fixation with pins or screws, once the swelling subsides. A below-knee, non-weightbearing cast is then applied (Fig. 15.68).

CUBOID FRACTURES

Fractures of the cuboid in children are uncommon. Cuboid fractures accounted for 1.1% of the fractures in one series.[152] Simonian and associates[153] described eight fractures of the cuboid in children younger than 4 years. These fractures are also known as "toddler's fracture." The common mechanism of compression fracture is a jump or fall from

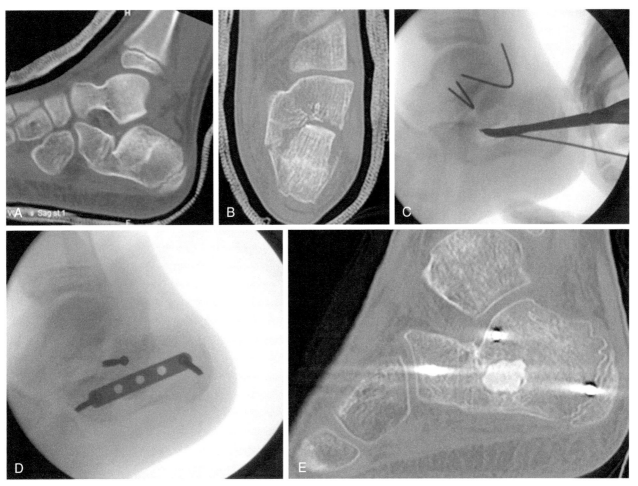

Fig. 15.65 (A and B) Computed tomography (CT) scan of a 9-year-old boy who sustained displaced fracture of the calcaneus following a zipline injury when his foot hit a tree. (C and D) During surgery through the lateral approach, the depressed posterior facet was elevated. The void was filled with bone cement. Final fixation included a screw and a buttress plate. (E) Postoperative CT scan shows adequate restoration of articular surface and Böhler angle.

a couch. It can sometimes be secondary to increased stress on the lateral border of the foot as the child is learning to walk. The parents may or may not have witnessed any injury. Initial radiographs may be normal. These occult fractures are diagnosed by point tenderness over the cuboid in a limping toddler and confirmed by the presence of sclerosis in the proximal cuboid on later radiographs (Fig. 15.69). A short-leg walking cast is the treatment of choice, primarily for comfort.

Another rare but severe type of cuboid fracture seen in older children and adolescents is termed the "nutcracker fracture."[154] Compared with toddler's fracture, which can be treated with benign neglect, the nutcracker fracture frequently requires surgical intervention. The mechanism of injury is forced abduction of the forefoot along with axial load, causing the cuboid to be compressed between the calcaneus and the fourth and fifth metatarsal. Ceroni et al reported four children who sustained this injury during horseback riding when the horse fell on them, with their foot caught in the stirrup.[155] Most often, these fractures are associated with other midfoot fractures or dislocations. CT scan would help to recognize the extent of injury. The fracture pattern may vary from intraarticular displacement to collapse of the cuboid with lateral wall extrusion and loss of lateral column length. Displaced fractures and those associated with loss of lateral column length should be treated by anatomic reduction and internal fixation. Prognosis is based on the extent of injury.

TARSOMETATARSAL (LISFRANC) INJURIES

These injuries are rare and may result from indirect injury, such as the violent plantar flexion and dorsiflexion found in toe walking or trying to break speed while sledding or tobogganing, or from direct injury, which is more common, secondary to an object falling onto the foot. The unique pattern of tarsometatarsal joint injuries described by numerous authors is related to the anatomic features of this joint complex and the mechanism of injury. The most relevant anatomic features are the fixed, mortised position of the base of the second metatarsal and the ligamentous attachment between the medial

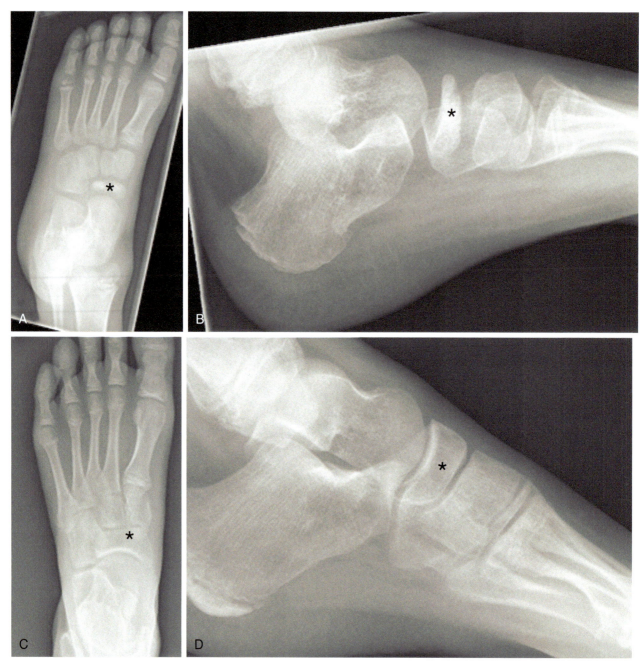

Fig. 15.66 Anteroposterior (A) and lateral (B) radiographs of a 7-year-old boy show the navicular bone (*asterisk*) to be sclerotic, fragmented and diminished in size, indicating Köhler disease. Patient was treated conservatively with symptomatic treatment. (C and D) Radiographs 4 years later show appropriate reconstitution and normal-appearing navicular bone.

cuneiform and base of the second metatarsal (Lisfranc ligament). This ligament is much stronger on its plantar aspect to resist the forces of body weight. The midfoot complex is responsible for maintaining the transverse and longitudinal arches of the foot. A fracture of the base of the second metatarsal is a sentinel feature of a tarsometatarsal joint injury. Lisfranc injuries without fractures occur because of disruption or sprain of the midfoot ligaments. These ligamentous Lisfranc injuries may be missed, and high degrees of clinical suspicion are required to diagnose them.

MECHANISM OF INJURY

Wiley[151] described three basic mechanisms of injury (Fig. 15.70):

Traumatic impact while in the tiptoe position. An example would be jumping from a height to the ground and landing on the toes. This mechanism usually causes forced plantar flexion of the forefoot, leading to metatarsal joint dislocation and fracture of the base of the second metatarsal.

Heel-to-toe compression. In this instance, the victim is in a kneeling position when the impact load strikes the heel. The second, third, fourth, and fifth metatarsals may be laterally dislocated, and the second metatarsal base may be fractured.

The fixed forefoot. In this situation, the patient falls backward while the forefoot is fixed to the ground by a heavy weight. The patient's heel resting on the ground becomes the fulcrum for the midfoot injury.

Most patients present with significant pain, swelling, and inability to bear weight on the involved side. Ecchymosis on the plantar aspect of midfoot may suggest injury to the Lisfranc ligament. There may not be obvious deformity, as spontaneous reduction of injury is common. The amount of swelling is noted, and the foot is watched for compartment syndrome.

MANAGEMENT

One should always obtain AP, lateral, and oblique radiographs. Although weightbearing radiographs are preferred, most patients with such injuries would not be able to bear weight. Fracture of the base of the second metatarsal should raise the suspicion of Lisfranc injury, although small osteochondral fractures may be missed. Based on measurements of normative values on a non-weightbearing AP radiograph of the foot in 352 children and adolescents, Knijnenberg et al reported that the normal distance between the base of first metatarsal and second metatarsal (<3 mm), as well as the distance between the medial cuneiform and the base of the second metatarsal (<2 mm), approached adult values after the age of 6 years. Before age 6 years, these distances measured more because of incomplete ossification.[156] The combination of a fracture at the base of the second metatarsal and fracture of the cuboid bone usually results from tarsometatarsal dislocation. CT scan or MRI are valuable in assessing patients who have normal results on plain radiographs after tarsometatarsal joint injury.[157] CT scan would also help in evaluation of joint surfaces, joint congruency, and assessment of comminuted fractures, to facilitate surgical planning in high-velocity injuries.

For undisplaced Lisfranc injuries, treatment consists of elevation of the extremity and compression, followed by a below-knee walking cast when the swelling has decreased and the patient is comfortable. Closed reduction should be performed for displaced fractures. The key to reduction involves aligning the base of the second metatarsal anatomically. Percutaneous pinning or cannulated screw

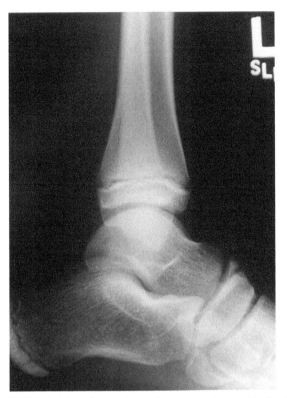

Fig. 15.67 This lateral foot radiograph shows a dorsal chip fracture of the navicular bone, which is the most common navicular fracture in children.

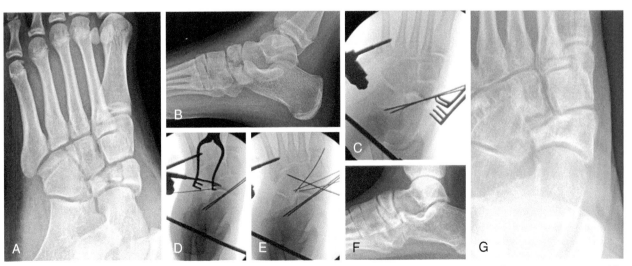

Fig. 15.68 (A and B) Comminuted fracture of navicular in a 12-year-old girl when her foot was run over by a car. (C) At surgery, an external fixator was used to distract the talonavicular joint, and then the medial aspect of the navicular was reduced to the talar head. (D and E) The remaining part of the navicular was "built" on to the medial side and stabilized with multiple K-wires. (F and G) Two years' postoperative radiographs show the healed navicular fracture and no degenerative changes.

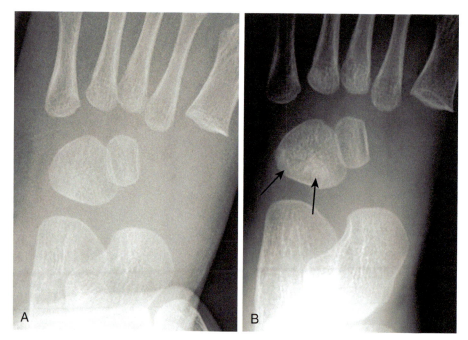

Fig. 15.69 (A) Normal foot radiograph of a 2-year-old boy who presented with a painful limp after a fall from a bed. Clinical evaluation demonstrated tenderness to palpation over the lateral border of foot. Cuboid toddler's fracture was suspected. (B) Repeat radiograph after 2 weeks shows increased sclerosis (*arrows*) in the proximal aspect of cuboid, suggesting healing fracture.

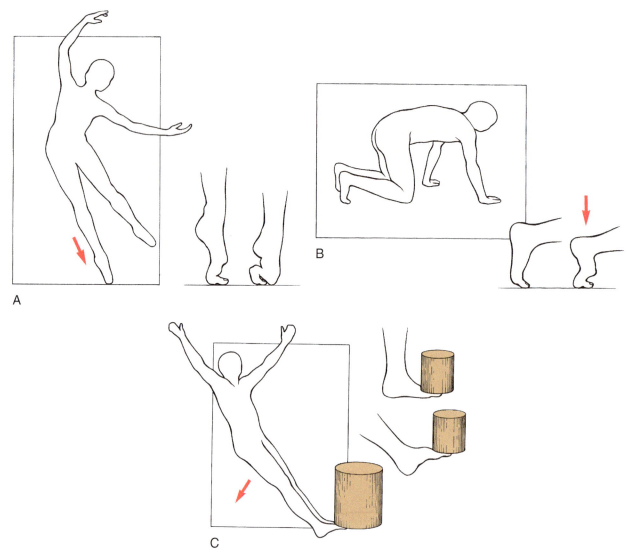

Fig. 15.70 Pathomechanics of tarsometatarsal injuries. (A) Illustration of tiptoe landing producing forced plantar flexion of the forefoot. (B) Illustration of the circumstances of sustaining a heel-to-toe compression injury of the foot. (C) Illustration of the circumstances of a backward fall with a pinned foot. (From Wiley JJ. Tarso-metatarsal injuries in children. *J Pediatr Orthop.* 1981;1:256.)

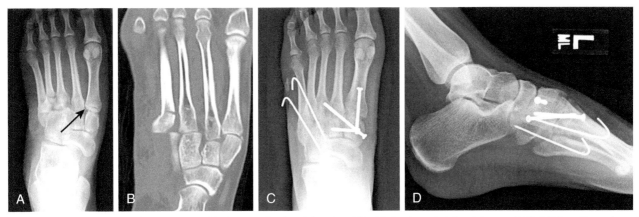

Fig. 15.71 (A) Foot radiograph of 16-year-old girl who sustained an injury to midfoot following a twisting injury and fall. A flake of bone (*arrow*) is seen between the metatarso-cuneiform joint, characteristic of a Lisfranc injury. (B) Computed tomography scan shows disruption and incongruity of first, second, and third tarsometatarsal joints and fracture of the fourth metatarsal. (C and D) At surgery, the medial column (1-3 tarsometatarsal joints) was stabilized using closed reduction and percutaneous cannulated screw fixation; the lateral column (4-5 tarsometatarsal joint) was stabilized by K-wires, which were removed in the clinic at 4 weeks.

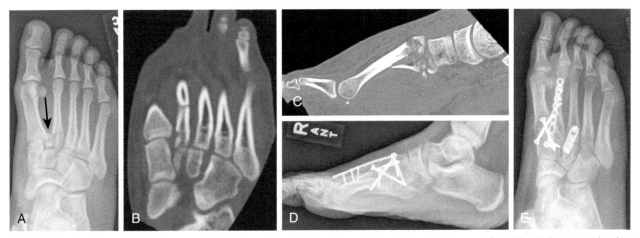

Fig. 15.72 (A) Foot radiograph of a 15-year-old girl who sustained injury to her midfoot after a fall from a height. The Lisfranc avulsion fracture from base of second metatarsal (*arrow*) can be appreciated. (B and C) Computed tomography (CT) scan shows comminuted fracture of the second metatarsal base and disruption of 1–3 tarsometatarsal joint. (D and E) Open reduction and internal fixation of the medial column using plate and screws.

fixation should be used to obtain stability of the reduction, followed by a short leg cast (Fig. 15.71). Failure to obtain anatomic reduction can cause persistent pain and swelling. This is usually the case in high-velocity, markedly disrupted, tarsometatarsal joint injuries. In such cases, open reduction and internal fixation using combination of K-wires, screws, and bridge plates may be required (Fig. 15.72). Removal of implants is controversial. Wiley[158] reported 18 tarsometatarsal injuries in children younger than 16 years; most of these patients were treated with casting or closed reduction and percutaneous pinning, which is in contrast to the usual adult treatment of Lisfranc injuries that are typically treated with open reduction and internal fixation or tarsometatarsal arthrodesis. Fourteen of 18 patients in the study were asymptomatic, and the remaining 4 of 18 patients had only minor pain 1 year postinjury. In a descriptive case series of pediatric Lisfranc injuries comprising 56 patients with a mean age of 14.2 years, 34% of the patients were treated operatively, and 66% were treated nonoperatively.[159] Open reduction and screw fixation was more common in patients with closed physis. At the authors' institution, 13 pediatric patients with

Lisfranc injuries completed outcomes questionnaires an average of 5 years after injury, and both nonoperative (8 out of 13) and operative treatment (5 out of 13) resulted in good/excellent long-term function and quality of life. Most pediatric Lisfranc injuries are treated nonoperatively with a below-knee cast for about 4 weeks. Older patients (over 12 years) with more complicated/displaced injuries are more likely to be treated operatively.[160]

METATARSAL FRACTURES

Metatarsal fractures accounted for 74% of the fractures of the foot seen in the study from our institution.[148] The injury usually occurs as a result of direct trauma from a falling object; indirect trauma after torsional stress may result in oblique fractures. In a study of 125 children with 166 metatarsal fractures, Singer et al noted that in children 5 years of age or less, the most common location of injury was in the house because of fall from height, and the first metatarsal fracture was most common. For those older than 5 years of age, injury occurred at sports facilities and involved the fifth metatarsal.[161] An avulsion fracture of the base of the fifth metatarsal is the most common isolated metatarsal injury in children. Stress fractures can occur in a foot subjected to repetitive trauma such as jogging and track-and-field activities. The injury occurs most commonly in the second metatarsal, although other metatarsals may be involved.

The necks of the metatarsals are rarely injured. The fracture pattern may be oblique, transverse, or linear. If the articular surface or condylar epiphysis is not injured, the injury usually resolves readily. Treatment consists of a below-knee walking cast for 3 weeks.

Metatarsal shaft fractures usually occur from a direct crushing blow, and solitary fractures are generally nondisplaced. Reduction of shaft injuries requires particular attention. Displacement of metatarsal fractures in medial-lateral plane is acceptable, although residual displacement of the border metatarsals (first and fifth) can lead to splaying of the foot. Residual dorsal or plantar angulation may be more problematic, as it may cause abnormal weight distribution. Malunion and nonunion are rare but may occur, although delayed union occurred in 15% of metatarsal fractures in a pediatric population in one study.[162]

Usually, the base of the metatarsal is injured in conjunction with other associated injuries, except for the bases of the first and fifth metatarsals. Isolated fracture of the first metatarsal base is not uncommon, and this injury may predispose to growth plate injury. The child's symptoms are usually swelling, pain, or ecchymosis across the forefoot. Evidence of fracture may or may not be seen on initial radiographs. Fractures of the base of the fifth metatarsal are more common in adolescent athletes involved in jumping sports.

Displaced fractures of the bases of the metatarsals are usually caused by strong, avulsive forces. It is important to appreciate the fibrous compartment of the interossei and short plantar muscles in patients with foot injuries, especially those with significant swelling. One should consider early fasciotomies, similar to those performed in the hand, in patients who have marked swelling with the skin stretched and taut or in those with significant venous congestion of the toes. One should be especially wary if multiple fractures are present and should not hesitate to perform fasciotomies.

Growth plate injuries to the metatarsals are rare but do occur under certain conditions: (1) the chondroepiphysis may be avulsed; (2) a fracture may extend into the epiphysis; or (3) the condylar surface of the secondary ossification center may be avulsed. Treatment of these injuries usually consists of a below-knee walking cast for 3 to 4 weeks. Growth inhibition is unusual; overgrowth is more common. Condylar fractures rarely require open reduction. Growth rates may be affected differently, depending on the type of injury.

TREATMENT

Significant displacement is rare. If swelling is present, one should refrain from the immediate use of a circular cast around the ankle, which would lead to dorsal pressure and a tourniquet effect. One should consider using a splint or a bulky dressing initially in all cases, even for those with minimal displacement. After reduction of swelling, a below-knee cast is applied. The treatment of multiple metatarsal fractures in children is controversial because of limited studies. Clear surgical indications include open fractures, displaced articular fractures, or metatarsal fractures associated with compartment syndrome. Based on the study of 98 patients with multiple metatarsal fractures (average age, 9.7 years, range: 1.3–17.9 years), Mahan et al reported that adolescents older than 14 years of age and having more than 75% displacement of at least one metatarsal fracture were more likely to undergo surgical stabilization.[163] Similarly, Robertson et al reported that in patients older than 12 years of age, multiple metatarsal fractures and increased translation at the fracture site (not angulation) were factors associated with surgical treatment (Fig. 15.73). No patients younger than 12 years of age required surgery.[162]

MANAGEMENT OF SPECIFIC INJURIES

First Metatarsal

The first metatarsal is often fractured. The injury occurs most frequently in the first decade, and as a result, the mechanism of injury is elusive. The child is seen with a limp, and the parents may simply state that the child "fell on the foot." The radiograph shows a buckle at the base of the metatarsal just distal to the physis (Fig. 15.74), similar to the torus radial forearm fracture. One should look carefully at the physis for evidence of injury. In contrast to the other metatarsals, the physis is located on the proximal end of the first metatarsal. A pseudoepiphysis may occur at the distal end. If the physis is injured, shortening may result and produce a deficiency on the longitudinal arch with further growth of the other bones. A buckle base injury may appear to be isolated on the initial radiograph; however, on follow-up, callus may be noted over other metatarsals, which is indicative of healing of nondisplaced fractures. A below-knee walking cast is all that is needed once the swelling has decreased.

Intraarticular fractures of the distal aspect of first metatarsal are uncommon and may or may not be associated with metatarsophalangeal dislocation. If displaced, these fractures are treated by anatomic reduction and internal fixation. Similar to other intraarticular fractures of the great toe, a cautious approach is recommended[164] (Fig. 15.75).

Second Metatarsal

Isolated fractures of the second metatarsal are rare. Fracture of this bone was associated with fractures of other metatarsals in 30 of 51 fractures of the lesser second through fifth metatarsals in the study from the Cincinnati Children's Hospital.[148] The most common mechanism of injury was indirect, such as jumping from a height of less than 5 feet. Other direct mechanisms included objects such as a rock, table, or chair falling on the foot. The fractures were rarely displaced, except in cases of severe trauma (e.g., foot run over by a car or a lawn mower). Most of these fractures can be treated with below-knee walking casts once the swelling has decreased.

The second metatarsal is more often subject to stress fracture. The injury occurs early in the second decade, is commonly called a march fracture, and usually occurs in runners. The authors have seen the injury in sedentary children who suddenly increase their walking or running activity. The child complains of persistent pain under the metatarsal arch. The initial radiographic results may be negative. MRI or bone scan could help with early diagnosis when clinical suspicion is high. Treatment most often consists of wearing a hard-soled shoe; rarely is a cast indicated. Displacement of

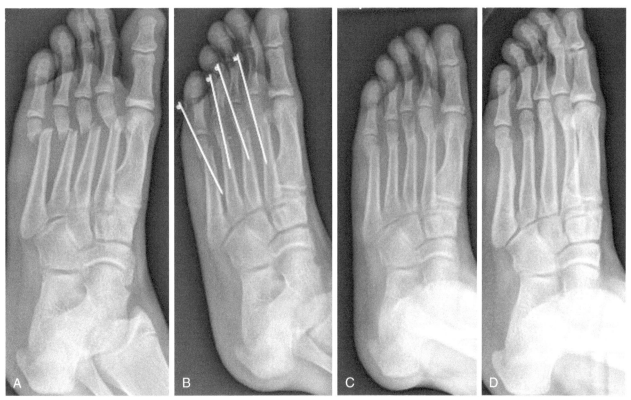

Fig. 15.73 A 12-year-old boy with direct blow from opponent's football helmet onto his left foot. (A) Oblique radiographs of 2-5 metatarsal neck fractures on day of injury. (B) One month after closed reduction and percutaneous pinning. (C) Near-complete healing 2 months postoperative; he returned to football and basketball 3.5 months postinjury. (D) Final 2-year follow-up with complete healing and remodeling and no pain.

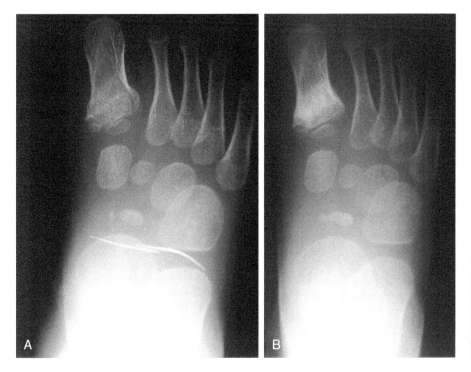

Fig. 15.74 Fractures of the base of the first metatarsal tend to buckle and have been termed *buckle base injuries;* these injuries heal uneventfully. (A) Initial anteroposterior (AP) radiograph showing a buckle fracture of the base of the first metatarsal. (B) Follow-up AP radiograph 3 weeks later; the fracture has healed, and remodeling is taking place.

the fragments is hardly ever seen. Periosteal cortical hypertrophy or new bone is generally present within 2 weeks after complaints of pain (Fig. 15.76).

Freiberg disease, or osteochondrosis of the second metatarsal head, may be confused with a fracture.[165] The second metatarsal is the longest and most rigidly fixed metatarsal

(Fig. 15.77). Repetitive trauma to the articular surface of the distal end of the second metatarsal may cause this injury. The injury usually occurs after intensive training for running sports and has been seen in avid young soccer players. Conservative treatment by rest or wearing a below-knee walking cast is recommended. Small osteochondral fragments

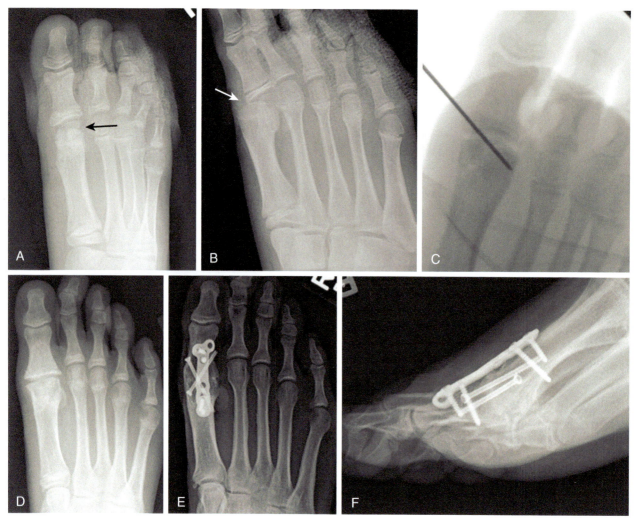

Fig. 15.75 (A and B) A 12-year-old boy with an open fracture-dislocation of the first metatarsophalangeal joint following fall of heavy weight on his foot. (C) He underwent open reduction and internal fixation of his articular fracture using K-wire. (D) Two years after his injury, he continued to have pain, and radiograph shows degenerative joint changes. (E and F) He eventually underwent first metatarsophalangeal arthrodesis. Patient remained asymptomatic 2 years after his fusion.

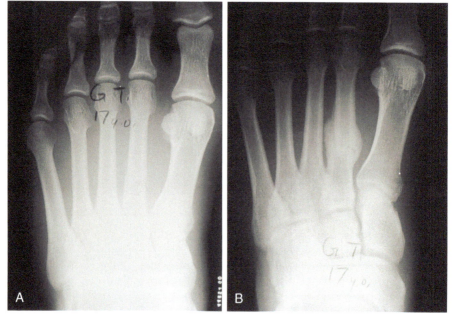

Fig. 15.76 Stress fracture of the second metatarsal. (A) The initial radiograph reveals a nondisplaced proximal second metatarsal fracture. (B) On follow-up, bulbous callus is noted around the fracture line at the base of the second metatarsal.

may be left in the second metatarsophalangeal joint. Open débridement with or without microfracture may be required for symptomatic patients who do not respond to conservative treatment; various other surgical procedures have been described in the literature.[166,167]

Fractures of the chondroepiphysis of the second metatarsal occur most frequently as Salter-Harris type II fractures of the neck. The injury is rarely displaced. Even fractures with plantar flexion tend to remodel. Condylar fractures are usually oblique Salter-Harris type IV fractures and rarely result in growth injuries (Fig. 15.78). Unless significantly displaced, these injuries are treated by below-knee casts and have resulted in good outcomes.

Fifth Metatarsal

The fifth metatarsal is a relatively common area of fracture. It was injured in 39 of 157 children and adolescents with metatarsal fractures; their average age was 12 years. The most common mechanism of injury was jumping during an athletic activity, such as basketball or volleyball.[148] The patient may complain of acute pain over the base of the lateral aspect of the foot and cease the activity immediately, or the child may be seen with a painful limp several days later. Initial radiographic findings may be negative and may show only soft tissue swelling over the lateral aspect of the foot. The presence of the apophysis (os vesalianum pedis) in this age group may cause it to be confused with a fracture. The

apophysis has longitudinal orientation, parallel to the metatarsal. A true fracture through the metatarsal usually has a transverse orientation (Fig. 15.79).

The intraosseous blood supply of the fifth metatarsal has been shown to be abundant in the region of the tuberosity, whereas the proximal diaphysis appears to depend on a longitudinal intramedullary blood supply derived from the nutrient artery.[168] This supports the vascular watershed concept often applied to the proximal metaphyseal-diaphyseal region of the fifth metatarsal and offers important anatomic support for fracture classification in this region. Thus, the

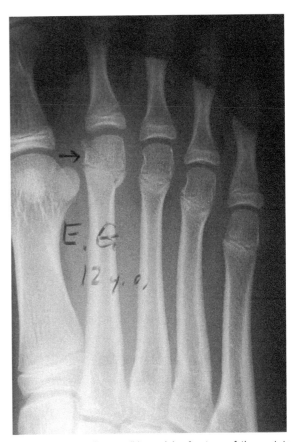

Fig. 15.78 Salter-Harris type IV condylar fracture of the metatarsal head. It healed uneventfully.

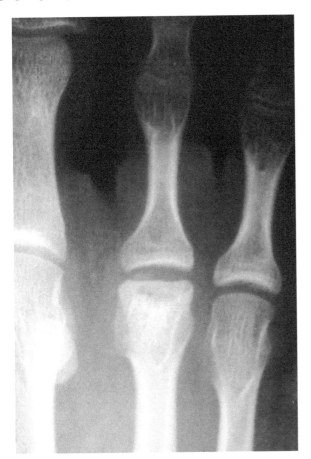

Fig. 15.77 This example of Freiberg disease was noted in an avid soccer player; the head of the second metatarsal of the right foot is flattened. A hard toeplate was inserted in the soccer shoe, and the patient continued playing with minimal difficulty.

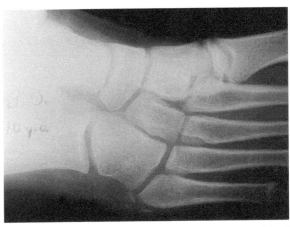

Fig. 15.79 Fracture of the os vesalianum pedis, an unusual fracture through the accessory apophysis.

spectrum of proximal fifth metatarsal fractures in children and adolescents includes apophyseal fractures, which have a very good prognosis for spontaneous healing, and fractures within the proximal watershed area, which have a rather guarded prognosis.[169] Ossification of the apophysis of the fifth metatarsal most commonly commences between 9 and 11 years of age in girls and between 11 and 14 years in boys.[170] Apophyseal closure (union with the shaft) typically follows 2 to 3 years after initiation of ossification.[170]

Incorporation of available anatomic and clinical data allows classification of proximal fifth metatarsal fractures in children and adolescents into at least six major categories: (1) apophyseal avulsions (involving either part or all of the variably ossified apophysis); (2) apophyseal stress fractures (Iselin disease); (3) tuberosity avulsion fractures; (4) Jones-type fractures through the metaphyseal-diaphyseal water-shaded area (typically a transverse fracture extending into the common articular facet of the fourth and fifth metatarsals);[171] (5) acute diaphyseal fractures; and (6) stress fractures of the diaphysis (Fig. 15.80). Most of these fractures (including the Jones-type fracture) heal rapidly in children after simple cast immobilization along with a variable period of protected weightbearing.

Older adolescents and teenagers may face adultlike challenges (slow healing or even nonunion) associated with Jones-type fracture (Fig. 15.81). At times, surgery is undertaken to either treat or minimize the risk of poor healing. Formal bone grafting of an established nonunion may be necessary. Cannulated screw fixation has become the norm for internal fixation of these fractures, especially in athletes. The general principle is that the largest screw accepted by the metatarsal should be used.[172–174] Refracture may occur after implant removal or even with an intramedullary screw in place.[175]

It is possible that the avulsion fracture that occurs in children is a result of the tendinous portion of the abductor digiti minimi and the tough lateral cord of the plantar aponeurosis inserting into the base. Most of these fractures can be treated by below-knee walking casts. Fractures with intraarticular displacement may require surgical treatment

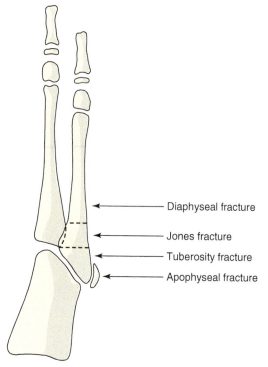

Diaphyseal fracture

Jones fracture

Tuberosity fracture

Apophyseal fracture

Fig. 15.80 Fifth metatarsal fractures in children.

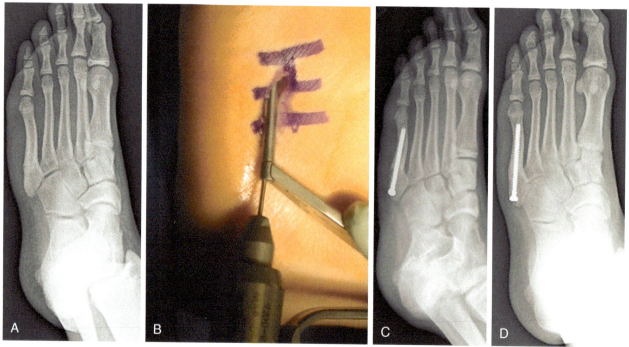

Fig. 15.81 (A) Fifth metatarsal base fracture at the meta-diaphyseal junction (Jones fracture). (B) Percutaneous cannulated screw placement to allow for adequate and timely healing of the fracture. The size and placement of the screw should be confirmed on two orthogonal fluoroscopic views. (C and D) Two months and 6 months postoperative, the fracture has healed.

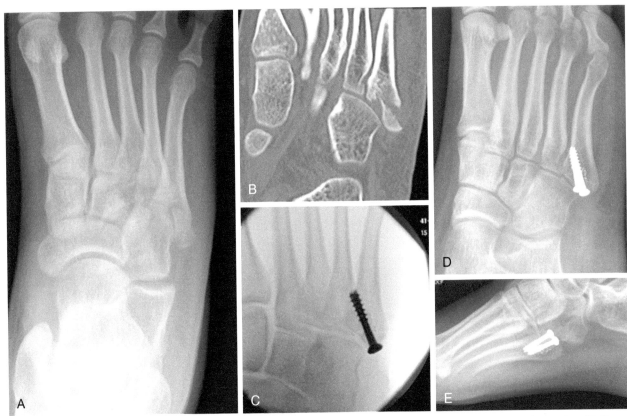

Fig. 15.82 (A) Fracture at the base of the fifth metatarsal involving the tuberosity in a 15-year-old girl following a fall while running. (B) Computed tomography scan shows disruption of the fifth tarsometatarsal joint. (C) The fracture was treated with open reduction and internal fixation. (D and E) Oblique and lateral radiographs, 1 year postoperative, show complete healing of the fracture.

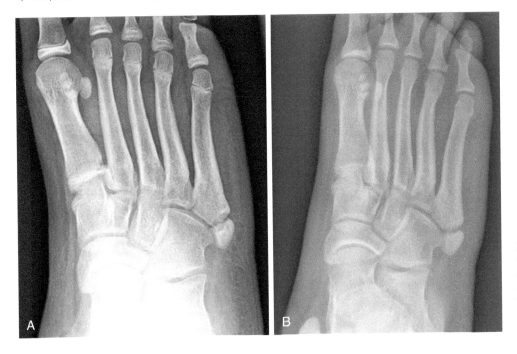

Fig. 15.83 (A) An 11-year-old girl with fracture of the fifth metatarsal tuberosity, which was treated conservatively. (B) Four years after initial injury, radiograph shows nonunion of the fracture; patient remained asymptomatic.

(Fig. 15.82). Nonunion is rare but can occur (Fig. 15.83). It occasionally may take longer than 4 to 6 weeks for radiographic bony union. Patients not showing union are immobilized only until they are pain free and are then allowed to return to their athletic activity.

Traction apophysitis at the base of the fifth metatarsal (Iselin disease) is common in active adolescents but it is either misdiagnosed or underreported.[176] A history of significant trauma is generally absent, although symptoms begin after an inversion injury. Children who are involved in sports that cause inversion stress on the forefoot appear to be especially prone. Examination shows the tuberosity to be larger than on the opposite side, with local soft tissue swelling and tenderness at the area of insertion of the peroneus brevis.

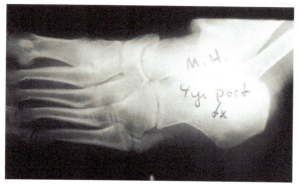

Fig. 15.84 Example of Iselin disease of the base of the fifth metatarsal. This condition is treated only until it is asymptomatic. The child was asymptomatic when seen for another problem approximately 4 years after his initial treatment.

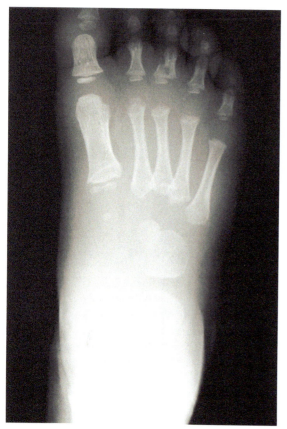

Fig. 15.85 A 3-year-old child with a third-ray proximal phalangeal fracture. These injuries may be buddy taped and tend to do well.

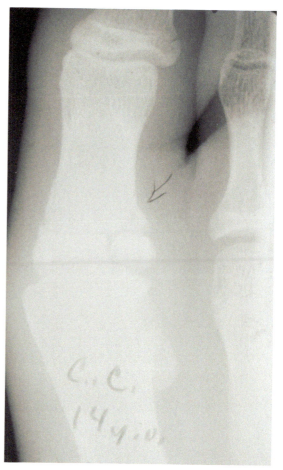

Fig. 15.86 Salter-Harris type III fracture through the articular surface of the proximal phalanx. Reduction and fixation are indicated if the fracture involves more than one-third of the articular surface and shows more than 2 mm of separation after reduction.

PHALANGEAL FRACTURES

Phalangeal fractures occurred in 31 of 175 children with fractures about the foot.[148] Twenty fractures (64%) occurred in the proximal phalanges, nine (29%) occurred in the middle, and two (6.4%) occurred in the distal phalanges. The usual mechanism of injury is either as a result of trauma from a falling object or because of stubbing of the unprotected toe against a hard surface. Rarely is operative reduction of a phalangeal fracture necessary; usually, traction, manipulative reduction, and buddy taping (i.e., taping the toe to an adjacent toe) after reduction is all that is needed (Fig. 15.85). In a young, active child, a below-knee cast may be applied past the toes for further protection for 3 to 4 weeks. In adolescents, a hard-sole or "postop" shoe is recommended for 3 to 4 weeks.

Fracture of the physis of the proximal phalanx of the great toe may involve the articular surface (Fig. 15.86). At times, the fracture may be confused with a normal vertical cleft in the physis; contralateral radiographs can help. The percentage of articular surface involved and its displacement determine the need for anatomic reduction. Anatomic reduction and internal fixation of the fragment are indicated when more than 30% of the articular surface is involved or when intraarticular displacement is greater than 2 mm. After anatomic reduction, the fragment should be stabilized with K-wires

Radiographs show enlargement of the apophysis and often fragmentation; in addition, the chondro-osseous junction may be widened (Fig. 15.84). Immobilization appears to help with the acute pain, and when the tenderness is completely resolved, physical therapy increases strength and coordination. Other conservative treatment modalities that have been successfully used include antiinflammatory medications, orthotics, relative rest, and activity modifications.[177] Bony union occurs in most patients. In a single reported case, conservative treatment failed, and surgical excision of the fragment was performed.[178] Early recognition and treatment would prevent long-term complications.

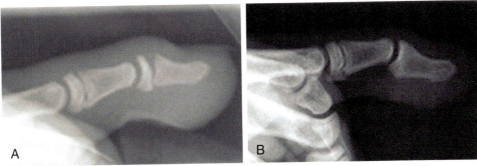

Fig. 15.87 (A) Radiograph showing Salter-Harris type II fracture of the distal phalanx in a 14-year-old boy who stubbed his toe and sustained a hyperflexion injury. Formal irrigation and débridement were performed. These injuries are frequently open injuries, and thus, open fracture management principles apply. The nail matrix may be interposed in the fracture site. Clinically, the angulation does not cause significant deformity. If reduction is required for increased angulation or deformity, these fractures remain stable after reduction, and internal fixation is usually not necessary. (B) Radiograph 6 months after injury shows that the physis had closed.

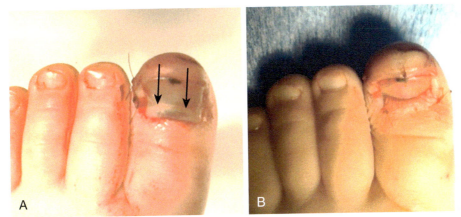

Fig. 15.88 (A) The laceration on the side of the nail was repaired in the emergency department, but the nail was on top of the eponychium instead of under it. A longer nail length or longer length of lunula (*arrows*) compared with contralateral side would indicate that the nail is positioned over the nail fold. (B) After removal of nail, repair of underlying nail bed laceration and repositioning of the nail under the eponychium. The nail would eventually fall off, but interposition of the nail between the eponychium and nail bed would prevent formation of adhesions between them, provide a biologic dressing, provide a mold for the nail bed, and act as a splint as underlying injuries heal.

or screws to prevent displacement. Closed reduction without fixation could allow persistent instability and a step-off of the fragments. Degenerative arthritis and hallux rigidus may occur. Rarely does incomplete reduction result in the formation of a bony bridge. In a series of 10 children (age range: 8.7–15.7 years) with displaced intraarticular fractures of great toe, open reduction (dorsal approach) and K-wire fixation was performed in nine cases. Seven fractures involved the base of proximal phalanx, of which four were Salter-Harris fractures through open physis; three fractures involved the neck. There were six significant complications: one suffered a refracture, one developed posttraumatic arthritis requiring interphalangeal joint fusion, one developed fibrous nonunion with AVN of the fragment, one had K-wire migration, and two underwent revision open reduction and internal fixation (one for postoperative displacement and one for painful nonunion).[164] The authors thus recommended a cautious approach for intraarticular fractures of the great toe.

A distal phalangeal epiphyseal fracture (Salter-Harris I or II) of the great toe could be an open fracture if there is any bleeding underneath or around the nail.[179] These "Pinckney" fractures represent the foot counterpart of the well-known Seymour fracture of the hand.[180] The typical mechanism of this injury is a stubbed toe because of

hyperflexion force causing an apex dorsal fracture through the physis (Fig. 15.87). Because of the close proximity of the distal phalangeal physis to the nail bed and matrix and because of thin skin at the base of the nail, it is common for these injuries to violate the soft tissue barrier, allowing for contamination of the fracture site. The proximal part of the nail may be lifted off to lie on the skin fold instead of under it (Fig. 15.88). These fractures should be treated with irrigation and débridement and early antibiotic administration. The fracture displacement is usually not severe enough to cause significant deformity or require reduction. Rarely, the fracture is unstable and may require fixation. If there is interposed nail matrix in the fracture site, it should be removed. The nail bed laceration should be repaired. The nail plate can be cleaned and replaced to serve as biologic dressing. Buddy taping and hard-sole shoe is sufficient to allow the injury to heal. As with any open fracture, infection and osteomyelitis are common when presentation is delayed or appropriate treatment is not administered (Fig. 15.89). Besides infection, the family should be counseled about other potential complications, including irregular nail, physeal arrest, and growth disturbances.

Besides these hyperflexion injuries, Park et al described four other mechanisms and specific injury patterns resulting from

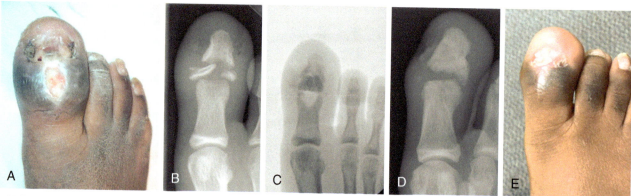

Fig. 15.89 (A and B) Infected great toe with osteomyelitis of the distal phalangeal physis in a 12-year-old boy, about 6 weeks after the injury. (C) The sequestered epiphysis was removed, and antibiotic-laden cement was placed in the dead space to control the fulminant infection. (D and E) Two months after initiation of treatment (cement removed in the interim), infection was under control, and the soft tissues/bone had healed.

barefoot stubbing injury of the great toe in 41 children.[181] These mechanisms included hyperextension, hyperabduction-flexion (most common), hyperabduction-extension, and hyperextension-adduction. The second most common mechanism was hyperabduction-extension injury in which avulsion fracture of the lateral volar condyle of the proximal phalanx was noted; this injury carried the worst prognosis with conservative treatment, and the authors recommended aggressive treatment.

Fractures of the proximal phalanges of the lateral four toes rarely require more than symptomatic treatment. They are seldom displaced enough to require operative treatment, and buddy taping tends to work well for these fractures. Fortunately, minor alignment disturbances hardly ever cause clinical problems. If these fractures are significantly displaced, closed or open reduction and internal fixation with K-wires may be necessary.

FOREFOOT DISLOCATIONS

Dislocations of the interphalangeal or metatarsophalangeal joints of the foot are extremely rare. Only four patients with dislocation of the joints of the foot were seen in 175 children with fractures and other injuries about the foot;[148] three of the four were older than 10 years. All except one sustained proximal interphalangeal joint dislocations of the second or third digits (Fig. 15.90). One child dislocated the metatarsophalangeal joint of the fifth ray (Fig. 15.91). Reductions of all the dislocations were uneventful; treatment consisted of buddy taping and a hard-soled shoe. A case of irreducible dislocation of proximal interphalangeal joint of second toe in a 6-year-old girl required open reduction and removal and repair of interposed medial collateral ligament.[182] Another case of proximal interphalangeal joint fracture-dislocation of fourth toe in a 10-year-old girl required open reduction and internal fixation of the plantar plate avulsion fracture from the middle phalanx.[183] Open dislocation of toe represents severe injury and would require prompt recognition, antibiotics, and surgical débridement (Fig. 15.92).

COMPARTMENT SYNDROME

Nine compartments of the foot have been identified. These include medial, lateral, superficial central, calcaneal (deep central), adductor, and four interossei compartments. Claw toe deformity attributed to missed compartment syndrome

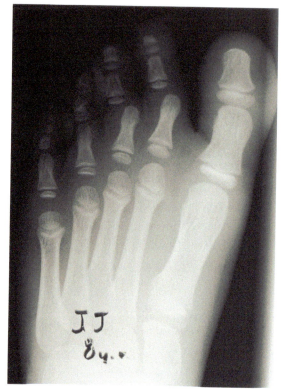

Fig. 15.90 Interphalangeal joint dislocations of the second and third toes. Reduction was easily accomplished by longitudinal traction and maintained by buddy taping.

of the foot is as a result of contracture of quadratus plantae muscle in the calcaneal compartment.[118] If compartment syndrome is suspected, pressure measurements should be obtained in the calcaneal and interossei compartments because they are more sensitive indicators of occult compartment syndrome of the foot.[184–186]

In a systematic review, Wallin et al summarized 11 studies that reported on 62 children with compartment syndrome of foot.[187] Of these, 59 cases had traumatic etiology, which included crush injuries, motor vehicle accidents, and compression force. History of high-velocity injury, swelling, and significant pain out of proportion are helpful in diagnosis of compartment syndrome but should not be used solely for diagnosis. Compared with compartment syndrome in other areas of the body, the signs and symptoms of compartment syndrome of foot are less reliable. Emergent compartment pressure measurements are indicated. Radiographic findings may be unremarkable due to lack of skeletal maturity. All patients underwent fasciotomies. Complications that were noted included muscle necrosis, arthritis, complex regional pain syndrome (CRPS), toe amputation, AVN of the growth plate, and hallux valgus. A high index of clinical suspicion, early recognition, and prompt treatment were critical in preventing morbidity and permanent disabilities.

Silas and colleagues[186] reviewed compartment syndrome of the foot in children. They found that the cause of compartment syndrome was a crush injury in six patients and a motor vehicle accident in one. All patients had swelling and pain with passive motion, but none had neurovascular deficits.

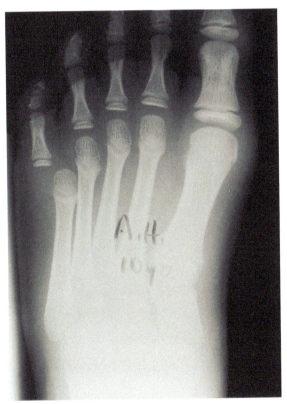

Fig. 15.91 Metatarsophalangeal dislocation of the fifth toe. Reduction and stabilization were achieved by traction and buddy taping.

Only the two oldest children had osseous injuries that necessitated open reduction and internal fixation, but all had elevated compartment pressure ranging from 38 to 55 mm Hg.

Fasciotomy to release all nine compartments is usually performed using the three-incision technique (Fig. 15.93). The incisions should be generous, and fascial release should extend down to the bone. Medial and lateral longitudinal incisions are made over the second and fourth metatarsals and are used to decompress the interossei and adductor compartments. The hindfoot incision is made over the medial portion of the heel at the glabrous skin border and is used to decompress the medial, central, and lateral compartments. The fasciotomy wounds are either packed open or a negative-pressure wound therapy unit is applied. K-wire fixation can be used to stabilize the bones but is rarely necessary. Delayed primary closure is performed in 5 to 7 days or once the swelling subsides (Fig. 15.94).

LAWN MOWER INJURIES

Lawn mowers remain a common source of serious injury and morbidity for children. An estimated 75,000 lawn mower–related injuries occur annually in the United States. The estimated annual cost for these injuries is $253 million, not including monetary damage for pain and suffering. It is estimated that 7 million new lawn mowers are purchased annually and that more than 30 million are used in the United States.[188]

Lawn mower injuries in children differ from comparable injuries in adults in several ways. First, a child's growth potential may be altered by direct injury to the physis, indirect stimulation of growth by the repair process, or inhibition of growth from neurovascular injury to that part. Second, vessel size may influence the choice of free tissue transplant,[189] the ability to repair a vessel, or both. Third, children in general tolerate prolonged immobilization better than adults do, and children tend to have better rehabilitative potential.[190]

These injuries represent some of the more contaminated injuries that one sees in pediatric orthopedics.[191] Dormans and colleagues[190] recommend that all patients be treated with fluid replacement, blood replacement (when appropriate), and intravenous triple antibiotics (i.e., penicillin, cefazolin, and an aminoglycoside).[190] Tetanus status should be evaluated, and appropriate coverage should be implemented. They further recommend that all wounds be débrided no fewer than two times and that early closure be avoided. Two types

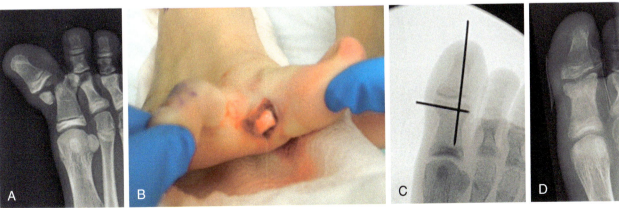

Fig. 15.92 (A and B) Open interphalangeal joint fracture-dislocation in a 10-year-old girl. (C) She underwent surgical débridement and internal fixation of the proximal phalangeal fracture and stabilization of the interphalangeal joint using K-wires. (D) Three months after injury, the fracture had healed, and patient was asymptomatic.

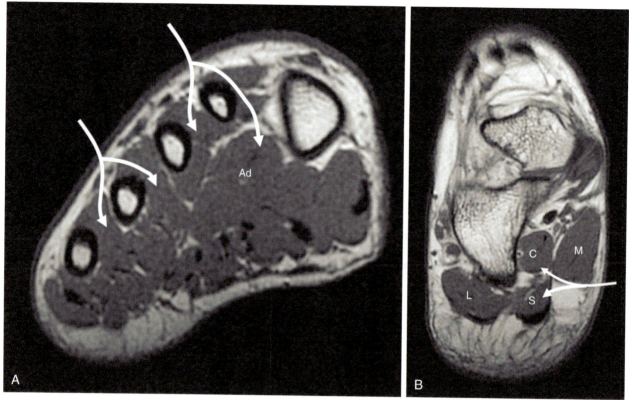

Fig. 15.93 (A) Magnetic resonance imaging (MRI) axial section through the forefoot. For fasciotomy of the foot, an incision over the second and the fourth metatarsal can help decompress all four interossei and adductor (*Ad*) compartments. (B) MRI axial section through the hindfoot. For fasciotomy, a medial approach can decompress all four compartments, including medial (*M*), lateral (*L*), superficial (*S*), and calcaneus (*C*) compartment.

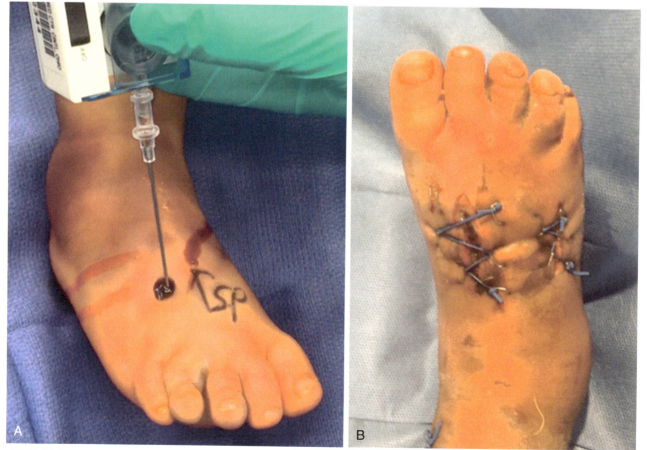

Fig. 15.94 (A) Compartment pressure measurement in a 4-year-old girl with suspected compartment syndrome. (B) Fasciotomy was performed and the incisions were closed 7 days later without the need for skin graft.

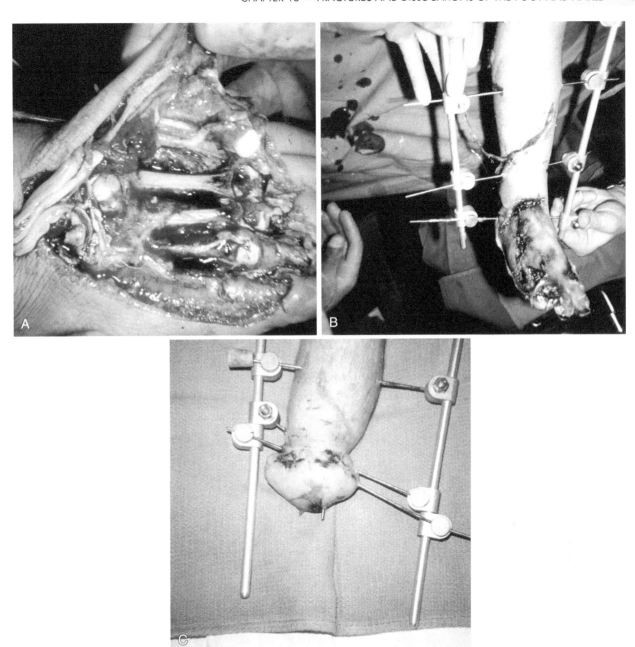

Fig. 15.95 Shredding injury. A severe contaminated lawn mower injury with comminuted tibial and fibular fractures was treated by external fixation and closure of the dorsal foot wound. The wound was closed, possibly injudiciously, but the parents refused to accept immediate amputation. After referral, the severe foot injury was treated definitively by Boyd-Syme amputation. (A) Initial clinical photograph showing complete destruction of the soft tissue over the dorsal lateral aspect of the foot. The wound was extensively débrided and closed. (B) At the time of referral, the dorsal soft tissue was completely necrotic. Because of the extensive loss of tendons and bone, a Boyd-Syme amputation was performed, with the plantar skin and heel pad maintained to allow weightbearing. Delayed primary closure was performed at 5 to 6 days. (C) Two threaded Steinmann pins were used to secure the weightbearing skin to the calcaneus. The fracture united uneventfully, and the child was able to fully ambulate on the stump.

of lawn mower injuries have been identified: a shredding injury, which is most common and either intercalary or distal (Fig. 15.95), and a paucilaceration type of injury (Fig. 15.96). The shredding injuries had the worst results. All patients with shredding type injury either required an amputation or had poor results with limb salvage; the authors recommended early amputation for these patients to prevent prolonged hospitalizations, higher incidence of surgical problems, and more complications. Patients with paucilaceration-type injury had excellent outcomes after limb salvage.[190]

Vosburgh and associates[192] found that riding mower injuries were more severe and resulted in a poorer functional outcome and more surgical procedures than did walk-behind mower injuries. All their cases of below-knee amputation, ankle disarticulation, and free vascularized grafting resulted from riding mower injuries. No patient sustaining an injury from a walk-behind mower required blood transfusion. They identified two areas that are somewhat controversial and in which their series differed from other reported series. The first was the conclusion that great toe amputation did not lead to severe disability in children. This statement is in contrast to Myerson and colleagues,[193] who concluded that amputation of the hallux proximal to the insertion of the flexor mechanism leads to instability of the first ray, loss of intrinsic strength, and lateral

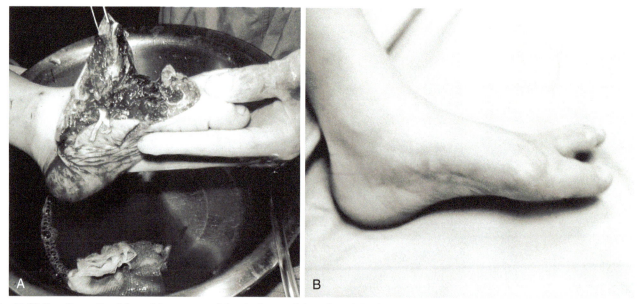

Fig. 15.96 Paucilaceration injury. A lawn mower injury to the medial portion of the forefoot severed the extensor hallucis longus, the extensor digitorum longus, and the brevis tendons and fractured the first metatarsal. It was treated by vigorous débridement and delayed primary closure. (A) At initial débridement, the extensor hallucis longus and extensor digitorum longus and brevis were all lacerated, and the first metatarsal bone was filleted. Aggressive débridement was performed, with a "second look" carried out in 3 days, at which time the long and short extensors were repaired, the fracture was pinned, and the wound was closed over a drain. (B) Six months after the injury, the wound is completely healed, and the child has excellent function, except for extension of the great toe. This type of result can be expected only in young children.

shift of forefoot pressure to the lesser toes. Because Vosburgh and colleagues' series[192] showed no significant problems, those authors found that heroic surgical measures to preserve the great toe were not required to ensure a satisfactory functional outcome for this particular foot injury.

The second area involves lacerations of the Achilles tendon. Vosburgh and associates[192] determined that it was more important to obtain a clean wound for closure than to consider repair and transfer early after Achilles tendon lacerations. They found that three of four patients with complete disruption and segmental loss of the Achilles tendon were able to ambulate independently without orthoses or special shoes when a "physiologic tendon" was permitted to develop by scar formation after irreparable laceration of the triceps surae.

In a multicenter study, Loder and colleagues[194] reported on gas-powered lawn mower injuries in 144 children with an average age at injury of 7 years. The child was the machine operator in 36 cases, a bystander in 84, and a passenger in 21. Amputations occurred in 67 children; the most common level was the toes (63%). Children injured by a riding lawn mower were typically younger, had a longer hospital stay, and required more surgery. Blood transfusions were given to 35 children. Fifty-six procedures were performed after initial hospital discharge. They reported that if children younger than 14 years had not been permitted around the lawn mowers, approximately 85% of the injuries in their report would have been prevented.

Lawn mower and threshing machine injuries are quite common in children in rural communities. Considerable judgment is required when managing these injuries. The force of injury causes soft tissue contamination by grass, shoe material, socks, and other debris. One should never make an early decision concerning the sterility or the ultimate viability of the tissue. The injury may involve the physis at multiple levels, possibly even excising the growth center. The injury may include loss of the articular surfaces and the collateral ligaments. Vigorous débridement and irrigation

are performed immediately. Avulsed tissue is usually less vital than it appears when first seen. This severe trauma may involve degloving of the bone and detachment of the perichondrial ring, with the subsequent development of a callus bridge between the epiphysis and metaphysis resulting in bar formation across the physes.[11] Early aggressive closure should be avoided until the issues of wound viability and sterility are resolved.

WOUND COVERAGE

The distal portion of the lower extremity is occasionally injured to the extent that either severe loss of soft tissue occurs or the injury results in nonviable tissue. This may result in extensive exposure of the fracture site, stripping of the periosteum, and exposure of bone, tendons, or neurovascular structures. In such cases, wound coverage is extremely important. The wound is thoroughly débrided of all necrotic and nonviable tissue. In the presence of underlying unstable fracture or dislocation, K-wires or an external fixator can be applied to achieve stability of the extremity and allow for wound management. A negative-pressure wound therapy (vacuum-assisted closure) has gained popularity and is widely used across all ages.[195] Repeated débridement at 48 to 72 hours interval may be required to completely resect nonviable or contaminated tissue and achieve healthy tissue margin. Wet to dry dressings or negative-pressure wound dressings can help form granulation tissue. Based on the size, depth, and location of the wound, definitive wound closure is planned. If secondary healing is not considered to be sufficient, then split-thickness skin grafting or free tissue transfer may be required for definitive wound closure. The preferred donor sources for free tissue transfer in children include the latissimus dorsi, the rectus abdominis, and the gracilis; these surgeries are preferably done by plastic surgeons (Fig. 15.97).

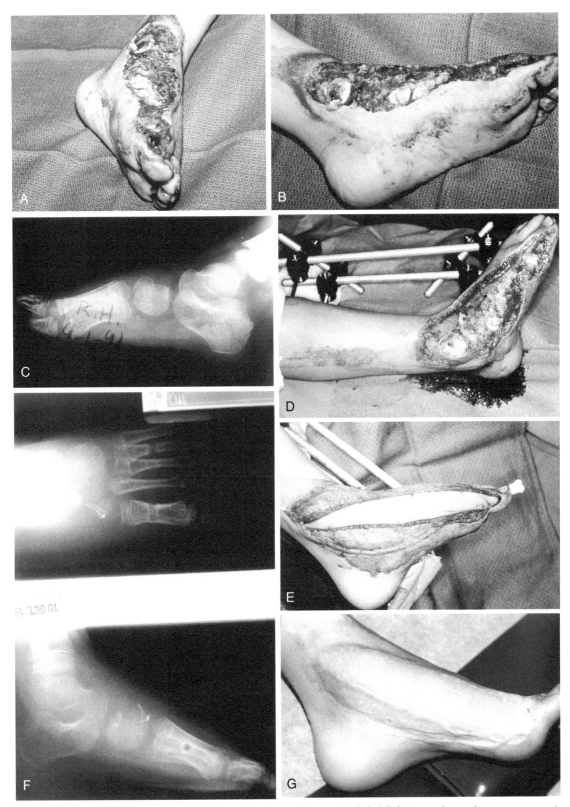

Fig. 15.97 This 4-year-old boy was in an auto accident in which the medial aspect of his left foot was dragged across a concrete surface; all the soft tissues overlying the medial malleolus, tarsals, metatarsal, and phalanges of the great toe were abraded. He underwent débridement and external fixation followed by free tissue transfer, skin grafting, and subsequent peroneus longus tendon transfer. (A) Soft tissue loss over the medial malleolus, tarsals, metatarsal, and phalanges of the great toe, with exposure of the underlying joints. The tibialis anterior and extensor hallucis longus tendons were abraded off. (B) Medial view. (C) Radiograph of the foot at the time of injury. No evidence of bony injury was noted. An external fixator was applied to allow for management of the wound while immobilizing the ankle to prevent deformity from asymmetric muscle forces. (D) After placement of an external fixator and initial débridement before reconstruction of the defect. (E) Closure of the defect with a free latissimus dorsi microvascular flap and split-thickness skin grafting. End-to-side reanastomosis was performed on the posterior tibial artery, high above the zone of injury. (F) Radiographs after peroneal tendon transfer for the anterior tibialis. (G) Four-year follow-up. (Courtesy Dr. David Billmire, Director of Plastic Surgery, Children's Hospital Medical Center, Cincinnati, OH.)

AMPUTATION

On occasion, the severity of an injury to an extremity is such that free tissue transfer, skin grafting, or replantation cannot be achieved (Fig. 15.95). In that case, amputation must be performed. An epidemiologic study on lower extremity amputations in children reported toe amputations to be the most common amputation, mostly caused by lawn mowers and machinery.[196] Foot and ankle amputations comprised about 6% of all amputations, and there was a six times higher likelihood of such amputations in children younger than 5 years of age than those 6 years of age and above. Loder had reported similar findings that 54 of 69 (78%) children with lawn mower–related amputations were younger than 5 years of age.[197] After 12 years of age, most amputations were related to motor vehicle crashes (25.6%) and pedestrian injuries (15.4%).

Amputations in children are occasionally performed at unconventional sites, as opposed to the ankle, Lisfranc joint, or Chopart joint. More often than not, every effort is made to maintain length. For foot amputations, the authors prefer a Boyd-Syme type of amputation. If the child has a shredding laceration that includes all of the dorsum of the foot, it is important to make an effort to preserve the plantar skin of the foot, which is good for weightbearing. The level of amputation is sometimes determined by the most viable proximal segment of tissue and bone. Transmetatarsal amputations are not necessarily as good as through-the-joint amputations (e.g., Chopart joint or Lisfranc joint) because of the possibility of stump overgrowth of the metatarsal segments, which may necessitate additional operations in the future. In a child younger than 10 years, when a midfoot amputation through the Chopart joint is a possibility, the authors recommend excising the talus, débriding the cartilage from the mortise as well as the dorsum of the calcaneus, and fusing the calcaneus to the mortise (Boyd technique). The malleoli will diminish in size over the years and will not present a problem for prosthetic fitting at the heel. It is important that balance of the anterior tibial or peroneal tendons be preserved; otherwise, it is possible that persistent plantar flexion contractures will develop secondary to overpull of the Achilles tendon. To prevent this, it is strongly recommended that a segment of no less than 1 inch of Achilles tendon be excised.

LACERATION INJURIES OF THE FOOT

Laceration of soft tissue structures may occur in association with open injuries or open fractures of the foot. One should carefully examine the limb for injury to nerves, vessels, or tendons. Besides infection and wound issues, laceration injuries of the foot may result in deformity, especially if the Achilles tendon, the anterior tibial tendon, or the posterior tibial tendon is involved and missed. These tendons are the only ones requiring immediate or delayed repair. Little indication exists for direct repair of the extensor hallucis longus, the long-toe flexor, or the long-toe extensors because little disability occurs after these injuries.

PUNCTURE WOUNDS

In children who have stepped on a nail, with or without shoes, the diagnosis is clear; in the absence of such a history, a radiograph to exclude a radiopaque foreign body is indicated. *Pseudomonas* is the most common organism cultured from children who have stepped on nails.[198] The age-old question of tennis sneaker glue harboring *Pseudomonas* has not been answered. Two cases of *Mycobacterium fortuitum* osteomyelitis secondary to a nail puncture wound in the foot have been described; one affected the cuboid, and the other affected the calcaneus. *Staphylococcus aureus* is also a common organism with puncture wounds.

These patients present with increasing pain, swelling, erythema or discharge after about 5 to 10 days of a penetrating injury. Based on the location and depth of the puncture wound, cellulitis, abscess, osteomyelitis, or septic arthritis should be considered (Fig. 15.98). The initial radiographs may be negative. If or when in doubt, an MRI may help to establish diagnosis. Tetanus toxoid and appropriate antibiotics should be promptly started. In presence of abscess, septic joint or foreign body, débridement is performed. The wound should be left open, or a drain should be inserted. The possibility of premature physeal arrest or AVN of the epiphysis should be considered. If the MTP joint is involved, early chondrolysis of the articular surfaces with fibrosis and subsequent arthritis may occur. The family should be informed of the possibility of growth plate involvement and be advised to continue follow-up examinations. Occasionally, older children are seen with short third or fourth toes and vague histories of stepping on nails or with occult foot injuries incurred at an earlier age. It appears in retrospect that osteomyelitis, AVN, and growth arrest occurred (Fig. 15.99).

FOREIGN BODY

If a child complains of pain and has a persistent limp with no clear history of injury, one has to consider the possibility of a retained foreign body. A small healed poke hole or induration may be appreciated on the plantar aspect of the foot. The object may or may not be visible on radiographs. Although CT and MRI have been used in the past to localize objects, the authors prefer ultrasonography. Ultrasonography discriminates between both radiodense and radiolucent lesions. The object may be localized and then marked or removed under ultrasonic control (Fig. 15.100). Occasionally, a foreign body such as a needle is seen in the foot of an asymptomatic patient who receives a radiograph for other reasons (Fig. 15.101). The authors do not recommend removal of these asymptomatic objects.

Shells from gunshot wounds are a notorious type of foreign body (Fig. 15.102). Most often, the wound is accidental, self-inflicted, and located in the forefoot. Depending on the size and caliber of the bullet, a large amount of soft tissue injury and debris such as shoe material and socks may be seen. Segmental loss of bone may also occur. The wound should be vigorously irrigated and débrided but not closed. Multiple dressing changes are performed, followed by mesh skin graft coverage. Reconstructive procedures should be considered only after all wounds are cleaned and closed, which might take 6 to 8 months.[199]

MISCELLANEOUS CAUSES OF FOOT PAIN

Foot pain and reluctance to bear weight with no direct history of trauma should lead one to consider other conditions,

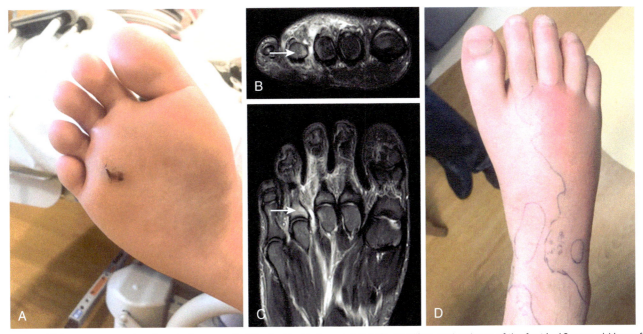

Fig. 15.98 (A) Puncture wound on the plantar aspect of the foot led to increasing pain, swelling, and redness of the foot in 16-year-old boy after stepping on a fire poker. (B and C) Magnetic resonance imaging shows evidence of osteomyelitis (*arrow*) of the proximal phalanx of the fourth toe. There was no abscess or septic joint. (D) Cellulitis extended on the dorsum of the foot and ankle. Patient responded well to parenteral antibiotics.

including infections, tarsal coalitions, stress fractures, tumors, and early inflammatory arthritis. The cause of the pain is usually age related. If plain radiographic findings are normal, and there is a strong index of suspicion, then an MRI may be indicated.

STRESS FRACTURES

Stress fractures usually occur after a sudden increase in activity in skeletally maturing adolescents who are starting to participate in intensive or repetitive sports training. The condition may be seen as early as 8 to 12 years of age. The most frequent sites are the proximal part of the tibia in 10- to 15-year-old patients, the distal end of the fibula in 2- to 5-year-old patients, and the second or third metatarsal in older adolescents (Fig. 15.76). In children, these fractures may be associated with foot deformities (e.g., cavus foot) or after correction of foot deformities, as weightbearing is transferred to the lesser metatarsals. Navicular stress fractures have also been reported in older adolescents and occur mainly in basketball players and runners.[200] Initial radiographs may be negative, and CT/MRI may be required to make a definitive diagnosis. If the fracture is nondisplaced, 4 to 6 weeks of below-knee cast is recommended. Healing is assessed on follow-up radiographs, which would likely show periosteal reaction around the fracture site. If displacement, delayed union beyond 12 weeks, or frank nonunion has occurred, internal fixation with bone grafting is indicated.[138] Internal fixation of certain stress fractures (navicular, fifth metatarsal) in athletes could allow earlier return to sports.

PATHOLOGIC OR FRAGILITY FRACTURES

Metabolic disease such as end-stage renal osteodystrophy may cause weakening of the bone at the metaphyseal-epiphyseal junction and subsequent fractures after trivial trauma.

In these same patients, brown tumors may also develop after secondary hyperparathyroidism, with resultant bone weakening (see Chapter 4). In addition, the bone may be undermined by constitutional disorders such as idiopathic juvenile osteoporosis, osteogenesis imperfecta, and congenital insensitivity to pain (Fig. 15.103) and by therapeutic procedures such as chemotherapy for leukemia or anticonvulsant medication such as phenytoin (Dilantin) for seizure disorders (Fig. 15.104).

Nonambulatory children with spina bifida, cerebral palsy, traumatic brain injury, or other neuromuscular disorders have a high risk of lower extremity fracture.[195,201] Such fractures are most common during early adolescence, with a reported annual incidence fracture rate of 29/1000.[202] In a study of 170 fractures in 92 patients with spina bifida, Akbar et al reported 10 (6%) fractures in the supramalleolar region, 5 (3%) fractures involving the distal tibial physis, and 1 (1%) fracture of the metatarsal.[203] The risk of fracture was sixfold higher in patients with thoracic level paralysis compared with those with sacral-level paralysis. Similarly, in another study, the risk of fracture was higher in patients with cerebral palsy whose Gross Motor Function Classification System (GMFCS) level was IV or V, when compared with those with GMFCS level I to III.[204] The increased risk of fracture can be explained by decreased bone density or osteoporosis due to reduced muscle activity in the affected limb with insufficient axial loading of the legs.[205] Such fractures can occur spontaneously or after orthopedic interventions, cast immobilization, or trivial trauma. Often, the initial presentation with swelling, erythema, and warmth, without a history of injury, may mimic infection or tumor. Radiographs show abundant callus formation, and the fracture tends to heal quickly. Immobilization with rigid cast should be minimized, as it can lead to further disuse

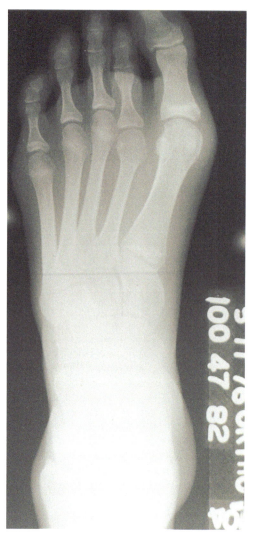

Fig. 15.99 This child was seen because a short second toe was developing. The history revealed that a nail had penetrated the child's foot when he was younger, and the toe became infected. It is believed that the retrospective history was that of osteomyelitis involving the physis, with subsequent growth arrest of the metatarsal.

osteopenia, and the vicious cycle of cast and fracture may continue. Treatment of these fractures should include bulky dressing, soft cast, or a splint for the shortest possible time. Prevention strategies have included calcium and vitamin D supplementation, bisphosphonates, and loading of the lower legs, although good-quality studies are lacking to support these recommendations.[206–208]

COMPLEX REGIONAL PAIN SYNDROME

CRPS is a syndrome characterized by severe regional pain with swelling, dysesthesia to light touch, and vasomotor instability that can lead to chronic trophic soft tissue changes, joint contractures, osteoporosis, and functional decline. In an attempt to classify patients by clinical signs and symptoms rather than pathophysiology, the term *reflex sympathetic dystrophy (RSD)* has been replaced by the new term *CRPS*, which is divided into two types: CRPS type I to replace RSD and CRPS type II to replace causalgia.[209]

In children, CRPS type I is much more common in girls, and a history of trauma (at times, trivial) is present in most cases. Lower extremity involvement is much more common than upper extremity involvement. In a group of 70 children treated for CRPSI, girls made up 84% of the affected patients, average age of onset was 12.5 years, and 87% had a lower extremity injury as the inciting event.[210] In a study of 24 children with CRPSI, 73% had specifically foot or ankle injuries.[211] Radiographic studies are not usually helpful in diagnosis. The spotty or patchy osteopenia typical of adults with CRPS is rare in children.[212] CRPS accounts for 11% of pediatric pain of uncertain origin.[213] Because the syndrome is relatively uncommon in children, diagnosis and treatment are often delayed. The delay in diagnosis prolongs the painful period and results in unnecessary and potentially morbid diagnostic and therapeutic interventions. Dysesthesia, vasomotor instability, and swelling of the affected area are found in most children with CRPS type I. Vasomotor instability (most commonly discoloration, temperature difference, and tache cérébrale) is present in almost all cases, and the diagnosis of CRPS should not be considered in its absence. Tache cérébrale

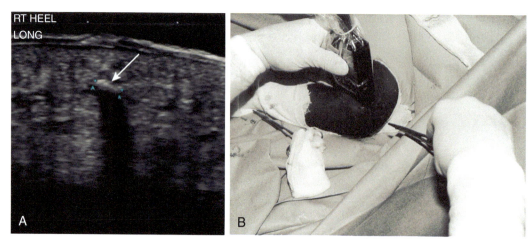

Fig. 15.100 Preoperative (A) and intraoperative (B) use of ultrasonography to remove foreign bodies allows the visualization of nonradiopaque and radiopaque objects. Its use is strongly recommended for prevention of the extensive dissection occasionally required to remove nonopaque foreign bodies.

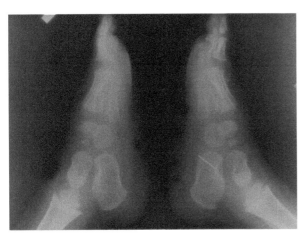

Fig. 15.101 A needle in the foot. This child was seen for another problem; the needle had apparently lodged in the foot several years earlier. Removal of an incidentally seen asymptomatic foreign body is contraindicated and is to be condemned.

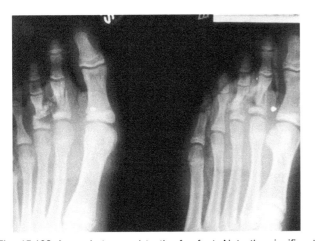

Fig. 15.102 A gunshot wound to the forefoot. Note the significant soft tissue swelling, phalangeal fractures, and metallic fragments. Most such injuries are self-inflicted through accident. They require extensive débridement, with the possibility of later skin grafting. Amputation is indicated for vascular compromise distal to the metatarsophalangeal joint.

is elicited by stroking the skin in the affected area with a blunt object, such as the head of a safety pin, and the contralateral limb is used as a control. Autonomic dysfunction is demonstrated by the appearance of an erythematous line 15 to 30 seconds after the stimulus; the line may persist as long as 15 minutes. This sign may be present before other signs of autonomic dysfunction appear.[213] The child may have a trivial injury to the lower extremity, followed by the full manifestations of CRPS type I. Dietz and colleagues[212] reported signs of vasomotor instability in 83% of CRPS cases, including color changes (60%), decreased temperature (58%), altered sweating (14%), and decreased pulses (16%). Local swelling was noted in 70% of their cases. The regional distribution was the foot and ankle (52%), arm (21%), knee (14%), hand (8%), and shoulder (5%). Limb-length discrepancy can develop in children secondary to altered blood flow and trophic changes.[209]

Early recognition and treatment of this disorder may provide the best prognosis. Some of these patients may have undergone extensive diagnostic testing as well as surgical procedures to address their pain. Most authors believe that physical therapy and mobilization are the best methods of treatment for this disorder; unfortunately, when most children complain of pain, immobilization is the first step in treatment, which may exacerbate CRPS type I.

Nonpharmacologic therapy has been successful in most cases reported in children. Children respond better to physical therapy and noninvasive treatments than adults but have higher rates of recurrence of symptoms.[210] Although children have reportedly had better outcomes after CRPS type I than adults, 54% of children in multidisciplinary treatment programs still have some CRPS type I symptoms 3 years after diagnosis.[214] Sherry and colleagues[215] reported on 103 children with CRPS type I. These patients were treated with an intense exercise therapy program for 14 days (daily 4 hours of aerobic and functionally directed exercise and 1 to 2 hours of hydrotherapy and desensitization). Seventy-seven percent were referred for psychologic counseling. Ninety-two percent of these patients recovered from all symptoms and regained full function. Recurrent episodes were seen in 31%, mostly within the first 6 months; the majority resolved with self-initiation of their exercise program.

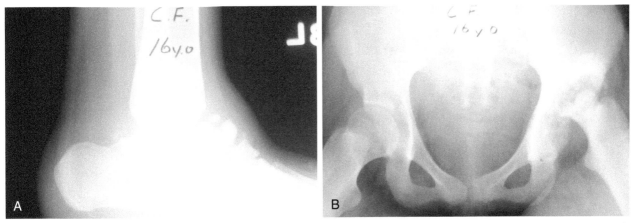

Fig. 15.103 This child has familial dysautonomia (congenital insensitivity to pain). (A) This lateral radiograph of the foot and ankle shows Charcot-like joints at the talonavicular cuneiform joints. (B) An anteroposterior view of the pelvis shows very similar Charcot-like changes in the hip with complete dissolution of the femoral head and marked distortion of the acetabulum.

A team approach to patients with chronic pain is important. The team should include an orthopedist, anesthesiologist, or rehabilitation medicine specialist, as well as physical and occupational therapist. A psychologist can also provide the necessary emotional and mental support. Early recognition may prevent a prolonged diagnostic encounter and morbidity. Practitioners who treat children should be familiar with CRPS and consider it when a child, usually female, is seen with considerable pain after trivial trauma that is out of proportion to the injury, especially when one is aware of potential psychologic disturbances or a dysfunctional family.

CHILDHOOD OBESITY AND FRACTURES

Obesity is an epidemic with an increased risk of musculoskeletal injuries. The association between young obese adults and severity of ankle fracture as well as loss of reduction after treatment of ankle fracture has been established.[216,217] Similar findings could be expected from childhood obesity and its association between ankle and foot fractures (Fig. 15.105), although there is paucity of literature related to it. Kessler et al investigated the relationship between childhood obesity and lower extremity fractures in a population-based cross-sectional study involving 913,178 patients aged 2 to 19 years.[218] Overweight, moderately obese, and extremely obese patients were 1.1 times, 1.2 times, and 1.4 times more likely to sustain a foot fracture when compared with normal-weight patients, respectively. Similarly, overweight, moderately obese, and extremely obese patients were 1.3 times, 1.3 times, and 1.5 times more likely to sustain a fracture of the ankle, knee, or leg when compared with normal-weight patients, respectively. The association was strongest in the 6- to 11-year-old age group. Two studies from level-1 trauma centers, including one from the authors' institution,

reported that obese children were significantly more likely to sustain lower extremity injuries than sustain head, face, or abdominal injuries than nonobese children, were more likely to need operative intervention, and had a higher risk of complications, including deep venous thrombosis and decubitus ulcers.[219,220]

APHORISMS FOR ANKLE AND FOOT INJURIES

Parents should be made aware of the possibility of a growth injury any time that an epiphysis is fractured. If the child is seen in the emergency department, the attending physician should impress on the parents how serious this issue is. The parents must be informed and made aware of the injury's potential to cause growth-related problems. The worst scenario is when growth arrest occurs and the parents were not even aware of the possibility.

Closed reduction is usually possible for most injuries around the foot and ankle. If the patient is under general anesthesia and anatomic reduction is accomplished, the authors strongly recommend percutaneous pinning or percutaneous use of an interfragmentary screw. Cannulated cancellous screws are optimal for this technique. The need for open reduction is minimal if the injuries are treated within 48 hours.

Soft tissue "goose egg" swelling over the distal end of the fibula usually represents a Salter-Harris type I growth plate injury. A fibular physeal fracture may or may not accompany a distal tibial physeal injury. After several weeks of treating an ankle sprain, the appearance of calcification around the distal fibular metaphysis or in the interosseous ligament is indicative of a previously unrecognized fracture.

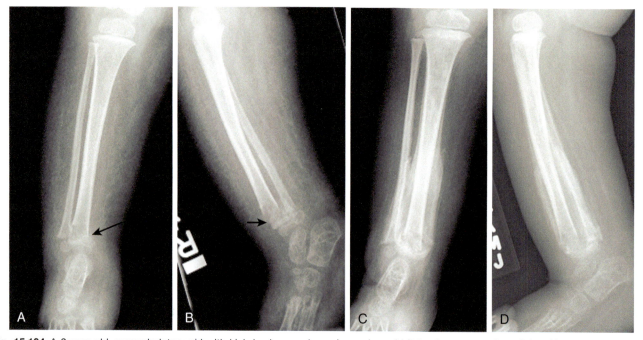

Fig. 15.104 A 2-year-old, nonambulatory girl with high lumbar myelomeningocele and bilateral cavovarus foot deformities was treated with ankle and foot orthoses braces. She was brought in for evaluation of a red, swollen ankle without any history of injury. Anteroposterior (A) and lateral (B) radiographs show osteopenia and insufficiency fractures involving the physis of distal tibia and fibula. Anteroposterior (C) and lateral (D) radiographs taken 3 weeks following application of soft cast show abundant callous formation.

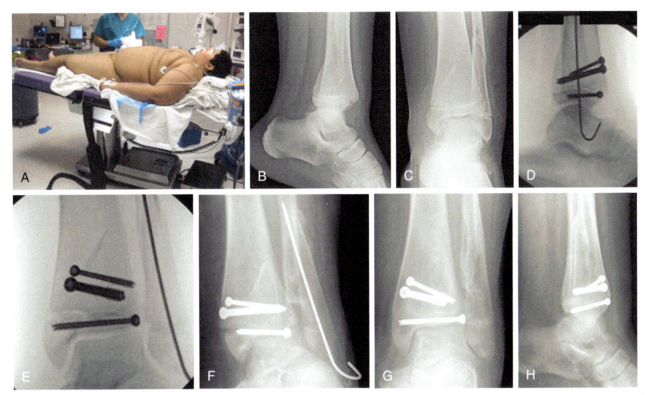

Fig. 15.105 (A) With increase in childhood obesity, it is not unusual to encounter patients weighing 380 lbs in a pediatric facility. The table had to be expanded using arm boards on either side to accommodate this 15-year-old boy who sustained a triplane ankle fracture with fibula fracture (B and C) after a dance twist and subsequent fall. Intraoperative fluoroscopic images (D and E) show anatomic reduction and internal fixation. (F) Radiograph taken 3 weeks after surgery show displacement of the fracture. There was a questionable history of fall and accidental weightbearing on the involved extremity. The fibular pin was removed, and the patient was treated with a well-molded below knee cast with satisfactory end result (G and H).

Epiphyseal injuries should be reduced within the first 24 to 48 hours; repeated manipulation after 5 or 6 days may be difficult and can cause epiphyseal damage. During reduction attempts, adequate muscle relaxation and traction should be used rather than forceful manipulation of the fracture. The authors would rather accept the malreduction after 1 week than risk injury to the growth plate.

The distal tibial and fibular ossification centers can vary, and sometimes these variants make the diagnosis of a fracture difficult. In most of these instances, the fracture is minor, with minimal displacement, and is adequately treated by simple immobilization. An MRI can differentiate an anomalous ossification pattern from a fracture.

Close attention must be paid to the direction of growth plate displacement after injury, especially the metaphyseal fragment. The direction of displacement of the metaphyseal fragment determines the mechanism of injury in most circumstances.

Epiphyseal articular fragment displacement of greater than 2 mm requires reduction. CT can be used not only to diagnose these injuries but also for surgical planning and to assess the reduction. It is more important that the articular cartilage rather than the metaphyseal-epiphyseal junction be anatomically reduced. The latter tends to remodel unless angulation is excessive or growth plate arrest has occurred.

An eccentric bony bridge is more likely to cause angular deformity than to significantly slow growth in a distal tibial injury because the central growth plate is too strong.

After injury, one should look closely at the growth arrest lines (Park-Harris) for evidence of bony bridging. These lines should be horizontal and parallel to the physis, and any tendency toward angulation into the fracture site indicates bony bridge formation.

A residual deformity with greater than 2 mm of displacement of the weightbearing articular surface after reduction is not compatible with a good result. Open reduction should be considered if manipulation under general anesthesia does not enable better apposition of the fragments. After having achieved anatomic reduction, one should be alert for possible instability; consequently, the authors strongly recommend a percutaneous pin or percutaneous interfragmentary screw to maintain stability.

Unrecognized damage to the articular cartilage at the time of injury may lead to chondrolysis and long-term symptoms in spite of adequate reduction and normal-appearing radiographic findings. The articular cartilage has poor remodeling potential, and injury tends to lead to arthritic changes.

Growth arrest is rare in triplane and Tillaux fractures. The child is usually an adolescent without much longitudinal growth remaining. The major residual problem is joint incongruity or an intraarticular gap greater than 2 mm, resulting in degenerative arthritis. All radiographs of the ankle should be made in no fewer than three planes; CT scan is recommended to determine the geometry of fracture fragments and to plan screw trajectory.

Mandatory follow-up of growth plate injuries for 1 year in children younger than 12 years is necessary. Managed healthcare plans are becoming more prevalent, and patients are constantly switching physicians as the plan dictates. This movement makes it extremely difficult to monitor patients who may or may not have a current problem but who have sustained a growth plate injury with a predictable future disability. One must be aware of "disappearing patients."

Angular deformity and shortening are usually asymptomatic. The patient returns because of deformity and not pain. Joint incongruity and articular cartilaginous injury leading to degenerative joint disease are more significant long-term problems that do cause pain.

The compartments of the foot are tight. Decompression is indicated for any persistent swelling, venous congestion, or taut skin or when multiple bones are involved. Compartment syndrome should be considered regardless of whether fractures are seen.

Displacement of metatarsal fractures is rare, but nonunion is not uncommon. There is a 15% rate of delayed union with metatarsal fractures, so patients should be followed until radiographic union. Medial or lateral displacement of the middle metatarsal (second through fourth) fracture fragments with varus or valgus angulation is acceptable, tends to remodel, and does not cause problems. Dorsal or plantar displacement is not acceptable because the resulting angular deformity alters the weightbearing pattern and leads to painful calluses.

A primary circular cast should be avoided for most ankle injuries because of the possibility of a tourniquet effect. It is recommended that a bulky dressing be used for initial management of these injuries. After several days, when the swelling has decreased, a well-molded cast is satisfactory.

Open reduction plus internal fixation of foot fractures is rarely indicated and should be avoided, if possible. Growth inhibition in and around the foot is unusual; overgrowth is more common. Usually, the only indications for open reduction of foot fractures are open injuries and significant soft tissue injury.

ACKNOWLEDGEMENT

The expertise and contribution of this chapter's prior authors (Drs. Alvin C. Crawford and Charles T. Mehlman) are greatly appreciated.

REFERENCES

The level of evidence (LOE) is determined according to the criteria provided in the Preface.

1. Galano G, Vitale MA, Kessler MW, et al. The most frequent traumatic orthopaedic injuries from a national pediatric inpatient population. *J Pediatr Orthop*. 2005;25:39–44. (**LOE II**).
2. Mann DC, Rajmaira S. Distribution of physeal and nonphyseal fractures in 2,650 long-bone fractures in children aged 0-16 years. *J Pediatr Orthop*. 1990;10:713–716. (**LOE IV**).
3. McNealy GA, Rogers LF, Hernandez R, et al. Injuries of the distal tibial epiphysis: systematic radiographic evaluation. *AJR Am J Roentgenol*. 1982;138:683–689. (**LOE IV**).
4. Kump WL. Vertical fractures of the distal tibial epiphysis. *Clin Orthop*. 1970;73:132–135. (**LOE IV**).
5. Ogden JA, Lee J. Accessory ossification patterns and injuries of the malleoli. *J Pediatr Orthop*. 1990;10:306–316. (**LOE V**).
6. Kramer DE, Cleary MX, Miller PE, Yen YM, Shore BJ. Syndesmosis injuries in the pediatric and adolescent athlete: an analysis of risk factors related to operative intervention. *J Child Orthop*. 2017;11(1):57–63. (**LOE IV**).
7. Dias LS, Tachdjian MO. Physeal injuries of the ankle in children: classification. *Clin Orthop Relat Res*. 1978;136:230–233. (**LOE IV**).
8. Kling TF Jr, Bright RW, Hensinger RN. Distal tibial physeal fractures in children that may require open reduction. *J Bone Joint Surg Am*. 1984;66:647–657. (**LOE IV**).
9. Peterson CA, Peterson HA. Analysis of the incidence of injuries to the epiphyseal growth plate. *J Trauma*. 1972;12:275–281. (**LOE IV**).
10. Spiegel PG, Cooperman DR, Laros GS. Epiphyseal fractures of the distal ends of the tibia and fibula. A retrospective study of 237 cases in children. *J Bone Joint Surg Am*. 1978;60:1046–1050. (**LOE IV**).
11. Rang M. *Children's Fractures*. Philadelphia: J.B. Lippincott. (**LOE V**).
12. Boutis K, Narayanan UG, Dong FFT, et al. Magnetic resonance imaging of clinically suspected Salter-Harris I fracture of the distal fibula. *Injury*. 2010;41:852–856. (**LOE IV**).
13. Kaye JJ, Bohne WH. A radiographic study of the ligamentous anatomy of the ankle. *Radiology*. 1977;125:659–667. (**LOE IV**).
14. Chande VT. Decision rules for roentgenography of clinical with acute ankle injuries. *Arch Pediatr Adolesc Med*. 1995;149:255–258. (**LOE III**).
15. Clark KD, Tanner S. Evaluation of the Ottawa ankle rules in children. *Pediatr Emerg Care*. 2003;19:73–78. (**LOE IV**).
16. Boutis K, Komar L, Jaramillo D, et al. Sensitivity of a clinical examination to predict need for radiography in children with ankle injuries: a prospective study. *Lancet*. 2001;358:2118–2121. (**LOE II**).
17. Vangsness CT Jr, Carter V, Hunt T, et al. Radiographic diagnosis of ankle fractures: are three views necessary? *Foot Ankle Int*. 1994;15:172–174. (**LOE III**).
18. Eisman EA, Stephan ZA, Mehlman CT, et al. Pediatric triplane ankle fractures: impact of radiographs and computed tomography on fracture classification and treatment planning. *J Bone Joint Surg*. 2015;97:995–1002. (**LOE III**).
19. Jones S, Phillips N, Ali F, et al. Triplane fractures of the distal tibia requiring open reduction and internal fixation: preoperative planning using computed tomography. *Injury*. 2003;34:293–298. (**LOE IV**).
20. Horn BD, Crisci K, Krug M, Pizzutillo PD, MacEwen GD. Radiologic evaluation of juvenile Tillaux fractures of the distal tibia. *J Pediatr Orthop*. 2001;21(2):162–164. (**LOE IV**).
21. Frush DP, Donnelly LF, Rosen NS. Computed tomography and radiation risks: what pediatric health care providers should know. *Pediatrics*. 2003;112:951–957. (**LOE V**).
22. Pugmire BS, Shailam R, Sagar P, et al. Initial clinical experience with extremity cone-beam CT of the foot and ankle in pediatric patients. *AJR Am J Roentgenol*. 2016;206(2):431–435. (**LOE IV**).
23. Lee TM, Mehlman CT. Hyphenated history: Park-Harris growth arrest lines. *Am J Orthop*. 2003;32:408–411. (**LOE V**).
24. Vahvanen V, Alto K. Classification of ankle fractures in children. *Arch Orthop Trauma Surg*. 1980;97:1–5. (**LOE IV**).
25. Leary JT, Handling M, Talerico M, et al. Physeal fractures of the distal tibia: predictive factors of premature physeal closure and growth arrest. *J Pediatr Orthop*. 2009;29:356–361. (**LOE III**).
26. Russo F, Moor MA, Mubarak SJ, Pennock AT. Salter-Harris II fractures of the distal tibia: does surgical management reduce the risk of premature physeal closure? *J Pediatr Orthop*. 2013;33:524–529. (**LOE V**).
27. Boutis K, Plint A, Stimec J, et al. Radiograph-negative lateral ankle injuries in children: occult growth plate fracture or sprain? *JAMA Pediatr*. 2016;170(1):e154114. (**LOE II**).
28. Gkiokas A, Brilakis E. Spontaneous correction of the partial physeal arrest: report of a case and review of the literature. *J Pediatr Orthop B*. 2012;21(4):369–372. (**LOE IV**).
29. Chadwick CJ. Spontaneous resolution of varus deformity at the ankle following adduction injury of the distal tibial epiphysis. A case report. *J Bone Joint Surg*. 1982;64(5):774–776. (**LOE V**).
30. Bostock SH, Peach BG. Spontaneous resolution of an osseous bridge affecting the distal tibia epiphysis. *J Bone Joint Surg Br*. 1996;78(4):662–663. (**LOE V**).
31. Cottalorda J, Beranger V, Louahem D, et al. Salter-Harris type III and IV medial malleolar fractures growth arrest: is it fate? A retrospective study of 48 cases with open reduction. *J Pediatr Orthop*. 2008;28:652–655. (**LOE IV**).
32. Charlton M, Costello R, Mooney JF 3rd, Podeszwa DA. Ankle joint biomechanics following transepiphyseal screw fixation of the distal tibia. *J Pediatr Orthop*. 2005;25(5):635–640. (**LOE N/A**).
33. Podeszwa DA, Wilson PL, Holland AR, Copley LA. Comparison of bioabsorbable versus metallic implant fixation for phy-

seal and epiphyseal fractures of the distal tibia. *J Pediatr Orthop.* 2008;28(8):859–863. **(LOE III)**.

34. Ashhurst AP, Bromer RS. Classification and mechanism of fractures of the leg bones involving the ankle. *Arch Surg.* 1922;4:51–129. **(LOE IV)**.

35. Carothers CO, Crenshaw AH. Clinical significance of a classification of epiphyseal injuries at the ankle. *Am J Surg.* 1955;89:879–887. **(LOE IV)**.

36. Barmada A, Gaynor T, Mubarak SJ. Premature physeal closure following distal tibia physeal fractures: a new radiographic predictor. *J Pediatr Orthop.* 2003;32(6):733–739. **(LOE IV)**.

37. Rohmiller MT, Gaynor TP, Pawelek J, Mubarak SJ. Salter-Harris I and II fractures of the distal tibia: does mechanism of injury relate to premature physeal closure? *J Pediatr Orthop.* 2006;26:322–328. **(LOE IV)**.

38. Ramsey PL, Hamilton W. Changes in tibiotalar area of contact caused by lateral talar shift. *J Bone Joint Surg Am.* 1976;58:356–357. **(LOE IV)**.

39. Thordarson DB, Motamed S, Hedman T, et al. The effect of fibular malreduction on contact pressures in an ankle fracture malunion model. *J Bone Joint Surg Am.* 1997;79:1809–1815. **(LOE IV)**.

40. Binkley A, Mehlman C, Freeh E. Salter-Harris II ankle fractures in children: does fracture pattern matter? *J Orthop Trauma.* 2019. **(epub) (LOE III)**.

41. Peterson HA, Burkhart SS. Compression injury of the epiphyseal growth plate: fact or fiction? *J Pediatr Orthop.* 1981;1:377–384. **(LOE V)**.

42. Salter RB, Harris WR. Injuries involving the epiphyseal plate. *J Bone Joint Surg Am.* 1963;45:587–622. **(LOE V)**.

43. Sugi MT, Tileston K, Krygier JE, Gamble J. Transepiphyseal (type VII) ankle fracture versus os subfibulare in pediatric ankle injuries. *J Pediatr Orthop.* 2018;38(10):e593–e596. **(LOE II)**.

44. Letts M, Davidson D, McCaffrey M. The adolescent pilon fracture: management and outcome. *J Pediatr Orthop.* 2001;21(1):20–26. **(LOE IV)**.

45. Kleiger B, Mankin HJ. Fracture of the lateral portion of the distal tibial epiphysis. *J Bone Joint Surg Am.* 1964;46:25–32. **(LOE IV)**.

46. Crawford AH. Ankle fractures in children. *Instr Course Lect.* 1995;44:317–324. **(LOE IV)**.

47. Crawford AH. Triplane and Tillaux fractures: is a 2 mm residual gap acceptable? *J Pediatr Orthop.* 2012;32:S69–S73. **(LOE V)**.

48. Ertl JP, Barrack RL, Alexander AH, Van Buecken K. Triplane fracture of the distal tibial epiphysis: long-term follow-up. *J Bone Joint Surg Am.* 1988;70:967–976. **(LOE IV)**.

49. Brown SD, Kasser JR, Zvrakowski D, et al. Analysis of 51 tibial triplane fractures using CT with multiplanar reconstruction. *AJR Am J Roentgenol.* 2004;183:1489–1495. **(LOE IV)**.

50. El-Karef E, Sadek HI, Nairn DS, et al. Triplane fracture of the distal tibia. *Injury.* 2000;31:729–736. **(LOE IV)**.

51. Rapariz JM, Ocete G, Gonzalez-Herranz P, et al. Distal tibial triplane fractures: long-term follow-up. *J Pediatr Orthop.* 1996;16:113–118. **(LOE IV)**.

52. Denton JR, Fischer SJ. The medial triplane fracture: report of an unusual injury. *J Trauma.* 1981;21:991–995. **(LOE IV)**.

53. Kärrholm J. The triplane fracture: four years of follow-up of 21 cases and review of the literature. *J Pediatr Orthop B.* 1997;6:91–102. **(LOE IV)**.

54. Von Laer L. Classification, diagnosis, and treatment of transitional fractures of the distal part of the tibia. *J Bone Joint Surg Am.* 1985;67:687–698. **(LOE IV)**.

55. Kärrholm J, Hansson LI, Laurin S. Computed tomography of intraarticular supination-eversion fractures in the ankle in adolescents. *J Pediatr Orthop.* 1981;1:181–187. **(LOE IV)**.

56. Spiegel PG, Mast JW, Cooperman DR, et al. Triplane fractures of the distal tibial epiphysis. *Clin Orthop Relat Res.* 1984;188:74–89. **(LOE V)**.

57. Feldman DS, Otsuka NY, Hedden DM. Extra-articular triplane fracture of the distal tibial epiphysis. *J Pediatr Orthop.* 1995;15:479–481. **(LOE IV)**.

58. Shin AY, Moran ME, Wenger DR. Intramalleolar triplane fractures of the distal tibial epiphysis. *J Pediatr Orthop.* 1997;17:352–355. **(LOE IV)**.

59. Kling TF Jr. Operative treatment of ankle fractures in children. *Orthop Clin North Am.* 1990;21:381–392. **(LOE IV)**.

60. Zelenty W, Yoon RS, Shabtai L, et al. Percutaneous versus open reduction and fixation for Tillaux and triplane fracture: a multicenter cohort comparison study. *J Pediatr Orthop B.* 2018;27:551–555. **(LOE III)**.

61. Choudhry IK, Wall EJ, Eismann EA, Crawford AH. Functional outcome analysis of triplane and Tillaux fractures after closed reduction and percutaneous fixation. *J Pediatr Orthop.* 2014;34(2):139–143. **(LOE III)**.

62. Lakomkin N, Fabricant PD, Cruz AI Jr, Brusalis CM, Chauvin NA, Lawrence JTR. Interrater reliability and age-based normative values for radiographic indices of the ankle syndesmosis in children. *JBJS Open Access.* 2016;2(1):e0004. **(LOE III)**.

63. Bozic KJ, Jaramillo D, DiCanzio J, Zurakowski D, Kasser JR. Radiographic appearance of the normal distal tibiofibular syndesmosis in children. *J Pediatr Orthop.* 1999;19(1):14–21. **(LOE IV)**.

64. Sung KH, Kwon SS, Moon SJ, Lee SY. Radiographic evaluation of the normal ankle joint in children and adolescent. *J Orthop Sci.* 2018;23(4):658–664. **(LOE IV)**.

65. Shore BJ, Kramer DE. Management of syndesmotic ankle injuries in children and adolescents. *J Pediatr Orthop.* 2016;36(suppl 1):S11–S14. **(LOE V)**.

66. Jarvis JG, Miyanji F. The complex triplane fracture: ipsilateral tibial shaft and triplane fracture. *J Trauma.* 2001;51:714–716. **(LOE IV)**.

67. Mubarak SJ. Extensor retinaculum syndrome of the ankle after injury to the distal tibial physis. *J Bone Joint Surg Br.* 2002;84:11–14. **(LOE IV)**.

68. Haumont T, Gauchard GC, Zabee L, et al. Extensor retinaculum syndrome after distal tibial fractures: anatomical basis. *Surg Radiol Anat.* 2007;29:303–311. **(LOE IV)**.

69. Moehring H, Tan RT, Marder RA, et al. Ankle dislocation. *J Orthop Trauma.* 1994;8:67–172. **(LOE IV)**.

70. Nusem I, Ezra E, Wientroub S. Closed posterior dislocation of the ankle without associated fracture in a child. *J Trauma.* 1999;46:350–351. **(LOE IV)**.

71. Peterson HA. Partial growth plate arrest and its treatment. *J Pediatr Orthop.* 1984;4:246–258. **(LOE IV)**.

72. Williamson RV, Staheli LT. Partial physeal growth arrest: treatment by bridge resection and fat interposition. *J Pediatr Orthop.* 1990;10:769–776. **(LOE IV)**.

73. Peterson HA. Physeal bar excision: a case report with a forty-two year follow-up. *J Bone Joint Surg Am.* 2011;93(14):e79. **(LOE IV)**.

74. Yoshida T, Kim WC, Tsuchida Y, et al. Experience of bone bridge resection and bone wax packing for partial growth arrest of distal tibia. *J Orthop Trauma.* 2008;22:142–147. **(LOE IV)**.

75. Carlson WO, Wenger DR. A mapping method to prepare for surgical excision of a partial arrest. *J Pediatr Orthop.* 1984;4:232–238. **(LOE IV)**.

76. Peterson HA. Growth plate injuries. In: Morrissy RT, ed. *Lovell and Winter's Pediatric Orthopaedics.* 3rd ed. Vol. 2. Philadelphia: J.B. Lippincott. **(LOE V)**.

77. Marsh JS, Polzhofer GK. Arthroscopically assisted central physeal bar resection. *J Pediatr Orthop.* 2006;26(2):255–259. **(LOE IV)**.

78. Langenskiöld A. Surgical treatment or partial closure of the growth plate. *J Pediatr Orthop.* 1981;1:3–11. **(LOE IV)**.

79. Petty W. The effect of methyl methacrylate on bacterial phagocytosis and killing by human polymorphonuclear leukocytes. *J Bone Joint Surg Am.* 1978;60:752–757. **(LOE IV)**.

80. Petty W. The effect of methyl methacrylate on chemotaxis of polymorphonuclear leukocytes. *J Bone Joint Surg Am.* 1978;60:492–498. **(LOE IV)**.

81. Berson L, Davidson RS, Dormans JP, et al. Growth disturbances after distal tibial physeal fractures. *Foot Ankle.* 2000;21:54–58. **(LOE IV)**.

82. Takakura Y, Takaoka T, Tanaka Y, et al. Results of opening-wedge osteotomy for the treatment of a post-traumatic varus deformity of the ankle. *J Bone Joint Surg Am.* 1998;80:213–218. **(LOE IV)**.

83. Foster BK, John B, Hasler C. Free fat interpositional graft in acute physeal injuries: the anticipatory Langenskiöld procedure. *J Pediatr Orthop.* 2000;20:282–285. **(LOE IV)**.

84. Jung ST, Wang SI, Moon YJ, Muarak SJ, Kim JR. Posttraumatic tibiofibular synostosis after treatment of distal tibiofibular fractures in children. *J Pediatr Orthop.* 2017;37(8):532–536. **(LOE IV)**.

85. Siffert RS, Arkin AM. Post-traumatic aseptic necrosis of the distal tibial epiphysis. *J Bone Joint Surg Am.* 1950;32:691–694. **(LOE IV)**.

86. Pugely AJ, Nemeth BA, McCarthy JJ, et al. Osteonecrosis of the distal tibia metaphysis after a Salter-Harris I injury: a case report. *J Orthop Trauma.* 2012;26:e11–e15. **(LOE IV)**.

87. Bhattacharjee A, Singh J, Mangham DC, Freeman R. Osteonecrosis of the distal tibial metaphysis after Salter-Harris type-2 injury: a case report. *J Pediatr Orthop B.* 2015;24(4):366–369. **(LOE V)**.

88. Mann RA. Biomechanics of the foot. In: American Academy of Orthopedic Surgeons. *Atlas of Orthotics. Biomechanical Principles and Applications.* C.V. Mosby: St. Louis; 257–266. **(LOE V).**

89. Morris JM. Biomechanics of the foot and ankle. *Clin Orthop.* 1977;122:10–17. **(LOE V).**

90. Tachdjian MO. *Pediatric Orthopedics.* 2nd ed. Philadelphia: W.B. Saunders. **(LOE V).**

91. Thermann H, Schratt HE, Hufner T, et al. Fractures of the pediatric foot. *Der Unfallchirurg.* 1998;101:2–11. **(LOE V).**

92. Peterson L, Romanus B, Dahlberg E. Fracture of the collum tali—an experimental study. *J Biomech.* 1976;9(4):277–279. **(LOE V).**

93. Mulfinger GL, Trueta J. The blood supply of the talus. *J Bone Joint Surg Br.* 1970;52:160–167. **(LOE IV).**

94. Canale ST, Kelly FB Jr. Fractures of the neck of the talus. Long-term evaluation of 71 cases. *J Bone Joint Surg Am.* 1978;60:143–156. **(LOE V).**

95. Eberl R, Singer G, Schalamon J, Hausbrandt P, Hoellwarth ME. Fractures of the talus—differences between children and adolescents. *J Trauma.* 2010;68(1):126–130. **(LOE IV).**

96. Hawkins LG. Fractures of the neck of the talus. *J Bone Joint Surg Am.* 1970;52:991–1002. **(LOE IV).**

97. Kruppa C, Snoap T, Sietsema DL, Schildhauer TA, Dudda M, Jones CB. Is the midterm progress of pediatric and adolescent talus fractures stratified by age? *J Foot Ankle Surg.* 2018;57:471–477. **(LOE IV).**

98. Zhang X, Shao X, Yu Y, Zhang Y, Zhang G, Tian D. Comparison between percutaneous and open reduction for treating paediatric talar neck fractures. *Int Orthop.* 2017;41(12):2581–2589. Erratum in: *Int Orthop.* 2017;41(12):2639. **(LOE II).**

99. Alimerzaloo F, Kashani RV, Saeedi H, Farzi M, Fallahian N. Patellar tendon bearing brace: combined effect of heel clearance and ankle status on foot plantar pressure. *Prosthet Orthot Int.* 2014;38(1):34–38. **(LOE N/A).**

100. Ogden J. The foot. In: Ogden J, ed. *Skeletal Injury in the Child.* New York: Springer Verlag; 2000:626–627. **(LOE N/A).**

101. Ibrahim MS, Jordan R, Lotfi N, Chapman AW. Talar head fracture: a case report, systematic review and suggested algorithm of treatment. *Foot (Edinb).* 2015;25(4):258–264. **(LOE V).**

102. Kirkpatrick DP, Hunter RE, Janes PC, et al. The snowboarder's foot and ankle. *Am J Sports Med.* 1998;26:271–277. **(LOE V).**

103. Wu Y, Jiang H, Wang B, Miao W. Fracture of the lateral process of the talus in children: a kind of ankle injury with a frequently missed diagnosis. *J Pediatr Orthop.* 2016;36(3):289–293. **(LOE IV).**

104. Mukherjee SK, Pringle RM, Baxter AD. Fracture of the lateral process of the talus. A report of thirteen cases. *J Bone Joint Surg Br.* 1974;56:263–273. **(LOE IV).**

105. Leibner ED, Simanovsky N, Abu-Sneineh K, Nyska M, Porat S. Fractures of the lateral process of the talus in children. *J Pediatr Orthop B.* 2001;10(1):68–72. **(LOE V).**

106. Smith JT, Curtis TA, Spencer S, Kasser JR, Mahan ST. Complications of talus fractures in children. *J Pediatr Orthop.* 2010;30(8):779–784. **(LOE IV).**

107. Talkhani IS, Reidy D, Fogarty EE, et al. Avascular necrosis of the talus after a minimally displaced neck of talus fracture in a 6 year old child. *Injury.* 2000;31:63–65. **(LOE IV).**

108. Letts RM, Gibeault D. Fractures of the neck of the talus in children. *Foot Ankle Int.* 1980;1:74–77. **(LOE IV).**

109. Gross R. Fractures and dislocations of the foot. In: Rockwood CA, Green DP, eds. *Fractures.* Philadelphia: J.B. Lippincott. **(LOE V).**

110. Grogan DP, Walling AK, Ogden JA. Anatomy of the os trigonum. *J Pediatr Orthop.* 1990;10:618–622. **(LOE IV).**

111. Nault ML, Kocher MS, Micheli LJ. Os trigonum syndrome. *J Am Acad Orthop Surg.* 2014;22(9):545–553. **(LOE V).**

112. Jones DM, Saltzman CL, El-Khoury G. The diagnosis of the os trigonum syndrome with a fluoroscopically controlled injection of local anesthetic. *Iowa Orthop J.* 1999;19:122–126. **(LOE IV).**

113. Berndt AL, Harty M. Transchondral fractures (osteochondritis dissecans). *J Bone Joint Surg Am.* 1959;41:988–1020. **(LOE IV).**

114. Canale ST, Belding RH. Osteochondral lesions of the talus. *J Bone Joint Surg Am.* 1980;62:97–102. **(LOE IV).**

115. Ogilvie-Harris DJ, Sarrosa EA. Arthroscopic treatment of osteochondritis dissecans of the talus. *Arthroscopy.* 1999;15:805–808. **(LOE IV).**

116. Stone JW. Osteochondral lesions of the talar dome. *J Am Acad Orthop Surg.* 1996;4:63–73. **(LOE V).**

117. Anderson DV, Lyne ED. Osteochondritis dissecans of the talus: case report on two family members. *J Pediatr Orthop.* 1984;4:356–357. **(LOE IV).**

118. Pick MP. Familial osteochondritis dissecans. *J Bone Joint Surg Br.* 1955;37:142–145. **(LOE IV).**

119. Schindler A, Mason DE, Allington NJ. Occult fracture of the calcaneus in toddlers. *J Pediatr Orthop.* 1996;16:201–205. **(LOE IV).**

120. White J. Osteochondritis dissecans in association with dwarfism. *J Bone Joint Surg Br.* 1957;39:261–267. **(LOE IV).**

121. Kessler JI, Jacobs JC Jr, Cannamela PC, Shea KG, Weiss JM. Childhood obesity is associated with osteochondritis dissecans of the knee, ankle, and elbow in children and adolescents. *J Pediatr Orthop.* 2018;38(5):e296–e299. **(LOE IV).**

122. Kessler JI, Weiss JM, Nikizad H, et al. Osteochondritis dissecans of the ankle in children and adolescents: demographics and epidemiology. *Am J Sports Med.* 2014;42(9):2165–2171. **(LOE IV).**

123. Rorbach BP, Paulus AC, Niethammer TR, et al. Discrepancy between morphological findings in juvenile osteochondritis dissecans (OCD): a comparison of magnetic resonance imaging (MRI) and arthroscopy. *Knee Surg Sports Traumatol Arthrosc.* 2016;24(4):1259–1264. **(LOE III).**

124. Higashiyama I, Kumai T, Takakura Y, et al. Follow-up study of MRI for osteochondral lesion of the talus. *Foot Ankle Int.* 2000;21:127–133. **(LOE IV).**

125. Taranow WS, Bisignani GA, Towers JD, et al. Retrograde drilling of osteochondral lesions of the medial talar dome. *Foot Ankle Int.* 1999;20:474–480. **(LOE IV).**

126. Perumal V, Wall E, Babekir N. Juvenile osteochondritis dissecans of the talus. *J Pediatr Orthop.* 2007;27(7):821–825. **(LOE IV).**

127. Kramer DE, Glotzbecker MP, Shore BJ, et al. Results of surgical management of osteochondritis dissecans of the ankle in the pediatric and adolescent population. *J Pediatr Orthop.* 2015;35(7):725–733. **(LOE IV).**

128. Weiss JM, Nikizad H, Shea KG, et al. The incidence of surgery in osteochondritis dissecans in children and adolescents. *Orthop J Sports Med.* 2016;4(3): 2325967116635515. **(LOE IV).**

129. Dolan AM, Mulcahy DM, Stephens MM. Osteochondritis dissecans of the head of the talus. *Foot Ankle Int.* 1997;18:365–368. **(LOE IV).**

130. Powell JH, Whipple TL. Osteochondritis of the talus. *Foot Ankle Int.* 1986;6:309–310. **(LOE IV).**

131. Liu Z, Zhao Q, Zhang L. Medial subtalar dislocation associated with fracture of the posterior process of the talus. *J Pediatr Ortho B.* 2012;21(5):439–442. **(LOE V).**

132. Dougherty CP, Nebergall RW, Caskey PM. Lateral subtalar dislocation in a 19-month-old female. *Am J Orthop.* 2003;32(12):598–600. **(LOE V).**

133. Hoexum F, Heetveld MJ. Subtalar dislocation: two cases requiring surgery and a literature review of the last 25 years. *Arch Orthop Trauma Surg.* 2014;134(9):1237–1249. **(LOE V).**

134. Essex-Lopresti P. The mechanism, reduction technique, and results in fractures of the os calcis. *Br J Surg.* 1952;39:395–419. **(LOE IV).**

135. Thomas HM. Calcaneal fracture in childhood. *Br J Surg.* 1969;56:664–666. **(LOE V).**

136. Matteri RE, Frymoyer JW. Fracture of the calcaneus in young children: report of 3 cases. *J Bone Joint Surg Am.* 1973;55:1091–1094. **(LOE IV).**

137. Schmidt TL, Weiner DS. Calcaneal fractures in children: an evaluation of the nature of the injury in 56 children. *Clin Orthop Relat Res.* 1982;171:150–155. **(LOE IV).**

138. Inokuchi S, Usami N, Hiraishi E, et al. Calcaneal fractures in children. *J Pediatr Orthop.* 1998;18:469–474. **(LOE IV).**

139. Brunet JA. Calcaneal fractures in children. Long-term results of treatment. *J Bone Joint Surg Br.* 2000;82:211–216. **(LOE IV).**

140. Ogden JA. *Skeletal injury in the child.* Philadelphia: Lea & Febiger. **(LOE V).**

141. Sanders R, Fortin P, DiPasquale T, Walling A. Operative treatment in 120 displaced intraarticular calcaneal fractures. Results using a prognostic computed tomography scan classification. *Clin Orthop Relat Res.* 1993;290:87–95. **(LOE III).**

142. Boyle MJ, Walker CG, Crawford HA. The paediatric Bohler's angle and crucial angle of Gissane: a case series. *J Orthop Surg Res.* 2011;10(6):2. **(LOE V).**

143. Cole JR, Brown HP, Stein RE, Pearce RG. Avulsion fracture of the tuberosity of calcaneus in children. *J Bone Joint Surg Am.* 1995;77:1568–1571. **(LOE IV).**

144. de Beer JD, Maloon S, Hudson DA. Calcaneal fractures in children. *S Afr Med J.* 1989;76:53–54. **(LOE IV)**.

145. Petit CJ, Lee BM, Kasser JR, Kocher MS. Operative treatment of intraarticular calcaneal fractures in the pediatric population. *J Pediatr Orthop.* 2007;27(8):856–862. **(LOE IV)**.

146. Tong L, Li M, Li F, Xu J, Hu T. A minimally invasive (sinus tarsi) approach with percutaneous K-wires fixation for intra-articular calcaneal fractures in children. *J Pediatr Orthop B.* 2018;27(6):556–562. **(LOE IV)**.

147. Feng Y, Yu Y, Shui X, Ying X, Cai L, Hong J. Closed reduction and percutaneous fixation of calcaneal fractures in children. *Orthopedics.* 2016;39(4):e744–748. **(LOE IV)**.

148. Crawford AH. *Fractures about the foot in children: a radiographic analysis.* The Children's Hospital Medical Center: Cincinnati.

149. Waugh W. The ossification and vascularisation of the tarsal navicular and their relation to Köhler's disease. *J Bone Joint Surg Br.* 1958;40:765–777. **(LOE IV)**.

150. Borges JL, Guille JT, Bowen JR. Köhler's bone disease of the tarsal navicular. *J Pediatr Orthop.* 1995;15:596–598. **(LOE IV)**.

151. Yamaguchi S, Niki H, Akagi R, Yamamoto Y, Sasho T. Failure of internal fixation for painful bipartite navicular in two adolescent soccer players: a report of two cases. *J Foot Ankle Surg.* 2016;55(6):1323–1326. **(LOE V)**.

152. Holbein O, Bauer G, Kinzl L. Fracture of the cuboid in children: case report and review of the literature. *J Pediatr Orthop.* 1998;18:466–468. **(LOE IV)**.

153. Simonian PT, Vahey JW, Rosenbaum DM, et al. Fracture of the cuboid in children. A source of leg symptoms. *J Bone Joint Surg Br.* 1995;77:104–106. **(LOE IV)**.

154. Ruffing T, Ruckauer T, Bludau F, et al. Cuboid nutcracker fracture in children: management and results. *Injury.* 2019;50(2):607–612. **(LOE IV)**.

155. Ceroni D, De Rosa V, De Coulon G, Kaelin A. Cuboid nutcracker fracture due to horseback riding in children: case series and review of the literature. *J Pediatr Orthop.* 2007;27(5):557–561. **(LOE IV)**.

156. Preidler KW, Brossmann J, Daenen B, et al. MR imaging of the tarsometatarsal joint: analysis of injuries in 11 patients. *AJR Am J Roentgenol.* 1996;167:1217–1222. **(LOE IV)**.

157. Knijnenberg LM, Dingemans SA, Terra MP, et al. Radiographic anatomy of the pediatric Lisfranc joint. *J Pediatr Orthop.* 2018;38(10):510–513. **(LOE III)**.

158. Wiley JJ. Tarsometatarsal joint injuries in children. *J Pediatr Orthop.* 1981;1:255–260. **(LOE IV)**.

159. Hill JF, Heyworth BE, Lierhaus A, Kocher MS, Mahan ST. Lisfranc injuries in children and adolescents. *J Pediatr Orthop.* 2017;26(2):159–163. **(LOE IV)**.

160. Denning JR, Butler L, Eismann EA et al. Functional outcomes and health-related quality of life following pediatric Lisfranc tarsometatarsal injury treatment. 2015 May, Pediatric Orthopaedic Society of North America Annual Meeting, paper 159. **(LOE N/A)**.

161. Singer G, Cichocki M, Schalamon J, Eberl R, Hollwarth ME. A study of metatarsal fractures in children. *J Bone Joint Surg Am.* 2008;90(4):772–776. **(LOE II)**.

162. Robertson NB, Roocroft JH, Edmonds EW. Childhood metatarsal shaft fractures: treatment outcomes and relative indications for surgical interventions. *J Child Orthop.* 2012;6:125–129. **(LOE III)**.

163. Mahan ST, Lierhaus AM, Spencer SA, Kasser JR. Treatment dilemma in multiple metatarsal fractures: when to operate? *J Pediatr Orthop PART B.* 2016;25:354–360. **(LOE IV)**.

164. Kramer DE, Mahan ST, Hresko MT. Displaced intra-articular fractures of the great toe in children: intervene with caution! *J Pediatr Orthop.* 2014;34(2):144–149. **(LOE IV)**.

165. Freiberg AH. Infraction of the second metatarsal bone, a typical injury. *Surg Gynecol Obstet.* 1914;19:191–193. **(LOE IV)**.

166. Schade VL. Surgical management of Freiberg's infraction: a systematic review. *Foot Ankle Spec.* 2015;8(6):498–519. **(LOE III)**.

167. Viladot A, Sodano L, Marcellini L. Joint debridement and microfracture for treatment late-stage Freiberg-Kohler's disease: long-term follow-up study. *Foot Ankle Surg.* 2018 Feb. **(LOE III)**.

168. Smith JW, Arnoczky SP, Hersh A. The intraosseous blood supply of the fifth metatarsal: implications for proximal fracture healing. *Foot Ankle Int.* 1992;13:143–152. **(LOE IV)**.

169. Herrera-Soto JA, Scherb M, Duffy MF, Albright JC. Fractures of the fifth metatarsal in children and adolescents. *J Pediatr Orthop.* 2007;27(4):427–431. **(LOE IV)**.

170. Dameron TB Jr. Fractures and anatomical variations of the proximal portion of the fifth metatarsal. *J Bone Joint Surg Am.* 1975;57(6):788–792. **(LOE IV)**.

171. Lawrence SJ. Technique tip: local bone grafting technique for Jones fracture management with intramedullary screw fixation. *Foot Ankle Int.* 2004;25:920–921. **(LOE IV)**.

172. Horst F, Gilbert BJ, Glisson RR, et al. Torque resistance after fixation of Jones fractures with intramedullary screws. *Foot Ankle Int.* 2004;25:914–919. **(LOE IV)**.

173. Porter DA, Duncan M, Heyer SJ. Fifth metatarsal Jones fracture fixation with 4.5 mm cannulated stainless steel screw in the competitive and recreational athlete: a clinical and radiographic evaluation. *Am J Sports Med.* 2005;33:726–733. **(LOE IV)**.

174. Reese K, Litsky A, Kaeding C, et al. Cannulated screw fixation of Jones fractures: a clinical and biomechanical study. *Am J Sports Med.* 2004;32:1736–1742. **(LOE IV)**.

175. Wright RW, Fischer DA, Shively RA, et al. Refracture of proximal fifth metatarsal (Jones) fracture after intermedullary screw fixation in athletes. *Am J Sports Med.* 2000;28:732–736. **(LOE IV)**.

176. Forrester RA, Eyre-Brook AI, Mannan K. Iselin's disease: a systematic review. *J Foot Ankle Surg.* 2017;56(6):1065–1069. **(LOE III)**.

177. Sylvester JE, Hennrikus WL. Treatment outcomes of adolescents with Iselin's apophysitis. *J Pediatr Orthop.* 2015;24(4):362–365. **(LOE IV)**.

178. Ralph BG, Barrett J, Kenyhercz C, et al. Iselin's disease: a case presentation of nonunion and review of the differential diagnosis. *J Foot Ankle Surg.* 1999;38:409–416. **(LOE IV)**.

179. Kensinger DR, Guille JT, Horn BD, Herman MJ. The stubbed great toe: importance of early recognition and treatment of open fractures of the distal phalanx. *J Pediatr Orthop.* 2001;21(1):31–34. **(LOE IV)**.

180. Pinckney LE, Currarino G, Kennedy LA. The stubbed great toe: a cause of occult compound fracture and infection. *Radiology.* 1981;138(2):375–377. **(LOE IV)**.

181. Park DY, Han KJ, Hah SH, Cho JH. Barefoot stubbing injuries to the great toe in children: a new classification by injury mechanism. *J Orthop Trauma.* 2013;27(11):651–655. **(LOE IV)**.

182. Nabi W, Kurup H. Irreducible dislocation of a proximal interphalangeal joint of the second toe in a six-year-old child: a case report. *J Bone Joint Surg Case Connect.* 2018;8(3):e66. **(LOE IV)**.

183. Neubauer T, Wagner M, Quell M. Interphalangeal dislocation of the fourth toe with avulsion-fracture in a child: report of a case. *Foot Ankle Int.* 1997;18(3):175–177. **(LOE V)**.

184. Manoli A 2nd, Weber TG. Fasciotomy of the foot: an anatomical study with special reference to release of the calcaneal compartment. *Foot Ankle Int.* 1990;10:267–275. **(LOE IV)**.

185. Myerson MS. Management of compartment syndromes of the foot. *Clin Orthop.* 1991;271:239–248. **(LOE IV)**.

186. Silas SI, Herzenberg JE, Myerson MS, et al. Compartment syndrome of the foot in children. *J Bone Joint Surg Am.* 1995;77:356–361. **(LOE IV)**.

187. Wallin K, Nguyen H, Russell L, Lee DK. Acute traumatic compartment syndrome in pediatric foot: a systematic review and case report. *J Foot Ankle Surgery.* 2016;55(4):817–820. **(LOE III)**.

188. Love SM, Grogan DP, Ogden JA. Lawn mower injuries in children. *J Orthop Trauma.* 1988;2:94–101. **(LOE IV)**.

189. Horowitz JH, Nichter LS, Kenney JG, et al. Lawn mower injuries in children: lower extremity reconstruction. *J Trauma.* 1985;25:138–146. **(LOE IV)**.

190. Dormans JP, Azzoni M, Davidson RS, et al. Major lower extremity lawn mower injuries in children. *J Pediatr Orthop.* 1995;15:78–82. **(LOE IV)**.

191. Letts RM, Mardirshah A. Lawn-mower injuries in children. *Can Med Assoc J.* 1977;116:1151–1153. **(LOE IV)**.

192. Vosburgh CL, Gruel CR, Herndon WA, et al. Lawn mower injuries in the pediatric foot and ankle: observations on prevention and management. *J Pediatr Orthop.* 1995;15:504–509. **(LOE IV)**.

193. Myerson MS, Mann RA, Coughlin MJ. Soft tissue trauma: acute and chronic management. In: Mann RA & Coughlin MJ, eds. *Surgery of the Foot and Ankle.* 6th ed. Philadelphia: C.V. Mosby; 1367–1410.

194. Loder RT, Brown KL, Zaleske DJ, et al. Extremity lawn-mower injuries in children: report by the Research Committee of the Pediatric Orthopaedic Society of North America. *J Pediatr Orthop.* 1997;17:360–369. **(LOE V)**.

195. Katz JF. Spontaneous fractures in paraplegic children. *J Bone Joint Surg Am.* 1953;35-A(1):220–226. **(LOE V)**.

196. Borne A, Porter A, Recicar J, Maxson T, Montgomery C. Pediatric traumatic amputations in the United States: a 5-year review. *J Pediatr Orthop.* 2017;37(2):e104–e107. (**LOE IV**).

197. Loder RT. Demographics of traumatic amputations in children. Implications for prevention strategies. *J Bone Joint Surg Am.* 2004;86-A(5):923–928. (**LOE IV**).

198. Miller EH, Semian DW. Gram-negative osteomyelitis following puncture wounds of the foot. *J Bone Joint Surg Am.* 1975;57:535–537. (**LOE IV**).

199. Stucky W, Loder RT. Extremity gunshot wounds in children. *J Pediatr Orthop.* 1991;11:67–71. (**LOE IV**).

200. Arendt EA. Orthopaedic knowledge update, sports medicine 2. *Rosemont, IL: American Academy of Orthopaedic Surgeons.*

201. Lock TR, Aronson DD. Fractures in patients who have myelomeningocele. *J Bone Joint Surg Am.* 1989;71(8):1153–1157. (**LOE IV**).

202. Dosa NP, Eckrich M, Katz DA, Turk M, Liptak GS. Incidence, prevalence, and characteristics of fractures in children, adolescents, and adults with spina bifida. *J Spinal Cord Med.* 2007;30(suppl 1): S5–9. (**LOE III**).

203. Akbar M, Bresch B, Raiss P, et al. Fractures in myelomeningocele. *J Orthop Traumatol.* 2010;11(3):175–182. (**LOE IV**).

204. Uddenfeldt WU, Nordmark E, Wagner P, Duppe H, Westbom L. Fractures in children with cerebral palsy: a total population study. *Dev Med Child Neurol.* 2013;55(9):821–826. (**LOE III**).

205. Khoury DJ, Szalay EA. Bone mineral density correlation with fractures in nonambulatory pediatric patients. *J Pediatr Orthop.* 2007;27(5):562–566. (**LOE IV**).

206. Sholas MG, Tann B, Baebler-Spira D. Oral bisphosphonates to treat disuse osteopenia in children with disabilities: a case series. *J Pediatr Orthop.* 2005;25(3):326–331. (**LOE IV**).

207. Mazur JM, Shurtleff D, Menelaus M, Colliver J. Orthopaedic management of high-level spina bifida. Early walking compared with early use of a wheelchair. *J Bone Joint Surg Am.* 1989;71(1):56–61. (**LOE IV**).

208. Marrieros H, Loff C, Calado E. Osteoporosis in paediatric patients with spina bifida. *J Spinal Cord Med.* 2012;35(1):9–21. (**LOE IV**).

209. Gellman H. Reflex sympathetic dystrophy: alternative modalities for pain management. *Instr Course Lect.* 2000;49:549–557. (**LOE V**).

210. Wilder RT, Berde CB, Wolohan M, et al. Reflex sympathetic dystrophy in children. Clinical characteristics and follow-up of 70 patients. *J Bone Joint Surg Am.* 1992;74(6):910–919. (**LOE IV**).

211. Sarrail R, Launay F, Marez M. Reflex dystrophy in children and adolescents. *J Bone Joint Surg Br.* 2004;86(suppl):23. (**LOE V**).

212. Dietz FR, Matthews KD, Montgomery WJ. Reflex sympathetic dystrophy in children. *Clin Orthop Relat Res.* 1990;258:225–231. (**LOE IV**).

213. Ehrlich MG, Zaleske DJ. Pediatric orthopaedic pain of unknown origin. *J Pediatr Orthop.* 1986;6:460–468. (**LOE IV**).

214. Wilder RT. Management of pediatric patients with complex regional pain syndrome. *Clin J Pain.* 2006;22(5):**443–438**. (**LOE V**).

215. Sherry DD, Wallace CA, Kelley C, et al. Short- and long-term outcomes of children with complex regional pain syndrome type I treated with exercise therapy. *Clin J Pain.* 1999;15:218–223. (**LOE IV**).

216. Murakami S, Yamamoto H, Furuya K, Tomimatsu T. Irreducible Salter-Harris type II fracture of the distal tibial epiphysis. *J Orthop Trauma.* 1994;8(6):524–526. (**LOE V**).

217. Bostman OM. Body-weight related to loss of reduction of fractures of the distal tibia and ankle. *J Bone Joint Surg Br.* 1995;77(1):101–103. (**LOE III**).

218. Kessler J, Koebnick C, Smith N, Adams A. Childhood obesity is associated with increased risk of most lower extremity fractures. *Clin Orthop Relat Res.* 2013;471(4):1199–1207. (**LOE III**).

219. Rana AR, Michalsky MP, Teich S, Groner JI, Caniano DA, Schuster DP. Childhood obesity: a risk factor for injuries observed at a level-1 trauma center. *J Pediatr Surg.* 2009;44(8):1601–1605. (**LOE III**).

220. Pomerantz WJ, Timm NL, Gittelman MA. Injury patterns in obese versus nonobese children presenting to a pediatric emergency department. *Pediatrics.* 2010;125(4):681–685. (**LOE III**).

Fractures and Dislocations about the Shoulder

16

James F. Mooney III | Robert F. Murphy

CLAVICLE

RELEVANT ANATOMY

The clavicle, or collar bone, is an S-shaped bone anterior to the base of the neck. Through articulations with the sternum medially and with the scapula at the acromion process laterally, it serves as an osseous connection between the axial skeleton and the upper extremity. In cross section, the medial portion of the clavicle is rounded or prismatic, and the lateral third is flattened. The entire anterosuperior aspect of the clavicle is subcutaneous without significant muscular coverage.

The clavicle acts as an origin for the pectoralis major on the medial two-thirds of its anterior surface and for the deltoid on the lateral third. Inferiorly, through its middle third, it provides an attachment for the subclavius muscle and its enveloping clavipectoral fascia while acting as a point of attachment for both portions of the coracoclavicular and the acromioclavicular ligaments laterally and for the costoclavicular ligament medially. Posteriorly, the clavicle provides an attachment in its lateral third for the trapezius and for the clavicular head of the sternocleidomastoid muscle medially. The subclavian vessels and brachial plexus lie posterior to the junction of the medial two-thirds and the lateral one-third of the bone.[1]

DEVELOPMENTAL ANATOMY

The clavicle is the first bone to begin ossification, which occurs from two primary centers that appear during the fifth or sixth week of fetal life.[2,3] It is one of the last to completely ossify, as its medial physis does not close completely until 24 to 26 years of age in many males.[4]

MEDIAL CLAVICLE FRACTURES AND STERNOCLAVICULAR JOINT DISLOCATIONS

INCIDENCE

A fracture of the medial portion of the clavicle occurs infrequently in children and accounts for only about 5% of all pediatric clavicular fractures.[5] Medial physeal fractures are more common than medial shaft fractures and may be mistaken for sternoclavicular joint dislocations.[5]

MECHANISM

The capsule of the sternoclavicular joint is more resistant to injury than is the physis of the medial portion of the clavicle. Because the physeal plate remains open until well into the young adult years,[1,4] children and adolescents are more likely to sustain a physeal injury rather than an actual dislocation of the sternoclavicular joint.[5–7] The most common mechanism of injury is axial compression of the shoulder toward the midline. Whether displacement of the lateral fragment occurs anterior or posterior to the sternum is determined by the secondary force vectors of this axial compression.[8] A direct anterior-to-posterior force can generate a fracture or dislocation of the medial segment of the clavicle; in such a case, displacement is always posterior.

DIAGNOSIS

The patient usually is seen with a history of either a blow to the medial part of the clavicle or the sternal area or, more commonly, after a direct axial compression through the shoulder. Physical examination reveals local swelling and tenderness about the medial part of the clavicle (Fig. 16.1). Anterior displacement presents with an obvious prominence in this area. When the displacement is posterior, symptoms of respiratory difficulty, dysphagia, dysphonia, or distended neck veins secondary to compression of adjacent structures may be present, although in some cases, no symptoms exist. Radiographs angled to minimize the effect of obscuring overlying tissues—for example, the "serendipity" view of Rockwood[8] (Fig. 16.2) or the Hobbs view,[9] with the medial part of the clavicle and the sternoclavicular joints visualized bilaterally for comparison—usually confirm the diagnosis. However, computed tomography (CT) of the sternoclavicular joint is the preferred modality because it delineates the direction and extent of displacement most clearly. In addition, CT provides information regarding the relationship of the displaced clavicular fragment to neighboring structures, particularly the trachea, the esophagus, and great vessels (Fig. 16.3).

TREATMENT

Nonoperative

Nondisplaced injuries of the medial portion of the clavicle or sternoclavicular joint can be managed symptomatically and have a good prognosis. A "bump" secondary to new callus should be expected and remodels to some extent with time, especially in a younger child. In many cases, anteriorly displaced fractures or dislocations require little treatment. Closed reduction can be attempted with longitudinal traction and direct pressure over the fracture.[10] Usually, reduction is easily obtained but difficult to maintain, and redisplacement is a common result. If reduction fails or

441

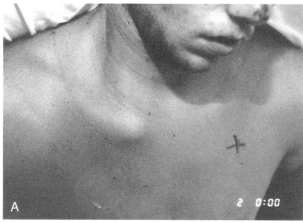

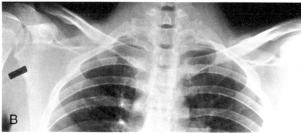

Fig. 16.1 Fracture of the medial portion of the clavicle. (A) This patient sustained multiple injuries; the prominence of the right medial clavicle is obvious. (B) A chest radiograph shows the asymmetry consistent with a medial physeal injury (the epiphysis is unossified). Incidental note is made of a contralateral first-rib fracture.

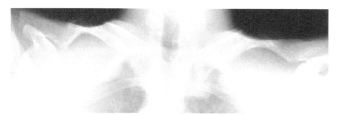

Fig. 16.2 A *serendipity,* or cephalic tilt, radiograph of a 14-year-old child. No fractures or dislocations are present. The film is obtained by placing a cassette behind the supine patient's head and neck and angling the beam cephalad 40 degrees from a distance of 45 to 60 inches.

redisplacement occurs, further intervention is rarely indicated. Some remodeling may be expected, and little, if any, morbidity is noted beyond a minor cosmetic defect from the residual prominence. However, some patients will present with persistent pain and instability after an anteriorly displaced fracture/dislocation.

A posteriorly displaced medial clavicular fracture or posterior sternoclavicular dislocation may be life-threatening, and because of the risk of potential respiratory distress, determination of the presence of an adequate airway should be an essential part of the patient's initial treatment. Closed reduction of these fractures can sometimes be attained by drawing the patient's shoulder posteriorly and into abduction; this maneuver is facilitated by placing the patient supine with a folded towel or another type of bump placed between the scapulae to abduct the shoulder girdles. In addition, longitudinal traction on the involved upper extremity may assist in the reduction. Posteriorly displaced fractures that fail to reduce with closed techniques

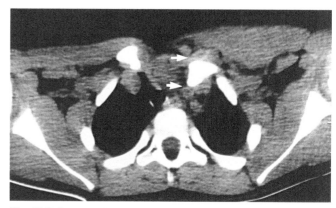

Fig. 16.3 Computed tomographic scan of an adolescent with a left posterior sternoclavicular dislocation *(arrows).* Note the impingement on the posterior structures.

may be amenable to percutaneous reduction. After suitable anesthesia and skin preparation, a sterile towel clip is used to control the medial part of the clavicular shaft and manipulate it to its reduced position. It is generally advised that a thoracic or cardiac surgeon be available for potential assistance whenever reduction of a posteriorly displaced fracture is undertaken, particularly in those cases with evidence of premanipulation respiratory or vascular compromise, although well-documented cases of catastrophic bleeding are not reported.

Posterior fractures or dislocations tend to be more stable than anteriorly displaced fractures after reduction as a result of the geometry of the medial clavicle and physis, as well as the associated capsular structures. As such, maintenance of closed reduction is more common if the initial displacement is posterior. In most cases, reduction can be maintained successfully with a figure-of-8 strap and an arm sling for approximately 4 weeks. The medial clavicular physis has excellent remodeling capacity, and late pain and deformity are rare after stable reduction of displaced medial clavicular fractures.

Operative

Primary open reduction should be reserved for open injuries requiring débridement, for posteriorly displaced fractures that adversely affect neighboring vital structures and have failed reduction by percutaneous methods, and for significant anterior displacements that cannot be reduced (and maintained) by closed techniques.[11–13] Internal fixation with Kirschner wires or smooth pins is inadvisable and has been associated with potentially serious complications.[14–16] Alternatively, sutures placed strategically through drill holes in the outer portion of the adjacent sternum or sternoclavicular ligament and the medial section of the clavicle should suffice to stabilize the reduction.[5] Waters and colleagues[17] demonstrated good results with a suturing technique using nonabsorbable material, and Goldfarb and colleagues[18] reported success with a figure-of-8 sternal wire after open reduction of posterior dislocations that had failed closed manipulation. Delayed operative reconstruction may be indicated in patients with pain and instability secondary to a prior anteriorly displaced injury.[11] Fixation methods, including reduction and suture techniques, are similar to those used in primary operative procedures.

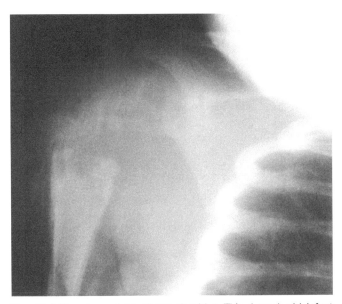

Fig. 16.4 Pseudoparalysis of the shoulder. This 4-week-old infant with pseudoparalysis after injury was treated for a clavicular fracture. The child was seen again in follow-up at 2.5 weeks, at which time the abnormal appearance of the proximal humeral metaphysis was apparent. Aspiration confirmed osteomyelitis. The differential diagnosis of pseudoparalysis in such a case is clavicular, proximal humeral, or scapular trauma; brachial plexus palsy; or sepsis of the joint, neighboring bone, or both.

PERINATAL CLAVICULAR SHAFT FRACTURES

INCIDENCE

The clavicle is the most commonly fractured bone in the newborn.[19] The incidence of birth fractures involving the clavicle ranges from 2.7 to 5.7 per 1000 term deliveries, and clavicular fractures account for 84% to 92% of all obstetric fractures.[20] Choi et al[21] reported an incidence of clavicle fractures complicating cesarean birth of 0.05% and felt that the primary risk factor in these patients was infant birthweight.

MECHANISM AND DIAGNOSIS

Clavicular injury at birth has been shown to correlate with increased birth weight of the infant,[21] lower head-to-abdominal circumference ratio of the infant, inexperience of the delivering physician, and forceps delivery.[22,23] In the vast majority of cases, the mechanism of fracture generation is secondary to axial compression of the shoulder girdle during passage through the birth canal. The most common fracture site is at the junction of the lateral and middle thirds of the bone. The fracture is usually minimally displaced; in many patients, it is unappreciated clinically and then discovered as a prominence over the shaft of the clavicle 7 to 10 days after birth as the fracture heals. Plain radiographs may be negative initially, but repeat images generally demonstrate periosteal reaction 7 to 14 days later. Kayser and associates[24] described using ultrasound to image suspected neonatal clavicular fractures with excellent success. Occasionally, the fracture is manifested by pseudoparalysis of the arm secondary to discomfort with motion (Fig. 16.4).[22] In this instance, the differential diagnosis includes fracture of the proximal end of the humerus, brachial plexus palsy, and sepsis of the shoulder joint.[19,25] It is important to remember that multiple diagnoses can coexist (e.g., fracture with brachial plexus palsy or fracture with infection). The presence of an asymmetric Moro reflex is useful

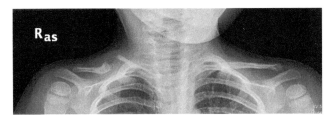

Fig. 16.5 2 years, 6 months-old boy with congenital pseudarthrosis of the right clavicle. The child was asymptomatic and treated with observation.

for differentiating a true paralysis (brachial plexus injury) from other causes of diminished spontaneous shoulder motion secondary to pain (pseudoparalysis).[26]

TREATMENT

In a patient in whom upper extremity movements appear painful or in those with pseudoparalysis most likely secondary to a clavicular fracture, splinting or binding the upper extremity to the chest wall with a stockinette stretch bandage or a similar soft, expandable material for approximately 10 days is appropriate.[8,27,28] Anecdotally, it may be easier and safer to clip the sleeve of the affected limb to the front of the infant's shirt or gown to avoid the potential problems of loose and shifting bandages (so-called "onesie pinning"). Clavicular fractures in this age group heal extremely quickly without long-term sequelae. Congenital pseudarthrosis of the clavicle should not be confused with an acute fracture and usually can be differentiated easily by physical examination, lack of symptomatology, and radiographic appearance (Fig. 16.5).

FRACTURE OF THE CLAVICULAR SHAFT IN CHILDHOOD

INCIDENCE

Fracture of the clavicle is one of the most frequent childhood fractures.[29] The most common fracture is the diaphyseal shaft, and such fractures account for approximately 85% of all childhood clavicular fractures.

MECHANISM AND ASSOCIATED INJURIES

The most common mechanism of a clavicular shaft fracture is a fall onto the shoulder. This mechanism accounted for 87% of the 150 prospectively studied cases carefully documented in the report by Stanley and colleagues.[29] Usually, the bone fractures where it changes shape (concave to convex and cross-sectionally from round to flat) within the middle third of the shaft. Less commonly, a direct blow may cause a clavicle fracture; this mechanism accounted for 7% of Stanley and colleagues' cases. The remaining 6% of patients sustained fractures secondary to a fall on an outstretched hand. High-energy trauma is associated with fracture comminution and greater fragment displacement and with a consequently higher likelihood of injury to surrounding nonosseous structures such as the brachial plexus, neighboring vessels, or apex of the lung.[30–32]

DIAGNOSIS

Characteristically, the child with an acute clavicular fracture holds the elbow of the affected limb with the opposite hand and tilts the head toward the affected side to minimize the pain associated with fracture displacement by the sternocleidomastoid and trapezius muscles. Radiographs at the time injury are often confirmatory, although for nondisplaced fractures, the results may initially be negative. The use of appropriate radiographic technique and careful attention to the periclavicular soft tissue shadow may detect subtle nondisplaced fractures. Overlying structures may obscure a medial physeal injury, and a Rockwood serendipity view[8] (40-degree cephalad-directed tube angle) or Hobbs projection[9] may be helpful. Children with appropriate histories and point tenderness over the clavicle but with negative primary radiographic results usually have callus at the site of injury on follow-up radiographs obtained 10 to 14 days after injury.

TREATMENT

Nonoperative

More than 200 methods of nonoperative management of a clavicular shaft fracture have been described.[33] Most commonly, these fractures are managed with an apparatus that draws the shoulder backward (e.g., a figure-of-8 wrap or bandage) or a simple sling. Generally, total time of immobilization is about 3 to 4 weeks, and a gradual increase in activities is allowed as discomfort lessens. Contact sports are not recommended for approximately 6 to 8 weeks.

A common residuum of the injury is a prominence or bump at the site of the fracture caused by healing callus. The child and parents should be made aware of this possibility at the initial visit. Characteristically, the bump becomes less distinct as the bone remodels over the next 6 to 9 months.[5] Long-term impairment as a consequence of a closed clavicular fracture managed by closed methods in childhood is rare.

Nonunion of a closed clavicle fracture in pediatric patients is extremely uncommon. Until recently, fewer than 15 cases had been described in the literature. In 2018, Pennock et al[34] reported the data regarding clavicular nonunions from a nine-hospital multicenter study group. The authors identified 25 patients with nonunions. Twenty-two of the 25 patients were treated nonoperatively for the original injury, whereas three had undergone attempted surgical fixation as the index procedure. The primary risk factor associated with nonunion was a clavicular refracture. In addition, older patient age, male gender, and greater fracture displacement were felt to have a role in this very uncommon complication.

Operative

Débridement followed by open reduction is indicated for the rare open clavicular shaft fracture. Internal fixation may be necessary to prevent impingement of displaced sharp bone ends on neighboring vital structures or to prevent them from protruding through the wound. A 3.5-mm or 2.7-mm reconstruction plate is appropriate internal fixation; one should avoid using smooth pins because of concerns regarding migration. Appropriate wound closure, based on the severity of contamination and soft tissue injury, and external support in a figure-of-8 bandage and a sling are indicated.

Open reduction may also be indicated for significantly displaced, irreducible fractures (e.g., those that have buttonholed through the trapezius or the fascia, with tenting and potential compromise of the skin).[35] Management of displaced clavicular fractures in adolescents without significant skin or soft tissue compromise has become more controversial, as surgeons have attempted to extend indications and results reported for adult patients to this younger population. Multiple authors have reported successful treatment of displaced fractures in adolescents. Kubiak and Slongo[36] reported good success using intramedullary titanium elastic nails in pediatric and adolescent patients requiring internal fixation of clavicular shaft fractures. Vander Have and associates[37] compared operative versus nonoperative treatment in adolescent patients and found a statistically significant lower time to radiographic union in those treated surgically. Five patients developed symptomatic malunions in the nonoperative group, but no nonunions or malunions occurred in the surgical cohort. Li et al[38] found that the overall complication rate after operative plate fixation of pediatric clavicle fractures was 86%, with implant prominence or irritation being the most common single complication. Hagstrom et al[39] reviewed outcomes of pediatric clavicle fractures managed with either surgical or nonoperative methods. The authors reported no difference in outcome scores, return to activity, or mean time to achieve full range of motion between the two groups. Overall, current opinion continues to favor nonoperative treatment of closed pediatric clavicular fractures. A survey of the Pediatric Orthopaedic Society of North America membership was undertaken, which presented four different case scenarios involving pediatric clavicle fractures to its members. In all situations, the majority of respondents preferred nonoperative treatment for closed fractures.[40] Despite these apparent opinions, as well as the high rate of reported complications in the literature, a review of medical records from a large, urban US pediatric medical center demonstrated a statistically significant increase in the percentage of midshaft clavicle fractures in patients aged 10 to 18 treated operatively with plate fixation from 1999 to 2011.[41]

DISTAL CLAVICULAR FRACTURE

RELEVANT ANATOMY

Two anatomic facts greatly enhance understanding of trauma to the distal end of the clavicle in children. The first is that the secondary ossification center at the distal end of the clavicle remains unossified until shortly before it unites with the diaphysis in the late teenage years. The second is that the thick periosteal sleeve surrounding the distal part of the clavicle and its epiphysis provides a strong attachment for the acromioclavicular and coracoclavicular ligaments. These anatomic relationships make it easier to understand why a physeal fracture in this region is much more common than dislocation of the acromioclavicular joint, similar to the pattern of injury seen at the medial end of the clavicle. Thus, when the distal end of the clavicle fractures in a child, there is generally an associated rent in the adjacent periosteal sleeve. With displacement, the ossified metaphysis herniates through the rent whereas the unossified epiphysis is retained in the sleeve. Because the epiphysis is cartilaginous and radiolucent, it gives the radiographic appearance of what would be, in an adult, an acromioclavicular joint dislocation. However, not all distal clavicular fractures involve the physis. True fractures of the distal clavicular metaphysis do occur but are relatively infrequent in children (Fig. 16.6).

INCIDENCE

The lateral aspect of the clavicle, including the acromioclavicular joint, accounts for 10% of fractures of the clavicle. These fractures occur with far greater frequency than do fractures at the medial end of the bone.[8,42]

MECHANISM OF INJURY

This injury is produced most frequently by a force on the apex of the shoulder—a fall or a blow. The patient is seen with pain and tenderness over the shoulder in the area of the acromioclavicular joint. If the fracture is displaced,

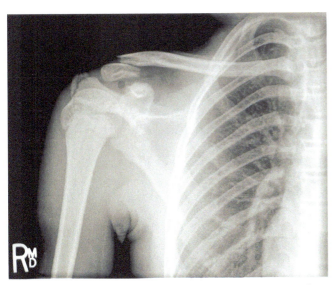

Fig. 16.6 Radiograph of a moderately displaced distal clavicular fracture in a 12-year-old patient.

deformity of the shoulder and tenting of the skin may be present. In the case of a displaced physeal fracture, radiographs of the shoulder may demonstrate a high-riding lateral clavicular metaphysis in relation to the neighboring acromion. Occasionally, an associated fracture of the base of the coracoid process may be present.[43]

CLASSIFICATION

Distal clavicular fractures have been classified into three types by Dameron and Rockwood.[8] Type I is a fracture without displacement, type II is a nonarticular displaced fracture, and type III is a fracture involving the acromioclavicular joint (Fig. 16.7). However, it should be noted that these classifications were formulated to describe fractures occurring in adults, and for the reasons discussed previously, fractures involving the joint itself are a rarity in the skeletally immature patient.

TREATMENT

In view of the tremendous remodeling potential (i.e., the osteogenic capacity of the retained periosteal sleeve), these injuries are almost universally managed nonoperatively. Treatment usually consists of a simple sling or Velpeau shoulder immobilization for 3 weeks, followed by gentle functional shoulder exercises. Several reports have described Y-shaped distal clavicular anatomy or distal clavicular duplication and ascribed them to developmental causes.[44,45] Ogden[5] suggested a traumatic cause, in which one limb of the Y is the original, now upwardly displaced, lateral clavicular metaphysis (Fig. 16.8), and the second limb is the bone that forms in the retained (nondisplaced) periosteal sleeve. The condition is asymptomatic and does not require treatment. As a rule, one should expect a normal-appearing and normally functioning shoulder after healing of a distal clavicular fracture in a child.

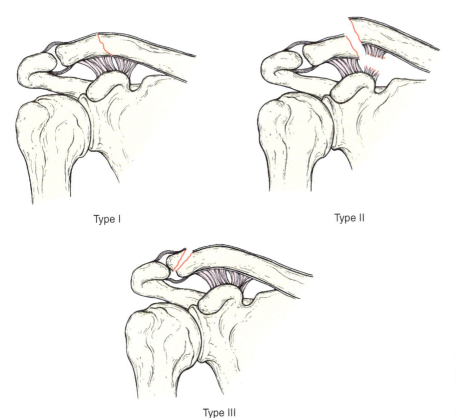

Type I

Type II

Type III

Fig. 16.7 Distal clavicular fractures classified into three types by Dameron and Rockwood.[35] Type I is nondisplaced and nonarticular, type II is displaced and nonarticular, and type III is intraarticular.

ACROMIOCLAVICULAR JOINT INJURY

As noted previously, a true injury to the acromioclavicular joint is rare in children but may be seen in older adolescents.[8] The mechanism of injury is the same as in adults: a blow to or a fall on the point of the shoulder. Allman[42] classified these injuries into three types: type I, a mild sprain of the acromioclavicular ligaments without subluxation of the joint; type II, a sprain of the acromioclavicular ligaments with subluxation of the joint but no disruption of the coracoclavicular ligament; and type III, dislocation of the joint with disruption of both ligaments, which is seen on anteroposterior (AP) radiographs as an increase in the coracoclavicular distance (Fig. 16.9).

Treatment of type I and II injuries consists of a simple form of immobilization such as a sling or shoulder Velpeau dressing for 3 to 4 weeks. The immobilization should be followed by functional shoulder exercises, and gradual progression of movement should be dictated by patient comfort. Type I injuries do well as a rule. Type II injuries are occasionally accompanied by late sequelae such as weakness and pain with shoulder movement. Affected individuals may be candidates for a reconstruction procedure when such an injury occurs in their late teen or early adult years. In those patients, an acromioclavicular ligament reconstruction may be indicated. Discussion in the adult literature has been abundant regarding the management of type III injuries; however, because of the rarity of the injury in pediatric patients, little exists in the literature on this subject in skeletally immature patients.

Indications for open treatment include acromioclavicular joint injuries in conjunction with scapulothoracic dissociation,[46] irreducible and widely displaced injuries in which the clavicle becomes subcutaneous and buttonholed through the fibers of the trapezius,[47] open injuries requiring débridement and irrigation, and patient and/or parent preference for early stabilization and mobilization. Early operative fixation may be most appropriate in high-level throwing or lifting athletes. These uncommon indications notwithstanding, nonoperative management[48,49] is the

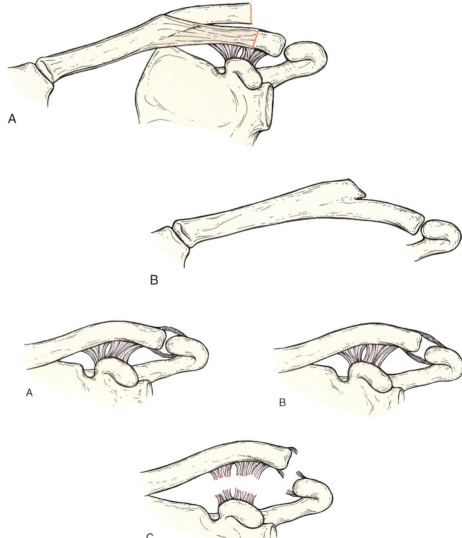

Fig. 16.8 (A) Distal clavicular fracture in an immature child with upward displacement. (B) Healing occurs within the retained periosteal sleeve.

Fig. 16.9 (A–C) Allman's three types of acromioclavicular joint injury.

treatment of choice for essentially all types of this injury in children and adolescents.

SCAPULA

DEVELOPMENTAL ANATOMY

The scapula begins to ossify from a single center at the eighth week of fetal life. The ossification center for the middle of the coracoid process forms at 1 year of age, and that for the base of the coracoid and upper portion of the glenoid at 10 years.[28] At puberty, two to five centers form in the acromion and fuse by 22 years of age; failure of any of these centers to fuse gives rise to the normal variant termed *os acromiale* (Fig. 16.10). A horseshoe-shaped secondary center at the inferior rim of the glenoid, a center for the medial border, and a center for the inferior angle form and later fuse with the remainder of the bone by approximately 22 years of age.[1,50,51]

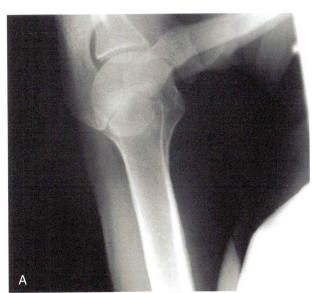

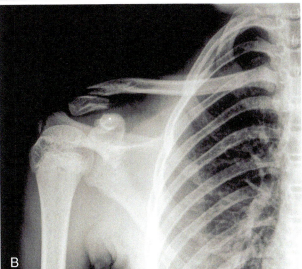

Fig. 16.10 (A) One of several possible patterns of os acromiale, which, in this case, was discovered incidentally on an axillary lateral projection of the glenohumeral joint. (B) Os acromiale noted incidentally in association with fracture of the distal clavicle.

ANATOMY

The scapula is a flat bone richly invested in muscle over the postero-superolateral aspect of the chest wall; there are multiple sites of muscle attachment ($n = 17$) on both its superficial and deep aspects, and only the dorsal edge of its spine and acromion are subcutaneous. It articulates with the clavicle at the acromioclavicular joint, with the humerus at the glenohumeral joint, and functionally with the chest wall through the scapulothoracic articulation (not a true joint). The muscles that invest the scapula participate in shoulder movements by rotating, stabilizing, and translating the scapula on the chest wall.[52] The articular surface of the glenoid is pear-shaped; the fibrocartilaginous labrum on its rim helps center the humeral head in the glenoid during function. The bony projections (i.e., the acromion and coracoid process) are oriented at 120 degrees to each other and to the axillary border of the scapula when viewed from the true lateral aspect of the bone (the so-called Y view of the scapula; Fig. 16.11).[53]

INCIDENCE AND CLASSIFICATION

Fractures of the scapula in children are rare and are classified according to the portion of the bone that is fractured: the body, glenoid, acromion, or coracoid.[54]

BODY FRACTURES

Scapular body fractures occur as a result of direct, significant trauma. With the large amount of surrounding muscle, clinical deformity is rarely evident. Clues on physical examination include abrasions, ecchymoses, neighboring wounds, swelling, and tenderness. True AP and lateral radiographic

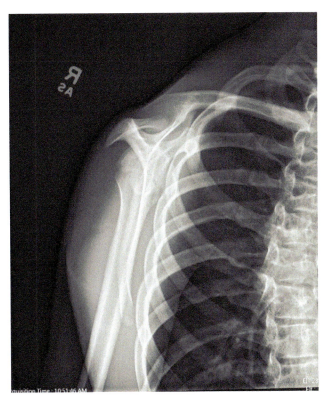

Fig. 16.11 A Y view of the glenohumeral joint.

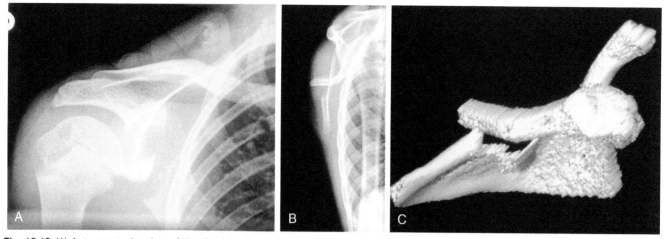

Fig. 16.12 (A) Anteroposterior view of the shoulder demonstrating displaced scapular body fracture. (B) Y view of the shoulder demonstrating the scapular body fracture. (C) Three-dimensional CT reconstruction of the scapular body fracture.

views are usually diagnostic, but opposite-side comparison views are sometimes necessary to detect subtle injuries in children. CT may be useful for delineating the true extent of the injury (Fig. 16.12).

In general, scapular body fractures, like scapulothoracic dissociations, imply absorption of a large amount of force, and associated injuries may have also occurred to the underlying chest as well as injury to neighboring neurovascular structures (e.g., subclavian and axillary vessels and the brachial plexus). In the vast majority of instances, pediatric scapular fractures are managed with sling immobilization of the shoulder for 2 to 3 weeks. This can be followed by gentle mobilization (e.g., pendulum exercises) and progression over a period of several weeks to full activity in accordance with patient comfort and findings on physical and radiographic examinations. There is little information in the literature regarding operative treatment of scapular body fractures in children.

Scapulothoracic dissociation can be diagnosed on an AP view of the chest. A search for associated injury to the brachial plexus,[55] vascular structures, and chest wall should be conducted.[46] Scapulothoracic dissociation has not been reported in newborns or very young children but has been reported twice in older children.[46,56]

GLENOID FRACTURES

Generally, fractures of the glenoid most commonly are the result of a direct force on the lateral aspect of the shoulder, and the humeral head is driven into the glenoid surface by that force. Some fractures of the glenoid are caused by forces transmitted by a fall on a flexed elbow.[35] Whether a posterior or an anterior rim fragment is associated with a corresponding subluxation of the humeral head is determined by the position of the arm at the time of injury. CT is especially useful in assessing the size and significance of these intraarticular fractures. If the fragment is large or if a significant amount of the joint surface is involved, the glenohumeral joint may become unstable, causing the humeral head to subluxate. In cases with associated glenohumeral dislocation, significant displacement of an associated glenoid rim fragment may occur.

For minimally displaced glenoid fragments not associated with humeral head subluxation or dislocation, the recommended treatment is sling immobilization for 3 weeks, followed by gentle functional shoulder exercises. For the uncommon situation of a large fragment associated with humeral head subluxation or dislocation, operative anatomic reduction with lag screw fixation (Fig. 16.13) or a small "hook" or "spring" plate and repair of associated capsular tears are indicated.[57,58] Careful preoperative planning is strongly recommended, and the surgical approach is dictated by the location of the fragment to be fixed. Postoperatively, the patient's arm is immobilized in a sling for 3 weeks, followed by gentle functional exercises. Screws or plates may be removed after 3 months, but there is no unanimity of opinion that exists regarding the issue of implant removal in this setting.[59] The severity of symptoms ascribed to retained implants may warrant their removal, but the symptoms should outweigh the risks associated with additional surgery.

ACROMION FRACTURES

Fractures of the acromion are rare but can result from a direct force on the point of the shoulder, or from obstetrical trauma (Fig. 16.14).[60] Failure of one of the several acromial epiphyses to fuse (i.e., os acromiale; see Fig. 16.10) is a normal developmental variant and should not be mistaken for a fracture. Comparison radiographs of the contralateral extremity may be helpful, as may reference to an appropriate radiographic atlas of normal skeletal variants.[61] The usual treatment consists of sling immobilization for 3 weeks, followed by early functional shoulder exercises.

CORACOID FRACTURES

Fracture of the coracoid process is uncommon in children.[5] The two fracture patterns seen when the injury does occur appear to represent an avulsion by the pull of either the acromioclavicular ligaments or the conjoined tendon of the coracobrachialis and short head of the biceps brachii.[62] The first type of fracture occurs through the physis at the base of the coracoid and the upper quarter of the glenoid,[63] and the second type occurs through the tip of the coracoid.[54] Coracoid fractures can accompany distal clavicular fractures, apparent acromioclavicular joint injuries,[64,65] and shoulder dislocations.[66,67] The injury can be demonstrated

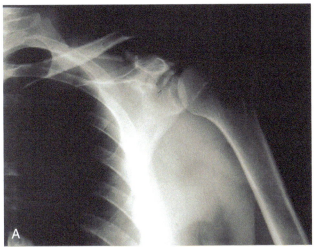

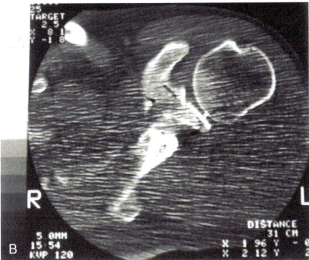

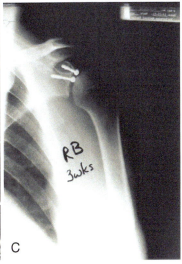

Fig. 16.13 (A) Intraarticular fracture of the glenoid with associated acromioclavicular separation and acromial fracture. (B) Computed tomography demonstrates the step-off displacement in the joint. (C) The articular fragment was repositioned anatomically via an anterior approach. The fragment was held in place by two lag screws.

by the Stryker notch view or by an axillary lateral view when the gantry is widened to include the coracoid on the film (Fig. 16.15). CT scans provide the most accurate view of a potential coracoid fracture. Treatment usually consists of sling immobilization of the shoulder for 3 weeks, followed by a functional shoulder exercise program.

GLENOHUMERAL JOINT DISLOCATION

DEVELOPMENTAL ANATOMY

Between 4 and 7 weeks' gestation, the proximal upper limb bud blastema differentiates into the scapula, the humerus, and an interzone. This interzone and its surrounding mesenchyme eventually give rise to the capsule and intraarticular structures of the glenohumeral joint.[68] Differentiation of these structures is complete by 7 to 8 weeks after fertilization.

ANATOMY

The glenohumeral articulation is a true synovial joint of the ball-and-socket variety. The joint comprises the shallow, pear-shaped glenoid and the spherical head of the humerus. The closely related capsule, its associated glenohumeral

ligaments, and its overlying rotator cuff tendons provide a mobile and dynamic extension of the glenoid cavity that centers and stabilizes the humeral head within that cavity and enables it to pass through a greater arc of motion than any other joint in the body. However, the glenohumeral joint's major reliance on soft tissue support for stability makes it susceptible to injury with resultant subluxation or dislocation.[69]

INCIDENCE

During childhood, because of the relative strength of the surrounding soft tissue structures, the growing proximal humeral physis is mechanically the weakest link in the glenohumeral articulation. Thus, traumatic force causing injury to this area is most often manifested as a proximal humeral physeal fracture. During the adolescent years, as the proximal humeral growth plate begins to close and strengthen compared with other parts of the glenohumeral articulation, the incidence of glenohumeral dislocation and associated capsular injuries rises. In the series reported by Rowe and colleagues[70–72] of 500 glenohumeral dislocations seen over a 20-year period, only eight (1.6%) occurred in children younger than 10 years, whereas 99 (19.8%) occurred in patients ages 10 through 20 years. Approximately half the injuries in the 10- to 20-year-old group (48 of 99) were

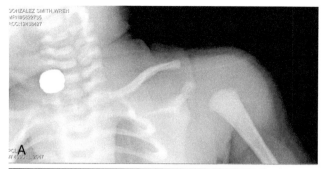

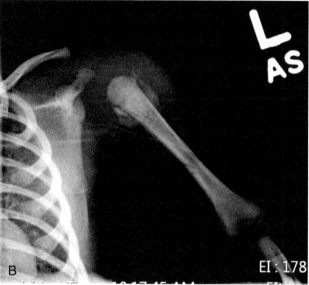

Fig. 16.14 Acromial fracture as a result of birth trauma in a neonate. One-day-old child presented with pseudoparalysis following a traumatic birth extraction. Radiographs demonstrated an acromial fracture (A). Note the widened joint space at the glenohumeral joint. (B) One month later, the acromial fracture healed. Note the abundant callus formation at the proximal humerus, indicating an associated proximal humerus fracture not well visualized at the time of injury.

recurrent dislocations. Recurrence rates ranged from 20% to 100% in children younger than 10 years and from 48% to 90% in patients between the ages of 10 and 20 years.[73] Dislocation of the shoulder during infancy is very rare but has been reported in association with brachial plexus palsy,[74] sepsis,[75] and congenital deformity.[76]

CLASSIFICATION

Glenohumeral dislocations may be classified according to the direction of the dislocation: anterior, posterior, or inferior (the latter two are much less frequent in all age groups). In addition, they may be classified according to cause, as shown in Fig. 16.16.

MECHANISM OF INJURY

Anterior glenohumeral dislocation is usually produced by a force on the outstretched hand with the shoulder in abduction, external rotation, and elevation—a position that causes anterior levering of the humeral head and secondary stretching of the anterior and inferior capsular tissues. Up to 85% of patients with an anterior dislocation demonstrate evidence of anterior and inferior soft tissue detachment from the glenoid—the so-called Bankart lesion.[77] Posterior dislocations are relatively uncommon but may be seen in patients after epileptic seizures or spasmodic muscle contractions. The mechanism of these injuries is explained by the powerful activity of the internal rotators, which act to lever the humeral head posteriorly.[78,79]

Many patients with a history of atraumatic dislocation can voluntarily subluxate or dislocate their shoulders. Those who perform this atraumatic, voluntary type of dislocation are more likely to be children or adolescents than adults. In the initial report by Rowe and colleagues,[71] 20 of 26 patients with voluntary dislocations (77%) were 16 years or younger; psychiatric factors were found to play an important role in these voluntary dislocations. Whether this ability is

Fig. 16.15 (A) The coracoid is adequately visualized on the axillary lateral projection when the gantry is wide. (B) The tip of the coracoid has been avulsed in this mature individual.

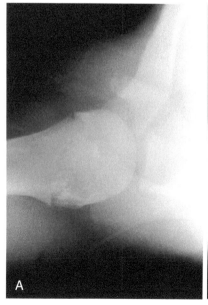
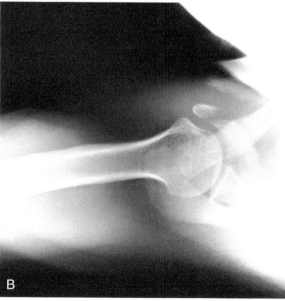

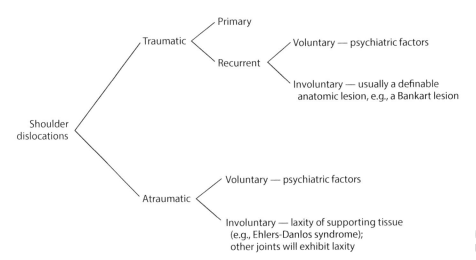

Fig. 16.16 Etiologic classification of glenohumeral dislocations.

spontaneous or acquired after an initial minimally traumatic injury is unclear. In this series, 11 patients could recall no specific episode of initial trauma; the remaining 15 could recall only minor injury or a fall.

DIAGNOSIS

Traumatic dislocation causes pain and swelling about the shoulder. In contradistinction, atraumatic dislocation causes little or minimal pain or swelling. The attitude of the arm at presentation is dependent on the direction of the dislocation. With an anterior dislocation, the arm is held abducted and usually slightly externally rotated; with a posterior dislocation, it is fixed in adduction and internal rotation; and with an inferior dislocation, it is classically held in abduction with the forearm lying on or behind the patient's head (the luxatio erecta position).

A careful neurovascular examination should be performed in all patients with a traumatic dislocation. Injury to the axillary nerve and tears of the rotator cuff tendons may be seen in association with glenohumeral dislocation and should be assessed. In their series of 226 anterior dislocations, Pasila and associates[80] reported an 11% incidence of brachial plexus injuries, 8% incidence of axillary nerve injuries, and 11% incidence of rotator cuff tears. The neighboring axillary artery and vein are also at risk of injury. The most common etiology of these injuries is as a result of excessively forceful attempts at shoulder reduction.[81]

Radiographic evaluation should include a "trauma series"[54] consisting of an AP and lateral view in the plane of the scapula. Because the overlying humeral head and chest wall can obscure subtle glenoid rim fractures (as well as a fracture of the lesser humeral tuberosity), an axillary lateral view or a modified axillary lateral view[82] should also be obtained.

TREATMENT

Reduction of an acute, traumatic dislocation can usually be accomplished safely by any of several classic methods. For immediate reduction of an acute dislocation (as in those witnessed and clinically apparent as dislocations and treated on an athletic field), slight abduction and derotation of the affected arm with minimal traction can be attempted

as described by O'Brien and associates.[69] The Hippocratic method consists of slow and gentle traction on the affected arm with gentle internal and external rotation to disengage the humeral head. With this technique, the physician may apply countertraction by placing a foot on the patient's chest wall (Fig. 16.17A) but not in the axilla. Alternatively, one can use a modification of this technique by placing a twisted sheet around the upper part of the patient's chest and having an assistant pull on the sheet to provide the desired countertraction (Fig. 16.17B).

The Stimson method calls for positioning the patient prone and allowing the affected arm to hang from the edge of the table with a weight (5–10 pounds) suspended from the end of the arm (Fig. 16.17C). This method is problematic because of the inherent difficulties in monitoring the sedated patient in the prone position. Numerous other methods have been described by various authors.[83–86] In general, the goal should be to perform the reduction in the least traumatic manner possible. Adequate sedation is essential in the pediatric patient population.

After reduction, the neurovascular examination should be repeated. A sling should be applied, followed by early motion; progression is dictated by patient comfort. The duration and method of immobilization after primary anterior dislocation remains unclear.[87] A period of enforced shoulder immobilization was not shown to influence the recurrence rate in a large prospective series by Hovelius.[88] In addition, multiple recent studies have shown no clear benefit of immobilization of the shoulder in external rotation versus internal rotation after primary dislocation.[89,90] What is clear is that both the patient and family should be informed of the high likelihood of recurrence in the pediatric and adolescent age group, the position of the arm and shoulder during activities that are likely to trigger it (for an anterior dislocation, it would be elevation with external rotation), and which sports should be considered high risk (for an anterior dislocation, it might be tennis or other overhead activities). Attempts may be made to increase the strength of the rotator cuff musculature, especially those involved with internal rotation, but this appears to be of limited benefit in this age group.

Most younger patients can be considered candidates for operative stabilization because of the high risk of repetitive instability, as data has shown that the recurrent dislocation

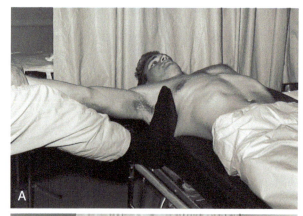

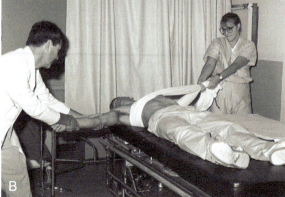

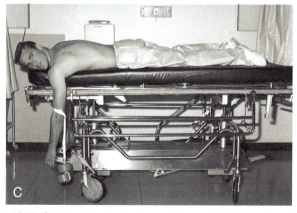

Fig. 16.17 Glenohumeral reduction techniques. (A) Hippocratic method. (B) Modified Hippocratic method. (C) Stimson method.

rate in this population can be lowered significantly with surgical intervention.[91–93] Patients with recurring dislocations, especially if associated with activities of daily living that are difficult to modify, are certainly candidates for a repair directed toward the specifically implicated disorder, such as a Bankart repair.[94] Surgical management can be performed by either open or arthroscopic techniques. Evaluation continues regarding recurrence and other sequelae for each type of approach. Arthroscopic stabilization has been shown to be successful in both overhead and contact athletes, and multiple studies have demonstrated acceptable outcome scores, and possibly a lower recurrent dislocation rate, utilizing open Bankart repairs in this age group.[95–99]

Patients with a history of voluntary dislocations are best managed initially by nonoperative means consisting of a rehabilitation program aimed at strengthening the rotator cuff and deltoid muscles.[71] When indicated, specific

counseling directed toward modifying any underlying attention-seeking behavior pattern should be pursued. If this counseling is successful, any recurring dislocations are often of the involuntary variety and may be multidirectional.[100] Surgical treatment with an appropriate capsular shift to correct this specific type of instability would then be indicated.[100,101]

PROXIMAL HUMERAL FRACTURES

DEVELOPMENTAL ANATOMY

The primary ossification center for the humerus appears around the sixth week of fetal development.[102] The ossification center for the humeral head appears at about the time of birth, that for the greater tuberosity between 7 months and 3 years, and of the lesser tuberosity 2 years later. These proximal secondary ossification centers coalesce between 5 to 7 years of age.[1,102] The proximal humeral growth plate closes between 14 and 17 years of age in females and between 16 and 18 years of age in males.[102,103]

ANATOMY

The proximal humeral physis is tent shaped, and its apex is located in the posteromedial aspect of the proximal end of the humerus on cross section (Fig. 16.18).[104] A small portion of the posterior proximal and medial metaphysis is intracapsular. The capsular attachment provides a strong tether just distal to this area. This anatomic characteristic, in addition to the relative thickness of the posteromedial periosteum and thinness of the anterolateral periosteum,[105] may explain the tendency for the metaphyseal fragment to buttonhole the periosteum anterolaterally when the proximal end of the humerus is fractured, whereas (in Salter-Harris type II injuries) a small posteromedial piece of metaphysis stays with the proximal fragment.

Salter-Harris type I and II fractures, which make up the vast majority of physeal injuries to the proximal humerus, typically pass through the zone of hypertrophy adjacent to the zone of provisional calcification. These types of fractures generally spare the embryonal cartilage cells within the germinal zone, thereby limiting the risk of growth disturbance to the proximal humeral physis.[105,106] The proximal humeral physis contributes 80% of the longitudinal growth of the humerus; thus, fractures at that site have great remodeling potential (Fig. 16.19).

INCIDENCE

Fractures involving the proximal humeral growth plate represent approximately 0.45% of all childhood fractures[107] and approximately 3% of all epiphyseal fractures.[108]

MECHANISM OF INJURY

The forces that bring about a proximal humeral fracture in children are most commonly indirect and result from a fall on the outstretched arm,[109] although a direct force, such as a blow on the posterolateral aspect of the upper part of the arm, has been implicated as a common mechanism.[108] Injury in the newborn is usually attributable to a

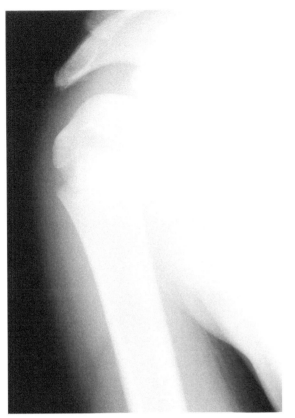

Fig. 16.18 Anteroposterior radiograph of a minimally displaced Salter-Harris type I fracture in a 14-year-old boy.

hyperextended and externally rotated position of the arm during vaginal delivery. This may result in an unusual traction injury, as the epiphysis fractures and dissociates from the metaphysis.[110,111]

DIAGNOSIS

In the neonate, diagnosis of proximal humerus fractures can be difficult. The findings may be subtle, such as irritability with arm movements, or more pronounced, such as pseudoparalysis. The differential diagnosis of pseudoparalysis or pain with passive motion includes septic arthritis, osteomyelitis of any bone of the shoulder girdle (see Figs. 16.4 and 16.14), clavicular injuries, and brachial plexus injury.[109] A history of prematurity, maternal sepsis, umbilical artery catheterization, or abnormal inflammatory markers may necessitate further evaluation to exclude joint sepsis or osteomyelitis. Plain radiographs of the proximal humerus should be obtained, along with comparison views of the opposite limb. In addition, ultrasonography[112] and magnetic resonance imaging (MRI) can be used to outline the position of the proximal (largely cartilaginous) fragment.

In older children, pain, splinting, and arm dysfunction are evident. Ecchymosis and swelling are variably present, and, in displaced fractures, the arm may be shortened and show prominence of the proximal metaphysis in the anterior aspect of the shoulder. Orthogonal plain radiographs should be obtained, including an AP view and an axillary lateral view (if possible).

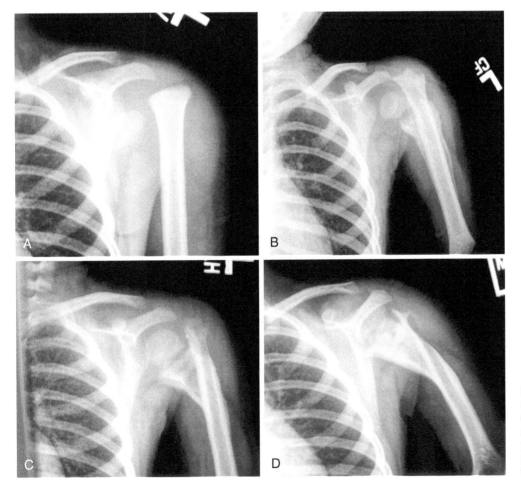

Fig. 16.19 (A) Acute Salter-Harris type I fracture in a 4-year-old child status postinjury without reduction. (B) Three weeks status postinjury. (C) Eight weeks status postinjury. (D) Twelve weeks status postinjury.

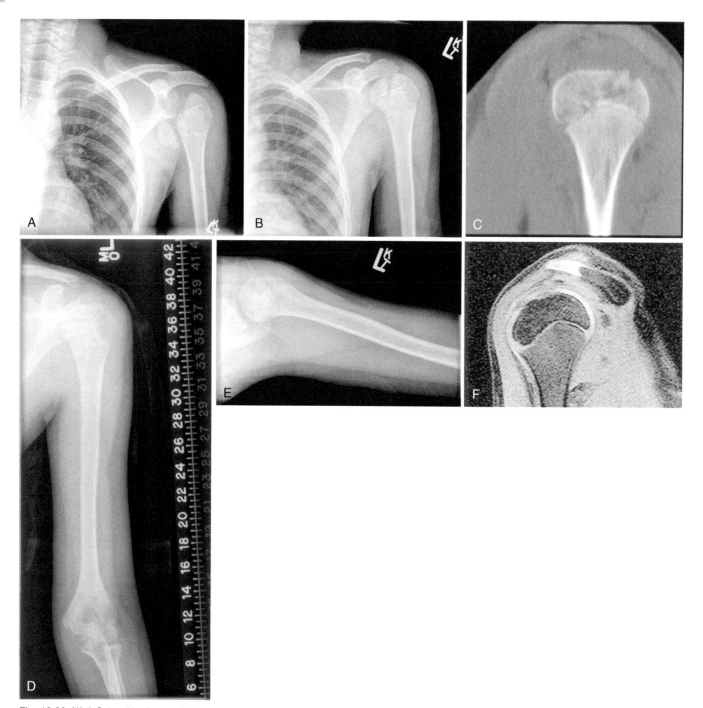

Fig. 16.20 (A) A Salter-Harris type IV fracture in a skeletally immature male. (B) Anteroposterior (AP) view after closed reduction. (C) Computed tomographic scan after closed reduction. (D) AP view 1 year status postfracture and reduction. (E) Lateral view 1 year status postfracture and reduction. (F) Magnetic resonance imaging 1year status postfracture demonstrates viable physis and no evidence of growth arrest.

CLASSIFICATION

The Salter-Harris classification has been applied to physeal injuries of the proximal end of the humerus.[113] Most of these fractures in children younger than 5 years are type I, 75% of fractures in children older than 11 years are type II, and most of the remainder are type I. Metaphyseal fractures predominate between ages 5 and 11 years. Salter-Harris types III, IV, and V injuries are rarely seen.[54,114,115] In addition, the authors have treated one patient with a Salter-Harris type IV injury that was amenable to closed reduction and immobilization (Fig. 16.20A–F).

Salter-Harris type II fractures of the proximal humerus have been subdivided further into four grades by Neer and Horwitz,[108] who used the extent of fracture displacement as classification criteria (Table 16.1). Note that within this classification system, grades III and IV are associated with varus angulation. In the Neer and Horwitz series, shortening of 1 to 3 cm was reported in 11% of group I and II patients and in 33% of group IV patients; no significant shortening resulted if the patient was younger than 11 years at the time of injury. Thus, the remodeling potential (in years) may play more of a role in determining the final outcome than the extent of displacement.

TABLE 16.1   Neer–Horwitz Classification of Proximal Humeral Fractures

Grade	Displacement
I	<5 mm
II	<1/3 shaft width
III	2/3 shaft width
IV	>2/3 shaft width

(From Neer CS, Horwitz BS. Fractures of the proximal humeral epiphyseal plate. *Clin Orthop Relat Res*. 1965;41:24.)

TABLE 16.2   Acceptable Alignment of Pediatric Proximal Humeral Fractures

Patient Age (years)	Allowable Displacement or Angulation
<5	Up to 70-degree angulation, 100% displacement
5–12	40- to 70-degree angulation
>12	Up to 40-degree angulation, 50% displacement

(Data from Beaty JH. Fractures of the proximal humerus and shaft in children. *Instr Course Lect*. 1992;41:369-372.)

TREATMENT

In the vast majority of cases, proximal humeral fractures in pediatric patients are managed by closed techniques. The need for reduction is determined by the extent of displacement and remodeling capacity, which is a function of skeletal maturity. Nondisplaced fractures at any age can be managed by sling-and-swathe immobilization followed by protected motion. When acceptable alignment cannot be achieved or when the reduction is lost as the arm is brought to the chest wall, a decision must be made regarding whether to accept malposition (usually varus with or without displacement), to make further attempts at reduction, or to use more elaborate immobilization methods. This decision should take into account the age of the patient (and thus the remodeling potential of the bone), as well as the fact that a functional shoulder can be expected in most cases, regardless of the method used.[8,106,116]

Sherk and Probst[117] determined minimal guidelines for an acceptable reduction: angulation of less than 20 degrees and displacement of less than 50%. When these criteria are met, an acceptable outcome can be expected. Beaty[118] delineated guidelines for acceptable fracture alignment that were stratified by patient age. In general, allowable displacement and angulation are related inversely to patient age because of the tremendous remodeling potential in younger patients (Table 16.2).

The options for treatment of displaced proximal humerus fractures include closed reduction and sling/swathe or hanging arm cast immobilization, closed or open reduction with percutaneous pinning, or open reduction with internal fixation.[119] A systematic review of the literature published in 2011[120] supports nonoperative treatment of most pediatric proximal humeral fractures. The authors of that review note that there is some evidence, albeit weak, that patients older than 13 years with widely displaced fractures may benefit from operative reduction and stabilization. Chaus et al[121] reviewed operative versus nonoperative management of proximal humerus fractures in a matched cohort of skeletally immature patients. They found there was no difference between either group. They did find a trend toward higher functional outcomes in those treated nonoperatively, but with less than desirable outcomes in patients older than 12 years of age treated nonoperatively.

In the older patient for whom adequate realignment of a proximal humerus fracture cannot be achieved under appropriate sedation, closed reduction under general anesthesia with fluoroscopic guidance and percutaneous pinning appears to be the treatment of choice.[122,123] Two or three smooth K-wires, or small-diameter Steinmann or Schanz pins with terminally threaded ends, are directed obliquely cephalad from the lateral metaphysis across the reduced physis and into the proximal epiphysis. Additional fixation with one or two wires placed antegrade from the proximal fragment may be indicated or desired. Stability of the fixation can then be evaluated under fluoroscopy (Fig. 16.21). The pins are cut and bent at the ends outside or just under the skin to minimize the risk of pin migration, and a sterile dressing is applied. Simple sling-and-swathe or collar-and-cuff immobilization is then applied to support the limb. Hutchinson and colleagues[124] compared patients who underwent closed reduction and either percutaneous pinning or retrograde intramedullary fixation with titanium flexible nails. They found similar functional results, but those patients who underwent stabilization with intramedullary nails had greater operating room time, higher blood loss, and the necessity of a second operative procedure for implant removal when compared with those undergoing percutaneous pin fixation.

Open reduction should be reserved for special circumstances, such as an open injury requiring surgical débridement, associated glenohumeral dislocation (in which forceful attempts at closed reduction may be hazardous to neighboring neurovascular soft tissue structures), associated vascular injuries, or in cases of irreducible fractures.[119,125,126] Traditionally, irreducibility of these fractures has been attributed to an interposed periosteal flap or entrapment of the long head of the biceps tendon within the fracture site.[127] However, Lucas and colleagues[128] reported MRI and cadaveric evidence that such entrapment may be much less common than previously thought. In addition, they demonstrated that it is extremely difficult to purposefully and manually generate such interposition or entrapment within the fracture site. If closed reduction cannot generate acceptable alignment, then open reduction and stabilization, with percutaneous pinning using smooth or terminally threaded pins, is generally recommended.

When percutaneous pins are used, the pins may be removed after 3 to 4 weeks, and the immobilization may be changed to a simple sling (Fig. 16.22). Periods of gentle motion out of the sling can start at that time. The fracture is usually healed by 6 weeks, at which point light activities are permitted. Vigorous activities involving the shoulder can be resumed in a gradual, stepwise fashion after completing a

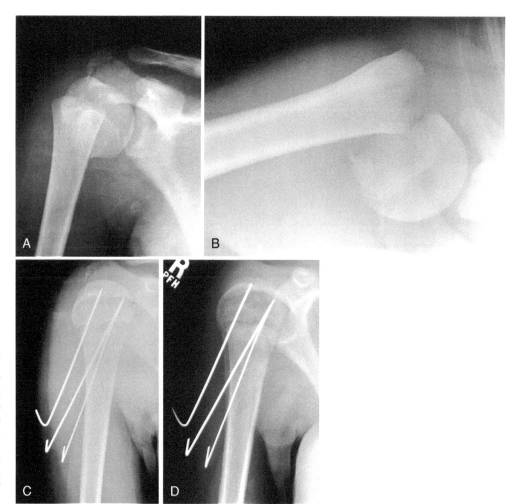

Fig. 16.21 (A and B) Radiographs of the proximal end of the humerus of a 14-year-old girl after a four-wheeler accident during which she sustained multiple traumatic injuries. (C) The fracture was managed with closed reduction and percutaneous pinning. (D) At follow-up 4 weeks later, the pins were removed; the patient quickly regained normal use of her shoulder.

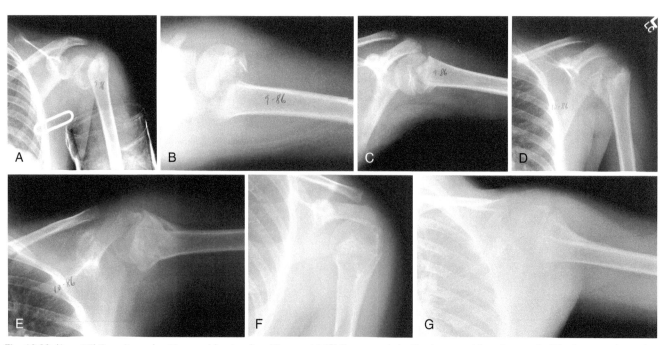

Fig. 16.22 (A and B) Type II proximal humeral fracture in a 12 year old. (C) Because abduction improved the alignment of the fracture, the patient was treated in abduction. (D) One month later, early healing is evident. (E) One month after (D), further healing is evident. (F and G) Radiographs 3 months later demonstrate more complete healing; the child had a normal clinical examination of the shoulder.

series of intermediate goals, including return of full-shoulder range of motion. The timetable depends on the individual and that person's healing capacity, the severity of the injury, and the type of stressful activity to be resumed.

SUBSCAPULARIS AVULSION (LESSER TUBEROSITY APOPHYSIS) FRACTURES

DEVELOPMENTAL ANATOMY

As noted previously, the lesser tuberosity is one of the three ossification centers of the proximal humerus. The three generally combine into a single epiphyseal segment between the ages of 5 and 7 years. The subscapularis muscle inserts on the lesser tuberosity.

INCIDENCE

A separate subset of proximal humeral fractures includes the subscapularis avulsion, which involves the avulsion of its insertion on the humerus along with a bony fragment of the lesser tuberosity. The fracture may be associated with glenohumeral dislocation. Isolated subscapularis avulsions are quite rare, with fewer than 40 cases reported in the English literature.[129,130]

MECHANISM OF INJURY

The most common mechanism appears to involve abduction, flexion, and external rotation of the shoulder; avulsion of the subscapularis occurs through a remnant of the apophysis of the lesser tuberosity. This mechanism is seen often as a result of high-energy sports injuries. In addition, a similar bony avulsion has been reported in throwing athletes.

DIAGNOSIS

Physical examination will demonstrate pain with passive external rotation of the shoulder and pain and weakness with active internal rotation. Plain radiographs of the shoulder with maximum internal rotation will usually reveal the bony fragment. MRI may be beneficial for assessing associated soft tissue injuries, particularly in cases of suspected intraarticular injury, soft tissue interposition, or instability (Fig. 16.23).[131]

TREATMENT

Results of nonoperative management of these injuries appear to be poor; thus operative treatment is recommended. Open reduction and internal fixation with multiple methods of stabilization have been reported.[129,130]

HUMERAL SHAFT FRACTURES

DEVELOPMENTAL ANATOMY

The humeral diaphysis begins to ossify during the sixth or seventh week of fetal life and is completely ossified by birth.[102] On cross section, the shaft is cylindrically shaped proximally and flattened distally in the coronal plane.[1] The posterior aspect of the bone provides the origin for the lateral head of the triceps

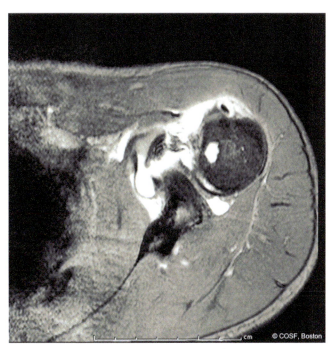

Fig. 16.23 Axial T2 image demonstrating avulsion of the lesser tuberosity of the humerus with subscapularis. (Image courtesy of D. Bae, MD. Copyrighted use with permission of the Children's Orthopaedic Surgery Foundation. All rights reserved.)

(superolaterally) and for its medial head (inferomedially), and the spiral groove lies in between. The radial nerve and its accompanying artery are in close relationship to the bone along this groove. Just proximal to its midpoint, the lateral aspect of the shaft provides the insertion for the deltoid muscle. Medially at this level is the attachment for the coracobrachialis. More proximally, the pectoralis major inserts into the lateral ridge of the intertubercular groove. The brachialis muscle has its origin from the distal half of the anterior aspect of the humeral shaft. An appreciation of these muscular attachments is essential for understanding the deforming forces acting on humeral shaft fracture fragments (Fig. 16.24).

INCIDENCE

The humeral shaft is fractured less frequently in children than in adults. Among the humeral shaft fractures of childhood, diaphyseal fractures are more common in children older than 12 or younger than 3 years. For children younger than 10 years, the incidence of shaft fractures is approximately 26 per 100,000 per year.[107] Overall, shaft fractures account for 2% to 5% of all fractures in children.[35] Traditionally, such fractures in patients 3 years or younger have been thought to correlate highly with child abuse. However, a 1997 review demonstrated that only 18% of humeral shaft fractures in a group of patients younger than 3 years could be classified as probable abuse, thereby raising doubts whether humeral shaft fractures are as commonly the result of nonaccidental injury, as previously suspected.[132] This information is somewhat confounded by a more recent review of 500 child abuse cases that demonstrated 2.3 times greater odds of a humeral shaft fracture being secondary to abuse, rather than accidental, if the patient is less than 18 months of age.[133]

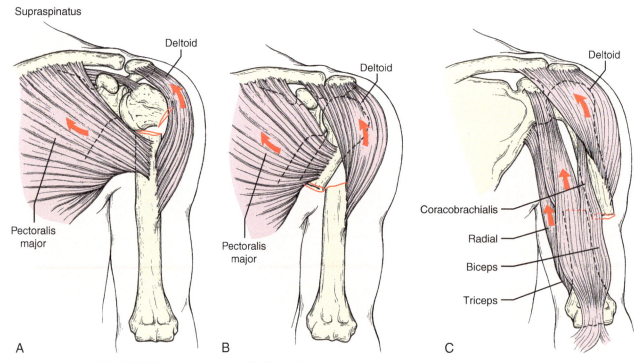

Fig. 16.24 Muscle attachments (A–C) that direct deforming forces in proximal humeral fractures.

MECHANISM OF INJURY

Transverse or short oblique fracture patterns are the result of direct trauma to the arm, which is the most common mechanism of injury. Indirect trauma (e.g., violent twisting) may result in a spiral or long oblique fracture pattern. This fracture pattern in any long bone, including the humerus, may be seen when child abuse is the cause,[103] but other fracture patterns do not rule out this etiology. It is essential to remember that any fracture pattern may occur as the result of child abuse.[134] If any injury is suspected to be nonaccidental, a full skeletal survey and report to the appropriate protective services agency are indicated.

Minor trauma may cause a previously unknown unicameral bone cyst of the humerus to fracture at the level of the cyst, which is the most common manifestation of this entity.[135] Symptomatic unicameral cysts are located most frequently in the metaphyseal/diaphyseal region of the proximal humerus.

Fracture at the junction of the middle and distal thirds of the shaft may be associated with injury to the radial nerve. Suspected radial nerve injury should be tested by asking the patient to extend the thumb. The vast majority of radial nerve injuries associated with a closed humeral shaft fracture will resolve without intervention.

DIAGNOSIS

Similar to proximal humeral fractures in neonates, neonatal humeral shaft fractures in this age group may present pseudoparalysis. Brachial plexus palsy, clavicular fracture, proximal humeral fracture, and infection should be part of the differential diagnosis. A child with a greenstick fracture of the humerus may have minimal symptoms and

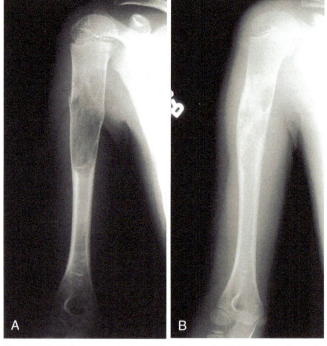

Fig. 16.25 (A) Anteroposterior (AP) radiograph at initial evaluation of a fracture through a unicameral (simple) bone cyst in the proximal end of the humerus of a 6-year-old girl. (B) AP radiograph 6 months after direct methylprednisolone injection reveals complete healing of the fracture and nearly complete resolution of the cyst.

tenderness. A pediatric patient with a displaced humeral shaft fracture usually has a history of significant trauma to the arm. The exception to this rule is a child with a fracture through a unicameral bone cyst that is brought about by otherwise trivial injury of the arm (Fig. 16.25).

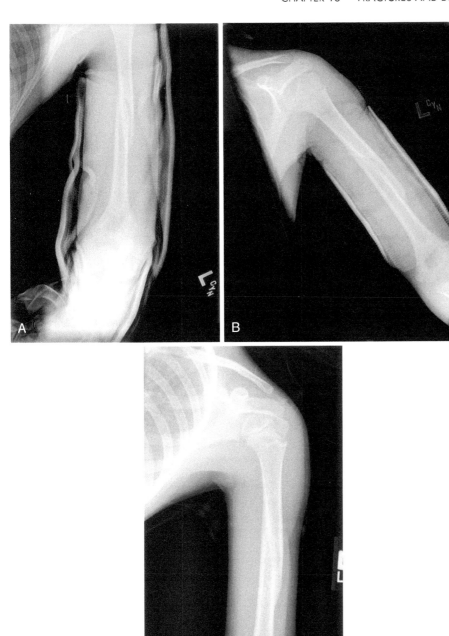

Fig. 16.26 (A) Humeral shaft fracture in a 9-year-old female treated initially with a long arm, hanging cast. (B) After acute swelling diminished, the fracture was managed in a nonremovable, functional brace, which allowed shoulder and elbow motion. (C) Healed fracture 9 weeks status postinjury.

Obvious deformity of the arm may be evident, and palpation elicits tenderness and crepitus over the area of the fracture. Plain radiographs in two orthogonal views are confirmatory.

TREATMENT

NONOPERATIVE

Isolated closed humeral shaft fractures are best managed by closed methods. One can take advantage of the stout surrounding periosteum by several methods, including a hanging arm cast or using the weight of the arm in a shoulder Velpeau dressing[136] or a collar-and-cuff bandage. Coaptation splints and, in older children and adolescents, prefabricated functional splints or braces can be used

(Fig. 16.26A–C). Prefabricated splints are best used after the period of acute swelling has passed, generally 10 to 14 days after injury. Humeral shaft fractures in a newborn associated with a traumatic delivery can be managed by splinting the arm to the chest wall with the arm of a long-sleeved shirt or "onesie" pinned to the chest portion of the clothing (Fig. 16.27).[137]

Remodeling in newborns and very young children is robust, and essentially any postfracture alignment is acceptable. In older patients, fracture angulation is most important for injuries of the distal half of the humerus. Less remodeling is expected for these fractures because of the distance from the proximal physis, which is responsible for up to 80% of the longitudinal growth of the humerus. As a guideline, alignment within 15° of anatomic

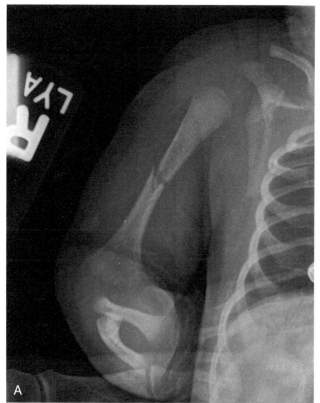

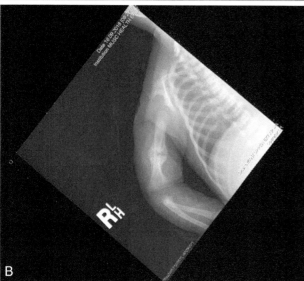

Fig. 16.27 Neonatal humeral shaft fracture. (A) One-day-old child with right humeral shaft fracture after difficult extraction. Child was treated with pinning the arm of the right onesie to the torso. (B) Six weeks later, note maintained alignment and abundant callus formation. Child had a full range of motion with normal motor examination.

should be maintained.[109] Bayonet apposition is acceptable in most cases, and some overgrowth of the humerus may occur.[35,138]

Most humeral shaft fractures develop sufficient callus to stabilize the fracture and permit limited range of motion at 3 to 4 weeks (2–3 weeks in newborns and very young children), and protected motion can then be started with brief periods out of the immobilization of choice. By 6 to 8 weeks (3–6 weeks in newborns and very young children), most fractures have healed well enough to go without support. Subsequent rehabilitation of the upper extremity is tailored to the demands of the individual. For a young child, rehabilitation can consist simply of the resumption of light play, with avoidance of activities that would risk a fall until the humerus has remodeled sufficiently.

Any associated radial nerve injuries should be observed for 16 to 20 weeks, as most will resolve spontaneously. The exception to this rule is a child who has intact radial nerve function at initial evaluation but loses it during or after an attempt at closed reduction. Under these circumstances, the radial nerve may be explored.[139] In patients with no sign of return of function after 4 to 6 months (the earliest returning motor function is that of the brachioradialis), the nerve should be explored, with neurolysis or neurorrhaphy as indicated by the intraoperative findings.

OPERATIVE

Open fractures require surgical irrigation and débridement. Subsequent to the application of a sterile dressing and the initiation of appropriate intravenous antibiotic therapy, the fracture fragments can be stabilized with a shoulder Velpeau dressing or similar technique. Internal fixation with either plate-and-screw constructs or flexible intramedullary nails may be used in these situations. External fixation should be reserved for severe open fractures with significant soft tissue injury for which frequent dressing changes may be required. Internal fixation as the primary method of management (Fig. 16.28) has a number of advantages in the polytraumatized child with either a closed or open injury, especially one with associated chest or severe head trauma.[122,140] These advantages include early functional use of the extremity, easier nursing care of the patient, and greater ease in mobilizing the patient. These advantages must be weighed against the enhanced potential for local infection and the need for later implant removal.[59] Although seldom necessary in children with an isolated humeral shaft fracture, internal fixation may be necessary in those with an associated vascular injury requiring repair or in those with nonunion of a shaft fracture. In the latter instance, bone grafting and rigid fixation with compression plating should be undertaken, and elbow and shoulder motion should be initiated in the immediate postoperative period.

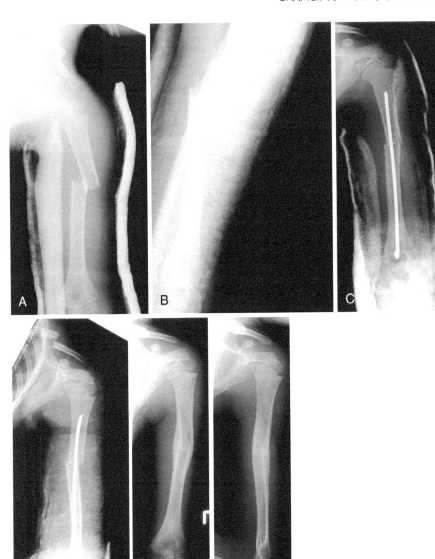

Fig. 16.28 (A and B) Anteroposterior (AP) and lateral radiographs of a closed humeral shaft fracture in a 5-year-old boy with an ipsilateral clavicular fracture, bilateral femoral fractures, severe closed head injury, and pulmonary contusion. (C and D) AP and lateral radiographs immediately after intramedullary fixation of the humeral fracture with a Rush rod performed at the time of operative stabilization of the femoral fractures. (E and F) AP and lateral radiographs 6 months after fixation and subsequent removal of the Rush rod. The patient had full active and passive range of motion of the elbow and shoulder.

REFERENCES

The level of evidence (LOE) is determined according to the criteria provided in the Preface.

1. H. G. *Anatomy of the Human Body*. Philadelphia: Lea & Febiger. **(LOE V)**.
2. Moseley HF. The clavicle: its anatomy and function. *Clin Orthop Relat Res*. 1968;58:17–27. **(LOE V)**.
3. Gardner E. The embryology of the clavicle. *Clin Orthop Relat Res*. 1968;58:9–16. **(LOE V)**.
4. Jit I, Kulkarni M. Times of appearance and fusion of epiphysis at the medial end of the clavicle. *Indian J Med Res*. 1976;64: 773–782. **(LOE IV)**.
5. J.A. O. *Skeletal Injury in the Child*. Philadelphia: WB Saunders. **(LOE V)**.
6. Lewonowski K, Bassett GS. Complete posterior sternoclavicular epiphyseal separation. A case report and review of the literature. *Clin Orthop Relat Res*. 1992;84–88. **(LOE IV)**.
7. Carmichael KD, Longo A, Lick S, Swischuk L. Posterior sternoclavicular epiphyseal fracture-dislocation with delayed diagnosis. *Skeletal Radiol*. 2006;35:608–612. **(LOE IV)**.
8. Dameron TB. Fractures and dislocations of the shoulder. In: *Fractures in Children*. Philadelphia: J.B. Lippincott;577–682. **(LOE V)**.
9. Hobbs DW. Sternoclavicular joint: a new axial radiographic view. *Radiology*. 1968;90:801. **(LOE V)**.
10. Yang J, al-Etani H, Letts M. Diagnosis and treatment of posterior sternoclavicular joint dislocations in children. *Am J Ortho*. 1996;25:565–569. **(LOE IV)**.
11. Bae DS, Kocher MS, Waters PM, Micheli LM, Griffey M, Dichtel L. Chronic recurrent anterior sternoclavicular joint instability: results of surgical management. *J Pediatr Orthop*. 2006;26:71–74. **(LOE IV)**.
12. Barth E, Hagen R. Surgical treatment of dislocations of the sternoclavicular joint. *Acta Orthop Scand*. 1983;54:746–747. **(LOE IV)**.
13. Eskola A. Sternoclavicular dislocation. A plea for open treatment. *Acta Orthop Scand*. 1986;57:227–228. **(LOE IV)**.
14. Clark RL, Milgram JW, Yawn DH. Fatal aortic perforation and cardiac tamponade due to a Kirschner wire migrating from the right sternoclavicular joint. *South Med J*. 1974;67:316–318. **(LOE IV)**.
15. Fowler AW. Migration of a wire from the sternoclavicular joint to the pericardial cavity. *Injury*. 1981;13:261–262. **(LOE IV)**.
16. Lyons FA, Rockwood Jr CA. Migration of pins used in operations on the shoulder. *J Bone Joint Surg Am*. 1990;72:1262–1267. **(LOE IV)**.
17. Waters PM, Bae DS, Kadiyala RK. Short-term outcomes after surgical treatment of traumatic posterior sternoclavicular fracture-dislocations in children and adolescents. *J Pediatr Orthop*. 2003;23:464–469. **(LOE IV)**.
18. Goldfarb CA, Bassett GS, Sullivan S, Gordon JE. Retrosternal displacement after physeal fracture of the medial clavicle in children treatment by open reduction and internal fixation. *J Bone Joint Surg Br*. 2001;83:1168–1172. **(LOE IV)**.
19. Rubin A. Birth injuries: incidence, mechanisms, and end results. *Obstet Gynecol*. 1964;23:218–221. **(LOE V)**.

20. Perlow JH, Wigton T, Hart J, Strassner HT, Nageotte MP, Wolk BM. Birth trauma. A five-year review of incidence and associated perinatal factors. *J Reprod Med.* 1996;41:754–760. (**LOE IV**).

21. Choi HA, Lee YK, Ko SY, Shin SM. Neonatal clavicle fracture in cesarean delivery: incidence and risk factors. *J Matern Fetal Neonatal Med.* 2017;30:1689–1692. (**LOE IV**).

22. Cohen AW, Otto SR. Obstetric clavicular fractures. A three-year analysis. *J Reprod Med.* 1980;25:119–122. (**LOE IV**).

23. Hsu TY, Hung FC, Lu YJ, et al. Neonatal clavicular fracture: clinical analysis of incidence, predisposing factors, diagnosis, and outcome. *Am J Perinatol.* 2002;19:17–21. (**LOE IV**).

24. Kayser R, Mahlfeld K, Heyde C, Grasshoff H. Ultrasonographic imaging of fractures of the clavicle in newborn infants. *J Bone Joint Surg Br.* 2003;85:115–116. (**LOE IV**).

25. Madsen ET. Fractures of the extremities in the newborn. *Acta Obstet Gynecol Scand.* 1955;34:41–74. (**LOE IV**).

26. Sanford HN. Moro reflex as a diagnostic aid in fracture of the clavicle in the newborn infant. *Am J Dis Child.* 1992;41:1304–1306. (**LOE IV**).

27. Blount WP. *Fractures in Children.* Baltimore: Williams & Wilkins; 1954. (**LOE V**).

28. Key JA, Conwell HE, Reynolds FC. *Key and Conwell's Management of Fractures, Dislocations, and Sprains.* 7th ed. St. Louis: Mosby; 1961. (**LOE V**).

29. Stanley D, Trowbridge EA, Norris SH. The mechanism of clavicular fracture. A clinical and biomechanical analysis. *J Bone Joint Surg Br.* 1988;70:461–464. (**LOE IV**).

30. Howard FM, Shafer SJ. Injuries to the clavicle with neurovascular complications. A study of fourteen cases. *J bone Joint surg Am.* 1965;47:1335–1346. (**LOE IV**).

31. Miller DS, Boswick Jr JA. Lesions of the brachial plexus associated with fractures of the clavicle. *Clini Orthop Relat Res.* 1969;64: 144–149. (**LOE IV**).

32. Tse DH, Slabaugh PB, Carlson PA. Injury to the axillary artery by a closed fracture of the clavicle. A case report. *J Bone Joint Surg Am.* 1980;62:1372–1374. (**LOE IV**).

33. Neviaser RJ. Injuries to the clavicle and acromioclavicular joint. *Orthop Clini N Am.* 1987;18:433–438. (**LOE V**).

34. Pennock AT, Edmonds EW, Bae DS, et al. Adolescent clavicle nonunions: potential risk factors and surgical management. *J Shoulder Elbow Surg.* 2018;27:29–35. (**LOE IV**).

35. Weber BG, Brunner CF, Freuler F. *Treatment of Fractures in Children and Adolescents.* Berlin; New York: Springer-Verlag; 1980. (**LOE V**).

36. Kubiak R, Slongo T. Operative treatment of clavicle fractures in children: a review of 21 years. *J Pediatr Orthop.* 2002;22:736–739. (**LOE IV**).

37. Vander Have KL, Perdue AM, Caird MS, Farley FA. Operative versus nonoperative treatment of midshaft clavicle fractures in adolescents. *J Pediatr Orthop.* 2010;30:307–312. (**LOE III**).

38. Li Y, Helvie P, Farley FA, Abbott MD, Caird MS. Complications after plate fixation of displaced pediatric midshaft clavicle fractures. *J Pediatr Orthop.* 2018;38(7):350-353. (**LOE IV**).

39. Hagstrom LS, Ferrick M, Galpin R. Outcomes of operative versus nonoperative treatment of displaced pediatric clavicle fractures. *Orthop.* 2015;38:e135–138. (**LOE III**).

40. Carry PM, Koonce R, Pan Z, Polousky JD. A survey of physician opinion: adolescent midshaft clavicle fracture treatment preferences among POSNA members. *J Pediatr Orthop.* 2011;31:44–49. (**LOE V**).

41. Suppan CA, Bae DS, Donohue KS, Miller PE, Kocher MS, Heyworth BE. Trends in the volume of operative treatment of midshaft clavicle fractures in children and adolescents: a retrospective, 12-year, single-institution analysis. *J Pediatr Orthop Part B.* 2016;25:305–309. (**LOE IV**).

42. Allman FL Jr. Fractures and ligamentous injuries of the clavicle and its articulation. *J Bone Joint Surg Am.* 1967;49:774–784. (**LOE IV**).

43. Eidman DK, Siff SJ, Tullos HS. Acromioclavicular lesions in children. *Am J Sports Med.* 1981;9:150–154. (**LOE IV**).

44. Golthamer CR. Duplication of the clavicle; (os subclaviculare). *Radiology.* 1957;68:576–578. (**LOE V**).

45. Twigg HL, Rosenbaum RC. Duplication of the clavicle. *Skeletal Radiol.* 1981;6:281. (**LOE V**).

46. An HS, Vonderbrink JP, Ebraheim NA, Shiple F, Jackson WT. Open scapulothoracic dissociation with intact neurovascular status in a child. *J Orthop Trauma.* 1988;2:36–38. (**LOE IV**).

47. Powers JA, Bach PJ. Acromioclavicular separations. Closed or open treatment? *Clini Orthop Relat Res.* 1974:213–223. (**LOE IV**).

48. Taft TN, Wilson FC, Oglesby JW. Dislocation of the acromioclavicular joint. An end-result study. *J Bone Joint Surg Am.* 1987;69:1045–1051. (**LOE IV**).

49. Larsen E, Bjerg-Nielsen A, Christensen P. Conservative or surgical treatment of acromioclavicular dislocation. A prospective, controlled, randomized study. *J Bone Joint Surg Am.* 1986;68:552–555. (**LOE I**).

50. McClure JG, Raney RB. Anomalies of the scapula. *Clini Orthop Relat Res.* 1975:22–31. (**LOE V**).

51. Samilson RL. Congenital and developmental anomalies of the shoulder girdle. *Orthop Clini N Am.* 1980;11:219–231. (**LOE V**).

52. Hollinshead WH. *Anatomy for Surgeons.* 3rd ed. Philadelphia: Harper & Row; 1982. (**LOE V**).

53. Rubin SA, Gray RL, Green WR. The scapular "Y": a diagnostic aid in shoulder trauma. *Radiol.* 1974;110:725–726. (**LOE V**).

54. Rockwood CA. *The Shoulder.* 4th ed. Philadelphia: Saunders/Elsevier; 2009. (**LOE V**).

55. Ebraheim NA, An HS, Jackson WT, et al. Scapulothoracic dissociation. *J Bone Joint Surg Am.* 1988;70:428–432. (**LOE IV**).

56. Nettrour LF, Krufky EL, Mueller RE, Raycroft JF. Locked scapula: intrathoracic dislocation of the inferior angle. A case report. *J Bone Joint Surg Am.* 1972;54:413–416. (**LOE IV**).

57. Mast J, Jakob R, Ganz R. *Planning and Reduction Technique in Fracture Surgery.* Berlin; New York: Springer-Verlag; 1989. (**LOE V**).

58. Zuelzer WA. Fixation of small but important bone fragments with a hook plate. *J Bone Joint Surg Am.* 1951;33-A:430–436. (**LOE IV**).

59. Schmalzried TP, Grogan TJ, Neumeier PA, Dorey FJ. Metal removal in a pediatric population: benign procedure or necessary evil? *J Pediatr Orthop.* 1991;11:72–76. (**LOE IV**).

60. McGahan JP, Rab GT, Dublin A. Fractures of the scapula. *J Trauma.* 1980;20:880–883. (**LOE V**).

61. Keats TE, Anderson MW. *Atlas of Normal Roentgen Variants that may Simulate Disease.* 7th ed. St. Louis: Mosby; 2001. (**LOE V**).

62. Kuhns LR, Sherman MP, Poznanski AK, Holt JF. Humeral-head and coracoid ossification in the newborn. *Radiol.* 1973;107:145–149. (**LOE IV**).

63. Heyse-Moore GH, Stoker DJ. Avulsion fractures of the scapula. *Skeletal Radiol.* 1982;9:27–32. (**LOE IV**).

64. Bernard Jr TN, Brunet ME, Haddad Jr RJ. Fractured coracoid process in acromioclavicular dislocations. Report of four cases and review of the literature. *Clini Orthop Relat Res.* 1983:227–232. (**LOE IV**).

65. Taga I, Yoneda M, Ono K. Epiphyseal separation of the coracoid process associated with acromioclavicular sprain. A case report and review of the literature. *Clini Orthop Relat Res.* 1986:138–141. (**LOE IV**).

66. Wong-Pack WK, Bobechko PE, Becker EJ. Fractured coracoid with anterior shoulder dislocation. *J Can Assoc Radiol.* 1980;31:278–279. (**LOE IV**).

67. Zilberman Z, Rejovitzky R. Fracture of the coracoid process of the scapula. *Injury.* 1981;13:203–206. (**LOE V**).

68. Gardner E. The prenatal development of the human shoulder joint. *Surg Clini N Am.* 1963;43:1465–1470. (**LOE V**).

69. O'Brien SJ, Warren RF, Schwartz E. Anterior shoulder instability. *Orthop Clini N Am.* 1987;18:395–408. (**LOE V**).

70. Rowe CR. Anterior dislocations of the shoulder: prognosis and treatment. *Surg Clini N Am.* 1963;43:1609–1614. (**LOE V**).

71. Rowe CR, Pierce DS, Clark JG. Voluntary dislocation of the shoulder. A preliminary report on a clinical, electromyographic, and psychiatric study of twenty-six patients. *J Bone Joint Surg Am.* 1973;55:445–460. (**LOE IV**).

72. Rowe CR, Zarins B, Ciullo JV. Recurrent anterior dislocation of the shoulder after surgical repair. Apparent causes of failure and treatment. *J Bone Joint Surg Am.* 1984;66:159–168. (**LOE IV**).

73. Asher MA. Dislocations of the upper extremity in children. *Orthop Clini N Am.* 1976;7:583–591. (**LOE V**).

74. Laskin RS, Sedlin ED. Luxatio erecta in infancy. *Clini Orthop Relat Res.* 1971;80:126–129. (**LOE V**).

75. Green NE, Wheelhouse WW. Anterior subglenoid dislocation of the shoulder in an infant following pneumococcal meningitis. *Clini Orthop Relat Res.* 1978:125–127. (**LOE IV**).

76. Haliburton RA, Barber JR, Fraser RL. Pseudodislocation: an unusual birth injury. *Can J Surg J Can de Chirurgie.* 1967;10:455–462. (**LOE IV**).

77. Bankart AS, Cantab MC. Recurrent or habitual dislocation of the shoulder-joint. *Clini Orthop Relat Res.* 1923;1993:3–6. (**LOE IV**).

78. Hawkins RJ, Koppert G, Johnston G. Recurrent posterior instability (subluxation) of the shoulder. *J Bone Joint Surg Am.* 1984;66:169–174. (**LOE V**).

79. Vastamaki M, Solonen KA. Posterior dislocation and fracture-dislocation of the shoulder. *Acta Orthop Scand*. 1980;51:479–484. **(LOE V)**.

80. Pasila M, Kiviluoto O, Jaroma H, Sundholm A. Recovery from primary shoulder dislocation and its complications. *Acta Orthop Scand*. 1980;51:257–262. (LOE V).

81. Blount WP. *Fractures in Children*. Huntington, NY: R. E. Krieger Pub. Co.;1977. (LOE V).

82. Bloom MH, Obata WG. Diagnosis of posterior dislocation of the shoulder with use of Velpeau axillary and angle-up roentgenographic views. *J Bone Joint Surg Am*. 1967;49:943–949. **(LOE IV)**.

83. Lacey T 2nd, Crawford HB. Reduction of anterior dislocations of the shoulder by means of the Milch abduction technique. *J Bone Joint Surg Am*. 1952;34-A:108–109. **(LOE V)**.

84. Russell JA, Holmes EM 3rd, Keller DJ, Vargas JH 3rd. Reduction of acute anterior shoulder dislocations using the Milch technique: a study of ski injuries. *J Trauma*. 1981;21:802–804. **(LOE IV)**.

85. Janecki CJ, Shahcheragh GH. The forward elevation maneuver for reduction of anterior dislocations of the shoulder. *Clini Orthop Relat Res*. 1982:177–180. **(LOE V)**.

86. Mirick MJ, Clinton JE, Ruiz E. External rotation method of shoulder dislocation reduction. *JACEP*. 1979;8:528–531. **(LOE V)**.

87. Beck JJ, Richmond CG, Tompkins MA, Heyer A, Shea KG, Cruz AI Jr. What's new in pediatric upper extremity sports injuries? *J Pediatr Orthop*. 2018;38:e73–e77. **(LOE V)**.

88. Hovelius L. Anterior dislocation of the shoulder in teen-agers and young adults. Five-year prognosis. *J Bone Joint Surg Am*. 1987;69:393–399. **(LOE IV)**.

89. Whelan DB, Kletke SN, Schemitsch G, Chahal J. Immobilization in external rotation versus internal rotation after primary anterior shoulder dislocation: a meta-analysis of randomized controlled trials. *Am J Sports Med*. 2016;44:521–532. **(LOE II)**.

90. Whelan DB, Litchfield R, Wambolt E, Dainty KN; Joint Orthopaedic Initiative for National Trials of the Shoulder. External rotation immobilization for primary shoulder dislocation: a randomized controlled trial. *Clini Orthop Relat Res*. 2014;472:2380–2386. **(LOE I)**.

91. Gigis I, Heikenfeld R, Kapinas A, Listringhaus R, Godolias G. Arthroscopic versus conservative treatment of first anterior dislocation of the Shoulder in adolescents. *J Pediatr Orthop*. 2014;34: 421–425. **(LOE III)**.

92. Longo UG, van der Linde JA, Loppini M, Coco V, Poolman RW, Denaro V. Surgical versus nonoperative treatment in patients up to 18 years old with traumatic shoulder instability: a systematic review and quantitative synthesis of the literature. *Arthroscopy*. 2016;32:944–952. **(LOE III)**.

93. Lin KM, James EW, Spitzer E, Fabricant PD. Pediatric and adolescent anterior shoulder instability: clinical management of first-time dislocators. *Curr Opini Pediatr*. 2018;30:49–56. **(LOE V)**.

94. Deitch J, Mehlman CT, Foad SL, Obbehat A, Mallory M. Traumatic anterior shoulder dislocation in adolescents. *Am J Sports Med*. 2003;31:758–763. **(LOE IV)**.

95. Cole BJ, L'Insalata J, Irrgang J, Warner JJ. Comparison of arthroscopic and open anterior shoulder stabilization. A two to six-year follow-up study. *J Bone Joint Surg Am*. 2000;82-A:1108–1114. **(LOE III)**.

96. Gartsman GM, Roddey TS, Hammerman SM. Arthroscopic treatment of anterior-inferior glenohumeral instability. Two to five-year follow-up. *J Bone Joint Surg Am*. 2000;82-A:991–1003. **(LOE IV)**.

97. Hatch MD, Hennrikus WL. The open Bankart repair for traumatic anterior shoulder instability in teenage athletes. *J Pediatr Orthop*. 2018;38:27–31. **(LOE IV)**.

98. Mohtadi NG, Chan DS, Hollinshead RM, et al. A randomized clinical trial comparing open and arthroscopic stabilization for recurrent traumatic anterior shoulder instability: two-year follow-up with disease-specific quality-of-life outcomes. *J Bone Joint Surg Am*. 2014;96:353–360. **(LOE I)**.

99. Shymon SJ, Roocroft J, Edmonds EW. Traumatic anterior instability of the pediatric shoulder: a comparison of arthroscopic and open Bankart repairs. *J Pediatr Orthop*. 2015;35:1–6. **(LOE III)**.

100. Neer CS 2nd. Involuntary inferior and multidirectional instability of the shoulder: etiology, recognition, and treatment. *Instr Course Lect*. 1985;34:232–238. **(LOE V)**.

101. Neer CS 2nd, Foster CR. Inferior capsular shift for involuntary inferior and multidirectional instability of the shoulder. A preliminary report. *J Bone Joint Surg Am*. 1980;62:897–908. **(LOE IV)**.

102. Gray DJ, Gardner E. The prenatal development of the human humerus. *Am J Anat*. 1969;124:431–445. **(LOE V)**.

103. Wenger DR, Pring ME, Pennock AT, Upasani VV, Rang M. *Rang's Children's Fractures*. 4th ed. Philadelphia: Wolters Kluwer Health; 2018. **(LOE V)**.

104. Ogden JA. *Skeletal Injury in the Child*. 2nd ed. Philadelphia: Saunders; 1990. **(LOE V)**.

105. Dameron TB Jr, Reibel DB. Fractures involving the proximal humeral epiphyseal plate. *J Bone Joint Surg Am*. 1969;51:289–297. **(LOE V)**.

106. Baxter MP, Wiley JJ. Fractures of the proximal humeral epiphysis. Their influence on humeral growth. *J Bone Joint Surg Br*. 1986;68:570–573. **(LOE V)**.

107. Rose SH, Melton LJ 3rd, Morrey BF, Ilstrup DM, Riggs BL. Epidemiologic features of humeral fractures. *Clini Orthop Relat Res*. 1982:24–30. **(LOE V)**.

108. Neer CS 2nd, Horwitz BS. Fractures of the proximal humeral epiphysial plate. *Clini Orthop Relat Res*. 1965;41:24–31. **(LOE V)**.

109. Hohl JC. Fractures of the humerus in children. *Orthop Clini N Am*. 1976;7:557–571. **(LOE V)**.

110. Campbell J, Almond HG. Fracture-separation of the proximal humeral epiphysis. A case report. *J Bone Joint Surg Am*. 1977;59:262–263. **(LOE IV)**.

111. Lemperg R, Liliequist B. Dislocation of the proximal epiphysis of the humerus in newborns. *Acta Paediatr Scand*. 1970;59:377–380. **(LOE IV)**.

112. Zieger M, Dorr U, Schulz RD. Sonography of slipped humeral epiphysis due to birth injury. *Pediatr Radiol*. 1987;17:425–426. **(LOE IV)**.

113. Salter RB. Injuries of the epiphyseal plate. *Instr Course Lect*. 1992;41:351–359. **(LOE V)**.

114. Gregg-Smith SJ, White SH. Salter-Harris III fracture-dislocation of the proximal humeral epiphysis. *Injury*. 1992;23:199–200. **(LOE V)**.

115. te Slaa RL, Nollen AJ. A Salter type 3 fracture of the proximal epiphysis of the humerus. *Injury*. 1987;18:429–431. **(LOE IV)**.

116. Beringer DC, Weiner DS, Noble JS, Bell RH. Severely displaced proximal humeral epiphyseal fractures: a follow-up study. *J Pediatr Orthop*. 1998;18:31–37. **(LOE IV)**.

117. Sherk HH, Probst C. Fractures of the proximal humeral epiphysis. *Orthop Clini N Am*. 1975;6:401–413. **(LOE V)**.

118. Beaty JH. Fractures of the proximal humerus and shaft in children. *Instr Course Lect*. 1992;41:369–372. **(LOE V)**.

119. Dobbs MB, Luhmann SL, Gordon JE, Strecker WB, Schoenecker PL. Severely displaced proximal humeral epiphyseal fractures. *J Pediatr Orthop*. 2003;23:208–215. **(LOE IV)**.

120. Pahlavan S, Baldwin KD, Pandya NK, Namdari S, Hosalkar H. Proximal humerus fractures in the pediatric population: a systematic review. *J Children's Orthop*. 2011;5:187–194. **(LOE III)**.

121. Chaus GW, Carry PM, Pishkenari AK, Hadley-Miller N. Operative versus nonoperative treatment of displaced proximal humeral physeal fractures: a matched cohort. *J Pediatr Orthop*. 2015;35:234–239. **(LOE III)**.

122. Loder RT. Pediatric polytrauma: orthopaedic care and hospital course. *J Orthop Trauma*. 1987;1:48–54. **(LOE IV)**.

123. King EC, Ihnow SB. Which proximal humerus fractures should be pinned? Treatment in skeletally immature patients. *J Pediatr Orthop*. 2016;36(suppl 1):S44–S48. **(LOE IV)**.

124. Hutchinson PH, Bae DS, Waters PM. Intramedullary nailing versus percutaneous pin fixation of pediatric proximal humerus fractures: a comparison of complications and early radiographic results. *J Pediatr Orthop*. 2011;31:617–622. **(LOE III)**.

125. Flynn JM. *Irreducible fracture of the proximal humerus*: American Academy of Orthopaedic Surgeons. (LOE V).

126. Wang P Jr, Koval KJ, Lehman W, Strongwater A, Grant A, Zuckerman JD. Salter-Harris type III fracture-dislocation of the proximal humerus. *J Pediatr Orthop Part B*. 1997;6:219–222. **(LOE IV)**.

127. Visser JD, Rietberg M. Interposition of the tendon of the long head of biceps in fracture separation of the proximal humeral epiphysis. *Neth J Surg*. 1980;32:12–15. **(LOE IV)**.

128. Lucas JC, Mehlman CT, Laor T. The location of the biceps tendon in completely displaced proximal humerus fractures in children: a report of four cases with magnetic resonance imaging and cadaveric correlation. *J Pediatr Orthop*. 2004;24:249–253. **(LOE IV)**.

129. Vezeridis PS, Bae DS, Kocher MS, Kramer DE, Yen YM, Waters PM. Surgical treatment for avulsion injuries of the humeral

lesser tuberosity apophysis in adolescents. *J Bone Joint Surg Am.* 2011;93:1882–1888. (**LOE IV**).

130. Garrigues GE, Warnick DE, Busch MT. Subscapularis avulsion of the lesser tuberosity in adolescents. *J Pediatr Orthop.* 2013;33:8–13. (**LOE IV**).
131. White PG, Mah JY, Friedman L. Magnetic resonance imaging in acute physeal injuries. *Skeletal Radiol.* 1994;23:627–631. (**LOE IV**).
132. Shaw BA, Murphy KM, Shaw A, Oppenheim WL, Myracle MR. Humerus shaft fractures in young children: accident or abuse? *J Pediatr Orthop.* 1997;17:293–297. (**LOE IV**).
133. Pandya NK, Baldwin K, Wolfgruber H, Christian CW, Drummond DS, Hosalkar HS. Child abuse and orthopaedic injury patterns: analysis at a level I pediatric trauma center. *J Pediatr Orthop.* 2009;29:618–625. (**LOE IV**).
134. Loder RT, Bookout C. Fracture patterns in battered children. *J Orthop Trauma.* 1991;5:428–433. (**LOE IV**).
135. Neer CS 2nd, Francis KC, Marcove RC, Terz J, Carbonara PN. Treatment of unicameral bone cyst. A follow-up study of one hundred seventy-five cases. *J Bone Joint Surg Am.* 1966;48:731–745. (**LOE IV**).

136. Gilchrist DK. A stockinette-Velpeau for immobilization of the shoulder-girdle. *J Bone Joint Surg Am.* 1967;49:750–751. (**LOE V**).
137. Astedt B. A method for the treatment of humerus fractures in the newborn using the S. von Rosen splint. *Acta Orthop Scand.* 1969;40:234–236. (**LOE IV**).
138. Hedstrom O. Growth stimulation of long bones after fracture or similar trauma. A clinical and experimental study. *Acta Orthop Scand Suppl.* 1969;122:1–134. (**LOE IV**).
139. Shaw JL, Sakellarides H. Radial-nerve paralysis associated with fractures of the humerus. A review of forty-five cases. *J Bone Joint Surg Am.* 1967;49:899–902. (**LOE IV**).
140. Garg S, Dobbs MB, Schoenecker PL, Luhmann SJ, Gordon JE. Surgical treatment of traumatic pediatric humeral diaphyseal fractures with titanium elastic nails. *J Children's Orthop.* 2009;3:121–127. (**LOE IV**).

Fractures and Dislocations about the Elbow

17

Megan E. Johnson | Gregory A. Mencio

INTRODUCTION

Fractures about the elbow are extremely common, and injuries about the elbow occur more frequently in the skeletally immature than they do in adults.[1,2] It is estimated that upper extremity injuries account for 65% of all fractures and dislocations in children and that fractures and dislocations about the elbow are second in frequency only to fractures of the distal end of the forearm.[3,4]

DISTAL HUMERAL ANATOMY

OSSIFICATION

Ossification of the distal end of the humerus progresses with age. At birth, the distal humeral metaphysis is ossified; however, none of the structures that constitute the epiphysis are ossified. The capitellum is the first structure to ossify and may be seen radiographically as early as 6 months of age, according to Silberstein and colleagues.[5] Haraldsson, in his classic article in 1959,[6] stated that the capitellum may ossify as early as 1 month of age; however, 6 months is probably the youngest age at which this ossification center is seen (Fig. 17.1). Although ossification of the capitellum may not take place until as late as 2 years of age, Silberstein and associates[5] state that it is invariably present by that time.

The medial epicondyle is the next ossification center to appear. It may be seen radiographically as early as 5 years of age in some but may not appear until 9 years in others. The medial epicondyle forms its own ossification center in the distal end of the humerus, whereas the capitellum, the trochlea, and the lateral epicondyle fuse to form a single ossification center. The trochlea, which appears next, may become ossified as early as 7 years of age, but more commonly, it begins to ossify between the ages of 9 and 10 years. The lateral epicondyle is the last portion of the distal humeral epiphysis to ossify. It may be identified radiographically as early as 8 to 9 years of age.

The capitellum and trochlea may fuse as early as the age of 10 years, but fusion usually begins by 12 years of age. This combined ossification center fuses to the lateral epicondyle at the same time to form the main body of the distal humeral epiphysis. The epiphysis fuses to the metaphysis of the humerus as early as 12 to 13 years of age, which signals the end of longitudinal growth of the distal humeral physis. Finally, the medial epicondyle fuses to the distal end of the humerus between 14 and 17 years of age.

VASCULAR ANATOMY

The collateral circulation about the elbow is rich and usually sufficient for maintaining adequate circulation to the forearm and hand, even if the main blood supply from the brachial artery is interrupted (Fig. 17.2). Although interruption of the brachial artery may not result in loss of the limb, it usually produces some signs of ischemia, such as claudication and cold intolerance.[7-11]

JOINT ANATOMY

The entire articular surface of the distal end of the humerus is intraarticular; however, the medial and lateral epicondyles are both extraarticular. The elbow capsule attaches to the ulna distal to the olecranon and coronoid process, so these structures are intraarticular. In addition, the entire radial head is located within the capsule, thus making it intraarticular. Two elbow fat pads are located between the capsule and the distal end of the humerus: one anterior and the other posterior. The radiographic appearance of these fat pads may aid in diagnosing injuries about the elbow; with an elbow effusion, one or both may become elevated from the distal humeral surface and can be seen as a lucent area on

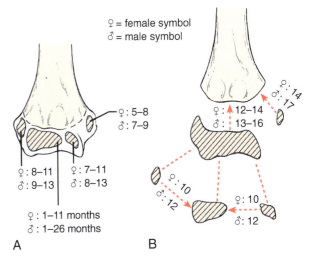

Fig. 17.1 Ossification and fusion of the growth centers of the distal end of the humerus. (A) Appearance of the distal humeral ossification centers in the early years. (B) Closure of the distal humeral ossification centers. (Modified from Haraldsson S. On osteochondrosis deformans juvenilis capituli humeri including investigation of intra-osseous vasculature in distal humerus. *Acta Orthop Scand Suppl.* 1959;38:1-232.)

lateral radiographs (Fig. 17.3).[12] De Beaux and associates[13] analyzed 45 cases of elbow trauma in children with one or two elevated fat pads and no radiographic evidence of a fracture. They found only 6% of those who underwent repeated radiographs 2 weeks later to have a fracture and concluded that routine repeated radiographs are not necessary unless children remain symptomatic. In a study by Skaggs and Mirzayan,[14] 76% of children with a visible posterior fat pad but no fracture on initial radiographs were subsequently found to have a fracture on follow-up radiographs at 2 to 3 weeks, as evidenced by periosteal reaction of the distal humerus, olecranon, or proximal radius.

RADIOGRAPHIC ANATOMY

Suspected elbow fractures are best evaluated on high-quality anteroposterior (AP) and lateral radiographs. On the AP view, the Baumann angle and the medial epicondylar epiphyseal angle are important landmarks for assessing

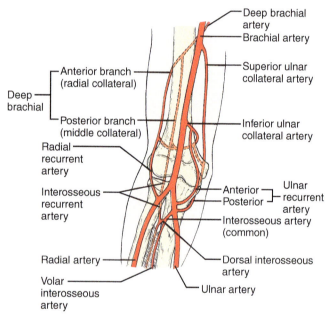

Fig. 17.2 The vascular supply about the elbow is rich and has excellent collateral circulation. The collateral circulation is usually sufficient to maintain viability of the extremity in the event of occlusion of the brachial artery.

supracondylar fractures. The Baumann angle is defined by the intersection of a line drawn along the physis of the capitellum and a line perpendicular to the longitudinal axis of the humerus on radiographs (Fig. 17.4). Williamson and associates[15] found the Baumann angle to be 72 degrees (standard deviation, 4 degrees), and 95% of normal elbows had a Baumann angle of 64 to 81 degrees. The Baumann angle is, however, dependent on the position of the elbow and is particularly affected by rotation.[16,17] Accuracy of measurement is assured by obtaining a true AP radiograph of the distal end of the humerus (Fig. 17.5). When the elbow cannot be fully extended, the x-ray beam and radiographic plate must be adjusted so that the beam is perpendicular to the distal end of the humerus and the plate parallel to the long axis of the humerus to avoid inadvertently obtaining a tangential view of the distal humerus and any parallax that might adversely affect measurement. Comparison of the Baumann angle of the contralateral uninjured elbow is often the best way to determine the adequacy of reduction of a supracondylar fracture,[18] with the caveat that radiographs of the distal ends of each humerus should be obtained in matched rotation and flexion to attempt to negate any variability in measurement caused by differences in position.[19]

The *medial epicondylar epiphyseal angle* may also be useful in determining the accuracy of reduction of supracondylar humeral fractures. This angle is formed by the intersection of lines drawn along the medial epicondylar growth plate and the longitudinal axis of the humerus. In younger children, in whom the medial epicondyle has not yet ossified, one can measure this angle by drawing a line along the medial metaphyseal border of the distal humerus and referencing it to a line drawn along the longitudinal axis of the humerus (Fig. 17.6).[20] As with the Bauman angle, comparison with the contralateral uninjured elbow is the best way to determine reduction.

On the lateral view, the *lateral capitellar angle* is measured by the intersection of a line parallel to the midpoint of the distal humeral shaft and one drawn through the midpoint of the capitellum. The normal inclination is approximately 30 degrees anterior (Fig. 17.7A). The *anterior humeral line* is a radiographic marker that is drawn along the anterior cortex of the humerus.[21] It should pass through the middle of the ossified capitellum. If this line passes anterior to the middle of the capitellum, the distal end of the humerus has been displaced posteriorly. Conversely, if it passes posterior

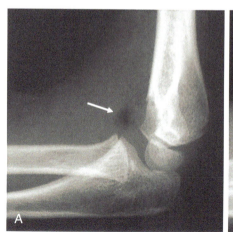

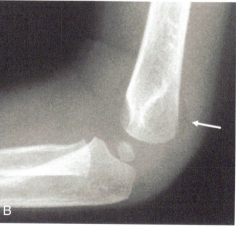

Fig. 17.3 Elevated fat pads anteriorly and posteriorly about the elbow indicate the presence of an elbow effusion. (A) This lateral radiograph of the elbow in a child who sustained a nondisplaced supracondylar fracture shows a markedly displaced anterior fat pad *(arrow)*. (B) A lateral elbow radiograph of a different child shows no obvious fracture, but both anterior and posterior elevated fat pads can be noted *(arrow)*. The child was treated for a supracondylar fracture that became evident 3 weeks later with the appearance of a periosteal reaction and a fracture line.

to the middle of the capitellum, the distal end of the humerus has been displaced anteriorly (Fig. 17.7B). This measurement is only accurate on a true lateral radiograph of the distal humerus. Skibo and Reed[22] showed that if the humerus is rotated even slightly, the anterior humeral line is not reliable and, in many instances, is falsely positive. More recently, Herman and associates[23] have shown that in children younger than 4 years, the line may lie in the anterior third of the capitellum. However, Murphy-Zane and Pyle have shown high intraobserver reliability in using this measurement to characterize posteriorly hinged supracondylar humerus fractures.[24] The *anterior coronoid line* is another sagittal radiographic marker. It is defined by a curvilinear line drawn along the coronoid and continued proximally, where it should just touch the anterior aspect of the capitellum. If the distal humerus is angled or displaced posteriorly, the capitellum will lie more posterior (Fig. 17.7C). Silberstein and colleagues[5] noted that the physis of the capitellum is wider posteriorly than anteriorly when viewed on a lateral radiograph. This appearance may be mistaken for an injury to the physis if one is not familiar with the normal radiographic anatomy (Fig. 17.8).

Comparison radiographs of the uninjured elbow have long been advocated as a way to assist in the diagnosis of subtle elbow trauma in children. However, in a study by Cheng and Shen,[25] in which orthopedic residents, emergency physicians, and a pediatric radiologist evaluated radiographs of injured and contralateral elbows in 3350 children, the authors found that comparison radiographs did not improve the diagnostic accuracy of elbow trauma in the pediatric emergency department.

Other means of evaluating elbow trauma include magnetic resonance imaging (MRI) and ultrasound. MRI has been shown to be a sensitive and accurate method in the diagnosis of occult fractures about the elbow and more accurate than conventional radiography in defining the fracture pattern and extent of articular disruption in fractures extending into the cartilaginous epiphysis.[26,27] Access to MRI in the acute setting and need for sedation in uncooperative children are two significant barriers to the use of MRI for the evaluation of elbow trauma. Ultrasonography has also been shown to be a sensitive study for diagnosing fractures of the elbow in children, especially the very young in whom ossification of the distal end of the humerus is minimal.[28] A

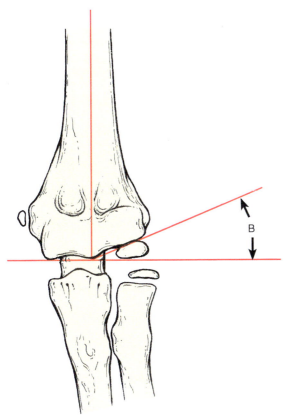

Fig. 17.4 The Baumann angle (B) is formed by the intersection of a line parallel to the metaphysis of the lateral aspect of the distal end of the humerus (i.e., the physis of the capitellum) and a line perpendicular to the longitudinal axis of the humerus. Deviation of more than 5 degrees compared with the contralateral side is abnormal.

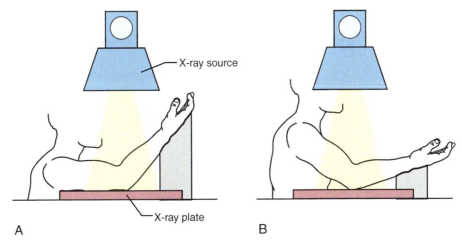

Fig. 17.5 True anteroposterior (AP) radiographs of the elbow are required to accurately assess injury and alignment after a reduction. If the elbow can be fully extended, the AP radiograph of the distal end of the humerus and an AP radiograph of the elbow will be identical. When the elbow is unable to be fully extended, it is necessary to obtain an AP radiograph of the distal humerus. (A) shows the proper orientation of the x-ray beam perpendicular to the distal portion of the arm that will give an undistorted AP rendering of the distal humerus. (B) shows the x-ray beam centered on the elbow. Because the elbow is flexed, the distal portion of the humerus will project tangentially, resulting in distortion of the bony architecture. (A and B, Modified from Camp J, Ishizue K, Gomez M, et al. Alteration of Baumann's angle by humeral position: implications for treatment of supracondylar humerus fractures. *J Pediatr Orthop.* 1993;13:522.)

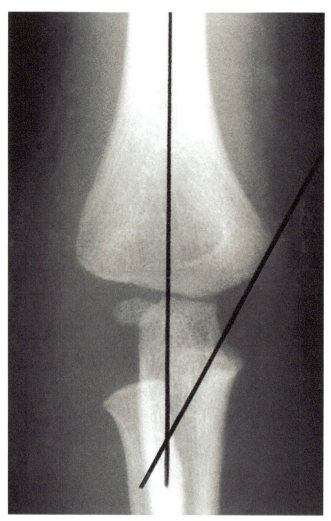

Fig. 17.6 The medial epicondylar epiphyseal angle is measured by the intersection of lines drawn along the medial epicondylar growth plate and the longitudinal axis of the humerus. In this radiograph, the medial epicondyle is not yet ossified; therefore, the line is drawn along the medial border of the distal humeral metaphysis.

recent prospective study of 130 patients showed that point-of-care ultrasonography performed by emergency department physicians was also highly sensitive in diagnosing elbow fractures in older children (mean age, 7.5 years).[29]

CARRYING ANGLE OF THE ELBOW

The carrying angle of the elbow is the clinical measurement of coronal (varus/valgus) angulation of the arm with the elbow fully extended and the forearm fully supinated. The intersection of a line along the midaxis of the upper part of the arm and a line along the midaxis of the forearm defines this angle. Beals has shown that the carrying angle varies widely among individuals.[30] The angle increases with age, and no consistent difference is seen between males and females. The carrying angle of a given elbow is best evaluated by comparison with the contralateral elbow.

SUPRACONDYLAR FRACTURES OF THE HUMERUS

INCIDENCE

Supracondylar fractures occur most often in the first decade of life and account for up to 17% of all pediatric fractures and 30% of all fractures in children younger than 7 years.[31–35] Extension injuries are the most common type, accounting for more than 95% of cases.

ANATOMY

The anatomy of the distal end of the humerus explains the susceptibility to injury in this location and instability of these types of fractures when they do occur. The medial and lateral columns of the distal humerus, which are relatively thick and strong, are connected by a thin wafer of bone that is only 1 mm thick in the central portion, separating the olecranon fossa posteriorly from the coronoid fossa anteriorly (Fig. 17.9).

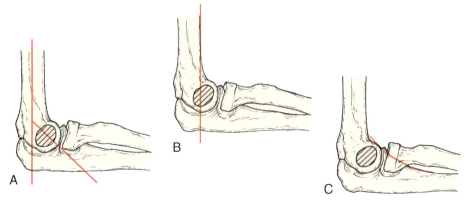

Fig. 17.7 Radiographic lines that may be demonstrated on a lateral radiograph of the elbow. (A) The *lateral capitellar angle* is measured by the intersection of a line parallel to the midpoint of the distal humeral shaft and one drawn through the midpoint of the capitellum. The normal inclination is approximately 30 degrees anterior. (B) The *anterior humeral line* is drawn along the anterior cortex of the distal end of the humerus. Distally, it should intersect the middle of the ossified capitellum. (C) The *anterior coronoid line* is drawn along the volar margin of the proximal ulna. As it is continued proximally, the line should just touch the anterior margin of the capitellum.

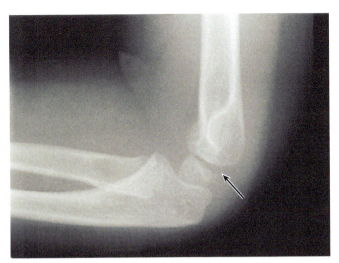

Fig. 17.8 Lateral radiograph of a normal elbow. The physis of the capitellum is normally slightly wider posteriorly than anteriorly *(arrow)*. This finding should not be confused with an injury to the physis.

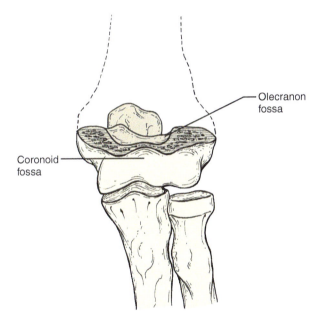

Fig. 17.9 Cross section of the distal end of the humerus at the level of the coronoid fossa. Note that the midportion of the humerus is extremely thin at this level, whereas the medial and lateral columns are thicker.

MECHANISMS OF INJURY

Supracondylar fractures of the humerus may be produced by either a hyperextension or a flexion mechanism. The *extension*-type fracture, resulting from a fall on an outstretched hand with the elbow hyperextended, is the more common pattern of injury. In this type of injury, the full force from the fall is directed to the anatomically weak olecranon fossa. Several studies have implicated the occurrence of supracondylar humeral fractures with the presence of ligamentous laxity and elbow hyperextension, both of which are common findings in children in the first decade of life when this injury is most common. Henrikson studied children who had sustained supracondylar humerus fractures and found that their uninjured elbows were capable of more than the average amount of hyperextension.[34] Others have correlated the relationship of ligamentous laxity and the site of upper extremity fractures, suggesting that children whose elbows are capable of hyperextension because of the presence of ligamentous laxity are more likely to sustain a supracondylar fracture as a result of a fall on an outstretched hand, whereas children without hyperextension of the elbow are more likely to fracture the distal forearm.[25,36] The less common *flexion*-type supracondylar fracture results from a fall on the olecranon with the elbow bent.

INJURY BIOMECHANICS

When the elbow is loaded in extension, the distal humerus begins to fail under tension. The anterior cortex of the distal humerus then fractures, and the anterior periosteum stretches over the fracture. If at this point, the hyperextension force ceases, a nondisplaced or minimally angulated fracture occurs. This injury has been termed a *stage I fracture* by Abraham and colleagues.[37] Radiographically, one may see only soft tissue swelling or possibly a decrease in the normal anterior inclination of the capitellum on a lateral view.

Continued application of an extension force leads to a *stage II fracture* that is characterized by further extension and angulation of the distal fragment but no translation. In a *stage III fracture*, the anterior periosteum is completely torn, and the distal fragment is displaced posteriorly, with translation. The periosteum is usually intact on the side to which the fracture is displaced, and can be used as a hinge to assist in reduction of the fracture. If the fracture is displaced posteromedially, which is generally the case, a posteromedial periosteal hinge is usually preserved. If the fracture is displaced posterolaterally, the intact periosteum is on the posterolateral side of the elbow. The location of the bruise in the antecubital fossa represents location of periosteal disruption and is another clue as to the direction of displacement of the fracture.

ASSOCIATED INJURIES

Ipsilateral fractures of the distal radius (so-called remote floating elbow) are most commonly caused by a similar injury mechanism (fall on an outstretched hand). Concomitant diaphyseal radial and ulnar fractures are less common but, when present, are associated with a higher risk of compartment syndrome.[38]

NERVE INJURIES

Supracondylar fractures of the humerus are associated with a relatively high risk of nerve injury (between 7% and 15.5%), although Campbell and associates[39] found that in 59 patients with type III supracondylar fractures, 24 (41%) had acute nerve injuries. A recent metaanalysis[40] indicated that nerve injuries occur in 11.3% of patients with supracondylar fractures. Garg and associates[41] reported a 12% incidence of nerve injury in the largest single center study of type III supracondylar humeral fractures (*n* = 872) reported to date.

Older reports showed that 45% of nerve injuries involved the radial nerve, and 32% involved the median nerve. Campbell and colleagues[39] found that anterior interosseous and/or median nerve injury was associated with posterolateral

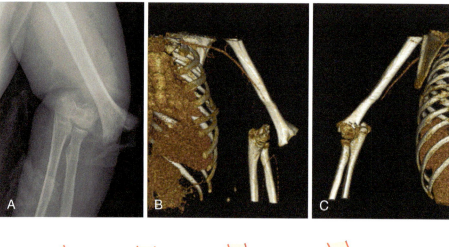

Fig. 17.10 Vascular injury associated with supracondylar humeral fracture. (A) Severely displaced supracondylar humeral fracture. (B and C) Anteroposterior and lateral three-dimensional computed tomographic angiograms demonstrating occlusion of the brachial artery. Note the distal runoff despite the vascular occlusion, emphasizing the robust collateral circulation about the elbow.

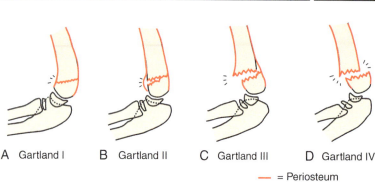

A Gartland I   B Gartland II   C Gartland III   D Gartland IV

— = Periosteum
— = Cortex

Fig. 17.11 Schematic of the Modified Gartland Classification. (A) Type I fractures are nondisplaced, and the anterior and posterior periosteum is intact. (B) Type II fractures are posteriorly impacted. The anterior cortex may be disrupted. The posterior cortex and periosteum are intact. (C) Type III fractures are characterized by complete disruption of the anterior and posterior cortices. The anterior periosteum is disrupted, but the posterior periosteum remains intact. (D) Type IV fractures are characterized by disruption of both anterior and posterior cortices. Both the anterior and posterior periosteum are torn, making these fractures very unstable.

displacement 87% of the time. The radial nerve was injured when the fracture became displaced in a posteromedial direction. The ulnar nerve is less commonly involved (23% of the time) and is more often associated with flexion-type supracondylar fractures. Although radial nerve injury was the most commonly reported in the older literature, more recent investigators have found the anterior interosseous branch to be the most commonly injured nerve.[39–43] As the metaphyseal fragment is displaced anteriorly, the median nerve is stretched. Anatomically, the anterior interosseous nerve (AIN) branch is at risk because it is tethered under the fibrous arch that arises from the deep head of the pronator teres. The AIN is a purely motor nerve; therefore, diagnosis of injury to it requires a specific examination of the flexor pollicis longus and flexor digitorum profundus of the index finger.[44,45] Concomitant loss of sensation would be suggestive of a median nerve injury, rather than just an AIN palsy.

VASCULAR INJURIES

Although the consequences of vascular injury associated with supracondylar humeral fractures may be significant, permanent vascular compromise of the extremity is rare. In a recent single-center study of 872 type III supracondylar humeral fractures, an absent pulse was found in 54 (6%), of which only five underwent vascular repair.[41] The brachialis muscle protects the brachial artery. With significant posterior displacement, the brachialis muscle may be torn by the metaphyseal fragment, compromising the protection it provides to the brachial artery (Fig. 17.10). The supratrochlear artery can also tether the brachial artery when there is significant displacement of the fracture, causing occlusion. Reducing the fracture usually relieves occlusion of the

artery unless it is physically present within the fracture gap. In this instance, the circulation is usually satisfactory until the fracture is manipulated and the artery is compressed by the fracture fragments, which results in loss of the radial pulse and compromised perfusion of the extremity. An entrapped brachial artery may be accompanied by the median nerve, which together may prevent reduction of the fracture. Whenever the inability to reduce a supracondylar humeral fracture perfectly is accompanied by absence/loss of the radial pulse, particularly in the presence of a median/AIN deficit, one should be aware of the strong possibility that the artery and (possibly) nerve are entrapped in the fracture and require open reduction to free the neurovascular structures.[46,47]

CLASSIFICATION

Supracondylar humeral fractures may be classified as extension or flexion-type injuries. Extension injuries are much more common (>95%) and are further defined as to the extent of displacement by the Gartland classification (Fig. 17.11).[48] Type I fractures are nondisplaced. The fracture line may be easily visible or indistinct. Good lateral views and observation of fat pad elevation help identify this fracture radiographically. Type II fractures are angulated but have an intact posterior periosteal hinge. Radiographically, the anterior angulation of the capitellum (normally 30 degrees) is diminished, and the anterior humeral line is positioned anterior to the middle of the capitellum (see Fig. 17.7). Type III fractures are completely displaced, with loss of all continuity between the two fragments. Displacement is most often posteromedial and less frequently posterolateral.

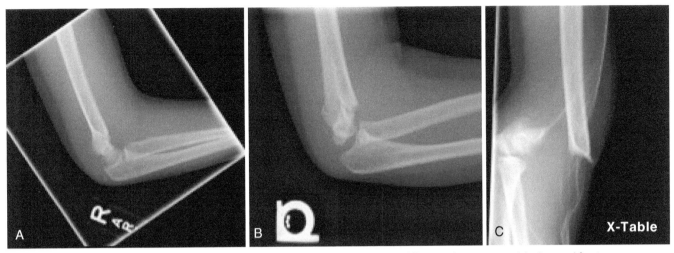

Fig. 17.12 Radiographs showing Gartland type I (A), type II (B), and type III (C) extension supracondylar humeral fractures.

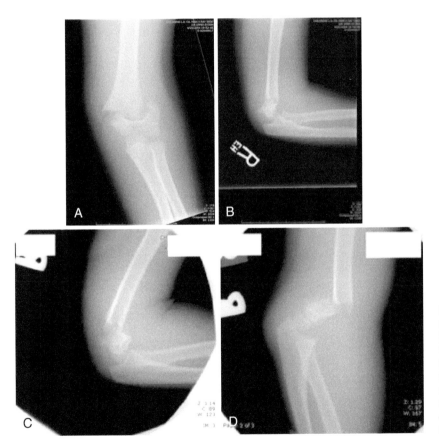

Fig. 17.13 (A and B) Injury radiographs of a multidirectionally unstable supracondylar humeral fracture. (C) Intraoperative image demonstrating fracture instability in flexion. (D) Intraoperative image demonstrating fracture instability in extension. (From Leitch KK, Kay RM, Famino JD, et al. Treatment of multidirectionally unstable supracondylar humeral fractures in children. A modified Gartland type-IV fracture. *J Bone Joint Surg Am.* 2006;88A(5):980-985. With permission.)

Wilkins modified the Gartland classification by dividing type II fractures into A and B subtypes. Type IIA fractures are extended but not rotated or translated; type IIB fractures have some component of rotational displacement or translation. Clinical implications are that IIA fractures are stable after manipulative reduction and may be treated closed, whereas IIB injuries are usually unstable and more likely to require reduction and fixation (Fig. 17.12).[11,49]

Leitch and colleagues proposed the addition of a type IV fracture to the original Gartland classification.[50] Type IV fractures are multidirectionally unstable in both flexion and extension because of complete loss of both anterior and posterior periosteal hinges and are thought to be caused by either excessive trauma or overzealous anteriorly directed force during attempted reduction of a type III fracture (Fig. 17.13).

EXTENSION-TYPE SUPRACONDYLAR FRACTURE

HISTORY AND PHYSICAL EXAMINATION

Children who are old enough to provide an adequate history usually describe a fall while running or from a height (typically playground equipment) and landing on an outstretched hand with the elbow extended. Children with supracondylar fractures have pain and swelling about the elbow, decreased range of motion, and variable amounts of deformity. Skin in the antecubital fossa is usually ecchymotic, and if the fracture is significantly displaced, it may cause tenting of the skin or puckering if the metaphyseal fragment is buttonholed through the brachialis muscle and fascia. A thorough assessment of skin integrity must be performed to be sure the fracture is not open, and an assessment of the rest of the upper extremity must be performed to be sure no other skeletal injury is present.

A complete neurologic evaluation of the arm is essential because of the frequency of nerve injuries associated with this fracture. The neurologic evaluation also establishes a baseline to compare to after treatment has been completed.[41] AIN injuries are most common, followed by injuries to the median, radial, and ulnar nerves. Ulnar nerve injury is usually associated with flexion-type fractures.[40] The neurologic examination should include motor and sensory assessment of the median, ulnar, and radial nerves. However, formal testing of nerve function is not always possible because of pain, anxiety, or lack of cooperation, and baseline assessment of nerve function often has to be made based on observation of spontaneous movement over several encounters with the child, particularly in the very young. In general, nerve deficits that are present immediately after the injury represent neurapraxia and will resolve spontaneously. In contrast, a change in neurologic status after treatment is more likely to be indicative of injury during manipulation, with pinning or by entrapment in the fracture site. This type of injury usually requires exploration and intervention.

Assessment of vascular status is also paramount. Assessment of perfusion of the hand is the most important indicator of vascular status of the extremity. The distal radial pulse should be palpated and, if not present, checked by Doppler ultrasonography. It is not uncommon for the radial pulse to be absent at the time of initial evaluation because of compression or tethering of the brachial artery over the anterior aspect of the proximal fragment of the fracture or arterial spasm. If the pulse is absent, the elbow should be flexed to relieve any pressure on the artery. Although absence of the radial pulse causes concern, the artery is rarely torn or damaged permanently.[40,41,51] The extensive collateral circulation around the elbow allows for sufficient perfusion to the forearm and hand in most instances to maintain viability, even if the artery is damaged. Regardless of whether the radial pulse is present, indicators of adequate distal perfusion include color ("pink"), temperature ("warm"), and normal capillary refill. The vascular status of the extremity can be described as normal, perfused (pink hand) but pulseless, or dysvascular (pulseless and white). Ischemia leading to compartment syndrome has been associated with this fracture and therefore should be carefully evaluated. Children with impending compartment syndrome may appear agitated and anxious and have increasing analgesic requirements long before the classic signs of ischemia—pain, paresthesia, pallor, paralysis (loss of motor function), and absent pulse—are evident. In patients in whom compartment syndrome is a concern, forearm compartment pressures should be measured. The risk of compartment syndrome is higher in patients with floating elbow injuries.[38,52]

RADIOGRAPHIC EVALUATION

Accurate radiographic diagnosis of a type III fracture of the supracondylar region of the distal end of the humerus is not usually difficult. Correct diagnosis of type I and occasionally type II fractures may be more difficult. As previously mentioned, use of the fat pad signs on lateral radiographs is helpful in localizing the trauma to the region of the elbow joint when no fracture line is clearly identified. In addition, on a lateral radiograph, one should look for any alteration in the intersection of the capitellum with the anterior humeral line; if this line crosses anterior to the middle of the capitellum, a type I or II supracondylar fracture is likely to be present.

MANAGEMENT

A patient with a supracondylar humeral fracture and a pale, pulseless hand requires emergent surgical attention. Closed supracondylar humeral fractures in children without associated neurovascular injury can be successfully managed by closed methods or surgery on an urgent basis. Surgical options include closed or open reduction and stabilization with Kirschner wires (K-wires). Specific treatment of extension-type supracondylar humeral fractures is determined by Gartland type.

Type I Fracture

Type I fractures are typically treated closed with 3 to 4 weeks of immobilization in a long arm cast with the elbow flexed to 90 degrees. If there is a large degree of swelling, a posterior splint may also be used. A small degree of posterior angulation of the distal fragment in a younger child may be accepted in anticipation of remodeling, although there may be hyperextension of the elbow and decreased elbow flexion until it does. Normally, the capitellum is angulated anteriorly about 30 degrees, and reduction is not required if the posterior angulation is 20 degrees or less, or if the anterior humeral line intersects any part of the capitellum.[2,53]

One pitfall in treating a type I fracture is not recognizing impaction of the medial column that, if left uncorrected, can result in a varus deformity, which will not correct with growth (Fig. 17.14). De Boeck and associates[54] identified 13 patients with medial compression of the distal end of the humerus in otherwise innocent-looking type I fractures that developed varus deformities. A type I fracture with medial compression must be reduced so to avoid development of cubitus varus. With the patient under general anesthesia, the fracture is reduced by application of longitudinal traction with the elbow in full extension. An assistant applies countertraction to the upper part of the arm. Valgus correction is obtained with the use of the forearm as a lever. Once reduced, the fracture may be treated in a long arm cast in extension or preferably, because the medial column may be inherently unstable, with crossed K-wires to prevent drift back into varus. Once the fracture is stabilized, the elbow may be flexed to 80 degrees to 90 degrees and immobilized for 3 weeks.

Type II Fracture

Management of type II fractures is controversial. Type IIA fractures, which are extended but have no rotation or translation, may be successfully treated with closed reduction and

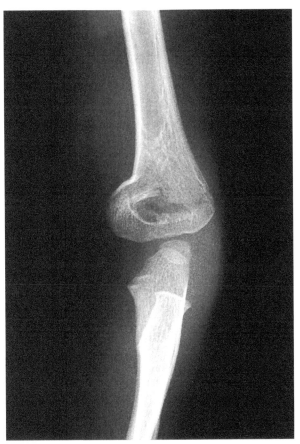

Fig. 17.14 Anteroposterior radiograph of the distal end of an elbow shows a nondisplaced supracondylar fracture with impaction of the metaphysis medially. The lateral column is intact. The deformity produced by this injury should be corrected to prevent persistent angular malalignment (cubitus varus) when the fracture heals.

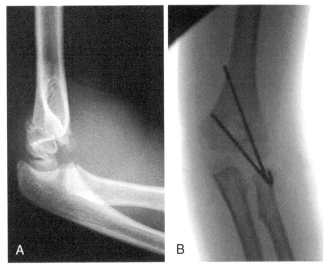

Fig. 17.15 Type II supracondylar humeral fracture. (A) Lateral radiograph of the elbow shows posterior angulation of the distal humeral fragment. The anterior humeral line does not intersect any part of the capitellum. The distal fragment is rotated. (B) Postreduction anteroposterior radiograph showing fixation with divergent lateral entry pins.

casting.[55] Alignment of these fractures does need to be closely monitored for loss of reduction, primarily in the coronal plane because varus or valgus angulation will not remodel. Residual posterior angulation can be expected to remodel with growth because the deformity is close to and primarily in the plane of motion of the joint. Two pitfalls in managing type IIA fractures closed are accepting reduction when the distal fragment is angulated too far posteriorly such that the capitellum is posterior to the longitudinal axis of the anterior humerus, and mistaking posterior translation of the distal fragment for angulation. In the former scenario, the patient may be left with a significant hyperextension deformity of the elbow that is more of a cosmetic problem than a functional one, and in the latter, the patient may have a significant flexion lag that can be a functional problem, particularly if it involves the dominant extremity. Type IIB fractures (Fig. 17.15) should be treated operatively with closed reduction and percutaneous pinning.[14,56]

Nonoperative Treatment. In all type II fractures, coronal angulation of the elbow must be carefully assessed. Clinical examination of the fully extended elbow under general anesthesia is the best means of accurately assessing the carrying angle. Type II fractures with posterior medial compression may be reduced and casted with the use of the technique described previously for type I fractures with impaction of the medial column. Reduction may be achieved by first extend-

ing the elbow and correcting the coronal plane deformity and then flexing the elbow while pronating the forearm to address sagittal plane angulation. Millis has shown that hyperflexion of the elbow to more than 120 degrees may be necessary to maintain reduction.[57] Despite techniques like the figure-of-eight cast described originally by Rang to avoid circumferential wrapping of the elbow to achieve this position, maintenance of hyperflexion carries a high risk of skin problems, neurovascular compromise, and compartment syndrome. Therefore, if there is significant soft tissue swelling, any question of vascular compromise, or fracture instability in any type II fracture, the fracture should be pinned percutaneously.

Operative Treatment. Type II fractures with translational or rotational deformity are unstable and are best treated in the same way as type III fractures (see next section). With the patient under general anesthesia and fluoroscopy available, the fracture may be reduced by application of a valgus force on the extended elbow to correct any medial compression/angulation. Next, the elbow is maximally flexed, and the olecranon is pushed anteriorly to reduce posterior angulation/translation. Pin fixation with K-wires is performed to maintain the reduction. Fixation with two lateral pins is generally sufficient for type II fractures, which are inherently more stable than type III fractures.[56,58] The arm is immobilized in a posterior splint or cast with the elbow at 60 to 80 degrees of flexion.

Type III Fracture

Type III fractures are best managed by closed reduction and percutaneous pin fixation. Type III fractures are more severe injuries that are associated with more significant swelling and soft tissue injury, are more difficult to reduce, and are more likely to have neurovascular injuries or complications. These fractures are completely displaced. In most instances, the proximal and distal bone fragments are not in contact, and only a small bridge of periosteum may be preserved posteriorly. These fractures are prone to developing

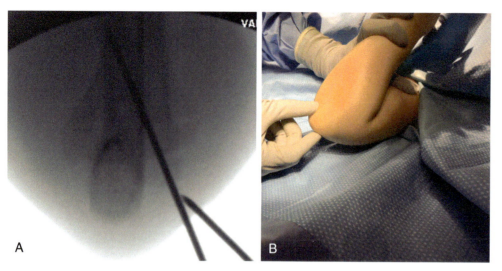

Fig. 17.16 The Jones view is an anteroposterior image of the distal humerus taken through the flexed, overlying forearm. (A) Intraoperative fluoroscopy image demonstrating the Jones view. This view allows for adequate assessment of the medial and lateral columns of the distal humerus and can be used intraoperatively for assessment of reduction and placement of pins. (B) Position of the arm to obtain a Jones view; the elbow is maximally flexed, and the image is taken through the overlying forearm. (Photos and radiographic images courtesy of Jonathan Schoenecker, MD, Vanderbilt University Medical Center, Nashville, TN.)

residual deformity, particularly cubitus varus, when treated by closed reduction and casting. In separate retrospective studies by Kurer and Regan[59] and Pirone and associates[60] of completely displaced supracondylar fractures, closed reduction and splinting or casting resulted in significantly fewer good results and more complications than traction or percutaneous pinning, which provided the best results. Based on the best current evidence and a systematic review of published studies as reported by Howard and associates,[61] closed reduction with percutaneous pinning is widely accepted as the best method of treatment for all type III fractures, as well as for any type II fractures that are not reducible or that are associated with neurovascular status changes during fracture reduction.

Type IV Fracture

Type IV fractures are unstable in both flexion and extension, have complete disruption of the periosteum both anteriorly and posteriorly, and need to be managed operatively (see Fig. 17.13). This fracture is inherently unstable and requires internal fixation. Leitch and colleagues [50] described a method of closed reduction and percutaneous fixation that involves placement of K-wires before reduction of the fracture and rotation of the fluoroscopy unit, rather than the extremity, to obtain orthogonal views. However, these fractures may need to be opened to obtain adequate reduction.

SPECIFIC TREATMENT

Closed Reduction and Cast Treatment

Accurate closed reduction of supracondylar humeral fractures is critical for preventing cubitus varus deformity, regardless of whether the fracture is treated closed or pinned. Reduction of the fracture is accomplished with the patient under general anesthesia and with fluoroscopic guidance. With the elbow extended, gentle longitudinal traction is applied to the supinated forearm while countertraction is applied to the upper part of the arm by an assistant. The distal fragment is then translated medially or laterally, depending on the position of displacement, by application of digital pressure to the appropriate condyle. Most of these fractures are displaced posteromedially, and reduction of this component of the deformity is achieved by having the surgeon flex

the patient's elbow to 120 degrees while simultaneously pronating the forearm and applying digital pressure with the thumb of the opposite hand to the olecranon to reduce the posterior displacement of the distal fragment. Pronating the forearm is thought to engage the intact posteromedial periosteum and allow the fracture to be reduced. Pronation also causes the wrist extensors and brachioradialis to tighten, which helps close down and stabilize the fracture laterally.[62] If the fracture is displaced posterolaterally, the forearm is supinated so that the intact posterolateral periosteal bridge can be used in a reciprocal manner.

The elbow must be flexed maximally so that reduction of the fracture is maintained while imaging is performed to assess alignment. A lateral view is relatively easily obtained by external rotation of the shoulder. Alternatively, if the reduction is tenuous, this view can be obtained by rotation of the fluoroscopy tube to a cross-table position so that the arm does not have to be moved. Adequate sagittal alignment can be assessed by the relationship of the capitellum to the anterior humeral line and the presence or absence of overlap of the ossification center of the capitellum on the olecranon. Coronal alignment of the fracture is assessed with the so-called *Jones view*, which is, in essence, an AP image of the distal humerus taken through the flexed, overlying forearm (Fig. 17.16). Although detail of the distal humerus is slightly obscured, the image is usually adequate for assessment of the alignment of the medial and lateral columns of the distal humerus and restoration of the olecranon fossa by slight internal and external rotation of the arm. The Baumann angle and the medial epicondylar epiphyseal angle can be measured on this view. Otsuka and Kasser[35] believed that the Baumann angle, the relationship of the capitellum to the anterior humeral line, and restoration of the normal anatomy of the olecranon fossa represented the best indicators of a satisfactory reduction.

Once the fracture has been reduced, immediate flexion of the elbow with either pronation (for posteromedial displacement) or supination (for posterolateral displacement) of the forearm is required to maintain reduction in a cast. The problem with this position is that immediate flexion of the elbow increases the tension in an already swollen extremity, thus increasing the risk of vascular compromise by reduction of arterial flow into and venous flow out of the

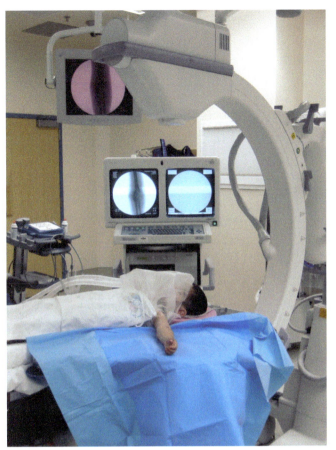

Fig. 17.17 The C-arm machine is draped sterilely so that it can be used as the operating table for reduction and pinning of supracondylar humeral fractures.

forearm. In a clinical study, Mapes and Hennrikus[63] showed that the Doppler pulse became weaker and even disappeared in patients with supracondylar humeral fractures whose elbows were flexed. The more the elbow was flexed, the weaker the pulse became. Because of the dilemma of potential vascular compromise with cast immobilization in the position necessary to prevent loss of reduction, percutaneous pinning has emerged as the treatment of choice for maintaining alignment after closed (or open) reduction of displaced supracondylar humeral fractures.

Closed Reduction and Percutaneous Pinning (Author's Preferred Treatment)

The modern era of treatment of this fracture began in 1948 with a description by Swenson of percutaneous pinning of distal humeral fractures in adults.[64] In 1961, Casiano[65] reported the use of this technique in children. Since this description, multiple reports of the use of percutaneous pinning for the maintenance of reduction of a displaced supracondylar fracture have appeared. Traditionally, a crossed pin configuration has been used to stabilize these fractures, but increasingly, the recent trend has been to stabilize only with lateral entry pins because of concerns of ulnar nerve injuries that have been reported in up to 10% of patients treated with a medial entry pin.[66]

Technique. Closed reduction and pinning are typically done with the child positioned supine and the injured limb suspended over the side of the table. This position allows free access to the C-arm, which is placed directly under the arm parallel to the operating table (Fig. 17.17). The procedure is usually done with sterile preparation and draping, with incorporation of the C-arm unit as the operating table. Alternatively, the procedure can be done in a semisterile fashion, as described by Lobst and associates.[67] Their technique does not require drapes or gowns, hence reducing operating room time and costs. In a series of more than 300 cases, there were no superficial or deep pin infections. Reduction of the fracture is carried out as described in the previous section.

Most fractures can be reduced with this technique; however, if the posterior periosteum is torn, the fracture will be completely unstable, as the hinge that the intact posterior periosteum provides for reduction is lost. Fracture reduction can also be hindered by soft tissue interposition in the fracture. If a spike of the proximal fragment penetrates the brachialis muscle, the muscle must be removed before the fracture is reduced. Peters and colleagues described a technique for dislodging the entrapped brachialis muscle by grasping the arm close to the axilla and gradually "milking" the anterior musculature in a proximal-to-distal direction toward the spike of the proximal fragment while an assistant applies countertraction through the axilla.[68] Pressure is placed primarily on the lateral side to avoid injury to the medial neurovascular structures. Freeing of the entrapped muscle may be accompanied by a palpable sensation of the bone disengaging the soft tissues. Once the brachialis muscle has been cleared, the reduction can usually be completed (Fig. 17.18). One must be cautious manipulating a supracondylar humeral fracture that is displaced in a posterolateral direction with buttonholing of the brachialis muscle, particularly when a neurologic deficit exists, because of the risk of further neurovascular injury. In 27 children with vascular deficits (22 of whom also had median nerve deficits) and posterolaterally displaced fractures, Rasool and Naidoo found that the neurovascular bundle was trapped just anterior to the metaphyseal spike in 18 patients, trapped behind the fracture in five, and separated by the fracture spike in four.[69]

Once obtained, fracture reduction is confirmed fluoroscopically. Sagittal alignment may be checked by either external rotation of the shoulder on the C-arm or, if the reduction is tenuous, by rotation of the C-arm to prevent loss of reduction. The Jones (transcondylar) view is used to assess coronal alignment with the elbow flexed, and alignment of the medial and lateral columns of the distal humerus can be further assessed by slight internal and external rotation of the arm. If reduction is satisfactory, percutaneous pinning is performed. It is debatable whether a medial entry pin should be used or whether two lateral pins are sufficient.[61] It has been shown that crossed pins are the most biomechanically stable[70–72]; however, in comparative clinical studies, the stability afforded by two lateral pins has been shown to be adequate for maintenance of reduction in type II and most type III fractures.[66,73–75] For type II fractures, the author uses two lateral pins, which afford ample stability (Fig. 17.19), and for type III fractures, the author adds a third pin, either lateral or medial entry, depending on fracture characteristics and surgeon preference, as recommended by Bloom and colleagues (Fig. 17.20).[76] In children younger than 4 years, 0.062-inch K-wires are adequate. In older children, 2-mm wires are more suitable.

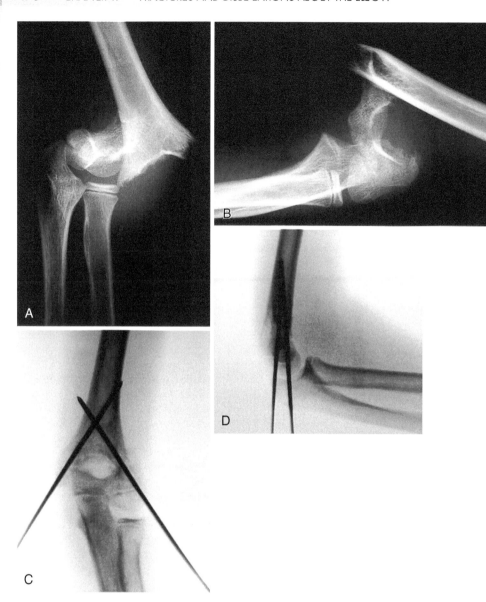

Fig. 17.18 Markedly displaced extension-type III supracondylar humeral fracture reduced with the "milking technique." (A and B) Anteroposterior (AP) and lateral radiographs show posteromedial displacement of the distal fragment. The anterior spike of the proximal fragment had penetrated through the brachialis muscle and was tenting the skin in the antecubital fossa. Neurovascular status of the extremity was intact. The fracture was reduced by closed means with a "milking technique" to massage the brachialis muscle off the end of the proximal fragment and then pinned percutaneously with the use of crossed medial and lateral entry pins. (C and D) Intraoperative AP and lateral radiographs show anatomic restoration of the distal humerus and the fracture stably fixed with pins crossing above the fracture site.

Pinning is performed with the elbow maximally flexed and resting on the C-arm tube. With the arm rotated to the neutral position and a small towel bump placed under the elbow to facilitate clearance from the C-arm, the first K-wire is inserted through the lateral condyle and across the distal humeral physis, ideally aiming up the lateral column of the metaphysis. The path of the pin in the coronal plane can be checked fluoroscopically with the use of the Jones (transcondylar) view. The position and direction of the pin in the sagittal plane can be checked by rotating the shoulder externally. The arm is then rotated back to neutral and the pin advanced to engage the opposite cortex. A second and, if necessary, a third lateral entry pin can be placed in similar fashion with the use of a parallel to slightly divergent path. The surgeon should attempt to achieve as much spread of the pins across the fracture site as possible, avoiding convergence or crossing at the fracture and engaging the cortices of both the lateral and medial columns.[31,77] A biomechanical study of pin configurations by Lee and colleagues[71] comparing crossed pins, parallel lateral pins, and divergent lateral pins found that the stability provided by divergent lateral pins exceeded that of parallel lateral pins and was similar to crossed pins in all but torsional loading; the study

prompted the recommendation for divergent placement for lateral entry pins so that stability could be maximized. If the fracture is comminuted or deemed to be very unstable, a medial entry pin may need to be placed. Zenios and colleagues performed prospective intraoperative evaluation of stability in 21 consecutive patients with type III fractures by taking lateral images of the elbow in external and internal rotation after pinning with two lateral pins; the authors found only six (28%) to be stable, necessitating placement of a third lateral or medial column pin in the remaining 15 fractures.[78] Similarly, Bauer and colleagues found internal rotation stress testing to be helpful in assessing alignment and need for additional fixation in type III supracondylar humerus fractures.[79]

There is no doubt that a crossed pin configuration is biomechanically the most stable construct and historically has been the technique of choice.[70] Zionts and colleagues studied the torsional strength of different pin configurations in displaced supracondylar humeral fractures and found that 37% less torque was required to produce 10 degrees of rotation with the use of two lateral pins than with the use of medial and lateral pins, and it was 80% less if the lateral pins were crossed at the fracture site.[72]

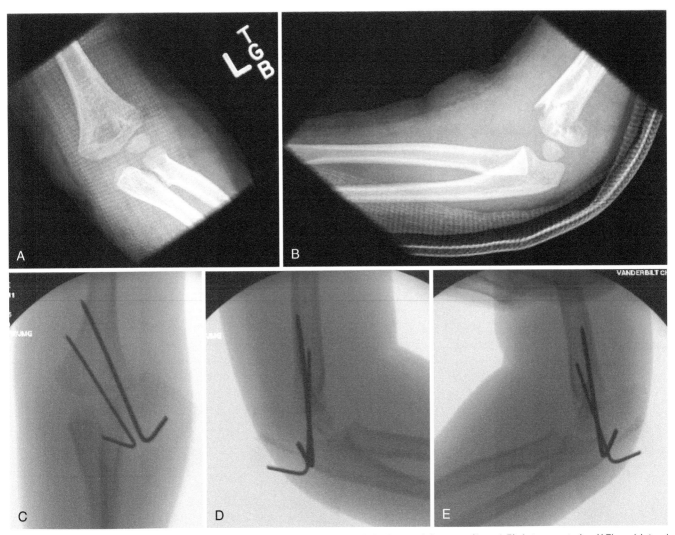

Fig. 17.19 A 4-year-old patient with a closed, extension-type II supracondylar humeral fracture. (A and B) Anteroposterior (AP) and lateral radiographs show posteromedial displacement with intact posterior cortex but with rotation of the distal fragment. (C and D) AP and lateral intraoperative fluoroscopic images after closed reduction and pin fixation with two lateral entry pins. Note the slight divergence of the pins and bicortical fixation, both of which are desirable for stability. (E) Internal rotation "stress" view shows a stable reduction with this pin configuration.

Despite the superior biomechanically stability of crossed pins, the use of this technique has fallen out of favor because of reports of ulnar nerve injury in up to 10% of patients treated with this pin configuration.[80] Injury to the ulnar nerve may occur by direct penetration, particularly when the nerve is unstable and subluxates in flexion.[81] Nerve injury can also occur by tethering if adjacent soft tissues are wrapped up as the pin is inserted, or by stretching around the pin when the elbow is flexed. These potential problems can be mitigated when the surgeon performs medial entry pin placement by extending the elbow to less than 80 degrees of flexion (permissible once fixation of the lateral column has been performed), allowing the ulnar nerve to move posteriorly away from the medial epicondyle. Additionally, a very small incision can be made over the medial epicondyle to allow direct placement of the K-wire on the bone, which ensures that the nerve is avoided during pin placement (Fig. 17.21).[56,79] The position of the medial pin is then checked with fluoroscopy and advanced through the lateral cortex of the humerus. The pins should cross proximal to the fracture for maximal stability. The elbow can then be extended so that the carrying angle and coronal alignment of the fracture can be

assessed on a true AP radiograph. The pins are padded and bent outside the skin, and the arm is splinted or placed in a bivalved cast with the elbow in 70 to 80 degrees of flexion. Using this technique, Green and associates[82] reported no ulnar nerve motor injuries and just one transient ulnar sensory neurapraxia in their single-cohort retrospective study of 71 consecutive children treated operatively for Gartland type II or III supracondylar humeral fractures.

Children should be hospitalized until they are comfortable, their neurologic status can be confirmed, and the risk of circulatory compromise is past. Perioperative ketorolac has been shown to decrease pain, opioid usage, and length of stay.[83] Alignment is checked with radiographs 1 week postoperatively, and the splint is converted to a long arm cast, or the bivalved cast is overwrapped. Pins may be removed and immobilization discontinued 3 to 4 weeks later if radiographs demonstrate adequate healing, although the utility of routine radiographs at this time, in the absence of clinical concerns, has been questioned.[84] Unprotected motion, with activity restrictions, is allowed. Formal physical therapy is not typically necessary because most children regain normal motion on their own.

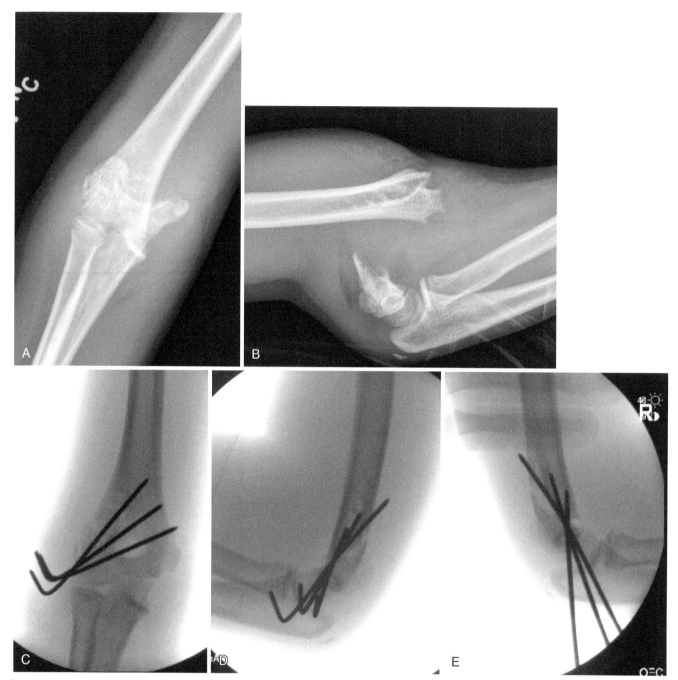

Fig. 17.20 An 8-year-old patient with a widely displaced extension-type III supracondylar humeral fracture that was treated by closed reduction and percutaneous fixation with three lateral entry pins. (A and B) Anteroposterior (AP) and lateral radiographs of the elbow show the fracture and extent of bony displacement and soft tissue disruption. (C and D) Intraoperative AP and lateral fluoroscopic views show a near-anatomic reduction. A third K-wire was placed based on the characteristics of this fracture. (E) Internal rotation "stress" view shows the reduction to be stable. Another fixation option would have been to use a medial entry pin. (Photos and radiographic images courtesy of Jonathan Schoenecker, MD, Vanderbilt University Medical Center, Nashville, TN.)

Pin Configuration and Alternate Techniques. The relative safety of medial entry pins has been addressed in several recent studies of type III supracondylar humeral fractures. A systematic review by Brauer and associates of 2054 children from 35 studies found the probability of iatrogenic nerve injury to be 1.84 times higher with medial pins.[85] Slobogean and associates performed a metaanalysis of 32 studies with 2639 patients and found a higher rate of ulnar nerve injury with crossed pinning and calculated the number needed to harm to be 28 (i.e., one ulnar nerve injury for every 28 patients treated with cross pinning).[86] In their analysis of

pooled data from 5154 fractures, Babal and associates found that medial entry pinning was associated with a 4% risk of injury to the ulnar nerve and that third lateral entry pins were associated with a 3% risk to the median nerve.[40] A prospective randomized clinical study by Kocher and colleagues in 2007 comparing lateral entry pins to medial and lateral entry pins found no statistically significant difference in the rate of ulnar nerve injury.[74] More recently, Garg and colleagues performed a retrospective comparative study of 872 patients with type III supracondylar humeral fractures, representing the largest single-center study of severe

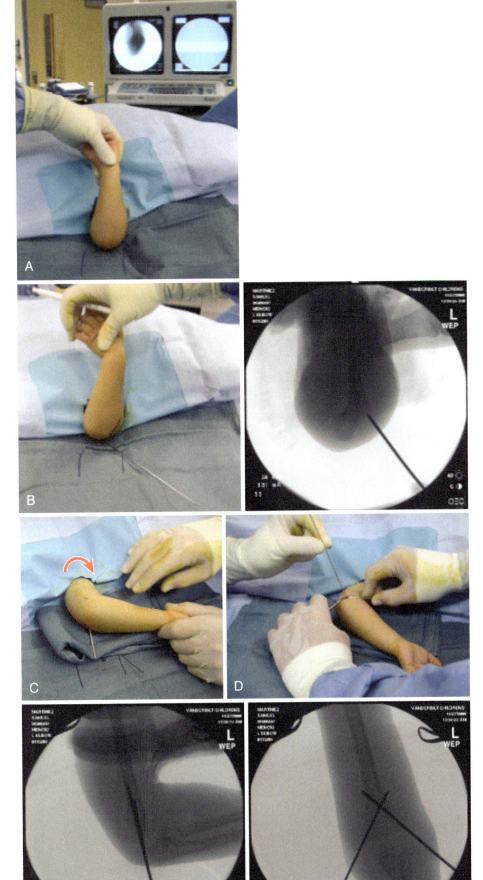

Fig. 17.21 Technique for placement of medial entry pin. (A) Patient is supine with arm draped free on the C-arm platform. (B) The lateral entry pin is placed first, and the fracture is provisionally stabilized. (C) The elbow can then be externally rotated and extended, which allows the ulnar nerve to move away from the medial epicondyle and permits access to the medial epicondyle. A 5-mm incision is made directly over the medial epicondyle, and soft tissue is swept away with a hemostat or elevator. (D) The K-wire can then be positioned directly on the medial epicondyle and driven up the medial column. (E) Anteroposterior and lateral radiographs showing pins crossing above the fracture site and bicortically engaged.

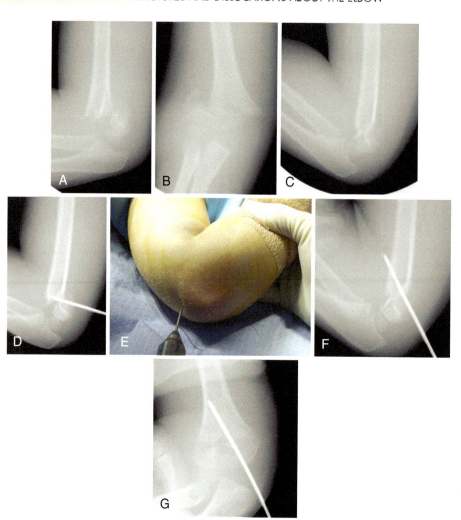

Fig. 17.22 Example of percutaneous leverage pinning to reduce a type III supracondylar humeral fracture. (A and B) Anteroposterior and lateral radiographs show a type III supracondylar humeral fracture. (C) Initial inability to obtain adequate closed reduction. (D) A 2-mm Kirschner wire is placed percutaneously through the triceps tendon, into the fracture site. (E) The surgeon moves hands distally, levering the fracture anteriorly, into more adequate alignment. (F and G) Once adequate alignment is obtained, the wire is advanced through the anterior cortex to maintain reduction. The surgeon can then proceed with lateral or medial pin placement. (Photos and radiographic images courtesy of Steven Lovejoy, MD, Vanderbilt University Medical Center, Nashville, TN.)

supracondylar humeral fractures (all type III), and found a slightly higher but statistically insignificant ($P > .5$) increase in the rate of ulnar nerve palsy with medial entry pins.[41] Specifically, 5 of 335 patients with medial pins and 4 of 537 patients without medial pins developed an ulnar nerve palsy.

Sawaizumi and colleagues described a technique referred to as "leverage pinning" to facilitate percutaneous reduction of displaced supracondylar humeral fractures that avoids the need for hyperflexion of the elbow.[87] In their original description, the authors positioned the patient laterally and placed the elbow in a reduction bracket attached to the operating room table with the forearm allowed to hang free. Under C-arm guidance, the medial and lateral alignment was corrected and confirmed on an AP view. Next, a 2-mm K-wire was introduced percutaneously through the triceps, in a proximal-to-distal direction, into the fracture site, engaging the proximal fragment just past the posterior cortex. The K-wire was then used as a "joystick" to lever the distal fragment in an anterior direction by movement of the pin distally. Once reduction was obtained, the K-wire was advanced through the anterior cortex of the humerus, thus stabilizing the fracture. An additional lateral pin was added to complete fixation. Another option is to place two lateral or medial and lateral pins and remove the reduction pin.

Yu and colleagues reported their experience with a similar technique, done with the patient supine, using a temporary 3-mm K-wire to facilitate reduction of type III supracondylar humeral fractures that could not be realigned with traditional

closed maneuvers (Fig. 17.22).[88] They used this technique in 42 of 118 patients and did not have to resort to open reduction of the fractures. Their results with this technique were similar to conventional closed reduction and cross pinning.

Open Reduction and Internal Fixation

The indications for open reduction of supracondylar fractures include fractures that cannot be reduced by closed methods, those that are not amenable to closed treatment because of intraarticular comminution, open fractures that require irrigation and débridement, and fractures with vascular compromise or neurologic loss after reduction that require exploration and possible repair of neurovascular structures. It is unusual for fractures to be irreducible by closed means; however, when it occurs, the most common cause is interposition of soft tissue or neurovascular structures. The brachialis is a common soft tissue impediment to reduction.[89] Entrapment of the brachial artery within the fracture may be heralded by vascular compromise after closed reduction. Fleuriau-Chateau and associates reported on 41 open reductions performed for irreducible supracondylar fractures.[90] The most common finding intraoperatively was buttonholing of the brachialis muscle by the distal end of the proximal fragment. They also found tethering of the median or radial nerve (or both), with or without the brachial artery, that was not expected on the basis of preoperative evaluation.

Failure to achieve adequate reduction is the most common cause of a poor outcome after supracondylar humeral fractures, and open reduction is preferable to repeated attempts at closed reduction or accepting suboptimal alignment. Results after open reduction compare favorably to closed reduction and pinning. Cramer and colleagues[91] found comparable results for open reduction with pin fixation and closed reduction with percutaneous pin fixation, despite the fact that the fractures in the open reduction group were more severe and were unable to be reduced by closed means. Ozkoc and colleagues[92] reported on 99 patients with displaced extension-type supracondylar fractures of the humerus. The first 44 were treated with open reduction and internal fixation because of a lack of an image intensifier. The next 55 patients were treated with closed reduction and percutaneous pin fixation. These authors found that the open surgical group had slightly worse functional outcomes. They lost an average of 6 degrees of extension and 8 degrees of flexion compared with 0.6 and 8 degrees, respectively, in the closed group. There were no cosmetic differences. This report confirms that closed reduction and percutaneous pinning is the preferred treatment but that open reduction also leads to very good results, when indicated.

Technique. Anterior, medial, lateral, and posterior surgical approaches to the distal humerus have all been described. A guiding principle in choosing an approach for supracondylar fractures is that it should be performed through the area of disrupted periosteum. The presence of a neurovascular deficit should also be considered when an approach is chosen.[31,35] An anterior approach through a transverse incision in the antecubital fossa provides access to the common soft tissue impediments to reduction and the best exposure of the neurovascular structures (Fig. 17.23). The scar runs parallel with the normal skin folds and, as such, is very cosmetic and avoids the contracture that can be associated with a longitudinal incision made across the flexor surface of the elbow. In addition, it can be converted to an extensile exposure by extending the incision proximally in a longitudinal fashion along the medial side of the brachium and/or distally along the radial side of the forearm as needed. The medial approach is preferred for flexion-type injuries in which the ulnar nerve is likely to be trapped in the fracture.[40]

Koudstaal and colleagues[93] reported their outcomes in 26 patients in whom the anterior approach was used and compared them with a historical group of their own patients whose fractures were treated through a lateral or combined medial and lateral approach. They used a transverse incision in the antecubital fossa. Results were evaluated with the use of Flynn's criteria, and no statistically significant difference was noted between the three approaches. Advantages of the anterior approach were as follows: (1) a more thorough hematoma evacuation from the antecubital fossa, (2) excellent fracture visualization with concurrent visualization of entrapped muscle and vascular and neural structures, and (3) the ability to directly palpate the medial and lateral epicondyles, which allows the surgeon to correct any residual displacement. Ay and colleagues[94] also performed a retrospective review of 61 children with displaced supracondylar humeral fractures who had open reduction and K-wire fixation via an anterior approach and found that all patients had either an excellent (73%) or good (27%) outcome by Flynn's criteria.

The medial approach is performed with the shoulder externally rotated. A 3- to 4-cm longitudinal incision is made on the medial side of the distal end of the humerus and elbow. Once the skin and subcutaneous fat have been incised, the fracture hematoma and the fracture are encountered.

The ulnar nerve is protected but does not have to be visualized. The periosteum over the anterior aspect of the proximal fragment is usually stripped by the injury. The fracture hematoma can be evacuated and the fracture explored by visual and digital inspection; this ensures that no neurovascular structures are trapped. Adequate visualization of the fracture is necessary to ensure anatomic reduction, but care must be taken not to disrupt the intact posteromedial periosteal hinge. The fracture is reduced and cross pinned. If anatomic reduction is not possible, a lateral approach is made to ensure a perfect reduction. The lateral incision, which is also longitudinal, is made over the lateral condyle of the distal end of the humerus; such an incision allows exposure of the lateral side of the fracture. As with closed reduction, the pins are left protruding from the skin and are bent over felt.

The posterior approach to the elbow is preferred when there is intraarticular extension or comminution of the distal humeral condyles in older patients. It is not generally indicated in young children with type III supracondylar fractures because it may compromise the only intact periosteum and blood supply to the distal humerus.

Postoperative discomfort is usually minimal, most likely attributable to decompression of the hematoma and neurovascular structures and stabilization of the fracture. Patients may typically be discharged from the hospital when they are comfortable, their neurologic status can be confirmed, and there is no concern for circulatory compromise. Follow-up care and course are the same as for closed pinning, with pin alignment check at 7 to 10 days and pin removal at 3 to 4 weeks after surgery.

TIMING OF SURGICAL INTERVENTION

Historically, closed reduction and pin fixation of type III supracondylar humeral fractures has been done on an emergent basis because of concerns about increased swelling, neurovascular compromise, compartment syndrome, and difficulty with closed reduction. It had been thought that early treatment enhances the likelihood of obtaining an anatomic reduction and reduces the risk of complications such as vascular compromise. The standard of care has evolved based on results of several studies indicating that these fractures can be treated on an urgent rather than emergent basis unless there is vascular compromise. Both Green[95] and Mehlman and colleagues[96] compared the effect of surgical timing on perioperative complications. Mehlman's group found no significant difference in fractures that were managed 8 hours or earlier after injury ($n = 52$) compared with those treated more than 8 hours after the injury ($n = 146$). Treatment of the fracture was delayed so that it could be undertaken during normal working hours. No increase in the incidence of cubitus varus, pin tract infection, or vascular complications was detected. There was no increased need for open reduction in the delayed-treatment group. Iyengar and colleagues[97] came to similar conclusions when comparing results of early versus delayed pinning of completely displaced supracondylar humeral fractures. Another report by Leet and colleagues[98] provides further support that delaying reduction in the operating room does not lead to further adverse events. Increased operative time, need to open the fracture site, hospital length of stay, and complications were not correlated with an increase in the time to surgical intervention. Likewise, Gupta and colleagues[99] compared 50 children with

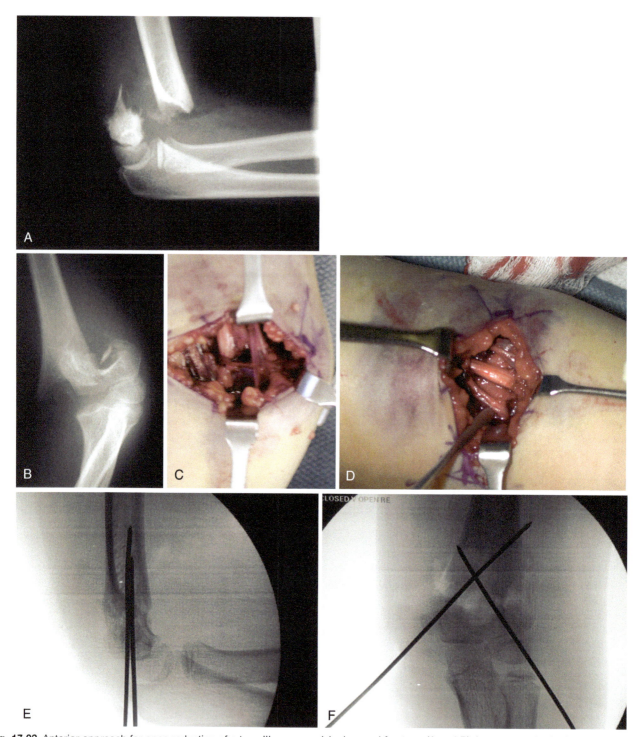

Fig. 17.23 Anterior approach for open reduction of a type III supracondylar humeral fracture. (A and B) Anteroposterior (AP) and lateral radiographs of a type III supracondylar humeral fracture in an 8-year-old patient with median nerve paresthesias and a decreased radial pulse. (C) Anterior approach through a transverse incision in the antecubital flexion crease shows entrapment of the median nerve and tethering of the brachial artery by the fracture. (D) Neurovascular structures were carefully decompressed and freed from the fracture site. The radial pulse improved almost immediately, which allowed the fracture to be reduced. (E and F) AP and lateral radiographs showing anatomic reduction of the fracture and crossed pin fixation. (Photos and radiographs courtesy of Gregory Mencio, MD, Vanderbilt University Medical Center, Nashville, TN.)

type III supracondylar humeral fractures treated in less than 12 hours with 100 children treated more than 12 hours after injury. They found no significant difference between groups in rates of open reduction, pin tract infections, compartment syndromes, vascular compromise, or nerve injuries.

More recently, a prospective study of 145 fractures showed no increase in the need for open reduction or the number of perioperative complications with a delay in surgical treatment up to 21 hours after injury.[100] In the study by Garg and associates,[41] the time from injury to surgical treatment for 872 severe (type III) supracondylar fractures averaged 16.3 hours. Patients were grouped into four cohorts based on time to surgery (<6 hours, 6–12 hours, 12–24 hours, >24 hours). The study found no increased rate of morbidity or complications with increased lengths of time from presentation to surgery. The authors of both of these studies emphasize the need for a thorough and accurate baseline assessment of neurovascular status, immobilization of the limb without fracture reduction, frequent neurovascular checks while awaiting surgery, and the availability of an operating room in an acceptable time frame.

COMPLICATIONS

There are numerous complications of supracondylar fractures and their treatment. Early complications are specifically related to the initial injury and treatment. They include vascular compromise, compartment syndrome, neurologic deficit, loss of reduction, and pin track infections; delayed problems include cubitus varus, elbow stiffness, myositis ossificans, nonunion, osteonecrosis of the epiphysis, and hyperextension deformity.

VASCULAR COMPROMISE

Vascular problems can be grouped into two types: acute, from occlusion of the brachial artery, and subacute, or Volkmann ischemia. Fortunately, acute vascular insufficiency is relatively uncommon, occurring in 5% to 12% of children with supracondylar humerus fractures.[35] The vascular status of the extremity can be assessed by color of the hand (pink or white), temperature of the extremity (warm or cold), neurologic status, amount of pain, and status of the radial pulse (presence or absent). The elbow has excellent collateral circulation that usually provides sufficient blood flow to the distal extremity, even if the brachial artery is damaged, hence the term *pink, pulseless hand.*[101]

The absence of the radial pulse on palpation is never normal, but it is not always an indication of a true arterial injury. In fact, the radial pulse may be absent because of spasm and may return after reduction of the fracture. Loss of the pulse during reduction may indicate obstruction from too much elbow flexion or entrapment of the artery in the fracture with reduction.[39,51,102–104] Although arterial exploration is always indicated in the event of a truly dysvascular extremity, the simple absence of the radial pulse with good peripheral circulation may not always be an indication for arterial exploration. When the radial pulse is absent (regardless of the perfusion status of the hand), fracture reduction with pin fixation and reassessment of the vascular status are the recommended treatment steps. If the radial pulse is absent but concomitant median or AIN palsy is present, immediate exploration may be warranted.[46] If the hand is perfused but remains pulseless after reduction, opinion is divided about the need for immediate arterial exploration in all children.

The persistent absence of a radial pulse after fracture reduction is always worrisome. Campbell and colleagues[39] studied 59 children with supracondylar humeral fractures in whom 11 (19%) had absent pulses; pulses returned after reduction in five patients and required no further treatment. The other six patients underwent exploration of the brachial artery. The artery was interposed in the fracture in one patient and lacerated in one, and one had an intimal tear. The other three patients were found to have spasm that resolved without other treatment. They recommend vascular exploration if the radial pulse is absent after reduction of the fracture.

Copley and colleagues[102] reviewed 128 children with grade III supracondylar fractures of the humerus. Seventeen of the children had absent or diminished (detected on Doppler but not on palpation) radial pulses on initial examination. A total of 14 of the 17 recovered pulses after fracture

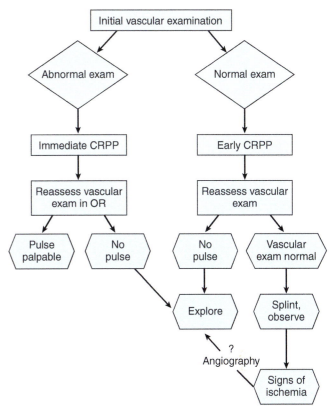

Fig. 17.24 Flowchart to guide decision-making in cases in which a possible vascular injury is associated with a displaced supracondylar humeral fracture. *CRPP,* Closed reduction and percutaneous pinning; *OR,* operating room. (Modified from Copley LA, Dormans JP, Davidson RS. Vascular injuries and their sequelae in pediatric supracondylar humeral fractures: toward a goal of prevention. *J Pediatr Orthop.* 1996;16:99-103.)

reduction, but the remaining three had persistent absence of the radial pulse. These patients underwent exploration of the brachial artery immediately, and a significant vascular injury requiring repair was found in each. In two of the 14 patients whose pulses returned after fracture reduction, progressive postoperative deterioration in their circulation developed during the first 24 to 36 hours after reduction, with loss of the radial pulse. In both, arteriography identified arterial injuries, and both underwent exploration and vascular repair. These investigators concluded that absence of the radial pulse after reduction of a supracondylar humeral fracture indicated the existence of a significant arterial injury requiring surgical exploration and vascular repair (Fig. 17.24).

Schoenecker and colleagues[104] agreed with these authors in recommending arterial exploration in the absence of a Doppler-detectable radial pulse. They performed surgical exploration in seven limbs without a radial pulse after a supracondylar fracture and found the brachial artery to be either kinked or entrapped in the fracture in four. They repaired three of the arteries.

On the other hand, Garbuz and associates[105] reviewed 326 patients with supracondylar fractures of the distal end of the humerus and found 22 whose radial pulses were absent on examination. Radial pulses returned in 15 patients after fracture reduction, and these extremities were monitored without exploration of the brachial artery. In seven patients, absence of the radial pulse persisted after reduction, and the hand was dysvascular. All of these patients underwent arterial exploration with arterial repair. Based on these results, the authors recommended that patients with an absent radial pulse but good circulation to the hand be observed after fracture reduction.

Sabharwal and colleagues[101] reviewed patients with supracondylar fractures of the humerus and found that 13 of 410 fractures did not have radial pulses. All patients without a radial pulse had adequate collateral circulation, as demonstrated by magnetic resonance angiography, duplex scanning, or both. They performed arterial exploration in all these patients and found arterial injuries in all of them. Arterial repair was performed in all patients; however, asymptomatic reocclusion and residual stenosis were observed in these patients at follow-up. They recommended observation of patients with supracondylar humeral fractures and an associated absence of a radial pulse. They reasoned that the collateral circulation is adequate for the normal survival and use of the upper extremity, and they further stated that if the brachial artery is repaired, it is likely to become occluded as a result of insufficient flow.

Choi and colleagues[106] determined that 2.6% of supracondylar fractures (33/1255) evaluated did not have a pulse. Of the 33 patients without radial pulses in this study, 24 were considered to be pulseless but well perfused at presentation, and all of these remained so immediately after reduction and internal fixation. Fourteen (58%) were also noted to have a palpable pulse postoperatively. Four more patients subsequently had return of a palpable pulse at an average of 8 weeks after surgery. In all, 75% of the perfused and pulseless limbs (18/24 patients) normalized after reduction and internal fixation. The other six patients in this group never had a documented return of pulse but sustained no known complications. Of the nine pulseless and poorly perfused limbs, only two had return of both pulse and perfusion, and another two regained perfusion but remained pulseless. The other five patients with pulseless, dysvascular limbs underwent exploration and repair at an average of 7.3 hours after injury and had good results. Garg and colleagues[41] observed restoration of a palpable pulse by the first postoperative visit in all of the children in their study of type III supracondylar fractures treated by closed reduction and pinning; these patients had initially been seen with absent palpable or Doppler-detected pulses but clinically perfused limbs.

More recent studies suggest that a "watchful, waiting" strategy for the pulseless, perfused limb after a supracondylar humeral fracture may underestimate the significance of the vascular injury. White and colleagues[51] performed a meta-analysis in which they studied pooled data for 313 pulseless supracondylar fractures. They found a 77% rate of true vascular injury in the setting of a pulseless, perfused supracondylar fracture and a 91% patent artery rate after brachial artery repair at 2 years' follow-up. Mangat and colleagues[46] found that 80% of patients with a pulseless, perfused hand had tethering or entrapment of the vessel when a concomitant nerve palsy (median or AIN) was present and recommended immediate arterial exploration in these circumstances. They also documented that all vessels repaired remained patent at follow-up. Reigstad and colleagues[107] performed exploration on five patients with type III supracondylar humeral fractures whose extremities remained pulseless with slow or absent capillary refilling after closed reduction and percutaneous pinning. All were found to have an entrapped brachial artery, of whom four required microvascular repairs, and two had entrapment of the median nerve. Normal function was documented at more than 1 year after exploration.

Blakey and colleagues[108] found that 23 of 26 patients with "pink, pulseless hands" who did not immediately undergo surgical exploration had some degree of ischemic contracture when they were examined at an average follow-up of 25 years (range, 4–26 years). These authors concluded that a pink, pulseless hand after fracture reduction is ischemic and that persistent and increasing pain with a deepening nerve lesion was indicative of critical ischemia. They recommended urgent surgical exploration when the pulse is absent to prevent the long-term sequelae observed in their study.

Consensus current practice for the management of displaced, type III supracondylar humeral fractures when the pulse is absent, regardless of the status of the vascularity of the hand, is to perform closed reduction and percutaneous pinning on an emergent basis. If the pulse returns, the extremity can be splinted, neurovascular status can be monitored to ensure that there is no deterioration, and the patient can be discharged when comfortable. Regardless of the status of the pulse, if the hand is well perfused, which indicates adequate distal circulation, observation is appropriate. Current evidence does not support exploring all limbs without a palpable radial pulse.[31] Findings by White and colleagues[51] and a poll of members of the Pediatric Orthopaedic Society of North America suggest that the common practice of watchful waiting for pulseless and perfused hands after supracondylar fractures should be questioned. There is, however, consensus that exploration of the brachial artery is indicated if the pulse returns but the vascular examination is equivocal, if the extremity is dysvascular, if there are signs of forearm ischemia, or if there is a concomitant median or AIN palsy. However a recent study by Harris et al of 71 patients from four trauma centers found that the presence of a pulseless extremities and concomitant anterior interosseous or median nerve palsy was not an absolute indication for open reduction.[47] Arteriography is rarely indicated preoperatively because the location of the lesion is at the level of the fracture, and an arteriogram is unlikely to reveal anything that is not already known and will only delay treatment that is otherwise necessary.

Compartment syndrome is a rare complication of supracondylar fractures of the humerus in children. Historically, Volkmann ischemia was more common after closed reduction and immobilization of the elbow in a hyperflexed position, which is a practice that has been largely abandoned in favor of current treatment with pin fixation that allows the elbow to be splinted in much less flexion. The rate of compartment syndrome in supracondylar humerus fractures is estimated to be 0.1% to 0.3%. The risk is highest in fractures with an absent radial pulse and dysvascular hand, even after successful vascular repair.[106] Posterolaterally displaced supracondylar fractures have a higher risk of vascular injury and compartment syndrome, whereas ipsilateral supracondylar and forearm fractures ("floating elbows") are a marker of significant trauma and have the highest risk of neurovascular injury and compartment syndrome.[109]

The traditional signs and symptoms of forearm ischemia in adults—pain, paresthesia, paralysis, pallor, and pulselessness—are less reliable in predicting the presence of impending compartment syndrome in children. Pain and paresthesia are early signs of ischemia and nerve compression. Paralysis, pallor, and an absent pulse are later findings of more prolonged ischemia and may reflect irreversible change. In children, the combination of increasing analgesic requirement plus anxiety and agitation, referred to as the *three As*, may be more predictive of impending compartment syndrome.[110] An increasing analgesic requirement is the most sensitive indicator of impending compartment syndrome in children, preceding changes in vascular status by more than 7 hours.[52] Progressively deteriorating neurologic status in the absence of pain or other "typical" clinical findings may also be a sign of an evolving compartment syndrome. This so-called "silent compartment syndrome" should be suspected particularly if a median nerve injury is present. In a young child, if there is suspicion of compartment syndrome, tissue pressure measurements should be obtained. This is best done emergently in the operating room. If compartment pressures are found to be elevated, a fasciotomy should be performed through an extensile volar approach extending from the elbow through the carpal tunnel. A fasciotomy performed within a mean of 30 hours from diagnosis has been shown to be effective in reducing the risk of permanent damage in 90% of children.

NEUROLOGIC INJURY

It has been shown that the risk of nerve injury after supracondylar humeral fractures increases with increasing fracture displacement.[111] Based on the findings of two recent studies—a metaanalysis of 5154 fractures by Babal and colleagues[40] and a single-institution, consecutive cohort study of 872 type III fractures by Garg and colleagues[41]—the incidence of neurologic injury after extension-type supracondylar humeral fractures is 12%. The most common nerve injured is the AIN, which is observed in one-third of cases, followed by injury to the radial nerve. Ulnar nerve injury was the least frequent.[40,41] Garg and colleagues[41] found a 28% rate of iatrogenic nerve injury but observed no difference with pin configuration.

Most nerve injuries that occur at the time of fracture are neurapraxias, regardless of the nerve injured. Motor recovery typically takes about 2 to 3 months, whereas sensory function may take up to 6 months[41,44,112] Routine (early) nerve exploration is not recommended unless no clinical or electromyographic evidence of recovery has been noted by 5 months.[44,113] Amillo and Mora[114] recommended that if nerve recovery is not seen within this time frame, nerve exploration should be undertaken as soon thereafter as possible because recovery is less predictable with further delay. Results were poor when exploration was performed beyond 1 year after injury. The outcomes of neurolysis are predictably good for chronic nerve palsies in which the nerve is in continuity. Early nerve exploration is indicated if nerve function deteriorates after closed reduction and pinning of the fracture because of the likelihood of nerve entrapment in the fracture site or iatrogenic injury. Extraction of the nerve from the fracture or from constricting soft tissue structures and removal of any compromising hardware should be performed as soon as the deficit is identified. Provided the nerve is not lacerated, observation is recommended for these iatrogenic injuries.

CUBITUS VARUS

Cubitus varus, defined as loss of carrying angle of more than 5 degrees compared with the contralateral elbow, is the most common late complication of displaced supracondylar humeral fractures and the most common angular deformity.[31,353] Historically, the incidence after closed treatment has been reported to be as high as 58%.[18,115–118] Pirone and colleagues[60] observed a 3% incidence of cubitus varus after pinning compared with 14% after closed treatment. It

is estimated that 5% to 10% of children with supracondylar fractures of the humerus will develop this complication, irrespective of the method of treatment.[117]

The prevailing thought is that cubitus varus is a malunion that occurs as a result of malreduction or loss of reduction of the fracture. The deformity is caused by internal rotation in the transverse plane, medial tilting coronally, and extension in the sagittal plane. Recognition of cubitus varus is often delayed until the elbow can be fully extended, perhaps fueling theories that the deformity develops after the fracture has healed. However, studies do suggest that growth disturbance, either medial arrest or lateral stimulation, caused by the fracture itself may play a role in the pathogenesis of the deformity.[81,119–122] Osteonecrosis of the trochlea is an uncommon cause of varus deformity.

Cubitus varus is usually not painful and has traditionally been regarded as a cosmetic problem. However, several studies have cast light on potential functional consequences of this deformity. Abe and colleagues[123] reported on 15 patients with tardy ulnar nerve palsy caused by cubitus varus deformity, at a mean interval of 15 years from fracture to the onset of symptoms. At operation they found compression of the ulnar nerve by a fibrous band running between the two heads of the flexor carpi ulnaris. Mitsunari and associates[124] postulated that internal rotation was a contributing factor in five patients with tardy ulnar nerve palsy and posttraumatic cubitus varus deformity. Spinner and associates[125] have observed ulnar neuropathy associated with cubitus varus caused by snapping of the medial portion of the triceps over the ulnar nerve.

Several biomechanical implications of residual cubitus varus have been identified. Davids and colleagues[126] identified a preexisting, posttraumatic cubitus varus deformity as a contributing factor in six children with lateral condyle fractures. They postulated that the presence of varus malalignment increases both the torsional moment and the shear force generated across the capitellar physis by a routine fall. Takahara and colleagues[127] have also found an increased incidence of fractures of the lateral condyle or distal humeral physis in patients with residual cubitus varus deformity. It therefore appears that a cubitus deformity may predispose a child to subsequent lateral condylar fracture.

More recently, O'Driscoll and colleagues[128] reported on tardy posterolateral rotatory instability of the elbow in patients with known cubitus varus. They identified 22 patients who were seen primarily with lateral elbow pain and signs of elbow instability two to three decades after having sustained supracondylar fractures that had healed in varus. Based on observations, they postulated that the presence of cubitus varus shifts the mechanical axis of the elbow medially, altering forces generated across the elbow by the triceps that, over time, lead to increased stress and eventual attenuation of the lateral collateral ligament.

The cosmetic issues and functional implications associated with significant cubitus varus underscore the importance of restoring anatomy and maintaining alignment when supracondylar fractures are initially treated and also support correction of residual deformity when it occurs. However, the timing of corrective osteotomy is best staged after the fracture has had a chance to heal and remodel, and elbow motion has plateaued. Ippolito and associates[120] found that the correction deteriorated with continued growth in young patients after osteotomy; thus, the authors recommended waiting until children were closer to skeletal maturity. Voss and colleagues[122] found that disruption of medial growth occurred in 11% of their patients with cubitus varus and was a potential cause of progressive deformity. They suggested waiting at least 1 year after injury before performing corrective osteotomy so that proper assessment of this potential problem could be undertaken. For all of the reasons just discussed, this author usually recommends waiting at least 1 year after injury before proceeding with surgery to correct residual cubitus varus. Many osteotomy techniques have been described, and discussion is beyond the scope of this chapter on acute injuries.

FLEXION-TYPE SUPRACONDYLAR FRACTURE

Flexion-type fractures are much less common than extension-type injuries. Wilkins[11] estimated the incidence to be about 2.5% of all supracondylar fractures; Fowles and Kassab[129] found the incidence to be slightly higher. This fracture occurs as the result of a fall on the flexed elbow. With this injury, the elbow is typically held flexed, in contrast to the position seen with extension-type supracondylar fractures. These injuries are thought to be more difficult to manage than extension-type fractures. Mahan and colleagues[130] reviewed the 10-year history of flexion-type supracondylar elbow fractures treated at one institution and compared them with an extension-type cohort collected during a similar period. The patients in the flexion-type group (mean age, 7.5 years) were older than those in the extension-type group (mean age, 5.8 years). The authors found no difference in the incidence of preoperative nerve symptoms; however, the flexion-type group had a significantly increased rate of ulnar nerve symptoms (19% vs. 3% in the extension-type group). In a review of pooled data of 5148 patients, Babal and colleagues[40] found a 17% rate of neurapraxia in flexion-type injuries (compared with 13% for extension-type fractures), 91% of which involved the ulnar nerve.

These injuries can be classified with the use of the Gartland classification, and treatment is similar to that of extension-type injuries. If the fracture is nondisplaced, simple immobilization is all that is necessary. If the distal fragment is angulated anteriorly but not displaced, reduction and immobilization with the elbow in extension, which takes advantage of the intact anterior periosteal hinge, is usually successful (Fig. 17.25). If the fracture is displaced, closed reduction and pinning should be attempted, and, if unsuccessful, open reduction and internal fixation should be performed through a medial approach. Mahan and colleagues[130] found that flexion-type injuries were more likely to require open reduction (31%) than those in the extension-type group (10%) and were more likely to have ulnar nerve entrapment requiring decompression. Green and colleagues[131] described the use of a transolecranon pin to add stability to unstable flexion-type supracondylar humerus fractures once reduction of the fracture in the sagittal plane is achieved. Rotational or angular malalignment in the coronal plane is then corrected, and then two to three lateral-based pins are placed to secure the fracture. The transolecranon pin is then removed.

FRACTURE-SEPARATION OF THE DISTAL HUMERAL PHYSIS

INCIDENCE

The exact incidence of this injury is not known, although it is probably underdiagnosed because of the rarity of the injury and high frequency of misdiagnosis.[132] DeLee and colleagues[133] reviewed three cases of infantile supracondylar fractures that had been reported by MacAfee and concluded that these were actually fracture-separations of the distal humeral physis. With increased awareness of this injury pattern, transphyseal fractures of the distal humerus are now being diagnosed more accurately and frequently because of increased awareness of the injury pattern.

MECHANISMS OF INJURY

Fracture-separations of the distal humerus typically occur in children less than 3 years of age by one of three mechanisms: birth trauma, fall on an outstretched hand with the elbow extended, or child abuse. In the neonate, differentiation must be made between separation of the distal humeral physis and brachial plexus birth palsy. Both injuries can be a cause of pseudoparalysis or true paralysis in an infant who will not move the affected arm. Brachial plexus injuries cause a true paralysis and are not associated with pain or swelling of the elbow. Both pain and swelling are associated with pseudoparalysis in a child with physeal separation of the distal humerus. In older children, this injury may occur as a result of a fall from a height, as reported by Holda and colleagues.[134] DeLee and colleagues[133] found child abuse, either proven or suspected, in six of their 16 patients. One must therefore rule out the possibility of child abuse if this fracture is seen in a young child.

CLASSIFICATION

DeLee and colleagues[133] reviewed a series of 16 patients with this injury and based their classification on the age of the child and the presence or absence of the capitellar ossification center. Type A fractures occur in infants from birth to 9 months. No ossification center is present in the capitellum at this age, and no metaphyseal bony fragment is attached to the epiphysis. Type B fractures occur in children 7 months to 3 years. The ossification center of the capitellum is present radiographically, and a fragment of the metaphysis (Thurston-Holland sign) may or may not be displaced with the epiphysis. Type C fractures occur in children 3 to 7 years. The capitellum is well ossified, and a large Thurston-Holland metaphyseal fragment is seen on the radiograph. In all 16 patients, the distal humeral physis was displaced posteromedially. Type C injuries can easily be confused with a lateral condyle fracture. Elbow arthrography performed in the operating room at the time of treatment will usually distinguish the two types of fractures.

DIAGNOSIS

Children with fracture-separations of the distal humeral physis have marked swelling about the elbow; the physical appearance of the joint resembles that of an elbow dislocation or infection. Gentle manipulation of the elbow reveals a muffled crepitus that is thought to be diagnostic of epiphyseal separation. It is the result of two cartilaginous surfaces rubbing together and should be distinguished from bony crepitus.

AP radiographs of the elbow in a child with physeal separation of the distal humerus show both the radius and ulna to be displaced in relation to the humerus while maintaining a normal relationship to one another. This injury must be distinguished radiographically from an elbow dislocation, a displaced fracture of the lateral condyle, and a true supracondylar

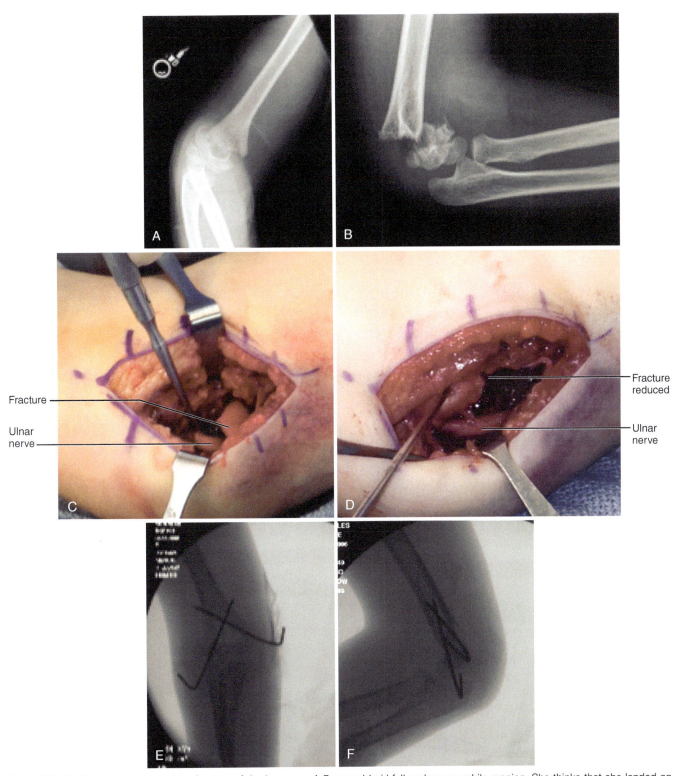

Fig. 17.25 Flexion-type supracondylar fracture of the humerus. A 7-year-old girl fell on her arm while running. She thinks that she landed on her arm with the elbow flexed. She has decreased ulnar sensation. (A and B) Anteroposterior (AP) and lateral radiographs show a flexion-type supracondylar humeral fracture. Closed reduction was unsuccessful. Open reduction was performed through a medial approach. (C) The ulnar nerve was found to be trapped in the fracture. (D) The nerve was freed, and the fracture was reduced and pinned with the elbow in extension with the use of a medial entry pin. The elbow was then flexed, and a lateral entry pin was placed to complete fixation. (E and F) Intraoperative AP and lateral fluoroscopic images showing reduction and pin configuration.

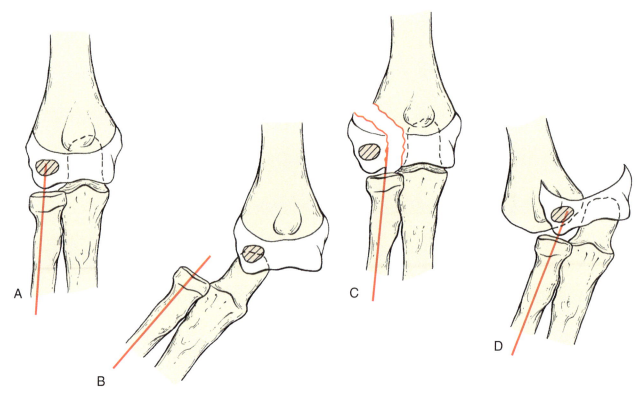

Fig. 17.26 Comparison of injuries about the distal end of the humerus. (A) Normal distal humeral relationships. (B) Dislocation of the elbow. A line drawn along the longitudinal axis of the radius no longer intersects the capitellum. The capitellum, however, maintains its normal relationship to the distal end of the humerus. (C) Displaced fracture of the lateral condyle. The longitudinal axis of the proximal part of the radius does not intersect the capitellum, and the capitellum is displaced from its normal position on the distal metaphysis of the humerus. (D) Fracture-separation of the distal humeral physis. The capitellum is displaced from its normal position on the lateral side of the distal humeral metaphysis but maintains its normal relationship with the radial head. (Modified from DeLee JC, Wilkins KE, Rogers KF, et al. Fracture-separation of the distal humeral epiphysis. *J Bone Joint Surg Am.* 1980;62:46.)

fracture. On an AP radiograph of a normal elbow, a line drawn along the longitudinal axis of the radius passes through the capitellum, regardless of the position of the elbow (Fig. 17.26A). If this line does not pass through the capitellum, either dislocation of the radius, elbow dislocation, or a displaced fracture of the lateral humeral condyle must have occurred.

In a fracture-separation of the distal humeral physis, the relationship of the radius to the capitellum is preserved (as it is in a supracondylar humeral fracture), but both the radius (along with the ulna) and capitellum are displaced, usually posteromedially (Fig. 17.26D). Before the appearance of the capitellar ossification center, the direction of displacement may be the only differentiator between physeal separations, which are almost always posteromedial, and elbow dislocations, which are generally displaced posterolaterally (Fig. 17.26B). A displaced fracture of the lateral condyle of the humerus may be distinguished by the fact that the radius and ulna retain their normal relationship with the humerus; however, because the capitellum is displaced, the radius does not properly align with it (Fig. 17.26C). Supracondylar fractures, which are uncommon in this age group, are distinguishable by a fracture line above the epiphysis.

In the very young child (before the capitellum has ossified), a fracture-separation is most easily confused with elbow dislocation. The latter is extremely uncommon in this age group and, as already mentioned, is usually displaced posterolaterally, whereas physeal separations almost always displace posteromedially. Ultrasound, MRI, and arthrography have

all been shown to help differentiate between pathologies, particularly before ossification of the capitellum.[123,135,136] Ultrasound (Fig. 17.27) requires technical expertise that may not be readily available in all settings, and MRI is also a limited resource that is expensive and requires children of this age group to be sedated. Arthrography (Fig. 17.28) also requires that the child be sedated but, if done in the operating room, affords the opportunity to assess the pattern of injury and manage it definitively, if indicated.

TREATMENT

Unlike a supracondylar fracture, a fracture-separation of the distal humerus physis is usually stable because it occurs through the thicker distal end of the humerus below the thin supracondylar region. It was initially reported that cubitus varus deformity is less likely to develop as a complication of this fracture than it is after a supracondylar fracture.[132,133] However, subsequent studies have found otherwise, citing an unacceptably high rate of cubitus varus with closed treatment.[123,133,134] The conclusion of two of these studies was that accurate reduction and pin fixation are necessary to prevent cubitus varus deformity.

DeLee and colleagues[133] recommended closed reduction if the fracture was diagnosed early and splinting/casting in situ if the diagnosis was delayed. Holda and colleagues[134] agreed with this approach because their results with more aggressive treatment were poor. Mizuno and associates,[137] however, obtained good results with open reduction through a posterior approach.

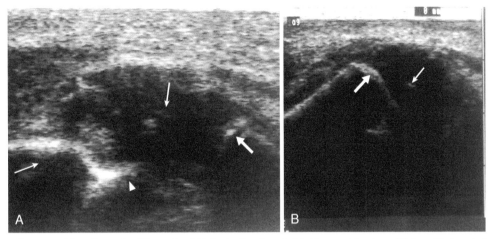

Fig. 17.27 Ultrasound images of the elbow of a 17-month-old infant with a type I distal humeral fracture. (A) A sagittal posterior sonogram shows a fracture *(arrowhead)* through the physis. The *thin arrow* on the left points to the distal end of the humerus. The *vertical arrow* points to the displaced capitellum. Ossification of the capitellum can be seen. The *heavy arrow* points to the head of the radius, which is articulating with the capitellum. (B) Posterolateral sonogram after reduction of the fracture. The *heavy arrow* points to the distal humeral physis. The capitellum can be seen in its normal position *(thin arrow)*. The distal end of the humerus is seen just underneath the *heavy arrow*. (Ultrasound images courtesy of R. S. Davidson, MD, Children's Hospital of Philadelphia, Philadelphia, PA.)

Author's Preferred Method of Treatment

With this injury, this author's preference is to first investigate the possibility of child abuse. If necessary, the child can be admitted to the hospital to facilitate this inquiry. If the fracture is not recent and the child has radiographic evidence of healing, simple immobilization is indicated (Fig. 17.29). If the fracture is displaced, closed reduction and percutaneous pinning is probably warranted because of the reported high incidence of cubitus varus deformity resulting from simple immobilization of this fracture. Closed reduction is achieved by gentle traction on the forearm. The medial displacement of the distal fragment is then corrected, any rotational abnormality is corrected, and the elbow is then flexed to 90 degrees and pinned as one does for a supracondylar fracture, using one or two smaller-diameter (0.062-inch) K-wires.

It can be challenging to judge the quality of the reduction intraoperatively because these injuries often occur before the capitellar ossification center is present. One method to help assess the adequacy of reduction is to use intraoperative arthrography to better define the anatomy of the distal humerus. This can be done either before or after reduction is performed. Chou and colleagues[138] developed radiographic parameters to help judge the adequacy of reduction in the operating room when no ossification centers are present in the distal humerus. The authors suggest the use of medial and lateral humeral lines drawn parallel to the medial and lateral humeral diaphysis. Adequate reduction is defined as reduction of the ulnar axis (line drawn along the long axis of the ulna) within the boundaries of the medial and lateral humeral lines (Fig. 17.30). Using this method, only 1 of the 13 (7.7%) patients developed cubitus varus, compared with the 25% to 71% incidence reported in the literature. Following reduction and pinning, the arm is casted or splinted for 2 to 3 weeks, after which the pin(s) are removed and unrestricted motion is allowed.

Fracture-separation of the distal humerus physis that occurs as a result of birth trauma in a newborn may be treated closed, even when displaced. Percutaneous pin fixation in a child who is only 1 to 2 days old is challenging, and with the tremendous remodeling potential of the distal humerus, closed treatment without reduction can be successful in this group of patients (Fig. 17.31).

T-CONDYLAR FRACTURE

INCIDENCE AND CLASSIFICATION

T-condylar fractures of the distal humerus are intraarticular fractures characterized by a central intercondylar split and extension of the fracture line proximally through both the medial and lateral columns. These injuries are caused by high-energy mechanisms that cause a direct blow to a flexed elbow or an axial load onto an outstretched arm. They occur more commonly in older children, adolescents, and teenagers with more mature physes.[139] They are uncommon in young children. Jarvis and D'Astous[140] reported on 16 patients with this injury whose average age was 12 years, 9 months. The authors classified the fractures into three groups. Type I is a nondisplaced fracture (however, they had no type I fractures in their series). Type II fractures are displaced with more than 1 mm of separation or step-off of the articular surface. A type III fracture is a fracture-dislocation and occurred only once in their series.

TREATMENT

Careful preoperative evaluation is necessary for identifying coexistent ipsilateral fractures and neurovascular compromise. Advanced imaging, including computed tomography (CT) and MRI, is often helpful for characterizing the fracture pattern, assessing intraarticular and extraarticular comminution, and quantifying displacement. The principles of treatment for T-condylar fractures are to restore both joint congruity and extraarticular fracture alignment. Fractures that are minimally displaced may be treated by closed reduction and percutaneous fixation with K-wires or screws.[141,142] If the joint surface is displaced, open reduction and internal fixation should be performed. Surgical principles for open reduction of fractures include performing an extensile

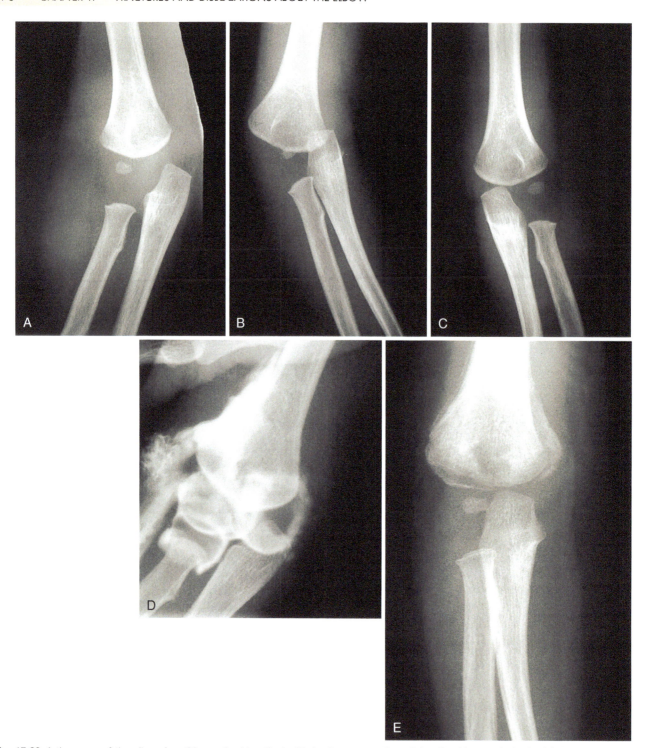

Fig. 17.28 Arthrogram of the elbow in a 20-month-old patient with fracture-separation of the distal humeral physis. (A) Anteroposterior (AP) radiograph of the injured extremity. The capitellum is displaced medially. (B) AP stress view of the same elbow demonstrating marked instability and further displacement of the capitellum medially. (C) AP view of the opposite extremity showing the normal relationship between the capitellum and the distal humeral metaphysis. (D) Arthrogram of the elbow outlining the distal humeral epiphysis, which is displaced medially. The proximal radius remains aligned. (E) An AP radiograph of the same elbow 3 weeks after injury shows healing of the physeal fracture with slight medial displacement.

surgical exposure that allows adequate visualization of the fracture and protection of the adjacent neurovascular structures. Restoration of articular congruity is the first priority, followed by reduction and stabilization of the reconstructed articular fragment to the proximal humerus. Comminuted distal humeral fractures require more extensive exposure.

When open reduction is performed, fixation of both columns of the distal humerus is preferable so that early motion of the elbow can be initiated.[143]

The surgical approach and choice of fixation are determined based on skeletal maturity and the fracture pattern. Minimally displaced fractures may be treated with closed

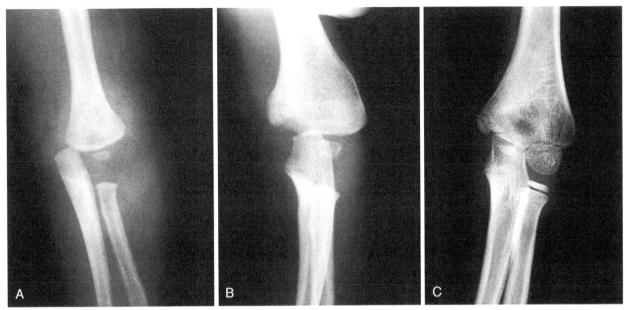

Fig. 17.29 Displaced fracture of the distal humeral physis. (A) An anteroposterior (AP) radiograph of the distal end of the humerus taken at the time of injury demonstrates medial displacement of the capitellum. Note that the longitudinal axis of the radius intersects the capitellum. (B) AP radiograph of the elbow 3 months after injury. The displacement was not corrected at the time of immobilization. (C) A follow-up radiograph 5 years after injury demonstrates remodeling of the distal end of the humerus. Clinically, the patient had full mobility of the elbow.

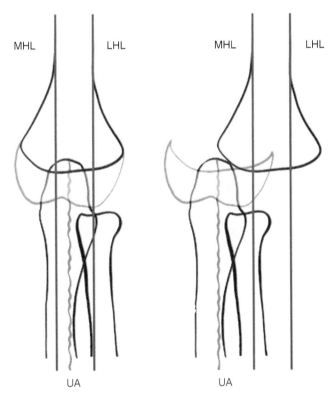

Fig. 17.30 Medial and lateral humeral lines in a normal elbow (left) and an elbow with a physeal separation of the distal humerus (right). *LHL,* Lateral humeral line; *MHL,* medial humeral line; *UA,* ulnar axis. In the physeal separation, the MHL and LHL are lateral to the UA. (From Chou ACC, Wong HYK, Kumar S, Mahadev A. Using the medial and lateral humeral lines as an adjunct to intraoperative elbow arthrography to guide intraoperative reduction and fixation of distal humerus physeal separations reduces the incidence of postoperative cubitus varus. *J Pediatr Orthop.* 2018;38(5):e262-e266. With permission.)

reduction and pin fixation in younger patients or with cannulated screw fixation in adolescents. Widely displaced or comminuted fractures require open reduction that may be performed through triceps-splitting, paratricipital or posteromedial (Bryan-Morrey) approaches in any age group; an olecranon osteotomy to visualize the distal humerus joint surface may be performed in older children who are skeletally mature (or nearly so). The triceps-splitting approach is performed through a posterior midline incision.[144] The triceps aponeurosis and muscle are divided in the midline, and the exposure is extended distally to the proximal ulna. The paratricipital approach is performed through the same midline incision and uses medial and lateral "windows" through the triceps and brachialis intervals. The triceps-sparing approach described by Bryan and Morrey[145] is a posteromedial approach in which the triceps is elevated off the distal humerus and subperiosteally off the proximal ulna. Re and colleagues[143] found that the posteromedial (Bryan-Morrey) and olecranon osteotomy approaches resulted in statistically significant better postoperative extension than the triceps-splitting approach. On the other hand, Remia and colleagues[146] found no statistically significant difference in function or range of motion between the Bryan-Morrey and triceps-splitting approaches. A recent systematic review of pediatric T-condylar humerus fractures found the highest outcome scores with the triceps-splitting approach, as well as the best arc of motion at follow-up. When the articular surface needed to be visualized, the Bryan-Morrey approach led to similar outcomes as an olecranon osteotomy, but with fewer approach-related complications.[147]

The choice of internal fixation is also age and fracture pattern dependent. Percutaneous K-wires (younger patients) or cannulated screws (adolescents and young teenagers) are often sufficient in minimally displaced, more stable

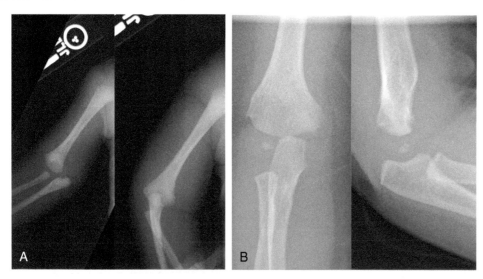

Fig. 17.31 Distal humerus physeal separation in a newborn. (A) Antero-posterior (AP) and attempted lateral radiograph of a distal humerus physeal birth fracture in a 3-day-old that was treated with casting only, no reduction. (B) AP and lateral radiographs of the same injury at 6 months demonstrating the remodeling potential of this injury. (Radiographic images courtesy of Gregory Mencio, MD, Vanderbilt University Medical Center, Nashville, TN.)

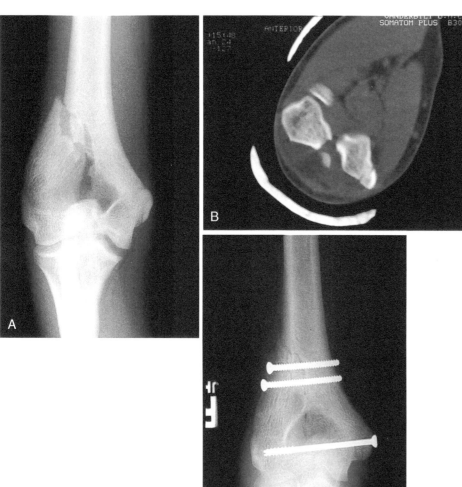

Fig. 17.32 T-condylar fracture of the distal end of the humerus in a 14-year-old boy with marked displacement of the articular surface. (A) An anteroposterior radiograph of the elbow demonstrates the displaced lateral condyle of the distal end of the humerus with a gap in the articular surface. (B) Computed tomography also reveals marked displacement of the distal humeral articular surface. (C) A postoperative radiograph of the distal end of the humerus shows anatomic restoration of the articular surface. The fracture was stabilized with three lag screws. Early motion was begun, and full function returned.

fractures. In either scenario, fixation may be achieved with the use of bicolumnar (Fig. 17.32) or "delta" configurations. In the latter, an interfragmental screw (3.5- or 4.0-mm diameter) or transverse K-wire is placed from lateral to medial, parallel to the articular surface of the distal humerus or just above the olecranon fossa, to hold intraarticular reduction of the fracture. Screws or K-wires can be placed up the medial and lateral columns of the distal humerus to complete the "delta" configuration (Fig. 17.33). In older patients, when open reduction is performed, an intercondylar screw and

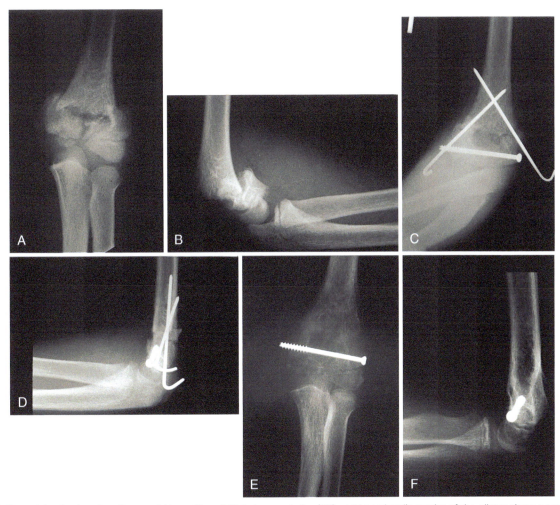

Fig. 17.33 T-condylar fracture in a 9-year-old boy. (A and B) Anteroposterior (AP) and lateral radiographs of the elbow show a supracondylar fracture with intercondylar extension. Separation of the capitellum and the trochlea is evident on the AP view (A). The distal fragments are flexed anteriorly (B). Open reduction was performed through a triceps-splitting approach. The distal fragments were reduced and stabilized with an interfragmental cannulated screw, which converted the comminuted fracture into a two-part supracondylar fracture that was then reduced and stabilized with percutaneous crossed pins. (C and D) Postoperative AP and lateral radiographs show restoration of the articular surface and reduction of the medial and lateral columns. The pins were removed in the office 4 weeks postoperatively. (E and F) Follow-up AP and lateral radiographs at 6 months after injury show healing of the fracture with no evidence of growth disturbance or avascular necrosis. The boy had full, painless range of motion of the elbow.

bicolumnar plates placed medially and posterolaterally provide rigid fixation and allow early motion (Fig. 17.34). Size matching may be an issue with periarticular plates designed for adults, so plates may need to be individually contoured to match the anatomy in some teenagers.

FLOATING ELBOW

Floating elbow injuries (distal humeral fractures with ipsilateral fractures of the forearm) are severe injuries that are usually the result of significant trauma and therefore have a higher potential for complications. They often require fixation of both fractures if they are displaced. Frequently, one or both of the fractures requires open reduction (Fig. 17.35). Children with these injuries must be evaluated carefully for associated vascular or neurologic injuries and monitored closely for signs of compartment syndrome.[109]

Although most of these injuries are treated by internal fixation of both fractures, a study of 47 floating elbows in children demonstrated the feasibility of treating the ipsilateral

forearm fracture by closed means.[148] Some 81% of ipsilateral forearm fractures in the study were treated by closed reduction after the elbow had been pinned. No patients had loss of reduction or required remanipulation. There were no cases of compartment syndrome.

PHYSEAL FRACTURES AND DISLOCATIONS ABOUT THE ELBOW

FRACTURE OF THE LATERAL CONDYLE OF THE HUMERUS

INCIDENCE

This fracture is relatively common and accounts for 12% to 20% of pediatric elbow fractures,[149] making it the second most common fracture about the elbow in children, with an annual incidence of 1.6 per 100,000.[150,151] These fractures occur most commonly in children between 5 and 10 years of age.

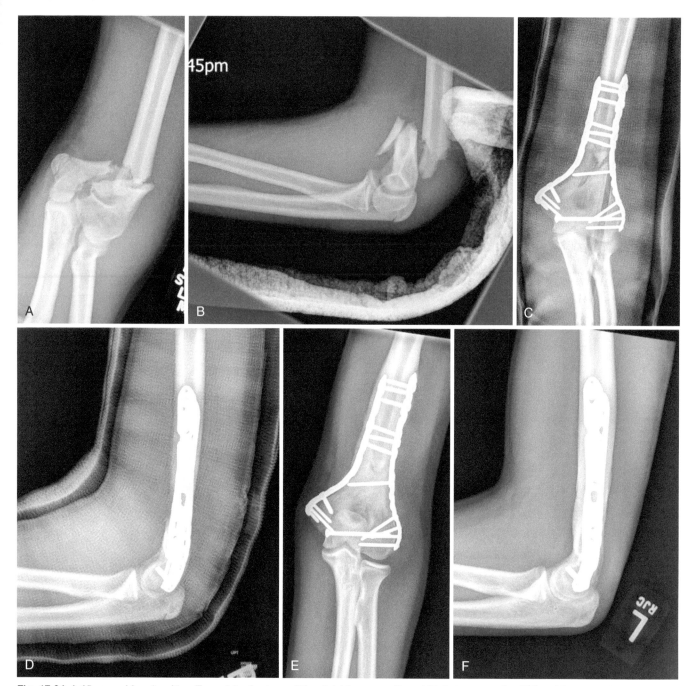

Fig. 17.34 A 15-year-old male with a T-condylar fracture of the distal humerus. (A and B) Anteroposterior (AP) and lateral radiographs show a comminuted intraarticular fracture of the distal humerus. Open reduction was performed through a paratricipital approach, and fixation was achieved with an intercondylar screw and bicolumnar, precontoured plates placed posterolaterally and medially. (C and D) AP and lateral radiographs immediately after surgery. The extremity was immobilized in a long arm cast for 2 weeks; then the patient was allowed to begin protected range of motion exercises. (E and F) AP and lateral radiographs at 6 months postoperatively. The fracture is healed. (Radiographic images courtesy of Christopher Stutz, MD, Vanderbilt University Medical Center, Nashville, TN.)

MECHANISMS OF INJURY

Two mechanisms for this fracture have been proposed. "Pull-off" or avulsion of the lateral condyle of the humerus may result from a fall on the outstretched hand with the forearm supinated. A varus force on the arm transmits through the forearm extensor muscles (extensor carpi radialis longus and brevis and brachioradialis), which attach to the lateral condyle, resulting in avulsion of the condyle.

Jakob and colleagues[152] were able to reproduce this injury in young cadavers consistently by adducting the supinated forearm with the elbow extended. Stimson, Fahey, and Milch,[150,153–155] however, believed that this fracture was the result of a "push-off" or compression injury because of a force directed upward and outward along the radius through the lateral condyle. Undoubtedly, both mechanisms of injury are possible.

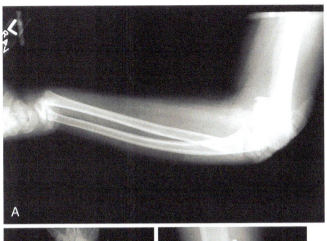

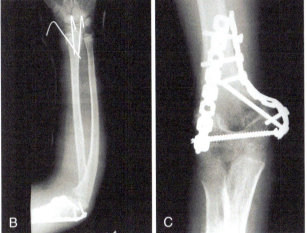

Fig. 17.35 Floating elbow injury. (A) Radiograph of the left upper extremity of a 12-year-old child showing a comminuted, intraarticular fracture of the distal humerus and ipsilateral fractures of the distal radius and ulna that were open. (B) The distal humerus was treated by open reduction through a paratricipital approach, and the fractures were stabilized with an intercondylar screw and bicolumnar plates that were custom contoured. The forearm fracture was débrided and stabilized with percutaneous K-wires. (C) Anteroposterior radiograph of the distal humerus demonstrates restoration of the articular surface of the elbow.

CLASSIFICATION

Milch[150,155] classified this fracture according to the location of the fracture line through the distal part of the humerus. In a type I injury, the fracture line tracks lateral to the capitello-trochlear groove, and the fracture may or may not become displaced. The elbow joint, however, does not dislocate (Fig. 17.36). The mechanism is thought to be impaction of the radial head on the capitellum. As long as some or all of the trochlea remains intact, it serves as a lateral buttress for the coronoid and prevents lateral displacement of the ulna (Fig. 17.37A). Type II fractures are thought to be caused by an avulsion mechanism and are characterized by a fracture line that extends into the trochlea. As a consequence of the loss of trochlear abutment, the ulna and radius may displace laterally (Fig. 17.37B–C). Although helpful in defining the mechanism of failure of the lateral condyle and perhaps the stability of the joint after injury, the Milch classification has been shown to be confusing and inaccurate in clinical application. Mirsky and colleagues[156] found that in more than half of patients, the Milch classification of preoperative radiographs did not correlate with intraoperative findings.

Jakob and colleagues[152] classified this fracture according to the amount of displacement (Fig. 17.38A). Stage I fractures are nondisplaced (<2 mm). The fracture line does not go through the entire cartilaginous epiphysis, and the articular surface is intact. A stage II fracture is complete. The fracture extends through the articular surface, and the fragment is displaced (>2 mm) but not rotated (Fig. 17.38B). A type III fracture is completely displaced, and the capitellum is rotated out of the joint. The normal relationship of the proximal end of the radius to the capitellum is completely disrupted (Fig. 17.38C). The practical implications of this classification are that if the articular cartilage is intact (stage I), the fracture is stable and may be treated closed, and if the fracture is complete (stage II or III) (i.e., extends to the articular surface), it is not and requires an operation.[151,152]

Because of the developmental anatomy of the distal humerus in children who sustain these fractures, it is often difficult to assess whether the articular surface is intact

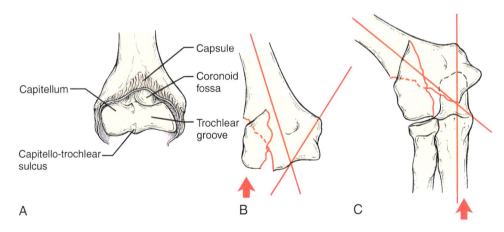

Fig. 17.36 (A) Drawing of the distal end of the humerus showing the trochlear groove and the capitello-trochlear sulcus. (B) Milch type I fracture of the lateral condyle. The fracture line exits lateral to the trochlear groove. The capitellum may be displaced partially or totally, but the elbow joint is stable because the trochlea is intact. (C) Milch type II fracture. The fracture line extends into the trochlear groove, which results in loss of the buttressing effect of the trochlea. The joint is potentially unstable, and the radius and ulna may displace laterally.

Capitellum
Capitello-trochlear sulcus
Capsule
Coronoid fossa
Trochlear groove

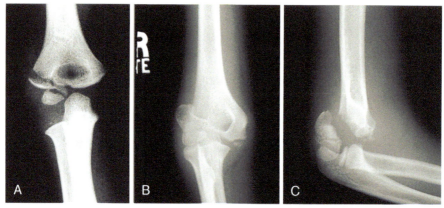

Fig. 17.37 Milch type I fracture of the lateral condyle of the distal end of the humerus. (A) Anteroposterior (AP) radiograph of the distal humerus demonstrates a lateral condylar fracture. Note that the fracture line extends through the distal humeral metaphysis and then exits the epiphysis through the capitellum. The fracture and capitellum are displaced, but the joint is stable, as evidenced by the normal relationship of the radius and ulna with the distal humerus. (B) and (C) Milch type II fracture of the lateral condyle. AP and lateral radiographs of the distal humerus also shows a fracture of the lateral condyle. The fracture line extends into the trochlea, and the joint is destabilized, as evidenced by lateral displacement of not only the lateral condylar fragment but also the proximal radius and ulna.

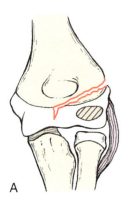 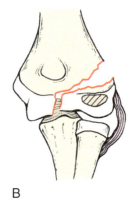 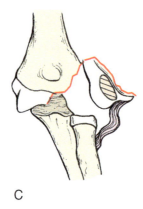

A   B   C

Fig. 17.38 Jakob classification of lateral condylar fractures according to the amount of displacement. (A) Stage I fracture. Note that the fracture line enters the cartilaginous surface of the distal end of the humerus between the capitellum and trochlea but that the fracture is not complete into the articular surface and is therefore nondisplaced. (B) Complete fracture (stage II). The fracture is complete through the articular surface but is not displaced from the elbow joint. (C) Complete fracture with displacement and rotation of the lateral condyle (stage III).

("non- or minimally displaced"), and therefore, it is difficult to know whether the fracture is stable. Finnbogason and colleagues[157] performed a prospective study to identify radiographic criteria that would predict displacement in otherwise innocuous-appearing fractures that they treated closed. They classified stage I "non- or minimally" displaced (<2 mm) lateral condylar fractures into three categories. Type A fractures have minimal or no fracture gap laterally, and the fracture line does not continue all the way to the epiphyseal cartilage (Fig. 17.39A). In type B fractures, the fracture line extends completely through the epiphyseal cartilage, and the lateral fracture gap is wider than the medial gap (Fig. 17.39B). Type C fractures also extend through the epiphysis, and the fracture gap is as wide medially as it is laterally (Fig. 17.39C). In this study, all 65 type A fractures healed uneventfully after closed treatment, but 17% of type B fractures and 42% of type C fractures displaced.

More recently, Song and colleagues[158,159] have proposed a more expanded classification that incorporates fracture patterns previously defined separately by Jakob and associates[152] and Finnbogason and associates.[157] The Song classification subdivides Jakob I fractures (i.e., those with <2 mm displacement) according to Finnbogason's criteria into those that are truly nondisplaced (stage I), those of indeterminate stability based on the presence of a lateral gap (stage II), and those that are likely unstable based on a fracture gap

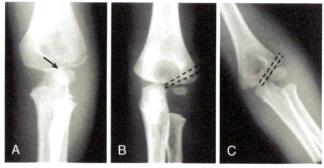

Fig. 17.39 Finnbogason classification of Jakob I non/minimally displaced (<2 mm) fractures of the lateral humeral condyle. (A) Type A fractures are incomplete. They have a minimal gap laterally but do not extend through the epiphysis. (B) Type B fractures extend through the epiphyseal cartilage, and the fracture gap is wider laterally than medially. (C) Type C fractures are complete, and the fracture gap is as wide medially as it is laterally.

that is as wide laterally as it is medially (stage III). In stage IV fractures, the displacement is greater than 2 mm (same as Jakob II), and in stage V, the fracture is displaced and rotated (as in Jakob III) (Fig. 17.40). The importance of the Song classification is that it can be used to guide treatment. The authors recommend closed treatment of type 1 fractures, in situ pin fixation of type 2 and some type 3 fractures,

Stage	Degree of displacement	Fracture pattern	Radiograph views used as basis	Stability
1	≤2 mm	Limited fracture line within the metaphysis	All 4 views	Stable
2	≤2 mm	Lateral gap	All 4 views	Indefinable
3	≤2 mm	Gap as wide laterally as medially	Any of 4 views	Unstable
4	>2 mm	Without rotation of fragment	Any of 4 views	Unstable
5	>2 mm	With rotation of fragment	Any of 4 views	Unstable

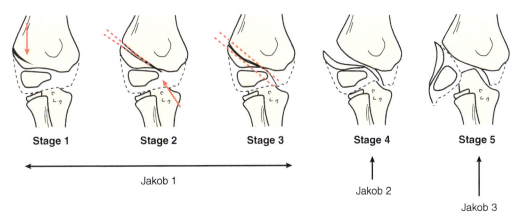

Fig. 17.40 Song classification of lateral condylar humeral fractures. This classification accounts for instability that can be seen in fractures with less than 2 mm of displacement by incorporating Finnbogason's classification of Jakob I fractures into those that are truly undisplaced (stage 1), those of indeterminate stability based on the presence of a lateral gap larger than the medial gap (stage 2), and those that are likely unstable based on a fracture gap that is as wide laterally as medially (stage 3); Song stage 4 are fractures that are displaced more than 2 mm (like Jakob II). Stage 5 fractures are, like Jakob III, widely displaced and rotated. (Modified from Song KS, Kang CH, Byung WM, et al. Closed reduction and internal fixation of displaced unstable lateral condylar fractures of the humerus in children. *J Bone Joint Surg Am.* 2008;90(12):2673–2681. With permission.)

and attempted closed reduction and percutaneous pin fixation of type 3, 4, and 5 fractures. For fractures that cannot be reduced via closed means, the authors recommend open reduction and internal fixation with K-wires.[158]

DIAGNOSIS

Clinically, swelling and pain about the elbow are most marked laterally. The fracture is usually easily identified radiographically if the capitellum is well ossified and if it is displaced. Internal oblique radiographs of the elbow may assist in the diagnosis of "non- or minimally" displaced fractures of the lateral condyle. Minimally displaced fractures may be difficult to differentiate from a fracture-separation of the distal humeral physis or from dislocation of the elbow, particularly if the fracture line is lateral to the trochlear groove and if the capitellum is not ossified. Even when the fracture is diagnosed, it may be difficult to tell whether the fracture extends to the articular surface or whether it is stable. CT, ultrasound, MRI, and arthrography may be helpful in further delineating the fracture pattern, displacement, and potential instability. CT has been shown to have excellent intraobserver reliability with regard to fracture classification and, in a prospective study of 10 patients, led to an alteration of treatment in two.[160] The presence of an intact cartilaginous hinge, which has been shown to correlate with stability of the fracture and healing without displacement, can be reliably demonstrated on both MRI[161,162] and ultrasound.[163] From a practical standpoint, MRI has some disadvantages because of the need for sedation and costs of the study, and ultrasonography is limited by the need for someone with technical proficiency to perform and interpret the study. None of

these advanced imaging modalities, however, affords the advantages of arthrography for assessing the fracture pattern and managing it definitively, if indicated.[158,159,164]

TREATMENT

Treatment decisions are based on initial displacement. Fractures with less than 2 mm of displacement and a fracture line limited to the metaphysis (Song types I and II) can be treated closed. Fractures in which the medial and lateral gaps are equally displaced (Song type III), even if less than 2 mm, and all fractures with greater than 2 mm of displacement (Song types IV and V) require operative treatment.

Closed Treatment

It has been this author's experience that nondisplaced fractures are less common than displaced fractures. One must be absolutely certain that the fracture is truly nondisplaced or, if displaced less than 2 mm, that the medial cartilaginous hinge is intact (Fig. 17.41). The extremity should be casted with the elbow flexed 90 degrees and the forearm supinated, and immobilization should be continued for a minimum of 6 weeks.[151] Frequent (weekly) radiographs must be obtained to ensure that displacement does not occur during the first 3 weeks of immobilization. Pirker and colleagues[165] reviewed 51 consecutive patients with "non- or minimally" displaced fractures of the lateral condyle and found five fractures (9.8%) that displaced during immobilization, for which internal fixation would have been recommended. In all cases, displacement occurred within 5 days, was detected on routine follow-up radiographs, and was successfully treated operatively. Similarly, Bast and colleagues[166] identified two of 95 patients with initial fracture displacement less than 2 mm whose fractures subsequently displaced during closed treatment; the patients were successfully diagnosed and treated operatively within 1 week after injury. Zale and colleagues[167] found the displacement and conversion rate from cast treatment to closed pinning for initially nondisplaced fractures to be 8.5%, with an average time to pinning of 13.2 days. Using the newer Song classification, Greenhill and associates[168] demonstrated that that 82% of Song type II fractures, whose initial stability was unknown, can be treated with casting alone. Some 18% of those fractures that displaced and required pin fixation did so within the first 2 weeks. These studies serve to underscore the importance of close, routine follow-up for detection of possible displacement of minimally displaced lateral condyle fractures of the humerus.

Closed Reduction and Percutaneous Pinning

Closed reduction and pin fixation should be considered if there is any doubt about stability in Jakob stage I fractures with less than 2 mm of initial displacement (Song stage II or III) and for fractures with greater than 2 mm

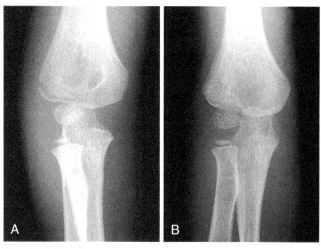

Fig. 17.41 Nondisplaced fracture of the lateral humeral condyle. (A) Anteroposterior radiograph of the elbow of a child who sustained a nondisplaced fracture of the lateral condyle. The fracture line has a minimal gap laterally, and the fracture line does not extend to the epiphyseal cartilage (Jakob I, Song I). (B) One month later, the fracture has healed after nonoperative cast treatment.

of displacement but minimal rotation (Jakob stage II; Song stage II–IV). Once reduction and pinning has been performed, arthrography may be performed through a posterior approach to assess reduction and assure that congruity of the articular surface has been anatomically restored (Fig. 17.42).[158,159,169] If the articular surface cannot be restored, open reduction and pinning must be performed to avoid articular malunion. Once the fracture is stabilized, the elbow is immobilized for 4 weeks in a long arm cast. The pins are removed, and the extremity is immobilized for another 2 weeks so that healing is ensured before motion is permitted.

Open Reduction and Pinning

Despite the successes reported with closed reduction for "less displaced" lateral condylar fractures, open reduction with pin fixation arguably remains the standard of care for any lateral condylar fracture displaced more than 2 mm and for all fractures that are rotationally unstable (Jakob stage III, Song stage V) (Fig. 17.43). Despite this, the author's own practice is to attempt closed reduction on all fractures, including rotationally unstable fractures (Song stage V) via the method described by Song and colleagues, and then move to open reduction if the articular surface cannot be restored.[158] Open reduction is performed with the patient supine and the arm positioned on a radiolucent table. A sterile tourniquet can be placed higher on the arm to minimize crowding around the surgical site. A headlight or lighted sucker (Electro Surgical, Rochester, NY) helps facilitate visualization. The fracture may be approached laterally through the triceps-brachioradialis interval or slightly more distally with a Kocher approach through the anconeus-wrist extensor interval. Care is taken to avoid soft tissue dissection posteriorly so that the blood supply to the trochlea is not disrupted and the risk of osteonecrosis is minimized. The joint is opened anteriorly, and the capsulotomy is extended distally to the radial head for adequate visualization of both the fracture and the distal humeral articular surface to the trochlea. Fracture reduction is performed with a digit, dental pick, K-wire, or modified dinner fork as described by Hennrikus and Millis.[170] The fracture is secured with two smooth K-wires that are inserted percutaneously and posterior to the incision. The pins may be configured in a parallel or divergent fashion to achieve bicortical fixation. Two pins provide adequate fixation for most fractures, but occasionally, in very unstable fractures with wide displacement or comminution, a third pin may be necessary.[9] Pins

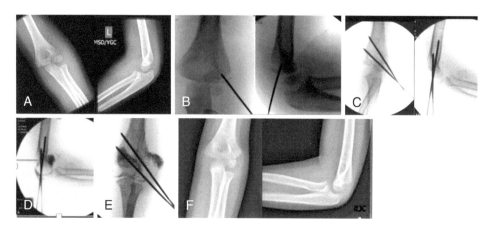

Fig. 17.42 (A) Lateral condylar humeral fracture in a 5-year-old female. The fracture is displaced less than 2 mm but demonstrates a gap that is as wide laterally as it is medially (Jakob I, Song III); thus, it is considered unstable. (B) The fracture was reduced closed. A K-wire was used as a "joystick" and percutaneously pinned (C-E) Arthrography was performed through a posterior approach confirming reduction of the fractures and restoration of joint congruity. (F) Two months later, the fracture is well healed.

may be left percutaneous and bent over felt or buried in the subcutaneous tissue. Exposed pins may be removed in the office, and studies have shown that they do not have a statistically significant higher rate of infection.[171,172] Cannulated screw fixation is also an option for treatment. A study of 336 patients showed a 100% union rate with cannulated screws versus 95% with K-wires. There was no significant difference in the rate of complications, although wound infection requiring débridement only occurred in the K-wire group.[173] Intraoperative radiographs are obtained to evaluate the quality of reduction. The elbow is immobilized for 4 weeks, after which the pins are removed, and the patient is placed back into a cast for an additional 2 weeks to ensure healing. Immobilization is then discontinued, and unrestricted motion is allowed.

Delayed Open Reduction

When presentation is delayed after lateral condylar fractures of the humerus (i.e., between 3 and 12 weeks), there is controversy about whether to treat these fractures operatively, despite the risk of nonunion, malunion, joint incongruity, elbow joint instability, stiffness, cubitus valgus or varus, and tardy ulnar nerve palsy with continued closed treatment. Those who believe that open reduction should not be performed point to the difficulty in achieving anatomic reduction because of soft tissue contracture and distortion of

landmarks caused by osteocartilaginous remodeling and the high risk of disrupting a precarious blood supply to the distal humerus, thus causing avascular necrosis (AVN).[6,152,174,175] Jakob and colleagues[152] recommend no treatment if the fracture is seen after 3 weeks. Dhillon and colleagues[174] also recommend that these fractures be left alone if not treated within 6 weeks of the time of injury.

However, despite the inherent risks associated with surgery, several reports in the literature have shown successful outcomes after open reduction and internal fixation of both late-presenting fractures and established nonunions of the lateral humeral condyle. Roye and associates[176] reported that delayed open reduction and internal fixation of these fractures could result in an excellent outcome. Gaur and associates[177] also reported good results with delayed fixation and recommended lengthening the aponeurosis of the common forearm extensor musculature because they believed that this muscle became contracted and was the main cause of difficulty in the late reduction of lateral condylar fractures. More recently, Saraf and Khare[178] reported their results in 22 patients with displaced fractures of the lateral condyle of the humerus seen up to 12 weeks postinjury. Their results were best in patients treated between 3 and 4 weeks postinjury and deteriorated slightly with increased duration from injury to treatment and degree of displacement. Agarwal and associates[179] reported a high rate of

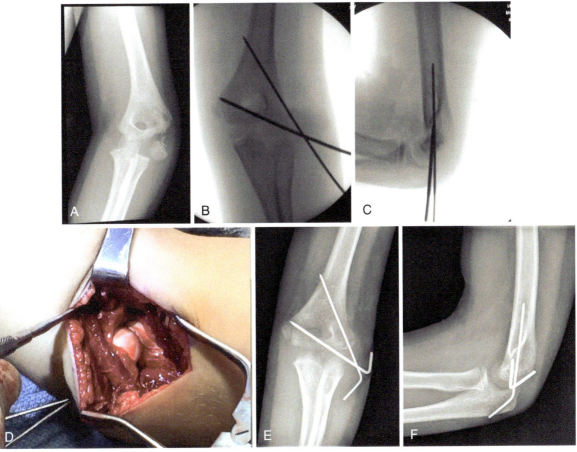

Fig. 17.43 (A) Anteroposterior (AP) radiograph of the elbow of an 8-year-old male shows a displaced and rotated lateral condylar humeral fracture. (B and C) Open reduction was performed through a lateral approach, and the fracture was stabilized with percutaneous K-wires. (D) Reduction of the fracture and articular surface of the lateral condyle is confirmed by visual inspection of the fracture through the anterior capsulotomy. (E and F) AP and lateral radiographs taken 4 weeks postoperatively before pin removal. The fracture is healed.

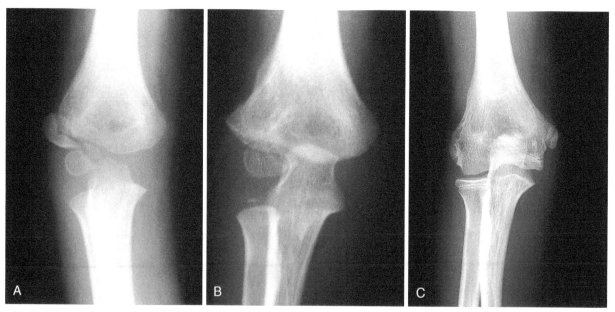

Fig. 17.44 (A) Anteroposterior radiograph of what was originally a Jakob I lateral condylar humeral fracture that has not healed and is now displaced after 6 weeks of cast treatment. Open reduction and internal fixation of the fracture were performed. (B) Four months after reduction and pin removal, the fracture is healed. (C) Seven years after reduction, the distal end of the humerus appears normal.

union (20 of 22 patients) and satisfactory elbow function in late presenting (>4 weeks) lateral condylar fractures in children after osteosynthesis.

This author's anecdotal experience with delayed treatment by open reduction and internal fixation in four patients between 6 and 12 weeks after injury has been favorable (Fig. 17.44) . The surgical approach to the lateral condyle when diagnosis has been delayed is the same as described for open reduction in an injury being treated immediately. The surgeon should approach the delayed union laterally and identify it by dissecting in a proximal-to-distal direction, keeping to the anterior aspect of the humerus and taking care to avoid stripping soft tissue from the lateral condylar fragment to avoid injury to the blood supply. Once the fracture is identified, the fibrous nonunion is opened carefully with a scalpel, and an osteotome is used to help strip the fibrous tissue from the fracture surface. Periosteum and soft tissue are carefully elevated from the margin of the fracture fragment to allow visualization of both sides of the fracture. Once mobilization of the fracture is complete, the two fracture surfaces are freshened, and the fracture is reduced and internally fixed. If the child is young and the metaphyseal fragment is small, the fracture is stabilized with smooth K-wires. On the other hand, if the child is older and the metaphyseal fragment is large enough, the fracture may be fixed with one or two screws inserted through the metaphysis of the fracture.

COMPLICATIONS

Nonunion

Nonunion is more common after lateral condyle fractures of the humerus than with other fractures in children. The rate of nonunion is reported to be anywhere from 1% to 5%.[171,180,181] Lateral condylar fractures are predisposed to nonunion because of exposure to synovial fluid as a result of the intraarticular location of the fracture, the pull of the common extensor mechanism that attaches to the lateral condyle, and poor blood supply to the epiphyseal fragment. Flynn and colleagues[151] have suggested that the presence of a fracture line more than 8 weeks after an injury is a cause for concern. Nonunion is more common after closed treatment[171] and may also result from a missed diagnosis of the fracture, particularly when displacement is minimal and the metaphyseal fragment is small. Flynn and associates reported that 35% of nonunions in their series were initially unrecognized.[151,182]

Treatment of established nonunions is controversial for the same reasons discussed in the previous section on delayed open reduction. Despite this, surgical treatment is recommended because of the fact that nonunions can become painful as a result of the mobility of the lateral condylar fragment and valgus instability of the elbow; they may also cause loss of motion.[183] Flynn and associates[151,182] have recommended that nonunions with less than 1 cm of displacement may be treated by stripping of fibrous tissue, curettage, grafting, and internal fixation of the metaphyseal fragment (Fig. 17.45). Masada and colleagues[184] found that such treatment of mobile nonunions generally resulted in some loss of elbow motion but that the tradeoff may be beneficial if pain and instability can be relieved and late sequelae like tardy ulnar nerve palsy can be prevented.

More recently, Tien and colleagues[185] have described a technique for in situ compression fixation of established lateral condylar nonunions in combination with a dome osteotomy to correct the cubitus valgus deformity through a posterior, triceps-splitting approach (Fig. 17.46). All eight of the lateral condylar nonunions in their series united, and valgus deformity was corrected from a mean of 31 degrees preoperatively to 5.5 degrees postoperatively.

Malunion

Approximately 20% of patients with lateral condylar humeral fractures develop cubitus varus deformity.[8] The etiology

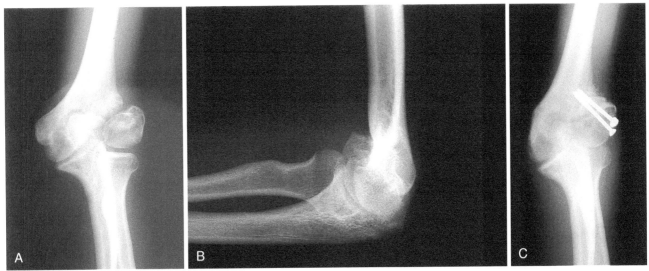

Fig. 17.45 (A) Anteroposterior (AP) radiograph demonstrates chronic nonunion of the lateral condyle. (B) Lateral radiograph of the elbow. The lateral condyle is freely mobile and moves proximally with elbow flexion and distally and posteriorly with elbow extension. (C) AP radiograph after open reduction and internal fixation with bone grafting of the nonunion.

of this deformity is not clear, and the functional significance is negligible. Loss of reduction with a medial tilt and lateral growth stimulation related to fracture healing and remodeling have been postulated as mechanisms. Cubitus valgus is less common, occurring in about 10% of patients after lateral condylar fractures, and is thought to be the result of a lateral physeal growth arrest. Skak and colleagues[186] identified premature closure of the capitellar physes in 4 of 28 patients with valgus deformity after lateral condylar fractures. Although this deformity may be associated with tardy ulnar nerve palsy, it usually does not progress and rarely causes functional or cosmetic problems.

Tardy Ulnar Nerve Palsy

Tardy ulnar nerve palsy is gradual paralysis of the ulnar nerve caused by stretching and is frequently seen as a long-term sequela of untreated, unstable lateral condylar nonunions and cubitus valgus. Ulnar nerve transposition is the treatment of choice.

FRACTURE OF THE CAPITELLUM

Fractures of the capitellum not involving the entire lateral condyle are rare injuries in children. These fractures are seen more commonly in adults but, in children, are almost always seen after 12 years of age. Capitellar fractures are thought to result from a shear mechanism caused by a fall on an outstretched hand with the elbow extended. These injuries were classified by Bryan and Morrey[145] as type I (Hahn-Steinthal fracture), which consists of a large fragment of cancellous bone off the articular surface of the capitellum and may also include a portion of the trochlea; type II (Kocher-Lorenz fracture), which is a largely cartilaginous articular fracture of the capitellum that may include a small fragment of subchondral bone; type III, which is a comminuted capitellar fracture; and type IV (McKee modification), which is a coronal shear involving the capitellum and trochlea.

Letts and colleagues[187] have shown that operative reduction of these fractures is usually successful in restoring normal elbow function. They reviewed capitellar fractures in seven adolescents with an average age of 14.7 years. Six of the seven fractures were type I fractures with a large anterosuperior fragment that required operative reduction and internal fixation in five cases. They used a variety of fixation devices, including K-wires, Herbert screws, and cannulated screws. De Boeck and Pouliart[188] also reported on six children between the ages of 11 and 15 years with this fracture, all of which were type I. All underwent operative reduction and internal fixation with one screw. Their results were excellent; no patients had AVN, and all had normal function. To the contrary, Onay and associates report decreased range of motion in four out of 13 (31%) patients with type IV fractures treated operatively. Two of the four went on to require further surgery to improve range of motion.[189] The surgical approach in this study was through a lateral incision, and fixation was performed with an interfragmental screw that entered the humerus posteriorly and was then directed anteriorly into the capitellar fragment. If a headless compression type of screw is used, it can be directed anterior to posterior, with the head buried under the articular cartilage. Another option, depending on the orientation of the fracture, is to place the screw in a lateral-to-medial direction (Fig. 17.47).

FRACTURE OF THE MEDIAL CONDYLE OF THE HUMERUS

Fractures of the medial humeral condyle are very uncommon and account for less than 2% of all elbow fractures in children.[190] As for lateral condylar fractures, fractures of the medial condyle can occur by either a "pull-off" or "push-off" mechanism.[191–193] The most common mechanism is through a fall on an outstretched hand with the elbow extended, leading to avulsion ("pull off") of the medial condyle by the flexor-pronator muscle group. Injuries can also occur by a fall on the olecranon, which is then driven into the trochlea, causing a fracture of the medial condyle ("push off").

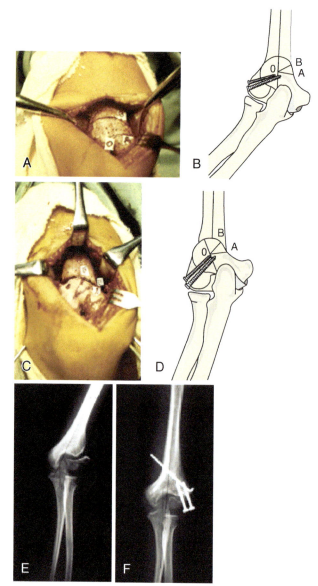

Fig. 17.46 Supracondylar dome osteotomy for cubitus valgus deformity associated with a lateral condylar nonunion. (A and B) Intraoperative photo and drawing demonstrating initial steps for correction of valgus. First, the lateral condylar nonunion undergoes screw fixation. Point *A* is the junction between the periosteum and perichondrium at the medial border of the distal humerus. Point *O* represents the intersection of the midline axis and upper border of the olecranon fossa and serves as the point of rotation for the "dome." The preoperatively determined angle of correction is measured and that is used to mark point *B*. (C and D) Segment *OB* is the dome radius, and the dome osteotomy is performed. The distal humeral segment is rotated so that point *A* aligns with point *B*. Crossed pins can then be placed to secure the osteotomy. (E) Preoperative radiograph demonstrating severe valgus and lateral condylar nonunion. (F) Postoperative radiograph demonstrating healed lateral condyle with improved coronal alignment. (From Tien YC, Chen JC, Fu YC, et al. Supracondylar dome osteotomy for cubitus valgus deformity associated with a lateral condylar nonunion in children. *J Bone Joint Surg Am.* 2005;87A(7):1456-1463. With permission.)

CLASSIFICATION

Kilfoyle[192] described a classification that is identical to the one used for lateral condylar fractures. A type I fracture is nondisplaced, and the fracture line does not go into the articular surface. The fracture line in a type II fracture goes through the articular surface, but displacement is less than 2 mm. A type III fracture is displaced and rotated. Bensahel and colleagues[190] used a similar classification system and noted that different injuries occur in different age groups. A type I injury occurs in children younger than 5 years, a type II fracture may be seen in any age group, and a type III fracture occurs in slightly older children, at a mean of 7 years.

DIAGNOSIS

This fracture may be difficult to diagnose because it is frequently seen before ossification of the trochlea begins. The diagnosis should be considered when a history of trauma and medial-sided elbow pain are present. In contrast to fractures of the medial epicondyle, which are often associated with elbow dislocation and are usually unstable to valgus stress, fractures of the medial condyle result in varus instability. When the medial condyle is markedly displaced, the fracture is readily diagnosed on routine AP and lateral radiographs (Fig. 17.48). Avulsion of a wafer of metaphyseal bone may be a subtle finding in children before ossification of the trochlea. Oblique views, arthrography, or MRI can be helpful in confirming the diagnosis.[194]

TREATMENT

The principles of treatment are similar to that of a lateral condylar fracture. Type I fractures (<2 mm of displacement) may be treated closed with cast immobilization; type II fractures with greater than 2 mm of displacement but no rotation may be treated by closed reduction and percutaneous pin fixation. If adequacy of the reduction is in question, open reduction should be performed to ensure congruency of the articular surface. Type III fractures, by definition, are displaced and rotated and require open reduction and pin fixation. The elbow should be immobilized for 4 weeks, followed by pin removal and immobilization for another 2 weeks. A retrospective study by Leet and colleagues[194] of 21 medial condylar fractures revealed a complication rate of 33%. Most of the minimally displaced fractures healed uneventfully with immobilization, although one patient developed AVN of the trochlea, and one patient developed a nonunion. Operative treatment was performed if more than 2 mm of displacement was present at the fracture site. Two of three fracture-dislocations lost reduction in the early postoperative period, requiring revision with more stable fixation. The authors emphasized the importance of adequate stabilization of the fracture and immobilization until radiographic evidence of healing is seen. A recent study of 14 children with medial condylar fractures demonstrated AVN of the trochlea leading to fishtail deformity in only two of the patients (14%). There was no significant loss of motion noted in any of the patients.[195]

FRACTURE OF THE MEDIAL EPICONDYLE

INCIDENCE

Medial epicondyle fractures of the humerus are relatively common injuries that account for approximately 10% to 20% of all children's elbow fractures. Most occur in adolescents (between 10 and 14 years of age), and approximately 60% occur in association with elbow dislocations.[196]

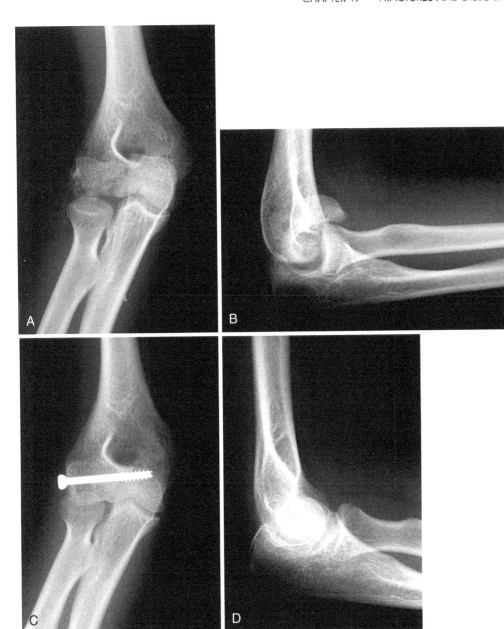

Fig. 17.47 Fracture of the capitellum in a 14-year-old female. (A and B) Anteroposterior (AP) and lateral radiographs of the elbow show fracture of the capitellum that is displaced anteriorly. (C and D) AP and lateral radiographs of the elbow 6 months after open reduction and internal fixation with an interfragmental screw demonstrating anatomic reduction of the capitellum and restoration of the radiocapitellar joint.

MECHANISM OF INJURY

Fractures of the medial epicondyle occur by one of three mechanisms: avulsion, direct trauma, or elbow dislocation. Injury from a direct blow is the least common of the three and one in which the medial epicondyle may be fragmented.[11] Avulsion is the most common mechanism and is caused by valgus stress and pulling at the flexor-pronator origin, typically as a result of a fall on an outstretched hand with the elbow extended and forearm supinated.[192,197–200] The third mechanism is elbow dislocation, in which the ulnar collateral ligament may cause avulsion of the epicondyle. In up to 25% of cases of elbow dislocation with fracture of medial epicondyle, the epicondylar fragment may be displaced and trapped within the joint.[194,196,200,201]

CLASSIFICATION

Most classification systems of this fracture are similar and are based on the amount of displacement of the fragment and whether it is entrapped in the elbow joint. The classification proposed by Wilkins[11] is comprehensive and takes into account patterns and degrees of displacement as well as chronicity (Table 17.1). Acute injuries are classified as nondisplaced, minimally displaced, or significantly displaced (>5 mm) fractures, with or without elbow dislocation; fractures in which the fragment is incarcerated in the joint; or fractures of the apophysis, with or without displacement. Chronic injuries are caused by repetitive stress (e.g., Little Leaguer's elbow).[11,196]

DIAGNOSIS

Diagnosis of this fracture is generally straightforward. The child has a history of a valgus injury to the arm, with pain and swelling localized to the medial side of the elbow. In the case of an elbow that is also dislocated but spontaneously reduced, generalized pain and swelling are often present, but the point tenderness is greatest medially. If entrapment of the medial epicondyle has occurred within the joint, the elbow may appear reduced, but elbow motion, usually

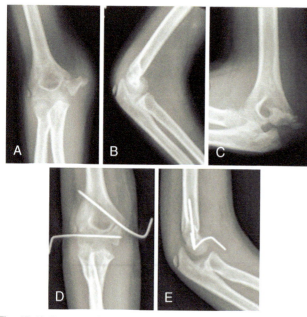

Fig. 17.48 Fracture of the medial humeral condyle. (A, B, and C) Displaced fracture of the medial condyle is evident on anteroposterior, lateral, and oblique radiographs of the elbow. Open reduction and internal fixation were performed through a medial approach. (D and E) AP and lateral radiographs demonstrating reduction and internal fixation with percutaneous smooth pins that were subsequently removed in the office.

TABLE 17.1	Classification of Fractures of the Medial Epicondyle
I	Nondisplaced
II	Minimally displaced (<5 mm)
III	Significantly displaced (>5 mm) Elbow not dislocated Elbow dislocated
IV	Fragment incarcerated in joint

extension, may be blocked. Medial stability of the elbow can be assessed by performance of a gravity stress test. This test is performed with the patient supine and resting on a rolled towel or small bolster and with the arm abducted 90 degrees, shoulder externally rotated 90 degrees, and the elbow flexed 15 degrees. Medial instability from gravity-induced valgus stress suggests the presence of secondary injuries to capsule-ligamentous structures and periarticular muscles.

IMAGING

Radiographic assessment of these injuries and their true degree of displacement remains controversial. Standard AP and lateral radiographs are usually sufficient for diagnosing this injury. In a "non- or minimally displaced" fracture, the physis of the medial epicondyle may appear wider than normal, the normally smooth margin of the physis may appear to be slightly irregular, and loss of the parallelism of the physis may be seen. The diagnosis may be difficult if the fracture occurs in a young child and the medial epicondyle is not fully ossified (Fig. 17.49). Comparison radiographs of the opposite elbow may be helpful in the diagnosis.[11,196]

This injury can be easily missed in a child with an elbow dislocation who undergoes closed reduction of the joint. Postreduction x-rays may show a concentric reduction of the elbow; however, one must take special care to inspect the medial side of the elbow to look for the presence of the medial epicondylar ossification center (if present based upon the patient's age) in the appropriate location along the medial condyle. If the medial epicondyle is not readily seen, then the radiograph must be scrutinized for the presence of the fragment in the joint or cross-sectional imaging obtained to locate the fragment. Failure to recognize an incarcerated medial epicondyle after elbow reduction can result in poor outcomes.

Medial instability may be assessed on stress radiographs as described originally by Woods and Tullos.[197] This test can be performed in the same way as described for the gravity-assisted valgus stress test with the patient supine and positioned over a bolster or the edge of the examination table and with the shoulder externally rotated and elbow slightly flexed. An AP radiograph of the elbow is taken in this position, and if the joint is unstable, medial widening will be seen.

Determination of the amount of displacement of the medial epicondylar fragment, arguably of importance in determining the need for surgical treatment, is unreliable on plain radiographs. Pappas and colleagues[202] have shown variable inter- and intraobserver agreement of fracture displacement on AP radiographs. Edmonds[203] has shown, using CT imaging, that "non- or minimally displaced" fractures, as characterized on AP and lateral radiographs, may actually be displaced as much as 1 cm anteriorly. He found that, compared with CT, AP radiographs overstated medial displacement, and anterior displacement was not measurable on lateral radiographs. In this and a subsequent cadaveric study,[204] it was shown that 45 degree internal oblique radiographs were reliable in measuring the true amount of displacement of these fractures and had high inter- and intraobserver agreement. Souder and colleagues[205] published on a novel imaging technique, the distal humeral axial view, to assess the true displacement of medial epicondyle fracture without the need for CT. Axial images were obtained by having the patient rest their elbow on the examination table with the humerus at a 45 degree angle from the vertical. The x-ray tube was then positioned with the central ray above the shoulder at about 25 degrees from the long axis of the humerus, centered on the distal humerus. The forearm can be propped up off the table so the elbow is at a 90 degree angle (Fig. 17.50). Using this technique, the axial images were found to more closely estimate the true amount of displacement with a mean 1.5-mm error in measurement for less than 10mm of displacement and 0.8 mm for greater than or equal to 10 mm of displacement. When compared with the axial view, AP, lateral and internal rotation views consistently underestimated the amount of true displacement of medial epicondyle humerus fractures (Fig 17.51).

TREATMENT

Nonsurgical management of these fractures consists of immobilization in a long arm cast with the elbow flexed to 90 degrees for up to 3 to 4 weeks, although some have advocated as short as 5 to 7 days so that stiffness does not become a problem.[206] Results of nonsurgical treatment of medial epicondylar fractures have been good to excellent,

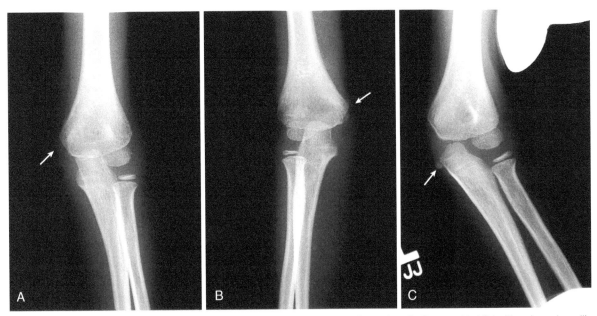

Fig. 17.49 Occult fracture of the medial humeral epicondyle. (A) Anteroposterior radiographs of a 5-year-old child with pain and swelling on the medial side of the elbow after a fall. The ossification center of the medial epicondyle, which is very small at this age, cannot be visualized. (B) Comparison radiograph of the opposite elbow reveals the medial epicondyle in its normal position *(white arrow)*. (C) A valgus stress radiograph demonstrates marked instability of the elbow and displacement of the medial epicondyle *(white arrow)*.

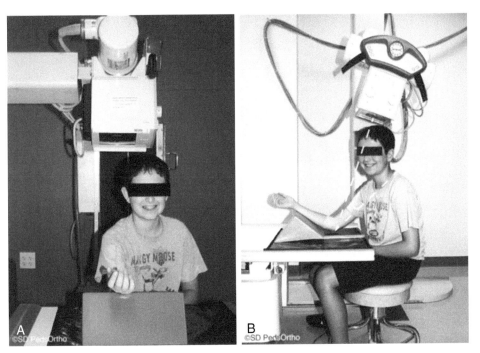

Fig. 17.50 (A) Patient positioning for distal humeral axial view. (B) X-ray beam projected 25 degrees anterior to the long axis of the humerus (dashed lines). (From Souder CD, Farnsworth CL, McNeil NP, Bomar JD, Edmonds EW. The distal humerus axial view: assessment of displacement in medial epicondyle fractures. *J Pediatr Orthop.* 2015;35(5):449-454. With permission.)

independent of the presence of bony union.[207–209] Ip and Tsang[210] found slightly better scores in patients treated nonoperatively, using the Mayo Clinic Performance Index, which emphasizes pain and activities of daily living. Bede and colleagues[211] reported good results in 79% of patients treated nonoperatively versus 62% treated operatively, and their definition of *good* was a pain-free, functional, stable, nondeformed elbow with less than 15 degrees loss of motion, less than 6 degrees cubitus valgus, and absence of ulnar nerve symptoms. Fowles and colleagues[129] reported less loss of motion (extension) in fractures treated nonsurgically.

Closed treatment of these fractures by cast immobilization is increasingly being replaced by operative fixation and early mobilization, which is a trend fueled by evolving knowledge of the role of the medial epicondyle and attached structures to elbow stability and by the increasing functional demands of pediatric patients who sustain these injuries. Woods and Tullos[197] showed that medial elbow stability depends on the integrity of the medial collateral ligament of the elbow and the forearm flexor muscles. The eccentric position of the medial epicondyle ensures that one of the three bands of the ulnar collateral ligament remains taut throughout the

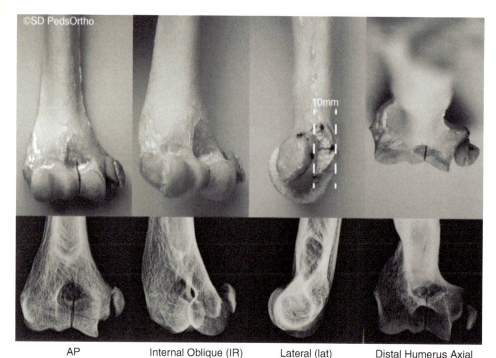

AP   Internal Oblique (IR)   Lateral (lat)   Distal Humerus Axial

Fig. 17.51 Comparison views of a medial epicondylar fracture with 10 mm of actual displacement. Photographs correspond with the x-ray directly below each photo. (From Souder CD, Farnsworth CL, McNeil NP, Bomar JD, Edmonds EW. The distal humerus axial view: assessment of displacement in medial epicondyle fractures. *J Pediatr Orthop.* 2015;35(5):449-454. With permission.)

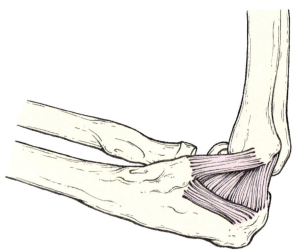

Fig. 17.52 Drawing of the ulnar collateral ligament of the elbow. Note the anterior, posterior, and oblique bands. Eccentric position of the medial epicondyle ensures stability because at least one of the bands is taut throughout the full range of elbow motion. The ligament becomes lax when the medial epicondyle is displaced.

full range of elbow motion (Fig. 17.52). When the medial epicondyle is displaced, the attached collateral ligament also becomes lax, which supports the argument for open reduction and internal fixation when valgus instability can be demonstrated (Fig. 17.53). Kamath and colleagues[209] performed a systematic review of the literature comparing operative versus nonoperative treatment of medial epicondylar fractures. Their analysis of pooled data of 498 patients from 14 studies showed that operative treatment afforded a significantly higher union rate (92.5%) compared with nonoperative management (49.2%), although they found no differences in pain or ulnar nerve symptoms. Lee and colleagues[200] found excellent outcomes (96.2 of a possible 100) after operative treatment, using the Japanese Orthopaedic Association Elbow Assessment Score.

Absolute indications for surgical intervention are an incarcerated fragment in the joint (Fig. 17.54) or an open fracture. Relative indications for surgical treatment include ulnar nerve entrapment, gross elbow instability, and fractures in athletes or other individuals who require high-quality upper extremity function. No consensus exists for the amount of fracture displacement that mandates surgical treatment,[199,206,212] although most consider more than 5 mm to be an indication for surgery.[196] Knapik and colleagues[213] studied 81 pediatric patients with medial epicondyle fractures, 42 of which had a fracture-dislocation of the elbow. All patients in the study were treated nonoperatively. Bony nonunion was seen in 69% of fracture-dislocations versus 49% of isolated fractures; however, there were minimal clinical or functional disabilities related to the bony nonunion at final follow-up. Some 43% in the fracture-dislocation group had decreased range of motion of the elbow versus 15% in the isolated fracture group. The authors of the study concluded that medial epicondyle fractures could be successfully treated by closed means even with a concomitant elbow dislocation.

Author's Preferred Method of Treatment

The author's preferred method is to perform closed treatment for simple, closed fractures of the medial epicondyle with less than 5 mm of displacement and to perform open reduction and internal fixation for all open injuries, for incarcerated fractures associated with elbow dislocations, and for fractures with more than 5 mm of displacement, particularly in high-demand patients.

In an adolescent or teenage patient, the fracture may be internally fixed with a cannulated screw (Fig. 17.55). The patient is positioned supine or prone on chest rolls with the operative extremity on a radiolucent hand table. Prone positioning allows for easy visualization of the medial elbow without the need for an assistant to hold the arm. A sterile tourniquet is used, which helps extend the surgical field by allowing the sterile drapes to be placed high on the arm.

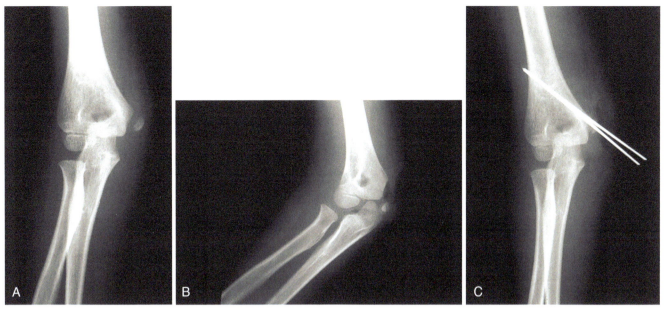

Fig. 17.53 Fracture of the medial epicondyle of the humerus in a 6-year-old child. (A) Anteroposterior radiograph of the right elbow shows a medial epicondylar fracture with more than 5 mm of displacement. (B) Further displacement of the medial epicondyle on valgus stress radiographs signifies significant instability. Open reduction and internal fixation were performed. (C) Postoperative radiograph of the elbow shows that the medial epicondyle is reduced and stabilized with two smooth pins.

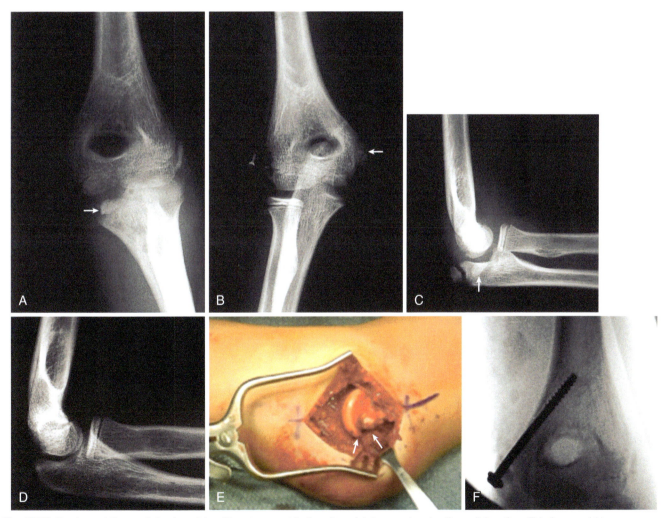

Fig. 17.54 Fracture of the medial epicondyle with entrapment in the elbow joint secondary to elbow dislocation. This 9-year-old boy was seen with a painful elbow after a fall. The elbow had dislocated and reduced spontaneously. (A) Anteroposterior (AP) radiograph of the injured elbow shows the absence of the medial epicondyle. The *arrow* points to the medial epicondyle entrapped within the elbow joint. (B) An AP radiograph of the opposite elbow shows the medial epicondyle *(arrow)* in its normal position. (C) A lateral radiograph of the injured elbow demonstrates widening of the elbow joint. The medial epicondyle can be seen within the elbow joint. It is overlying the olecranon *(arrow)*. (D) A comparison lateral radiograph of the opposite elbow shows that the elbow joint is not widened as it is on the opposite side. (E) Intraoperative picture shows the flexor pronator mass incarcerated in the ulnohumeral joint *(white arrows)*. (F) AP radiograph of the injured elbow after open reduction of the fracture. The medial epicondyle was removed from the joint, replaced in its normal position, and stabilized with a cannulated screw.

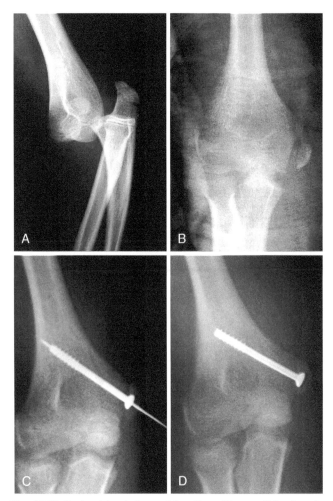

Fig. 17.55 Posterolateral elbow dislocation with a medial epicondylar fracture. (A) Lateral radiograph of a 15-year-old patient showing posterior elbow dislocation. (B) An anteroposterior radiograph of the elbow after reduction of the dislocation demonstrates a fracture of the medial epicondyle with 5 mm of displacement. The elbow was unstable on stress testing, and open reduction and screw fixation were performed. (C) Intraoperative radiograph shows insertion of a cannulated screw across the reduced fracture. (D) Postoperative radiograph of the elbow shows fracture healing.

A curvilinear incision is made over the medial epicondyle to allow exposure of the fracture and visualization of the ulnar nerve. If the fragment is incarcerated, it is retrieved from the joint at this point. Soft tissue is cleared from the fragment, the fracture bed is prepared, and the medial epicondyle is reduced. Reduction may be facilitated by flexion of the wrist and pronation of the forearm to reduce tension in the flexor pronator mass. A dental pick or small K-wire may be helpful for stabilizing the reduction. A guidewire is placed in antegrade fashion through the medial epicondyle and across the fracture. The position of the wire and alignment of the fractures are confirmed fluoroscopically. The guidewire is overdrilled with a cannulated drill bit. A second, smaller K-wire may be placed to provide rotational stability of the fragment while drilling is done. An alternative technique is for the surgeon to predrill the epicondylar fragment in a retrograde fashion before reducing it, then proceeding as described for the antegrade technique. Fixation is performed with a 3.5- or 4.0-mm cannulated screw.

Bicortical purchase is not necessary to achieve adequate compression of the fracture and, in fact, is contraindicated. Marcu and colleagues[214] have reported two cases of radial nerve injury while drilling the far (lateral) cortex in an attempt at bicortical screw placement. If the fracture is comminuted or largely cartilaginous, a washer may be used to increase the surface area of the screw contact on the fragment, so penetration/fragmentation is prevented as the fracture is compressed. In a study of 17 patients undergoing operative fixation of medial epicondyle fractures, 12 were treated with a screw and washer and five with a screw alone. There were no episodes of fragmentation or penetration of the epicondylar fragment. No patient treated with screw alone requested hardware removal, versus 58% in whom a washer was used.[215] Following fixation, the arm is immobilized in a posterior splint or cast for 2 weeks, at which point motion is initiated to prevent stiffness. A hinged elbow brace may be helpful for protecting the repair and allowing mobilization of the joint.

In younger, skeletally immature patients, the fracture may be fixed with two smooth pins. The pins are left exposed through the skin and are either bent or capped so that pin migration is prevented. The pins are removed at 3 to 4 weeks, and motion is started.

FRACTURE OF THE LATERAL EPICONDYLE

Fracture of the lateral epicondyle is an extremely uncommon injury. More commonly, the lateral epicondylar ossification center, which is the last to appear and close, may be mistaken for an acute injury. In the rare event of injury, the mechanism is either a direct blow to the lateral side of the elbow or avulsion by the wrist extensors, although the latter is more likely to cause a lateral condylar fracture. Treatment of these rare injuries is simple immobilization for comfort and early motion.

PROXIMAL RADIAL FRACTURE

INCIDENCE

Fractures about the proximal end of the radius represent about 8% of all elbow fractures in children.[11] In contrast to adults, who sustain fractures of the radial head, children more commonly have fractures of the proximal radius that involve the neck and physis. The majority occur in children between the ages of 9 and 12 years.[216,217] Associated injuries, especially of the olecranon and medial epicondyle, are common.

ANATOMY

The proximal end of the radius normally angulates about 15 degrees laterally and approximately 5 degrees anteriorly. This angulation may be mistaken for a fracture.[218]

MECHANISM OF INJURY

Fractures of the proximal radius occur as the result of a fall on an outstretched hand with the elbow extended or in association with posterior dislocation of the elbow. In the former mechanism, force is transmitted through the shaft of the radius as the momentum of the body drives the capitellum against the lateral half of the radial head, causing it to tilt and displace. If the forearm is fully supinated on impact,

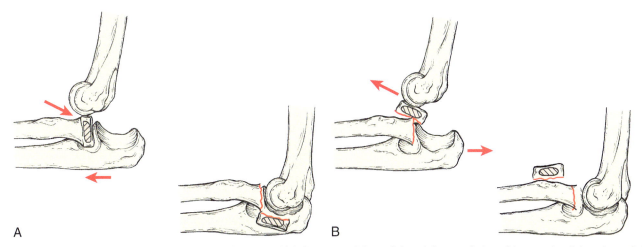

Fig. 17.56 This illustration depicts the two mechanisms by which fractures of the radial neck in association with posterior dislocations of the elbow are thought to occur. (A) Fracture of the radial neck and displacement of the head occurs during reduction, so the radial head is displaced posteriorly. (B) Fracture and displacement of the epiphysis occur during dislocation, resulting in an anteriorly displaced radial head and neck. (A, From Jeffery C. Fractures of the head of the radius in children. *J Bone Joint Surg Br.* 1950;32:314–324.[136] B, From Neuman JH. Displaced radial neck fractures in children. *Injury* 1977;9:114.[205])

the radial head displaces laterally, and if the forearm is neutral, the displacement is posterior. Fractures may involve the physis or just the metaphysis. When this fracture occurs in association with elbow dislocation, the epiphysis is displaced posteriorly if the fracture occurs as the elbow is reduced.[219] If the fracture occurs at the time of dislocation, rather than during reduction, the radial epiphysis is knocked off as it exits the joint and is displaced anteriorly (Fig. 17.56).[216]

CLASSIFICATION

Chambers[220] classified fractures of the radial head and neck into three groups based on injury pattern and mechanism. In group I, the radial head is primarily displaced; in group II, displacement primarily occurs through the radial neck; and in group III, injuries to the radial head or neck are caused by repetitive stress. Group I injuries are subdivided mechanistically by those that occur as a result of a valgus load (types A, B, and C) and those that are associated with elbow dislocations (types D and E). The valgus injuries are defined further by the location and type of fracture: type A is a Salter-Harris type I or II injury, type B is a Salter-Harris type IV fracture, and type C is a metaphyseal fracture. Regardless of the particular fracture pattern, the radial head can be angulated, translated, or completely displaced. Fractures associated with elbow dislocation are further divided based on the original descriptions of Jeffrey[219] and Newman[216] into two additional types. In both, the radial head is completely displaced: in type D, fracture of the radial neck and displacement of the head occurs during reduction, so the radial head is posterior; in type E, fracture and displacement of the epiphysis occur during dislocation, resulting in an anteriorly displaced radial head (Table 17.2). Group II consists of injuries in which primary displacement occurs through the radial neck. This pattern of failure may be seen in Monteggia-equivalent injuries.[221] In these injuries, radioulnar joint congruence is maintained, and treatment involves reducing the radial neck to the radial head. Group III injuries are caused by chronic, repetitive stress and may manifest as osteochondritis dissecans of the radial head or angular deformity of the radial neck.

TABLE 17.2 Classification of Proximal Radial Fractures

I	Valgus fractures
	Type A: Salter-Harris types I and II
	Type B: Salter-Harris type IV
	Type C: fracture of the radial metaphysis only
II	Fractures related to elbow dislocation
	Type D: reduction injuries
	Type E: dislocation injuries

(From Wilkins KE. Fractures and dislocations of the elbow region. In Rockwood CH, Wilkins KE, King RE, eds. *Fractures in Children*. Philadelphia: J.B. Lippincott; 1984.)

DIAGNOSIS

The history, mechanism of injury, and clinical examination of the patient should alert one to the diagnosis of a possible fracture of the proximal radius. The child typically has tenderness over the radial head, and rotation of the forearm produces pain in the lateral aspect of the elbow that may radiate distally into the forearm. The diagnosis of a displaced fracture of the neck of the radius is usually easily made on routine AP and lateral radiographs. Nondisplaced fractures may be difficult to visualize radiographically, and rotational views of the proximal end of the radius may be helpful. If the forearm cannot be rotated, the radiocapitellar view described by Greenspan and Norman[222] may be helpful for visualizing the proximal radius. This view is an oblique lateral performed with the forearm in neutral rotation, and the x-ray beam is directed 45 degrees proximally so that it projects the radial head anterior to the distal humerus. In young children, before ossification of the radial head, the only finding of a displaced fracture may be irregularity of the metaphysis. Ultrasound, MRI, and arthrography may be necessary to fully define the extent of the injury.[223,224]

MANAGEMENT

Regardless of the treatment method or final alignment, loss of motion is common after this injury. Factors that may affect prognosis include initial and postreduction angulation and displacement of the fracture, the presence of other in-juries like elbow dislocations or fractures of the olecranon or medial epicondyle, the age of the child, and the timing of surgery. Authors disagree about the need for reduction of angulated fractures of the radial neck in children. It is known that these fractures remodel and that the remodel-ing potential is considerable because of the degree of move-ment of the radiohumeral and radioulnar joints. Although some authors recommend aggressive treatment of angu-lated radial neck fractures, accepting no more than 10 to 15 degrees of angulation,[218,225,226] most agree that up to 30 degrees of angulation is acceptable[154,219,227,228]; some even suggest that up to 45 degrees is tolerable.[80,229]

Nonoperative Treatment

Most surgeons currently believe that fractures with up to 30 degrees of angulation may be treated by immobilization with the use of a sling, posterior splint, or cast primarily for comfort with mobilization as soon as symptoms permit but ideally within 14 days. If the angulation is more than 30 degrees, closed manipulation of the fracture should be attempted. Several maneuvers have been described for re-duction of these fractures, which suggests that none works universally; thus, having some familiarity with more than one may be beneficial.

Patterson[230] described a maneuver for reduction of this fracture with the elbow in extension. With an assistant pro-viding countertraction on the upper part of the arm, the surgeon supinates the forearm and applies longitudinal traction. At the same time, the assistant forces the elbow into varus. The forearm is then rotated until the position of maximal tilt of the radial head is directed laterally,[219] at which point the radial head can be reduced by application of direct digital pressure with a thumb.

Kaufman described a maneuver called the *Israeli technique* that is performed with the elbow in flexion and the forearm supinated. The surgeon applies direct pressure to the radi-al head with his or her thumb, and the forearm is pronat-ed to effect reduction.[231] Neher and Torch[232] described a two-person technique wherein the assistant places a laterally directed force on the radial neck, and the surgeon applies a varus force to the elbow with one hand and attempts to digitally reduce the radial head with the thumb of the oth-er. Chambers[220] described a "milking" technique using an elastic bandage (Ace wrap or Esmarch bandage) wrapped in a distal-to-proximal direction that effectively compresses the soft tissue envelope in the proximal forearm and indi-rectly reduces the radial head. The goal of closed reduction, by whatever method, is to achieve postreduction angula-tion that is less than 30 degrees, with less than 3 to 4 mm of translation, and preservation of a minimum of 50 degrees of pronosupination.

Operative Treatment

If there is more than 30 degrees to 45 degrees of angula-tion, more than 4 mm of translation, or restricted motion, operative methods should be considered. In 1981, Ange-lov[233] described a method of percutaneous reduction of the angulated radial neck using a double-pronged instrument to push the head of the radius back into an acceptable po-sition. Others have reported variations of this technique (Fig. 17.57).[234,235] Dormans[235] described a percutaneous

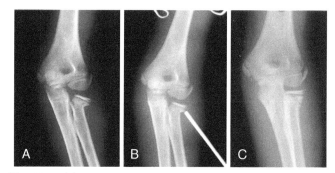

Fig. 17.57 (A) Anteroposterior (AP) radiograph of the elbow shows a fracture of the radial neck that is angulated 45 degrees and trans-lated 4 mm. (B) AP radiograph showing a percutaneously inserted Steinmann pin that was used to push the radial head back into an acceptable position. (C) The fracture has been reduced, and an AP radiograph shows complete correction of fracture translation and an-gulation.

technique using a Steinmann pin to reduce the fracture and arthrography to help assess the amount of angulation and adequacy of reduction. Wallace[236] has described yet another modification of percutaneous reduction in which a perios-teal elevator is inserted through a small incision just distal to the level of the bicipital tuberosity, over the lateral subcu-taneous border of the ulna, to act as a lever to stabilize or reduce the distal portion of the fracture while the head is reduced with digital pressure or a Steinmann pin. With any of these percutaneous approaches, pronating the forearm and using a more posterior entry with the pin can help avoid the posterior interosseous nerve, which runs volar and distal to the radial head.

Another technique that avoids opening the fracture has been described by Metaizeau and colleagues[237] and Sessa and colleagues[258] and involves retrograde insertion of an elastic intramedullary nail across the fracture site to capture, reduce, and stabilize the radial head. Under fluoroscopic guidance, the nail is inserted into the radius through an entry point in the distal radial metaphysis. The nail is advanced up the intramedullary canal to the level of the fracture. The curved tip of the nail is used to capture the displaced radial epiphysis, then a "T-handle chuck" (or similar proprietary tool) is used to rotate the nail so that the radial head is placed back into position. Once re-duced, the fracture is usually stable; however, most authors recommend leaving the nail in place for internal fixation (Fig. 17.58).[237,238] Reproducibility of this technique has been demonstrated in several large series with the use of both elastic nails, as originally described, and K-wires and Ilizarov wires for fixation.[239–241]

Most agree that avoiding open treatment of the fracture is preferable, even if a perfect anatomic reduction is not possible by closed means, because of the risk of stiffness and AVN of the radial head.[80,227,242] Open reduction is, howev-er, indicated if the fracture cannot be reduced satisfactorily by closed or percutaneous manipulation or intramedullary pinning. If the radial head is completely displaced, it may be irreducible. In addition, authors have reported the head flipping 180 degrees during attempts at closed or percuta-neous reduction such that the articular surface is opposed to the metaphysis.[17,107] The radial head and neck may be accessed through a lateral Kocher approach to the elbow.

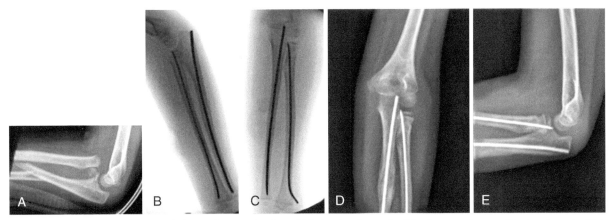

Fig. 17.58 A 6-year-old female with a grade I open forearm fracture. (A) Lateral radiograph of the forearm shows a Monteggia variant injury with a fracture of the ulna and displaced fracture of the radial neck. She underwent débridement and intramedullary fixation of the ulna and then reduction of the radial neck fracture with the use of the flexible titanium intramedullary nail technique described by Metaizeau. (B and C) Antero-posterior and lateral radiographs show anatomic reduction of both fractures and healing at 2 months (D and E).

Care must be taken to avoid injury to the radial nerve by pronation of the forearm, which moves the posterior interosseous nerve in a volar and medial direction away from the working area.[2,225,243] The skin incision is centered laterally over the radial head, and the deep interval is developed between the anconeus and extensor carpi ulnaris. The capsule is opened longitudinally, and the proximal fragment is identified and reduced under direct and fluoroscopic visualization. If the fracture appears stable after reduction, the surgeon has the option not to perform internal fixation.[53,244] There is, however, evidence to support the argument that if the fracture requires open reduction, internal fixation should be performed to ensure maintenance of reduction.[219,225]

Pins are the most common fixation option and may be inserted obliquely from the articular margin of the radial head in the safe zone[245] to cross the fracture obliquely (Fig. 17.59). Transcapitellar pins are not recommended because they provide poor fixation and are prone to breakage at the joint.[216] Suture fixation has been described.[246] Headless screws and mini T-plates may be an option in skeletally mature individuals. Radial head excision should be avoided in children because of predictably poor results related to the development of cubitus valgus and longitudinal instability of the forearm.[80,225] Even if the fracture is old, surgical reduction should be performed if forearm motion is significantly restricted.

Postoperative Care

Postoperatively, the elbow should be immobilized at 90 degrees. The length of immobilization depends on the nature of the fracture and the treatment. If the fracture is minimally angulated and no reduction is necessary, the elbow may be immobilized for comfort for 5 to 7 days and rapidly mobilized thereafter so that loss of motion does not occur. If the fracture has been reduced, immobilization for 3 weeks is usually sufficient. If pins are used for fixation, they should not be removed until there is radiographic evidence of healing. For this reason, it may be preferable to bury the pins rather than to place them percutaneously in the event of delayed union. Motion should not be started until the pins are removed.

COMPLICATIONS

The most common complications of radial neck fractures are loss of motion, which is to be expected regardless of the treatment modality; overgrowth of the radial head, which occurs in 40% of cases and can contribute to loss of motion[227]; nonunion, which has been reported most commonly with open reduction after failed attempts at closed treatment[247]; osteonecrosis, which has been reported in up to 20% of cases, 70% of which occur after open reduction[80,216]; and radioulnar synostosis, which is rare (<10%) and is usually the result of delayed open treatment and extensive soft issue dissection, although it can occur after closed or percutaneous reduction.[216,234,248]

OLECRANON FRACTURE

INCIDENCE

Olecranon fractures are relatively uncommon in children. They constitute approximately 5% of all fractures about the elbow and, overall, only about 25% of all olecranon fractures. Newell[249] reported on 40 cases seen over a 40-year period, most of which were minimally displaced. Up to 70% may be associated with another injury about the elbow, most commonly a fracture of the proximal radius or elbow dislocation.[250–254] It is estimated that less than 20% require surgical treatment.[11]

MECHANISM OF INJURY

Fractures of the olecranon may occur as the result of direct trauma but are more commonly caused by a force transmitted up the forearm after a fall on an outstretched hand with a variable degree of elbow extension and forearm rotation.[220,250] The force may be valgus or varus, depending on the fall, and the resulting fracture is commonly an oblique fracture through the metaphysis, the direction of which may vary according to the degree of elbow flexion. Fractures through the apophysis and the growth plate are much less common, although they probably arise from similar mechanisms. Mechanistically, a fall with the elbow flexed usually results in failure on the tension (dorsal) side of the bone or apophysis, which causes a transverse fracture that is variably

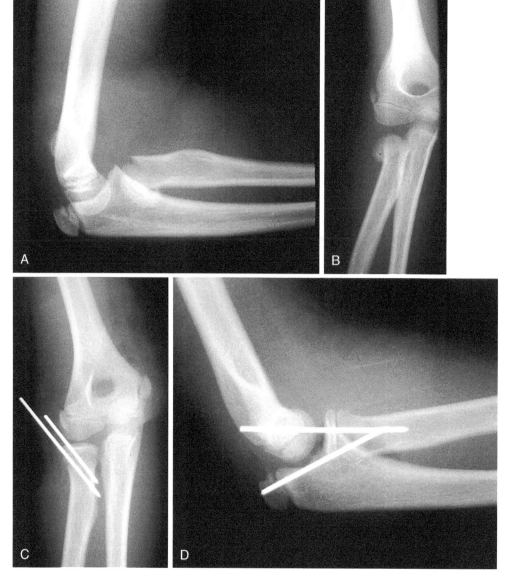

Fig. 17.59 Angulated fracture of the radial neck. A 9-year-old child fell and sustained a fracture of her radial neck. (A and B) Anteroposterior (AP) and lateral radiographs of the elbow of a 9-year-old child showing a fracture of the radial neck that is angulated laterally and displaced posteriorly. After failed attempts at closed and percutaneous reduction, open reduction was performed, and the fracture was stabilized with K-wires. (C and D) Wires were inserted obliquely from the margin of the radial head as seen on the postoperative AP and lateral radiographs before hardware removal. The fracture is reduced and has healed.

displaced, depending on the force of the injury. A fall with the elbow extended results in a more longitudinal fracture pattern that is usually incomplete (i.e., greenstick). If there is associated valgus loading, a concomitant fracture of the proximal radius (Monteggia variant) or medial epicondyle may ensue, whereas varus loading may cause lateral dislocation of the radial head (type III Monteggia).[255] A direct blow to the proximal ulna results in failure on the volar side of the olecranon.

Olecranon fractures are common in pediatric patients with osteogenesis imperfecta (OI). In a series of 358 patients with OI, 8.1% had an olecranon fracture at a mean age of 11.9 years. Of those patients, 41.4% fractured the contralateral side at an average of 5 months after their first fracture. These types of fractures occurred mainly in children with type I OI.[256]

CLASSIFICATION

Several classification systems have been proposed for fractures of the olecranon in children. Chambers'[220] classification

is based on the mode of injury. Graves and Canale[252] and Gaddy and colleagues[251] classified these fractures by extent of displacement. Papavasiliou and colleagues[257] classified the injuries according to joint involvement and displacement. Matthews[254] incorporated displacement and associated injuries into his classification. The classification of Evans and Graham[250] is the most comprehensive, incorporating the anatomic site and pattern of the fracture, amount of displacement, and the presence of associated injuries (Table 17.3). This classification is based on the pathoanatomic features, the consideration of which can be used as a basis for determining treatment.

TREATMENT

In general, regardless of the anatomic site or fracture configuration, the type of treatment is dictated by the amount of intraarticular displacement and extensor mechanism disruption. Minimally displaced or nondisplaced fractures account for 80% of all olecranon fractures and may be managed with immobilization. Oblique metaphyseal fractures are the most

TABLE 17.3   Classification of Fractures of the Olecranon

Anatomic site	1. Apophyseal
	  a. Extraarticular
	  b. Intraarticular
	2. Physeal (Salter-Harris equivalent)
	3. Metaphyseal
	  a. Juxtaphyseal
	  b. True metaphyseal
	4. Combined olecranon-coronoid process fracture

Fracture configuration	1. Transverse (<30 degrees) 2. Oblique (30–60 degrees) 3. Longitudinal (>60 degrees)
Intraarticular displacement	1. <2 mm 2. 2–4 mm 3. >4 mm
Associated injuries (ipsilateral)	1. Radial head/neck fracture 2. Radial head subluxation/dislocation 3. Lateral humeral condyle fracture 4. Medial humeral epicondyle injury 5. Supracondylar humeral fracture 6. Distal radius/ulna fracture

(From Evans MC, Graham HK. Olecranon fractures in children. Part 1: clinical review; Part 2: a new classification and management algorithm. *J Pediatr Orthop.* 1999;19(5):559–569.)

common injury and, in teenagers, may be treated satisfactorily with tension-band wiring as is performed in adults (Fig. 17.60). In younger children, the technique described originally by Gortzak and colleagues,[258] using an absorbable or nonabsorbable suture for the tension band, is effective and obviates the need for reoperation for hardware removal. The pins may be removed at 4 weeks, and the absorbable suture is left behind (Fig. 17.61). Fractures of the radial neck are commonly associated injuries and may be treated closed or open, depending on their individual characteristics. For fractures that are more oblique and those that are longitudinally oriented, interfragmental screw fixation may be the more appropriate method of internal fixation. The presence of associated fractures usually signifies a more severe injury mechanism (Fig. 17.62). Precontoured periarticular plates can be used in older children with comminuted fractures. In many cases, these implants need to be removed once the fracture is healed because of implant prominence.

DISLOCATIONS OF THE ELBOW JOINT

Elbow dislocations in children are classified as posterior, anterior, medial, or lateral based on the position of the proximal radius and ulna relative to the distal humerus. They are also classified as divergent (rare) if the proximal radioulnar articulation is disrupted or translocated in the extremely rare event that the proximal radius and ulna are reversed in their normal relationship to each other and the distal humerus.

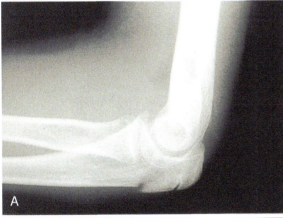

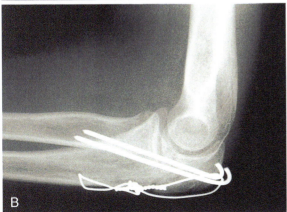

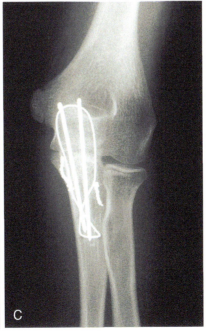

Fig. 17.60 Displaced fracture of the olecranon in a 13-year-old girl. (A) A lateral radiograph of the elbow demonstrates a fracture of the olecranon with 3 mm of displacement. (B) A lateral radiograph of the elbow 4 weeks after surgery shows union of the fracture. The fracture was stabilized with two pins and a tension band. Early active elbow motion was begun, and the patient had nearly full elbow flexion and extension at the time of this radiograph. (C) Anteroposterior radiograph of the fracture 4 weeks after open reduction of the fracture shows figure-of-8 tension band fixation technique.

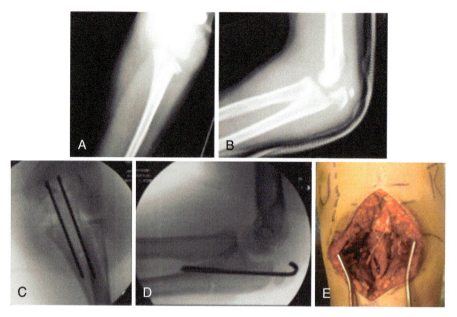

Fig. 17.61 A 9-year-old child with transverse olecranon and radial neck fractures. (A and B) Anteroposterior and lateral radiographs showing displaced fractures of the olecranon and radial neck. (C and D) Intraoperative fluoroscopic images after open reduction and internal fixation of the olecranon fracture and closed treatment of the radial neck. (E) Intraoperative picture showing the nonabsorbable suture used for the tension band.

POSTERIOR DISLOCATION OF THE ELBOW JOINT

Incidence

Dislocation of the elbow is a rare injury in children. Henrikson[34] found 45 elbow dislocations among 1579 elbow injuries in children, which yielded an incidence of about 3%. Although these injuries may occur at any age, the peak incidence is during the second decade of life.[69,259–261] Posterior dislocations are most common. Pure dislocations are relatively uncommon because most elbow dislocations are associated with fractures around the elbow, of which the medial epicondyle (33%) is most common.[69,259,261] Less frequently, injuries may involve the radial neck, coronoid process, trochlea, lateral condyle, and, rarely, disruption of the proximal radioulnar joint (divergent dislocation).[262–264] Anterior dislocations are usually associated with avulsion or fractures of the olecranon.[265]

Mechanism of Injury

Posterior dislocation usually results from a fall on an outstretched hand with the forearm supinated and elbow extended or partially flexed. The coronoid process, which normally acts as a buttress to resist posterior displacement of the ulna, is relatively small in children and may not be fully ossified. As a result, when the force of impact tears the anterior elbow joint capsule, the coronoid may not be sufficient to prevent dislocation of the ulna. If all force is directed posteriorly, a straight posterior dislocation of the elbow occurs (Fig. 17.63). If a valgus load is combined with the posteriorly directed force at impact, fracture of the medial epicondyle may occur (Fig. 17.64). Rarely, in cases of high-energy trauma, the axial forces directed along the long axis of the forearm may cause disruption of the interosseous membrane and annular ligament, resulting in a divergent dislocation. If the forearm is markedly pronated on impact, translocation of the proximal radius and ulna may ensue because the radial head dislocates medially into the coronoid fossa or even further, followed by posterior displacement of the olecranon. This very rare injury is called *proximal radioulnar translocation.*

Treatment

Closed reduction is usually successful in treating posterior dislocations and should be performed as soon as possible, before there is significant soft tissue swelling. Royle[266] has demonstrated that outcomes after early reduction were better than outcomes of reductions done later. Before any treatment, a complete evaluation of the neurovascular status of the extremity must be made because injury to the brachial artery and the median and, less commonly, the ulnar nerves may occur at the time of dislocation. Adequate sedation in the emergency room or general anesthesia is necessary to facilitate relaxation of the musculature about the elbow so that the reduction can be performed.

With the patient supine, supinating the forearm reduces tension in the biceps and unlocks the coronoid and radial head from behind the humerus. Lateral translation should be corrected at this point to minimize the risk of median nerve entrapment.[267] While an assistant stabilizes the torso, the surgeon initiates reduction by applying longitudinal traction to the forearm, just below the elbow, in line with the long axis of the humerus to overcome the deforming forces of the triceps and brachialis. The surgeon then completes the reduction by pulling the radius and ulna distally, in line with the longitudinal axis of the forearm,[197] and the olecranon forward while completing the reduction. Hyperextending the elbow before initiating reduction should be avoided because of the risk of further injury, including rupture, of the brachialis muscle.[268]

After reduction, stability of the elbow and concentricity of the reduction need to be confirmed. If the elbow is stable after reduction, it may be immobilized in a posterior splint with the elbow flexed to 90 degrees for 1 to 3 weeks.[197,266,269] Studies in adults have shown improved functional outcomes with a sling and early motion. This author prefers 1 week of immobilization to allow for resolution of pain and swelling followed by rapid mobilization. If the elbow is unstable after reduction, it should be immobilized in the position of stability for a minimum of 3 weeks. After that time, a removable splint or hinged brace should be worn. Although motion is encouraged, full extension is not attempted until 6 weeks after the injury.

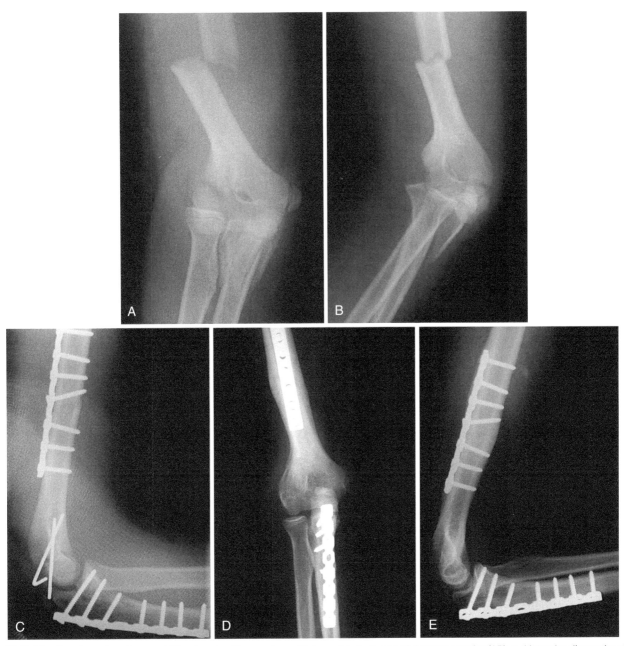

Fig. 17.62 Floating elbow in a 9-year-old boy involved in a motor vehicle accident. (A and B) Anteroposterior (AP) and lateral radiographs of the elbow demonstrating a comminuted fracture of the olecranon, a transverse fracture of the humerus shaft, and a supracondylar humeral fracture. (C) Lateral radiograph of the elbow 3 weeks after open reduction of the fractures. The humeral fracture was exposed through a posterior triceps-splitting incision that was then extended to allow access to the olecranon. The humerus was stabilized with a 3.5-mm compression plate, the supracondylar fracture was fixed with two lateral entry pins (0.062 in.), and the olecranon fracture was stabilized with a plate and screws with interfragmental compression of the fracture. (D and E) AP and lateral radiographs of the elbow 6 months after the injury. The fractures are healed. The patient has full flexion and extension of the elbow and full pronation and supination of the forearm.

Absolute indications for open reduction are open fractures, nonconcentric reductions, and the presence of osteochondral fractures or incarceration of the medial epicondyle. Entrapment of the medial epicondyle should be suspected if the elbow is unstable after reduction or if the reduction is not concentric after closed treatment. Careful inspection of the radiographs will often reveal the position of the medial epicondyle. If it is within the elbow joint after reduction, it must be removed by either manipulation or, more commonly, open reduction and fixation (Fig. 17.65). The presence of associated extraarticular fractures is a relative indication for surgical treatment. Several studies have shown better results with surgical treatment of these concomitant injuries.[129,197,259,270]

Complications

Complications of elbow dislocation occur both early and late. Early complications are usually related to the injury itself and include neurologic and vascular compromise. Complications that manifest later are consequences of the healing process and include joint stiffness, heterotopic ossification, myositis ossificans, radioulnar synostosis, and recurrent instability.

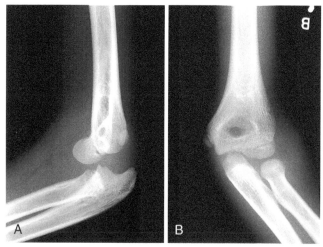

Fig. 17.63 Posterior dislocation of the elbow. (A and B) Anteroposterior and lateral radiographs of the elbow showing the ulna and radius displaced posteriorly.

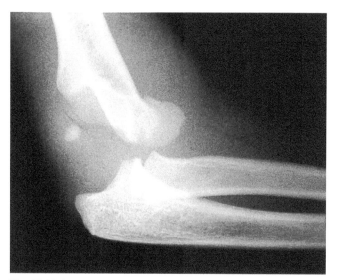

Fig. 17.64 Lateral radiograph demonstrating dislocation of the elbow with avulsion of the medial epicondyle, suggesting a combined posterior and valgus load at impact.

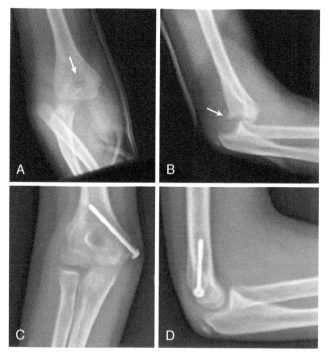

Fig. 17.65 Posterior elbow dislocation in a 10-year-old boy. (A and B) Anteroposterior (AP) and lateral radiographs of the elbow demonstrating posterior dislocation. The medial epicondyle is displaced and incarcerated in the joint. The dislocation could not be reduced closed. Open reduction was performed through a medial approach. The epicondyle was extracted, reduced, and stabilized with a cannulated screw. (C and D) AP and lateral radiographs of the elbow after open reduction and fixation.

Vascular. Stans[271] estimated a 3% incidence of arterial injuries in a combined series of 317 children and adolescents with posterior elbow dislocations.[260,261,266,272] Compression, spasm, or entrapment of the brachial artery is not uncommon after posterior elbow dislocations and usually resolves after reduction of the elbow.[259] True disruption of the brachial artery (i.e., thrombosis or rupture) is, fortunately, a much less common occurrence.[8,10] Entrapment of the brachial artery after reduction has also been reported.[273] Brachial artery injury is more common with open dislocations in which distal perfusion can be severely compromised by disruption of the collateral circulation about the elbow.[10] Whenever vascular compromise is associated with elbow dislocation, the joint should be reduced emergently and vascular status should be reassessed. Arterial exploration and repair should be performed in all open injuries and in any circumstances in which ischemia persists or distal perfusion is questionable after reduction.[10,273–275]

Neurologic Injury. Both ulnar and median nerve injuries have been reported to occur with dislocation of the elbow. In Stans's[271] analysis of 317 patients pooled from four series of posterior elbow dislocations, injuries to the ulnar nerve were most common (32 patients), followed by isolated injuries to the median nerve (seven patients), and then combined median and ulnar nerve injuries (four patients).[260,261,266,272] Injuries to the radial nerve are extremely rare.[265]

Injuries to the ulnar nerve comprise more than two-thirds of all nerve injuries after posterior elbow dislocations and have been associated with valgus dislocation and avulsion of the medial epicondyle. These nerve lesions are usually transient.[272,276] Median nerve injuries are much less common than ulnar injuries; when they do occur, however, the consequences are often profound and are related to nerve entrapment within the elbow joint. Hallett[277] described three mechanisms (which he attributed to Fourier) by which the median nerve may become entrapped within the elbow joint. In the first type, the nerve becomes entrapped within the joint after a valgus dislocation in which the medial epicondyle is avulsed or the forearm flexor muscles are detached, along with tearing of the ulnar collateral ligaments. The nerve slips behind the humerus during the dislocation and becomes entrapped within the joint after the reduction. In the second type, the nerve is encased by the healing fracture of the medial epicondyle and may form a neuroforamen. In the third type, the nerve becomes looped anteriorly in the joint. A fourth type that is actually a combination of the first and second types has also been described.[278,279]

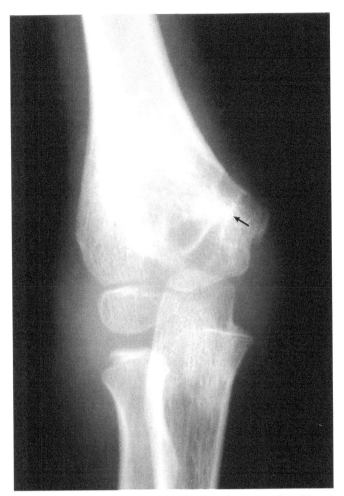

Fig. 17.66 Anteroposterior radiograph taken 4 months after dislocation of the elbow. Note the cortical depression in the distal end of the humerus just proximal to the medial epicondyle *(arrow)*. This depression marks the location of the median nerve that became entrapped in the elbow joint after dislocation.

The diagnosis of median nerve injury may be difficult to make because of the absence of pain; thus, the diagnosis is often delayed.[277] Fortunately, excellent recovery can be expected, even with late recognition and repair of the problem. Green[280] published a case report of a 7-year-old female who had dislocated her elbow 4 months previously and continued to have pain and inability to extend her arm, and eventually developed a complete median nerve palsy. The nerve was found to be looped around the distal humerus and entered the elbow joint posteriorly. Radiographically, evidence was seen of a cortical depression in the ulnar side of the distal end of the humerus caused by the nerve, as described by Matev[281] (Fig. 17.66). The damaged portion of the nerve trapped within the joint was resected and directly repaired. The patient regained nearly total normal motor function and almost normal sensation in the median nerve distribution.

Recurrent Dislocation. Because recurrent dislocations of the elbow are uncommon (<1%) after posterior dislocations, few reports of this complication are available.[271] Residual capsuloligamentous laxity and osteocartilaginous defects have been implicated etiologically. Osborne and Cotterill[282] propose that the primary problem is that recurrent sublux-

ation leads to the development of secondary osteocartilaginous depressions in the capitellum and radial head. These alterations in the articular surface then predispose to further instability.[283–285] O'Driscoll and colleagues[128] identified two pediatric patients with posterolateral rotatory instability caused by laxity of the ulnar band of the radial collateral ligament.

Treatment of recurrent dislocation of the elbow requires repair of the lax posterolateral structures of the elbow. Osborne and Cotterill[282] described a method of reattachment of the capsule and lateral collateral ligaments to restore elbow stability. These structures are incised in line with their fibers, beginning at the humeral epicondylar ridge. The incision is continued distal to the annular ligament. The bone of the lateral epicondyle is roughened, and the capsule and collateral ligament are reattached to the bone with sutures.

TRANSVERSE DIVERGENT ELBOW DISLOCATION

This type of elbow dislocation is uncommon. The injury is usually caused by higher-energy mechanisms, and there may be associated injuries of the proximal radius, ulna, and distal humerus. The probable mechanism is an axial load on the elbow with the forearm pronated, which results in both posterior elbow dislocation and disruption of the proximal radioulnar articulation. For this injury pattern to occur, the ligamentous stabilizers of the elbow and the proximal portion of the interosseous membrane must be disrupted.[286] Despite the significant soft tissue disruption, these injuries can usually be treated closed. The elbow joint is reduced first, and then the divergence of the radius and ulna is reduced by pronation of the forearm, followed by compression of the proximal radius and ulna (Fig. 17.67).

RADIAL HEAD DISLOCATION

Incidence

Isolated traumatic dislocation of the radial head is extremely rare and often missed or misdiagnosed.

Mechanism of Injury

The annular ligament stabilizes the head of the radius and prevents dislocation. This ligament may be torn with forced pronation of the forearm.[287,288] The radial head may not appear displaced at presentation. Spontaneous reduction after initial injury and then subsequent dislocation of the radial head has been reported.[289] More commonly, this injury is associated with fracture or plastic deformation of the ulna and may be overlooked on initial radiographs (a missed Monteggia lesion).[290–292] Lincoln and Mubarak[292] described the "ulnar bow sign" to assist in the proper recognition of the often subtle deformity of the ulna in this injury pattern.

Differentiation from Congenital Dislocation of the Radius

Frequently, the patient or the family does not notice symptoms related to congenital dislocation of the radial head because the arm functions normally. Then, when a child sustains a relatively minor injury to the elbow, prominence of the radial head is observed. Differentiation from a true acute injury may be made by careful examination of the extremity. Although a child with a congenital dislocation and recent trauma may have pain, it is usually less severe than

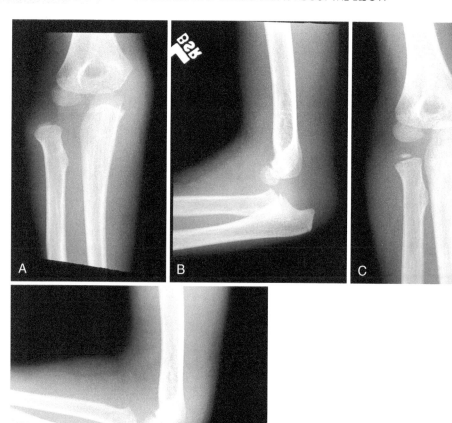

Fig. 17.67 Divergent dislocation of the elbow. (A) An anteroposterior (AP) radiograph of the elbow demonstrates the separation between the radius and the ulna. (B) Lateral radiograph of the elbow shows that the radius and ulna are posteriorly dislocated. (C and D) AP and lateral radiographs after closed reduction demonstrating restoration of the normal anatomy of the elbow. (From Holbrook JL, Green NE. Divergent pediatric elbow dislocation. A case report. *Clin Orthop Relat Res.* 1988;234:72.)

one would expect with traumatic dislocation. The elbow motion, especially in rotation, is most likely greater than expected. Radiographically, the radial head is dislocated, but characteristic dysplastic changes of the radiohumeral joint are present. The capitellum may be hypoplastic, and the radial head may be dome shaped, without its normal central depression. These findings clearly distinguish this entity from a traumatic dislocation of a normal radial head.[293–295] (Fig. 17.68).

Management

Surgical treatment of true congenital dislocation of the head of the radius is not warranted in children because attempts at reduction have not been rewarding. A child with essentially normal elbow function is likely to lose elbow motion and function after surgical reduction. Neglected traumatic dislocation, in contrast, has been treated with open reduction with good results, even when the interval between the trauma and the surgical reduction has been more than 3 years.[296,297] Careful analysis and correction of any ulnar bowing is mandatory. The use of a strip of the triceps tendon for reconstruction of the annular ligament has been advocated.[296]

SUBLUXATION OF THE RADIAL HEAD

INCIDENCE

Although subluxation of the radial head is the most accurate description of this injury, it is also known by the terms *pulled*

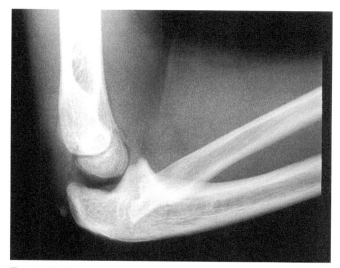

Fig. 17.68 Congenital dislocation of the radial head. On this lateral radiograph, the radial head is displaced posteriorly and has migrated proximally. The radial neck is narrow and dysplastic, indicative of a long-standing dislocation.

elbow and *nursemaid's elbow.* It is probably the most common traumatic elbow injury in children. Radial head subluxation has been estimated to occur in 15% to 27% of all elbow injuries in children younger than 10 years.[298,299] The average age at injury is between 2 and 4 years, but it may occur in older children.

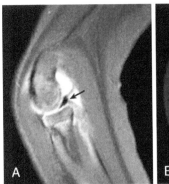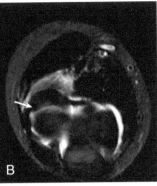

Fig. 17.69 Magnetic resonance image of "pulled elbow." (A) Sagittal proton-density fat-saturated image shows that the annular ligament is subluxated and located at the joint line *(arrow)*. (B) Axial T2 fat-saturated image shows the ligament to be subluxated *(arrow)*. Posterior attachment of the capsule is not well visualized, which suggests that it is torn *(arrow)*. Joint effusion and edema are present on both images.

MECHANISM OF INJURY

This injury is produced with the forearm in pronation. The radial head is an ovoid structure, and in pronation, the lateral edge of the radial head is more flat than it is in supination, where it is more defined.[300] When longitudinal traction is applied to the pronated forearm, the annular ligament slips over the more narrow, rounded lateral portion of the radial head. In the process, it may tear at its attachment. The head of the radius moves distally, and as the traction is released, the annular ligament becomes caught between the radial head and the capitellum[298-300] (Fig. 17.69). With a large tear, more of the annular ligament may become entrapped in the radiocapitellar joint, which makes the reduction difficult. This injury is not seen in older children because the attachments of the annular ligament to the radial neck become thicker with age and more resistant to disruption. Salter and Zaltz[300] claim that this injury is rare after the age of 5 years because ligamentous laxity is also thought to be a factor in the pathogenesis of this problem. Amir and colleagues[301] found an increased incidence of hypermobility in children with nursemaid's elbow compared with a cohort of healthy children.

The typical clinical scenario in which radial head subluxation occurs is when a child is lifted or swung by the wrist or when a child reaches up to grab something to break a fall, recreating the pathomechanical scenario of elbow extension, forearm pronation, and longitudinal traction.

MANAGEMENT

A child with radial head subluxation holds the arm flexed at the elbow with the forearm pronated. The initial pain quickly subsides, and the child may return to play but will not use the injured extremity. An infant may simply be seen with pseudoparalysis of the extremity, raising concerns of infection or other occult trauma. Careful examination of the arm reveals pain in the elbow only. If the history is not consistent with radial head subluxation, radiographs should be obtained to exclude another injury. The physician can perform reduction by supinating the forearm with the elbow flexed approximately 60 degrees, applying a medially directed force to the radial head with the thumb, and then maximally flexing the elbow.[299] Reduction of the radial head is usually accompanied by a tactile and sometimes audible click as the annular ligament slides back over the lateral edge of the radial head. Typically, the child begins to use the arm almost immediately after reduction, and successful treatment is confirmed by demonstration of full elbow flexion and extension and forearm pronosupination. Young children (< 5 years) may be at risk of recurrent subluxations because of increased ligamentous laxity and pliability of the annular ligament and its attachments to the radial neck.[302,303]

ACKNOWLEDGMENT

The authors would like to acknowledge and thank Dr. Neil E. Green and Dr. Nathan L. Van Zeeland for their contributions to the previous versions of this chapter.

REFERENCES

The level of evidence (LOE) is determined according to the criteria provided in the Preface.

1. Buhr AJ, Cooke AM. Fracture patterns. *Lancet.* 1959;1(7072):531–536. **(LOE V)**.
2. Rang M, ed. *Children's Fractures.* JB Lippincott; 1983. **(LOE N/A)**.
3. Hanlon CR, Estes J WL. Fractures in childhood, a statistical analysis. *Am J Surg.* 1954;87(3):312–323. **(LOE IV)**.
4. Lichtenberg RP. A study of 2,532 fractures in children. *Am J Surg.* 1954;87(3):330–338. **(LOE IV)**.
5. Silberstein MJ, Brodeur AE, Graviss ER, et al. Some vagaries of the medial epicondyle. *J Bone Joint Surg Am.* 1981;63(4):287–291. **(LOE IV)**.
6. Haraldsson S. On osteochondrosis deformans juvenilis capituli humeri including investigation of intra-osseous vasculature in distal humerus. *Acta Orthop Scand Suppl.* 1959;38:1–232. **(LOE IV)**.
7. Kamal AS, Austin RT. Dislocation of the median nerve and brachial artery in supracondylar fractures of the humerus. *Injury.* 1980;12(2):161–164. **(LOE IV)**.
8. Kilburn PS J, Silk F. Three cases of compound posterior dislocation of the elbow with rupture of the brachial artery. *J Bone Joint Surg Br.* 1982;44:119–121. **(LOE V)**.
9. Liddell W. Neurovascular complications in widely displaced supracondylar fractures of the humerus. *J Bone Joint Surg Br.* 1967;49:1631–1636. **(LOE IV)**.
10. Louis DS, Ricciardi JE, Spengler DM. Arterial injury: a complication of posterior elbow dislocation. A clinical and anatomical study. *J Bone Joint Surg Am.* 1974;56(8):1631–1636. **(LOE IV)**.
11. Wilkins K. Fractures and dislocations of the elbow region. In: Rockwood C, King R, eds. *Fractures in Children.* Philadelphia: J.B. Lippincott; 1984:363–450. **(LOE N/A)**.
12. Murphy WA, Siegel MJ. Elbow fat pads with new signs and extended differential diagnosis. *Radiology.* 1977;124(3):659–665. **(LOE II)**.
13. de Beaux AC, Beattie T, Gilbert F. Elbow fat pad sign: implications for clinical management. *J R Coll Surg Edinb.* 1992;37(3):205–206. **(LOE IV)**.
14. Skaggs D, Mirzayan R. The posterior fat pad sign in association with occult fracture of the elbow in children. *J Bone Joint Surg Am.* 1999;81(10):1429–1433. **(LOE IV)**.
15. Williamson D, Coates C, Miller R, Cole W. Normal characteristics of the Baumann (humerocapitellar) angle: an aid in assessment of supracondylar fractures. *J Pediatr Orthop.* 1992;12(5):636–639. **(LOE III)**.
16. Dodge H. Displaced supracondylar fractures of the humerus in children. Treatment by Dunlop's traction. *J Bone Joint Surg Am.* 1972;54(7):1408–1418. **(LOE IV)**.
17. Reinaerts HH, Cheriex EC. Assessment of dislocation in the supracondylar fracture of the humerus, treated by overhead traction. *Reconstr Surg Traumatol.* 1979;17:92–99. **(LOE IV)**.
18. Aronson DD, Prager BI. Supracondylar fractures of the humerus in children. A modified technique for closed pinning. *Clin Orthop Relat Res.* 1987;219:174–184. **(LOE IV)**.

19. Camp J, Ishizu K, Gomez M, et al. Alteration of Baumann's angle by humeral position: implications for treatment of supracondylar humerus fractures. *J Pediatr Orthop.* 1993;13(4):521–525. (**LOE IV**).

20. Biyani A, Gupta SP, Sharma JC. Determination of medial epicondylar epiphyseal angle for supracondylar humeral fractures in children. *J Pediatr Orthop.* 1993;13(1):94–97. (**LOE IV**).

21. Rogers LF, Malave Jr S, White H, et al. Plastic bowing, torus and greenstick supracondylar fractures of the humerus: radiographic clues to the obscure fractures of the elbow in children. *Radiology.* 1978;128(1):145–150. (**LOE III**).

22. Skibo L, Reed MH. A criterion for a true lateral radiograph of the elbow in children. *Can Assoc Radiol J.* 1994;45(4):287–291. (**LOE III**).

23. Herman M, Boardman M, Hoover J, Chafetz R. Relationship of the anterior humeral line to the capitellar ossific nucleus: variability with age. *J Bone Joint Surg Am.* 2009;91(9):2188–2193. (**LOE III**).

24. Murphy-Zane MS, Pyle L. Reliability of the anterior humeral line index compared with the Gartland classification for posteriorly hinged supracondylar humerus fractures. *Orthopedics.* 2018;41(4):e502–e505. (**LOE IV**).

25. Cheng JC, Lam TP, Shen WY. Closed reduction and percutaneous pinning for type III displaced supracondylar fractures of the humerus in children. *J Orthop Trauma.* 1995;9(6):511–515. (**LOE IV**).

26. Pudas T, Hurme T, Mattila K, Svedström E. Magnetic resonance imaging in pediatric elbow fractures. *Acta Radiol.* 2005;46(6):636–644. (**LOE V**).

27. Beltran J, Rosenberg ZS, Kawelblum M, et al. Pediatric elbow fractures: MRI evaluation. *Skeletal Radiol.* 1994;23(4):277–281. (**LOE IV**).

28. Davidson RS, Markowitz RI, Domans J, et al. Ultrasonographic evaluation of the elbow in infants and young children after suspected trauma. *J Bone Joint Surg Am.* 1994;76(12):1804–1813. (**LOE III**).

29. Rabiner J, Khine H, Avner J, Friedman L, Tsung J. Accuracy of point-of-care ultrasonography for diagnosis of elbow fractures in children. *Ann Emerg Med.* 2013;61(1):9–17. (**LOE III**).

30. Beals RK. The normal carrying angle of the elbow. A radiographic study of 422 patients. *Clin Orthop Relat Res.* 1976;119:194–196. (**LOE III**).

31. Abzug J, Herman M. Management of supracondylar humerus fractures in children: current concepts. *J Am Acad Orthop Surg.* 2012;20:69–77. (**LOE V**).

32. Cheng J, Ng B, Ying S, Lam P. A 10-year study of the changes in the pattern and treatment of 6,493 fractures. *J Pediatr Orthop.* 1999;19(3):344–350. (**LOE II**).

33. Cheng JC, Shen WY. Limb fractures pattern in different pediatric age groups: a study of 3,350 children. *J Orthop Trauma.* 1993;7(1):15–22. (**LOE II**).

34. Henrikson B. Supracondylar fracture of the humerus in children. A late review of end-results with special reference to the cause of deformity, disability and complications. *Acta Chir Scand Suppl.* 1966;369:1–72. (**LOE III**).

35. Otsuka N, Kasser J. Supracondylar fractures of the humerus in children. *J Am Acad Orthop Surg.* 1997;5(1):19–26. (**LOE V**).

36. Nork SE, Hennrikus WL, Loncarich DP, et al. Relationship between ligamentous laxity and the site of upper extremity fractures in children: extension supracondylar fracture versus distal forearm fracture. *J Pediatr Orthop B.* 1999;8(2):90–92. (**LOE III**).

37. Abraham E, Powers T, Witt T, et al. Experimental hyperextension supracondylar fractures in monkeys. *Clin Orthop Relat Res.* 1982;171:309–318. (**LOE V**).

38. Blakemore L, Cooperman D, Thompson G, Wathey C, Ballock R. Compartment syndrome in ipsilateral humerus and forearm in children. *Clin Orthop Relat Res.* 2000;376:32–38. (**LOE IV**).

39. Campbell C, Waters P, Emans J, et al. Neurovascular injury and displacement in type III supracondylar humerus fractures. *J Pediatr Orthop.* 1995;15(1):47–52. (**LOE III**).

40. Babal J, Mehlman C, LKlein G. Nerve injuries associated with pediatric supracondylar humeral fractures. A meta-analysis. *J Pediatr Orthop.* 2010;30(3):253–263. (**LOE II**).

41. Garg S, Weller A, Larson M, et al. Clinical characteristics of severe supracondylar humerus fractures in children. *J Pediatr Orthop.* 2013;34(1):34–39. (**LOE II**).

42. Cramer KE, Green NE, Devito DP. Incidence of anterior interosseous nerve palsy in supracondylar humerus fractures in children. *J Pediatr Orthop.* 1993;13(4):502–505. (**LOE IV**).

43. Dormans JP, Squillante R, Sharf H. Acute neurovascular complications with supracondylar humerus fractures in children. *J Hand Surg Am.* 1995;20(1):1–4. (**LOE IV**).

44. Jones ET, Louis DS. Median nerve injuries associated with supracondylar fractures of the humerus in children. *Clin Orthop Relat Res.* 1980;150:181–186. (**LOE IV**).

45. Spinner M, Schreiber SN. Anterior interosseous nerve paralysis as a complication of supracondylar fractures of the humerus in children. *J Bone Joint Surg Am.* 1969;51(8):1584–1590. (**LOE V**).

46. Mangat K, Martin A, Bache C. The "pulseless pink" hand after supracondylar fracture of the humerus in children: the predictive value of nerve palsy. *J Bone Joint Surg Br.* 2009;91(11):1521–1525. (**LOE III**).

47. Harris LR, Arkader A, Broom A, et al. Pulseless supracondylar humerus fracture with anterior interosseous nerve or median nerve injury–an absolute indication for open reduction? *J Pediatr Orthop.* 2019;39(1):e1–e7. (**LOE IV**).

48. Gartland JJ. Management of supracondylar fractures of the humerus in children. *Surg Gynecol Obstet.* 1959;109(2):145–154. (**LOE IV**).

49. O'Hara L, Barlow J, Clark N. Displaced supracondylar fractures of the humerus in children. Audit changes practice. *J Bone Joint Surg Br.* 2000;82(2):204–210. (**LOE III**).

50. Leitch K, Kay R, Famino J. Treatment of multidirectionally unstable supracondylar humeral fractures in children. A modified Gartland type-IV fracture. *J Bone Joint Surg Am.* 2006;88(5):980–985. (**LOE III**).

51. White L, Mehlman C, Crawford A. Perfused, pulseless, and puzzling: a systematic review of vascular injuries in pediatric supracondylar humerus fractures and results of a POSNA questionnaire. *J Pediatr Orthop.* 2010;30(4):328–335. (**LOE II**).

52. Bae D, Kadiyala R, Waters P. Acute compartment syndrome in children: contemporary diagnosis, treatment, and outcome. *J Pediatr Orthop.* 2001;21(5):680–688. (**LOE IV**).

53. Rang M, Moseley CF, Roberts JM, et al. Symposium: management of displaced supracondylar fractures of the humerus. *Contemp Orthoped.* 1989;18:497–535. (**LOE V**).

54. De Boeck H, De Smet P, Penders W, et al. Supracondylar elbow fractures with impaction of the medial condyle in children. *J Pediatr Orthop.* 1995;15(4):444–448. (**LOE IV**).

55. Parikh S, Wall E, Foad S, Wiersma B, Nolte B. Displaced type II extension supracondylar humerus fractures: do they all need pinning? *J Pediatr Orthop.* 2004;24(4):380–384. (**LOE III**).

56. Gordon J, Patton C, Luhman S, Bassett G, Schoenecker P. Fracture stability after pinning of displaced supracondylar distal humerus fractures in children. *J Pediatr Orthop.* 2001;21(3):313–318. (**LOE III**).

57. Millis MB, Singer IJ, Hall JE. Supracondylar fracture of the humerus in children. Further experience with a study in orthopaedic decision-making. *Clin Orthop Relat Res.* 1984;188:90–97. (**LOE IV**).

58. Skaggs D, Sankar W, Albrektson J, Vaishna S, Choi P, Kay R. How safe is the operative treatment of Gartland type 2 supracondylar humerus fractures in children? *J Pediatr Orthop.* 2008;28(2):139–141. (**LOE III**).

59. Kurer M, Regan M. Completely displaced supracondylar fracture of the humerus in children. *Clin Orthop Relat Res.* 1990;256:205–214. (**LOE IV**).

60. Pirone A, Graham H, Krajbich J. Management of displaced extension-type supracondylar fractures of the humerus in children. *J Bone Joint Surg Am.* 1988;70:641–650. (**LOE IV**).

61. Howard A, Mulpuri K, Abel M, et al. The treatment of pediatric supracondylar humerus fractures. *J Am Acad Orthop Surg.* 2012;20:320–327. (**LOE II**).

62. Arnold JA, Nasca RJ, Nelson CL. Supracondylar fractures of the humerus: the role of dynamic factors in prevention of deformity. *J Bone Joint Surg Am.* 1977;59(5):589–595. (**LOE IV**).

63. Mapes RC, Hennrikus WL. The effect of elbow position on the radial pulse measured by Doppler ultrasonography after surgical treatment of supracondylar elbow fractures in children. *J Pediatr Orthop.* 1998;18(4):441–444. (**LOE III**).

64. Swenson A. The treatment of supracondylar fractures of the humerus by Kirschner wire transfixion. *J Bone Joint Surg Am.* 1948;993–997. **(LOE IV).**

65. Casiano E. Reduction and fixation by pinning "banderillero"-style fractures of the humerus at the elbow in children. *Mil Med.* 1961;125:262–264. **(LOE IV).**

66. Skaggs D, Hale J, Bassett J, Kaminsky C, Kay V. Operative treatment of supracondylar fractures of the humerus in children. The consequences of pin placement. *J Bone Joint Surg Am.* 2001;83(5):735–740. **(LOE III).**

67. Iobst C, Spurdle C, King W, Lopez M. Percutaneous pinning of pediatric supracondylar humerus fractures with the semisterile technique: the Miami experience. *J Pediatr Orthop.* 2007;27(1):17–22. **(LOE III).**

68. Peters CL, Scott SM, Stevens PM. Closed reduction and percutaneous pinning of displaced supracondylar humerus fractures in children: description of a new closed reduction technique for fractures with brachialis muscle entrapment. *J Orthop Trauma.* 1995;9(5):430–434. **(LOE IV).**

69. Rasool MN, Naidoo KS. Supracondylar fractures: posterolateral type with brachialis muscle penetration and neurovascular injury. *J Pediatr Orthop.* 1999;19(4):518–522. **(LOE IV).**

70. Herzenberg J, Koreska J, Carroll N, Rang M. Biomechanical testing of pinfixation techniques for pediatric supracondylar humerus fractures. *Orthopaedic Transactions.* 1988;12(12):678–679.

71. Lee SS, Mahar AT, Miesen D, et al. Displaced pediatric supracondylar humerus fractures: biomechanical analysis of percutaneous pinning techniques. *J Pediatr Orthop.* 2002;22(4):440–443. **(LOE V).**

72. Zionts LE, McKellop HA, Hathaway R. Torsional strength of pin configurations used to fix supracondylar fractures of the humerus in children. *J Bone Joint Surg Am.* 1994;76(2):253–256. **(LOE V).**

73. Topping RE, Blanco JS, Davis TJ. Clinical evaluation of crossed-pin versus lateral-pin fixation in displaced supracondylar humerus fractures. *J Pediatr Orthop.* 1995;15(4):435–439. **(LOE III).**

74. Kocher M, Kasser J, Waters P, et al. Lateral entry compared with medial and lateral entry pin fixation for completely displaced supracondylar humeral fractures in children. A randomized clinical trial. *J Bone Joint Surg Am.* 2007;89(4):713–717. **(LOE I).**

75. Gaston R, Cates T, Devito D, et al. Medial and lateral entry pin versus lateral entry pin fixation for type 3 supracondylar fractures in children: a randomized, surgeon randomized study. *J Pediatr Orthop.* 2010;30(8):799–806. **(LOE I).**

76. Bloom T, Robertson C, Mahar A, Newton P. Biomechanical analysis of supracondylar humerus fracture pinning for slightly malreduced fractures. *J Pediatr Orthop.* 2008;28:766–772.

77. Sankar W, Hebela N, Skaggs D, Flynn J. Loss of pin fixation in displaced supracondylar humeral fractures in children: causes and prevention. *J Bone Joint Surg Am.* 2007;89(4):713–717. **(LOE III).**

78. Zenios M, Ramachandran M, Milne B, Little D, Smith N. Intraoperative stability testing of lateral-entry pin fixation of pediatric supracondylar humeral fractures. *J Pediatr Orthop.* 2007;27:695–702. **(LOE III).**

79. Bauer JM, Stutz CM, Schoenecker JG, Lovejoy SA, Mencio GA, Martus JE. Internal rotation stress testing improves radiographic outcomes of type 3 supracondylar humerus fractures. *J Pediatr Orthop.* 2019;39(1):8–13. **(LOE III).**

80. D'Souza S, Vaishya R, Klenerman L. Management of radial neck fractures in children: a retrospective analysis of one hundred patients. *J Pediatr Orthop.* 1993;13(2):232–238. **(LOE III).**

81. Eren A, Güven M, Erol B, Akman B, Özkan K. Correlation between posteromedial or posterolateral displacement and cubitus varus deformity in supracondylar humerus fractures in children. *J Child Orthop.* 2008;2(2):85–89. **(LOE IV).**

82. Green DW, Widmann RF, Frank JS, et al. Low incidence of ulnar nerve injury with crossed pin placement for pediatric supracondylar humerus fractures using a mini-open technique. *J Orthop Trauma.* 2005;19(3):158–163. **(LOE III).**

83. Adams AJ, Buczek MJ, Flynn JM, Shah AS. Perioperative ketorolac for supracondylar humerus fracture in children decreases postoperative pain, opioid usage, hospitalization cost, and length-of-stay. *J Pediatr Orthop.* 2019.

84. Karalius VP, Stanfield J, Ashley P, et al. The utility of routine postoperative radiographs after pinning of pediatric supracondylar humerus fractures. *J Pediatr Orthop.* 2017;37(5):e309–e312. **(LOE IV).**

85. Brauer C, Lee B, Bae D, Waters P, Kocher M. A systematic review of medial and lateral entry pinning versus lateral entry pinning for supracondylar fractures of the humerus. *J Pediatr Orthop.* 2007;27(2):181–186. **(LOE V).**

86. Slobogean B, Jackman H, Tennant S, Slobogean G, Mulpuri K. Iatrogenic ulnar nerve injury after the surgical treatment of displaced supracondylar fractures of the humerus: number needed to harm, a systematic review. *J Pediatr Orthop.* 2010;30(5):430–436. **(LOE II).**

87. Sawaizumi T, Takayama A, Ito H. Surgical technique for supracondylar fracture of the humerus with percutaneous leverage pinning. *J Shoulder Elbow Surg.* 2003;12(6):603–606. **(LOE IV).**

88. Yu SW, Su JY, Kao FC, et al. The use of the 3-mm K-Wire to supplement reduction of humeral supracondylar fractures in children. *J Trauma.* 2004;57(5):1038–1042. **(LOE IV).**

89. Archieck M, Scott S, Peters C. Brachialis muscle entrapment in displaced supracondylar humerus fractures: a technique of closed reduction and report of initial results. *J Pediatr Orthop.* 1997;17:298–302. **(LOE IV).**

90. Fleuriau-Chateau P, McIntyre W, Letts WM. An analysis of open reduction of irreducible supracondylar fractures of the humerus in children. *Can J Surg.* 1998;41(2):112–118. **(LOE III).**

91. Cramer KE, Devito DP, Green NE. Comparison of closed reduction and percutaneous pinning versus open reduction and percutaneous pinning in displaced supracondylar fractures of the humerus in children. *J Orthop Trauma.* 1992;6(4):407–412. **(LOE III).**

92. Ozkoc G, Gonc U, Kayaalp A, et al. Displaced supracondylar humeral fractures in children: open reduction vs. closed reduction and pinning. *Arch Orthop Trauma Surg.* 2004;124(8):547–551. **(LOE III).**

93. Koudstaal MJ, De Ridder VA, De Lange S, et al. Pediatric supracondylar humerus fractures: the anterior approach. *J Orthop Trauma.* 2002;16(6):409–412. **(LOE III).**

94. Ay S, Akinci M, Kamiloglu S, et al. Open reduction of displaced pediatric supracondylar humeral fractures through the anterior cubital approach. *J Pediatr Orthop.* 2005;25(2):149–153. **(LOE IV).**

95. Green NE. Overnight delay in the reduction of supracondylar fractures of the humerus in children. *J Bone Joint Surg Am.* 2001;83–A(3):321–322. **(LOE V).**

96. Mehlman CT, Strub WM, Roy DR, et al. The effect of surgical timing on the perioperative complications of treatment of supracondylar humeral fractures in children. *J Bone Joint Surg Am.* 2001;83–A(3):323–327. **(LOE III).**

97. Iyengar S, Hoffinger S, Townsend D. Early versus delayed reduction and pinning of type III displaced supracondylar fractures of the humerus in children: a comparative study. *J Orthop Trauma.* 1999;13(1):51–55. **(LOE III).**

98. Leet AI, Frisancho J, Ebramzadeh E. Delayed treatment of type 3 supracondylar humerus fractures in children. *J Pediatr Orthop.* 2002;22(2):203–207. **(LOE IV).**

99. Gupta N, Kay RM, Leitch K, et al. Effect of surgical delay on perioperative complications and need for open reduction in supracondylar humerus fractures of the elbow in children. *Clin Orthop Relat Res.* 2004;71:112–117. **(LOE III).**

100. Bales J, Spencer H, Wong M, Fong Y, Zionts L, Silva M. The effects of surgical delay on the outcome of pediatric supracondylar humeral fractures. *J Pediatr Orthop.* 2004;30(8):785–791. **(LOE III).**

101. Sabharwal S, Tredwell S, Beauchamp R, et al. Management of pulseless pink hand in pediatric supracondylar fractures of humerus. *J Pediatr Orthop.* 1997;17(3):303–310. **(LOE III).**

102. Copley LA, Dormans JP, Davidson RS. Vascular injuries and their sequelae in pediatric supracondylar humeral fractures: toward a goal of prevention. *J Pediatr Orthop.* 1996;16(1):99–103. **(LOE III).**

103. Eilert R, Epps H, Frick S, Mehlman C, Skaggs D. Supracondylar fractures in children: current concepts and treatment considerations (round table). *Orthopedics Today.* 2011;31(11):50–57. **(LOE V).**

104. Schoenecker PL, Delgado E, Rotman M, et al. Pulseless arm in association with totally displaced supracondylar fracture. *J Orthop Trauma.* 1996;10(6):410–415. **(LOE III).**

105. Garbuz DS, Leithch K, Wright JG. The treatment of supracondylar fractures in children with an absent radial pulse. *J Pediatr Orthop.* 1996;16(5):594–596. **(LOE III).**

106. Choi P, Melikian R, Skaggs D. Risk factors for vascular repair and compartment syndrome in the pulseless supracondylar humerus fracture in children. *J Pediatr Orthop.* 2010;30(1):50–56. **(LOE III).**

107. Reigstad O, Thorkildsen R, Grimsgaard C, et al. Supracondylar fractures with circulatory failure after reduction, pinning, and entrapment of the brachial artery: excellent results more than 1 year after open exploration and revascularization. *J Orthop Trauma.* 2011;25(1):26–30. **(LOE IV).**

108. Blakey CM, Biant LC, Birch R. Ischaemia and the pink, pulseless hand complicating supracondylar fractures of the humerus in childhood: long-term follow-up. *J Bone Joint Surg Br.* 2009;91(11):1487–1492. **(LOE IV).**

109. Roposch A, Reis M, Molina M, et al. Supracondylar fractures of the humerus associated with ipsilateral forearm fractures in children: a report of forty-seven cases. *J Pediatr Orthop.* 2001;21:307–312. **(LOE IV).**

110. Noonan K, McCarthy J. Compartment syndromes in the pediatric patient. *J Pediatr Orthop.* 2010;30(S96–S101). **(LOE IV).**

111. Kiyoshige Y. Critical displacement of neural injuries in supracondylar humeral fractures in children. *J Pediatr Orthop.* 1999;19(6):816–817. **(LOE III).**

112. McGraw JJ, Akbarnia BA, Hanel DP, et al. Neurological complications resulting from supracondylar fractures of the humerus in children. *J Pediatr Orthop.* 1986;6(6):647–650. **(LOE IV).**

113. Culp R, Osterman A. Neural injuries associated with supracondylar fractures of the humerus in children. *J Bone Joint Surg Am.* 1990;72:1211–1215. **(LOE IV).**

114. Amillo SG, Mora G. Surgical management of neural injuries associated with elbow fractures in children. *J Pediatr Orthop.* 1999;19(5):573–577. **(LOE IV).**

115. Arino VL, Lluch EE, Ramirez AM, et al. Percutaneous fixation of supracondylar fractures of the humerus in children. *J Bone Joint Surg Am.* 1977;59(7):914–916. **(LOE IV).**

116. DeRosa GP, Graziano GP. A new osteotomy for cubitus varus. *Clin Orthop Relat Res.* 1988;236:160–165. **(LOE IV).**

117. Flynn J, Sarwark J, Waters P, Bae D, Lemke L. The operative management of pediatric fractures of the upper extremity. *J Bone Joint Surg Am.* 2002;84:2078–2089. **(LOE V).**

118. Mann TS. Prognosis in supracondylar fractures. *J Bone Joint Surg Br.* 1963;45:516–522. **(LOE IV).**

119. Bakalim G, Wilppula E. Supracondylar humeral fractures in children. Causes of changes in the carrying angle of the elbow. *Acta Orthop Scand.* 1972;43(5):366–374. **(LOE III).**

120. Ippolito E, Moneta M, D'Arrigo C. Post-traumatic cubitus varus. Long-term follow-up of corrective supracondylar humeral osteotomy in children. *J Bone Joint Surg [Am].* 1990;72(5):757–765. **(LOE IV).**

121. Theruvil B, Kapoor V, Fairhurst J, Taylor G. Progressive cubitus varus due to a bony physeal bar in a 4-year-old girl following a supracondylar fracture: a case report. *J Orthop Trauma.* 2005;19(9):669–672. **(LOE V).**

122. Voss F, Kasser J, Trepman E, Simmons E, Hall J. Uniplanar supracondylar humeral osteotomy with preset Kirschner wires for posttraumatic cubitus varus. *J Pediatr Orthop.* 1994;14(471–478). **(LOE IV).**

123. Abe M, Ishizu T, Shirai H, et al. Tardy ulnar nerve palsy caused by cubitus varus deformity. *J Hand Surg Am.* 1995;20(1):5–9. **(LOE IV).**

124. Mitsunari A, Muneshige H, Ikuta Y, et al. Internal rotation deformity and tardy ulnar nerve palsy after supracondylar humeral fracture. *J Shoulder Elbow Surg.* 1995;4(1Pt 1):23–29. **(LOE IV).**

125. Spinner RJ, O'Driscoll SW, Davids JR, et al. Cubitus varus associated with dislocation of both the medial portion of the triceps and the ulnar nerve. *J Hand Surg Am.* 1999;24(4):718–726. **(LOE V).**

126. Davids JR, Maguire MG, Mubarak SJ, et al. Lateral condylar fracture of the humerus following posttraumatic cubitus varus. *J Pediatr Orthop.* 1994;14(4):466–470. **(LOE III).**

127. Takahara M, Sasaki I, Kimura T, et al. Second fracture of the distal humerus after varus malunion of a supracondylar fracture in children. *J Bone Joint Surg Br.* 1998;80(5):791–797. **(LOE V).**

128. O'Driscoll SW, Spinner RJ, McKee MD, et al. Tardy posterolateral rotatory instability of the elbow due to cubitus varus. *J Bone Joint Surg Am.* 2001;83–A(9):1358–1369. **(LOE V).**

129. Fowles JV, Slimane N, Kassab MT. Elbow dislocation with avulsion of the medial humeral epicondyle. *J Bone Joint Surg Br.* 1990;72(1):102–104. **(LOE IV).**

130. Mahan S, May C, Kocher M. Operative management of displaced flexion supracondylar humerus fractures in children. *J Pediatr Orthop.* 2007;27(5):551–556. **(LOE III).**

131. Green BM, Stone JD, Bruce Jr RW, Fletcher ND. The use of a transolecranon pin in the treatment of pediatric flexion-type supracondylar humerus fractures. *J Pediatr Orthop.* 2017;37(6):e347–e352. **(LOE IV).**

132. Dameron Jr TB. Transverse fractures of distal humerus in children. *Instr Course Lect.* 1981;30:224–235. **(LOE V).**

133. DeLee JC, Wilkins KE, Rogers KF, et al. Fracture-separation of the distal humeral epiphysis. *J Bone Joint Surg Am.* 1980;62(1):46–51. **(LOE IV).**

134. Holda M, Manoli A 2nd, LaMont R. Epiphyseal separation of the distal end of the humerus with medial displacement. *J Bone Joint Surg [Am].* 1980;62(1):52–57. **(LOE IV).**

135. de Jager LT, Hoffman EB. Fracture-separation of the distal humeral epiphysis. *J Bone Joint Surg Br.* 1991;73(1):143–146. **(LOE IV).**

136. Markowitz RI, Davidson RS, Harty MP, et al. Sonography of the elbow in infants and children. *AJR Am J Roentgenol.* 1992;159(4):829–833. **(LOE III).**

137. Mizuno K, Hirohata K, Kashiwagi D. Fracture-separation of the distal humeral epiphysis in young children. *J Bone Joint Surg Am.* 1979;61(4):570–573. **(LOE IV).**

138. Chou ACC, Wong HYK, Kumar S, Mahadev A. Using the medial and lateral humeral lines as an adjunct to intraoperative elbow arthrography to guide intraoperative reduction and fixation of distal humerus physeal separations reduces the incidence of postoperative cubitus varus. *J Pediatr Orthop.* 2018;38(5):e262–e266. **(LOE IV).**

139. Popkin CA, Rosenwasser KA, Ellis Jr HB. Pediatric and adolescent T-type distal humerus fractures. *J Am Acad Orthop Surg Glob Res Rev.* 2017;1(8):e040. **(LOE V).**

140. Jarvis J, D'Astous J. The pediatric T-supracondylar fracture. *J Pediatr Orthop.* 1984;4(6):697–699. **(LOE IV).**

141. Kanellopoulos A, Yiannakopoulos C. Closed reduction and percutaneous stabilization of pediatric T-condylar fractures of the humerus. *J Pediatr Orthop.* 2004;24(13–16). **(LOE IV).**

142. Ruiz A, Kealey W, Cowie H. Percutaneous pin fixation of intercondylar fractures in young children. *J Pediatr Orthop B.* 2001;10:211–213. **(LOE III).**

143. Re P, Waters P, Hresko T. T-condylar fractures of the distal humerus in children and adolescents. *J Pediatr Orthop.* 1999;19(3):313–318. **(LOE III).**

144. Kasser J, Richards K, Millis M. The triceps-dividing approach to open reduction of complex distal humerus fractures in adolescents: a Cybex evaluation of triceps function and motion. *J Pediatr Orthop.* 1990;10:93–96. **(LOE III).**

145. Bryan R, Morrey B. Extensive posterior exposure of the elbow. A triceps-sparing approach. *Clin Orthop Relat Res.* 1982;166:188–192. **(LOE IV).**

146. Remia L, Richards K, Waters P. The Bryan-Morrey triceps-sparing approach to open reduction of T-condylar humeral fractures in adolescents: cybex evaluation of triceps function and elbow motion. *J Pediatr Orthop.* 2004;24:615–619. **(LOE III).**

147. Anari JB, Neuwirth AL, Carducci NM, Donegan DJ, Baldwin KD. Pediatric T-condylar humerus fractures: a systematic review. *J Pediatr Orthop.* 2017;37(1):36–40. **(LOE V).**

148. Blumberg TJ, Bremjit P, Bompadre V, Steinman S. Forearm fixation is not necessary in the treatment of pediatric floating elbow. *J Pediatr Orthop.* 2018;38(2):82–87. **(LOE IV).**

149. Tejwani N, Phillips D, Goldstein R. Management of lateral humeral condylar fracture in children. *J Am Acad Orthop Surg.* 2011;19:350–358. **(LOE V).**

150. Milch H. Fractures and fracture dislocations of the humeral condyles. *J Trauma.* 1964;15:592–607. **(LOE IV).**

151. Flynn JC, Richards Jr JF, Saltzman RI. Prevention and treatment of non-union of slightly displaced fractures of the lateral humeral condyle in children. An end-result study. *J Bone Joint Surg Am.* 1975;57(8):1087–1092. **(LOE III).**

152. Jakob R, Fowles J, Rang M, et al. Observations concerning fractures of the lateral humeral condyle in children. *J Bone Joint Surg [Br].* 1975;57(4):430–436. **(LOE IV)**.
153. Stimson LA. *A Practical Treatise on Fractures and Dislocations*, 1900. **(LOE V)**.
154. Fahey JJ. Fractures of the elbow in children. *Instr Course Lect.* 1960;17:13–46. **(LOE V)**.
155. Milch H. Fractures of the external humeral condyle. *J Am Med Assoc.* 1956;160(8):641–646. **(LOE IV)**.
156. Mirsky EC, Karas EH, Weiner LS. Lateral condyle fractures in children: evaluation of classification and treatment. *J Orthop Trauma.* 1997;11(2):117–120. **(LOE III)**.
157. Finnbogason T, Karlsson J, Lindberg L, et al. Nondisplaced and minimally displaced fractures of the lateral humeral condyle in children: a prospective radiographic investigation of fracture stability. *J Pediatr Orthop.* 1995;15(4):422–425. **(LOE III)**.
158. Song K, Kang C, Byung W, Bae K, Cho C, Lee J. Closed reduction and internal fixation of displaced unstable lateral condylar fractures of the humerus in children. *J Bone Joint Surg Am.* 2008;90A(12):2673–2681. **(LOE II)**.
159. Song K, Shin Y, Chang W, Bae K, Cho C. Closed reduction and internal fixation of completely displaced and rotated lateral condyle fractures of the humerus in children. *J Orthop Trauma.* 2010;24(7):434–439. **(LOE II)**.
160. Chapman V, Grottkau B, Albright M, Salamipour H, Jaramillo D. Multidetector computed tomography of pediatric lateral condylar fractures. *J Comput Assist Tomogr.* 2005;29(6):842–846. **(LOE II)**.
161. Horn B, Herman M, Crisci K, Pizzitullo P, MacEwen G. Fractures of the lateral humeral condyle: role of the cartilage hinge in fracture stability. *J Pediatr Orthop.* 2002;22(1):8–11. **(LOE III)**.
162. Kamegaya M, Shinohara Y, Kurokawa M, Ogata S. Assessment of stability in children's minimally displaced lateral condyle fracture by magnetic resonance imaging. *J Pediatr Orthop.* 1999;19(5):570–572. **(LOE II)**.
163. Vocke-Hell A, Schmid A. Sonographic differentiation of stable and unstable lateral condyle fractures of the humerus in children. *J Pediatr Orthop B.* 2001;10(2):138–141. **(LOE II)**.
164. Marzo J, d'Amato C. Usefulness and accuracy of arthrography in management of lateral humeral condyle fractures in children. *J Pediatr Orthop.* 1990;10(3):317–321. **(LOE III)**.
165. Pirker ME, Weinberg AM, Hollwarth ME, et al. Subsequent displacement of initially nondisplaced and minimally displaced fractures of the lateral humeral condyle in children. *J Trauma.* 2005;58(6):1202–1207. **(LOE III)**.
166. Bast SC, Hoffer MM, Aval S. Nonoperative treatment for minimally and nondisplaced lateral humeral condyle fractures in children. *J Pediatr Orthop.* 1998;18(4):448–450. **(LOE IV)**.
167. Zale C, Winthrop ZA, Hennrikus W. Rate of displacement for Jakob Type 1 lateral condyle fractures treated with a cast. *J Child Orthop.* 2018;12(2):117–122. **(LOE IV)**.
168. Greenhill DA, Funk S, Elliot M, Jo CH, Ramo BA. Minimally displaced humeral lateral condyle fractures: immobilize or operate when stability is unclear? *J Pediatr Orthop.* 2018. **(LOE III)**.
169. Mintzer CM, Waters PM, Brown DJ, et al. Percutaneous pinning in the treatment of displaced lateral condyle fractures. *J Pediatr Orthop.* 1994;14(4):462–465. **(LOE III)**.
170. Hennrikus W, Millis M. The dinner fork technique for treating displaced lateral condylar fractures of the humerus in children. *Orthop Rev.* 1993;22(11):1278–1280. **(LOE IV)**.
171. Launay F, Leet A, Jacopin S, Bollini G, Sponseller P. Lateral humeral condyle fractures in children: a comparison of two approaches to treatment. *J Pediatr Orthop.* 2004;18(4):448–450. **(LOE III)**.
172. Chan L, Siow H. Exposed versus buried wires for fixation of lateral humeral condyle fractures in children: a comparison of safety and efficacy. *J Child Orthop.* 2011;5(5):329–333. **(LOE III)**.
173. Ganeshalingam R, Donnan A, Evans O, Hoq M, Camp M, Donnan L. Lateral condylar fractures of the humerus in children. *Bone Joint J.* 2018;100-B(3):387–395. **(LOE IV)**.
174. Dhillon KS, Sengupta S, Singh BJ. Delayed management of fracture of the lateral humeral condyle in children. *Acta Orthop Scand.* 1988;59(4):419–424. **(LOE III)**.
175. Mehserle WL, Meehan PL. Treatment of the displaced supracondylar fracture of the humerus (type III) with closed reduction and percutaneous cross-pin fixation. *J Pediatr Orthop.* 1991;11(6):705–711. **(LOE III)**.
176. Roye DP Jr, Bini SA, Infosino A. Late surgical treatment of lateral condylar fractures in children. *J Pediatr Orthop.* 1991;11(2):195–199. **(LOE IV)**.
177. Gaur SC, Varma AN, Swarup A. A new surgical technique for old ununited lateral condyle fractures of the humerus in children. *J Trauma.* 1993;34(1):68–69. **(LOE IV)**.
178. Saraf S, Khare G. Late presentation of fractures of the lateral condyle of the humerus in children. *Indian J Orthop.* 2011;45(1):39–44. **(LOE IV)**.
179. Agarwal A, Qureshi N, Gupta N, et al. Management of neglected lateral condyle fractures of humerus in children: a retrospective study. *Indian J Orthop.* 2012;46(6):698–704. **(LOE IV)**.
180. Thomas D, Howard A, Cole W, Hedden D. Three weeks of Kirschner wire fixation for displaced lateral condylar fractures of the humerus in children. *J Pediatr Orthop.* 2001;21(5):565–569. **(LOE III)**.
181. Pace JL, Arkader A, Sousa T, Broom AM, Shabtai L. Incidence, risk factors, and definition for nonunion in pediatric lateral condyle fractures. *J Pediatr Orthop.* 2018;38(5):e257–e261. **(LOE IV)**.
182. Flynn J. Nonunion of slightly displaced fractures of the lateral humeral condyle in children: an update. *J Pediatr Orthop.* 1989;9(6):691–696. **(LOE III)**.
183. Wattenbarger J, Gerardi J, Johnston C. Late open reduction internal fixation of lateral condyle fractures. *J Pediatr Orthop.* 2002;22(3):394–398. **(LOE III)**.
184. Masada K, Kawai H, Kawabata H, et al. Osteosynthesis for old, established non-union of the lateral condyle of the humerus. *J Bone Joint Surg Am.* 1990;72(1):32–40. **(LOE IV)**.
185. Tien YC, Chen JC, Fu YC, et al. Supracondylar dome osteotomy for cubitus valgus deformity associated with a lateral condylar nonunion in children. *J Bone Joint Surg Am.* 2005;87(7):1456–1463. **(LOE IV)**.
186. Skak S, Olsen S, Smaabrekke A. Deformity after fracture of the lateral humeral condyle in children. *J Pediatr Orthop Br.* 2001;10(2):142–152. **(LOE IV)**.
187. Letts M, Rumball K, Bauermeister S, et al. Fractures of the capitellum in adolescents. *J Pediatr Orthop.* 1997;17(3):315–320. **(LOE IV)**.
188. De Boeck H, Pouliart N. Fractures of the capitellum humeri in adolescents. *Int Orthop.* 2000;24(5):246–248. **(LOE IV)**.
189. Onay T, Gumustas SA, Baykan SE, Akgulle AH, Erol B, Irgit KS. Mid-term and long-term functional and radiographic results of 13 surgically treated adolescent capitellum fractures. *J Pediatr Orthop.* 2018;38(8):e424–e428. **(LOE IV)**.
190. Bensahel H, Csukonyi Z, Badelon O, et al. Fractures of the medial condyle of the humerus in children. *J Pediatr Orthop.* 1986;6(4):430–433. **(LOE IV)**.
191. Fowles JV, Kassab MT. Displaced fractures of the medial humeral condyle in children. *J Bone Joint Surg Am.* 1980;62(7):1159–1163. **(LOE IV)**.
192. Kilfoyle RM. Fractures of the medial condyle and epicondyle of the elbow in children. *Clin Orthop Relat Res.* 1965;41:43–50. **(LOE III)**.
193. Varma BP, Srivastava TP. Fracture of the medial condyle of the humerus in children: a report of 4 cases including the late sequelae. *Injury.* 1972;4(2):171–174. **(LOE IV)**.
194. Leet A, Young C, Hoffer M. Medial condyle fractures of the humerus in children. *J Pediatr Orthop.* 2002;22(1):2–7. **(LOE IV)**.
195. Fernandez FF, Vatlach S, Wirth T, Eberhardt O. Medial humeral condyle fracture in childhood: a rare but often overlooked injury. *Eur J Trauma Emerg Surg.* 2018. **(LOE IV)**.
196. Gottschalk H, Eisner E, Hosalkar H. Medial epicondyle fractures in the pediatric population. *J Am Acad Orthop Surg.* 2012;20(4):223–232. **(LOE V)**.
197. Woods GW, Tullos HS. Elbow instability and medial epicondyle fractures. *Am J Sports Med.* 1977;5(1):23–30. **(LOE IV)**.
198. Smith FM. Children's elbow injuries: fractures and dislocations. *Clin Orthop Relat Res.* 1967;50:7–30. **(LOE V)**.
199. Smith FM. Medial epicondyle injuries. *JAMA.* 1950;142(6):396–402. **(LOE IV)**.
200. Lee H, Shen H, Chang J, Wu S. Operative treatment of displaced medial epicondyle fractures in children and adolescents. *J Shoulder Elbow Surg.* 2005;14(2):178–185. **(LOE IV)**.
201. Smith F. Displacement of the medial epicondyle of the humerus into the elbow joint. *Ann Surg.* 1946;12:410–425. **(LOE IV)**.

202. Pappas N, Lawrence J, Donegan D, Ganley T, Flynn J. Intraobserver and interobserver agreement in the measurement of displaced medial epicondyle fractures in children. *J Bone Joint Surg Am.* 2010;92(2):322–327. (**LOE II**).

203. Edmonds E. How displaced are "nondisplaced" fractures of the medial humeral epicondyle in children? Results of a three-dimensional computed tomography analysis. *J Bone Joint Am.* 2010;92(17):2785–2791. (**LOE II**).

204. Gottschalk H, Bastrom T, Edmonds E. Reliability of internal oblique elbow radiographs for measuring displacement of medial epicondyle humerus fractures: a cadaveric study. *J Pediatr Orthop.* 2013;33(1):26–31. (**LOE II**).

205. Souder CD, Farnsworth CL, McNeil NP, Bomar JD, Edmonds EW. The distal humerus axial view: assessment of displacement in medial epicondyle fractures. *J Pediatr Orthop.* 2015;35(5):449–454.

206. Bernstein SMK, Sanderson RA. Fractures of the medial epicondyle of the humerus. *Contemp Orthoped.* 1981;12:637–641. (**LOE IV**).

207. Farsetti P, Potenza V, Caterini R, Ippolito E. Long-term results of treatment of fractures of the medial humeral epicondyle in children. *J Bone Joint Surg Am.* 2001;83(9):1299–1305. (**LOE III**).

208. Josefsson P, Danielsson G. Epicondylar elbow fracture in children: 35 year follow-up of 56 unreduced cases. *Acta Orthop Scand.* 1986;57(4):313–315. (**LOE II**).

209. Kamath A, Baldwin K, Horneff J, Hosalkar H. Operative versus nonoperative management of pediatric medial epicondyle fractures: a systematic review. *J Child Orthop.* 2009;3(5):345–357. (**LOE III**).

210. Ip D, Tsang W. Medial humeral epicondylar fracture in children and adolescents. *J Orthop Surg (Hong Kong).* 2007;15(2):170–173. (**LOE IV**).

211. Bede WB, Lefebvre AR, Rosman MA. Fractures of the medial humeral epicondyle in children. *Can J Surg.* 1975;18(2):137–142. (**LOE IV**).

212. Peterson HA. Physeal injuries of the distal humerus. *Orthopaedics.* 1986;15(7):799–808. (**LOE IV**).

213. Knapik DM, Fausett CL, Gilmore A, Liu RW. Outcomes of nonoperative pediatric medial humeral epicondyle fractures with and without associated elbow dislocation. *J Pediatr Orthop.* 2017;37(4):e224–e228. (**LOE II**).

214. Marcu D, Balts J, McCarthy J, Kozin S, Noonan K. Iatrogenic radial nerve injury with cannulated fixation of medial epicondyle fractures in the pediatric humerus: a report of 2 cases. *J Pediatr Orthop.* 2011;31(2):e13–e16. (**LOE IV**)

215. Pace GI, Hennrikus WL. Fixation of displaced medial epicondyle fractures in adolescents. *J Pediatr Orthop.* 2017;37(2):e80–e82. (**LOE IV**).

216. Newman JH. Displaced radial neck fractures in children. *Injury.* 1977;9(2):114–121. (**LOE IV**).

217. Reidy JA, Vangorder GW. Treatment of displacement of the proximal radial epiphysis. *J Bone Joint Surg Am.* 1963;45:1355–1372. (**LOE IV**).

218. Vahvanen V, Gripenberg L. Fracture of the radial neck in children. A long-term follow-up study of 43 cases. *Acta Orthop Scand.* 1978;49(1):32–38. (**LOE III**).

219. Jeffery C. Fractures of the head of the radius in children. *J Bone Joint Surg (Br).* 1950;32:314–324. (**LOE IV**).

220. Chambers H. Fractures of the proximal radius and ulna. In: Kasser J, Beaty J, eds. *Rockwood and Wilkins' Fractures in Children.* 5th ed. Philadelphia: Lippincott, Williams and Wilkins; 2001:483–528.

221. Olney B, Menelaus M. Monteggia and equivalent lesions in childhood. *J Pediatr Orthop.* 1989;9:219–223. (**LOE III**).

222. Greenspan A, Norman A. The radial head-capitellum view: useful technique in elbow trauma. *Am J Roentgenol.* 1982;138:1186–1188. (**LOE III**).

223. Javed A, Guichet J. Arthrography for reduction of a fracture of the radial neck in a child with a nonossified radial epiphysis. *J Bone Joint Surg Br.* 2001;83:542–543. (**LOE IV**).

224. Lazar R, Waters P, Jaramillo D. The use of ultrasonography in the diagnosis of occult fracture of the radial neck. A case report. *J Bone Joint Surg Am.* 1998;80:1361–1364. (**LOE V**).

225. Jones E, Esah M. Displaced fractures of the neck of the radius in children. *J Bone Joint Surg Br.* 1971;53(3):429–439. (**LOE IV**).

226. Salter R, Harris W. Injuries involving the epiphyseal plate. *J Bone Joint Surg Am.* 1963;45:587–592. (**LOE III**).

227. Tibone JE, Stoltz M. Fractures of the radial head and neck in children. *J Bone Joint Surg Am.* 1981;63(1):100–106. (**LOE IV**).

228. McBride EM, Monnet J. Epiphyseal fracture of the head of the radius in children. *Clin Orthop.* 1960;16:264–271. (**LOE IV**).

229. Vocke A, Von Laer L. Displaced fractures of the radial neck in children: long term results and prognosis of conservative treatment. *J Pediatr Orthop B.* 1998;7:217–222. (**LOE II**).

230. Patterson R. Treatment of displaced transverse fractures of the neck of the radius in children. *J Bone Joint Surg Am.* 1934;16:695–698. (**LOE IV**).

231. Kaufman B, Rinott M, Tanzman M. Closed reduction of fractures of the proximal radius in children. *J Bone Joint Surg Br.* 1989;71(66–67). (**LOE IV**).

232. Neher C, Torch M. New reduction technique for severely displaced pediatric radial neck fractures. *J Pediatr Orthop.* 2003;23:626–628. (**LOE IV**).

233. Angelov A. A new method for treatment of the dislocated radial neck fracture in children. In: Chapchal G, ed. *Fractures in Children.* 1981:192–194. (**LOE N/A**).

234. Steele JA, Graham HK. Angulated radial neck fractures in children. A prospective study of percutaneous reduction. *J Bone Joint Surg Br.* 1992;74(5):760–764. (**LOE II**).

235. Dormans JP. Arthrographic-assisted percutaneous manipulation of displaced and angulated radial neck fractures in children. *J Orthop Techn.* 1994;2:77–81. (**LOE IV**).

236. Kocialkowski A, Wallace WA. Closed percutaneous K-wire stabilization for displaced fractures of the surgical neck of the humerus. *Injury.* 1990;21(4):209–212. (**LOE IV**).

237. Metaizeau JP, Lascombe P, Lamelle JL, et al. Reduction and fixation of displaced radial neck fractures by closed intramedullary pinning. *J Pediatr Orthop.* 1993;13(3):355–360. (**LOE III**).

238. Sessa S, Lascombes P, Prevot J, et al. Fractures of the radial head and associated elbow injuries in children. *J Pediatr Orthop B.* 1996;5(3):200–209. (**LOE IV**).

239. Nawabi D, Kang N, Curry S. Centromedullary medullary pinning of radial neck fractures: length matters! *J Pediatr Orthop.* 2006;26:278–279. (**LOE IV**).

240. Prathapkumar K, Garg N, Bruce C. Elastic stable intramedullary nail fixation for severely displaced fractures of the neck of the radius in children. *J Bone Joint Surg Br.* 2006;88:358–361. (**LOE IV**).

241. Schmittenbecher P, Haevernick B, Herold A, et al. Treatment decision, method of osteosynthesis, and outcome of radial neck fracture in children: a multicenter study. *J Pediatr Orthop.* 2005;25:45–50. (**LOE III**).

242. Steinburg EL, Golomb D, Salama R, et al. Radial head and neck fractures in children. *J Pediatr Orthop.* 1988;8(1):35–40. (**LOE III**).

243. Strachan J, Ellis B. Vulnerability of the posterior interosseous nerve during radial head dissection. *J Bone Joint Surg Br.* 1971;53:320–323. (**LOE III**).

244. O'Brien PI. Injuries involving the proximal radial epiphysis. *Clin Orthop Relat Res.* 1965;41:51–58. (**LOE IV**).

245. Caputo A, Mazzocca A, Santoro V. The nonarticulating portion of the radial head: anatomic and clinical correlations for internal fixation. *J Hand Surg.* 1998;23(6):1082–1090.

246. Chotel F, Valiese P, Parot R, Laville J, Hodgkinson I, et al. Complete dislocation of the radial head following fracture of the radial neck in children: the Jeffery type II lesion. *J Pediatr Orthop Br.* 2004;13(4):268–274. (**LOE IV**).

247. Waters P, Stewart S. Radial neck fracture nonunion in children. *J Pediatr Orthop.* 2001;21:570–576. (**LOE III**).

248. Henrikson B. Isolated fracture of the proximal end of the radius in children. *Acta Orthop Scand.* 1969;40:246–260. (**LOE III**).

249. Newell RL. Olecranon fractures in children. *Injury.* 1975;7(1):33–36. (**LOE IV**).

250. Evans M, Graham H. Olecranon fractures in children: Part 1: a clinical review; Part 2: a new classification and management algorithm. *J Pediatr Orthop.* 1999;19(5):559–569. (**LOE II**).

251. Gaddy B, Strecker W, Schoenecker P. Surgical treatment of displaced olecranon fractures in children. *J Pediatr Orthop.* 1997;3(321–324). (**LOE III**).

252. Graves S, Canale S. Fractures of the olecranon in children. Long-term follow-up. *J Pediatr Orthop.* 1993;13:239–241. (**LOE III**).

253. Landin L, Danielsson L. Elbow fractures in children: an epidemiological analysis of 589 cases. *Acta Orthop Scand.* 1986;57:309–312. (**LOE II**).

254. Matthews JG. Fractures of the olecranon in children. *Injury.* 1980;12(3):207–212. (**LOE IV**).

255. Bado JL. The Monteggia lesion. *Clin Orthop Relat Res.* 1967;50:71–86. (**LOE III**).

256. Tayne S, Smith PA. Olecranon fractures in pediatric patients with osteogenesis imperfecta. *J Pediatr Orthop.* 2019. (**LOE IV**).

257. Papavasiliou V, Beslikas T, Nenopoulos S. Isolated fractures of the olecranon in children. *Injury.* 1987;18:100–102. (**LOE IV**).

258. Gortzak Y, Mercado E, Atar D, et al. Pediatric olecranon fractures: open reduction and internal fixation with removable Kirschner wires and absorbable sutures. *J Pediatr Orthop.* 2006;26(1):39–42. (**LOE III**).

259. Carlioz H, Abols Y. Posterior dislocation of the elbow in children. *J Pediatr Orthop.* 1984;4:8–12. (**LOE IV**).

260. Neviaser JS, Wickstrom JK. Dislocation of the elbow: a retrospective study of 115 patients. *South Med J.* 1975;70(2):172–173. (**LOE III**).

261. Roberts PH. Dislocation of the elbow. *Br J Surg.* 1969;56(11):806–815. (**LOE IV**).

262. DeLee J. Transverse divergent dislocation of the elbow in a child: a case report. *J Bone Joint Surg Am.* 1981;63:322–323. (**LOE IV**).

263. Holbrook J, Green N. Divergent pediatric elbow dislocation. A case report. *Clin Orthop Relat Res.* 1988;234:72–74. (**LOE V**).

264. Sovio O, Tredwell S. Divergent dislocation of the elbow in a child. *J Pediatr Orthop.* 1986;6:96–97. (**LOE V**).

265. Rasool M. Dislocations of the elbow in children. *J Bone Joint Surg Br.* 2004;86(7):1050–1058. (**LOE IV**).

266. Royle S. Posterior dislocation of the elbow. *Clin Orthop Relat Res.* 1991;269:201–204. (**LOE IV**).

267. Steiger R, Larrick R, Meyer T. Median nerve entrapment following elbow dislocation: a report of 2 cases. *J Bone Joint Surg Am.* 1969;51(2):381–385. (**LOE V**).

268. Loomis L. Reduction and after treatment of posterior dislocation of the elbow. *Am J Surg.* 1944;63:56–60. (**LOE IV**).

269. Ross G, McDevitt E, Chronister R, et al. Treatment of simple elbow dislocation using an immediate motion protocol. *Am J Sports Med.* 1999;27:308–311. (**LOE III**).

270. Wheeler D, Linscheid R. Fracture dislocations of the elbow. *Clin Orthop Relat Res.* 1967;20:95–106. (**LOE IV**).

271. Beaty J, Kasser J, eds. *Rockwood and Wilkins' Fractures in Children.* 7th ed. Philadelphia: Lippincott, Williams, & Wilkins; 2010. (**LOE N/A**).

272. Linscheid RL, Wheeler DK. Elbow dislocations. *JAMA.* 1965;194(11):1171–1176. (**LOE IV**).

273. Hennig K, Franke D. Posterior displacement of the brachial artery following closed elbow dislocation. *J Trauma.* 1980;20:96–98. (**LOE IV**).

274. Hofammann KE 3rd, Moneim M, Omer G. Brachial artery disruption following closed posterior elbow dislocation in a child. A case report with review of the literature. *Clin Orthop Relat Res.* 1984;184:145–149. (**LOE V**).

275. Wilmshurst A, Millner P, Batchelor A. Brachial artery entrapment in closed elbow dislocation. *Injury.* 1989;20:240–241. (**LOE IV**).

276. Galbraith KA, McCullough CJ. Acute nerve injury as a complication of closed fractures or dislocations of the elbow. *Injury.* 1979;11(2):159–164. (**LOE IV**).

277. Hallett J. Entrapment of the median nerve after dislocation of the elbow. A case report. *J Bone Joint Surg Br.* 1981;63-B(3):408–412. (**LOE V**).

278. al-Qattan, Zuker R, Weinberg M. Type 4 median nerve entrapment after elbow dislocation. *J Hand Surg.* 1994;19(5):613–615. (**LOE V**).

279. Oxkoc G, Akpinar S, Hersekli M, et al. Type 4 median nerve entrapment in a child after elbow dislocation. *Arch Orthop Trauma Surg.* 2003;123:555–557. (**LOE V**).

280. Green NE. Entrapment of the median nerve following elbow dislocation. *J Pediatr Orthop.* 1983;3(3):384–386. (**LOE V**).

281. Matev I. A radiological sign of entrapment of the median nerve in the elbow joint after posterior dislocation. A report of two cases. *J Bone Joint Surg Br.* 1976;58(3):353–355. (**LOE V**).

282. Osborne G, Cotterill P. Recurrent dislocation of the elbow. *J Bone Joint Surg Br.* 1966;48(2):340–346. (**LOE IV**).

283. Hassman G, Brunn F, Nerr C. Recurrent dislocation of the elbow. *J Bone Joint Surg Am.* 1975;57(8):1080–1084. (**LOE III**).

284. Symeonides P, Paschaloglu C, Stavrou Z, et al. Recurrent dislocation of the elbow. Report of three cases. *J Bone Joint Surg Am.* 1975;57:1084–1086. (**LOE IV**).

285. Trias A, Comeau Y. Recurrent dislocation of the elbow in children. *Clin Orthop Relat Res.* 1974;100:74–77. (**LOE IV**).

286. Altuntas A, Balakumar J, Howells R, et al. Posterior divergent dislocation of the elbow in children and adolescents: a report of three cases and a review of the literature. *J Pediatr Orthop.* 2005;25:317–321. (**LOE IV**).

287. Wiley JJ, Galey JP. Monteggia injuries in children. *J Bone Joint Surg Br.* 1985;67(5):728–731. (**LOE III**).

288. Wiley JJ, Pegington J, Horwich JP. Traumatic dislocation of the radius at the elbow. *J Bone Joint Surg Br.* 1974;56B(3):501–507. (**LOE IV**).

289. Weisman DS, Rang M, Cole WG. Tardy displacement of traumatic radial head dislocation in childhood. *J Pediatr Orthop.* 1999;19(4):523–526. (**LOE IV**).

290. Stitgen A, McCarthy J, Nemeth B, Garrels K, Noonan K. Ulnar fracture with late radial head dislocation: delayed Monteggia fracture. *Orthopedics.* 2012;35(3):e434–e437. (**LOE V**).

291. Hamilton W, Parkes JC 2nd. Isolated dislocation of the radial head without fracture of the ulna. *Clin Orthop Relat Res.* 1973;97:94–96. (**LOE IV**).

292. Lincoln T, Mubarak S. "Isolated" traumatic radial head dislocation. *J Pediatr Orthop.* 1994;14:454–457. (**LOE II**).

293. Almquist EE, Gordon LH, Blue AI. Congenital dislocation of the head of the radius. *J Bone Joint Surg Am.* 1969;51(6):118–127. (**LOE IV**).

294. Mardam-Bey T, Ger E. Congenital radial head dislocation. *J hand Surg Am.* 1979;4(4):316–320. (**LOE IV**).

295. McFarland B. Congenital dislocation of the head of the radius. *Br J Surg.* 1936;24(41–49). (**LOE V**).

296. Bell Tawse AJ. The treatment of malunited anterior Monteggia fractures in children. *J Bone Joint Surg Br.* 1965;47:718–723. (**LOE IV**).

297. Lloyd-Roberts GB, Bucknill T. Anterior dislocation of the radial head in children. *J Bone Joint Surg Br.* 1979;59:402–407. (**LOE IV**).

298. Corrigan AB. The pulled elbow. *Med J Aust.* 1965;17:187–189. (**LOE IV**).

299. Snellman O. Subluxation of the head of the radius in children. *Acta Orthop Scand.* 1959;28:311–315. (**LOE IV**).

300. Salter RB, Zaltz C. Anatomic investigations of the mechanism of injury and pathologic anatomy of "pulled elbow" in young children. *Clin Orthop Relat Res.* 1971;77:134–143. (**LOE V**).

301. Amir D, Frankl U, Pogrund H. Pulled elbow and hypermobility of joints. *Clin Orthop Relat Res.* 1990;257:94–99. (**LOE III**).

302. Taha A. The treatment of pulled elbow: a prospective randomized study. *Arch Orthop Trauma Surg.* 2000;120:336–337. (**LOE II**).

303. Teach S, Schutzman S. Prospective study of recurrent radial head subluxation. *Arch Pediatr Adoles Med.* 1986;150:164–166. (**LOE II**).

18 Fractures and Dislocations of the Forearm, Wrist, and Hand

Chris Stutz

INTRODUCTION

Upper extremity injury is one the most common presenting complaints after trauma in the pediatric population. Fractures of the forearm represent 40% of fractures in all age groups of children.[1–3] Upper extremity fractures and dislocations are slightly more common in boys than in girls. There is a higher incidence from ages 4 to 14 years as children begin to independently interact with their environment and participate in recreational and competitive sporting activities.[4–6] The most common injuries are to the distal metaphyseal and physeal region of the forearm.[7] Diaphyseal fractures remain more common in prepubescent children, whereas physeal injuries are more common among adolescents. Fractures of the carpus are far less common. Frequently, these are subtle injuries that are initially overlooked. Hand injuries remain common and are most often caused by direct trauma, such as crush injuries in the young and sports injuries in the school-age and adolescent athlete.[8–11]

MECHANISM OF INJURY/BIOMECHANICS

It is important to understand the mechanism of injury and regional anatomy of the injured upper extremity to appreciate the resultant deformity and make appropriate treatment decisions. This understanding is necessary for correcting the deformity and preventing complications. In fractures of the distal radius and ulna, the three-dimensional location of the torn periosteum influences reduction maneuvers. In the diaphyseal forearm, the angular and rotational deformities guide reduction techniques. Interposed periosteum, muscle, or tendon may block reduction of fractures.

MECHANISM OF DIAPHYSEAL FOREARM FRACTURES

Fractures of the forearm in children often result from a fall on an outstretched hand. This results in forceful axial loading with resultant bony failure in compression and bending. These forces can cause plastic deformation, partial (greenstick) fracture, or complete fractures, usually of both the radius and ulna. Any fracture of a single bone of the forearm from a fall should be considered unusual and is highly suggestive of an associated injury to the proximal or distal radioulnar articulations or plastic deformation of the other bone.[12–16] Single-bone injuries are more characteristic of a direct blow, such as striking the ulna with an object such as a baseball bat. In addition to excessive axial loading, falls on

an outstretched hand also result in forceful rotation of the forearm with resultant rotational deformity.[17–19] This usually results in a supination deformity and apex volar angulation. The rotational malalignment may be unappreciated and undertreated. It is generally accepted that rotational deformities have little to no potential for remodeling, even in very young children. Thus, a failure to diagnose and correctly treat rotational malalignment is the most common cause of permanent loss of forearm rotation in children.

MECHANISM OF FRACTURES OF THE DISTAL RADIUS

Fractures of the distal radius comprise approximately one-third of all fractures in children.[20] Since 1980, their incidence has increased, likely secondary to increased participation in sports or increased body weight.[21,22] The mechanism of injury is usually a fall on an outstretched hand, similar to diaphyseal forearm fractures.

MECHANISM OF CARPAL FRACTURES

Carpal fractures are uncommon in children. Similar to adults, the scaphoid remains the most fractured carpal bone in children, representing only 0.45% of all fractures in the pediatric population.[23] Also similar to adult distributions, the scaphoid waist fracture is the most common (71%), followed by distal pole fractures representing 23% and proximal pole fractures comprising the remaining 6%.[24] Carpal fractures are often missed in children on initial presentation secondary to the cartilaginous nature of the bones; hence, the treating physician must maintain a high index of suspicion to accurately make the diagnosis in a timely fashion. The mechanism of injury remains a fall on an outstretched hand.

MECHANISM OF HAND FRACTURES

Multiple mechanisms are responsible for hand fractures in children. Phalangeal fractures are the most common hand fractures in children;[1] metacarpal fractures are relatively rare. The most common mechanisms for hand fractures in children include jamming injuries in sports, crush injuries, and direct blow injuries.[9–10,25]

EVALUATION

Obtaining a thorough history is critical for the accurate diagnosis of these injuries. This can be difficult in small children, thus making an interview with parents or any witnesses to the injury essential. Unwitnessed injuries in nonverbal children may yield no available history. Clear details on the mechanism of injury are integral to understanding the deformity, energy of the injury, and the likelihood of associated injuries. To protect children in cases of abuse, physicians should always consider the plausibility and consistency of the history.

EXAMINATION

Physical examination is an integral part of deformity assessment. In addition to angular deformities, subtle rotational deformities should not be overlooked, and comparison with the unaffected limb is essential. In addition to the known site of injury, thorough examination of the shoulder, elbow, wrist, and hand must be completed to rule out concomitant injuries. Assessment of the soft tissues is important, particularly in higher-energy and open fractures. Serial evaluations over several days may be necessary to fully appreciate the extent of associated soft tissue injuries in rare, major trauma situations. Compartment syndrome must be considered in all fractures and instances of severe soft tissue injury, such as crush or burn injuries. The three As of compartment syndrome in children—agitation, anxiety, and analgesics—should be evaluated in all injuries at risk of development of compartment syndrome.[26,27] Measurement of compartment pressures may be necessary in nonverbal or obtunded children. A careful prereduction and postreduction neurovascular assessment is mandatory, and frequent serial assessment is prudent.[28] Open fractures and concomitant fractures of the same limb have the highest risk.[29–31]

IMAGING

Plain radiography remains the gold standard for musculoskeletal evaluation and should be completed in all patients with a physical examination suggestive of a fracture or dislocation. Biplanar radiographs demonstrate most fractures and dislocations. However, the limitations of two-dimensional evaluation of three-dimensional deformities are real and can result in a failure to clearly illustrate nondisplaced fractures, subtle dislocations, and malrotation injuries.[32,33] Oblique radiographs can greatly aid in such diagnoses. Rotational deformities can be especially difficult to assess by plain radiography. Loss of anatomic bow or cortical diameter mismatches may suggest such deformity.[34] True anteroposterior and lateral views are necessary,[19,33] whereas oblique and specially tailored views often aid in diagnosis. At a minimum, the joint above and below the injury should be clearly imaged. Suboptimal films are not acceptable and must be repeated. Magnetic resonance imaging (MRI) has emerged as a useful adjunct for evaluating soft tissues, diagnosing occult fractures (e.g., scaphoid fractures), and assessing cartilaginous injuries to the immature skeleton. Computed tomography (CT) remains the study of choice for detailed evaluation of bony anatomy, such as intraarticular fractures. MRI and CT arthrograms can be invaluable in evaluation of joints, particularly in small children whose nonossified epiphyses can be difficult to evaluate by plain radiographs.

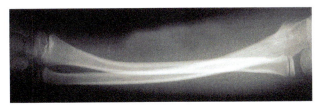

Fig. 18.1 Lateral radiograph of a plastic deformation fracture of the forearm. This degree of deformation often results in a cosmetic serpentine appearance and a mechanical block to forearm rotation. Forceful closed reduction under anesthesia is necessary for realignment.

CLASSIFICATION

Pediatric upper extremity fractures are typically described on the basis of (1) which bone or bones are involved, (2) fracture location (e.g., diaphyseal, metaphyseal, epiphyseal), (3) direction of displacement (e.g., apex volar), (4) physeal involvement (e.g., Salter-Harris classification), (5) articular involvement, and (6) failure mode (e.g., plastic deformation, partial or greenstick fracture, or complete fracture).

The biomechanical properties of bone in children differ from that in adults. Immature bone is more elastic and has a greater ability to deform without fracture. As a result, excessive mechanical loading of immature bone can result in a spectrum of pathologic change, including plastic deformation, greenstick fracture, and complete fracture. Each of these can result in clinically significant deformity. Combinations of these injuries are common and must be recognized (e.g., complete fracture of the radius with concomitant greenstick fracture of the ulna).

PLASTIC DEFORMATION

Immature bone has greater elasticity. In children, bone may deform under loading with a resultant angular deformity but no actual cortical disruption (Fig. 18.1).[35,36] Thus the fracture may not be obvious radiographically. Rather, only the contour of the bone has changed. These injuries can range in severity from subtle and clinically insignificant to a complete loss of anatomic bow with permanent loss of forearm rotation if left untreated. Such deformities can be easily overlooked by the untrained eye and must always be suspected, particularly in cases of single-bone forearm fractures. Generally, a plastic deformation injury with restricted forearm pronation and supination requires a reduction with conscious sedation or general anesthesia. Considerable reduction force is required and applied over a solid bolster for several minutes (Fig. 18.2).

PARTIAL (GREENSTICK) FRACTURES

The elasticity of bone in children also explains its greater tendency for partial or unicortical fracture. Greenstick fractures are characterized by incomplete cortical fracture with angulation and rotation through plastic deformation of the remaining intact cortex. These fractures are commonly seen in children and are often noted in conjunction

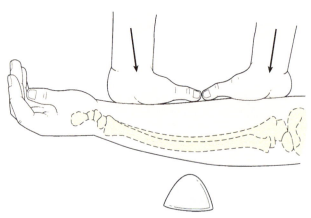

Fig. 18.2 Method of reducing plastic deformity of the forearm. (From Price C. Fractures of the forearm. In: Letts R, ed. *Management of Pediatric Fractures*. New York: Churchill-Livingstone; 1994:329.)

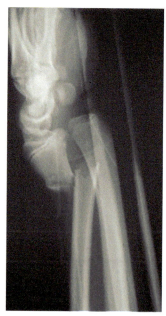

Fig. 18.4 Oblique view of the wrist revealing an isolated displaced distal radius fracture. This injury also represents a displacement of the distal radioulnar joint, a Galeazzi fracture-dislocation.

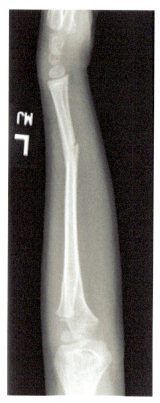

Fig. 18.3 Lateral radiograph of a diaphyseal forearm fracture with an apex volar supination deformity in a young child. Treatment is usually by closed reduction and initial long arm cast immobilization under conscious sedation in the emergency department.

with a complete fracture of the other bone of the forearm. Diaphyseal fractures of the forearm are usually apex volar supination injuries (Fig. 18.3)[36]. Greenstick fractures are primarily a rotational deformity, although the radiographs are commonly misinterpreted as an angular deformity. As with any fracture, the degree of angular and rotational deformity must be assessed and treated accordingly. Apex volar fractures are supination deformity injuries requiring pronation for reduction. Conversely, less common apex dorsal fractures are pronation deformity injuries requiring supination for reduction. Greenstick fracture patterns are inherently more stable than complete fracture patterns after reduction. As such, they are usually treated with cast immobilization in the appropriate corrective rotation with molding to maintain the interosseous space and a straight ulnar border.

The greater mechanical stability of greenstick fractures may also result in greater difficulty when a reduction is required. In the case of both-bone forearm fractures, greenstick fracture of the ulna in association with a complex fracture of the radius may act not only as a contributor to the deformity but also as a potential block to reduction. Several authors have advocated "completion" of the greenstick fracture to facilitate the ease of reduction.[37] Others have suggested that this is not necessary and adds unwanted instability to the fracture.[3,38] Long-term data on this subject are lacking, and this approach remains controversial. Most would agree that the completion of greenstick fractures is acceptable and appropriate when necessary for achieving an anatomic reduction.

COMPLETE FRACTURES

Greater force of injury results in the complete disruption of cortical bone. In the forearm, this typically involves both bones but may involve a single bone in conjunction with greenstick fracture or plastic deformation of the other. True single-bone forearm fractures do occur and are typically the result of a direct blow. Single-bone forearm fractures in the setting of an axial load are rare and should raise the suspicion of an injury to the proximal or distal radioulnar joint (e.g., Monteggia or Galeazzi fracture, respectively) (Fig. 18.4). Complete fractures usually occur in older children and are inherently more unstable after reduction.

MANAGEMENT

DIAPHYSEAL FOREARM FRACTURES

EMERGENT TREATMENT

The need for emergent treatment of diaphyseal forearm fractures is rare. Those fractures that are associated with a neurovascular injury or are complicated by a developing compartment syndrome qualify for true emergent treatment. Otherwise, most forearm fractures can be treated with appropriate urgency to stabilize the injury. This can be completed temporarily with a splint in the emergency department before evaluation for definitive management. Recently, some have advocated for the treatment of Gustilo grade I open fractures with local débridement, administration of antibiotics, and closed reduction and casting in the emergency room forgoing the typical formal operative irrigation and débridement.[39]

INDICATIONS FOR DEFINITIVE CARE

The goals of treatment include the safe and expedient correction of bone length, angulation, and rotation to as anatomic a position as possible within acceptable standards of anticipated remodeling; anatomic reductions of joint dislocations; maintenance of reduction until adequate healing has occurred; and appropriate treatment of soft tissue injuries. Nondisplaced stable fractures are treated with brief immobilization for comfort and prevention of recurrent injury during the healing phase.[40] Displaced fractures and dislocations in the forearm are most often treated with closed reduction and cast immobilization.[40,41] Operative intervention is indicated when adequate reduction cannot be achieved or maintained by closed means. Frequently used methods depending on the clinical situation include closed reduction and percutaneous pinning, percutaneous or open intramedullary rodding, and open reduction-internal fixation with the use of plates and screws. External fixation is less commonly used in children.

NONOPERATIVE TREATMENT

The majority of fractures and dislocations involving the forearm can be treated nonoperatively. The rapid healing, the remodeling potential of children's bones in the planes of motion of the adjacent joints, and their tolerance for immobilization make cast-splint management the treatment of choice in most cases. Proper technique in reduction and immobilization is critical for successful treatment.

Displaced fractures, dislocations, and fracture-dislocations require reduction before immobilization. Manual manipulation of the extremity can range from gentle traction to vigorous and forceful re-creation of the injury mechanism for deformity correction, depending on the fracture location and degree of deformity. Determining whether a fracture reduction is necessary is of paramount importance. This decision is based on acceptable standards reported in the literature for expected specific injury outcomes as they relate to fracture displacement, joint dislocation or subluxation, fracture location (i.e., metaphyseal, diaphyseal, or epiphyseal), and the potential for remodeling (i.e., skeletal age of the patient, proximity to an open physis, and the plane of deformity relative to that of the proximate joints).

Once the determination has been made that the present fracture alignment is unacceptable, the patient is prepared for a reduction maneuver. In most children, this requires some level of anesthesia. In smaller children, this may be in the form of conscious sedation administered in the emergency department setting. This usually entails a combination of analgesic and amnestic medications such as ketamine, narcotics, and/or benzodiazepines.[42–44] Conscious sedation should only be administered to children in a monitored setting by an experienced pediatrician or anesthesiologist who is certified in pediatric advanced life support. Oxygen, reversal agents, and equipment for emergency airway management must be made available before administration of sedation. For more complex cases or anticipated prolonged procedures, formal administration of a general anesthetic in the operating room is considered to be safer and a more controlled option. Adolescents approaching adulthood may not require sedation for closed reductions, particularly of distal radial metaphyseal and physeal fractures. A hematoma block or intrafracture local anesthetic injection may suffice for closed reductions in the emergency department in this age group.

Once the patient is adequately and safely sedated or anesthetized, the reduction maneuver is performed. Proper technique is essential for a successful reduction. The techniques used for reduction maneuvers vary greatly, depending on the specific injury pattern. However, some general principles apply to all reduction maneuvers. The patient must be positioned in such a way as to provide the surgeon optimal mechanical advantage and access to the extremity. Aid from a qualified assistant can be invaluable and should be sought if and when resources allow. Prereduction and postreduction neurovascular examination and documentation should be considered part of every reduction maneuver. Portable image intensification should be used when available. Casting or splinting materials should be collected and prepared as completely as possible before reduction. Some surgeons prefer to apply stockinette or even cast padding before reduction in an effort to minimize the risk of loss of reduction during cast application. The surgeon must then be prepared to safely apply the necessary amount of force to achieve reduction. This may range from only gentle axial traction to forceful manipulation. An understanding of the exact amount of force that is both necessary and safe is gained only by practical experience and reduction maneuvers performed under supervision whenever possible. In children, a partially intact layer of periosteum may act as a tether that indirectly blocks reduction, necessitating the re-creation of the injury mechanism with intentional exaggeration of angulation to "unhook" the fracture. This allows subsequent unfettered rotation at the fracture site around a hinge of intact periosteum. When the correct technique is used to unhook the fracture, this hinge of periosteum can act as an aid in reduction by preventing complete displacement, guiding the reduction to a more anatomic position, and adding stability to the injury pattern as a tension band. Attempts should be made to keep any remaining periosteum intact. The "three-point" cast molding technique exploits the fulcrum created by the partially intact periosteum to provide added stability to the reduction and subsequent immobilization. Muscle spasm and contracture may contribute to fracture deformity. Relaxation can be achieved by steady longitudinal traction applied over time, which eventually results in muscle fatigue and gradual lengthening. Older children may tolerate elevation in finger traps with 5 to 10 pounds of weight suspended around the upper arm. Intravenous muscle relaxants are rarely necessary. The goal of closed reduction is anatomic alignment with correction of translation, malrotation, and angulation. This lessens the risk of unacceptable loss of reduction over the ensuing 3 to 4 weeks of fracture healing.

Unacceptable reduction is generally considered to be greater than 20 degree angulation with 2 years or less of growth remaining. However, in the proximal forearm, malalignment of greater than 10 to 15 degrees may not remodel and may thus impair forearm rotation permanently. Bayonet apposition has been thought to be acceptable up to 8 to 10 years of age, as long as angulation and malrotation are corrected. In the case of unexpectedly difficult reductions, the surgeon must entertain the possibility of interposed tissues such as periosteum, muscle, tendon, or neurovascular structures. Interposed structures may render anatomic reduction impossible, necessitating surgical exploration. Particular caution is necessary when reduction of displaced physeal fractures is attempted. This should be limited to one or two gentle closed reduction attempts, and forceful manipulation of the physis should be avoided, if possible. Repeated attempts at reduction of physeal injuries may result in iatrogenic physeal injury and growth arrest.

The majority of forearm fractures, whether proximal or diaphyseal, should be immobilized in a long arm cast or splint. Important molding characteristics include (1) well-contoured supracondylar humeral molds, (2) well-contoured interosseous forearm molds, (3) three-point molding techniques, (4) allowance of appropriate elbow flexion, and (5) a straight ulnar border. If circumferential casting is the preferred immobilization technique, the author prefers to bivalve the cast to decrease pressure and allow for swelling without compromising the maintenance of the reduction.[45,46] Poor casting technique can result in unnecessary loss of reduction and can place the patient at higher risk of cast-related complications such as skin breakdown and cast-saw burns (Fig. 18.5).

Nondisplaced fractures should be casted with the elbow in 90 degrees of flexion and the forearm in neutral rotation. Displaced fractures requiring reduction should also be casted with the elbow flexed 90 degrees, but forearm rotation may be one of supination or pronation (more common), depending on the fracture pattern and the stable position after reduction. Cast immobilization is usually continued for 4 to 6 weeks, depending on evidence of radiographic healing. Frequent radiographs, usually weekly for up to 3 weeks, should be obtained for fractures requiring reduction so that acceptable alignment is maintained.

SURGICAL TREATMENT

Surgical treatment of forearm fractures is reserved for those fractures that are irreducible by closed means or that fail closed management because of loss of reduction, open fracture type, refracture, segmental injury pattern, ipsilateral humerus fractures ("floating elbow" injuries), or compartment syndrome complications.

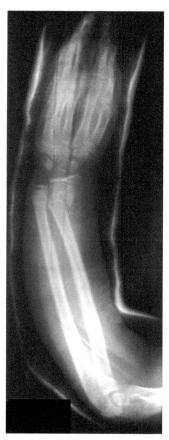

Fig. 18.5 Note the "banana cast" in this radiograph without a straight ulnar border, appropriate interosseous mold, and distal humeral mold in this long arm cast. As a consequence, there is loss of reduction of the fracture.

Surgical Anatomy

Development. A thorough understanding of the development of the radius and ulna and their articulation is essential for treating injuries to the growing forearm. Familiarity with normal ages of ossification and locations of all secondary growth centers, as well as the expected growth potential and age at fusion of all physes, is also essential for the protection of the immature physis and nonossified epiphyses when injuries are being treated. It is important to note that epiphyses form initially as cartilaginous structures, only to ossify secondarily with further growth. It is critical to remain cognizant of the fact that these structures can be significantly injured before ossification with little radiographic evidence of injury.

The radius and ulna form from primary ossification centers that appear during the eighth week of gestation. Secondary ossification centers, or epiphyses, later begin to ossify at the proximal end of the radius in the fifth to seventh year and in the proximal ulna in the ninth to tenth years. The distal epiphysis of the radius ossifies during the first year in girls and shortly after 1 year in boys.[13,47] The distal ulnar epiphysis, however, does not begin to ossify until approximately age 6 in boys and girls (Table 18.1). Note that either the distal radial or ulnar epiphyses may occasionally develop from two distinct ossification centers and should not be mistaken for fracture of the radial or ulnar styloids. Distal radial and ulnar physes typically fuse in the sixteenth to eighteenth year. Girls' physes generally fuse earlier than boys' physes.

TABLE 18.1 Expected Chronologic Age in Years of Growth Center Ossification and Physeal Closures of the Radius and Ulna in Boys and Girls

Growth center	Ossification		Physeal Closure	
	Boys	Girls	Boys	Girls
Proximal radius	5–7	5–7	16–18	16–18
Distal radius	1–1.5	<1	18–19	17
Proximal ulna	9–10	9–10	16–18	16–18
Distal ulna	6	6	17–18	16–17
Primary radius	8 weeks	8 weeks		
Primary ulna	8 weeks	8 weeks		

Osteology. The forearm is composed of the radius and ulna. They articulate with one another at both the proximal (PRUJ) and distal radioulnar joints (DRUJ). The interosseous membrane provides a fibrous attachment between the two bones along their length (Fig. 18.6).[48–50] At the elbow, the radius and ulna articulate with the capitellum and the trochlea of the humerus, respectively. At the wrist, the radius and ulna articulate with the proximal row of the carpus (i.e., scaphoid, lunate, and triquetrum from radial to ulnar). In cross section, the radius is cylindrical proximally, becomes triangular in its middle third, and is broader and more elliptical distally. The radius has a physiologic bow in the radial and posterior direction with the forearm in supination, which creates the interosseous space and is critical for forearm rotation.[51,52] It is stabilized proximally by the annular ligament, the PRUJ and the quadrate ligament, proximal fibers of the interosseous membrane, lateral collateral ligaments of the elbow, and the osseous constraints of the radiocapitellar joint. The radial head and radial styloid are palpable proximally and distally, respectively. Just distal to the radial neck, the biceps tendon attaches to the bicipital tuberosity, which points anteriorly in supination and posteriorly in pronation. This can be a useful landmark radiographically for assessing rotational deformities and loss of the anatomic bow.[53] Lister's tubercle is a dorsal prominence on the distal aspect of the radius, which can also serve as a useful landmark clinically and radiographically. The extensor pollicis longus (EPL) passes ulnar to Lister tubercle and can be injured by fracture fragments or internal fixation techniques. The ulna is triangular in cross section and has a straight border and small posterior bow in its proximal third. It is statically stabilized proximally by the osseous constraints of the trochlea, the PRUJ, and the medial and lateral collateral ligaments of the elbow. The coronoid and olecranon processes form the trochlear notch of the ulna, providing the osseous stability of the ulnohumeral articulation. Distally, the ulna is stabilized by the DRUJ and the attachments of the triangular fibrocartilage complex (TFCC).[54] The ulnar styloid is a palpable prominence at the distal ulnar aspect of the ulna.

Proximal Radioulnar Joint. The head of the radius sits in the radial notch of the ulna. It is stabilized in this position by the annular ligament, which encases the radial head nearly circumferentially and has fibrous attachments both to the ulna and to the medial and lateral collateral ligaments of the elbow. The joint capsule and the oblique cord, which runs from the base of the coronoid process to just distal to the radial tuberosity, provide additional stability. The quadrate ligament is a stout and flat band that lies deep to the annular ligament on the anterior aspect of the PRUJ, extending from the base of the coronoid to the radial neck.[55] Similar to the interosseous membrane, it tightens with supination of the radius, stabilizing the radial head in the notch of the ulna. Finally, during supination, the broadest area of the radial head is in contact with the radial notch of the ulna. It is for these reasons that the PRUJ is most stable in forearm supination. Injury to these structures can be seen in Monteggia fractures, elbow dislocations, and radial head fracture-dislocations.

Interosseous Membrane. This flat, fibrous layer runs from the medial border of the radius to the lateral border of the ulna. It extends from a level 1 cm distal to the radial tuberosity distally to the DRUJ. The obliquely oriented fibers run from the radius directed distally to the ulna at an angle of approximately 60 degrees. The membrane is most taut in neutral to 30 degrees of supination and relaxes in pronation and terminal supination.[32,50,56–58] The interosseous membrane is important in the mechanics of forearm rotation, stabilization of the PRUJ, and in resistance of proximal migration of the radius relative to the ulna. It also serves as a useful surgical landmark for demarcating the anterior and posterior compartments of the forearm. The Essex-Lopresti lesion is characterized by radial head fracture with associated rupture of the interosseous membrane. In these injuries, the DRUJ can be injured or unstable because of loss of bone and soft tissue constraints related to proximal migration of the radius.

Distal Radioulnar Joint. The volar and dorsal radioulnar ligaments, the ulnar collateral ligament of the wrist, and the attachments of the TFCC stabilize the DRUJ. The carpal ligaments contribute stability to the DRUJ and will be discussed under anatomy of the wrist. It is important to understand the relationship between the DRUJ and the TFCC and to recognize that an injury to one often suggests an injury to the other.

The TFCC consists of the triangular fibrocartilage and the ulnocarpal ligaments, serving as an important stabilizer of the DRUJ and ulnar aspect of the wrist.[54] It also serves as a cushion to ulnotriquetral impaction during ulnar deviation of the wrist. The TFCC is a fibrocartilaginous disk similar to the meniscus of the knee. It is thicker and more vascular at its periphery but thinner and relatively avascular near its center. It has strong attachments to the volar and dorsal radioulnar ligaments and the ulnar collateral ligament of the wrist. At the periphery, it has attachments to the joint capsule. It spans the DRUJ, separating the carpal articular surface from the notch of the ulna. Extending from the ulnar aspect of the radial articular surface, it covers the distal aspect of the ulna with peripheral attachments at the joint capsule, the base of the ulnar styloid, and the ulnar collateral ligament of the wrist.

Injuries to the DRUJ may occur in isolation or may be seen in combination with a fracture such as in a Galeazzi fracture (DRUJ dissociation with radial shaft fracture)[14,16,59,60] or Essex-Lopresti lesions (DRUJ injury in association with radial head fracture and interosseous membrane disruption).

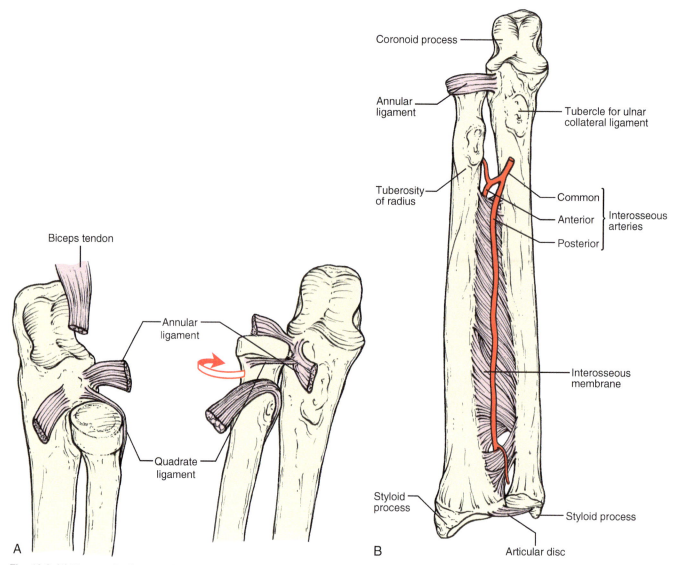

Fig. 18.6 (A) The annular ligament is the major stabilizing structure of the proximal radioulnar articulation. When the forearm is supinated, the anterior border of the quadrate ligament becomes taut and draws the radial head snugly against the radial notch of the ulna. (B) The interosseous membrane. (A, from Spinner M, Kaplan EB. The quadrate ligament of the elbow–its relationship to the stability of the proximal radio-ulnar joint. *Acta Orthop Scand.* 1970;41:632-647.) (From Grant JCB. *An Atlas of Anatomy.* 7th ed. Baltimore: Williams & Wilkins; 1988: Fig. 6.51.)

Forearm Rotation. With forearm rotation, the radius rotates, or "radiates," around the ulna and around a longitudinal axis centered through the radiocapitellar joint proximally and the center of the ulna distally. Rotation of the radius about the ulna has been described as forming a half-cone of approximately 150 to 180 degrees. The radial head pivots within the annular ligament. With forearm supination, the quadrate ligament tightens across the anterior aspect of the PRUJ, and the volar radioulnar ligament tightens across the DRUJ.

It is critical to understand the significance of the interosseous space and membrane in forearm rotation. Cadaveric studies have shown that the diameter of the interosseous space and the tension across the interosseous membrane change with forearm rotation. At neutral to 30 degrees of supination, the interosseous space is at its greatest diameter, and the membrane is most taut. The interosseous space decreases with pronation and at extremes of supination, and the membrane tension decreases accordingly. The radial

bow is normally in the radial and dorsal direction. A loss of this anatomic bow can effectively decrease the diameter of the interosseous space (Fig. 18.7).[61–63] As a result, significant pronation may be lost secondary to radioulnar impingement at terminal pronation. The most common cause of loss of range of motion after a forearm fracture is a loss of rotation secondary to a failure to restore the anatomic bow of the radius.[17–19] In malreduced proximal fractures, the bicipital tuberosity may impinge on the ulna.

Positioning Techniques. For procedures performed on the forearm, the patient is best positioned supine on the operating room table with the injured extremity extended onto a hand table. A tourniquet is useful for obtaining a bloodless operative field. Surgeon preference denotes the use of a sterile versus a nonsterile tourniquet across the upper brachium. The image intensifier is often placed perpendicular to the operating room table and parallel to the operative extremity to allow the surgeon and an assistant unimpeded access to the operative field.

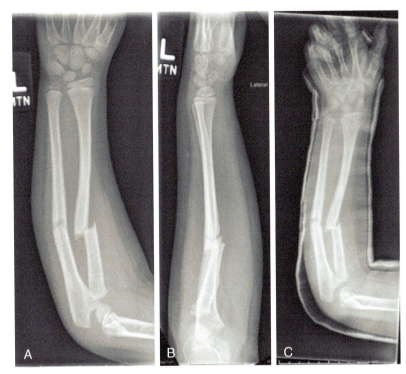

Fig. 18.7 Anteroposterior (A) and lateral (B) radiographs of a complete diaphyseal forearm fracture in a 7-year-old patient. There is overlap of the fracture fragments. Attempted closed reduction with long arm cast immobilization (C) reveals pending malunion. The loss of radial bow proximally will be a problem if not corrected. Current practice is to treat this type of fracture with internal fixation.

TABLE 18.2   Anterior (Henry) Approach to the Radius

Approach	Muscular Interval	Internervous Plane	Dangers
Anterior radius	Proximal: pronator teres and brachioradialis	Median and radial nerves	PIN, superficial radial nerve, radial artery
	Distal: FCR and brachioradialis		

FCR, Flexor carpi radialis; *PIN*, posterior interosseous nerve.

Surgical Approach

Anterior (Henry) Approach to the Radius. The anterior approach to the forearm, also commonly referred to as the Henry approach (Table 18.2), is a workhorse for the upper extremity surgeon (Fig. 18.8).[64,65] This extensile approach provides excellent exposure of the radius from the wrist to the elbow. It may also be extended across the elbow and carried proximally in the anterior approach to the upper arm and shoulder. Theoretically, the upper extremity osseous structures can be exposed from the wrist to the shoulder through one incision with the use of this approach. Five muscles must be detached from the anterior aspect of the radius to expose it in its entirety. From proximally to distally, they are the supinator, pronator teres, flexor digitorum superficialis (FDS), flexor pollicis longus (FPL), and pronator quadratus.

The anterior approach to the forearm exploits the internervous plane between the median and radial nerves.

Proximally, this plane lies between the pronator teres (median nerve) and brachioradialis (radial nerve) muscles. Distally, the plane is between the flexor carpi radialis (FCR) (median nerve) and the brachioradialis. For incision location, the brachioradialis muscle and mobile wad are palpated on the radial forearm. Just medial to the brachioradialis and lateral to the biceps tendon, a linear longitudinal incision is initiated just distal to the elbow flexion crease and is carried distally toward the insertion of the FCR tendon, in line with the radial shaft. The dissection is carried down to the subcutaneous fascia. The lateral antebrachial cutaneous nerve may be visualized in the proximal aspect of the wound and must be protected.

In the proximal third, the interval between the pronator teres and the brachioradialis is identified. The fascia is incised in line with these fibers, and the interval is bluntly defined. A collateral branch of the radial artery, known as the recurrent leash of Henry, is often encountered in this interval and must be ligated so that the brachioradialis can be mobilized laterally. The radial artery can then be retracted medially. The next muscle encountered is the supinator, which is easily identified by the transverse course of its fibers. Great care must be taken during this portion of the exposure to avoid injury to the posterior interosseous nerve (PIN). The radial nerve, which runs between the brachialis and brachioradialis muscles in the distal humerus, branches just below the elbow into the superficial (sensory) and posterior interosseous (motor) branches. The superficial branch continues distally between the brachioradialis and extensor carpi radialis longus (ECRL) muscles and should be mobilized laterally with the brachioradialis. It pierces the fascia to become subcutaneous roughly 5 to 7 cm above the wrist. The PIN travels medially and posteriorly, passing under the fibrous leading edge of the supinator, known as the arcade of Frohse, and splitting the two heads of the supinator muscle. Not all patients have two heads of the supinator muscle; thus, the nerve can lie directly on the periosteum, where it is at greatest risk of injury. It then traverses the muscle, wrapping posteriorly around the radial neck and proceeding distally across the origin of the abductor pollicis longus (APL) muscle along the posterior aspect of the interosseous membrane. It is also at this level that the PIN is at greatest risk of injury during the anterior approach. It runs in very close proximity to the radius at this level and may be difficult to visualize through the supinator. Supination of the forearm will move the PIN radially and posteriorly, displacing it from the incision and protecting it. The insertion of the supinator on the radius is then identified and elevated in a subperiosteal fashion, moving circumferentially from medial to lateral, and carefully posteriorly around

the radial neck. It is critical that the supinator be elevated subperiosteally to protect the PIN. Even gentle retraction of the supinator on the radial aspect of the radius can result in neuropraxia of the PIN and should be avoided whenever possible. Blind placement of retractors on the radial and posterior aspect of the proximal radius puts the nerve at risk and is not recommended. Subperiosteal exposure of the radius can then be safely carried distally.

The anterior middle third of the radius is covered by the insertion of the pronator teres and the origin of the FDS tendons. Pronation of the forearm at this point exposes the lateral insertion of the pronator on the radius. The pronator and FDS can then be elevated from proximal to distal in a subperiosteal fashion. Distal to the pronator teres insertion

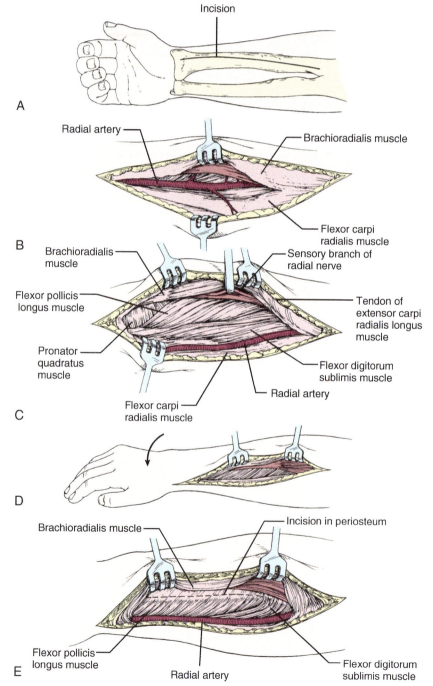

Fig. 18.8 Anterior approach to the radius (Henry approach). (A) Skin incision. (B) Fascia is incised. Brachioradialis is retracted laterally and flexor carpi radialis medially. (C) Sensory branch of the radial nerve is within the fascia, beneath the brachioradialis. These are retracted together laterally. The radial artery deep to the brachioradialis is mobilized and retracted medially, along with the flexor carpi radialis. This exposes the flexor pollicis longus, the flexor digitorum sublimis, and distally, the pronator quadratus. (D) The forearm is pronated to expose the radius lateral to the origins of the pronator quadratus and flexor pollicis longus. (E) Periosteum is incised along the broken line, and the flexor pollicis longus and pronator quadratus are reflected by subperiosteal dissection. (From Crenshaw AH. General principles. In: Crenshaw AH, ed. *Campbell's Operative Orthopedics.* 8th ed. St. Louis: C.V. Mosby; 1992:108-109.)

the superficial plane lies between the brachioradialis and the FCR. Many surgeons incise the floor of the sheath of the FCR tendon longitudinally. The radial artery is identified and usually mobilized laterally. This reveals the pronator quadratus and FPL attachments to the anterior aspect of the distal radius. With the forearm once again in supination, these muscles can be detached subperiosteally from the lateral aspect of the radius and retracted medially, providing excellent exposure of the distal third of the radius. A cuff of tissue should be preserved to allow repair of these muscles, whenever possible.

Anterior Exposure of the Ulnar Nerve. Occasionally, exploration of the ulnar nerve may be necessary in the forearm (Table 18.3 and Figs. 18.9 and 18.10). It is useful for the upper extremity surgeon to be comfortable with this approach and to be knowledgeable of the course of the major nerves in the forearm. This approach exploits the space between the flexor carpi ulnaris (FCU) (ulnar nerve) and the FDS (median nerve). The ulnar nerve provides motor innervation to the FCU and the ulnar half of the flexor digitorum

profundus (FDP) in the forearm and can be found lying between these two muscles running medial to the ulnar artery. Proximally in the upper arm, the ulnar nerve pierces the intermuscular septum from anterior to posterior to travel posterior to the medial epicondyle at the elbow, traveling beneath the leading edge of the FCU. Distally at the wrist, the ulnar nerve traverses the wrist through Guyon's canal.

TABLE 18.3	Anterior Approach to the Ulnar Nerve		
Approach	**Muscular Interval**	**Internervous Plane**	**Dangers**
Ulnar nerve, anterior	FCU and FDS	Ulnar and median nerves	Ulnar nerve and artery

FCU, Flexor carpi ulnaris; *FDS,* flexor digitorum superficialis.

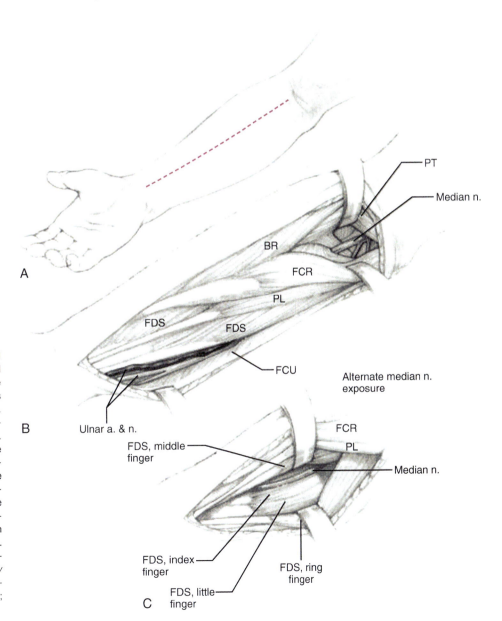

Fig. 18.9 Approach to the median and ulnar nerves. (A) Incision. (B) Proximal exposure of the median nerve is in the interval between the pronator teres *(PT)* and the flexor carpi radialis *(FCR).* This space may be most easily identified at their distal zone of separation. The ulnar nerve is found in the space between the flexor digitorum superficialis *(FDS)* of the little finger and the flexor carpi ulnaris *(FCU).* (C) The distal aspect of the median nerve may be identified beneath the FDS to the middle finger and in the space between the FDS of the middle and ring fingers. *BR,* Brachioradialis; *PL,* pollicis longus. (From Doyle B. *Surgical Anatomy of the Hand and Upper Extremity.* Philadelphia: Lippincott Williams & Wilkins; 2003:442-443.)

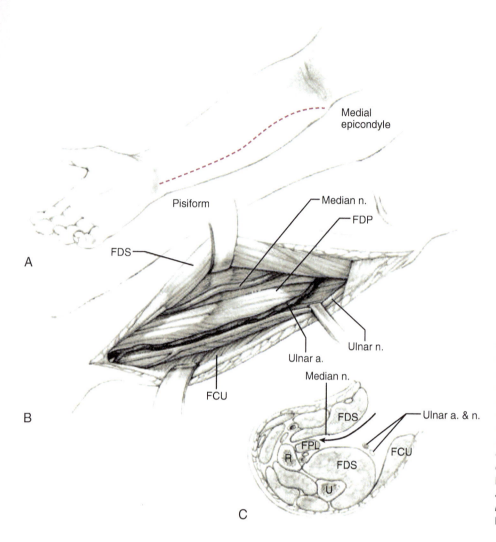

Fig. 18.10 The McConnell approach to the median nerve. (A) Incision. (B and C) The space between the flexor digitorum superficialis *(FDS)* and flexor carpi ulnaris *(FCU)* is used to expose the median nerve, which travels as a "satellite" on the undersurface of the FDS. This approach also provides excellent exposure of the ulnar nerve and artery. *FDP,* Flexor digitorum profundus; *FPL,* flexor pollicis longus; *R,* radius; *U,* ulna. (From Doyle B. *Surgical Anatomy of the Hand and Upper Extremity.* Philadelphia: Lippincott Williams & Wilkins; 2003:442-443.)

TABLE 18.4	Posterior (Thompson) Approach to the Radius		
Approach	**Muscular Interval**	**Internervous Plane**	**Dangers**
Radius, posterior	ECRB and EDC	Radial nerve and PIN	PIN

ECRB, Extensor carpi radialis brevis; *EDC,* extensor digitorum communis; *PIN,* posterior interosseous nerve.

Posterior (Thompson) Approach to the Radius. The posterior approach to the radius, also known as the Thompson approach (Table 18.4), is another useful and commonly used approach to the radius (Fig. 18.11).[66–68] This approach is particularly useful for fractures of the proximal third of the radius because it allows enhanced exposure and visualization of the PIN, which is at risk in these fractures. It also provides exposure of the tension side of the bone, which is the optimal position for plate application. This approach exploits the internervous plane between the radial and posterior interosseous nerves because the dissection is performed proximally between the extensor carpi radialis brevis (ECRB) (radial

nerve) and the extensor digitorum communis (EDC) (PIN). Distally, the plane lies between the ECRB and the EPL. A linear incision is made from just distal to the lateral epicondyle of the humerus, extending distally in line with the radius, and terminating on the ulnar side of the Lister tubercle of the radius. The fascia is split in line with its fibers. The interval between the ECRB and EDC is then identified. This plane can be more easily defined distally where the muscles of the first dorsal compartment (APL and extensor pollicis brevis) travel between the two. Dissection is carried from distal to proximal. Blunt dissection in the proximal aspect of the space reveals the underlying supinator muscle and its associated PIN. As in the anterior approach at this level, the PIN is at risk and must be protected. In contrast to the anterior approach, in the Thompson approach, the PIN is typically identified and dissected free. This is achieved with the forearm positioned in pronation. The nerve is then identified proximally or distally as it enters or exits between the deep and superficial heads of the supinator. The nerve exits approximately 1 cm proximal to the distalmost extent of the supinator. It may be necessary to detach the origins of the ECRB and ERCL so that the PIN may be visualized entering the supinator proximally. Once the nerve has been identified and protected, the forearm is supinated, and the supinator is elevated off the anterior aspect of the radius in

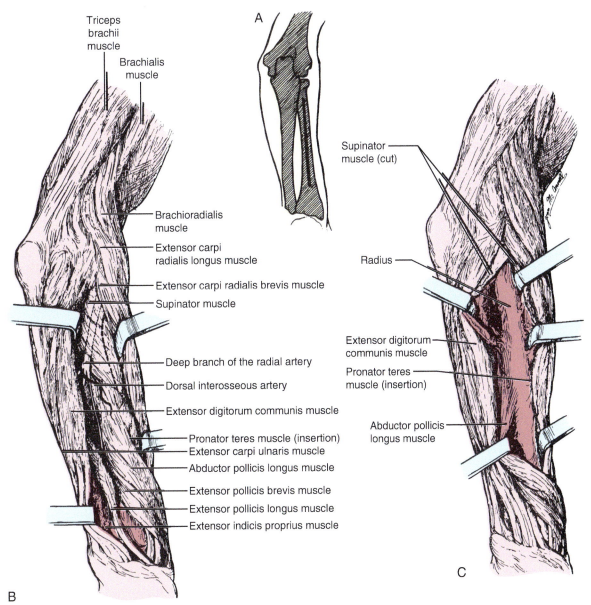

Triceps brachii muscle

Brachialis muscle

A

Brachioradialis muscle

Extensor carpi radialis longus muscle

Extensor carpi radialis brevis muscle

Supinator muscle

Deep branch of the radial artery

Dorsal interosseous artery

Extensor digitorum communis muscle

Pronator teres muscle (insertion)
Extensor carpi ulnaris muscle

Abductor pollicis longus muscle

Extensor pollicis brevis muscle

Extensor pollicis longus muscle

Extensor indicis proprius muscle

B

Supinator muscle (cut)

Radius

Extensor digitorum communis muscle

Pronator teres muscle (insertion)

Abductor pollicis longus muscle

C

Fig. 18.11 Posterior approach to the radius (Thompson approach). (A) Skin incision along a line from the lateral epicondyle of the humerus to the Lister tubercle on the dorsal aspect of the radius. (B) The fascia is incised between the extensor radialis brevis and extensor digitorum communis. The abductor pollicis and extensor pollicis brevis cross the plane of dissection in the distal third. (C) The radius is exposed by reflecting the abductor pollicis longus and extensor pollicis brevis. (From Crenshaw AH. General principles. In: Crenshaw AH, ed. *Campbell's Operative Orthopedics.* 8th ed. St. Louis: C.V. Mosby; 1992:105.)

a subperiosteal fashion, similar to that used in an anterior approach. Distally, the interval between the ECRB and EPL is exposed deep to the overlying APL and EPB. The distal radius can then be safely exposed in a subperiosteal fashion. The crossing APL and EPB can be mobilized proximally or distally to facilitate exposure of the interval and the underlying radius.

Posterolateral (Boyd) Approach to the Proximal Radius and Ulna. The Boyd approach (Table 18.5) is unique because it allows the simultaneous exposure of the proximal radius and ulna (Fig. 18.12).[69] This distal extension of the posterolateral (Kocher) approach to the elbow is most useful for the treatment of Monteggia fractures and equivalent injuries.[70] Proximally, it exploits the interval between the anconeus (radial nerve) and the extensor carpi ulnaris (ECU)

TABLE 18.5 Posterolateral (Boyd) Approach to the Proximal Radius and Ulna

Approach	Muscular Interval	Internervous Plane	Dangers
Radius and ulna, posterolateral	Proximal: anconeus and ECU Middle: FDS and ECU Distal: FCU and ECU	Radial nerve and PIN Median nerve and PIN Ulnar nerve and PIN	PIN, median nerve, brachial artery

ECU, Extensor carpi ulnaris; *FCU,* flexor carpi ulnaris; *FDS,* flexor digitorum superficialis; *PIN,* posterior interosseous nerve.

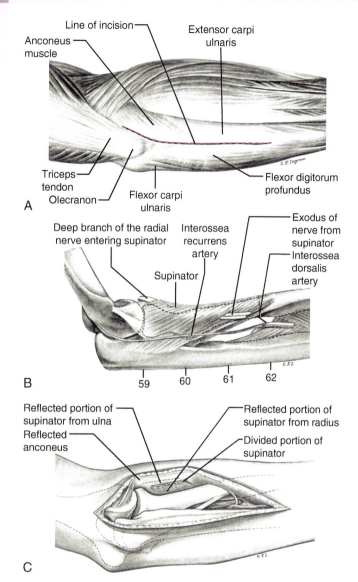

Fig. 18.12 The Boyd approach. (A) Line of the incision. (B) Pathway of the radial nerve. (C) Complete exposure of the upper third of the ulna, upper fourth of the radius, and radiohumeral articulation. (From Boyd HB. Exposición quirúrgica de la ulna y del tercio proximal del radio a través de una incisión. *Surg Gynecol Obstet.* 1940;71:81-88.)

TABLE 18.6 Medial Approach to the Ulna

Approach	Muscular Interval	Internervous Plane	Dangers
Ulna, medial	ECU and FCU	PIN and ulnar nerve	Ulnar nerve

ECU, Extensor carpi ulnaris; *FCU,* flexor carpi ulnaris; *PIN,* posterior interosseous nerve.

are safely anterior in the interval between the brachialis and the brachioradialis muscles.

Medial Approach to the Ulna. Exposure of the ulna is typically performed through a separate incision (Table 18.6). The ulna is largely subcutaneous at its ulnar border, thus facilitating its rapid and safe exposure. In addition, neither the anterior nor the posterior approaches to the radius afford adequate exposure for safe and effective fixation of fractures of the ulna. The ulna can easily be exposed in its entirety along its subcutaneous border. This approach exploits the internervous plane between the FCU (ulnar nerve) and the ECU (PIN). A longitudinal incision is made over the subcutaneous border of the ulna. The plane between the FCU and ECU is confirmed, and the incision is carried directly down to the periosteum on the ulnar aspect of the bone. The ulna is then exposed in a subperiosteal fashion. Care must be taken not to inadvertently dissect on the lateral side of the FCU muscle. It is here that the ulnar nerve and artery travel in the space between the FCU and FDP muscles and are at risk of injury. These structures are also at risk during dorsal-to-volar–directed drilling and screw placement in the ulna and must be protected with careful subperiosteal retractor placement around the ulna.

Technique of Forearm Compartment Release. Compartment syndrome of the forearm can be a complication in the pediatric trauma patient. High-risk injuries include floating elbows (supracondylar humerus and forearm fractures), segmental fractures, and open forearm fractures. Pinning of both the distal humerus and distal radius and application of a loose dressing and splint is most often the treatment for a floating elbow to lessen the risk of a compartment syndrome,[29,31] but the necessity of forearm fixation has been questioned.[71]

The surgeon must always be prepared to identify and deal with compartment syndromes in a safe, expeditious, and effective manner before permanent ischemic injury occurs. Clinical examination for a compartment syndrome follows classic signs of the five *P*s: pain, pallor, paresthesias, pulselessness, and paralysis. Pain on passive stretching of the involved compartment is considered a classic sign, but in children, it may be difficult to distinguish fracture and muscle injury pain from compartment syndrome pain. Increasing analgesic requirement, anxiety, and agitation (the three *A*s) precede the more dramatic signs of neuromuscular ischemia in children postoperatively.[26] The degree of compartment swelling and tenseness is assessed with removal of constrictive dressings and casts in any suggestive case. Compartment pressure measurements are performed by standard techniques in equivocal cases. Unquestioned cases of compartment

(PIN) muscles. The dissection can be extended distally along the border of the ulna, with use of the space between the ECU (PIN) and the FDP (median nerve) and the FCU (ulnar nerve) more distally. Pronation of the forearm moves the PIN anteriorly and radially, displacing it from the wound and protecting it. The supinator can then be elevated from the ulna and retracted anteriorly and radially with the PIN safely protected in its substance. Vigorous retraction of the supinator and blind placement of retractors around the radius should be avoided. At this point, the annular ligament and anterior capsule of the elbow joint are exposed. Fractures of the proximal radius, ulna, or both may be treated at this point. Open reduction of the radial head and repair or reconstruction of the annular ligament may be performed. The surgeon must be aware of the close proximity of the median nerve and brachial artery as they cross the elbow joint on the anterior surface of the joint capsule medial to the biceps tendon. The radial nerve and its superficial branch

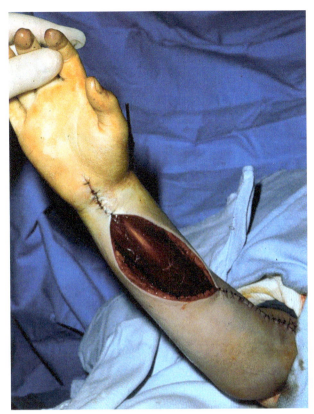

Fig. 18.13 Intraoperative photograph after volar fasciotomy of a forearm compartment syndrome.

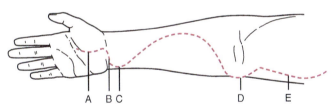

Fig. 18.14 The authors' preferred skin incision for performing a volar forearm fasciotomy, beginning at A and ending at E. (From Green DP, Hotchkiss RN, Pederson WC, et al. *Green's Operative Hand Surgery*. 5th ed. New York: Churchill-Livingstone; 2005:1991.)

syndrome are treated emergently with surgery. The treatment of choice for an established compartment syndrome remains emergent surgical decompression of all affected muscle compartments by open fasciotomy (Fig. 18.13). In the forearm, this has classically required longitudinal volar and dorsal incisions providing the exposure necessary for fascial release of the deep and superficial muscles of the anterior and posterior forearm, the mobile wad, and the carpal tunnel. More recently, the authors have used a single volar incision because this generally decompresses both volar and dorsal compartments with reduced pressures (Fig. 18.14). The dorsal compartment pressure is then remeasured after volar release; if it remains elevated, a dorsal compartment release is also performed. Presently, the authors have used a vacuum-assisted device over the open wound with serial trips to the operating room until delayed primary closure can be performed. With this technique, the use of skin grafts or flaps for coverage has decreased markedly.

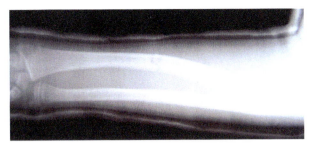

Fig. 18.15 Anteroposterior radiograph of a forearm after closed reduction and long arm cast immobilization. Note the restoration of the radial bow and the straight ulna as desired.

Reduction Techniques

Most plastic deformation and incomplete diaphyseal radial and ulnar fractures in the skeletally immature can be treated by closed reduction and cast immobilization techniques.[35–36] Plastic deformation fractures with significant deformity can limit forearm rotation and have a serpentine cosmetic appearance that does not remodel if closed reduction is not performed (see Fig. 18.1). Correction of a plastic deformation usually requires the application of a high degree of force, often with bolster or across-knee techniques. Therefore, reduction is usually performed in the operating room under general anesthesia. This allows for pain-free testing of forearm rotation to be certain the reduction is adequate.

Greenstick or incomplete fractures are generally treated with closed reduction techniques. These fractures have predominantly rotational malalignment, although the radiographs can be misinterpreted as showing mostly malangulation. The principle of closed reduction is therefore correction of the malrotation. Most are apex volar supination deformity fractures (see Fig. 18.3), which are reduced first with pronation, then by three-point molding (Fig. 18.15).[40,72] Less often, diaphyseal incomplete fractures are apex dorsal, pronation deformity fractures treated with supination reduction.[73] These fractures are generally stable after reduction; thus, cast immobilization is used.

Fixation Techniques

Closed Reduction and Percutaneous Pinning. In unstable fracture patterns, an acceptable reduction may be achieved via closed manipulation but may be difficult or impossible to maintain with traditional noninvasive forms of immobilization, such as a cast. Percutaneous smooth Kirschner (K)- or C-wire fixation has been used as a relatively noninvasive means for providing necessary stabilization to unstable distal radial fractures. Pin fixation is generally less mechanically stable than intramedullary or plate fixation, but it has been considered an acceptable or preferred treatment option for specific fractures.[74–78] The procedure is performed in the operating room under general anesthesia with use of intraoperative imaging. After anatomic reduction, pins are advanced under power with the use of fluoroscopic guidance. Utilization of an adequate incision and pin guide protection is recommended whenever tendons or neurovascular structures are at risk. Pin size, number, and configuration are determined by the fracture location and pattern. A minimum of two parallel or divergent pins is optimal for rotational control but may not always be possible. Fracture

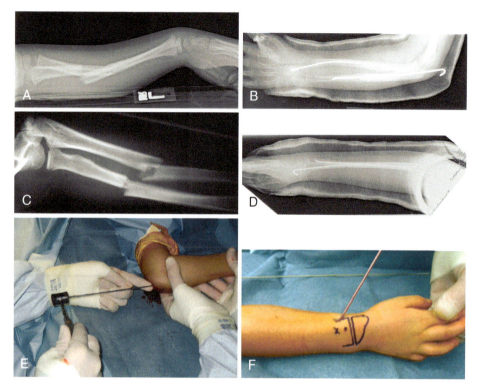

Fig. 18.16 Technique for intramedullary fixation of radial and ulnar diaphyseal fractures. Case examples include parts (A, B, C and D). (A) through (D) represent preoperative and postoperative radiographs of a diaphyseal forearm fracture fixed with intramedullary nails. (E and F) illustrate insertion techniques. (E) illustrates transapophyseal ulna insertion. The pin is tapped down the intramedullary canal by a mallet after power insertion through the proximal cortex. (F) illustrates metaphyseal insertion in the radius with care taken to avoid injury to the physis, extensor tendons, and radial sensory nerve.

reduction, stability, and pin position are then confirmed radiographically. The pins are then bent, cut at the tip, and may be buried or left above the skin. Most often, the authors leave them out of the skin for easy removal in the office setting. Supplementation with cast immobilization is standard in children. The pins are typically removed in 3 to 4 weeks, after adequate healing has occurred.

Intramedullary Fixation. Unstable complete diaphyseal forearm fractures in the skeletally immature are often now treated with intramedullary fixation (Fig. 18.16).[79–84] This allows for acceptable alignment of the fracture(s) by percutaneous or minimal surgical exposure. Closed reduction of a fracture in the operating room is performed with fluoroscopic guidance. If acceptable reduction can be obtained, percutaneous fixation is performed, generally with elastic stable intramedullary nailing, as introduced by Lascombes and colleagues.[85] Small-diameter nails (1.5–2.5 mm) are contoured so that the apex of the bow in the nail matches the fracture site. For the radius, insertion usually involves a distal-to-proximal insertion. The distal radial physis is radiographically identified and protected. Insertion in the metaphysis can be radial, central, or ulnar. With radial insertion, care is taken to protect the radial sensory nerve and the extensor tendons of the first and second dorsal compartments. Central insertion is performed proximal to the Lister tubercle while the thumb (EPL) and digital (EDC) extensors are protected. Ulnar-sided insertion can also be performed between the fourth and fifth dorsal compartments while the EDC and extensor digiti quinti (EDQ) are protected. For the author, the radial rod is inserted from the radial metaphysis beneath the insertion of the brachioradialis tendon through a protective skin incision for the extensor tendons and radial sensory nerve. The wire is prebent into an *S* or *C* shape. A drill hole is made proximal to the physis, and insertion into the medullary canal is performed bluntly to avoid impingement or penetration of the

volar or ulnar cortex. Rotation of the rod with proximal passage is performed so that the proximal aspect of the nail is in the radial neck and the apex of the nail bow is at the fracture site. Passage across the fracture site can be difficult, especially if anatomic reduction does not take place. For the ulna, most surgeons use a proximal-to-distal insertion technique (Fig. 18.17). The wire can usually be passed across the proximal ulnar apophysis without consequence. This is the author's preferred insertion technique. It allows for a straight passage of the wire. A small incision is made over the olecranon apophysis, blunt dissection is carried down to the apophysis, and drill entry is performed into the medullary canal. Care is taken not to create a false passage through the opposite cortex. Blunt passage of the wire to and across the fracture site is performed. The other alternative is to enter the ulnar metaphysis just distal to the apophysis. This avoids the theoretical worry about growth problems but requires a bend in the pin on insertion. Rods left for a longer period of time may do better if buried under soft tissues in the metaphyseal region.

Once the rods are safely in the diaphysis, they are passed to and across the fracture sites in sequence (Fig. 18.18). Most often, this can be achieved with fracture manipulation by hand, by reduction, or by intramedullary wire adjustments. The F-tool is designed to assist with reduction while avoiding unnecessary radiation to the surgeon's hands. However, prolonged, repetitive manipulations of the fracture site and wire passage attempts can lead to an increased risk of compartment syndrome.[28,86,87] Therefore, if passage is difficult percutaneously, open reduction and wire passage are advocated. This may be necessary in 10% to 30% of fractures to limit complications.

Single-bone intramedullary fixation is indicated in some young children (usually ages 8–12 years) with unstable fractures.[37,88] Most often, this is performed by intramedullary fixation of the ulna and closed reduction of the radius, but

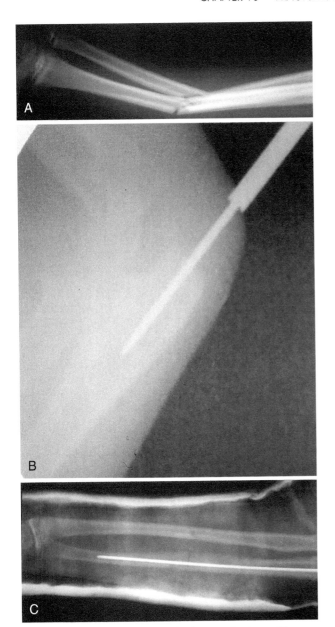

Fig. 18.17 (A) Lateral radiograph of a forearm fracture with an apex volar supination deformity in a young child. On occasion, this can be unstable after closed reduction. Single-bone fixation has been used as noted in (B). This provided ulnar stability and allowed closed reduction of the radial deformity. The entry site proximally through the apophysis is noted in (C). A metaphyseal entry site can also be used.

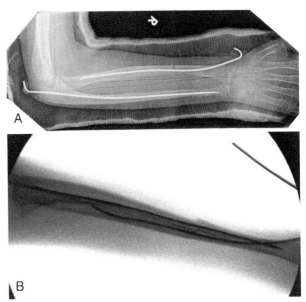

Fig. 18.18 (A) Intramedullary fixation of both bones. This has become a more common treatment for complete fractures in the older child. These wires were left out of the skin. Most are buried until complete healing, but care must be taken to avoid injury to the extensor tendons distally. (B) Intraoperative lateral fluoroscopic radiograph of intramedullary fixation of the radius and ulna with elastic titanium nails.

fixation of the radius with closed reduction of the radius also retains some clinical usefulness. It is important to test stability in the operating room with rotation and stress. If the fractured bone without fixation tends to displace, then dual fixation is advocated.

Plate and Screw Fixation. Standard adult treatment of diaphyseal radial and ulnar fractures is indicated in skeletally mature adolescents to provide stable fixation without immobilization and to allow for early motion to prevent contracture development.[89,90] Operative exposure of the radius is usually by a standard Henry approach, and exposure of the ulna is by a direct medial approach. Anatomic reduction and compression plating techniques are performed. Correction of malrotation and restoration of the radial bow is critical to successful treatment. Immobilization postoperatively is brief until the patient is comfortable. Protected rehabilitation is performed until full fracture healing and restoration of motion and strength are achieved. Unless the hardware is irritating, plate removal is usually not performed because of the risks of neurovascular compromise and refracture.

PITFALLS/AVOIDANCE OF COMPLICATIONS

Good technique, attention to detail, and appropriate and timely follow-up are the keys to minimizing complications. Inadequate reduction and loss of reduction can result from poor casting technique or acceptance of a marginal reduction.[76–78,91] Failure to recognize the rotational component of deformity can result in loss of the normal anatomic alignment and joint motion. Concomitant injuries to neurovascular structures must be recognized and dealt with appropriately.[92–94] Attention to detail and good technique in cast application is necessary to avoid preventable complications such as cast-saw burns and skin breakdown. Compartment syndromes must be ruled out in all traumatic injuries to the extremity, including open fractures. A high level of suspicion and a low threshold for prophylactic compartment release can help avoid the devastating complication of Volkmann ischemic contracture. Traumatic and iatrogenic physeal injuries are unique to children, and, if unrecognized or left untreated, they can result in partial or complete growth arrest with resultant limb length discrepancy or progressive angular deformity.[60,95,96] Appropriate and timely antimicrobial therapy, organism culture, when indicated, and meticulous wound management limit infections.

POSTOPERATIVE CARE AND REHABILITATION

The postoperative care after fixation of forearm fractures varies depending on several factors. Diaphyseal fractures managed by closed means are generally treated in a long arm cast with the elbow flexed to 90 degrees and appropriate forearm rotation for a period of 4 to 6 weeks based on radiographic evidence of healing. Those fractures managed with closed reduction and pin fixations are treated in a similar manner. After intramedullary nail fixation of fractures, some surgeons allow the child to move immediately postoperatively, whereas others prefer to immobilize the child. The length of postoperative immobilization in a cast and timing of wire removal varies widely among surgeons. The issues involved in these decisions are risk of stiffness, pin problems, and possibility of refracture. Some surgeons do not cast at all, and others cast until healing. Some remove the wires when the bone is healed at 6 to 12 weeks; others leave them in place for up to a year after fracture treatment. In addition, some surgeons have advocated for leaving the intramedullary implants exposed through the skin for ease of removal immediately after fracture healing.[97] The clear indications for removal are pin problems or infections. The risk of refracture is present for up to a year after injury; thus, the timing of removal and sports participation need to take this into account for each case.

Rehabilitation is an important component of the treatment of any fracture or dislocation. However, the necessity for a formal physical or occupational therapy program varies greatly by injury type, location, chronicity, duration of immobilization, and the age of the patient. Younger children have a greater tolerance for prolonged periods of immobilization than do adolescents and young adults. Contracture secondary to cast immobilization is much less of a problem in children, often obviating the need for formal therapy. Gradual return to normal play often provides the strengthening and range of motion necessary for full recovery. Conversely, adolescents approaching skeletal maturity may behave similarly to an adult. Formal therapy may be necessary to prevent the development of a permanent elbow contracture, for example, after even a brief period of long arm casting. The need for formal therapy should be decided on a case-by-case basis.

COMPLICATIONS

NONUNION OR DELAYED UNION

Nonunion of pediatric forearm fractures is a relatively rare complication after treatment. Intramedullary nail fixation has been implicated in delayed union of forearm fractures, especially when the fracture site is distracted by too thick a pin.[98–100] The incidence of nonunion or delayed union has been associated with age greater than 10 years, open reduction, and open fractures. The ulna is more commonly affected than the radius. Treatment can include additional time in immobilization or activity limitations for delayed unions and revision fixation with or without bone grafting for established nonunions.

MALUNION

The definition of acceptable alignment when treating pediatric diaphyseal forearm fractures depends on the surgeon's interpretation of the existing literature. Malunions with symptomatic loss of forearm function, usually secondary to loss of pronosupination, are indications for a corrective osteotomy. The osteotomy is usually performed at the level of the previous fracture or at the apex of deformity. Fixation of the osteotomy can be rigid with

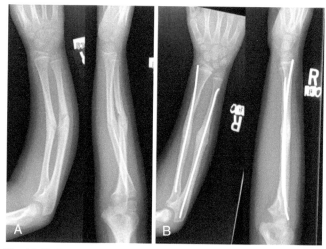

Fig. 18.19 Forearm malunion in a 7-year-old female treated with osteotomy and intramedullary nail fixation. (A) Preoperative malalignment. (B) Postoperative corrected position.

plate-and-screw fixation or semirigid with intramedullary nail fixation (Fig. 18.19). The choice of fixation depends on the child's age; younger children are more amenable to semirigid fixation.

REFRACTURE

Refracture after closed treatment of pediatric forearm fractures is common. It has been reported to occur at a rate of 1.4% to 8%.[101–103] Refracture has been attributed to greater residual angulation of the fracture (<15 degrees).[103] A refracture should be treated by the same principles outlined for the treatment of primary pediatric forearm fractures.

RADIOULNAR SYNOSTOSIS

Radioulnar synostosis is a rare complication of treatment of pediatric forearm fractures and is most commonly associated with mechanisms involving high-energy trauma.[99,104] There have been cases reported after both intramedullary fixation and plate-and-screw fixation of diaphyseal fractures.[68,99,105] Synostoses resulting in functional limitations have been treated successfully with surgical resection of the aberrant union.

Special Circumstances

Monteggia Fracture-Dislocations. Monteggia fracture-dislocations can lead to dire consequences if the injury is not recognized immediately or stable reduction that prevents redisplacement is not provided.[12,106,107] Any fracture of the forearm should be assessed for dislocation of the PRUJ and radiocapitellar joint. Appropriate anteroposterior and lateral radiographs of the wrist, forearm, and elbow are necessary for exact injury definition. Despite extensive literature about the risk of a missed Monteggia lesion and the difficulties of chronic Monteggia fracture-dislocation reconstruction, this lesion is still missed by otherwise competent orthopedic surgeons, radiologists, and emergency and primary care physicians. Simplistically, the radius needs to be in anatomic alignment with the capitellum in all radiographic views.[106,108] If this relationship cannot be adequately seen, more radiographs need to be obtained in the acute care setting.

Pediatric Monteggia lesions are classified by the direction of displacement of the radial head (i.e., anterior, posterior, or lateral)[12] and by the type of forearm fracture. Isolated ulnar fractures constitute the majority of forearm fractures associated with radial head dislocations. These isolated ulnar fractures are categorized as plastic deformation, incomplete, and complete fractures, similar to other diaphyseal forearm fractures. Complete fractures are further classified as transverse, short oblique, long oblique, and comminuted fractures.[109] This subclassification of ulnar fractures aids the surgeon in determining both the stability of the ulnar fracture and appropriate treatment. Other forearm fractures associated with a radial head dislocation are called Monteggia equivalents, and there are many of these.[110–113] Therefore, the treating clinician needs to be aware of the possibility of an unstable or dislocated proximal radioulnar and radiocapitellar joint with any forearm fracture. All forearm fracture radiographs should be scrutinized for proximal radioulnar and radiocapitellar joint dislocations.

Successful treatment of a pediatric Monteggia fracture-dislocation depends on anatomic reduction and stabilization of the ulna.[109] With plastic deformation and incomplete fractures, reduction and stabilization can usually be obtained by closed manipulation. The problem with plastic deformation and incomplete fractures is more often the failure to recognize the injury immediately rather than the loss of reduction after successful closed manipulation. With complete fractures, the complication is more often the failure to maintain reduction. Treatment by closed means for displaced transverse, short oblique, long oblique, and comminuted ulnar fractures associated with proximal radial dislocations has an increasing risk of loss of reduction by fracture type with cast immobilization. Reduction and stabilization of the ulnar fracture are recommended in many of these cases, but successful closed reduction and casting can be accomplished with the requirement of close follow-up to ensure maintenance of reduction.[114] Transverse and short oblique fractures are best treated with intramedullary ulnar stabilization (Fig. 18.20).[12,107–109,112,115] Long oblique and comminuted fractures of the ulna are best treated with plate-and-screw fixation after anatomic reduction.[109]

For intramedullary fixation, the elastic nail or K-wire is inserted through a proximal insertion site in the olecranon apophysis similar to the method described and illustrated in the forearm fracture section. The pin is left exposed and removed with fracture healing, usually at 4 to 6 weeks. Elastic nails require removal in the day surgery unit under anesthesia, whereas the stainless steel wire left exposed through the skin can be removed in the office without sedation. Successful reduction and appropriate stabilization of ulnar fractures almost always lead to an anatomic and stable reduction of the radial head. Rare situations, however, require open reduction of the PRUJ and repair of the disrupted annular ligament.[108] The surgeon needs to be certain during early treatment and follow-up that the radial head is anatomically reduced in relationship to the capitellum and proximal ulna on all radiographic views. After reduction and stabilization, stress testing of the radial head reduction in the operating room is advised. Postoperative cast immobilization is usually for 4 to 6 weeks in a long arm cast with forearm supination to aid in reduction of the radial head and healing of the injured annular ligament. Protected mobilization is initiated after radiographic

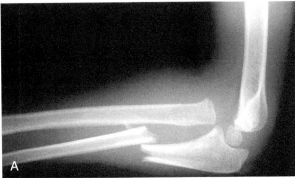
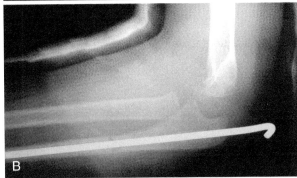

Fig. 18.20 (A) Lateral radiograph of a displaced Monteggia fracture-dislocation. This is the most common Bado I anterior dislocation of the radial head. (B) After closed reduction and pin stabilization of the ulnar fracture, the radial head is anatomically reduced.

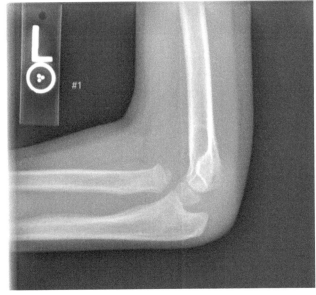

Fig. 18.21 Lateral radiograph of a missed Monteggia fracture-dislocation. This is a more complex reconstruction than acute care of the recognized injury.

fracture healing is demonstrated. The intramedullary pins are removed in the office or day surgery setting, depending on implant type and placement. Plates and screws are removed at the discretion of the surgeon and the patient.

Care of chronic Monteggia fracture-dislocations is complicated (Fig. 18.21). Opinion varies about the natural history of an untreated chronic Monteggia lesion from limited disability to progressive, painful deformity.[116–122] The

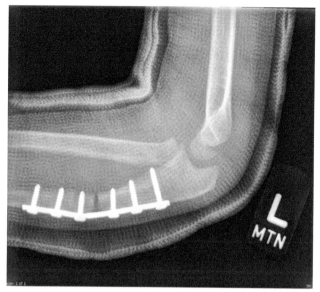

Fig. 18.22 Postoperative radiograph after chronic Monteggia fracture reconstruction with an ulnar osteotomy and correction of the radiocapitellar joint alignment.

spectrum of results from the published small series of retrospective case analyses includes full recovery to a high incidence of complications. Thus, the decision to intervene when a chronic Monteggia fracture is diagnosed is multifactorial and includes consideration of the time elapsed since the initial injury, the degree of deformity and functional limitations, and the surgeon's clinical preferences and experience. This is not an operation for the uninitiated. Relatively recent injuries with radiographic evidence of progressive dislocation of the proximal radius and clinical pain are clear candidates for surgery performed by an experienced practitioner. Long-standing dislocations with minimal limitation of motion or function may be better treated with observation and serial radiographs. This is even clearer when plain radiographic or MRI evidence indicates loss of the normal concave radial head-convex capitellar anatomic relationship. Surgical reconstruction always requires an ulnar osteotomy. No consensus exists regarding open reduction of the joint and annular ligament reconstruction (Fig. 18.22). Radial nerve decompression and prophylactic forearm fasciotomies may be warranted to limit neurovascular complications. Some authors recommend 3 to 6 weeks of radiocapitellar pin fixation to maintain reduction during ligamentous healing. However, pin migration or breakage is of concern with this technique. Of note, the pin cannot substitute for an inadequate ligament reconstruction or joint reduction. Recurrent subluxation or dislocation has occurred with all of the various techniques of reconstruction. Resultant limitations of motion and function, at times associated with pain, are disappointing. Thus, the patient, family, and surgeon must be aware of the real risk of failure with reconstruction of a chronic Monteggia fracture-dislocation.

FRACTURES OF THE DISTAL RADIUS

Distal fractures of the radius and ulna are the most common forearm injuries. These fractures are classified as torus or buckle fractures, incomplete or greenstick fractures, and complete fractures. Most complete fractures involve both the ulna and radius, whereas most torus fractures are isolated injuries to the radius. Increased participation in sports, particularly extreme sports, has led to a rise in the incidence of distal radial and ulnar fractures seen in children.[123,124] Obesity, poor postural balance, ligamentous laxity, and decreased bone mineralization place children at increased risk of distal radial and ulnar fractures.[125–128]

EMERGENT TREATMENT

Emergent treatment for distal radial fractures is reserved for open fractures, those fractures that involve a concomitant neurovascular injury, and those complicated by compartment syndrome or acute carpal tunnel syndrome.[129] Treatment of open fractures of the distal radius is similar to the treatment of other open fractures, requiring timely irrigation, débridement, and reduction of the deformity. Those fractures associated with neurovascular compromise require emergent reduction of the deformity and serial examinations. Continued neurovascular compromise requires emergent surgical exploration and repair or decompression of injured structures. Similar to other fractures, those distal radial fractures complicated by compartment syndrome and/or acute carpal tunnel syndrome require emergent surgical fasciotomy and carpal tunnel release.

INDICATIONS FOR DEFINITIVE CARE

Torus fractures of the radius are stable injuries and require limited immobilization for comfort and for prevention of early reinjury that could result in a displaced fracture. The majority of the complete fractures displace into extension with apex volar angulation of the distal fragment. These metaphyseal fractures are juxtaphyseal and have a high degree of remodeling potential, especially in the flexion-extension plane of motion of the wrist joint. Thus, in the skeletally immature with more than 2 years of growth remaining, closed reduction and cast immobilization is usually the treatment of choice for both metaphyseal and physeal displaced fractures.

Clear evidence in the published literature shows that complete distal radial and ulnar fractures are unstable injuries.[34,76–78] Loss of reduction is common, even under the ideal circumstances of an experienced surgeon, appropriate anesthesia, fluoroscopic image control, and a well-molded cast. Failure to completely reduce the angulation and translation increases the risk of subsequent loss of alignment with cast treatment. Similarly, an inadequate cast has been shown to be a factor in loss of reduction.[34,38] A well-molded short arm cast may be as effective as a long arm cast in maintaining reduction and is preferred by patients for functional activities.[130] Malunion is a risk in these fractures. Patients treated with closed reduction and cast immobilization need close radiographic follow-up in the first 3 to 4 weeks after reduction. Up to one-third of these injuries eventually displace and require repeated reduction to prevent malunion. Minor degrees of flexion-extension malalignment remodel with growth. Because of the risk of malunion secondary to loss of reduction with closed treatment, many surgeons advocate closed reduction and percutaneous pin fixation for displaced metaphyseal injuries in the older child.[34,76–78] Data indicate that closed reduction and pin fixation are equivalent at 2-year follow-up, provided that the principles

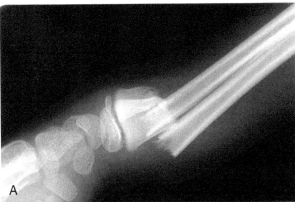

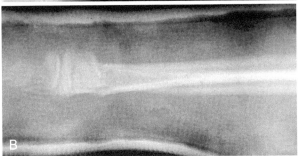

Fig. 18.23 (A) Lateral radiograph of a completely displaced distal radial metaphyseal fracture. (B) Closed reduction to anatomic position is noted in the cast by this lateral radiograph. This fracture may have approximately a 30% risk of loss of reduction in the ensuing 3 weeks and needs close radiographic follow-up to prevent malunion.

of treatment are followed in each case. In general, more than 20 degrees of residual angulation after reduction in a pediatric patient with less than 2 years' growth remaining is an indication for repeated reduction or pin fixation. In addition, any child with a floating elbow injury is a candidate for pin fixation of both the elbow region and radius fracture to lessen the risk of compartment syndrome.[131,132]

NONOPERATIVE TREATMENT

Closed reduction and casting or splinting can treat the majority of distal radial fractures in children. Reduction can be performed with a local anesthesia hematoma block, under conscious sedation in the emergency department, or even with general anesthesia, depending on the local practice setting and expertise. Reduction of the common hinged, extension fractures requires distraction and flexion to restore alignment. Reduction of the metaphyseal fracture with overlap of the distal fragment dorsally on the volar proximal fragment requires hyperextension of the deformity to untether the periosteum before flexion reduction (Fig. 18.23). This is a more difficult reduction and requires adequate analgesia, muscle relaxation, and clinician experience to be successful in the ambulatory setting. Excessive attempts at closed reduction can result in marked swelling, increased risk of compartment syndrome, and failure to successfully treat this fracture with a closed technique, even in the operating room. Longitudinal traction with increasing weights similar to adult fracture reduction is not indicated because this will further tighten the dorsal periosteum and prevent reduction.

After acceptable closed reduction, the extremity is immobilized in a long or short arm cast or splint. Some evidence questions the need for long arm immobilization. Studies have highlighted the efficacy of short arm cast immobilization, including no statistical differences in the rate of loss of reduction and improved patient satisfaction with short arm immobilization.[130] Regardless of the immobilization technique used, the fracture should be observed closely for the first 3 to 4 weeks to identify cases of loss of reduction. Fracture healing is generally evident 4 to 6 weeks after the injury, and immobilization can be discontinued when radiographic healing is evident.

Torus or buckle fractures represent compression injuries that are inherently stable. They do not require a reduction. Treatment should consist of short-term immobilization—2 to 4 weeks—to prevent further injury and assist in pain control. Immobilization in a removable orthosis or a short arm cast has been shown to provide equivalent satisfactory outcomes.[133,134]

Distal radial physeal injuries have great potential to remodel when sufficient growth remains. Malreduced physeal injuries can result in permanent deformity when they occur close to skeletal maturity. Nondisplaced physeal injuries are adequately treated with cast immobilization. Displaced fractures can be treated with gentle closed reduction and casting. Multiple attempts at reduction should be avoided because of the risk of physeal injury resulting in growth arrest. Similarly, late reduction—longer than 7 to 10 days after the injury—should be avoided.[135] Physeal injuries should be followed up closely to identify those cases of loss of reduction in an effort to avoid permanent deformity in patients close to skeletal maturity.

SURGICAL TREATMENT

Surgical Anatomy

The appearance of the distal radial epiphysis usually occurs by 2 years of age, trending toward earlier appearance in girls than in boys.[136] The epiphysis of the distal ulna generally appears by 7 years of age. Physeal closure of the ulna happens at approximately 16 years of age in girls and 17 years of age in boys. The closure of the distal radius follows shortly thereafter.[137,138] The DRUJ serves as the platform supporting the carpus and the hand. The DRUJ is stabilized by the TFCC and its complex association of volar and dorsal ligaments. The TFCC spans from the sigmoid notch of the radius, across the head of the ulna, to insert in the fovea at the base of the ulnar styloid. The ulna remains relatively immobile as the radius rotates around it. This complex articulation allows for 120 degrees of flexion and extension of the wrist, 50 degrees of radial and ulnar deviation, and 150 degrees of forearm rotation.[139] The length relationship between the radius and ulna is defined as ulnar variance. This relationship can be used to determine the adequacy of reduction and restoration of appropriate length.[140] Variance measurements depend on the position of the forearm; hence, radiographs should be taken with the forearm in neutral rotation with the elbow flexed and shoulder abducted 90 degrees to allow for standardized measurements.[141,142] Comparison with the uninjured side is useful. The normal force transmission across the wrist joint is 80% through the radiocarpal joint. The ulnocarpal joint bears the additional 20%. Changes in variance can affect this relationship, as seen in cases of fracture, TFCC tears (associated with positive ulnar variance), and Kienböck disease (associated with negative ulnar variance).[143,144]

Positioning Techniques

The patient is positioned supine on the operating room table with the arm outstretched on a hand table for both open and closed treatments of distal radial fractures. If an open technique is anticipated, the use of a brachial pneumatic tourniquet assists in the acquisition of a bloodless operative field. The image intensifier is positioned perpendicular to the operating table and parallel to the operative extremity so that the surgeon and an assistant have adequate exposure to the operative field.

SURGICAL APPROACH

Volar Approach to the Distal Radius. The volar approach to the distal radius, as described by Henry,[65] allows for complete exposure of the distal radial metaphysis with an option for extension proximally, if needed. The incision is centered over the FCR tendon. Distally, the incision begins at the proximal wrist flexion crease and extends proximally an adequate distance to ensure full exposure of the fracture. The dissection is taken through the floor of the FCR tendon sheath, exposing the underlying FPL proximally and pronator quadratus distally. The radial artery lies radial to the FCR tendon and should be identified and protected throughout the exposure. The FPL is retracted in an ulnar direction, revealing the pronator quadratus on the volar surface of the radial metaphysis. The pronator quadratus is released sharply from its radial insertion and elevated in subperiosteal fashion in an ulnar direction. This allows the surgeon full exposure to the metaphyseal portion of the distal radius.

Dorsal Approach to the Distal Radius. The dorsal exposure of the distal radius allows for extensile exposure of the distal radial metaphysis, while also allowing for direct visualization of the distal radial articular surface, exposure of the DRUJ and distal ulna, and access to the ulnocarpal joint. Understanding the anatomy of the sensory branches of the radial nerve is necessary for safe exposure of the dorsal distal radius. The sensory branch of the radial nerve becomes subcutaneous 5 to 10 cm proximal to the ulnar styloid, emerging between the ECRL and the brachioradialis tendons. It then bifurcates into palmar and dorsal branches. The dorsal branch passes radial to the Lister tubercle and continues distally to supply sensation to the first and second web spaces. The palmar branch passes within 2 cm of the first dorsal compartment tendons, directly over the EPL tendon, on its way to providing sensation to the dorsolateral aspect of the thumb.

Deep dissection requires identification of the EPL tendon as it emerges from the distal aspect of the retinaculum ulnar to the Lister tubercle. Once identified, proximal dissection releasing the EPL from the retinaculum allows for retraction of the tendon in a radial direction. The floor of the third dorsal compartment can then be entered sharply, cutting through periosteum, to the distal radial metaphysis. Subperiosteal exposure in both radial and ulnar directions provides adequate exposure of the distal radius for fracture reduction while protecting the overlying extensor tendons. Care should be taken to preserve the dorsal radioulnar ligaments stabilizing the DRUJ.

If exposure of the distal radial articular surface is necessary, the dorsal wrist capsule can be incised transversely from its attachment to the distal radius; a cuff of tissue should be left intact for later repair.

Injuries requiring exposure of the distal ulna can also be treated from the dorsal approach. The dorsal cutaneous branch of the ulnar nerve arises from the ulnar nerve deep to the FCU tendon. It becomes subcutaneous on the ulnar border of the forearm, approximately 5 cm from the proximal border of the pisiform.[145] The distal ulnar, DRUJ, and TFCC should be approached through the floor of the fifth dorsal compartment. The retinaculum overlying the EDQ should be incised sharply and retracted radially. A capsular flap should be raised from the distal ulna with care taken to protect the TFCC and dorsal DRUJ ligaments.

Medial Approach to the Distal Ulna. The medial approach to the distal ulna can be useful for treatment of distal ulnar fractures irreducible by closed means. The exposure is a distal extension of the proximal exposure used for reaching ulnar shaft fractures. The interval between the flexor and extensor compartments of the forearm can be entered sharply, and subperiosteal exposure of the volar and dorsal surfaces of the ulna can be easily accomplished. Care should be taken in the distalmost portion of the wound to avoid injury to the dorsal sensory branch of the ulnar nerve that traverses the subcutaneous tissues from volar to dorsal on its way to innervate the dorsal skin on the ulnar side of the hand. The nerve crosses the subcutaneous border of the ulna at or near the ulnar head.

Carpal Tunnel Release. Release of the carpal tunnel can be indicated in the setting of forearm compartment syndrome, carpal dislocation, or the presence of foreign body within the anatomic space. The carpal tunnel is approached through the volar side of the hand and wrist. The incision is outlined just radial to the hook of the hamate and can be extended across the proximal wrist flexion crease with the use of a zigzag-type incision if the procedure is associated with a forearm compartment release. When an extensile approach to the carpal tunnel is used, care should be taken to avoid injury to the palmar cutaneous branch of the median nerve, arising from the median nerve approximately 6 cm proximal to the wrist flexion crease and running ulnar to the FCR tendon. The incision is deepened sharply through the palmar fat and the superficial palmar fascia to the level of the transverse carpal ligament. The transverse carpal ligament is released from its ulnar attachment to the hook of the hamate to avoid injury to the recurrent motor branch of the median nerve. The ligament is released distally until the palmar fat pad is visualized. The superficial palmar arch is intimately associated within the palmar fat; hence, dissection should be approached carefully in this location. The proximal portion of the ligament is released with the leading edge of the antebrachial fascia. This can become continuous with the fascial release of the forearm, if necessary.

Reduction Techniques

The most common pattern of injury results in dorsal displacement of distal radial fragments and apex volar angulation. Gentle traction with re-creation of the injury and translation of the distal fragment is usually sufficient for reduction of the fracture deformity. When rotational malalignment is present, pronation or supination of the forearm may assist in anatomic alignment of the fracture. Occasionally, interposed muscle or periosteum may block the surgeon's ability to adequately reduce the fracture by closed means.

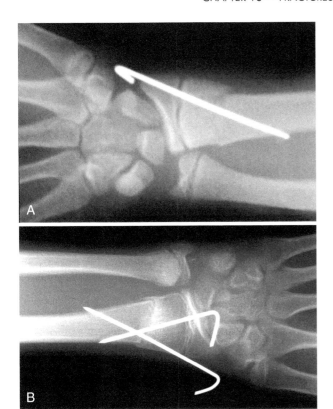

Fig. 18.24 An alternative treatment to closed reduction of a completely displaced distal radial metaphyseal fracture is reduction and percutaneous pin fixation. A single oblique pin from the radial side (A) or crossed pins (B) may be appropriate, depending on fracture stability. Care must be taken to avoid injury to the radial sensory nerve or extensor tendons with insertion.

Percutaneous techniques have been described to assist in the reduction by use of a K-wire or small elevator inserted into the fracture from a dorsal approach, levering the distal fragment onto the proximal metaphysis.[146–149]

When closed reduction fails to achieve acceptable alignment of a distal radial fracture, open reduction is performed with the use of one of the aforementioned approaches, depending on the fracture pattern and suspected blocks to reduction.

Fixation Techniques

One or two oblique pin(s) from the radial side or crossed pins placed from distal to proximal are sufficient for pediatric distal radial fracture fixation (Fig. 18.24). Care is taken to avoid the extensor tendons and radial sensory nerve with use of an appropriately sized incision and pin insertion guides for the protection of soft tissues in all cases. If possible, the pin(s) is placed in the metaphysis, thus avoiding physeal injury. If necessary, smooth, small-diameter pins are placed across the distal radial physis for a short duration. Threaded pins should be avoided because of the risk of injury to the physis and the difficulty of removal. Pins are removed in the office when there is sufficient healing, generally at 4 to 6 weeks. Cast or splint immobilization is used in conjunction with pin fixation until sufficient healing occurs to begin rehabilitation. Adding a thumb spica component to the immobilization helps prevent pin irritation in the snuff-box area.

Pitfalls/Avoidance of Complications

Achievement of an acceptable reduction, early identification of associated injuries, appropriate cast application, and serial follow-up will eliminate many of the factors associated with poor outcomes in the treatment of distal radial fractures in children. Special attention to protecting the growth potential of the distal radial and ulnar physes should remain a foremost priority when these injuries are treated. The use of small-caliber, smooth pins when fixation is necessary and avoidance of late manipulation minimize the risk of iatrogenic injury to physeal integrity.

Postoperative Care and Rehabilitation

Distal radial fractures in children usually heal within 4 to 6 weeks after injury. When radiographic union is confirmed, discontinuation of immobilization is appropriate. Children rarely require formal therapy to regain motion and return to unimpeded function and activity. The fractures with physeal involvement should be followed with a radiograph at 6 months after healing to ensure physeal growth has resumed.

Special Circumstances

Galeazzi Fracture-Dislocations. Pediatric Galeazzi injuries are rare. Radiographically, they are recognized as displaced distal radial fractures associated with a DRUJ dislocation or displaced ulnar physeal injury (Galeazzi equivalent).[150,14,59] In addition, rare minor fractures of the radius are occasionally associated with an unstable DRUJ, which must be recognized clinically. Treatment of the pediatric Galeazzi injury requires anatomic reduction of both the radius fracture and DRUJ dislocation. In the young with a greenstick radius fracture, closed reduction restores anatomic alignment and is usually stable.[14–15,59] Long arm treatment in the position of rotational stability is sufficient for healing of both fracture and DRUJ disruption. These fracture-dislocations are usually stable in supination; however, in some instances, the dislocation occurs in the opposite direction, and pronation is required for reduction and stabilization. This is best assessed after reduction with volar-dorsal stress to the DRUJ in the neutral position, in supination, and in pronation. In the older child in whom this fracture-dislocation is most common, open reduction internal fixation of the radial metaphyseal-diaphyseal fracture is recommended.[15,151] A volar approach to the fracture through the floor of the FCR tendon sheath with elevation of the pronator quadratus is the preferred surgical approach. Plate fixation is used to achieve stable, anatomic fixation. Stress testing of the DRUJ after fixation of the radius is performed in all positions of forearm rotation. Generally, the DRUJ is stable in supination after plate fixation of the radius, and long arm cast immobilization is used in that position for 4 to 6 weeks. If the joint is unstable in all planes, the author uses two pins across the distal radius and ulna protruding from each bone for ease of removal in the case of pin fracture. An irreducible DRUJ is very rare but requires an open reduction to remove interposed tendon or periosteum.[152]

Failure to recognize an irreducible dislocation early makes successful late reconstruction much more difficult. Injuries to the TFCC do occur with distal radial fractures, even in children and adolescents.[153] The exact incidence of injury and percentage of complete healing with cast immobilization for fracture treatment is unknown. Patients with

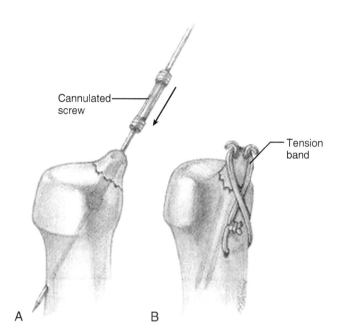

Cannulated screw

Tension band

A   B

Fig. 18.25 (A and B) Several methods are available to fix an ulnar styloid fracture depending partly on the size of the styloid fragment. (A) A cannulated screw can be used to fix larger ulnar styloid fragments. (B) Smaller fragments can be fixed with the use of a tension band technique. (Modified from Trumble TE, Culp R, Hanel DP, et al. Intra-articular fractures of the distal aspect of the radius. *Instr Course Lect.* 1999;48:465-480.)

displaced base-of-the-ulnar-styloid fractures are at greater risk of TFCC injuries.[153–155] Treatment with an early tension band technique is recommended for the rare, unstable displaced base-of-the-styloid fracture (Fig. 18.25). Exposure is performed by a straight ulnar incision. The ulnar sensory nerve is protected. With fluoroscopic guidance, dissection is carried down to the displaced styloid. Reduction is performed with bone-holding clamps. A single oblique pin is placed from the distal ulnar styloid across the fracture with penetration of the proximal radial cortex of the ulna. Drill holes are placed proximal to the fracture, and a polyester suture is used as a tension band through the drill holes and twisted into a figure eight around the distal bent wire. Immobilization in a long arm cast is required until fracture healing at 4 to 6 weeks. The percutaneous pin is removed in the office.

Patients seen with long-standing ulnocarpal pain with wrist ulnar deviation on forearm rotation after a distal radial fracture should be evaluated clinically and radiographically for a chronic TFCC tear. A nonunion of the ulnar styloid, hypertrophic healed ulnar styloid fracture, or positive ulnar variance are risk factors for ulnocarpal impaction and a TFCC tear.[156,157] MRI scans or arthrograms may be diagnostic. Wrist arthroscopy is definitive for diagnosis and usually appropriate for treatment. At times, complex reconstruction of the TFCC and DRUJ is necessary for chronic instability.

Physeal Fractures. Distal radial and ulnar physeal fractures are usually extension injuries. They occur most commonly in the preadolescent growth spurt. Radial physeal injuries occur more commonly than ulnar physeal injuries.[1,158–160] These injuries are classified by Salter-Harris criteria,[161] and type II injuries are the most common displaced fractures.

The common nondisplaced Salter-Harris type I injuries are apparent clinically by tenderness or swelling over the physeal region.[162,163] Rare types III and IV injuries require careful analysis of the plain radiographs and usually CT examination to make diagnosis and treatment decisions.[96,164,165] Failure to recognize and anatomically reduce a type III or IV injury can lead to articular incongruity and physeal arrest. For displaced radial types I and II physeal injuries, the risk of growth arrest is low, in the 3% to 5% range, for the fracture and subsequent treatment. Recurrent or late reductions of radial physeal fractures beyond 5 to 10 days have a higher risk of radial growth arrest (Fig. 18.26).[164,166,167] Displaced ulnar physeal injuries have a much higher risk of growth arrest, in the 20% to 50% range (Fig. 18.27).[168–170] Because 70% to 80% of growth of the radius and ulna comes from the distal physeal region, an arrest of one of the bones leads to progressive deformity in the forearm and wrist.[153–155]

Brief immobilization until resolution of discomfort is advocated for stable, nondisplaced type I injuries. Closed reduction and cast immobilization is the treatment of choice for almost all displaced types I and II physeal injuries. Reduction is performed with appropriate analgesia to lessen the risk of iatrogenic injury to the physis. The physeal displacement can generally be reduced with gentle distraction and dorsal-to-volar pressure for the common extension fracture. Long or short arm well-molded cast immobilization is required for 4 to 6 weeks. Repeated reduction is not advocated for the skeletally immature patient with loss of anatomic reduction in the first 1 to 3 weeks after fracture reduction (Fig. 18.28). Fortunately, as long as the physis is not impaired, marked remodeling can occur in the young patient with an extension malunion (Fig. 18.29).[40,41] For the near mature adolescent, anatomic alignment is necessary for prevention of malunion that will not remodel because of insufficient growth remaining (Fig. 18.30).[16,52] These fractures, along with those associated with neurovascular compromise or a floating elbow, are the ones most often treated with closed reduction and pinning. In the case of malunion, corrective osteotomy with a bone graft and internal fixation is necessary for treatment of instability and impaction pain and prevention of the risk of long-term arthrosis.

Pin fixation is advised for patients with excessive swelling or associated neurovascular compromise.[171] This lessens the risk of compartment syndrome, along with circumferential cast immobilization. This is particularly true for patients with median neuropathy on presentation. Single, small-diameter, smooth transphyseal pin fixation is usually adequate. If necessary for rotational stability, crossed pin fixation is used. Again, care is taken to avoid the extensor tendons or radial sensory nerve injury with pin placement. The pins are removed in the office at 3 to 6 weeks, and mobilization is begun with fracture healing. Follow-up radiographs are advised at 6 to 12 months to identify the rare physeal arrest. This allows for timely treatment decisions before marked deformity occurs.

Types III and IV physeal injuries require anatomic reduction of both the joint and physeal cartilage. This can usually be performed percutaneously, but the surgeon should be prepared for an open reduction if persistent joint incongruity is suspected. Arthroscopically assisted reduction is helpful at times.[172] Smooth, small-diameter pin fixation may be adequate. External fixation may be necessary for stabilization

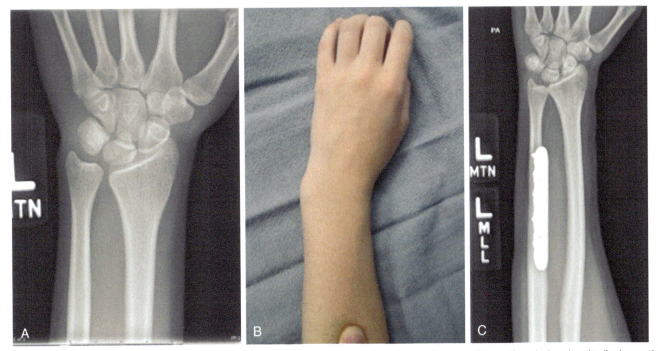

Fig. 18.26 (A) Anteroposterior (AP) radiograph revealing radial growth arrest after physeal fracture with continued ulnar longitudinal growth. Symptomatic ulnocarpal impaction was present in this patient. (B) Clinical photograph of radial deviation deformity and prominent distal ulna. (C) AP fluoroscopic radiograph of ulnar shortening osteotomy to neutral variance.

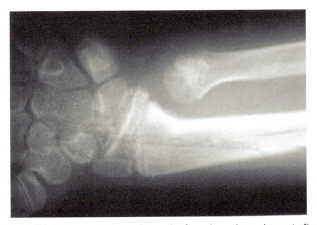

Fig. 18.27 Anteroposterior radiograph of an ulnar physeal arrest after Galeazzi-equivalent injury. The radial physeal deformity is progressive because of the ulnar tether.

and also avoids the use of more extensive hardware in the physeal region (Fig. 18.31). Ulnar physeal injuries have such a high risk of growth arrest that anatomic reduction and stabilization of the physis are recommended. Care is taken to avoid additional physeal injury with operative exposure and fixation. Careful follow-up of all these injuries is necessary for early recognition, evaluation, and treatment of growth- and joint-related problems.

COMPLICATIONS

MALUNION

Malunion of distal radial fractures is an uncommon complication. Given the growth potential of the distal radial physis, malunions in children with significant growth remaining often correct over time. The malunited fracture should be followed closely over the ensuing 6 to 12 months

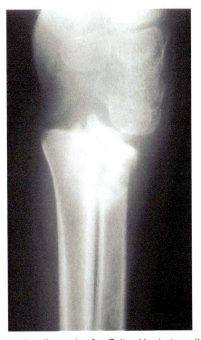

Fig. 18.28 Lateral radiograph of a Salter-Harris type II distal radial malunion. Repeated reduction now is not advised because of (1) the risk of iatrogenic growth arrest, and (2) the probability that this will most likely correct with growth.

to verify remodeling. In the setting of persistent, symptomatic malunion, distal radial osteotomy can be used to correct malalignment and restore function.

PHYSEAL ARREST

The incidence of radial growth arrest after a fracture has been reported as 4% to 5%.[21,164,168] Physeal arrest can be secondary to the trauma of the index injury or from iatrogenic causes, such as late reduction (>7 days) of a physeal injury. Early diagnosis of physeal arrest is key to successful treatment. After a physeal fracture of the distal radius, radiographs should be taken at 6 and 12 months to screen for the development of a physeal arrest. Depending on the growth potential

remaining, the arrest can be treated with epiphysiodesis of the remaining distal radial physeal growth potential, epiphysiodesis of the distal ulnar physis for maintenance of the relationship of the DRUJ, or resection of the physeal bar.[173,174]

CARPAL FRACTURES

EMERGENT TREATMENT

Few indications exist for emergent treatment of carpal injuries. Skeletally mature adolescents may mimic an adult injury pattern and sustain fracture-dislocations of the carpus requiring urgent reduction, but a perilunate fracture-dislocation injury pattern is exceedingly rare in the young child. High-energy injuries with involved carpal pathology may be at risk of compartment syndrome, but again, this would be the exceptional situation.

INDICATIONS FOR DEFINITIVE CARE

Scaphoid fractures are commonly missed at the time of injury. This can be attributed to the failure of the patient to be seen for care early or the diagnosis of the injury as a sprain rather than a fracture. Radiographic results may be interpreted as normal at initial presentation. A high degree of clinical suspicion should be maintained based on the mechanism of injury and the physical examination because missed fractures often result in nonunion and are a chronic source of pain and instability. Physical examination findings that may indicate a scaphoid fracture include tenderness over the scaphoid, pain with radial deviation, and pain with active wrist range of motion.[175] The scaphoid is palpable in three distinct areas of the wrist. The proximal pole is palpated approximately 1 cm distal to the Lister tubercle on the dorsum of the wrist. The scaphoid waist is examined through the anatomic snuff-box. Finally, the distal pole of the scaphoid is palpable on the volar aspect of the palm beneath the trapezial ridge at the base of the thumb. Pain with axial compression of the thumb is the most reliable physical examination finding.

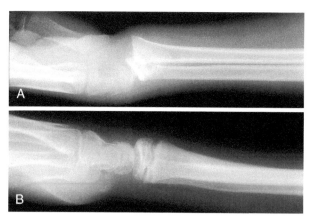

Fig. 18.29 (A) Lateral radiograph of a healed distal radial physeal malunion with late presentation. No corrective action was taken. (B) Lateral radiograph 6 months later after an accelerated growth spurt. Note the correction to anatomic alignment by natural history.

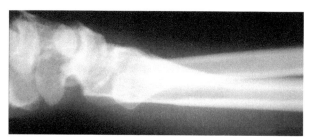

Fig. 18.30 Lateral radiograph of a distal radial metaphyseal malunion. This patient was too old to remodel the malalignment that was present after closed reduction. Corrective osteotomy will be necessary to prevent long-term radiocarpal problems.

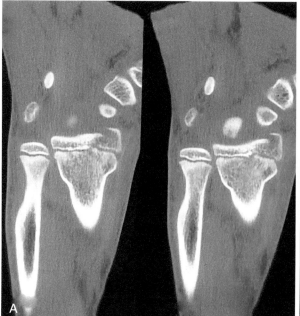

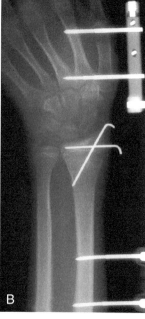

Fig. 18.31 (A) Computed tomography reveals a triplane fracture of the distal radius with epiphyseal and metaphyseal displacement. (B) Reduction and stabilization were performed with a combination of smooth, small-diameter pins to avoid injury to the physis and a distraction technique with an external fixator.

Scaphoid fractures are classified by the degree of displacement, as well as the location and direction of the fracture. Distal pole, waist, and proximal fractures all occur in children. Waist fractures are now the most common scaphoid fracture, even in the pediatric patient.[24] Displacement beyond 1 to 2 mm is a risk for malunion or nonunion, similar to the circumstance in adults.[176] CT or MRI evaluation is important in determining the degree of displacement and in guiding treatment of these fractures.[177–179] Avascular necrosis does occur in children, especially in displaced proximal waist and pole fractures.[180] Displaced fractures of the scaphoid waist and distal pole and displaced and nondisplaced fractures of the proximal pole are indications for surgical treatment, which will decrease the incidence of nonunion.[24]

NONOPERATIVE TREATMENT

Nondisplaced distal pole and scaphoid waist fractures can be treated by nonoperative means. Nondisplaced distal pole fractures usually heal without complication.[181–184] Close inspection of the plain radiographs, or, if appropriate, CT scan is performed to detect distal intraarticular extension or displacement. Long or short arm thumb spica cast immobilization for up to 6 weeks is recommended for protected healing in the distal pole fracture. Nondisplaced waist fractures are treated with cast immobilization in a child or adolescent. CT is indicated to establish three-dimensional anatomic alignment. Cast immobilization is required until complete healing. Some evidence indicates that initial long arm casting is more efficacious.[182,185] At times, CT is required to confirm healing. The risk of both nonunion and avascular necrosis exists, even with nondisplaced waist fractures. Recently, percutaneous interosseous screw fixation has been used more commonly in adults with nondisplaced scaphoid fractures because of concerns about prolonged immobilization, nonunion, and complications of avascular necrosis.[186,187] This technique has now carried over to the educated adolescent patient and family who desire earlier mobilization. At present, this treatment is not recommended as the standard of care for the nondisplaced waist fracture.

SURGICAL TREATMENT

SURGICAL ANATOMY

The scaphoid is positioned as the radial-most bone in the proximal carpal row. The scaphoid ossific nucleus appears in males around age 6 years and slightly earlier in females, between the ages of 4 and 5 years. Its formation is complete by age 13 to 14 years.[188] The radial artery serves as the blood supply for the scaphoid, and a dorsal branch enters through the dorsal ridge, supplying the majority of the nourishment to the scaphoid body and proximal pole. A volar arterial branch from the radial artery supplies the distal pole of the scaphoid.[189] There is evidence for the formation of bipartite scaphoid formation in the absence of trauma.[190,191]

The scaphoid serves as the link between the proximal and distal rows of the carpus. Disruption of this link serves to promote degeneration of carpal kinematics such that a well-delineated pattern of wrist degeneration develops in adults.[192]

POSITIONING TECHNIQUES

Surgical fixation of the scaphoid is performed with the patient in the supine position on the operating table with the operative extremity outstretched onto a hand table. A pneumatic brachial tourniquet is used to achieve a bloodless operative field. The image intensifier is positioned perpendicular to the operating table and parallel to the operative extremity so that the surgeon and an assistant have unimpeded access to the surgical limb.

SURGICAL APPROACH

VOLAR APPROACH TO THE SCAPHOID

This approach (Fig. 18.32) is best used for fixation of distal pole fractures, scaphoid waist fractures, and the treatment of scaphoid waist nonunions. The incision is made from the base of the first metacarpal extending proximal to the junction of the FCR tendon and the proximal wrist flexion crease. It is then carried proximal on the radial aspect of the FCR tendon sheath. The incision is deepened through the subcutaneous tissue, which raises a laterally based skin flap. Identification of the radial artery in the radial aspect of the exposure is begun proximally and carried distally to allow retraction of the structure throughout the operation. A volar branch of the artery is reliably found traversing the operative field at the level of the FCR tunnel. This branch can be preserved with a vesi-loop or safely ligated, exposing the underlying palmar carpal ligaments. Sharp incision of the palmar carpal ligaments allows for structural repair at the conclusion of the case. In the distal portion of the exposure, the origin of the thenar musculature should be elevated from the scaphotrapezial joint, which will allow access to the joint capsule. Protection of the first compartment tendons and radial sensory nerve branches is important. Incision of the scaphotrapezial joint capsule allows for subluxation of the joint and access to the distal aspect of the scaphoid, which is necessary to obtain the correct starting point for placement of an intraosseous headless compression screw.

Dorsal Approach to the Scaphoid

This approach is used for the treatment of scaphoid fractures without flexion deformity and proximal pole scaphoid fractures. The longitudinal incision is made in line with the Lister tubercle, extending distally in line with the third metacarpal. The incision is deepened bluntly through the subcutaneous tissues with care taken to protect the dorsal sensory branches of the radial nerve. The EPL tendon is identified as it turns around the distal end of the Lister tubercle. The most distal portion of the extensor retinaculum is incised, which allows for radial retraction of the EPL tendon. The wrist capsule is identified between the tendons of the second and fourth dorsal compartments. The tendons of these compartments are retracted in radial and ulnar directions, respectively. The capsule is then incised transversely from the distal radius, which leaves a cuff of tissue for later repair. Making a longitudinal cut in the capsule distally while taking care to protect the scapholunate interosseous ligament can widen the exposure. The entrance of the perforating vessel into the dorsal ridge limits radial exposure of the scaphoid. Every precaution should be taken to protect this dorsal vascular supply. Flexion of the wrist allows access to the proximal pole of the scaphoid and visualization of the starting point for placement of an interosseous headless compression screw.

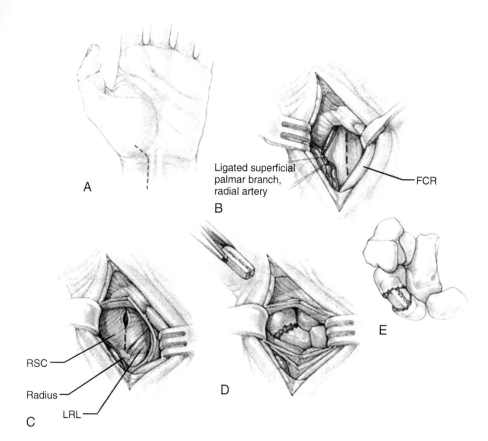

Fig. 18.32 Original Russe bone graft technique. (A) The incision. (B) The flexor carpi radialis *(FCR)* tendon is retracted to expose the volar capsule. (C) The volar capsule is divided longitudinally to expose the radioscaphocapitate *(RSC)* and long radiolunate *(LRL)* ligaments. Care should be taken to minimize ligament injury. (D) An egg-shaped cavity is created distal and proximal to the fracture line. A corticocancellous bone graft, usually obtained from the ipsilateral iliac crest, is fashioned to fit snugly into this cavity. (E) The corticocancellous bone graft has been wedged into the cavity of the scaphoid. The stability of the graft and the fracture fragments should be satisfactory. If not, additional fixation with one or two Kirschner wires is recommended. (From Green DP, Hotchkiss RN, Pederson WC, et al. *Green's Operative Hand Surgery.* 5th ed. New York: Churchill-Livingstone; 2005:730.)

REDUCTION TECHNIQUES

Reduction of scaphoid fractures can be challenging. Manipulation of the wrist position can be helpful in reducing the fracture through ligamentotaxis. Ulnar deviation of the wrist will elongate the carpus and can be used to obtain length for shortened or flexed fractures. Direct control of the proximal and distal fragments can be obtained through the placement of K-wires in each fragment, which can then be used as joysticks for fracture reduction. At times, transradial styloid pinning of the lunate in anatomic neutral alignment aids in scaphoid reduction.

FIXATION TECHNIQUES

Smooth wire or intraosseous screw fixation is used after anatomic reduction. The authors' preference is cannulated interosseous screw fixation. Arthroscopically assisted reduction and fixation have been performed for acutely displaced scaphoid fractures.[193] This is more technically demanding. Arthroscopic inspection and manipulation of the fracture site to anatomic alignment for cannulated pin and screw placement are performed under both fluoroscopic guidance and arthroscopic visualization.

PITFALLS/AVOIDANCE OF COMPLICATIONS

Preserving the blood supply of the scaphoid is of paramount importance in treating scaphoid fractures. Limited dissection dorsally to avoid damage to the perforating vessel of the dorsal ridge minimizes this risk.

In addition, placement of an intraosseous compression screw can be difficult. Before overdrilling, the surgeon should confirm that the guidewire is in the center of the scaphoid. Multiple intraoperative fluoroscopic views should be used to ensure its proper placement. Small proximal pole fragments are at risk of iatrogenic fracture during placement of the screw; hence, the appropriate screw size should be chosen before placement. Additionally, the torque required to properly set the interosseous compression screw may rotate the fracture fragments, effectively causing a malreduction. The placement of an eccentric derotational wire can avert this problem.

Proximal pole scaphoid fractures are at high risk of avascular necrosis and nonunion. Percutaneous screw fixation before fracture displacement or fragmentation may be most useful in this rare adolescent fracture. Perfect placement of the screw is necessary in this situation to lessen the risk of complications. Usually the screw is placed from dorsal proximal to volar distal with fluoroscopic guidance. This is now becoming the authors' preferred treatment for these complicated proximal pole fractures before they displace or collapse. Established proximal pole nonunions with displacement may require reduction, vascularized grafting, and internal fixation to achieve healing. (Fig. 18.33)[180,194] Standard nonvascularized grafting and fixation have a high incidence of failure in that situation.

Postoperative Care and Rehabilitation

Postoperative splint or cast immobilization is used as deemed necessary by the surgeon to prevent excessive stress on the healing fracture while motion is maximized. Proximal pole fractures may take as long as 3 months to

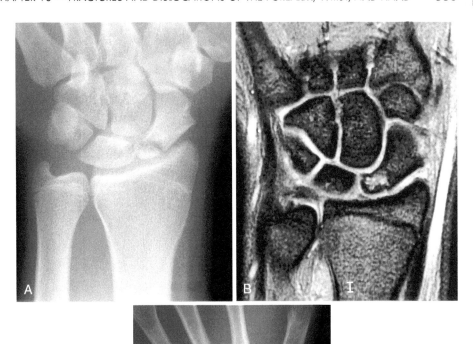

Fig. 18.33 (A) Radiograph of a proximal pole scaphoid nonunion. This injury is rare in children and adolescents but is at high risk of avascular necrosis (AVN) and continued nonunion. (B) Magnetic resonance image revealing proximal pole AVN. (C) Pedicle vascularized bone grafting and pin fixation treatment leading to union.

heal. Generally, postfracture stiffness from prolonged immobilization is not as much of a risk in adolescents as in adults with a healed scaphoid fracture. Once radiographic and clinical healing is confirmed, the patient is allowed to return to activity. Formal therapy for range of motion and strengthening can be used to expedite return to activity.

COMPLICATIONS

NONUNION

Nonunion is a well-documented complication of treatment of scaphoid fractures. Although uncommon, nonunion of a scaphoid fracture can have severe consequences if left untreated. Scaphoid waist nonunions are often treated with autologous bone grafting and interosseous screw fixation. Severe humpback deformities may require tricortical iliac crest grafting to correct the flexion deformity (Fig. 18.34). Nonunions of the proximal pole complicated by avascular necrosis may be better treated with vascularized bone grafting with the use of one of many well-described techniques.[180]

HAND FRACTURES

MALUNION

Hand Fractures

The hand is the most commonly injured body part in a child. In the toddler, injuries are often caused by a crush injury, such as in a door.[10,11,25,195,196] In the older child, the fractures are usually primary to recreational sports. Fortunately, most of these injuries heal without complications (70%–80%).[197] However, subsets of fractures, dislocations, and soft tissue injuries have dire consequences if not treated appropriately in the acute care setting.

EMERGENT TREATMENT

Emergent treatment of hand injuries is centered on the presence of open injuries or injuries to the tendons and neurovascular structures. Failure to perform isolated tendon and nerve testing can result in a delayed or missed diagnosis. Wrist lacerations often involve multiple lacerations to tendons and, at times, major nerves or blood vessels. Early operative exploration and repair are recommended in a young child because of limits of the preoperative examination.

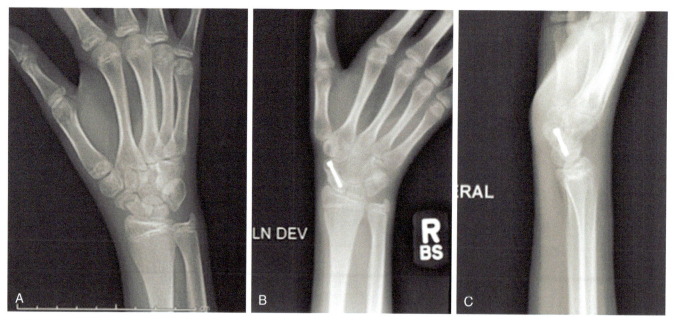

Fig. 18.34 (A) Radiograph of a waist-region scaphoid nonunion in an adolescent athlete. Late presentation of an initial missed diagnosis is not uncommon. (B and C) Surgical treatment with tricortical anterior iliac crest bone graft and intraosseous headless compression screw.

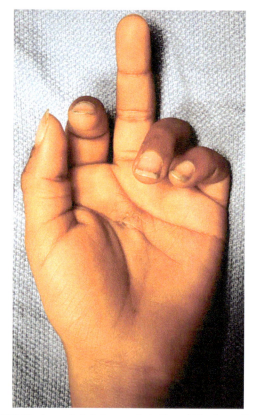

Fig. 18.35 The loss of digital cascade in the middle finger illustrated here should be indicative of a flexor tendon laceration without further examination. The small glass laceration in the palm accounts for the profundus laceration. Too often, these children are seen late because of a missed diagnosis.

Palmar or digital lacerations also require careful examination to detect partial or complete nerve, tendon, or arterial lacerations (Fig. 18.35). Obviously, an avascular digit is an operative emergency. Too often, digital nerve or isolated

flexor tendon injuries are missed in the early period. Delay in repair of up to 2 to 3 weeks can be uncomplicated, but beyond that, the long-term prognosis becomes an increasing concern. Microscopic digital nerve repairs in the child and adolescent generally regain full discriminatory sensibility. Postoperative protection is only necessary for approximately 2 weeks. Flexor tendon outcome is more complicated but generally better than in adults. Debate exists about cast immobilization versus protected mobilization. Cast immobilization for 4 weeks has a favorable total active arc of motion result with a lower incidence of tendon rupture compared with protected flexor tendon mobilization protocols in published results in children.[198,199] However, information is limited.

A complete amputation in a child proximal to the level of the trifurcation of the digital arteries is considered an indication for replantation. Crush injury amputations, such as occur from exercise equipment, have a higher failure rate for replantation than sharp lacerations. Microscopic repair that results in prompt capillary refill and instantaneous restoration of arterial flow intraoperatively is a positive sign for long-term viability. The techniques of replantation in a child are the same as in an adult. Digital survival after replantation is most favorable with sharp amputations, body weight greater than 11 kg, more than one vein repaired, bone shortening and interosseous wire fixation, and vein grafting of arteries and veins, as needed.

Complete distal tip amputations are treated with various techniques, depending on the surgeon's experience and preference and the size and orientation of the defect.[200–203] If the skin loss is minimal, irrigation and débridement and sterile dressing coverage with white petrolatum and 3% bismuth tribromophenate (Xeroform) are appropriate. Healing by secondary intention is relatively rapid and uncomplicated in the young. Because the proximal physis has not been violated, longitudinal growth will be unimpaired and length will be near normal subsequently. At times, early treatment requires minimal débridement of exposed bone with a rongeur followed by dressing changes. More extensive loss can be treated with composite grafting with the use of the amputated part, pedicle grafting such as an advancement or thenar flap, or skin or composite grafting from distant donor sites. Attachment of the amputated part as a composite graft can be performed immediately in the emergency department after débridement of both the part and the amputation site. Healing is more prolonged by this technique than local dressings alone but may result in greater bulk and less risk of nail deformity in the extensive injury. Flap or donor grafting is usually performed shortly thereafter when it is clear that it is required.

INDICATIONS FOR DEFINITIVE CARE

Distal Phalangeal Injuries

Distal Tip Crush Injuries. Crush injuries to the distal aspect of the finger are the most common injury in a toddler. Partial or complete distal tip amputations may occur. Nail bed and plate injuries are usually associated with distal phalangeal fractures that range from minor avulsions to comminuted open fractures. Fortunately, the growth plate is usually not involved, except in the case of a Seymour fracture (distal phalangeal physeal separation and interposed nail bed). Most distal tip injuries in the child can be cared for in the emergency department with local anesthesia or conscious sedation. The more complicated injuries require general anesthesia. With partial amputations, the dorsal skin, nail bed, and eponychial regions are usually lacerated and have an intact, viable volar skin bridge to the distal fingertip. Repair in the emergency department is aided by loupe magnification to anatomically and delicately repair the nail bed with absorbable suture after nail plate removal.[204,205] In the long term, most of these injuries heal without nail deformity.

Mallet Fingers. Mallet fingers in children are similar to those in adults with disruption of the terminal tendon as it inserts onto the distal phalanx dorsally. The terminal tendon inserts on the epiphysis in children with open physes. The volar FDP inserts on the metaphysis distal to the physis, and these forces account for the flexion deformity through the physis in a child. Mallet injuries occur either with a bony avulsion or an intrasubstance tendon injury. Both can be treated with an extension splint for 6 weeks, immobilizing the distal interphalangeal joint while allowing motion of the proximal interphalangeal joint (Fig. 18.36). Successful healing with splint treatment is expected if the patient is compliant with splint wear. This even includes treatment of the chronic mallet finger. In rare cases, chronic mallet injuries require tenodermodesis reconstruction to achieve improved active extension.[206] The risk of this procedure is loss of flexion or nail plate deformity.

Seymour Fracture. Some flexion injuries in children result in a physeal separation between the dorsal terminal tendon and volar FDP insertion: a Seymour fracture.[207] The germinal matrix of the nail bed can become interposed in the physeal fracture site and prevent reduction (Fig. 18.37). Often the resultant flexed digit is misinterpreted as a mallet finger and treated with dorsal splinting. The open wound can subsequently become infected if left without appropriate treatment. Recognition of the injury early is imperative. Treatment involves removal of the nail plate, delicate removal of the entrapped germinal matrix from the physis, débridement and reduction of the fracture, and nail bed

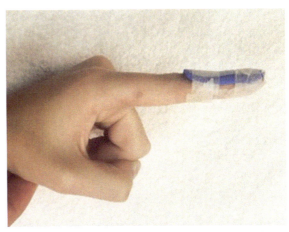

Fig. 18.36 The custom mallet splint depicted fits on the dorsum of the finger, keeping the distal interphalangeal joint (DIP) slightly hyperextended. The paper tape allows for daily changing of the splint following showers. The dorsum of the DIP joint is monitored carefully for skin breakdown during treatment period.

repair.[208] Usually the phalangeal fracture is stable after soft tissue repair. Replacing the nail plate can add stability to the fracture. At times, pin fixation of the distal phalanx and interphalangeal joint for 3 to 4 weeks is protective of the nail bed repair and maintains fracture alignment.

Phalangeal Neck Fractures

Injuries to the subchondral region of the proximal or middle phalanges are common with more proximal crush injuries, such as those from closure of a door on the child's finger in the proximal and middle phalangeal region. As the child attempts to extract the digit from the door, the greatest force is across the subchondral region and it fractures. The resultant phalangeal neck fracture can displace dorsally and into extension (Fig. 18.38).[209] Radiographically, the distal fragment appears small because, in the young, much of the intraarticular surface is cartilaginous. The severity of displacement and its effect on adjacent interphalangeal joint motion can be underappreciated. Failure to treat this injury with anatomic reduction and pin stabilization can result in a malunion that limits digital flexion. At the proximal interphalangeal joint, the loss of the subcondylar fossa can result in marked loss of digital motion. The fracture may also exhibit an element of malrotation. It is imperative that these injuries be recognized early. They are usually unstable injuries that redisplace after closed reduction and cast immobilization, which is an occurrence that is difficult to appreciate with in-cast radiographs. Closed reduction and pin stabilization with a distal-to-proximal oblique pin(s) for 3 to 4 weeks is recommended. Children who are seen with an incipient malunion can frequently be treated with either a percutaneous pin reduction and stabilization (Fig. 18.39)[210] or a careful open reduction that protects the blood supply to the distal fragment through the collateral ligaments. Treatment of an established malunion is more complex. In the very young, it may remodel with growth, especially at the middle phalanx.[211,212] However, remember that the physis is proximal; thus, this process will be slow (1–2 years), and patience by the surgeon and family is required. If remodeling is not sufficient, subchondral fossa reconstruction via a volar approach improves but does not normalize motion.[213]

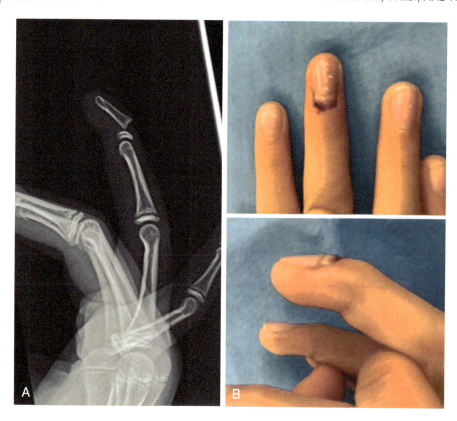

Fig. 18.37 (A) Radiographic lateral view of a displaced physeal fracture. The terminal tendon is intact here with insertion onto the nondisplaced epiphysis. The germinal matrix can become entrapped in the physeal fracture site. (B) Clinical appearance of a Seymour fracture with physeal displacement and entrapment of the germinal matrix. The nail plate and eponychium are noted to be displaced. This requires repair of the nail bed and reduction of the physis.

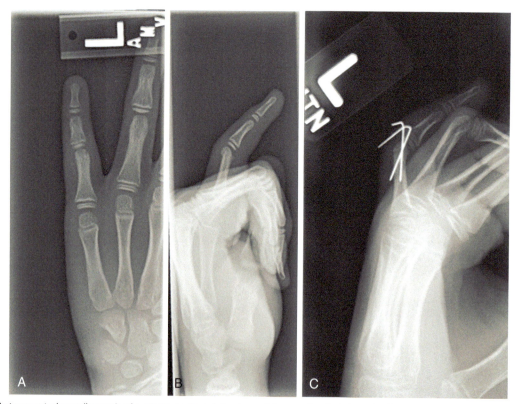

Fig. 18.38 (A) Anteroposterior radiograph of a phalangeal neck fracture of the proximal phalanx is often subtle in appearance and can be often overlooked. (B) The lateral radiograph adequately represents the displacement of the fracture. The subchondral fossa is blocked by the extension displacement of the condylar fragment. If untreated, this will lead to a flexion block at the interphalangeal joint. (C) Closed reduction and percutaneous pin fixation restore the anatomic alignment of the condyles while the fracture heals.

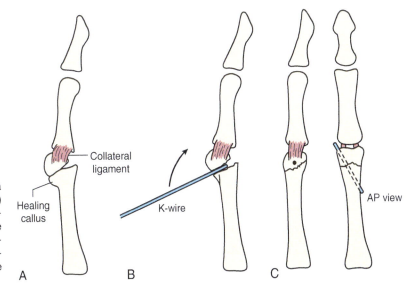

Fig. 18.39 (A) Illustration of technique. Lateral view of a partially healed, malaligned phalangeal neck fracture. (B) A percutaneous Kirschner (K) wire is introduced dorsally through the fracture callus into the fracture site. The K-wire is used to lever the distal fragment back into anatomic alignment. (C) The reduced fracture is percutaneously pinned obliquely from distal to proximal with one or two K-wires. *AP,* Anteroposterior.

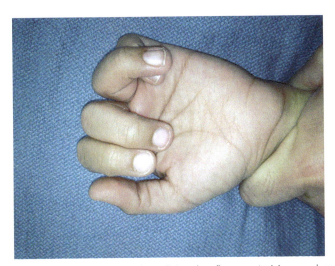

Fig. 18.40 Clinical malrotation of the ring finger noted by passive tenodesis examination.

Clearly, the best option in this injury is accurate recognition and treatment in the acute care setting.

Malrotated Fractures

Any phalangeal or metacarpal fracture can result in digital malrotation (Fig. 18.40). It is imperative to perform a clinical examination of the injury by inspection of wrist tenodesis for digital alignment and assessment of active motion alignment if the level of pain allows it. Passive wrist extension results in passive digital flexion and allows for inspection of digital alignment. Asymmetric convergence or divergence of the fractured digit is apparent even in the acute care setting with a tenodesis examination. All malrotated digits require anatomic reduction and operative stabilization. Most commonly, oblique phalangeal and metacarpal fractures are evident on radiographs, and treatment is by smooth pin stabilization or internal fixation (Fig. 18.41). However, physeal, transverse, intraarticular, and minor fractures may appear well aligned on two-dimensional radiographs but can lead to malrotation. A high index of suspicion and careful clinical examination are critical for prevention of malunion.

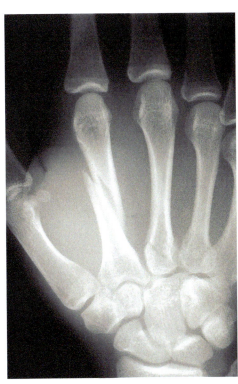

Fig. 18.41 Anteroposterior radiograph of an oblique fracture of an index metacarpal. This fracture is at risk of malrotation. Clinical examination by passive tenodesis and active motion is important in preventing malunion. Reduction and fixation are often necessary for this fracture.

Intraarticular Fractures

Any intraarticular fracture requires anatomic alignment and stability during healing. Some injuries are nondisplaced and stable and can be treated with a closed technique. However, careful follow-up clinically and radiographically during the healing phase is necessary to ensure that no loss of alignment occurs. Displaced fractures require reduction and pin or screw stabilization.[9] At the middle phalanx, these injuries can involve central osteochondral fragmentation. Careful operative dissection and

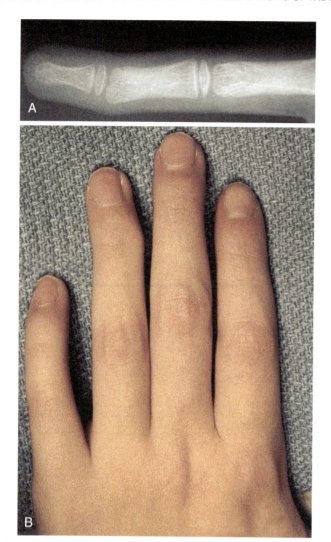

Fig. 18.42 (A) Anteroposterior radiograph of intraarticular malunion of a middle phalangeal unicondylar fracture. This fracture requires reduction and fixation in the acute care setting. (B) Clinical appearance of the malunion with ulnar deviation of the ring finger through the distal interphalangeal joint.

anatomic reduction are necessary to lessen the already real risk of avascular necrosis with these fractures. At times, immediate bone grafting is necessary for stability of comminuted intraarticular fractures. The olecranon distal to the apophysis is a reasonable source of cortical bone in a child. Intraarticular injuries can be unicondylar, bicondylar, or comminuted. The interphalangeal joint is always at risk of permanent loss of motion with any juxta-articular or intraarticular injury. Permanent articular incongruity clearly increases that risk. Anatomic reduction by closed or open techniques followed by pin or screw stabilization is the treatment of choice for displaced, unstable injuries. Most often in the pediatric population, this can be performed with percutaneous pin reduction and fixation. Extreme comminution that would require distraction treatment is rare in children and adolescents.[214] Postoperative rehabilitation to regain interphalangeal motion is necessary to lessen the risk of a flexion contracture. Intraarticular malunions are a difficult problem because loss of motion, pain, and the risk of arthrosis are common (Fig. 18.42). Unfortunately, late

intraarticular osteotomies often produce less than desired results in terms of motion, even when the radiographs indicate improvement or anatomic alignment.

Displaced Salter-Harris type III intraarticular fractures of the thumb are the pediatric equivalent of the adult gamekeeper thumb.[215,216] Rather than injuring the ulnar collateral ligament of the metacarpal phalangeal joint with a fall, such as occurs in downhill skiing, the epiphysis fractures. A displaced epiphyseal fracture of the proximal phalanx results in articular and physeal incongruity. Open reduction and pin fixation are required (Fig. 18.43). Surgical dissection into the joint is distal to the intact ulnar collateral ligament insertion via the fracture site. When anatomically realigned, these injuries heal in 4 to 6 weeks without complication. When unrecognized or left malreduced, they can result in a nonunion or malunion that is painful and limits motion and function. Similarly, displaced intraarticular fractures of the base of the metacarpal (Bennett [Fig. 18.44] or Rolando fractures [Fig. 18.45]) require anatomic articular reduction and pin stabilization. The oblique ligament between the first and second metacarpal holds the ulnar basilar fragment in place while the APL dynamically displaces the larger radial fragment. Reduction involves restoring length and correcting the angulation and malrotation. Two or three percutaneous pins into the adjacent index metacarpal base and carpus provide stability until the fracture is healed. The rare comminuted intraarticular fracture requires careful open reduction. Severe injuries that are best treated with distraction techniques in the adult are almost nonexistent in the child.

Dislocations

Most interphalangeal joint injuries are "jammed fingers" at the proximal interphalangeal joint secondary to a hyperextension force such as occurs from catching a basketball. This results in a volar plate injury and, at times, a minor avulsion fracture of the volar middle phalanx epiphysis. These injuries can be overtreated with immobilization that can result in subsequent interphalangeal joint stiffness. Complete dislocations can usually be reduced with distraction and reduction without complication (Fig. 18.46). If the joint is reduced and stable with motion, treatment involves brief splint protection and early mobilization. Buddy taping is frequently used for protection, and active and passive mobility should be encouraged. The rare pediatric base-of-the-middle-phalanx avulsion that results in a displaced, unstable joint is drastically different (Fig. 18.47). This injury requires joint reduction and mobilization only within the stable flexion-extension arc. Fluoroscopic examination is necessary to determine the safe arc of motion. Dorsal splint or pin extension blocking is used to prevent joint subluxation. Progressive extension as stability is restored with healing is performed carefully to maintain joint reduction while achieving maximum interphalangeal motion. These injuries heal over 6 weeks, and subsequent therapy can be prolonged.

Most interphalangeal joint dislocations are uncomplicated. Dorsal dislocations are most common and often are treated at the site of injury with reduction by the patient, trainer, parent, or coach with gentle distraction. These injuries are usually stable after reduction as long as another hyperextension force is avoided during volar plate and collateral ligament healing. Early, protected mobilization is advocated to lessen the risk of long-term stiffness. Metacarpophalangeal

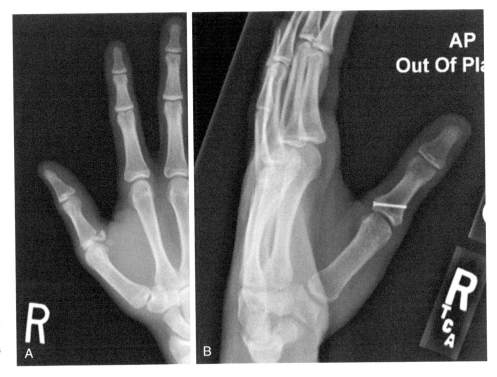

Fig. 18.43 (A) Radiograph of a displaced Salter-Harris type III intraarticular fracture of the proximal phalanx of the thumb. This is a pediatric equivalent of gamekeeper thumb. (B) Open reduction and internal fixation are indicated to restore articular and physeal congruity and joint stability. anteroposterior radiograph reveals screw fixation.

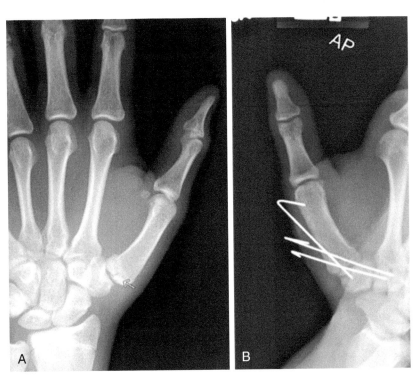

Fig. 18.44 (A) Radiograph of a displaced Bennett fracture. The distal fragment is rotated and pulled proximally by the insertion of the abductor pollicis longus. (B) Closed reduction of the displaced fracture and fixation with smooth Kirschner wires allows bony healing in anatomic position.

(MCP) joint dislocations are more likely to be irreducible ("complex dislocation").[217,218] Irreducible dorsal dislocation of either the interphalangeal or MCP joint is usually secondary to volar plate entrapment. In the MCP joint, this may be evident radiographically by sesamoid interposition or bayonet apposition alignment (Fig. 18.48). Closed reduction is not feasible. Open reduction by either a volar approach[217,219–221] or a dorsal approach is necessary. If a volar

approach to an irreducible MCP joint dislocation is used, extreme care should be taken with the skin incision to protect the displaced radial digital neurovascular pedicle. For the uninitiated, the dorsal approach is safer. The authors usually operatively reduce these with a volar approach but are extremely cautious regarding the neurovascular bundles. Protected mobilization early is important to lessen the risk of stiffness.[220,221]

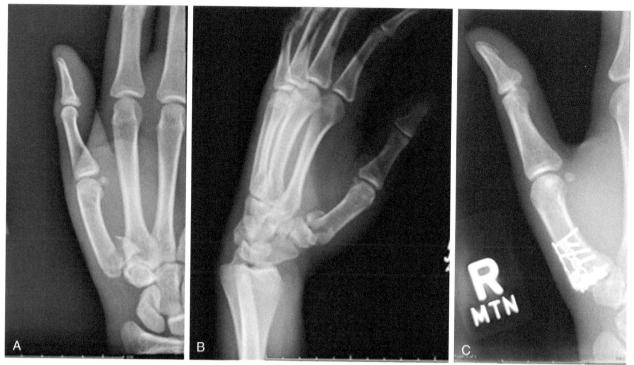

Fig. 18.45 (A and B) Radiograph of a displaced Rolando fracture. The articular base of the first metacarpal is in three separate pieces. (C) Open reduction and internal fixation of the fracture fragments allows for restoration of joint congruity.

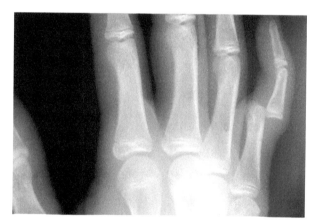

Fig. 18.46 Typical proximal interphalangeal joint dislocation in extension. Distraction and flexion reduction are usually concentric and stable. Reduction is often performed on the field.

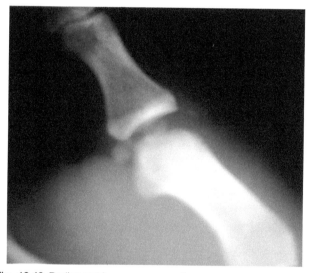

Fig. 18.48 Radiographic appearance of an entrapped sesamoid in the metacarpophalangeal joint of the thumb in an irreducible dislocation.

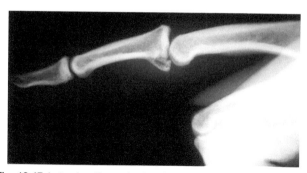

Fig. 18.47 Lateral radiograph of an incomplete reduction of this volar intraarticular fracture-dislocation. Congruent reduction needs to be achieved in this injury, and the arc of stable motion needs to be determined.

REFERENCES

The level of evidence (LOE) is determined according to the criteria provided in the Preface.

1. Landin LA. Fracture patterns in children. Analysis of 8,682 fractures with special reference to incidence, etiology and secular changes in a Swedish urban population 1950-1979. *Acta Orthop Scand Suppl.* 1983;202:1–109. (**LOE IV**).
2. Lawton L. Fractures of the distal radius and ulna in management of pediatric fractures. In: Letts M, ed. *Management of pediatric fractures.* New York: Churchill-Livingstone; 345–368.
3. Thomas EM, Tuson KW, Browne PS. Fractures of the radius and ulna in children. *Injury.* 1975;7(2):120–124. (LOE IV).
4. Chung KC, Spilson SV. The frequency and epidemiology of hand and forearm fractures in the United States. *J Hand Surg.* 2001;26(5):908–915. (LOE IV).
5. Landin LA. Epidemiology of children's fractures. *J Pediatr Orthop B.* 1997;6(2):79–83. (**LOE IV**).
6. Naranje S, Erali R, Warner W Jr, et al. Epidemiology of pediatric fractures presenting to emergency departments in the United States. *J Pediatr Orthop.* 2016;36(4):e45–e48. (**LOE III**).
7. Bailey DA, Wedge JH, McCulloch RG, et al. Epidemiology of fractures of the distal end of the radius in children as associated with growth. *J Bone Joint Surg Am.* 1989;71(8):1225–1231. (**LOE IV**).
8. Bhende MS, Dandrea LA, Davis HW. Hand injuries in children presenting to a pediatric emergency department. *Ann Emerg Med.* 1993;22(10):1519–1523. (**LOE IV**).
9. Hastings H 2nd, Simmons BP. Hand fractures in children. A statistical analysis. *Clin Orthop Relat Res.* 1984;188:120–130. (**LOE IV**).
10. Worlock PH, Stower MJ. The incidence and pattern of hand fractures in children. *J Hand Surg Br.* 1986;11(2):198–200. (**LOE IV**).
11. Worlock P, Stower M. Fracture patterns in Nottingham children. *J Pediatr Orthop.* 1986;6(6):656–660. (**LOE IV**).
12. Bado JL. The Monteggia lesion. *Clin Orthop Relat Res.* 1967;50:71–86. (**LOE V**).
13. Bley L, Seitz WH Jr. Injuries about the distal ulna in children. *Hand Clin.* 1998;14(2):231–237. (**LOE V**).
14. Letts R. Monteggia and Galeazzi fractures. In: Letts R, ed. *Management of Pediatric Fractures.* New York: Churchill-Livingstone; 313–321.
15. Mikic ZD. Galeazzi fracture-dislocations. *J Bone Joint Surg Am.* 1975;57(8):1071–1080. (**LOE V**).
16. Walsh HP, McLaren CA, Owen R. Galeazzi fractures in children. *J Bone Joint Surg Br.* 1987;69(5):730–733. (**LOE IV**).
17. Holdsworth BJ, Sloan JP. Proximal forearm fractures in children: residual disability. *Injury.* 1982;14(2):174–179. (**LOE IV**).
18. Matthews LS, Kaufer H, Garver DF, Sonstegard DA. The effect on supination-pronation of angular malalignment of fractures of both bones of the forearm. *J Bone Joint Surg Am.* 1982;64(1):14–17. (**LOE III**).
19. Trousdale RT, Linscheid RL. Operative treatment of malunited fractures of the forearm. *J Bone Joint Surg Am.* 1995;77(6):894–902. (**LOE IV**).
20. Cheng JC, Shen WY. Limb fracture pattern in different pediatric age groups: a study of 3,350 children. *J Orthop Trauma.* 1993;7(1):15–22. (**LOE IV**).
21. Bae DS, Waters PM. Pediatric distal radius fractures and triangular fibrocartilage complex injuries. *Hand Clin.* 2006;22(1):43–53. (**LOE V**).
22. Khosla S, Melton LJ 3rd, Dekutoski MB, et al. Incidence of childhood distal forearm fractures over 30 years: a population-based study. *JAMA.* 2003;290(11):1479–1485. (**LOE IV**).
23. Christodoulou AG, Colton CL. Scaphoid fractures in children. *J Pediatr Orthop.* 1986;6(1):37–39. (**LOE IV**).
24. Gholson JJ, Bae DS, Zurakowski D, Waters PM. Scaphoid fractures in children and adolescents: contemporary injury patterns and factors influencing time to union. *J Bone Joint Surg Am.* 2011;93(13):1210–1219. (**LOE III**).
25. Fischer MD, McElfresh EC. Physeal and periphyseal injuries of the hand. Patterns of injury and results of treatment. *Hand Clin.* 1994;10(2):287–301. (**LOE V**).
26. Bae DS, Kadiyala RK, Waters PM. Acute compartment syndrome in children: contemporary diagnosis, treatment, and outcome. *J Pediatr Orthop.* 2001;21(5):680–688. (**LOE IV**).
27. Noonan KJ, McCarthy JJ. Compartment syndromes in the pediatric patient. *J Pediatr Orthop.* 2010;2(suppl 30):S96–S101. (**LOE V**).
28. Yuan PS, Pring ME, Gaynor TP, et al. Compartment syndrome following intramedullary fixation of pediatric forearm fractures. *J Pediatr Orthop.* 2004;24(4):370–375. (**LOE IV**).
29. Blakemore LC, Cooperman DR, Thompson GH, et al. Compartment syndrome in ipsilateral humerus and forearm fractures in children. *Clin Orthop Relat Res.* 2000;376:32–38. (**LOE IV**).
30. Haasbeek JF, Cole WG. Open fractures of the arm in children. *J Bone Joint Surg Br.* 1995;77(4):576–581. (**LOE IV**).
31. Ring D, Waters PM, Hotchkiss RN, Kasser JR. Pediatric floating elbow. *J Pediatr Orthop.* 2001;21(4):456–459. (**LOE IV**).
32. Creasman C, Zaleske DJ, Ehrlich MG. Analyzing forearm fractures in children. The more subtle signs of impending problems. *Clin Orthop Relat Res.* 1984;188:40–53. (**LOE IV**).
33. Price CT, Scott DS, Kurzner ME, Flynn JC. Malunited forearm fractures in children. *J Pediatr Orthop.* 1990;10(6):705–712. (**LOE IV**).
34. McLauchlan GJ, Cowan B, Annan IH, Robb JE. Management of completely displaced metaphyseal fractures of the distal radius in children. A prospective, randomised controlled trial. *J Bone Joint Surg Br.* 2002;84(3):413–417. (**LOE I**).
35. Mabrey JD, Fitch RD. Plastic deformation in pediatric fractures: mechanism and treatment. *J Pediatr Orthop.* 1989;9(3):310–314. (**LOE IV**).
36. Sanders WE, Heckman JD. Traumatic plastic deformation of the radius and ulna. A closed method of correction of deformity. *Clin Orthop Relat Res.* 1984;188:58–67. (**LOE IV**).
37. Flynn JM, Waters PM. Single-bone fixation of both-bone forearm fractures. *J Pediatr Orthop.* 1996;16(5):655–659. (**LOE IV**).
38. Chess DG, Hyndman JC, Leahey JL, et al. Short arm plaster cast for distal pediatric forearm fractures. *J Pediatr Orthop.* 1994;14(2):211–213. (**LOE IV**).
39. Godfrey J, Choi P, Shabtai L, et al. Management of pediatric type I open fractures in the emergency department or operating room: a multicenter perspective. *J Pediatr Orthop.* 2017 [epub ahead of print]. (**LOE III**).
40. Rang M. *Children's fractures.* 2nd ed. Philadelphia: Lippincott;.
41. Kasser J. Forearm fractures. In: MacEwen G, Heinrich S, eds. *Pediatric Fractures: A Practical Approach to Assessment And Treatment.* Baltimore: Williams and Wilkins; 165–190.
42. Kennedy RM, Porter FL, Miller JP, Jaffe DM. Comparison of fentanyl/midazolam with ketamine/midazolam for pediatric orthopedic emergencies. *Pediatrics.* 1998;102(4 Pt 1):956–963. (**LOE II**).
43. Snodgrass WR, Dodge WF. Lytic/"DPT" cocktail: time for rational and safe alternatives. *Pediatr Clin North Am.* 1989;36(5):1285–1291. (**LOE IV**).
44. Yaster M, Nichols DG, Deshpande JK, Wetzel RC. Midazolam-fentanyl intravenous sedation in children: case report of respiratory arrest. *Pediatrics.* 1990;86(3):463–467. (**LOE IV**).
45. Levy J, Ernat J, Song D, et al. Outcomes of long-arm casting versus double-sugar-tong splinting of acute pediatric distal forearm fractures. *J Pediatr Orthop.* 2015;35(1):11–17. (**LOE II**).
46. Zaino C, Patel M, Arief M, Pivec R. The effectiveness of bivalving, cast spreading, and webril cutting to reduce cast pressure in a fiberglass short arm cast. *J Bone Joint Surg Amer.* 2015;4(97):374–380. (**LOE II**).
47. Ogden JA, Beall JK, Conlogue GJ, Light TR. Radiology of postnatal skeletal development. IV. Distal radius and ulna. *Skeletal Radiol.* 1981;6(4):255–266. (**LOE IV**).
48. Manson TT, Pfaeffle HJ, Herdon JH, et al. Forearm rotation alters interosseous ligament strain distribution. *J Hand Surg.* 2000;25(6):1058–1063. (**LOE III**).
49. Markolf KL, Lamey D, Yang S, et al. Radioulnar load-sharing in the forearm. A study in cadavera. *J Bone Joint Surg Am.* 1998;80(6):879–888. (**LOE III**).
50. Skahen JR 3rd, Palmer AK, Werner FW, Fortino MD. Reconstruction of the interosseous membrane of the forearm in cadavers. *J Hand Surg.* 1997;22(6):986–994. (**LOE III**).
51. Firl M, Wunsch L. Measurement of bowing of the radius. *J Bone Joint Surg Br.* 2004;86(7):1047–1049. (**LOE III**).
52. Sage FP. Medullary fixation of fractures of the forearm. A study of the medullary canal of the radius and a report of fifty fractures of the radius treated with a prebent triangular nail. *J Bone Joint Surg Am.* 1959;41-A:1489–**1516**. (**LOE IV**).

53. McGinley JC, Hopgood BC, Gaughan JP, et al. Forearm and elbow injury: the influence of rotational position. *J Bone Joint Surg Am.* 2003;85-A(12):2403–2409. (**LOE IV**).

54. Palmer AK, Werner FW. The triangular fibrocartilage complex of the wrist—anatomy and function. *J Hand Surg.* 1981;6(2):153–162. (**LOE IV**).

55. Kaplan EB. The quadrate ligament of the radio-ulnar joint of the elbow. *Bull Hosp Joint Dis.* 1964;25:126–130. (**LOE V**).

56. DeFrate LE, Li G, Zayontz SJ, Herndon JH. A minimally invasive method for the determination of force in the interosseous ligament. *Clin Biomech (Bristol, Avon).* 2001;16(10):895–900. (**LOE IV**).

57. Gabriel MT, Pfaeffle HJ, Stabile KJ, et al. Passive strain distribution in the interosseous ligament of the forearm: implications for injury reconstruction. *J Hand Surg.* 2004;29(2):293–298. (**LOE IV**).

58. Nakamura T, Yabe Y, Horiuchi Y. In vivo MR studies of dynamic changes in the interosseous membrane of the forearm during rotation. *J Hand Surg Br.* 1999;24(2):245–248. (**LOE III**).

59. Letts M, Rowhani N. Galeazzi-equivalent injuries of the wrist in children. *J Pediatr Orthop.* 1993;13(5):561–566. (**LOE IV**).

60. Peterson HA. Physeal fractures: part 3, classification. *J Pediatr Orthop.* 1994;14(4):439–448. (**LOE IV**).

61. Dumont CE, Thalmann R, Macy JC. The effect of rotational malunion of the radius and the ulna on supination and pronation. *J Bone Joint Surg Br.* 2002;84(7):1070–1074. (**LOE III**).

62. Kasten P, Krefft M, Hesselbach J, Weinberg AM. How does torsional deformity of the radial shaft influence the rotation of the forearm? A biomechanical study. *J Orthop Trauma.* 2003;17(1):57–60. (**LOE III**).

63. Tynan MC, Fornalski S, McMahon PJ, et al. The effects of ulnar axial malalignment on supination and pronation. *J Bone Joint Surg Am.* 2000;82-A(12):1726–1731. (**LOE III**).

64. Bass RL, Stern PJ. Elbow and forearm anatomy and surgical approaches. *Hand Clin.* 1994;10(3):343–356. (**LOE V**).

65. Henry A. *Extensile Exposure.* 2nd ed. Edinburgh: Churchill-Livingstone.

66. Mekhail AO, Ebraheim NA, Jackson WT, Yeasting RA. Vulnerability of the posterior interosseous nerve during proximal radius exposures. *Clin Orthop Relat Res.* 1995;315:199–208. (**LOE III**).

67. Strauch RJ, Rosenwasser MP, Glazer PA. Surgical exposure of the dorsal proximal third of the radius: how vulnerable is the posterior interosseous nerve? *J Shoulder Elbow Surg.* 1996;5(5):342–346. (**LOE III**).

68. Wyrsch B, Mencio GA, Green NE. Open reduction and internal fixation of pediatric forearm fractures. *J Pediatr Orthop.* 1996;16(5):644–650. (**LOE IV**).

69. Crenshaw A. Surgical approaches. In: Canale S, ed. *Campbell's Operative Orthopaedics.* St. Louis: CV Mosby; 107–109.

70. Mih PM. Fractures of the distal radius and ulna. In: Rockwood CA, Wilkins KE, Beatty E, eds. *Rockwood and Wilkins' Fractures in Children.* Philadelphia: Lippincott Williams and Wilkins.

71. Blumberg T, Bremjit P, Bompadre V, Steinman S. Forearm fixation is not necessary in the treatment of pediatric floating elbow. *J Pediatr Orthop.* 2018;38(2):82–87. (**LOE IV**).

72. Boyer BA, Overton B, Schrader W, et al. Position of immobilization for pediatric forearm fractures. *J Pediatr Orthop.* 2002;22(2):185–187. (**LOE I**).

73. Griffin PP. Forearm fractures in children. *Clin Orthop Relat Res.* 1977;129:320–321. (**LOE IV**).

74. Calder PR, Achan P, Barry M. Diaphyseal forearm fractures in children treated with intramedullary fixation: outcome of K-wire versus elastic stable intramedullary nail. *Injury.* 2003;34(4):278–282. (**LOE III**).

75. Guero S. Fractures and epiphyseal fracture separation of the distal bones of the forearm in children. In: Cooney PS, ed. *Fractures of the Distal Radius.* 3rd ed. Philadelphia: Lippincott.

76. Mani GV, Hui PW, Cheng JC. Translation of the radius as a predictor of outcome in distal radial fractures of children. *J Bone Joint Surg Br.* 1993;75(5):808–811. (**LOE IV**).

77. Miller BS, Taylor B, Widmann RF, et al. Cast immobilization versus percutaneous pin fixation of displaced distal radius fractures in children: a prospective, randomized study. *J Pediatr Orthop.* 2005;25(4):490–494 (**LOE I**).

78. Proctor MT, Moore DJ, Paterson JM. Redisplacement after manipulation of distal radial fractures in children. *J Bone Joint Surg Br.* 1993;75(3):453–454. (**LOE IV**).

79. Griffet J, Baby M, el Hayek T. Intramedullary nailing of forearm fractures in children. *J Pediatr Orthop B.* 1999;8(2):88–89. (**LOE IV**).

80. Myers GJ, Gibbons PJ, Glithero PR. Nancy nailing of diaphyseal forearm fractures. Single bone fixation for fractures of both bones. *J Bone Joint Surg Br.* 2004;86(4):581–584. (**LOE IV**).

81. Richter D, Ostermann PA, Ekkernkamp A, et al. Elastic intramedullary nailing: a minimally invasive concept in the treatment of unstable forearm fractures in children. *J Pediatr Orthop.* 1998;18(4):457–461. (**LOE IV**).

82. Shah MH, Heffernan G, McGuinness AJ. Early experience with titanium elastic nails in a trauma unit. *Irish Med J.* 2003;96(7):213–214. (**LOE IV**).

83. Till H, Huttl B, Knorr P, Dietz HG. Elastic stable intramedullary nailing (ESIN) provides good long-term results in pediatric long-bone fractures. *Eur J Pediatr Surg.* 2000;10(5):319–322. (**LOE IV**).

84. Toussaint D, Vanderlinden C, Bremen J. [Stable elastic nailing applied to diaphyseal fractures of the forearm in children]. *Acta Orthop Belg.* 1991;57(2):147–153. (**LOE IV**).

85. Lascombes P, Prevot J, Ligier JN, et al. Elastic stable intramedullary nailing in forearm shaft fractures in children: 85 cases. *J Pediatr Orthop.* 1990;10(2):167–171. (**LOE IV**).

86. Blackman AJ, Wall LB, Keeler KA, et al. Acute compartment syndrome after intramedullary nailing of isolated radius and ulna fractures in children. *J Pediatr Orthop.* 2014;34(1):50–54. (**LOE IV**).

87. Flynn JM, Jones KJ, Garner MR, Goebel J. Eleven years experience in the operative management of pediatric forearm fractures. *J Pediatr Orthop.* 2010;30(4):313–319. (**LOE IV**).

88. Dietz JF, Bae DS, Reiff E, et al. Single bone intramedullary fixation of the ulna in pediatric both bone forearm fractures: analysis of short-term clinical and radiographic results. *J Pediatr Orthop.* 2010;30(5):420–424. (**LOE IV**).

89. Ortega R, Loder RT, Louis DS. Open reduction and internal fixation of forearm fractures in children. *J Pediatr Orthop.* 1996;16(5):651–654. (**LOE IV**).

90. Van der Reis WL, Otsuka NY, Moroz P, Mah J. Intramedullary nailing versus plate fixation for unstable forearm fractures in children. *J Pediatr Orthop.* 1998;18(1):9–13. (**LOE III**).

91. Gibbons CL, Woods DA, Pailthorpe C, et al. The management of isolated distal radius fractures in children. *J Pediatr Orthop.* 1994;14(2):207–210. (**LOE IV**).

92. Clarke AC, Spencer RF. Ulnar nerve palsy following fractures of the distal radius: clinical and anatomical studies. *J Hand Surg Br.* 1991;16(4):438–440. (**LOE IV**).

93. Vance RM, Gelberman RH. Acute ulnar neuropathy with fractures at the wrist. *J Bone Joint Surg Am.* 1978;60(7):962–965. (**LOE IV**).

94. Wolfe JS, Eyring EJ. Median-nerve entrapment within a greenstick fracture; a case report. *J Bone Joint Surg Am.* 1974;56(6):1270–1272. (**LOE IV**).

95. Fodden DI. A study of wrist injuries in children: the incidence of various injuries and of premature closure of the distal radial growth plate. *Arch Emerg Med.* 1992;9(1):9–13. (**LOE IV**).

96. Peterson HA. Physeal fractures: part 2. Two previously unclassified types. *J Pediatr Orthop.* 1994;14(4):431–438. (**LOE IV**).

97. Kelly B, Miller P, Shore B, et al. Exposed versus buried intramedullary implants for pediatric forearm fractures: a comparison of complications. *J Pediatr Orthop.* 2014;34(8):749–755. (**LOE III**).

98. Fernandez FF, Eberhardt O, Langendorfer M, Wirth T. Nonunion of forearm shaft fractures in children after intramedullary nailing. *J Pediatr Orthop B.* 2009;18(6):289–295. (**LOE IV**).

99. Martus JE, Preston RK, Schoenecker JG, et al. Complications and outcomes of diaphyseal forearm fracture intramedullary nailing: a comparison of pediatric and adolescent age groups. *J Pediatr Orthop.* 2013;33(6):598–607. (**LOE IV**).

100. Schmittenbecher PP, Fitze G, Godeke J, et al. Delayed healing of forearm shaft fractures in children after intramedullary nailing. *J Pediatr Orthop.* 2008;28(3):303–306. (**LOE IV**).

101. Fiala M, Carey TP. Paediatric forearm fractures: an analysis of refracture rate. *Orthop Trans.* 1995;18:1265–1266. (**LOE IV**).

102. Litton LO, Adler F. Refracture of the forearm in children: a frequent complication. *J Trauma.* 1963;3:41–51. (**LOE IV**).

103. Tisosky A, Werger M, McPartland T, Bowe J. The factors influencing the refracture of pediatric forearms. *J Pediatr Orthop.* 2015;35(7):677–681. **(LOE IV)**.

104. Vince KG, Miller JE. Cross-union complicating fracture of the forearm, part II: children. *J Bone Joint Surg Am.* 1987;69(5):654–661. **(LOE IV)**.

105. Cullen MC, Roy DR, Giza E, Crawford AH. Complications of intramedullary fixation of pediatric forearm fractures. *J Pediatr Orthop.* 1998;18(1):14–21. **(LOE IV)**.

106. Smith FM. Monteggia fractures; an analysis of 25 consecutive fresh injuries. *Surg Gynecol Obstet.* 1947;85(5):630–640. **(LOE IV)**.

107. Wiley JJ, Galey JP. Monteggia injuries in children. *J Bone Joint Surg Br.* 1985;67(5):728–731. **(LOE IV)**.

108. Storen G. Traumatic dislocation of the radial head as an isolated lesion in children; report of one case with special regard to roentgen diagnosis. *Acta Chir Scand.* 1959;116(2):144–147. **(LOE IV)**.

109. Ring D, Waters PM. Operative fixation of Monteggia fractures in children. *J Bone Joint Surg Br.* 1996;78(5):734–739. **(LOE IV)**.

110. Kristiansen B, Eriksen AF. Simultaneous type II Monteggia lesion and fracture-separation of the lower radial epiphysis. *Injury.* 1986;17(1):51–52. **(LOE IV)**.

111. Letts M, Locht R, Wiens J. Monteggia fracture-dislocations in children. *J Bone Joint Surg Br.* 1985;67(5):724–727. **(LOE IV)**.

112. Olney BW, Menclaus MB. Monteggia and equivalent lesions in childhood. *J Pediatr Orthop.* 1989;9(2):219–223. **(LOE IV)**.

113. Ravessoud FA. Lateral condylar fracture and ipsilateral ulnar shaft fracture: Monteggia equivalent lesions? *J Pediatr Orthop.* 1985;5(3):364–366. **(LOE IV)**.

114. Foran I, Upasani V, Wallace C, et al. Acute pediatric Monteggia fractures: a conservative approach to stabilization. *J Pediatr Orthop.* 2017;37(6):e335–e341. **(LOE IV)**.

115. Dormans JP, Rang M. The problem of Monteggia fracture-dislocations in children. *Orthop Clin North Am.* 1990;21(2):251–256. **(LOE IV)**.

116. Best TN. Management of old unreduced Monteggia fracture dislocations of the elbow in children. *J Pediatr Orthop.* 1994;14(2):193–199. **(LOE IV)**.

117. Hurst LC, Dubrow EN. Surgical treatment of symptomatic chronic radial head dislocation: a neglected Monteggia fracture. *J Pediatr Orthop.* 1983;3(2):227–230. **(LOE IV)**.

118. Oner FC, Diepstraten AF. Treatment of chronic post-traumatic dislocation of the radial head in children. *J Bone Joint Surg Br.* 1993;75(4):577–581. **(LOE IV)**.

119. Rodgers WB, Waters PM, Hall JE. Chronic Monteggia lesions in children. Complications and results of reconstruction. *J Bone Joint Surg Am.* 1996;78(9):1322–1329. **(LOE IV)**.

120. Stoll TM, Willis RB, Paterson DC. Treatment of the missed Monteggia fracture in the child. *J Bone Joint Surg Br.* 1992;74(3):436–440. **(LOE IV)**.

121. Tajima T, Yoshizu T. Treatment of long-standing dislocation of the radial head in neglected Monteggia fractures. *J Hand Surg.* 1995;20(3 Pt 2):S91–S94. **(LOE IV)**.

122. Thompson JD, Lipscomb AB. Recurrent radial head subluxation treated with annular ligament reconstruction. A case report and follow-up study. *Clin Orthop Relat Res.* 1989;246:131–135. **(LOE IV)**.

123. de Putter CE, van Beeck EF, Looman CW, et al. Trends in wrist fractures in children and adolescents, 1997-2009. *J Hand Surg.* 2011;36(11):1810–1815.e2. **(LOE IV)**.

124. Wood AM, Robertson GA, Rennie L, et al. The epidemiology of sports-related fractures in adolescents. *Injury.* 2010;41(8):834–838. **(LOE IV)**.

125. Faulkner RA, Davison KS, Bailey DA, et al. Size-corrected BMD decreases during peak linear growth: implications for fracture incidence during adolescence. *J Bone Miner Res.* 2006;21(12):1864–1870. **(LOE III)**.

126. Goulding A, Jones IE, Taylor RW, Manning PJ, et al. More broken bones: a 4-year double cohort study of young girls with and without distal forearm fractures. *J Bone Miner Res.* 2000;15(10):2011–2018. **(LOE III)**.

127. Goulding A, Jones IE, Taylor RW, Williams SM, et al. Bone mineral density and body composition in boys with distal forearm fractures: a dual-energy x-ray absorptiometry study. *J Pediatr.* 2001;139(4):509–515. **(LOE III)**.

128. Pullagura M, Gopisetti S, Bateman B, van Kampen M. Are extremity musculoskeletal injuries in children related to obesity and social status? A prospective observational study in a district general hospital. *J Child Orthop.* 2011;5(2):97–100. **(LOE II)**.

129. Van Meir N, De Smet L. Carpal tunnel syndrome in children. *Acta Orthop Belg.* 2003;69(5):387–395. **(LOE IV)**.

130. Hendrickx RP, Campo MM, van Lieshout AP, et al. Above- or below-elbow casts for distal third forearm fractures in children? A meta-analysis of the literature. *Arch Orthop Trauma Surg.* 2011;131(12):1663–1671. **(LOE IV)**.

131. Papavasiliou V, Nenopoulos S. Ipsilateral injuries of the elbow and forearm in children. *J Pediatr Orthop.* 1986;6(1):58–60. **(LOE IV)**.

132. Stanitski CL, Micheli LJ. Simultaneous ipsilateral fractures of the arm and forearm in children. *Clin Orthop Relat Res.* 1980;153:218–222. **(LOE IV)**.

133. Bae DS, Howard AW. Distal radius fractures: what is the evidence?. *J Pediatr Orthop.* 2012;32(Suppl 2):S128–S130. **(LOE V)**.

134. Kuba M, Izuka B. One brace: one visit: treatment of pediatric distal radius buckle fractures with a removable wrist brace and no follow-up visit. *J Pediatr Orthop.* 2018;38(6):e338–e342. **(LOE IV)**.

135. Stutz C, Mencio GA. Pediatric fractures of the distal radius and ulna: metaphyseal and physeal injuries. *J Pediatr Orthop.* 2010;30(suppl 2):S85–**S89**. **(LOE V)**.

136. Garn SM, Rohmann CG, Silverman FN. Radiographic standards for postnatal ossification and tooth calcification. *Med Radiogr Photogr.* 1967;43:45–66. **(LOE IV)**.

137. Mino DE, Palmer AK, Levinsohn EM. Radiography and computerized tomography in the diagnosis of incongruity of the distal radio-ulnar joint. A prospective study. *J Bone Joint Surg Am.* 1985;67(2):247–252. **(LOE III)**.

138. Pyle WG. *Radiographic Atlas of Skeletal Development of the Hand and Wrist.* Stanford: Stanford University Press.

139. Fernandez DL. Fractures of the distal radius. In: Green D, Peterson W, eds. *Green's Operative Hand Surgery.* New York: Churchill-Livingstone; 929–985.

140. Hafner R, Poznanski AK, Donovan JM. Ulnar variance in children—standard measurements for evaluation of ulnar shortening in juvenile rheumatoid arthritis, hereditary multiple exostosis and other bone or joint disorders in childhood. *Skeletal Radiol.* 1989;18(7):513–516. **(LOE III)**.

141. Epner RA, Bowers WH, Guilford WB. Ulnar variance—the effect of wrist positioning and roentgen filming technique. *J Hand Surg.* 1982;7(3):298–305. **(LOE III)**.

142. Steyers CM, Blair WF. Measuring ulnar variance: a comparison of techniques. *J Hand Surg.* 1989;14(4):607–612. **(LOE III)**.

143. Ekenstam F. Anatomy of the distal radioulnar joint. *Clin Orthop Relat Res.* 1992;275:14–18. **(LOE IV)**.

144. Gelberman RH, Salamon PB, Jurist JM, Posch JL. Ulnar variance in Kienbock's disease. *J Bone Joint Surg Am.* 1975;57(5):674–676. **(LOE III)**.

145. Watson JT, Boyer MI. Operative exposure. In: Gelberman R, ed. *The wrist.* 3rd ed. Philadelphia: Wolters Kluwer Lippincott Williams and Wilkins; 1–16.

146. Greatting MD, Bishop AT. Intrafocal (Kapandji) pinning of unstable fractures of the distal radius. *Orthop Clin North Am.* 1993;24(2):301–307. **(LOE IV)**.

147. Guichet JM, Moller CC, Dautel G, Lascombes P. A modified Kapandji procedure for Smith's fracture in children. *J Bone Joint Surg Br.* 1997;79(5):734–737. **(LOE IV)**.

148. Parikh SN, Jain VV, Youngquist J. Intrafocal pinning for distal radius metaphyseal fractures in children. *Orthopedics.* 2013;36(6):783–788. **(LOE IV)**.

149. Walton NP, Brammar TJ, Hutchinson J, et al. Treatment of unstable distal radial fractures by intrafocal, intramedullary K-wires. *Injury.* 2001;32(5):383–389. **(LOE IV)**.

150. Landfried MJ, Stenclik M, Susi JG. Variant of Galeazzi fracture-dislocation in children. *J Pediatr Orthop.* 1991;11(3):332–335. **(LOE IV)**.

151. Mohan K, Gupta AK, Sharma J, et al. Internal fixation in 50 cases of Galeazzi fracture. *Acta Orthop Scand.* 1988;59(3):318–320. **(LOE IV)**.

152. Ooi LH, Toh CL. Galeazzi-equivalent fracture in children associated with tendon entrapment—report of two cases. *Ann Acad Med Singapore.* 2001;30(1):51–54. **(LOE IV)**.

153. Terry CL, Waters PM. Triangular fibrocartilage injuries in pediatric and adolescent patients. *J Hand Surg.* 1998;23(4):626–634. **(LOE IV)**.

154. Palmer AK, Glisson RR, Werner FW. Relationship between ulnar variance and triangular fibrocartilage complex thickness. *J Hand Surg.* 1984;9(5):681–682. **(LOE III)**.

155. Waters PM, Bae DS, Montgomery KD. Surgical management of posttraumatic distal radial growth arrest in adolescents. *J Pediatr Orthop.* 2002;22(6):717–724. **(LOE IV)**.

156. DiFiori JP, Puffer JC, Aish B, Dorey F. Wrist pain, distal radial physeal injury, and ulnar variance in young gymnasts: does a relationship exist? *Am J Sports Med.* 2002;30(6):879–885. **(LOE IV)**.

157. Maffulli N, Fixsen JA. Painful hypertrophic non-union of the ulnar styloid. *J Hand Surg Br.* 1990;15(3):355–357. **(LOE IV)**.

158. Mizuta T, Benson WM, Foster BK, et al. Statistical analysis of the incidence of physeal injuries. *J Pediatr Orthop.* 1987;7(5):518–523. **(LOE IV)**.

159. Peterson HA, Madhok R, Benson JT, et al. Physeal fractures: Part 1. Epidemiology in Olmsted County, Minnesota, 1979-1988. *J Pediatr Orthop.* 1994;14(4):423–430. **(LOE IV)**.

160. Stansberry SD, Swischuk LE, Swischuk JL, Midgett TA. Significance of ulnar styloid fractures in childhood. *Pediatr Emerg Care.* 1990;6(2):99–103. **(LOE IV)**.

161. Salter RB. Injuries of the epiphyseal plate. *Instr Course Lect.* 1992;41:351–359. **(LOE IV)**.

162. Musharafieh RS, Macari G. Salter-Harris I fractures of the distal radius misdiagnosed as wrist sprain. *J Emerg Med.* 2000;19(3):265–270. **(LOE IV)**.

163. Pershad J, Monroe K, King W, et al. Can clinical parameters predict fractures in acute pediatric wrist injuries? *Acad Emerg Med.* 2000;7(10):1152–1155. **(LOE II)**.

164. Lee BS, Esterhai JL Jr, Das M. Fracture of the distal radial epiphysis. Characteristics and surgical treatment of premature, post-traumatic epiphyseal closure. *Clin Orthop Relat Res.* 1984;185:90–96. **(LOE IV)**.

165. Peterson HA. Triplane fracture of the distal radius: case report. *J Pediatr Orthop.* 1996;16(2):92–194. **(LOE IV)**.

166. Horii E, Tamura Y, Nakamura R, Miura T. Premature closure of the distal radial physis. *J Hand Surg Br.* 1993;18(1):11–16. **(LOE IV)**.

167. Valverde JA, Albinana J, Certucha JA. Early posttraumatic physeal arrest in distal radius after a compression injury. *J Pediatr Orthop B.* 1996;5(1):57–60. **(LOE IV)**.

168. Cannata G, De Maio F, Mancini F, Ippolito E. Physeal fractures of the distal radius and ulna: long-term prognosis. *J Orthop Trauma.* 2003;17(3):172–179; **discussion 179–180. (LOE IV)**.

169. Golz RJ, Grogan DP, Greene TL, et al. Distal ulnar physeal injury. *J Pediatr Orthop.* 1991;11(3):318–326. **(LOE IV)**.

170. Nelson OA, Buchanan JR, Harrison CS. Distal ulnar growth arrest. *J Hand Surg.* 1984;9(2):164–170. **(LOE IV)**.

171. Waters PM, Kolettis GJ, Schwend R. Acute median neuropathy following physeal fractures of the distal radius. *J Pediatr Orthop.* 1994;14(2):173–177. **(LOE IV)**.

172. Waters PM. Fractures of the distal radius and ulna. In: Rockwood CA, Wilkins KE, Beatty E, eds. *Rockwood and Wilkins' Fractures in Children.* Philadelphia: Lippincott Williams and Wilkins.

173. Langenskiöld A. Surgical treatment of partial closure of the growth plate. *J Pediatr Orthop.* 1981;1(1):3–11. **(LOE IV)**.

174. Langenskiöld A, Österman K. Surgical treatment of partial closure of the epiphyseal plate. *Reconstr Surg Traumatol.* 1979;17:48–64. **(LOE IV)**.

175. Evenski AJ, Adamczyk MJ, Steiner RP, et al. Clinically suspected scaphoid fractures in children. *J Pediatr Orthop.* 2009;29(4):352–355. **(LOE IV)**.

176. Mintzer CM, Waters PM. Surgical treatment of pediatric scaphoid fracture nonunions. *J Pediatr Orthop.* 1999;19(2):236–239. **(LOE IV)**.

177. Brydie A, Raby N. Early MRI in the management of clinical scaphoid fracture. *Br J Radiol.* 2003;76(905):296–300. **(LOE IV)**.

178. Dorsay TA, Major NM, Helms CA. Cost-effectiveness of immediate MR imaging versus traditional follow-up for revealing radiographically occult scaphoid fractures. *AJR Am J Roentgenol.* 2001;177(6):1257–1263. **(LOE III)**.

179. Mack MG, Keim S, Balzer JO, et al. Clinical impact of MRI in acute wrist fractures. *Eur Radiol.* 2003;13(3):612–617. **(LOE IV)**.

180. Waters PM, Stewart SL. Surgical treatment of nonunion and avascular necrosis of the proximal part of the scaphoid in adolescents. *J Bone Joint Surg Am.* 2002;84-A(6):915–920. **(LOE IV)**.

181. Burge P. Closed cast treatment of scaphoid fractures. *Hand Clin.* 2001;17(4):541–552. **(LOE V)**.

182. Gellman H, Caputo RJ, Carter V, et al. Comparison of short and long thumb-spica casts for non-displaced fractures of the carpal scaphoid. *J Bone Joint Surg Am.* 1989;71(3):354–357 **(LOE II)**.

183. Hambidge JE, Desai VV, Schranz PJ, et al. Acute fractures of the scaphoid. Treatment by cast immobilisation with the wrist in flexion or extension? *J Bone Joint Surg Br.* 1999;81(1):91–92. **(LOE I)**.

184. Yanni D, Lieppins P, Laurence M. Fractures of the carpal scaphoid. A critical study of the standard splint. *J Bone Joint Surg Br.* 1991;73(4):600–602. **(LOE III)**.

185. Kaneshiro SA, Failla JM, Tashman S. Scaphoid fracture displacement with forearm rotation in a short-arm thumb spica cast. *J Hand Surg.* 1999;24(5):984–991. **(LOE III)**.

186. Adolfsson L, Lindau T, Arner M. Acutrak screw fixation versus cast immobilisation for undisplaced scaphoid waist fractures. *J Hand Surg Br.* 2001;26(3):192–195. **(LOE II)**.

187. Yip HS, Wu WC, Chang RY, So TY. Percutaneous cannulated screw fixation of acute scaphoid waist fracture. *J Hand Surg Br.* 2002;27(1):42–46. **(LOE IV)**.

188. Stuart HC, Pyle SI, Cornoni J, Reed RB. Onsets, completions and spans of ossification in the 29 bonegrowth centers of the hand and wrist. *Pediatrics.* 1962;29:237–249. **(LOE IV)**.

189. Gelberman RH, Menon J. The vascularity of the scaphoid bone. *J Hand Surg.* 1980;5(5):508–513. **(LOE III)**.

190. Doman AN, Marcus NW. Congenital bipartite scaphoid. *J Hand Surg.* 1990;15(6):869–873. **(LOE IV)**.

191. Louis DS, Calhoun TP, Garn SM, et al. Congenital bipartite scaphoid—fact or fiction?. *J Bone Joint Surg Am.* 1976;58(8):1108–1112. **(LOE IV)**.

192. Vender MI, Watson HK, Wiener BD, Black DM. Degenerative change in symptomatic scaphoid nonunion. *J Hand Surg.* 1987;12(4):514–519. **(LOE IV)**.

193. Slutsky DJ, Trevare J. Use of arthroscopy for the treatment of scaphoid fractures. *Hand Clin.* 2014;30(1):91–103. **(LOE V)**.

194. Kollitz K, Pulos N, Bishop A, Shin A. Primary medial femoral condyle vascularized bone graft for scaphoid nonunions with carpal collapse and proximal pole avascular necrosis. *J Hand Surg Eur.* 2019;44(6):600–606. **(LOE IV)**.

195. Mahabir RC, Kazemi AR, Cannon WG, Courtemanche DJ. Pediatric hand fractures: a review. *Pediatr Emerg Care.* 2001;17(3):153–156. **(LOE V)**.

196. Rajesh A, Basu AK, Vaidhyanath R, Finlay D. Hand fractures: a study of their site and type in childhood. *Clin Radiol.* 2001;56(8):667–669. **(LOE IV)**.

197. Kozin SH. Fractures and dislocations of the hand and carpus in children. In: Rockwood CA, Wilkins KE, Beatty E, eds. *Rockwood and Wilkins' Fractures in Children.* Philadelphia: Lippincott Williams and Wilkins.

198. Piper S, Wheeler L, Mills, et al. Outcomes after primary repair and staged reconstruction of zone I and II flexor tendon injuries in children. *J Pediatr Orthop.* 2019;39(5):263–267. **(LOE IV)**.

199. Sikora S, Lai M, Arneja J. Pediatric flexor tendon injuries: a 10-year outcome analysis. *Can J Plast Surg.* 2013;21(3):181–185. **(LOE IV)**.

200. Atasoy E, Ioakimidis E, Kasdan ML, et al. Reconstruction of the amputated finger tip with a triangular volar flap. A new surgical procedure. *J Bone Joint Surg Am.* 1970;52(5):921–926. **(LOE IV)**.

201. Clayburgh RH, Wood MB, Cooney WP 3rd. Nail bed repair and reconstruction by reverse dermal grafts. *J Hand Surg.* 1983;8(5 Pt 1):594–598. **(LOE IV)**.

202. Kappel DA, Burech JG. The cross-finger flap. An established reconstructive procedure. *Hand Clin.* 1985;1(4):677–683. **(LOE IV)**.

203. Zook EG, Russell RC. Reconstruction of a functional and esthetic nail. *Hand Clin.* 1990;6(1):59–68. **(LOE V)**.

204. Sandzen SC, Oakey RS. Crushing injury of the fingertip. *Hand.* 1972;4(3):253–256. **(LOE IV)**.

205. Zook EG, Guy RJ, Russell RC. A study of nail bed injuries: causes, treatment, and prognosis. *J Hand Surg.* 1984;9(2):247–252. **(LOE IV)**.

206. Kardestuncer T, Bae DS, Waters PM. The results of tenodermodesis for severe chronic mallet finger deformity in children. *J Pediatr Orthop.* 2008;28(1):81–85. **(LOE IV)**.

207. Seymour N. Juxta-epiphysial fracture of the terminal phalanx of the finger. *J Bone Joint Surg Br.* 1996;48(2):347–349. **(LOE IV)**.

208. Krusche-Mandl I, Kottstorfer J, Thalhammer G, et al. Seymour fractures: retrospective analysis and therapeutic considerations. *J Hand Surg.* 2013;38(2):258–264. **(LOE IV)**.

209. Dixon GL Jr, Moon NF. Rotational supracondylar fractures of the proximal phalanx in children. *Clin Orthop Relat Res.* 1972;83:151–156. **(LOE IV)**.

210. Waters PM, Taylor BA, Kuo AY. Percutaneous reduction of incipient malunion of phalangeal neck fractures in children. *J Hand Surg.* 2004;29(4):707–711. **(LOE IV)**.

211. Cornwall R, Waters PM. Remodeling of phalangeal neck fracture malunions in children: case report. *J Hand Surg.* 2004;29(3):458–461. **(LOE IV)**.

212. Hennrikus WL, Cohen MR. Complete remodelling of displaced fractures of the neck of the phalanx. *J Bone Joint Surg Br.* 2003;85(2):273–274. **(LOE IV)**.

213. Simmons BP, Peters TT. Subcondylar fossa reconstruction for malunion of fractures of the proximal phalanx in children. *J Hand Surg.* 1987;12(6):1079–1082. **(LOE IV)**.

214. Schenck RR. Dynamic traction and early passive movement for fractures of the proximal interphalangeal joint. *J Hand Surg.* 1986;11(6):850–858. **(LOE IV)**.

215. Mintzer CM, Waters PM. Late presentation of a ligamentous ulnar collateral ligament injury in a child. *J Hand Surg.* 1994;19(6):1048–1049. **(LOE IV)**.

216. White GM. Ligamentous avulsion of the ulnar collateral ligament of the thumb of a child. *J Hand Surg.* 1986;11(5):669–672. **(LOE IV)**.

217. Light TR, Ogden JA. Complex dislocation of the index metacarpophalangeal joint in children. *J Pediatr Orthop.* 1988;8(3):300–305. (LOE IV).

218. Smith RJ. Post-traumatic instability of the metacarpophalangeal joint of the thumb. *J Bone Joint Surg Am.* 1977;59(1):14–21. **(LOE IV)**.

219. Becton JL, Christian JD Jr, Goodwin HN, Jackson JG 3rd. A simplified technique for treating the complex dislocation of the index metacarpophalangeal joint. *J Bone Joint Surg Am.* 1975;57(5):698–700. **(LOE IV)**.

220. Kaplan EB. Dorsal dislocation of the metacarpophalangeal joint of the index finger. *J Bone Joint Surg Am.* 1957;39-A(5):1081–1086. **(LOE IV)**.

221. McLaughlin HL. Complex "locked" dislocation of the metacarpophalangeal joints. *J Trauma.* 1965;5(6):683–688. **(LOE IV)**.

19 Skeletal Trauma in Young Athletes

Eric W. Edmonds | Nathan L. Grimm | Aleksei B. Dingel | Kevin G. Shea

INTRODUCTION

In the words of Mercer Rang, "children are not small adults."[1]

EPIDEMIOLOGY OF YOUTH SPORTS

The popularity of youth sports continues to grow and increasing participation of children at younger ages is being seen. Approximately 30 to 44 million preadolescents and adolescents are involved in organized sports, and an estimated 7.6 million students are involved in high school athletics.[2,3] This participation is beneficial to the overall health of these children but is not without risk.[3] Previous surveys estimated the annual number of injuries resulting from participation in sports and recreational activities to be 4,379,000; of these, 1,363,000 were classified as serious (i.e., requiring hospitalization, surgical treatment, missed school, or a half day or more in bed).[4,5] A recent analysis of high school athletes demonstrated an estimated 446,715 severe injuries involving the knee (29%), ankle (12.3%), and shoulder (10.9%) most commonly. Of these injuries, 36% were fractures. Slightly more than half of the severe sports injuries resulted in medical disqualification for the season, and approximately a quarter of the injuries required surgical intervention.[6]

In a separate study, Swenson and colleagues[7] found an incidence of 10% fractures in high school athletes, and an increased proportion of fractures were inversely associated with maturity of the player. Fracture rates were highest in football, ice hockey, and lacrosse, and the hand/finger (32.1%), lower leg (10.1%), and wrist (9.5%) were affected most commonly.

INFLUENCE OF GENDER

Enacted in 1972, Title IX legislation was designed to increase participation of females in sports, which it has done. The increase in female sports participation has brought a disproportionate increase in female injuries, and in gender-comparable sports, girls have a higher injury rate than boys.[8] In sports that involve running and cutting, jumping, and landing, females have been shown to sustain higher rates of knee injuries than males. Moreover, Frisch and colleagues[9] also found an association with sports injury and previous injury between the two genders, but highlighted that girls were more likely to sustain an injury in team sports compared with boys in racquet sports. Although they found no difference in the severity of sports injuries between genders, they did find an increased incidence of foot and ankle injuries in girls. Girls may have a higher risk of injury; thus, this gender is often targeted by injury prevention programs to help reduce sports injury risk,[10–19] although some recent research has questioned the effectiveness of some of these programs.[20]

ANATOMY OF THE SKELETALLY IMMATURE JOINT AND LIGAMENTS

The physis is specialized cartilaginous tissue interposed between the metaphysis and the epiphysis in the long bones of children.[21] The physis is a multilayered structure that physiologically transcends zones of cartilaginous matrix to complete ossification, resulting in increased length of the bone. Both sides of the physis are active in the process of bone formation: proximally (intramembranous), resulting in both cylinderization and funnelization, and distally, directly beneath the articular cartilage layer (endochondral formation), resulting in hemispherization.[22] The open physes are easily seen on magnetic resonance imaging (MRI), as shown in the sagittal view of the knee (Fig. 19.1). The region of greatest risk for injury is the area between the hypertrophic cells and the region of calcification.[23] The physeal cartilage adds unique biomechanical character to the pediatric skeleton. This tissue is more viscoelastic than bone; thus, it is more likely to fail in traumatic situations, particularly in rotation.[1,24–26] In many types of pediatric injuries, the physeal cartilage will fail before the surrounding ligaments or osseous tissues.[27]

Pediatric joints have a higher percentage of cartilage than adult joints because of the physis and nonossified regions of the epiphysis, and this may explain the higher incidence of physeal and apophyseal fractures in the skeletally immature joints, such as the knee. Although occasionally seen in adults, tibial eminence avulsion injuries are relatively rare compared with midsubstance anterior cruciate ligament (ACL) injuries. Tibial eminence avulsion injuries are commonly seen in skeletally immature patients and may represent the fact that the epiphyseal region of the tibial plateau is composed of a relatively high percentage of cartilage compared with the adult knee (Fig. 19.2).[28–30] Avulsion injuries of the posterior cruciate ligament (PCL) are also seen in skeletally immature patients.

Pediatric bone is more flexible and less brittle than adult bone because of its decreased density.[1,24,25,31] These different mechanical properties are evidenced by the unique fracture types seen in children, including buckle, bowing, and greenstick deformities.[1,31]

Many studies of pediatric trauma have supported the concept that the physis is weaker than ligaments and that the physeal structure is more likely to fail than ligaments, especially under conditions of high-energy transfer. The weakest area of the physis is thought to be the zone of hypertrophy,[32–35] although fractures can occur in other regions.[36] Examples of fractures of this type include a medial epicondylar avulsion of the elbow, triplane fractures of the distal tibia, and traumatic displacement of the proximal femoral physis. These fractures are complicated by the susceptibility to growth disturbance after an injury, especially when physeal fractures are involved.[37–41] Although these fracture patterns are relatively common in skeletally immature athletes, ligamentous injuries similar to those in adults can still occur in the skeletally immature.

Biomechanical studies of the physis and ligaments have shown that failure modes are related to the magnitude and rate of load application.[33] Ligaments are more likely to fail at lower rates of load application, whereas physeal fractures are more likely to occur at higher rates of load application.[33,42] The cartilaginous physes are approximately one-third as strong as their associated ligaments, and this difference becomes more disparate during growth spurts.[43] As the child becomes older, the physis becomes stiffer and may make the incidence of a ligamentous injury more likely than a physeal injury.[24,33,44–46]

PRINCIPLES OF EXAMINATION AND TREATMENT OF THE PEDIATRIC AND ADOLESCENT PATIENT

The principles of examination (for the pediatric patient) are similar to those used for adults. Establishing trust and rapport with the child during the history (taking) will make the examination of a painful injury easier. It is often best to start away from the most painful site and work toward the injured area. Although serious injuries are rare, especially in smaller children, physeal and ligamentous injuries should always be considered. Thus, knowledge of physeal anatomy and the specific location of symptoms is needed to accurately diagnose these injuries. Often, the pediatric examination may be easier because of smaller joints and very distinct ligamentous end points. Some children naturally have increased laxity; therefore, comparison with the contralateral side is important. With knee examinations, Lachman test excursions may be easier to detect and quantify compared with adult patients. Specialized pediatric equipment, such as a KT-1000 Junior (MEDmetric, San Diego, California), may be helpful for these examinations. Historically, a complete examination was not thought to be possible without the use of sedation or anesthesia in some injuries. Because of the availability of current imaging technology, specifically MRI and computed tomography (CT), the need for examination under anesthesia is rarely necessary anymore.

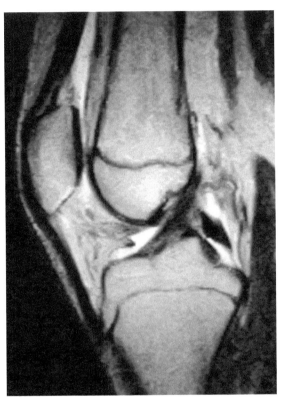

Fig. 19.1 Sagittal magnetic resonance imaging of pediatric knee.

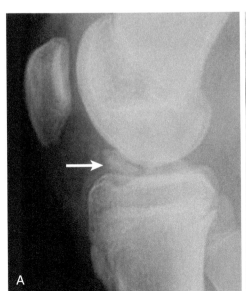
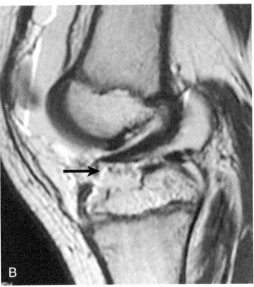

Fig. 19.2 Radiograph (A) and magnetic resonance image (B) of a displaced tibial spinal fracture.

Treating pediatric and adolescent patients is less complicated than treating adults in some respects. Children's injuries tend to heal more quickly and are less apt to develop arthrofibrosis than adults. Younger patients generally require a shorter period of immobilization because of rapid healing. Adolescents and older patients with serious knee and other joint injuries are usually mobilized early to reduce the risk of arthrofibrosis. When arthrofibrosis does occur, in the authors' experience, it tends to respond better to nonoperative measures in children than in adults. Thus, the treating physician may observe younger patients somewhat longer before considering surgical intervention in a stiff joint. In cases of severely ankylosed knees, Cole and Ehrlich[47] described a successful approach for functional restoration in children.[47] When manipulation is considered, caution is warranted because of the risk of physeal injury.

DIAGNOSTIC IMAGING

Diagnostic imaging is useful for serious injuries in young patients. Plain radiographs can identify osseous injuries, although they are inadequate for the evaluation of certain acute injuries such as a knee with hemarthrosis.[48,49] Comparison views can be invaluable aids when physeal irregularities are being assessed. MRI seems to have replaced stress and nonstress radiographs in differentiating a physeal injury from a ligamentous injury.[37,50,51]

MRI has been assessed as a mode of evaluation for the sports injury, especially in the knee.[37,50,51] Imaging in children younger than 5 to 7 years may be limited because of the small size of the knee.[51–53] The indications for MRI in children are still being established, although many clinicians rely on MRI for diagnosis.[54] MRI is a very sensitive tool for the evaluation of physeal, osseous, and ligamentous structures. One significant limitation of MRI in skeletally immature patients is in the evaluation of meniscal tears: interpretation of meniscal tissue intrasubstance signal variation can be difficult because these younger patients frequently have variations in the meniscal signal, particularly in the posterolateral horn of the meniscus, that can suggest an injury in the setting of normal meniscal tissue.[53,55] Kocher and colleagues and others have questioned the effectiveness and necessity of MRI for the routine evaluation of knee injuries in children,[53,54,56,57] although imaging studies may help identify occult fracture[58] or ligamentous injuries.[55]

With regard to the rate of injuries found with the use of MRI, a recent study[59] on the knee demonstrated that preadolescent patients with an effusion had patellar dislocations (36%), ACL tears (22%), and isolated meniscal tears (15%). Adolescent patients had slightly different rates of injury with knee effusion: ACL tears (40%), patellar dislocations (28%), and isolated meniscal tears (13%).

SPORT INJURIES TO THE UPPER EXTREMITY

SHOULDER INJURIES

Shoulder pain is a common complaint among young athletes who perform overhead activities such as pitching, throwing, and swimming.[60,61] The pain is usually located anteriorly, but lateral and posterior pain is not uncommon (especially as the dermal nerve distribution all comes from the axillary nerve). The pain is typically described as a dull ache, which occurs when they are performing their activities.

Examination of the shoulder consists of range-of-motion testing, a thorough neuromuscular assessment (particularly strength of the rotator cuff muscles), and specific diagnostic tests. Limits in range of motion may signal an acute injury, fracture, or dislocation. Occasionally, passive or active motion may help the child localize the pain. Weakness in a specific nerve distribution may indicate a cervical cause as the pain generator (either by radiculopathy or muscle imbalance). Weakness of the rotator cuff muscles will often lead to shoulder pain, especially with background joint laxity, because of excessive motion of the humerus in the glenohumeral joint. A differential diagnosis can usually be formulated after acquiring the history and performing the initial physical examination.

The sensitivity and specificity of clinical tests for superior labrum anterior/posterior (SLAP) lesions may be limited when used individually, but the diagnostic value may improve when several tests are used. In the assessment of SLAP tears, the O'Brien test, Biceps Load II test, Dynamic Labral Shear test (O'Driscoll test), Speed test, and the labral tension test have been assessed for predictability with very low yield to identify this injury pattern.[62] Once the physical examination is complete, then confirmatory diagnostic testing may be performed.

Diagnostic testing involves plain radiographs of the shoulder that include anteroposterior (AP) and lateral projections. Depending on the differential diagnoses involved, this might include an axillary view, Velpeau axillary view, scapular Y view, AP shoulder with humerus internal and external rotation, Grashey view (true glenoid AP), or a serendipity view of the clavicle.[63] After plain radiographs, there may be an indication for obtaining either MRI or CT scans. CT scans would be appropriate if a more detailed reconstruction of the bony architecture is required; however, for soft tissue injuries that cannot be evaluated by either a CT scan or a plain film, MRI is the diagnostic modality of choice, and often they are performed with an arthrogram to improve visualization of labral tears and partial undersurface tears of the rotator cuff tendon in children.

SHOULDER DISLOCATION AND INSTABILITY

Shoulder injuries in the pediatric athlete are often because of instability, especially in sports with overhead movements and contact, such as football, rugby, wrestling, and basketball. Repeated overhead motions can stretch the joint capsule and allow excessive motion of the humeral head and contact to an actively abducted and externally rotated humerus places the glenohumeral joint at risk. Acute shoulder dislocation may result in stretching of the joint capsule or other glenohumeral pathology, such as labral tears (Perthes lesions), bony Bankart, glenolabral articular disruption lesions, partial articular sided rotator cuff tears (PASTA, or subscapularis tears), humeral avulsions of the glenohumeral ligaments, and anterior labroligamentous periosteal sleeve avulsions.[64]

Historically, individuals 11 to 20 years old demonstrate approximately the same incidence of glenohumeral joint dislocation as their more mature counterparts 51 to 60 years old.[65] However, this younger cohort may have more than a 70% chance of recurrent dislocation without surgical intervention.[66] Pediatric dislocations are believed to stretch the capsule more than adult dislocations and diminish the capsule's ability to provide the support needed for proper articulation. Surgical treatment for instability is generally successful[67,68] and is often recommended, but the rate of recurrence in the adolescent population after either open or arthroscopic surgical repair may be as high as 10% to 24% at 2 years, with a 5-year survivability curve suggesting as high as 50% recurrent instability.[69,70,71] The results of multidirectional instability surgery may be similar to pure anterior instability, with a recurrence of about 24% after surgical intervention in a young adult population.[72] Isolated posterior instability fares no better in terms of outcomes, with 90% of children remaining stable after surgical intervention; but only about two-thirds able to return to preinjury level of play.[73]

Physical examination and diagnostic testing may demonstrate the concomitant injuries of a Bankart lesion (anterior bony or labral tear), SLAP tear, Kim lesions (posterior sublabral pathology), Hill-Sachs (posterolateral humeral head compression fracture) lesions, rotator cuff muscle tears, and subscapularis or lesser tubercle avulsions.[74–76] Recent evidence in the pediatric population suggests that preoperative evaluation and MRI underestimate the full extent of labral pathology seen at the time of arthroscopy.[77]

An associated pathology to instability of the shoulder is internal impingement. There is a distinct difference between external impingement syndrome (formerly "impingement syndrome" of the shoulder) and internal impingement syndrome, with the former occurring in a more mature athlete or sedentary adult and the latter occurring almost exclusively in a younger athletic shoulder.[78] The cause of internal impingement is believed to be multifactorial but occurs predominantly in overhead athletes (baseball, softball, volleyball, tennis, water polo, and swimming). Instability of the shoulder (even microinstability), especially with associated weakness to rotator cuff and periscapular stabilizers, posterior capsule contracture, and scapular dyskinesis, will cause scapulohumeral hyperangulation, scapular protraction, and ultimately contact of the humerus on the posterosuperior glenoid during activity. This contact then may result in partial articular surface tearing of the supraspinatus and infraspinatus tendon at their insertion on the humerus, as well as posterosuperior labral fraying and tearing. Early arthroscopic findings may be hypertrophic synovitis. MRI has been shown to underestimate the potential pathology seen in this overuse type injury, and therefore, inability to improve with conservative management may indicate surgical intervention.[79]

Treatment

In the acute care setting, dislocated shoulders should undergo closed reduction as quickly as possible. As previously discussed, children tend not to have favorable outcomes after shoulder dislocation: only 10% to 30% have success without surgical intervention. Surgical treatment for shoulder laxity, in the form of anterior, posterior, or multidirectional instability, may be delayed until a several-month period of physical therapy and activity modification has been attempted without significant clinical improvement.[80] Should the child fail conservative management or have secondary laxity

to a shoulder dislocation, at least a capsulorrhaphy may be required to create a stable glenohumeral joint.[81] Other surgical treatments can be added à la carte, depending on the specific pathology present in each case. Recognition of osseous abnormality in the humeral head and/or glenoid may be an important factor associated with recurrent instability after surgery.[82]

Suture anchors and plication of the redundant capsule appear to have the best outcomes from an arthroscopic approach. An open capsular shift through a standard deltopectoral approach remains the technique with the greatest reproducibility and results in the most postoperative stability. Outcomes for open procedures result in reported recurrent dislocation rates of 2.7% to 3.5% in adults[83,84] as compared with arthroscopic results that range from 3.4% to 40%, depending on the study.[85,86] Bottoni and colleagues[87] conducted a randomized clinical trial of 66 patients and found comparable clinical outcomes between open and arthroscopic techniques for treating recurrent anterior shoulder instability. However, Lenters and colleagues[88] published a systematic review and meta-analysis of reports comparing open and arthroscopic repairs for recurrent anterior shoulder dislocation and found that arthroscopic repairs were associated with significantly higher rates of recurrent instability, recurrent dislocation, and reoperation.

If the patient has bony defects in the glenoid or a Hill-Sachs lesion, these defects may be addressed by one of several procedures. These procedures include the Bristow procedure, the Latarjet procedure,[89] and iliac crest bone grafting.[90,91] To reduce the morbidity associated with autografting, recent techniques have used allograft from the femoral head[92] and the distal tibia.[81] These procedures are typically performed through an anterior open approach to the shoulder. Current techniques for arthroscopic Latarjet procedures have been developed[93] but are technically demanding.[93,94] Complications associated with the Latarjet procedure may be higher than those for arthroscopic procedures and include infection, neurologic injury, and recurrent dislocation.[95]

Recent research is also studying the impact of humeral head defects, which, in some cases, may be a significant problem.[96–99] Hill-Sachs deformities can also contribute to significant shoulder instability that cannot be addressed with a more traditional soft tissue and anterior Bankart repair. Techniques have been developed to prevent this posterior humeral defect from engaging the glenoid, which can cause shoulder disability and recurrent dislocation.[100–103] These approaches address the humeral head defect by treating the osseous defects with bone supplementation.[104] Techniques include allografting, humeral osteotomy,[105] humeroplasty, and resurfacing arthroplasty.[103] Soft tissue techniques have also been used and may include mobilizing the posterior aspect of the capsule and the infraspinatus tendon[106] to fill the defect, termed "remplissage." In cases of a traditional Bankart lesion combined with a significant Hill-Sachs deformity, this remplissage procedure may be combined with a Bankart repair via an arthroscopic approach (Fig. 19.3). The presence of a significant glenoid defect may be a contraindication for this procedure, and other approaches may be necessary.[103,107]

Future research comparing the outcomes of different osseous-based procedures will continue, and future

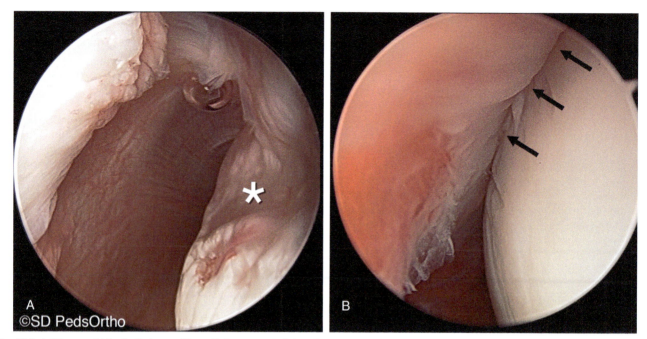

Fig. 19.3 A 17-year-old football player with multiple recurrent dislocation events and a large Hill-Sachs lesion (A) seen in an arthroscopic photo *(asterisk)*, and (B) the same photograph after remplissage procedure brings the infraspinatus and posterior capsule into the defect *(arrows)*.

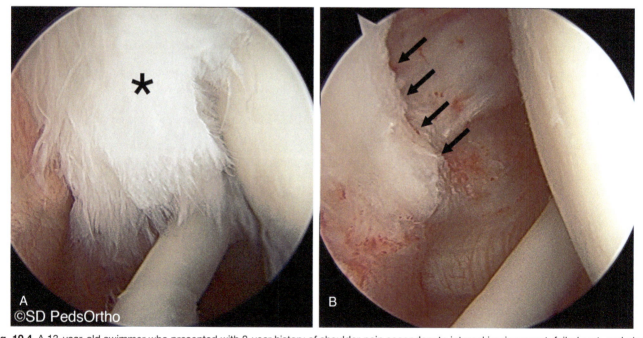

Fig. 19.4 A 13-year-old swimmer who presented with 2-year history of shoulder pain secondary to internal impingement, failed rest, and physical therapy to resolve pain. (A) Arthroscopic photo demonstrating a 4-mm supraspinatus articular tear *(asterisk)*. (B) Arthroscopic photo after debridement to stable edges *(arrows)*. She further underwent posterior capsulorrhaphy for instability to resolve and prevent further symptoms.

arthroscopic techniques may eventually allow for correction of osseous and soft tissues deficits. A higher complication rate associated with these osseous procedures is a concern.

Internal impingement syndrome is treated with physical therapy that focuses on range of motion, periscapular strengthening, and activity-specific training that is integral to treatment and later prevention of reinjury in these young, aggressive athletes. Initial management should include activity modification in the form of rest, plus cryotherapeutic modalities and nonsteroidal antiinflammatory agents. If conservative management fails, then surgical treatment may be considered. The surgical treatment options vary based on the intraoperative findings and the suspected source of the internal impingement (instability, posterior capsular contracture, etc.).[108] Either way, arthroscopy is the treatment of choice for débridement of PASTA tears less than 7 mm thickness, repairs of rotator cuff tears that are larger, débridement or repair of posterior labral pathology or synovitis, plus capsulorrhaphy in the setting of instability (anterior, posterior, or multidirectional) or capsular release for posterior contracture. (Fig. 19.4)

OVERUSE INJURIES

Adams[109] was the first to describe *Little Leaguer's shoulder* in boys 9 to 15 years of age. In the original description, the pathology was believed to be consistent with osteochondrosis of the proximal humeral epiphysis secondary to "an abnormal whip-like action, which places a forceful repetitious traction strain on the shoulder joint." Since that time, a biomechanical study has demonstrated that 12-year-old baseball pitchers are able to consistently create 215 N of shoulder distraction force (about 50% of body weight) at ball release and 18 Newton-(N) meters of peak external rotation torque at the late arm-cocking phase.[110] These forces, when consistently applied during the pitching motion of a young baseball player, are large enough to create deformation of the proximal physeal cartilage.

A stress fracture through the physeal plate may be the actual source of this Little Leaguer's shoulder and the source of the symptomatic changes in the proximal physis of the humerus with repetitive baseball pitching. The first stage of this fracture is demonstrated by osteochondrosis, or epiphysiolysis, followed by widening of the physeal plate, and ultimately callus formation around the perichondral ring of LaCroix secondary to stripping of the periosteum.[110,111] Advanced imaging techniques are consistent with biomechanical failure of the proximal humeral physis.[76,112]

Stress fractures may occur along the entire shaft of the humerus, not just at the proximal growth plate. These metaphyseal and diaphyseal stress fractures are more likely to develop in adolescent overhead athletes, who have limited or no growth potential in their proximal humeral growth plate but who continue to have immature bone.[113] The risk of development of this type of injury may also be increased by a concurrent period of rapid growth. An antecedent finding of stress fracture, or possibly a distinct entity, is humeral periostitis.[114]

Little Leaguer's shoulder, humeral periostitis, and humeral stress fractures have overlapping signs and symptoms, and pain of the proximal humerus and shoulder is often aggravated by the specific overhead activity that caused the pain and relieved with activity modification. The most common radiographic finding in Little Leaguer's shoulder is widening of the proximal humeral epiphysis. Other findings may be demineralization, sclerosis, or fragmentation of the proximal humeral metaphysis.[115] Stress fractures and periostitis may require a bone scan or MRI for definitive diagnosis, although the authors prefer the use of MRI because it avoids the use of radiation and offers much greater anatomic detail.

TREATMENT

The treatment for Little Leaguer's shoulder and stress fractures of the humerus is activity modification.[116] Most often this involves rest and cessation of the offending activity for at least 4 weeks, followed by gradual resumption of pain-free activities over the next 4 to 8 weeks.[111,113] Occasionally, physical therapy may be helpful for range of motion (in the form of teaching good throwing mechanics) and strengthening of the shoulder girdle musculature. If the child is not able to return to preinjury activity without pain, then the recommendation should be to stop that specific activity. This may mean cessation of the overhead sport or changing positions (on a baseball team) to one that is less demanding of the young athlete's shoulder. Repeated imaging to confirm the health of the pathologic proximal humerus is debatable, if all symptoms have been resolved.

ELBOW INJURIES

The young overhead athlete is vulnerable not only to shoulder injuries but also to traumatic and overuse elbow injuries. Injuries to the elbow are not limited to the overhead athlete, such as those engaged in throwing and swimming, but also include gymnasts, whose elbows, being weight-bearing joints during the sport, are also at risk.[117] The elbow joint comprises three major articulations: radiocapitellar, ulnohumeral, and proximal radioulnar. Before understanding pathologic changes in the elbow, it is important to understand the normal ossification of the elbow through the six secondary centers. All of the ossification centers except the medial and lateral epicondyles are intraarticular. Injuries of the immature elbow have a predilection for involving the weaker growth plates, as compared with the bony or ligamentous structures.

The physical examination of the young elbow is most often led by the location of pain. Many of the structures involved in youth injuries are nearly subcutaneous, and the examination should include palpation of the medial epicondyle, olecranon, lateral epicondyle, and the radial head. Passive and active range of motion (i.e., flexion, extension, supination, and pronation) should be assessed, as well as varus and valgus stressing. Loss of motion, especially mild flexion contractures, occurs frequently. The elbow averages a clinical carrying angle of 7 degrees of valgus alignment. Muscle strength and any neurologic deficits should be recorded.

Radiographic findings are based on the standard AP, lateral, and oblique films of the elbow and often require contralateral elbow films for comparison. From AP radiographs, one can measure the Baumann angle (the angle created at the bisection of the capitellar physeal line and a line perpendicular to the humeral shaft), which should be within 8 degrees of the contralateral elbow.[118] The lateral films should demonstrate a normal humerocapitellar angle of 30 to 40 degrees of flexion. More importantly, a line drawn along the anterior humeral shaft should bisect the center of the capitellum. Any view should be evaluated for fractures or dislocations, especially widening of the growth plates.

MRI studies of asymptomatic high school baseball players have demonstrated asymmetric anterior band ulnar collateral ligament thickening, mild sublime tubercle/anteromedial facet edema, and posteromedial subchondral sclerosis of the ulnotrochlear articulation, including posteromedial ulnotrochlear osteophytes and ulnotrochlear chondromalacia.[119]

Fleisig and colleagues[120] estimated that valgus forces at the elbow reach 64 N meters during late cocking and early acceleration phases of throwing, based on their biomechanics testing. Simultaneously, the compressive forces at the lateral radiocapitellar articulation, as the elbow arcs from 110 to 20 degrees of flexion at velocities of 3000 degrees/sec, may reach 500 N. The combination of these forces across the elbow joint may create a valgus extension overload that may become pathologic with repetitive throwing events.[121]

Valgus extension overload can result in most overhead sport-related injuries of the elbow because of the way the significant valgus loads, coupled with rapid elbow extension, produce tensile stress of the medial restraints, compression stress of the lateral compartment, and shear stress in the posterior compartment.

Medial elbow pain may represent an injury to the ulnar collateral ligament, flexor-pronator mass, medial epicondyle apophysis, or the ulnar nerve. In many cases of overuse elbow injuries, several of these injuries may coexist. Lateral elbow pain more likely represents an injury to the radial head or neck, lateral epicondyle apophysis, or capitellum. Posterior elbow pain usually represents an injury to the posteromedial tip of the olecranon or the trochlear and olecranon fossa.

TRAUMATIC ELBOW INJURIES

ELBOW DISLOCATIONS AND MEDIAL EPICONDYLE FRACTURES

Fractures of the medial epicondyle are more common than dislocations and account for approximately 10% of elbow fractures in children.[122] Because of the physeal anatomy of the skeletally immature elbow, the ulnar collateral ligament and flexor muscles frequently avulse a fragment from the medial epicondyle. Elbow dislocations and fractures of the medial epicondyle are usually the result of falling with the forearm supinated and the elbow in full or partial extension.[123] Nearly 50% of medial epicondyle fractures are associated with dislocation of the elbow, and often the displaced fragment becomes trapped in the joint,[124] interfering with closed reduction of the dislocated elbow (Fig. 19.5).

Medial epicondyle fractures and dislocations of the elbow are frequently seen in young gymnasts.[125] Isolated medial epicondyle fractures are occasionally seen in adolescent pitchers. These injuries typically occur during the act of pitching and may be preceded by symptoms of medial epicondylitis. Both dislocations and overuse injuries can result in an ulnar collateral ligament injury.

A direct correlation of injury to the anterior bundle of the medial ulnar collateral ligament (ABMUCL) over years of extreme utilization (pitching since an early age) has been elucidated by ultrasound studies.[126]

TREATMENT

Evaluation and treatment of medial epicondyle elbow fractures continues to evolve.[127] Radiographic analysis of fracture displacement has limitations, and more advanced imaging modalities may assist clinical decision-making.[128,129] Treatment of medial epicondyle fractures is controversial, especially for minimally displaced fractures.[130] Nondisplaced fractures are typically treated with casting, but displaced fractures may require surgery.[130] In athletes who put high demand on their elbows (e.g., throwers, gymnasts, and wrestlers), anatomic reduction of medial epicondyle fractures may be important for future athletic performance; however, current literature suggests no difference in outcomes between surgical and nonsurgical cohorts.[131]

Evidence has shown that ulnar collateral ligament reconstructions do well in the adolescent population,[132] but there may be some evidence that success may be achieved with a direct repair in this younger population.[133,134] The technique of reconstruction does not differ significantly in this age group compared with the skeletally mature; however, the technique for humeral fixation does need to take into account the open, or closing, medial epicondyle apophysis. Docking techniques can still be used, but it is the authors' opinion that screw fixation is best so that it minimizes risk of disrupting the apophysis at its weakest time without anything more than suture fixation through a tunnel (Fig. 19.6).

OVERUSE ELBOW INJURES

Overuse injuries of the immature elbow can all fall under one name, *Little Leaguer's elbow*, and happen in 75% to 80% of all children playing baseball, with nearly one-third reporting psychological effects (not having fun) from the pain and 50% of them being encouraged to play through the pain.[135] Klingele and Kocher[136] described the various injuries that may be called Little Leaguer's elbow, on the basis of the common etiology of repetitive microtrauma of the immature elbow (Table 19.1).

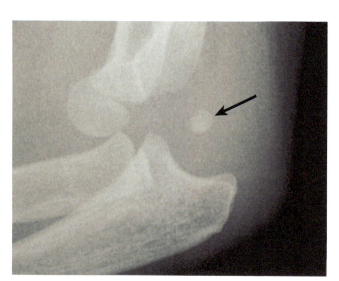

Fig. 19.5 Radiograph of a posterior elbow dislocation. The medial epicondyle is displaced and incarcerated in the joint.

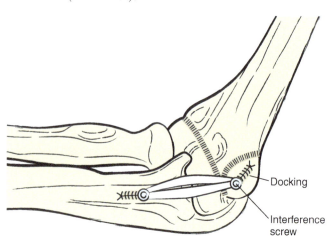

Docking

Interference screw

Fig. 19.6 Line drawing demonstrating the medial anatomy of the skeletally immature elbow with a double-docking screw fixation technique controlling the apophysis of the medial epicondyle during fixation of the proximal end of the medial ulnar collateral ligament reconstruction.

Pain at the medial side of the elbow may be medial epicondyle apophysitis or an avulsion fracture. Radiographs will usually demonstrate physeal widening but may also demonstrate fragmentation of the ossification center. The elbow may appear to have a growth disturbance, represented by delayed ossification, or, contrarily, accelerated growth, marked by premature physeal closure. Occasionally, the physis is not the location of the pathology; instead, the injury may be to the ulnar collateral ligament or common flexor origin (golfer's elbow in adults) or may be ulnar neuritis.

The lateral aspect of the elbow appears to demonstrate injuries involving the radiocapitellar joint rather than the lateral epicondyle (the source of "tennis elbow"). The capitellum may be the source of pain from osteochondrosis (Panner disease) or osteochondritis dissecans (OCD). It is important to differentiate between these two pathologic processes. The former occurs in younger children (<10 years) and is self-limited, and complete resolution is the norm after activity modification. The latter most often represents an osteochondral fracture in the older child or adolescent and often requires surgical intervention to achieve healing of the OCD and return to play.

If the capitellum is not the source of pain of the lateral elbow, then the radial head may be the cause. The radial head may also be subject to OCD lesions, which may be difficult to assess on plain radiographs. The radial neck may be subject to deformation that can lead to poor elbow mechanics and pain.[137]

Posterior elbow pain most often represents an injury to the olecranon apophysis, an avulsion fracture, or delay of apophyseal fusion.[138] Comparison of contralateral films may be helpful. MRI has proven itself nearly essentially in the workup in elbow pathology, because of the complex anatomy. The ability to determine the characteristics of an OCD lesion within the capitellum is almost impossible without an MRI, in that it can help determine the precise location of the lesion on the capitellum (is it a "shoulder lesion"?), and it can discern the stability of the lesion.[139] This information greatly influences the recommended treatment and is essential to preoperative planning. With valgus extension overload, the compression stress on the posteromedial olecranon can create osteophytes. The osteophytes may then lead to bony extension contracture; it is important to realize that the osteophytes are a by-product of the pathology.

On occasion, Little Leaguer's elbow may include anterior elbow pain and pathology that is secondary to the valgus extension overload. This usually comes in the form of anterior-based capsular contractures that cause a flexion contracture of the elbow.

Treatment

Initial management of Little Leaguer's elbow is conservative and nonsurgical unless the diagnosis is that of a fracture. Activity restrictions, therapy, and change to another position that requires less throwing are all options that help with healing. Medial epicondyle fractures or olecranon stress fractures, for example, may require open reduction and internal fixation (ORIF) for predictable outcomes in some athletes.[118,140,141] The other scenario that calls for initial management to be operative is the finding of loose bodies within the joint, because the pain is unlikely to resolve without excision.[118,136]

The initial nonoperative management, whether started for medial epicondyle apophysitis, an ulnar collateral ligament injury, or any of the other manifestations of valgus extension overload syndrome, is the same regimen independent of the diagnosis. The first step in management is cessation of provocative activities for at least 4 to 6 weeks, with concurrent cryotherapeutic and antiinflammatory modalities. Cessation of all throwing until the elbow is asymptomatic with reassessment of throwing mechanics and number of pitches thrown is essential.[118,142] During the rest from throwing activities, a transition into physical therapy that begins with regaining motion and strengthening the shoulder girdle, scapular stabilizers, and rotator cuff musculature should be started.[118] Poor mechanics of the shoulder may increase the pathologic stresses across the elbow during the throwing motion. Once the symptoms of pain begin to wane with this physical therapy program, strengthening of the medial flexor-pronator muscles may commence. Finally, with complete resolution of pain, a controlled regimen of activity-specific exercises, plyometrics, and an interval throwing program is undertaken before return to competitive activities.[117,118,136] The duration of this program often extends beyond 4 to 6 months if done appropriately (with the throwing program itself taking 3 to 4 months to complete). Families should be encouraged to stay true with the program for the health of their child's elbow. Plus, the concept of pitch counts often requires re-education (it includes every league played concurrently and the use of a pitching coach).

It is important to realize that nonoperative treatment of ABMUCL injuries is generally indicated in nonthrowing

TABLE 19.1 Little League Elbow	
Little League Elbow Pathology	**Diagnostic/Examination Findings**
Medial epicondylar apophysitis	Tenderness at epicondyle
Osteochondritis dissecans (capitellum/ radial head)	Pain laterally, radiographic evidence
Traumatic and/or chronic avulsion of medial epicondyle	Pain at epicondyle, radiographic evidence
Anterior medial bundle ulnar collateral ligament injury	Pain with milking maneuver, pain at epicondyle or the sublime tubercle
Ulnar nerve subluxation/neuritis	Positive Tinel's or evidence of subluxation with elbow flexion
Panner disease	<10 years of age

athletes because good outcomes can be achieved; in contrast, patients who are involved in high-demand overhead sports (throwing, volleyball, tennis, javelin) do not respond as well to nonoperative management. Therefore, differentiating between a true ligament tear and incompetency versus medial epicondyle apophysitis or avulsion is important.[118] If, indeed, the child is given a diagnosis of a tear in the ABMUCL and still wishes to continue competitive pitching, then the treatment of choice after failed conservative management may be ulnar collateral ligament reconstruction.[143,144]

The best treatment for many of these injuries may actually be prevention. This means teaching children good mechanics and, in throwing sports, limiting the number of pitches. Current recommendations for the number of pitches per game differ with the age of the child: 7- to 8-year-old athletes are limited to 50 pitches, 9- to 10-year-old athletes are limited to 75 pitches, 11- to 12-year-old athletes are limited to 85 pitches, 13- to 16-year-old athletes are limited to 95 pitches, and 17- to 18-year-old athletes are limited to 105 pitches.[145]

Lateral elbow pain is treated in the same manner as medial and posterior elbow pain. Nonoperative management with activity modifications and physical therapy directed in a similar fashion to the medial elbow should be attempted first, and the focus should initially be on the shoulder, but then followed by the lateral forearm extensor mass. Failure of this regimen may require arthroscopic débridement, chondroplasty, microfracture, or removal of loose bodies, as needed, especially if an OCD lesion with a loose fragment is the cause.[146] The utilization of osteochondral plugs to replace the diseased part of the capitellum has been met with success and return to sports, especially for unstable capitellum OCD[147,148] (Fig. 19.7).

Posterior elbow pain, especially in the form of a stress fracture or olecranon apophysitis, can be treated successfully with surgery. A technique that percutaneously places a screw across the apophysis, creating compression, has been demonstrated to have success and achieve early return to sports.[140] But initial nonoperative management (as discussed above) should still be considered first-line treatment in this injury pattern to avoid the complications of surgery and need for secondary surgery to remove the implant.

WRIST INJURIES

Wrist pain in an overhead-throwing athlete is not as common as that of pain in the elbow or shoulder. In contrast to throwers, gymnasts have a much higher incidence of wrist pathology. Chronic wrist pain is estimated to affect nearly 80% of all child gymnasts at one time or another because of the way that the wrist becomes a weight-bearing joint. The younger the child begins training for gymnastics, the more likely that the growth plates surrounding the wrist are potential sites of injury.[149]

Other children at risk of developing wrist pain are those using bats, rackets, or their hands to strike a ball. Most often, these injuries are considered acute and may involve fractures of the carpal bones, especially the scaphoid and hook of the hamate. Repetitive striking of the volleyball has been implicated as a potential cause of Keinböck avascular necrosis of the lunate.[150]

Examination of the wrist should involve a thorough neuromuscular assessment, evaluation of range of motion, and location of the pain. Pain in the anatomic snuff box may indicate a scaphoid fracture, pain over the radial styloid is more consistent with distal radial pathology, and pain near the ulnar styloid may represent a tear of the triangular fibrocartilage complex (TFCC).

Radiographs should consist of AP and lateral wrist or hand views, as well as specialized views depending on the differential diagnosis; these may include a carpal tunnel view to evaluate the hook of the hamate and contralateral wrist views to help assess growth plate injuries. Depending on the differential diagnosis, MRI may be performed to exclude nondisplaced fractures or osteonecrosis of the carpals. Furthermore, MRI or a CT scan, depending on the information desired, may be obtained to better evaluate wrist pathology. Often, TFCC tears and chondral lesions may be missed even on MRI.

GYMNAST WRIST

Gymnast wrist has been defined as chronic radial pain with the following radiographic findings: growth plate widening with "haziness" or ill-defined borders, metaphyseal cyst formation, and epiphyseal beaking.[151] Some evidence has

Fig. 19.7 A 16-year-old basketball player with recalcitrant capitellum osteochondritis dissecans. (A) Preoperative magnetic resonance imaging (MRI) (sagittal SPGR FS) demonstrating articular cartilage breakdown *(arrow)*, and (B) 3 months' postoperative MRI with healed osteochondral allograft plug *(asterisk)* and restored articular cartilage surface (sagittal three-dimensional MERGE). *SPGR*, Spoiled gradient-recalled echo.

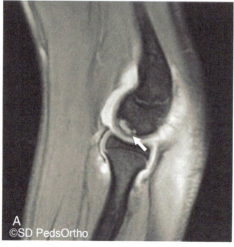
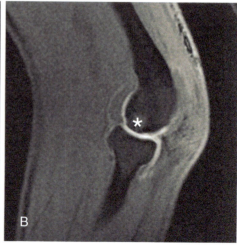

©SD PedsOrtho

shown that these changes may result in premature physeal closure of the distal radius.[152] Albanese and colleagues[152] further postulated through a summary of previous studies that some repetitive compression loading of a physis may result in increased growth, whereas too much repetitive compression loading will inhibit growth and possibly result in physeal arrest. Therefore, the etiology of gymnast risk is unclear (given the widening of the physis but the risk of arrest) in this population of athletes who are using their wrists in a weight-bearing fashion.[153] It is important to note that 70% of all gymnasts will experience some form of wrist pain in their young careers.

Past MRI study demonstrated that not all gymnasts sustain classic gymnast wrist. Dwek and colleagues[154] did find chronic physeal changes consistent with gymnast wrist, but more importantly, they discovered focal lunate osteochondral defects, TFCC tears, scapholunate ligament tears, and metacarpal head flattening and necrosis in the group of adolescent teenagers they studied.

Scaphoid fractures have also been reported to occur in gymnasts, and surgical treatment may be necessary in some cases.[155]

TREATMENT

The mainstay of treatment of gymnast wrist is activity modification, specifically cessation of wrist weight-bearing activities. Physical therapy with cryotherapy and antiinflammatory management may be undertaken during this period of rest in an effort to accelerate recovery time and ensure prevention of reinjury. Children should not be allowed to return to competitive activities unless they are pain free and are able to remain that way during activity.

If nonoperative management fails, then a few operative choices may be considered. Depending on the preoperative findings, an ulnar shortening osteotomy may be performed if positive ulnar variance is found; a chondroplasty or arthroscopic débridement of loose bodies or synovitis may also be done to alleviate symptoms.[149] The results of operative management are good in terms of pain relief,

but oftentimes the symptoms will return with competitive activities.

TRIANGULAR FIBROCARTILAGE COMPLEX INJURIES AND ULNAR-SIDED WRIST PAIN

Gymnasts and other athletes are also prone to ligamentous injuries and injuries to the TFCC because of repetitive weight-bearing on the wrist, as mentioned above in the imaging studies. Other young athletes (such as those participating in basketball, lacrosse, or baseball) may also be susceptible to these soft tissue injuries. Tears of the TFCC may result in further damage to the adjacent articular cartilage if the offending activity is not stopped. Chondromalacia has been found to involve the ulnolunate, ulnotriquetral, and radiocarpal joints.[156]

A recent study on ulnar-sided wrist pain demonstrated many possible causes in the athletic population.[157] Fractures of the ulnar styloid, hamate, pisiform, and base of the fifth metacarpal may be present; in addition, soft tissue injuries consistent with ulnar impaction syndrome, extensor carpi ulnaris disorder, or even flexor carpi ulnaris disorders may be causes.

TREATMENT

Once again, initial management of this condition is activity modification, antiinflammatory medications, cryotherapy, and occupational therapy. If this initial effort fails to produce significant improvement of the symptoms after 4 to 6 weeks, then immobilization may be used. The wrist is casted or braced depending on the child, and complete cessation of gymnastic activities is ordered for another 6 weeks. If pain continues, then the next step is to obtain an MRI to better prepare for surgical treatment. Operative treatment consists of arthroscopic débridement and possible repair of the TFCC tear (Fig. 19.8).[156] Surgical treatment in the athletic population appears to be predictably good, but perhaps not excellent, in that return to activities occurs at approximately 3 months.[158]

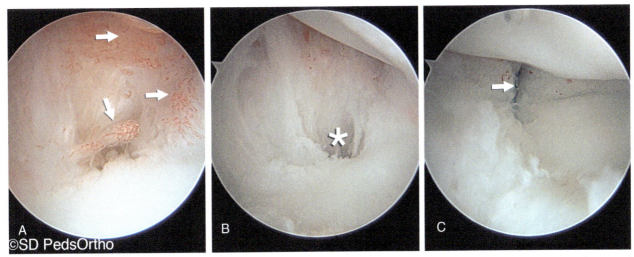

Fig. 19.8 A 10-year-old girl, level 7 gymnast, with 1-year history of ulnar-sided wrist pain treated unsuccessfully with rest and occupational therapy. Arthroscopic images: (A) view toward ulnar styloid with synovitis *(arrows)*, (B) after débridement reveals small tear *(asterisk)* causing a slack in the triangular fibrocartilage complex (TFCC) sling, and (C) after repair *(arrow)* of the TFCC back to the ulnar styloid (note the reduction in joint space after repair). Child returned to gymnastics the following season without issues.

PELVIC AND HIP INJURIES

APOPHYSEAL AVULSIONS OF THE PELVIS

Among the acute injuries of the pelvic region, apophyseal avulsions are the most common.[159] An apophysis is the point on the bone at which a muscle attaches, and occasionally the muscle wholly or partially dislodges a fragment of bone. Apophyseal avulsions are usually caused by a sudden or violent muscle contraction.[160,161] Common sites for apophyseal avulsions in pediatric and adolescent athletes include the ischial tuberosity (hamstrings), pubis (adductors), lesser trochanter (iliopsoas),[162] anterior superior iliac spine (tensor fascia lata), anterior inferior iliac spine (rectus femoris), and the iliac crest (gluteus medius) (Fig. 19.9)[163] Although certain apophyseal avulsions have traditionally been uncommon in the pediatric population, rates of this injury have been increasing in recent years, presumably because of the increase in competitive sports involvement and improvements in imaging techniques. Sudden or violent muscle activity is typically seen in sports such as gymnastics, tackle football, sprinting, field events in track and field, soccer, and any activity involving quick or powerful muscle contractions.[164]

The athlete typically reports having felt a sudden "pop" or "letting go" near the site of the injury, followed immediately by considerable pain and loss of function. In many respects, these injuries mimic muscle strains and are often initially misdiagnosed as such. Careful physical examination differentiates muscle strains from apophyseal avulsions. The initial evaluation should include a history of the activity immediately preceding the injury and palpation of the painful area. Functional testing should include manual muscle testing of the suspected muscle group, and attention should be paid to increases in pain or significant weakness. Point tenderness is demonstrated, and pain may also be referred to another region of the hip.[164] Walking with a limp indicates a more severe injury.[165]

Treatment

Initial treatment for apophyseal avulsions includes rest, ice, compression, and elevation. The athlete should be fitted with crutches to limit weight-bearing and then referred to a physician for a more complete medical evaluation. Radiographic evaluation confirms the diagnosis; however, this injury can be difficult to visualize because of its size and location.[166,167] Definitive treatment is usually nonoperative and includes rest, ice, and pain management, followed by a gradual return to activity concomitant with a general strength and flexibility program.[168] Surgical intervention is rarely required because most injuries involve minimal displacement of the avulsed fragment.[161] However, recent literature suggests that surgery may be necessary to ensure the best outcomes for some of these injuries, especially for large displaced fragments.[164,168–171]

KNEE INJURIES

PHYSEAL FRACTURES OF THE KNEE

Physeal fractures of the knee are commonly associated with youth sports and involve either the distal femoral or proximal tibial physeal plate. The injury usually results from a valgus stress, similar to the mechanisms commonly associated with tears of the ACL and medial collateral ligament (MCL) in adults.[160] Fractures of the distal femoral physis occur 10 times more frequently than proximal tibial physeal fractures and are most common in boys ages 10 to 14 years.[172] Pain at the physis is a sign of a femoral physeal injury. A physeal fracture of the knee may also present with apparent ligament laxity.[173] When this injury is suspected, one should be careful not to apply excessive force when performing a drawer test or a valgus or varus stress test because this may cause displacement through a physeal fracture. The evaluation should be restricted to a gradually applied force testing for relative laxity compared with the uninjured knee.

Although less likely, injuries of the proximal tibial physis do occur. The mechanism typically is direct trauma, such as a blow to the anterior aspect of the knee.[171] With proximal tibial physeal fractures, symptoms include pain on weight-bearing and point tenderness in the region of the joint line and just distal to it, directly over the region of the proximal tibial physis.

Radiographic evidence is necessary to confirm a diagnosis of physeal fracture; however, the diagnosis may be elusive because some of these injuries spontaneously reduce, and specialized imaging techniques may be required. Historically, stress or oblique radiographs have been used,[159] but MRI is a better diagnostic tool. Increasingly, MRI may be the imaging tool of choice if the radiographic results are normal and the clinical suspicion of a physeal injury is high. Treatment for physeal injuries ranges from closed reduction

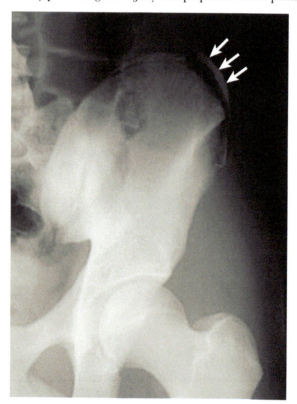

Fig. 19.9 Avulsion of iliac crest *(arrows)* in athlete with sudden onset anterior hip pain following twisting injury during a batting session in baseball.

with casting, to percutaneous pinning, to ORIF. More information on treatment of these injuries is in the chapters on distal femoral and proximal tibial injuries.

LIGAMENTOUS INJURIES OF THE KNEE

As recently as 40 years ago, some suggested that ligamentous injuries about the knee did not occur in the skeletally immature or were exceptionally rare.[174] Historically, injuries about the knee in children were thought to consistent mainly of fractures and physeal injuries, although a growing body of literature supports the concept of serious ligamentous knee injuries in pediatric and adolescent patients and athletes. The increase in knee injuries in skeletally immature patients may reflect several phenomena. The increased use of MRI and its ability to detect soft tissue injuries may play a role,[175] in addition to increased participation in sports.

In addition to athletic injuries, trauma studies have also demonstrated ligamentous injuries in skeletally immature subjects,[173,176–178] and it is recommended that patients be screened for ligamentous injuries of the knee when fractures or effusion are present about the knee.

Historically, an ACL intrasubstance injury was thought to be less common than tibial spine or tibial eminence fractures.[160,179] More recent research suggests that ACL tears are becoming more common in pediatric and adolescent patients.[180] A recent epidemiologic study of knee injuries in high school athletes indicated a rate of 0.56 ACL injuries per 10,000 athletic exposures (AEs).[181] An ACL injury was the third most common knee injury in high school athletes, behind an MCL ligament injury (0.80 injuries per 10,000 AEs) and a patella/patellar tendon injury (0.65 injuries per 10,000 AEs). The ACL pulls a fragment of bone from its tibial insertion, the tibial eminence (also referred to as the *intercondylar eminence*). Although tibial eminence avulsions are more frequent, evidence suggests that ACL tears without tibial eminence involvement seem to be increasingly common.[182] Interestingly, females, especially those of high school age, are at higher risk of ACL injuries relative to males.[183,184]

Most of the ligaments and capsular structures of the knee attach to the epiphysis. This anatomic configuration is probably the underlying biomechanical explanation for the higher risk of a physeal injury versus a ligamentous injury about the knee. With the exception of the distal MCL, the ligaments of the knee are contained within the epiphyseal/physeal envelope, which has been described by Stanitski[172] (Fig. 19.10)

ANTERIOR CRUCIATE LIGAMENT INJURY

The ACL originates from the epiphyseal portion of the lateral femoral condyle below the femoral physis and inserts on the epiphyseal portion of the tibia.[124,185,186] During torsional force application to the knee, the ligamentous and capsular tissues transfer the forces to the epiphysis, contributing to a physeal injury.

The mechanisms of injury that produce ACL tears in the pediatric and adolescent athlete population are probably similar to those of adults. Two general categories of mechanisms exist: contact and noncontact. Noncontact injuries typically involve landing from a jump with a hyperextended

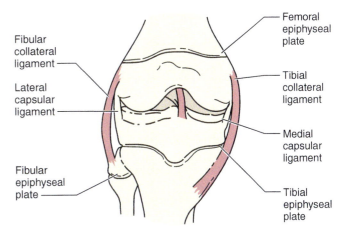

Fig. 19.10 Knee ligament anatomy in the skeletally immature. The anterior cruciate ligament, posterior cruciate ligament, lateral collateral ligament, and posterolateral complex are contained within the "physeal envelope" of the knee. The medial collateral ligament extends below the tibial physis and attaches to the tibial metaphysis. (From Delee JC. Ligamentous injury of the knee. In: Staniski CL, Delee JC, Drez DJ Jr., eds. *Pediatric and Adolescent Sports Medicine*. Philadelphia: W.B. Saunders; 1994:406-432.)

knee or with the knee out of position relative to the body's center of mass; this produces a valgus stress on the knee combined with axial rotation. Noncontact ACL injuries can also be caused by rapid deceleration or when running. Despite extensive research, a consensus group concluded that the precise mechanism of injury for noncontact ACL injuries is still to be determined.[187,188]

A child reporting a pop or snap within the joint at the time of injury raises the level of suspicion for a major ligamentous injury. Increased laxity of the major ligaments is normal in females of this age group.[56] As such, it is critical to compare all examinations with the uninjured, contralateral knee. The knee should be evaluated for all the major ligamentous restraints with use of standard functional tests. When significant laxity is found, imaging studies are necessary to determine the specific nature of the injury (i.e., true ligamentous rupture versus avulsion of the tibial eminence because tibial eminence fractures are readily identified on radiographs). MRI may be helpful for evaluating knee injuries because of its unique ability to visualize soft tissues such as the ACL and the menisci (Fig. 19.11).

The decision regarding conservative treatment versus surgical repair of a complete ACL tear in a child is complex because both surgical and nonsurgical treatments have potential complications. Long-term absence of the ACL subsequent to the injury can result in meniscal damage, osteoarthritis, and poor outcomes.[189–193] Moreover, several recent studies have shown that delayed reconstruction can lead to chondral and meniscal injuries.[194–196] Because of concerns that transphyseal drilling during traditional ACL reconstruction would result in growth disturbance or axis deviations, several authors have reported successful physeal-sparing techniques.[197–199] Recent reports have also shown good results with transphyseal reconstructions in skeletally immature patients as they approach skeletal maturity.[200–202]

A limited number of published studies support surgical (intraarticular) reconstruction of the ACL in pediatric and adolescent athletes who intend to return to their preinjury

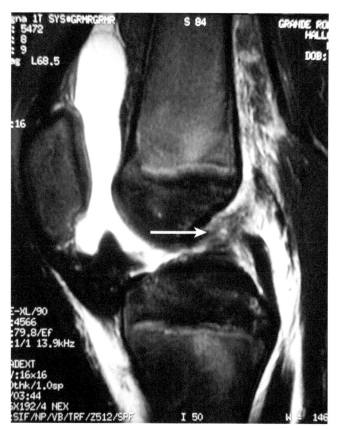

Fig. 19.11 Sagittal magnetic resonance imaging scan of midsubstance anterior cruciate ligament tear in a skeletally immature athlete.

activity level.[190,191,193] Most concerns related to surgical reconstruction focus on avoiding intrusion into the distal femoral or proximal tibial physes, which can lead to physeal arrest and result in leg length discrepancies or angular deformities.[203] Despite these concerns, it appears that reconstructions can be successful[189,192,204,205] when the placement of hardware and transphyseal tunnels is taken into account. Nonetheless, ACL reconstruction remains a controversial topic among pediatric orthopedists, and growth plate complications from this procedure have been reported.[206–208] Different surgical techniques may be considered, based on the age of the patient, amount of growth remaining, and presence of other injuries.[209]

Recently, a systematic review and meta-analysis by Frosch and colleagues[210] of 55 articles and a total of 935 patients evaluated the outcomes of ACL reconstructions in children and adolescents. The meta-analysis found overall low rates of complications and also found that physeal-sparing techniques were associated with more leg length differences and axis deviations, whereas transphyseal techniques had a higher risk of rerupture.

TIBIAL EMINENCE AVULSION

Tibial eminence avulsions, usually seen only in children, are the result of mechanisms that would lead to an ACL tear in an adult.[211] Tibial eminence avulsion fractures are classified based on relative radiographic displacement.[212] Type I fractures are nondisplaced and are treated conservatively with immobilization in a long leg cast for 4 to 6 weeks.

Type II fractures are minimally displaced, and type III are completely displaced. Type II and type III tibial eminence avulsions may be secured with internal fixation placed either arthroscopically or with open reduction.[213] Reports of meniscal entrapment with more displaced fractures are concerning, and these patients may be best treated with arthroscopic evaluation.[207] The meniscus and transverse meniscal ligament can be impediments to reduction of these fractures.[214] Recent reports have also shown a significant incidence of meniscal tears with these fractures.[215] Treatment of tibial spine fractures depends on the degree of displacement. Nondisplaced fractures can be treated with casting. Fractures with significant displacement may require surgery. Numerous recent investigators have demonstrated excellent outcomes with arthroscopic repair of these fractures. Different techniques have been published for repair of these injuries, including the use of suture-based techniques,[216–218] buttons,[219] and screw fixation[214,220,221]; in addition, biomechanical studies have also been conducted to analyze these repair techniques.[222] Arthroscopic repair also allows for evaluation of meniscal pathology, such as entrapment or a tear.[207] One significant complication of these injuries is postoperative arthrofibrosis; early motion may help reduce the risk of this complication.[223]

MEDIAL COLLATERAL LIGAMENT

ANATOMY AND BIOMECHANICS OF THE MEDIAL COLLATERAL LIGAMENT

The medial aspect of the knee has been described as three distinct layers.[175,224–227] The second layer includes the superficial MCL, originating from the medial femoral epicondyle, anterior to the adductor tubercle and below the distal femoral physis. The insertion of the MCL is located distal to the tibial physis. In the third and deepest layer of the medial aspect of the knee, the MCL is a continuation of the joint capsule. This structure is intimately associated with the medial meniscus; thus, injuries to this layer of the MCL are often associated with medial meniscal injuries.

These structures act as a complex sleeve of tissues that is both a dynamic and a static stabilizer of the knee (Fig. 19.12A,B). The static stabilizers include the superficial MCL, the posterior oblique ligament, and the deep MCL.[225] In concert with the MCL, the ACL also plays a role in resisting valgus forces about the knee.[228,229] The dynamic stabilizers include the vastus medialis and the semimembranosus muscles.[230] The MCL is the primary static knee stabilizer with respect to valgus stress,[224,226] and both the deep and superficial MCLs contribute resistance.[229,231] The posterior oblique ligament works in concert with the superficial MCL as a medial stabilizer. The MCL and posterior oblique ligament also resist external rotation of the tibia.[224,226,230] The posterior fibers of the MCL-posterior oblique complex tighten as the knee extends (Fig. 19.13). The MCL fibers extend well below the tibial physis in the skeletally immature knee (Fig. 19.14).

EVALUATION AND TREATMENT OF A MEDIAL COLLATERAL LIGAMENT INJURY

There have been relatively few descriptions of MCL injuries in skeletally immature athletes. These injuries are rare in young athletes with completely open growth plates, but they

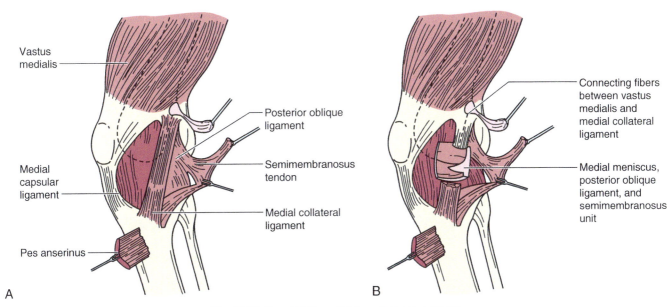

Fig. 19.12 (A and B) Superficial medial knee anatomy.

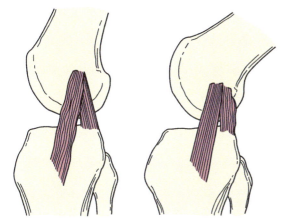

Fig. 19.13 Posterior fibers of the medial collateral ligament posterior oblique; image on left is in extension, and the posterior band is under tension, whereas in the image on the right, the knee is in flexion, and the anterior band is under tension.

do occur (Fig. 19.15). An MCL injury is probably more common in adolescents as they approach skeletal maturity.[232] The possibility of a physeal fracture always needs to be considered in these pediatric and adolescent patients, especially those with open physes.[37] Fractures can occur through the distal femoral physeal scar and may mimic an MCL injury. In addition, MCL injuries can also occur with epiphyseal fractures[233] or with an avulsion-type injury.[175] Bradley and colleagues[234] described a series of pediatric patients with serious knee injuries and reported a small number of MCL injuries. In 40 pediatric patients 16 years or younger with hemarthrosis, Eiskjaer and colleagues[235] identified two isolated ruptures of the MCL.

The history of the event is an important factor for evaluation of MCL injuries. An injury to the MCL most often occurs as a result of a valgus stress but may also be seen with excessive external rotation of the knee. In many sports-related cases, these injuries involve contact with another athlete. This mechanism of injury is very common in American football and soccer, although it can be seen with any

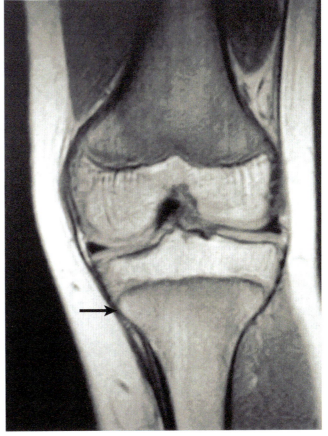

Fig. 19.14 Magnetic resonance image of knee showing medial collateral ligament (MCL) and tibial physis. The MCL insertion extends below the epiphysis, attaching to the tibial metaphysis.

contact sport. As a general rule, younger and more skeletally immature patients have a higher risk of sustaining physeal fractures, whereas older more skeletally mature adolescents have a higher probability of soft tissue MCL injuries.

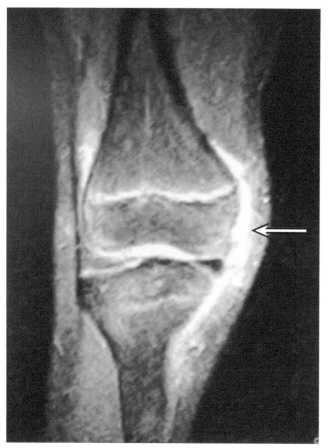

Fig. 19.15 Magnetic resonance imaging (MRI) scan of medial collateral ligament injury in 9-year-old with wide open physes. The MRI shows significant edema around the medial capsular structures of the knee.

The physical examination is important for distinguishing an MCL injury from a physeal fracture. For most isolated MCL injuries, an effusion, if present, is likely to be small. Palpation of the medial aspect of the knee is important for localizing the area of injury and for determining whether the physis is involved. Tenderness may be localized to the region of the MCL, including the femoral, joint-line, or tibial regions. If an MCL injury is suspected, the knee should be subjected to valgus stress testing at full extension and at 30 degrees of flexion. In cases of an isolated MCL injury, the knee will be stable to stress at full extension because of the integrity of the posteromedial capsular structures and the cruciate ligaments. If laxity is demonstrated in full extension, a more serious soft tissue injury or physeal fracture needs to be considered. In these cases, the patient can be evaluated under anesthesia or by MRI. In flexion, the posteromedial capsular structures are relaxed, which will allow isolated evaluation of the MCL. The degree of laxity should be quantified and compared with the uninjured knee.

Because the literature on MCL injuries in pediatric and adolescent athletes is limited, the adult literature and treatment recommendations, which have evolved over the last 30 years, provide guidance for management of these injuries in young athletes. Kennedy[236] described a surgical procedure for MCL reconstruction in young athletes in the late 1970s, although limited clinical information was available for follow-up evaluation. Bradley and colleagues[234] gathered data

over 15 years and described 6 children, ages 6 to 11 years, who underwent operative repair of the MCL after traumatic rupture. Patients were treated with open suture repair of the torn MCL and 5 to 6 weeks of immobilization. Subjective and clinical results were excellent to good for five patients and fair for one, who also had an associated ACL tear. An isolated MCL injury from an automobile accident has been reported in a 4-year-old child.[237] In this case, primary repair with sutures and 4 weeks of immobilization produced an excellent result.

Although surgical treatment of MCL injuries has been advocated in adults,[238,239] recent trends have been toward more conservative, nonoperative treatment even for high-grade isolated MCL injuries.* Although some have suggested that nonoperative treatment of a grade III MCL injury will result in a poor outcome,[240,241] the current literature supports conservative treatment for most isolated grade III injuries.[242–244]

Some rehabilitation protocols include immobilization, either in full extension or 90 degrees of flexion,[225,245,246] whereas others have advocated early motion (without a period of casting or immobilization).[247,248] In patients treated with early mobilization and weight-bearing as tolerated, a low-profile knee brace with a medial and lateral hinge will provide some support to the MCL while healing. A brief period of immobilization may be necessary in patients with significant discomfort. In a study of 51 athletes managed with an active rehabilitation program involving full or partial mobilization, athletes with grade I sprains returned to full participation after an average of 10.6 days, and those with grade II sprains returned after 19.5 days.[249]

MCL injuries and ACL injuries may occur simultaneously in young athletes. Recent studies have shown that early bracing of grades II and III MCL injuries, followed by ACL reconstruction in young athletes, results in excellent clinical outcomes.[250]

THE LATERAL COLLATERAL LIGAMENT AND THE POSTEROLATERAL CORNER

ANATOMY AND BIOMECHANICS OF THE LATERAL COLLATERAL LIGAMENT AND POSTEROLATERAL CORNER

The lateral and posterolateral aspects of the knee have been described by Andrew and associates[163] as the "dark side of the knee" because less was known about this region compared with other areas.[251] Recent studies have defined the anatomy and biomechanics of this region. Seebacher and colleagues[252] have described the posterolateral aspect of the knee using a three-layer model in which the lateral collateral ligament (LCL) is within layer III, the deepest layer (Fig. 19.16). The LCL originates from a ridge on the lateral femoral epicondyle, between the origins of the lateral head of the gastrocnemius and the tendon of the popliteus.[253] The pear-shaped insertion of the LCL is on the V-shaped epiphyseal portion of the superolateral aspect of the fibula, proximal to the physis. Anatomic variability of the posterolateral corner is high: absence of the arcuate or fabellofibular ligament occurs in 20% and 13% of the population, respectively.[253] Although anatomic variability is seen in the posterolateral corner, the popliteus complex (popliteus muscle and popliteofibular ligament) and LCL are consistent anatomic findings.

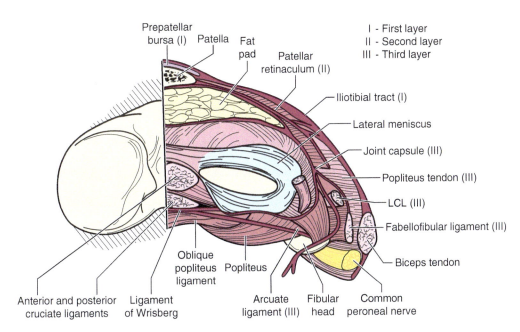

Fig. 19.16 Anatomic layers of the posterolateral knee. (From Seebacher JR, Inglis AE, Marshall JL, et al. The structure of the posterolateral aspect of the knee. *J Bone Joint Surg Am.* 1982;64(4):536-541.) *LCL,* Lateral collateral ligament.

Numerous dynamic and static stabilizing structures, in addition to the LCL and the PCL, contribute to the stability of the posterolateral corner. The static structures of the posterolateral corner include the LCL, the popliteofibular ligament, posterolateral joint capsule, arcuate ligament complex, and the fabellofibular ligament. Several dynamic structures exist, including the popliteus, iliotibial band, lateral head of the gastrocnemius, and biceps femoris tendon. The LCL and the popliteus complex are likely the most important structures with respect to posterolateral knee stability.

The posterolateral structures of the knee are normally subjected to greater forces and are generally stronger than those of the medial aspect of the knee.[254] The role of the posterolateral ligament complex in determining knee stability continues to be investigated. Several studies have concluded that the LCL and popliteus complex are two of the major structures that resist lateral opening and varus stress. In addition, recent studies by Pasque and colleagues[255] and Ullrich and colleagues and others[251,256,257] have documented the importance of both the popliteus complex and LCL in providing tibial rotational stability.

INCIDENCE AND MECHANISM OF LATERAL COLLATERAL LIGAMENT AND POSTEROLATERAL CORNER INJURIES

LCL and posterolateral corner injuries are rare in skeletally immature patients, and the literature contains little research on this age group. Thus, treatment principles for these injuries must partially rely on insight from adult studies. For adult patients, an injury to the lateral and posterolateral structures of the knee is much less common than MCL or ACL injuries. Even though the incidence of an isolated posterolateral corner injury is probably less than 2% to 3% of all knee injuries,[254] a growing number of studies in adult patients have focused on these injuries.[258–262] An isolated injury to the LCL is extremely uncommon, and an injury to the posterolateral structures is usually seen with other injuries such as strains of the lateral fascia and iliotibial tract, biceps femoris tendon, or PCL.[263,264] The orthopedic

literature contains limited information concerning the frequency of these injuries in pediatric or adolescent populations. LCL or posterolateral corner injuries are rarely found in studies of knee injuries in children.[173,265,266] Swenson and colleagues[181] reported the epidemiology of knee injuries among high school athletes. This study identified LCL and PCL injury rates of 0.17 and 0.05 per 10,000 AEs, respectively. Kovack and colleagues[267] recently described an avulsion injury of the posterolateral corner of the knee in the skeletally immature.

An injury to the posterolateral corner or LCL may occur from athletic competition, motor vehicle accidents, or knee dislocations.[213,268] When an injury to the LCL and posterolateral corner occurs, it is usually because of a medial blow to the extended knee and may involve external rotation. LCL and posterolateral injuries may also occur from noncontact hyperextension and external rotation or from forceful deceleration with the lower leg planted.[171,254] With injuries to the proximal fibular physis, laxity resembling LCL or posterolateral injuries may also be present.[269] In cases of a displaced fracture through the fibular physis, surgery may be necessary.[269]

CLINICAL EXAMINATION OF THE PATIENT WITH SUSPECTED LATERAL COLLATERAL LIGAMENT OR POSTEROLATERAL CORNER INJURIES

Evaluation of the patient's gait and lower extremity alignment is important for both adults and skeletally immature patients. Adult patients may exhibit gait deviations, which include varus thrust and hyperextension of the knee.[254,263,264] The overall alignment of the lower extremity should be evaluated because genu varum may increase the likelihood of a poor outcome. A newly injured knee may exhibit ecchymosis and pain over the posterolateral aspect or in the popliteal fossa region (Fig. 19.17). A careful evaluation of neurovascular status is important because LCL and posterolateral corner injuries may be associated with peroneal nerve injuries.[254] The possibility of a spontaneously reduced knee dislocation should always be considered, and a thorough neurovascular examination is essential.

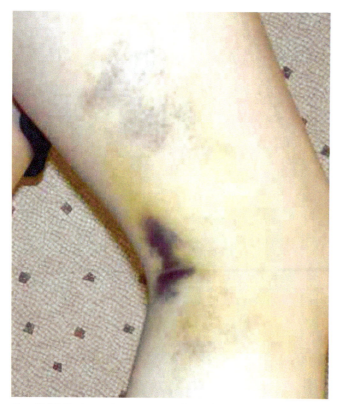

Fig. 19.17 Ecchymosis over posterolateral/popliteal fossa region on newly acutely injured knee.

Numerous tests have been described for assessing laxity of the posterolateral knee complex. These tests evaluate the integrity of the LCL, the posterolateral corner, and the PCL, and include the evaluation of translation, varus position, laxity, and external rotation. Each test should be compared with the contralateral knee in all patients.[254] This is especially important because pediatric and adolescent patients often have physiologic laxity.[270] A posterolateral corner injury will demonstrate increased varus laxity, external tibial rotation, and posterior translation. In cases of an isolated posterolateral injury with an intact PCL, posterior translation will be most obvious at 20 to 30 degrees of flexion but will decrease significantly when the knee is flexed to 90 degrees. With combined posterolateral corner and PCL injuries, significant posterior subluxation will occur at 90 degrees of flexion.[254] Varus stress testing at 0 degrees and 30 degrees will demonstrate laxity with LCL and posterolateral corner injuries.[271,272] A significant amount of varus laxity should raise suspicion of other injuries, including injuries to the PCL and ACL.[212,268]

In the posterolateral drawer test, the knee is placed in 80 to 90 degrees of flexion, with the foot in fixed position of 15 degrees of external rotation. A force is exerted over the proximal anterolateral tibia so that posterior movement and outward tibial rotation can be assessed.[271,272] The sensitivity and specificity of this test are limited, and other tests as well as imaging may be necessary to fully assess the knee.[254,273,274]

Another examination, the external rotation recurvatum test,[275,276] is performed with the patient in a supine position. The great toe of each leg is elevated by the examiner, and the posture of the knee is evaluated. The knee will demonstrate varus, hyperextension, and external rotation of the tibia if a significant injury to the posterolateral corner is present. Other injuries may also be present, including injuries to the ACL, PCL, or both.

The tibial external rotation test is performed with the patient in a supine or prone position. An outward rotation moment is applied to both feet at 30 and 90 degrees. A difference of outward rotation of more than 10 degrees is significant. A positive test at 30 degrees is considered more specific for a posterolateral corner injury, whereas a positive test at 90 degrees suggests a combined posterolateral corner and PCL injury.[254,261–264]

The reverse pivot shift test can also be used to evaluate the posterolateral corner, although comparison with the other extremity is important. This test may also be positive in a significant number of patients without injuries, so the results of this test should be interpreted with caution.[232,268] Several descriptions of this test exist. With the foot held in external rotation and the knee flexed to 90 degrees, the knee is extended. A palpable shift or jerk near full extension may occur as the posteriorly subluxated tibial plateau shifts anteriorly.[271,272]

TREATMENT OF LATERAL COLLATERAL LIGAMENT AND POSTEROLATERAL CORNER INJURIES

An LCL injury is often associated with other ligamentous injuries, such as posterolateral corner injuries or ACL and PCL tears.[254] An injury to the posterolateral corner or PCL is extremely rare in children; thus, few reports of treatment exist for this injury. The natural history of LCL and posterolateral corner injuries has not been well-defined in skeletally immature patients. In pediatric patients, cast immobilization is probably a reasonable treatment option until studies support operative intervention. A report of a 4-year-old child with an LCL tear and a femoral fracture treated with a spica cast indicated a good outcome.[176]

Treatment for the adolescent patient with this injury should follow the protocols established for adult patients. Some patients with low-grade injuries may return to activities with little or no disability.[254,277] Low-grade injuries with minimal laxity may be treated with immobilization for 2 to 4 weeks, followed by a rehabilitation program.[254] In adults, Kannus[277] demonstrated good outcomes for conservative treatment of grade II injuries but poor outcomes for nonsurgically treated grade III injuries.

For grade III injuries, nonoperative treatment may yield poor outcomes, and recent research has focused on early surgical reconstruction in these cases. Several authors have suggested that early reconstruction or primary repair of a posterolateral corner injury yields better results than reconstructions that have been delayed.[57,263,264] Numerous techniques have focused on reconstruction of the LCL and popliteus complex,[278–280] but no technique has emerged as the gold standard. In recent studies of adults, an emphasis has been placed on anatomic reconstruction, and the focus has been on recreating the natural anatomy and biomechanics of the posterolateral corner, LCL, or both.

Primary repair of injured structures or reduction of avulsed fragments should be the first objective of surgical repair[254]; although this may not be possible in the chronically injured knee, it may be a reasonable option in a skeletally immature patient. Early repair of a periosteal avulsion has been described.[267] Early intervention after the injury may allow for anatomic repair of injured and avulsed structures. In older or chronic injuries, these structures may not be readily identified, and soft tissue reconstruction procedures may be more appropriate. Tibial avulsions of the popliteus can be reduced by simple screws or suturing,[263,264] whereas avulsions of the femoral origins of the LCL and popliteus may require sutures through transosseous drill holes.[254] Fibular disruption of the LCL or popliteofibular ligament can be addressed with sutures and reinforcement with the fabellofibular ligament, if present.[263,264]

More complex procedures to address posterolateral corner and LCL injuries have been described. These include augmentation of a severely torn popliteus tendon with use of a portion of the iliotibial tract, fixed to the tibia via sutures passed through a drill hole.[261,262] Reconstruction of the popliteofibular ligament can be accomplished with the use of a portion of the biceps femoris tendon fixed to the lateral femoral condyle.[263,264]

Advancement of the arcuate complex, if intact, has been used by some authors with fair to good results. With this technique, the structures of the lateral aspect of the knee, including the lateral head of the gastrocnemius, the popliteus tendon, the arcuate ligament, and the LCL, are advanced proximally on the femur in line with the LCL so that tension is restored. The disadvantage of this procedure is that it may produce nonanatomic changes in the ligament biomechanics, which may lead to stretching and failure over time.[254]

Combination repairs of the LCL and popliteus have been described by Veltri and Warren.[263,264] In this technique, reconstruction of the popliteus uses a single drill hole in the lateral femoral condyle and a split patellar tendon graft. The proximal aspect of the graft is secured in the femoral hole and fixed distally in two locations: on the posterior tibia and lateral fibula. This creates a reconstruction that approximates the anatomic course of the popliteus. For reconstruction of the LCL, a portion of the biceps femoris tendon is released proximally, rerouted to the lateral femoral condyle, and attached at the approximate isometric point on the lateral femoral condyle. This method is advantageous because it approximates normal anatomy and biomechanics.[254]

Isolated LCL rupture has been addressed by numerous authors, and techniques have been described to reconstruct this ligament with the use of the biceps femoris tendon,[263,264] bone-tendon-bone autografts,[280] Achilles allografts,[263,264,281] semitendinosus autografts,[282] and quadriceps tendon autografts.[278,279] With the exception of procedures using the biceps femoris tendon, these techniques use a cephalocaudal-oriented drill hole in the fibular head and a transverse drill hole on the femur. Fixation is achieved with interference screws, sutures, or both. These studies of reconstruction of the LCL have had good results in adults but are limited by their lack of pediatric and adolescent subjects.

Injuries to the posterolateral corner or PCL are likely to occur at or near skeletal maturity, and the concern about physeal arrest may not be a significant clinical problem.[283] In adolescent cases, the use of standard adult techniques, which may use drill holes at or near the physeal region, are probably appropriate because the risk of physeal arrest is less in these older patient groups. Although the authors do not have significant personal experience with these rare injuries in the skeletally immature, primary repair and reduction of avulsions of the LCL or popliteal complex could

likely be performed in skeletally immature patients if care is taken to avoid placement of hardware or drill holes across the physis. For LCL reconstruction, techniques that use the attachment of the biceps femoris tendon have an advantage in that they do not require a drill hole in the proximal fibula. Anderson and Anderson[284] reported a case of intraarticular PCL and extraarticular posterolateral corner reconstruction in an adolescent with good outcomes. Knowledge of the anatomy of the ligaments to be reconstructed, along with their relation to the physes, is helpful in avoiding iatrogenic growth disturbance. The reconstructive drill holes used for LCL and posterolateral corner reconstruction should be relatively small, thus reducing the risk of producing a significant physeal injury. Drill hole positioning should consider the location of the femoral, tibial, and fibular physeal regions. If drill hole placement avoids the physis, surgical reconstructive techniques for addressing LCL and posterolateral corner injuries may be successful, but this has yet to be demonstrated in clinical or animal studies. Adolescents at or close to skeletal maturity can be safely treated as adults with minimal risk of growth complications. Recent studies of ACL reconstruction have demonstrated the potential for growth plate complications, and these issues will need to be discussed thoroughly with the patient and family before any reconstructive procedure for the ACL, PCL, or other ligaments of the knee.

THE POSTERIOR CRUCIATE LIGAMENT

ANATOMY OF THE POSTERIOR CRUCIATE LIGAMENT

The PCL originates from the anteromedial region of the intercondylar notch of the femur and courses posterolaterally to the posterior tibia. Anatomic studies have shown that the PCL has a large oblong femoral insertion, spanning nearly 3 cm in the adult.[285,286] The PCL attaches posteriorly to the tibial eminence, approximately 10 mm to 15 mm inferior to the posterior tibial plateau, and extends distally toward the proximal tibial physis.[287] The PCL is 20% to 50% larger in cross section than the ACL and fans out at its origin and insertion—so much so that the area of attachment is five times the size of the midsubstance cross-sectional area. The midsubstance of the PCL is asymmetric in that larger diameters are on the femoral end of the ligament.[288,289]

The PCL has been described as having two functional units: the posteromedial bundle and the anterolateral bundle (Fig. 19.18). These two nonisometric parts of the PCL have slightly different roles in providing knee stability. From studies in adults, it was found that the anterolateral bundle is twice as large in cross section and is stiffer and stronger than the posteromedial bundle.[288–290]

INCIDENCE AND NATURAL HISTORY OF POSTERIOR CRUCIATE LIGAMENT INJURIES

PCL disruption is less common than ACL injuries, and studies in adults have identified PCL injuries in 3% to 20% of patients with knee injuries.[213,268] Reports of isolated PCL injuries are rare in children. Because of the limited number of PCL injuries in skeletally immature patients, the natural history of this injury in pediatric populations is not well defined. There have been limited case reports in the literature of various PCL injuries, including isolated PCL injuries,[291,292] PCL tears in combination with other injuries,[177,233]

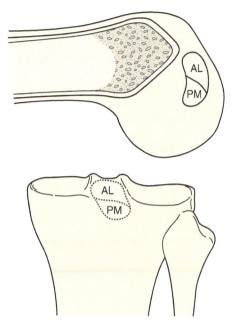

Fig. 19.18 Origin and insertion of posterior cruciate ligament anterolateral (*AL*) and posteromedial bands (*PM*). (From Harner CD, Hoher J. Evaluation and treatment of posterior cruciate ligament injuries. *Am J Sports Med.* 1998;26(3):471-482.)

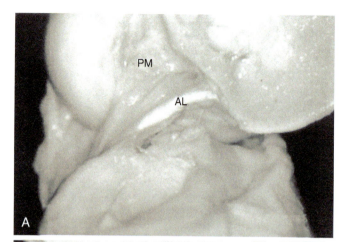

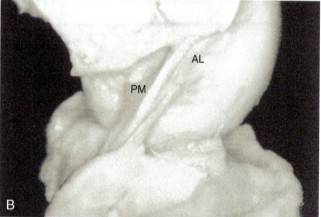

Fig. 19.19 (A) Anatomic pictures of anterolateral (AL) and posteromedial (PM). (B) Bundles of posterior cruciate ligament.

or avulsions of the tibial[293–295] or femoral attachments.[296–298] An incomplete avulsion of the origin of the PCL has also been reported in an adolescent.[299]

Studies of the natural history of isolated PCL injuries in adult patients are conflicting because some have reported good outcomes,[300–302] whereas others have demonstrated poor long-term knee function.[303–306] Shelbourne and colleagues[307] found that in athletically active patients with PCL injuries at an average of 5.4 years after injury, half were able to return to the same or higher level of sports, one-third returned to a lower level of competition, and one-sixth did not return to the same sport. Parolie and Bergfeld,[301] in a study with an average patient follow-up time of 6.2 years, reported on 25 patients who had sustained isolated PCL injuries and were treated nonoperatively. They found that 80% were satisfied with their knees and that 84% had returned to their previous sport (68% at the same level of performance and 16% at a decreased level of performance). Interestingly, they found that patients who were unable to regain 100% of preinjury quadriceps strength were more likely to have a poor outcome and fail to return to preinjury levels of activity. Complications because of chronic PCL deficiency are not clearly defined but are understood to possibly include functional limitations,[306] pain and articular degeneration,[303] and articular cartilage defects.[305]

Reports of the natural history of PCL injuries in children are rare and consist of limited case reports and small series (Fig. 19.19). One case report of nonoperative treatment in a 6-year-old boy showed an excellent functional outcome, despite clinical PCL laxity, which suggests that at least short-term conservative management in children may be appropriate.[291] Another case report of PCL deficiency in a 6-year-old patient reported chronic instability after an initial asymptomatic period lasting more than 4 years.[292] At a follow-up examination 5 years after the injury, the boy reported acute anterior knee pain as well as occasional instability.

A tear of the medial meniscus was found on MRI. These two case reports suggest that short-term conservative treatment may be appropriate but that complications may eventually develop. Kocher and colleagues[308] reported a recent series of 25 skeletally immature patients with PCL injuries. Partial tears or nondisplaced avulsion injuries had good outcomes. Surgical repairs also produced good outcomes with minimal complications in those in whom nonoperative treatment failed.

EVALUATION AND MANAGEMENT OF POSTERIOR CRUCIATE LIGAMENT INJURIES

Examination of the knee for PCL deficiency includes tests described for posterolateral corner and LCL injuries. If the PCL is torn, varus laxity, external tibial rotation, and posterior translation will be present at 90 degrees of flexion.[270] The posterior drawer test at 90 degrees of flexion is very useful for evaluation of the PCL. Laxity or subluxation should be graded and compared with the contralateral knee because pediatric patients often have physiologic laxity. With PCL examination, identification of starting points and end points is important because an unsuspected PCL injury can produce a false-positive anterior drawer result if the tibia is sagging posteriorly. The end point quality of the ligamentous structures should be graded in addition to the overall laxity or displacement. In the normal knee, the tibial condyle is usually 10 mm anterior to the femoral condyle with the knee at 90 degrees of flexion.

TREATMENT OF POSTERIOR CRUCIATE LIGAMENT INJURIES IN CHILDREN

Because of the limited data available concerning treatment of pediatric PCL injuries, the adult literature serves as a useful guide. Veltri and Warren[270] have developed algorithms for the approach to PCL injuries in adults. Isolated acute PCL tears with less than 10 mm of posterior laxity at 90 degrees of flexion should be treated with aggressive physical therapy and rehabilitation. Reconstruction should be done for severe tears with more than 10 to 15 mm of laxity or PCL injuries in the knee with multiple other injuries. In adults, chronic PCL injuries initially should be treated with aggressive physical therapy and rehabilitation. Most authors advocate repair of all PCL avulsions in children,[287,294,297,309] although casting for nondisplaced fractures has shown good results.[310]

Treatment of midsubstance tears of the PCL may present problems unique to the immature skeleton. Standard adult procedures may result in iatrogenic damage to the physis, leading to premature growth arrest. However, Lobenhoffer and colleagues[297] performed a repair of an avulsion of the femoral attachment of the PCL in a child with use of transphyseal tunnels and sutures, and no complications were reported. In pediatric and adolescent patients, the risks of causing growth disturbances must be weighed against known complications of chronic PCL deficiency. From the few published case reports and case series, it is advisable to treat PCL tears in children conservatively until skeletal maturity is approached, although intervention may be warranted if symptoms and instability persist.[284,308,311]

The unique biomechanical properties of the PCL pose a challenge to reconstruction because a single graft is unlikely to mimic natural anatomy. Evidence exists that single-bundle grafts result in increased laxity,[312,313] presumably because of their inability to approximate the natural PCL. Some authors have advocated a single graft placed in the approximate position of the anterolateral bundle only.[289,312,314] With single-graft techniques, precise placement of the femoral tunnel is closely tied to functional outcome, more so than location of the tibial tunnel.[315] Single-graft reconstructions are frequently performed with allografts, but bone-tendon-bone and hamstring grafts are also used. Because of concerns about physeal damage to the tibial tubercle, bone-tendon-bone autografts are probably not a desirable choice for the skeletally immature.

Double-tunnel techniques, with a single tibial tunnel and two femoral tunnels, have been described.[316–319] This style of graft is thought to better approximate the natural biomechanics of the PCL, and there is evidence that these may be superior to single grafts.[317,319] Paulos[318] advocates the outside-in technique so that the tunnels for the anterolateral and posteromedial bundles can be oriented to be collinear with their maximum tension vectors. Graft choices for the double bundle are numerous: semitendinosus, gracilis autograft,[318,319] hamstring allograft,[318,319] anterior tibialis allograft,[316] or quadriceps tendon.[254] Regardless of the technique, in a double-tunnel reconstruction, each graft must be tensioned separately. Despite its biomechanical advantages, there are limits to the double-tunnel procedure, including a steep learning curve, a more prolonged surgical procedure, and the need for precise placement of each grafted

bundle. The double-tunnel technique is more complex, but its superiority has been suggested in the literature.[317,320] The use of single- versus double-bundle grafts for PCL injuries continues to be an active area of research, and many questions remain unanswered. Double-bundle ACL reconstruction techniques have been shown to increase the volume of growth plate damage for the distal femur,[321] and a similar phenomenon may also occur with pediatric double-bundle PCL surgery.

Treatment of an isolated PCL injury is still evolving in adults. Recent descriptions of techniques to treat pediatric PCL injuries have been described,[308,311,322] although nonoperative treatment may offer excellent outcomes in patients with isolated injuries. All-epiphyseal PCL reconstruction has been described.[311,323] A recent series of skeletally immature patients with isolated PCL injuries demonstrated good outcomes at short-term follow-up with nonoperative treatment.[308]

PATELLAR DISLOCATIONS

EPIDEMIOLOGY

Patellar dislocation is a common injury in the skeletally immature[324] and is one of the most common causes of acute hemarthrosis in young athletes.[43,56,325,326] Studies have demonstrated an annual incidence of this injury at 5.8/100,000, and studies in pediatric patients have shown a higher incidence of 43/100, 000.[327] Some studies have suggested that males and females have equal rates of dislocation,[328,329] whereas others have demonstrated the highest rate of dislocation to be in females younger than 18 years.[330–332] Although seen in association with underlying diseases, these injuries are very common in the young athlete. These injuries are frequently seen with sports that involve rapid directional changes or cutting.[328,333]

ANATOMY

Most dislocations occur in a lateral direction and are associated with an injury to the medial retinacular tissues and the medial patellofemoral ligament (MPFL).[334,335] Medial and superior dislocation can also occur,[336–339] and rare cases of intraarticular dislocation have also been reported.[340] The patellofemoral joint is complex, and the path of the patella during knee motion is a complex combination of motion in multiple planes.[341] At full extension, the patella assumes a slightly lateral relationship to the femoral groove, and in this position, the patella may assume the most lateral displacement.[342] During the first 30 degrees of flexion, the patella begins to engage the femoral sulcus.[337,342] In patients with patella alta, the patella may not engage the trochlear groove until additional flexion occurs, which may contribute to an increased risk of patellar instability.[324,328,329,343]

ANATOMIC RISK FACTORS

Although these injuries may be seen in association with anatomic conditions,[344–347] increased genu valgum, patella alta,[348–350] lower extremity torsion abnormalities,[351–354] trochlear dysplasia, increased quadriceps angle,[355] foot pronation, and patellar tilt,[356,357] among others, the relationship between these physical findings and patellar instability is not clearly defined.[328,329,358–360] Recent studies have increasingly focused on the tibial tubercle and trochlear groove relationship, which may have a significant impact on patellar instability.[164,361] Patellar dislocations occur in otherwise healthy individuals,[328,329] although soft tissue laxity may be a significant risk factor.[328,329,362] Recent studies of trochlear dysplasia have attempted to define the relationship between trochlear morphology and patellar dislocation.[363–366] Some of these studies have suggested that trochlear dysplasia may have a genetic basis,[363,364] and other studies have suggested that the risk of dislocation may be higher in some families.[330–332]

MECHANISM OF INJURY

Several different mechanisms of injury have been proposed, including direct and indirect mechanisms.[367] The indirect mechanism involves a position of internal rotation of the femur, knee valgus, and a planted foot in combination with a quadriceps contraction.[329,337] The direct mechanism involves a laterally directed force to the medial aspect of the patella. Combinations of these mechanisms can occur.[367]

MEDIAL PATELLOFEMORAL LIGAMENT

Although the medial retinacular tissues limit the lateral displacement of the patella, the MPFL is one of the primary restraints preventing patellar dislocation (Fig. 19.20). Injury to this ligament is common during patellar dislocation.[334,335,368] This structure originates from the adductor tubercle region of the femoral condyle, travels transversely, and attaches to the upper two-thirds of the medial patellar border.[334,335,369,370] Biomechanical studies have shown this to be one of the main soft tissue structures preventing lateral patellar dislocations. Other structures contribute to the stability of the patella with respect to lateral subluxation, including the meniscopatellar and tibiopatellar ligaments, and dynamic contribution is produced by the vastus medialis obliquus muscle.[123,371]

The location of the injury to the MPFL can be clearly seen on MRI. Recent research demonstrates that the location of the injury can be at the MPFL origin, insertion, or midsubstance. The majority of these injuries may occur at the MPFL origin on the adductor tubercle region of the femur.[372]

In the skeletally immature, controversy surrounds the location of the femoral origin of the MPFL and its relationship to the distal femoral physis. Shea and colleagues[373] used a technique[374] to approximate the origin's location on radiographs and found the center of the origin at a location several millimeters proximal to the physis based on analysis of the lateral radiographs. On the basis of the height of the MPFL, this study suggests that the MPFL origin extends slightly above and below the physis. Nelitz and colleagues[375] used a combination of two previously described techniques[374,376] to approximate the origin's location on radiographic images but found the MPFL origin distal to the physis. Kepler and colleagues[377] reviewed MRI scans of children and adolescents with confirmed MPFL tears. They identified the MPFL origin's mean location to be 5 mm distal to the physis, but the range was from 7.5 mm proximal to 16 mm distal to the physis. Given these discrepant results, further research should be done to clarify the location of the MPFL origin in children and adolescents.

OSTEOCHONDRAL INJURIES

In addition to disruption of the medial restraints and the MPFL, which occurs during acute lateral patellar dislocation, osteochondral fractures and contusions are seen in 40% to 76% of patients. During the dislocation, the osteochondral fragments may originate from the lateral femoral condyle or the medial patella facet. Many of these injuries can be significant and may not be recognized on plain radiographs.[378] These injuries may result from a shearing force during the patellar dislocation. In some cases, the osteochondral injury of the lateral femoral condyle may be in a more posterior region, in areas of significant weight-bearing during full extension.[379]

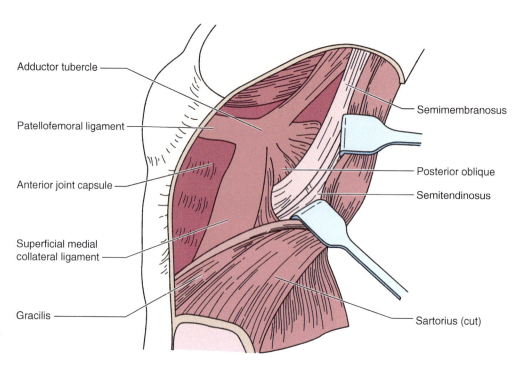

Fig. 19.20 Medial soft tissue restraints of the knee.

Adductor tubercle

Patellofemoral ligament

Anterior joint capsule

Superficial medial collateral ligament

Gracilis

Semimembranosus

Posterior oblique

Semitendinosus

Sartorius (cut)

NATURAL HISTORY

Several studies have attempted to define the natural history of this injury in adult and skeletally immature athletes. Additional long-term studies will be necessary to assess the incidence of osteoarthritis, define subgroups that have a higher risk of secondary dislocations, and determine the effectiveness of nonoperative and operative treatment regimens.[330–332] Additional studies in younger athletes will also help better clarify the natural history of this injury. Studies have demonstrated redislocation rates of 13% to 52% for nonsurgical treatment. Significant knee dysfunction may persist, even in patients who do not have secondary dislocation episodes.[328,380]

Previous studies on patellar dislocation demonstrate a small number of prospective designs. These study designs may best identify the natural history of this condition and determine which patients need operative or nonoperative treatment regimens. A limited number of prospective studies have evaluated the natural history of patellar dislocations, with a specific focus on secondary dislocation and other dysfunction.[330–332,381,382]

In a well-designed prospective cohort study, Fithian and colleagues[330–332] followed up 189 patients for 2 to 5 years. The group with the highest risk of dislocations was females 10 to 17 years of age. Approximately 61% of dislocations occurred during sports, and 9% occurred during dancing. The risk of recurrent patellar instability/dislocation appeared to be significantly higher in females. Young age at the time of the first dislocation was also a significant risk factor for future dislocation/subluxation events.

Clinical Evaluation

Patients with a first-time patellar dislocation may recall a specific dislocation event, which may have spontaneously reduced or may have required a reduction at the scene of the injury or in the emergency department. In other cases, patients may describe a significant "pop" or other major mechanical sensation or event, although they may not realize that a dislocation occurred. The dislocation-relocation sequence may occur very quickly. The history, examination, and image evaluation will determine whether patellar dislocation occurred.

Athletes with a first-time patellar dislocation usually are seen with significant effusion. Many patients have been evaluated in the emergency department and have been placed in a knee immobilizer and have been advised to use crutches. Patients may be quite uncomfortable and apprehensive, and the examiner should work to help the patient relax as much as possible. This will facilitate a more complete examination. The examination should include a thorough evaluation and a search for other injuries, including ligamentous injuries such as those to the ACL or MCL, osteochondral injuries, and meniscal tears. Injuries to the medial retinacular restraints and the MPFL may produce tenderness in the region of the MCL. Gentle valgus stress maneuvers with the knee near full extension, and in 30 to 45 degrees of flexion, should help determine if an MCL injury has occurred.

Observation of the patient's gait and rotational profiles of the lower extremity are important elements in the evaluation. This may be limited in the acute injury setting, especially the review of the gait. Review of the torsional profile of the femur and tibia are important physical examination findings because these may contribute to recurrent instability episodes.[383] For patients with significant rotational abnormalities of the femur and tibia, CT will allow for appropriate estimation of both tibial and femoral torsion.

With regard to the examination of the patellofemoral joint, the examiner should palpate the medial retinacular structures, looking for evidence of disruption of these tissues. Significant ecchymosis or palpable defects could be evidence of major structural damage to these tissues. This palpation should be done very gently because it will not require much pressure to produce discomfort at the site of the traumatized structures. Palpation should also include the entire medial and superomedial border of the patella and the vastus medialis. These areas may be tender because of medial retinacular avulsion, avulsion injury of the vastus medialis, and/or the presence of an osteochondral injury from the medial aspect of the patella. The lateral femoral condyle should also be palpated: areas of tenderness suggest an underlying chondral injury.

The evaluation of patellar stability, especially with regard to significant lateral laxity because of traumatized medial restraints, may be challenging in the first 1 to 15 days after the dislocation. Patellar mobilization after the initial injury may be quite uncomfortable for the patient, and more information may be obtained after the knee has had several weeks of recovery and therapy. Comparison of the injured knee to the uninjured knee can provide very useful information when the degree of laxity of the patellofemoral joint is determined.

Many patients, especially female patients, may have other signs of soft tissue laxity or other anatomic issues that predispose them to primary and secondary dislocations.[330–332] Stanitski[319] has emphasized the importance of evaluating patients for signs of soft tissue laxity. Evaluating the patients for genu recurvatum, hyperextension of the elbows, and soft tissue laxity of the wrist, thumbs, and fingers may also be helpful during the evaluation and subsequent treatment.

Imaging Evaluation

AP, lateral, and Merchant view radiographs can evaluate patella alta, patella baja, or osteochondral fractures of the patella or the intercondylar groove or lateral femoral condyle. Avulsion injuries of the medial aspect of the patella may be best seen on Merchant view radiographs.[367] Radiographs have limited utility in identifying osteochondral injuries.[326,380,384] In addition to radiographic evaluation for the presence of osteochondral injuries, radiographic studies have also been used to assess patellofemoral malalignment.[385] Numerous radiographic and CT measures of patellofemoral dysplasia have been described in the literature, including measures of congruence,[109,386] sulcus angles,[387] patellar tilt,[356,388,389] dysplasia,[363,364] subluxation, and hyperlaxity, among others. Future studies that use dynamic measurement methods may provide more insight into normal patellofemoral mechanics.[390]

In the authors' own practice, plain radiographs are routinely evaluated for the presence of patellofemoral alignment, other anomalies, or the presence of significant osteochondral injuries. Most patients come from the emergency department with films available for review. For skeletally immature subjects, the patellar height can be evaluated with the method described by Koshino and Sugimoto (Fig. 19.21).[391]

Although the indications for MRI after patellar dislocation may require further clarification in the literature, MRI can provide significant information with regard to the location and magnitude of soft tissue and osteochondral injuries and the anatomy of the trochlea.[334,335,369,392] Several MRI studies have demonstrated significant injuries missed on the initial radiographic evaluation.[326,362,380,384] MRI sequences have also been used in the evaluation of anatomic parameters associated with patellar dislocation, including vastus medialis insertion,[393] patellar tilt,[394] and the sulcus angle.[395]

For athletes, the authors obtain MRI studies early in the evaluation process. This may allow for the identification of trochlear dysplasia, as well as evidence of significant osteochondral injuries or intraarticular fragments (Fig. 19.22). This information can be useful during the evaluation and counseling about possible treatment options, both surgical and nonsurgical. For nonathletes or individuals in lower-demand activities, the authors may not obtain an MRI study initially. They counsel these patients that future knee dysfunction may warrant further imaging evaluation. Even in patients in lower-demand activities, an MRI study may be obtained if concerns exist about a significant osteochondral injury or intraarticular fragments.

Treatment

Treatment protocols for patellar dislocation in athletes continue to evolve, and both operative and nonoperative modalities have been recommended for first-time dislocations. In a recent systematic review of the literature, the superiority of surgical versus nonsurgical treatment was not demonstrated, although surgical treatment for recurrent dislocation may provide better outcomes in some patient groups.[161] A large cases series demonstrated that young patients with first-time patellar dislocations had a recurrent dislocation rate of 38%. Patients with trochlear dysplasia and open physes had a dislocation recurrence rate of 69%.[396]

Historically, nonoperative treatment programs advocated several weeks of immobilization, followed by therapy to recover motion and strength.[333,359,360,397,398] Because of concerns that immobilization may lead to problems with

arthrofibrosis, atrophy of cartilage, muscle, ligaments, and bone, several recent studies have advocated early rehabilitation programs emphasizing range of motion, strengthening, and the use of patellar buttress braces.[325,329,399]

A limited number of prospective studies have compared operative and nonoperative treatment protocols for patellar dislocation. Nikku and colleagues[397] studied 126 patients. Part of the study group underwent operative treatment, and the other group was treated by nonoperative means. The patients were followed for 2 years. The subjective and objective outcome measures did not differ significantly for these groups. The follow-up period was short, but many studies have demonstrated dislocation after 2 years' follow-up. A secondary study of this same patient group at 7 years' follow-up did not demonstrate improved outcomes in patients who underwent surgery for primary patellar dislocation.[381] Both of these studies had significant limitations, including a nonrandomized design.

Recently, Bitar and colleagues[233] reported on 39 patients (41 knees) with primary acute patellar dislocations who were randomly assigned to either nonoperative treatment with immobilization and physiotherapy or MPFL reconstruction. Patients were followed up for a minimum of 2 years. The surgically treated group had overall better outcomes and no reports of recurrences or subluxations. The nonoperative group had seven recurrences/subluxations (35% of cases).

In a retrospective study, Buchner[325] evaluated 126 patients at 8.1 years of follow-up. The study evaluated two groups: those managed with or without surgery. The functional and subjective results were good overall, but the recurrence rate was high in both surgical and nonsurgical groups. Although this study had several limitations, including variation in surgical procedures, the author suggested that many patients might not do better with surgery, although surgery was still indicated in some cases.

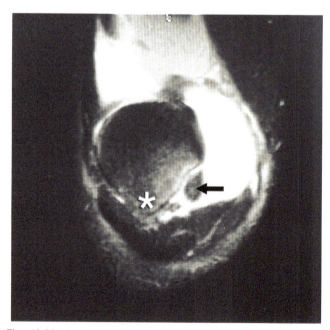

Fig. 19.22 Magnetic resonance image identifying injury to patella. T2-weighted coronal image (inferior pole marked by asterisk) demonstrating a bony fragment (arrow).

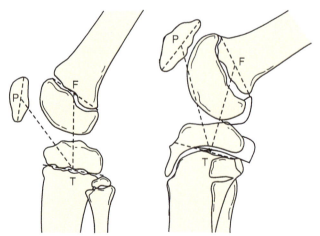

Fig. 19.21 Koshino and Sugimoto method for evaluating patellar height.

Palmu and colleagues[400] conducted a clinical trial of 71 patients younger than 17 years, randomly assigned to either operative or nonoperative treatment. Patients were seen at a 2-year follow-up and contacted by telephone at 6 and 14 years. Subjective and functional results were good for most patients at long-term follow-up. However, a high rate of recurrent dislocation was noted for both groups: 71% and 67% for the nonoperative and operative groups, respectively.

A plethora of operative treatment protocols exist for the treatment of patellar dislocations, which makes review of the literature even more challenging. Over the past 50 years, well over 100 operations have been described to address patellar dislocation. These procedures have ranged from less invasive procedures to more invasive procedures and include open or arthroscopic lateral release, soft tissue repair/augmentation,[401] soft tissue proximal realignment with lateral release,[402,403] medial tissue imbrications,[404] tubercle osteotomy with/without soft tissue procedure,[405] thermal shrinkage of medial retinaculum and lateral release,[406] transfer of the patellar tendon to the MCL,[407,408] MPFL reconstruction,[334,335,409–411] and distal transposition of the patellar tendon in cases of patella alta.[349]

Work by Fithian and Paxton and the International Patellofemoral Study Group[287] has suggested that the indications for lateral release for the treatment of patellar dislocation or instability are very limited, and these procedures appear to be much less popular than in the past.[330–332] Other authors have also suggested that the results of lateral release for the treatment of patellar dislocation are not predictable, and this isolated procedure is rarely indicated for this condition.[412–414]

Physeal Considerations in Skeletally Immature Patients

The operative treatment options in skeletally immature athletes are somewhat different than those available in adults because of concerns about potential physeal injury to the distal femoral or proximal tibial physis or apophysis. Procedures that violate these structures or the surrounding perichondral ring can produce complications of altered growth, including coronal plane angular deformity, leg length discrepancy, and recurvatum.[415,416] For these reasons, soft tissue procedures are more likely to be appropriate in children or adolescents with significant growth remaining. Numerous soft tissue procedures have been described, and these procedures range from those with extensive exposure to those with arthroscopic or minimally invasive approaches.

Reconstruction of the MPFL has been described in children,[417] although the close association between the distal femoral physis and the origin of this ligament warrant caution during surgical procedures in this area.[373]

Tubercle osteotomy procedures used in adults are contraindicated in those with significant growth remaining. Procedures that involve transfer of the patellar tendon, such as the Roux-Goldthwait patellar tendon transposition, may play a role in some patients with patellar dislocation.[418,419] Another approach to medializing a portion of the patellar tendon without damaging the physis includes the technique described by Oliva and colleagues,[420] in which a medial section of the patellar tendon is mobilized medially and attached to the proximal tibia.

With respect to the authors' practice, the following treatment protocols for nonoperative and operative management will be described.

Nonoperative Treatment Protocol

Whether surgical or nonsurgical treatment protocols are chosen, the authors usually start all patients on an early treatment regimen with several goals: (1) reduction of swelling; (2) early mobilization, strengthening, and proprioception for minimization of weakness and associated dysfunction of all major muscle groups of the lower extremity, especially the thigh musculature; and (3) early return to sports and other exercise.

Aspiration is performed on some patients, especially those with large effusions. In the authors' experience, a very large effusion may interfere with a rehabilitation program, although many young patients seem to respond to rehabilitation programs earlier than adults. The effusion may prolong the period of motion recovery and may also have deleterious effect on quadriceps and hamstring activation about the knee.

By the time of arrival to the clinic, most of our patients have spent 2 to 10 days in a knee immobilizer with protected weight-bearing. This treatment protocol is almost universal in primary care clinics and emergency departments. The patients have significant quadriceps and vastus medialis obliquus atrophy, which develops rapidly after an injury, especially in patients who have been placed in a knee immobilizer. Cryotherapy is used several times daily for the first several days to weeks to help decrease swelling. In some cases, a short course of oral antiinflammatory drugs may also be used to assist with the effusion. A patellar sleeve is also provided to the patient as the swelling decreases.

All of these patients are referred to a formal physical therapy program. This program emphasizes active contraction of the quadriceps and hamstrings, isometrics, straight leg raises, and return to early full weight-bearing. The patient is quickly advanced to riding an exercise bike, first with a light load on the injured leg. The load on the injured leg is increased as the patient is capable of assuming more demands on the lower extremity. As recovery progresses, patients are encouraged to "stand in the saddle" on the exercise bike, to place more proprioceptive and coordination demands on the knee. If patients have access to a pool, they are encouraged to swim laps with a kickboard. The kickboard program is done in both a prone and supine position because the prone position focuses on the hip flexors and quadriceps and the supine position focuses on the gluteals and hamstrings.

Return to running activity is also managed closely, with a stepwise return to activity. Athletes will start with easy jogging and slowly increase their speed. Cutting and directional change activity is started at slow speed in a controlled noncompetitive environment, and the speed is slowly increased. The patient will then begin work on sports-specific activity. An emphasis on strengthening and stretching is emphasized throughout the recovery program.

For patients with first-time dislocations, the usual protocol is to have them complete their rehabilitation program and return to their sport. The time to return to the sport is 6 to 16 weeks, depending on the age of the patient, rate of progression with the physical therapy program, presence of significant clinic signs of instability/apprehension on the examination, and higher versus lower demand athletic activity. Patients must demonstrate full range of motion, excellent strength, and evidence of coordinated lower extremity function appropriate for their highest demand sport activity before being cleared to return to sports or unlimited activity.

Patients are followed up closely for the development of symptoms such as pain, mechanical symptoms arising from the patellofemoral joint, or new subluxation events. Patients are counseled about the possibility of future problems with respect to subluxation, dislocation, and cartilage problems.

Operative Treatment Protocol

The treatment protocols for patellar dislocation continue to evolve.[329] Over the last 10 years, a growing number of studies have looked at the medial patellar restraints, the MPFL, and the configuration of the trochlea. As these anatomic and clinical follow-up studies continue, the authors anticipate continued modification to their treatment protocols.

In most cases of first-time dislocation, the authors do not recommend surgical intervention unless a displaced osteocartilaginous fragment is present.[421] In cases with significant laxity and soft tissue disruption or a significant osteochondral injury in association with an intraarticular fragment, operative intervention may be discussed with the patient and family after the first dislocation. In most cases, a rehabilitation program will be initiated. Modification of sports activities or switching to lower risk sports can be considered, but in the authors' experience, most young athletes and their parents are not particularly interested in changing to other sports or giving up one sport altogether.

Significant osteochondral injuries will usually be approached arthroscopically. Recent studies have demonstrated good outcomes for repair of significant osteochondral injuries.[422] Lesser injuries, those with bone contusions without significant chondral defects, or those without obvious free fragments will be observed. Free fragment removal and microfracture treatment of chondral defects are usually performed. The athlete and the family will be counseled about the significance of a chondral injury and the potential for long-term problems with osteoarthritis. Although some of the osteochondral fragments are not amenable to repair, larger fragments may be repaired in an arthroscopically assisted and/or mini-open manner.

In the authors' experience, MRI sequences will usually identify significant free fragments or damage that may indicate early surgery.[378] On occasion, MRI may miss these fragments, or these fragments may detach later and lead to mechanical symptoms; thus, surgery may be performed at a later date. The authors routinely counsel patients about the possibility of future symptoms, as well as the possibility of future surgery to address these symptoms.

If patients are seen with a history of previous dislocations or subluxations or if a previous nonoperative rehabilitation program has failed to help them, athletes and their families will be counseled about surgical options. In some cases, the presence of significant soft tissue laxity or other risk factors may be an indication for surgery after a first-time dislocation. Although patients are examined for anatomic factors that may predispose them to dislocations, the authors find that young athletes who are seen at their clinic do not have obvious osseous deformities such as torsional abnormalities, genu valgum, or patella alta.

Although more recent research has looked at the tibial tubercle and trochlear groove distance, historical studies have also included the quadriceps (Q) angle in clinical and preoperative evaluation.[123] Problems with reproducibly measuring this parameter exist. Tibial tuberosity and trochlear groove distance have received significant attention as important factors in patellar instability. These values can change with weight-bearing, knee position, and rotation.[424,425] MRI has been used to evaluate other factors that contribute to patellar instability, including trochlear groove configuration and distance, patellar tilt and height, and tibial tuberosity. Trochlear dysplasia may be one of the most important factors.[426] All of these factors may play a role in recurrent patellar instability.[427]

Fithian and colleagues[330–332] identified several historical and anatomic risk factors for predicting secondary dislocations: young age at presentation, female gender, a history of a previous dislocation or subluxation, a family history of dislocation or subluxation, developmental hip dysplasia, increased Q angle, and torsional malalignment.

Hinton and Sharma[329] have outlined the main indications for surgery in young athletes, and the authors believe that their surgical algorithm is appropriate for most patients. The relative indications for surgery include the following:

1. failure to improve with nonoperative care;
2. concurrent osteochondral injury;
3. continued gross instability;
4. palpable disruption of the MPFL and the vastus medialis obliquus; and
5. high-level athletic demands coupled with mechanical risk factors and an initial injury mechanism not related to contact.

For patients who undergo surgery, the authors perform a thorough examination of both knees under anesthesia. The degree of patellar laxity is assessed for both the normal and abnormal knee. In some cases, both knees will be prepared during the procedure because this will allow comparison of both knees for assessment of the appropriate tension of the retinacular tissues on the repaired side.

For many patients with recurrent dislocations or subluxations, the authors first evaluate the MPFL structures. If the patients do not have other significant anatomic issues, they may undergo primary repair and advancement of the medial retinacular tissues, although in most cases, the authors use other complementary procedures. The use of supplemental tissue, such as semitendinosus autograft or allograft, may be determined preoperatively or intraoperatively.[346,347,410,417,428] If the medial tissues are of questionable quality, supplemental tissue may be used for formal MPFL reconstruction.

A lateral release may be performed in cases of significant tightness of the lateral retinacular tissues;[343] however, it is rare in the authors' surgical practice to do so. Lateral release is not without complications, and medial patellar instability has been reported.[330–332,429–431] Long-term follow-up of lateral release in patellar instability has not demonstrated good outcomes.[432] In addition to reconstruction and tightening of the static medial restraints, the medial retinaculum, and the MPFL, the authors may also perform a distal advancement or a repair of the damaged or avulsed vastus medialis obliquus.

Furthermore, additional soft tissue reconstruction may be done in select cases.[420] This may be most appropriate in patients with excessive soft tissue laxity, previous surgery, or other factors that suggest a higher rate of surgical failure. These patients may have additional reconstruction of the patellotibial ligaments with the use of an autograft or allograft.[433] Similar to Hinton and Sharma,[329] the authors do not routinely reconstruct the patellotibial ligament.

Surgery on the tibial tubercle in those with significant growth remaining may cause complications of physeal disturbance, including recurvatum.[329,415,416] Although these procedures may have a significant impact on recurrent patellar instability, the authors urge caution in younger patients. In these patients, a modified Roux-Goldthwait procedure may be an option,[434] as would be a medialization of a portion of the patellar tendon without an osteotomy.[420]

Recent studies of patellofemoral sulcus dysplasia have attempted to define normal and pathologic anatomy of the patellofemoral joint. Although the authors have very limited experience with procedures that attempt to modify the configuration or depth of the sulcus, they follow these anatomic and surgical studies closely. These procedures would have the potential to damage the distal femoral physis; therefore, they may be best delayed until the patient is close to or is at skeletal maturity. Trochlear osteotomies or trochleoplasties can be very difficult to perform, and concerns about surgical complications and osteoarthritis are legitimate. A recent systematic review comparing trochleoplasty and MPFL reconstruction showed reasonable outcomes in both groups, although the follow-up periods of the review were limited.[435]

Regardless of the surgical procedure performed, a closely supervised physical therapy program is started early after surgery. The program is modified to account for patient variables, such as significant soft tissue laxity. Prolonged immobilization is best avoided because of concerns about arthrofibrosis, cartilage atrophy, and significant muscle atrophy. With the use of a hinged knee brace, motion is progressed so that early recovery of motion of the knee and patellofemoral joint can be achieved. Patellofemoral mobilization modalities are also implemented so that the risk of arthrofibrosis of the patellofemoral joint is reduced. Patients are slowly returned to sports-specific activity with use of a protocol similar to that described in the previous section.

OSTEOCHONDRITIS DISSECANS

The condition involving loose bodies of the knee was first described in 1840 by Paré, further characterized as a "quiet necrosis" in 1870 by Paget, and later termed OCD by König in 1888.[169,436–438] OCD is a focal, idiopathic alteration of subchondral bone with the risk of instability and disruption of adjacent articular cartilage that may result in premature osteoarthritis.[439] The spectrum of disease is further categorized between juvenile and adult forms depending on the skeletal maturity of the patient; closed physes foreshadow a worse outcome with likely development of early knee arthritis.[131,142,440] Furthermore, in children, conservative or nonoperative treatment has been shown to facilitate healing

in the majority of patients, although those with larger lesions, swelling, and mechanical symptoms are not as likely to heal.[135] Many hypotheses have been postulated concerning the cause of OCD lesions of the knee, including trauma, genetics, vascular pathology, and constitutional factors, but the etiology remains elusive.[131,142,211,441,442]

OCD can affect any joint in the body but most commonly affects the medial femoral condyle.[443] A recent epidemiologic study of OCD in children and adolescents by Kessler and colleagues[444] found that those with the greatest odds ratio for developing OCD were non-Hispanic black-ethnicity adolescents 12 to 19 years of age (compared with children 6–11 years of age) and males. Kessler and colleagues also identified that the overall incidence for OCD in children and adolescents 6 to 19 years of age was 22.6 and 9.9 for males and females, respectively. OCD has been found to occur more frequently in children and adolescents than in adults.[445]

Diagnostic Imaging

Radiographic identification of OCD lesions is the first step for every patient, and the lesion can often be visualized with plain radiographs that include AP, lateral, Merchant, and notch views. For assessment of the stability of the lesion and the articular cartilage, an MRI study can also be obtained (Figs. 19.23 and 19.24). Several studies have identified signs of lesion instability on MRI; these include high T2 signal rims, surrounding cysts, high T2 signal fracture lines, and fluid-filled osteochondral defects.[446] Studies have reported up to 100% correlation of these signs of instability on MRI with instability as determined at the time of arthroscopy.

In some cases involving the femoral condyle of younger, skeletally immature patients, it can be difficult to differentiate between a diagnosis of OCD and a benign variation in femoral condylar ossification. Jans and colleagues[447]

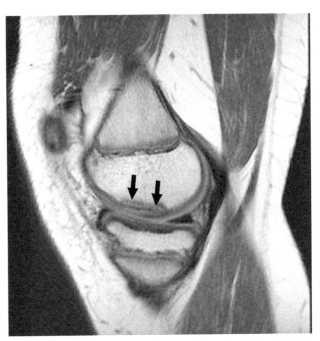

Fig. 19.23 Magnetic resonance image of T1-weighted sagittal view showing osteochondritis dissecans lesion (*arrows*).

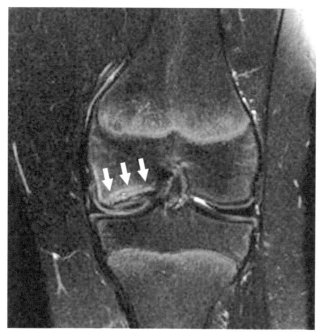

Fig. 19.24 Magnetic resonance image of T2-weighted coronal view showing osteochondritis dissecans lesion (*arrows*).

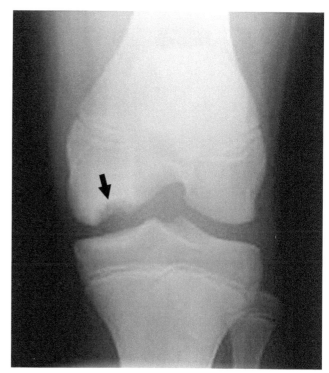

Fig. 19.25 Plain radiograph coronal view showing osteochondritis dissecans lesion (*arrow*).

reviewed MRI studies of 315 patients and identified 165 with OCD lesions and 150 with ossification variations. Among other findings, they identified that ossification variation did not occur in girls older than 10 years and boys older than 13 years and that OCD did not occur in children younger than 8 years.

Treatment

Early authors demonstrated good results with nonoperative management of OCD lesions of the femoral condyles, especially in skeletally immature patients[440,448,449]; however, more recent literature suggests that conservative management does not reliably protect patients from early knee arthritis later in life.[440,442,450] Numerous operative techniques described in the literature have shown good results in affecting the natural history of OCD lesions, including open drilling, open fixation, arthroscopic fixation, arthroscopic drilling, open and percutaneous extraarticular drilling, bone pegging, fragment excision, crater trimming with bone penetration, and osteochondral bone grafting. In some cases, the authors use transarticular drilling, although some may prefer extraarticular and intraepiphyseal drilling (retroarticular) for OCD lesions with intact articular cartilage (Figs. 19.25 and 19.26), bioabsorbable fixation of delaminated cartilage after arthroscopic drilling, or débridement with arthroscopic drilling for those lesions completely denuded of articular cartilage.

In 2010, the American Academy of Orthopaedic Surgeons created an evidence-based clinical practice guideline (CPG) on the diagnosis and treatment of OCD of the knee.[451,452] This CPG was unable to make any good or strong recommendations because of the weak and inconclusive evidence for many clinical areas of this disorder. This document did identify several promising areas of future research, which should clarify treatment options in the future.

ANKLE INJURIES

For high school-aged athletes, the most commonly injured body region is the ankle when looking at all sports in aggregate.[453] Furthermore, when looking at each individual sport independently, ankle injuries are the number one most commonly injured body region for female soccer, basketball, and volleyball and are the number one for male basketball as well.[454] Moreover, in the skeletally immature athlete, the open or closing physis presents unique biological and mechanical characteristics that portend unique fracture patterns in these athletes. Because of these unique fracture patterns and the need to respect the physis in a growing athlete, these patients require unique surgical techniques to preserve the physis.

Using a working definition of ankle injuries as those occurring distal to the tibial and fibular metaphysis,[455] the aim of this section is to review the germane, traumatic injuries of the ankle that are frequently seen in the skeletally immature athlete.

TILLAUX FRACTURES

A Tillaux fracture (Figs. 19.27 and 19.28) is an isolated Salter-Harris type III fracture of the distal tibial epiphysis. These fractures account for 3% to 5% of pediatric ankle fractures.[456] These fractures occur typically because of an external rotation force of the ankle in a skeletally immature subject. Given the predictable physeal closure pattern of the distal tibial physis—central, medial, and then lateral—these injuries tend to occur in young athletes that are close to physeal closure with the lateral-most physis closing but not completely closed. The anterior inferior tibiofibular ligament (AITFL) is of particular importance for this fracture.

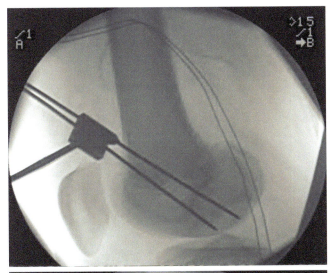

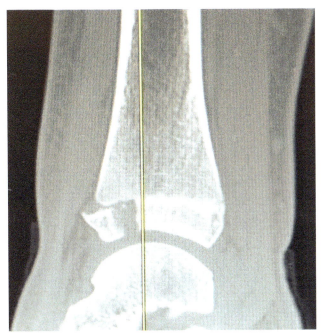

Fig. 19.27 Tillaux fracture.

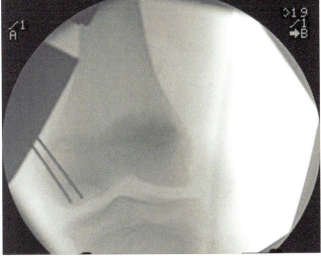

Fig. 19.26 Intraoperative fluoroscopy of osteochondritis dissecans (OCD) lesion with guide pin placed center-center within the lesion and a second drilling K-wire perforating the sclerotic rim of the OCD.

The AITFL is one of the three ligaments that makes up the syndesmotic complex: AITFL, posterior inferior tibiofibular ligament, and the interosseous ligament, respectively.[457] The AITFL attaches obliquely from the fibula to the tibia approximately 5 mm proximal to the articular surface with a width range of 7 to 12 mm on the fibular side and 9 to 22 mm on the tibial side.[457]

Given the attachment site, although the AITFL is the weakest of the three syndesmotic ligaments, in the skeletally immature athlete, the tensile strength overcomes the strength of the lateral aspect of the distal tibia where the physis has remained patent. As such, an external rotation force will avulse this bony fragment from its origin, causing a fracture line, which extends horizontally through the open physis and then vertically through the epiphysis of the tibia.[456]

TREATMENT

Given that this fracture pattern is technically an intraarticular fracture, special attention should be paid to achieving an anatomic reduction while respecting the physis. It is accepted that fractures with less than 2 mm may have a

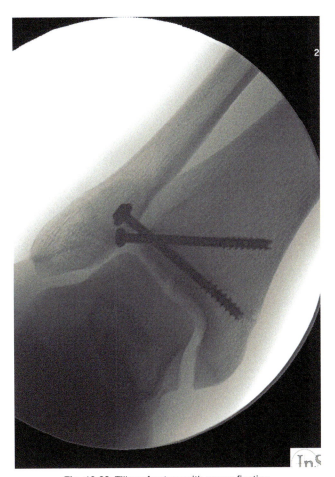

Fig. 19.28 Tillaux fracture with screw fixation.

better tolerance for nonoperative treatment; however, there is no consensus on this. Typically, if the fracture is thought to be more than 2 mm of displacement, based on x-ray, a

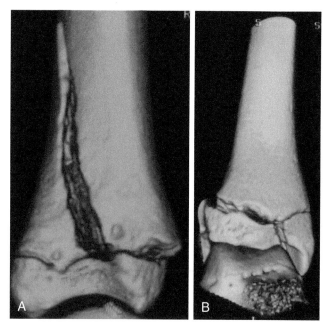

Fig. 19.29 Triplane fracture. (A) Sagittal plane three-dimensional reconstruction shows posterior metaphyseal component of fracture. (B) Coronal plane reconstruction shows intraepiphyseal component of the fracture. The axial plane of the fracture extends through the physis.

CT may be beneficial for surgical planning and fracture characterization.

For the minimally displaced (<2 mm) Tillaux fracture, nonoperative treatment may consist of non-weight-bearing in a simple long leg cast for 4 to 6 weeks. Internal rotation of the ankle may help with reduction of the fracture fragment to a more anatomic location. Weekly radiographs are recommended to evaluate for interval loss of reduction, which may necessitate surgical intervention. The authors recommend a transition to a walking boot after cast removal in 4 to 6 weeks with initiation of non-weight-bearing passive and active range of motion with physical therapy for 2 to 3 weeks.

For fractures with significant displacement (>2 mm), surgery is typically recommended. Several surgical treatment options are available and include closed reduction internal fixation (CRIF),[458] ORIF,[459,460] and arthroscopic-assisted reduction and internal fixation (ARIF).[461,462,463] Excellent results have been found with ORIF,[459] and some advocate ORIF over CRIF because of concerns for potential interposed periosteal tissue, which can potentially increase risk for nonunion. Whether ORIF, CRIF, or ARIF methods are chosen for treatment, the fixation method should consist of a single all-epiphyseal lag screw or two, which should be placed using AO principles to achieve primary bone healing through compression of the fragment.

TRIPLANE FRACTURES

Similar to the Tillaux fracture, a triplane fracture (Figs. 19.29 and 19.30) is unique in that it is also one of the so-called *transitional fractures*. It is "transitional" in the sense that the physis is in the process of transitioning from an open to a closed status. Given this transitional position, the ankle is in a unique position, as the physis may act as an additional weak link for fractures to propagate through. This particular fracture pattern is consistent with a Salter-Harris type IV fracture with three planes of fracture propagation: coronal, sagittal, and transverse. These injuries occur in young athletes in up to 65% of some series[464] and are concerning, as insults to the distal tibial physis can result in growth arrest or aberrancies, as the distal tibial physis is responsible for approximately 45% of the overall growth of the tibial.[465]

Standard, radiographic three views of the ankle, including an AP, Mortise, and lateral view, should be carefully evaluated. Although an MRI will show superior anatomic soft tissue details of the ankle, a CT is useful in characterizing the fracture pattern and is important for determining the amount of displacement. Eismann et al evaluated the utility of using a CT in a cohort of patients with triplane fractures.[466] These authors showed there was a 41% change in the treatment plan when a CT scan was used when compared with only x-rays in the same cohort being used.[466]

The argument against obtaining a CT scan for these fractures is that there is a theoretical uncertain morbidity associated with increased radiation with each exposure to ionizing radiation. However, it is important to note that CT scans of this region of the lower extremity are among the lowest radiation dose used.[467]

TREATMENT

Principles of intraarticular fracture management apply to these fractures given the epiphyseal component of this fracture type. Broadly speaking, a tolerance of 1 to 2 mm of step-off is the threshold for nonoperative treatment. Beyond this, most surgeons would consider operative management. In those fractures that are minimally displaced (< 2 mm) closed reduction, long leg cast application and a period of 4 to 6 weeks of non-weight-bearing is recommended. Reduction maneuver is achieved with axial traction and internal rotation.[455]

ORIF is typically recommended for those who fail closed reduction or those who have an intraarticular fracture displacement greater than 2 mm. For those who fail closed reduction, interposed tissue has been found to be the issue in up to 75% of cases.[464] The approach for ORIF of the triplane fracture can involve a two-incision approach utilizing lag screws to capture the metaphyseal fracture fragment to achieve adequate reduction and compression. This also allows for visualization of the joint surface to confirm reduction of the epiphyseal fragment. The epiphyseal fragment can be reduced and fixed utilizing a lag screw through a small, medially based incision.

OSTEOCHONDRAL LESIONS OF THE TALUS

Although König has been credited for first describing OCD in 1888, the original description was in the knee.[468] However, not long after this others had found what appeared to be OCD lesions in the talus.[423,469] Although both traumatic and atraumatic etiologies have been suggested for OCD, a traumatic etiology is favored, as this is commonly seen in athletic individuals. Because of the discrepancies in proposed etiologies this entity has been referred to, in the literature, as an *osteochondral lesion* of the talus (OLT) (Fig. 19.31). This term is broad and encompasses other lesions, including avascular necrosis and osteochondral fractures, as well.[470]

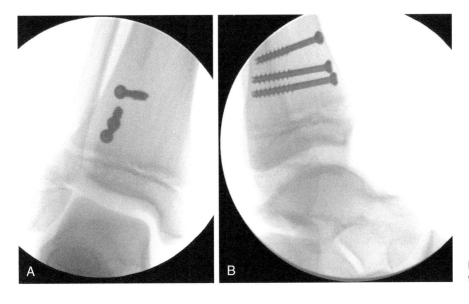

Fig. 19.30 Triplane fracture with screw fixation. Anteroposterior (A) and lateral (B) views.

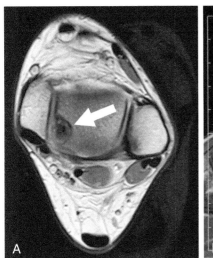

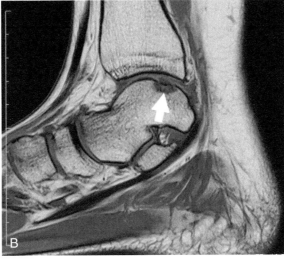

Fig. 19.31 Osteochondral lesions of the talus (OLT): (A) axial view, and (B) sagittal view (arrow pointing to the OLT).

Most series have described OCD of the talus in a mix of adult and pediatric patients; however, publications of an exclusively adolescent population have been described.[471,472] Although the exact incidence is not clear, the proportion of these lesions seem to occur on the medial aspect of the talus and to a lesser degree on the lateral aspect of the talus.[472] These lesions are painful for the young athlete, with pain and ankle swelling being the most common complaints.[470,472] Additionally, these lesions can occur in several different stages along a continuum.[473] Berndt and Harty attempted to classify these lesions based on radiographic characteristics in 1959.[473] They can exist in a form with overlying cartilage intact and a mild depression of the subchondral bone to a lesion, which is fragmented and completely ex situ from its bony bed as a loose body within the joint.[473] This variability within the stage of the lesion therefore makes it challenging to treat, as each stage may be approached with variable nonsurgical or surgical options for treatment.

TREATMENT

Most authors agree that treatment of the majority of OCD lesions of the talus should start with a trial of nonoperative treatment.[470,472] There is variability in what nonoperative treatment should consist of. Some authors recommend non-weight-bearing for 6 weeks,[471] whereas others recommend weight-bearing as tolerated in a cast for 5 to 8 weeks.[472,474] Sport restriction is recommended for up to 6 months.[470] The authors' preferred nonoperative treatment consists of non-weight-bearing for 6 weeks followed by sport restriction for a minimum of 3 months with follow-up radiographs or evidence of healing. Because of increased healing potential in younger children, Bruns et al recommend longer periods of nonoperative treatment in these patients and earlier surgical intervention in the older child or young adult.[475]

Indications for operative treatment include mechanical symptoms in the setting of radiographic evidence of an OLT, failure of conservative treatment, and displaced fragments that are ex situ.[470,476] The surgeon should consider the stage of the lesion, the status of the overlying cartilage, size of lesion, the amount of subchondral bone on the progeny fragment, as well as the location of the lesion on the talus—medial versus lateral—as these factors will help guide the surgeon toward the most appropriate surgical intervention.

For lesions in which the fragment is stable, in situ and the overlying cartilage is intact, a transarticular or retroarticular drilling technique should be considered. Both methods involve a theoretical marrow stimulation of the underlying necrotic bone, which will stimulate the healing of the lesion.[477] The advantage of a retroarticular approach is that there is no compromise of the overlying cartilage of the lesion. Taranow et al describe a retroarticular approach via the sinus tarsi for medial sided talar lesions with 88% healing at 7 months of follow-up.[478] One technical difficulty with drilling lesions in children is the small ankle joint in this population. However, newer arthroscopic instrumentation has been refined to adjust for smaller joint size.

Lesions that have fissuring of the overlying cartilage, are mobile to probing, and have 2 to 3 mm of subchondral bone on the fragment may be amenable to rigid fixation with metallic screws, bioabsorbable products, or biologics such as cortical bone pegs.[479] However, in the majority of cases, these lesions may not be amenable to fixation, and some recommend curettage and bone marrow stimulation such as microfracture as a first next step.[480] If this treatment option fails, more invasive procedures include osteochondral autograft transfer, typically from the ipsilateral femoral condyle, osteochondral allograft transplantation as plugs or as a larger unit depending on the size of the lesion, and cell-based therapies such as autologous chondrocyte transplantation techniques.

REFERENCES

The level of evidence (LOE) is determined according to the criteria provided in the Preface.

1. Rang M, Thompson GH. Children's fractures: principles and management. *Reconstr Surg Traumatol.* 1979;17:2–15. **(LOE N/A).**
2. Foundation NRaE. *Request for Proposals: Epidemiology Study Pediatric Sports Health Care;* 2001. **(LOE N/A).**
3. Gottschalk AW, Andrish JT. Epidemiology of sports injury in pediatric athletes. *Sports Med Arthrosc Rev.* 2011;19(1):2–6. **(LOE IV).**
4. Bijur PE, Trumble A, Harel Y, Overpeck MD, Jones D, Scheidt PC. Sports and recreation injuries in US children and adolescents. *Arch Pediatr Adolesc Med.* 1995;149(9):1009–1016. **(LOE III).**
5. Dalton SE. Overuse injuries in adolescent athletes. *Sports Med.* 1992;13(1):58–70. **(LOE II).**
6. Darrow CJ, Collins CL, Yard EE, Comstock RD. Epidemiology of severe injuries among United States high school athletes: 2005-2007. *Am J Sports Med.* 2009;37(9):1798–1805. **(LOE III).**
7. Swenson DM, Henke NM, Collins CL, Fields SK, Comstock RD. Epidemiology of United States high school sports-related fractures, 2008-09 to 2010-11. *Am J Sports Med.* 2012;40(9):2078–2084. **(LOE III).**
8. Rechel JA, Collins CL, Comstock RD. Epidemiology of injuries requiring surgery among high school athletes in the United States, 2005 to 2010. *J Trauma.* 2011;71(4):982–989. **(LOE III).**
9. Frisch A, Seil R, Urhausen A, Croisier JL, Lair ML, Theisen D. Analysis of sex-specific injury patterns and risk factors in young high-level athletes. *Scand J Med Sci Sports.* 2009;19(6):834–841. **(LOE III).**
10. Caraffa A, Cerulli G, Projetti M, Aisa G, Rizzo A. Prevention of anterior cruciate ligament injuries in soccer. A prospective controlled study of proprioceptive training. *Knee Surg Sports Traumatol Arthrosc.* 1996;4(1):19–21. **(LOE I).**
11. Hewett TE, Ford KR, Myer GD. Anterior cruciate ligament injuries in female athletes: part 2, a meta-analysis of neuromuscular interventions aimed at injury prevention. *Am J Sports Med.* 2006;34(3):490–498. **(LOE I).**
12. Hewett TE, Lindenfeld TN, Riccobene JV, Noyes FR. The effect of neuromuscular training on the incidence of knee injury in female athletes. A prospective study. *Am J Sports Med.* 1999;27(6):699–706. **(LOE II).**
13. Hewett TE, Myer GD, Ford KR. Decrease in neuromuscular control about the knee with maturation in female athletes. *J Bone Joint Surg Am.* 2004;86-A(8):1601–1608. **(LOE III).**
14. Hewett TE, Myer GD, Ford KR. Reducing knee and anterior cruciate ligament injuries among female athletes: a systematic review of neuromuscular training interventions. *J Knee Surg.* 2005;18(1):82–88. **(LOE III).**
15. Hewett TE, Myer GD, Ford KR, Slauterbeck JR. Preparticipation physical examination using a box drop vertical jump test in young athletes: the effects of puberty and sex. *Clin J Sport Med.* 2006;16(4):298–304. **(LOE III).**
16. Hewett TE, Paterno MV, Myer GD. Strategies for enhancing proprioception and neuromuscular control of the knee. *Clin Orthop Relat Res.* 2002;(402):76–94. **(LOE V).**
17. Hewett TE, Stroupe AL, Nance TA, Noyes FR. Plyometric training in female athletes. Decreased impact forces and increased hamstring torques. *Am J Sports Med.* 1996;24(6):765–773. **(LOE III).**
18. Junge A, Rosch D, Peterson L, Graf-Baumann T, Dvorak J. Prevention of soccer injuries: a prospective intervention study in youth amateur players. *Am J Sports Med.* 2002;30(5):652–659. **(LOE III).**
19. Soderman K, Werner S, Pietila T, Engstrom B, Alfredson H. Balance board training: prevention of traumatic injuries of the lower extremities in female soccer players? A prospective randomized intervention study. *Knee Surg Sports Traumatol Arthrosc.* 2000;8(6):356–363. **(LOE I).**
20. Grimm NL, Shea KG, Leaver RW, Aoki SK, Carey JL. Efficacy and degree of bias in knee injury prevention studies: a systematic review of RCTs. *Clin Orthop Relat Res.* 2013;471(1):308–316. **(LOE II).**
21. Edwards TB, Greene CC, Baratta RV, Zieske A, Willis RB. The effect of placing a tensioned graft across open growth plates. A gross and histologic analysis. *J Bone Joint Surg Am.* 2001;83-A(5):725–734. **(LOE N/A).**
22. J.G. G. Development and maturation of the neuromusculoskeletal system. In: Morrissey RT, Weinstein SL, eds. *Lovell and Winter's Pediatric Orthopaedics.* **(LOE N/A).**
23. Guy J. ML. Pediatric and adolescent athletes. In: Schenck RC Jr, ed. *Athletic Training and Sports Medicine.* Rosemont, IL: American Academy of Orthopaedic Surgeons. **(LOE N/A).**
24. Bright RW, Burstein AH, Elmore SM. Epiphyseal-plate cartilage. A biomechanical and histological analysis of failure modes. *J Bone Joint Surg Am.* 1974;56(4):688–703. **(LOE II).**
25. Bright RW, Elmore SM. Physical properties of epiphyseal plate cartilage. *Surg Forum.* 1968;19:463–464. **(LOE N/A).**
26. Poland J. *Traumatic Separation of the Epiphysis.* Smith and Elder: London. **(LOE N/A).**
27. Koester MC. Adolescent and youth sports medicine: a "growing" concern. *Athlet Ther Today.* 2002;7(6):6–12. **(LOE V).**
28. Clanton TO, DeLee JC, Sanders B, Neidre A. Knee ligament injuries in children. *J Bone Joint Surg Am.* 1979;61(8):1195–1201. **(LOE IV).**
29. DeLee JC, Curtis R. Anterior cruciate ligament insufficiency in children. *Clin Orthop Relat Res.* 1983;(172):112–118. **(LOE IV).**
30. Eady JL, Cardenas CD, Sopa D. Avulsion of the femoral attachment of the anterior cruciate ligament in a seven-year-old child. A case report. *J Bone Joint Surg Am.* 1982;64(9):1376–1378. **(LOE IV).**
31. Currey JD, Butler G. The mechanical properties of bone tissue in children. *J Bone Joint Surg Am.* 1975;57(6):810–814. **(LOE IV).**
32. Bright RW. Physeal injury. In: Rockwood CA, Wilkins KE, King R, eds. *Fractures in Children.* J.B. Lippincott: Philadelphia;87–172. **(LOE N/A).**
33. DeLee JC. Ligamentous injury of the knee. *Pediatric and Adolescent Sports Medicine.* 3:406–432.
34. Ogden JA. Injury to the growth mechanisms of the immature skeleton. *Skeletal Radiol.* 1981;6(4):237–253. **(LOE V).**
35. Ogden JA, Tross RB, Murphy MJ. Fractures of the tibial tuberosity in adolescents. *J Bone Joint Surg Am.* 1980;62(2):205–215. **(LOE IV).**
36. Williams JL, Vani JN, Eick JD, Petersen EC, Schmidt TL. Shear strength of the physis varies with anatomic location and is a function of modulus, inclination, and thickness. *J Orthop Res.* 1999;17(2):214–222. **(LOE N/A).**
37. Close BJ, Strouse PJ. MR of physeal fractures of the adolescent knee. *Pediatr Radiol.* 2000;30(11):756–762. **(LOE V).**
38. Futami T, Foster BK, Morris LL, LeQuesne GW. Magnetic resonance imaging of growth plate injuries: the efficacy and indications for surgical procedures. *Arch Orthop Trauma Surg.* 2000;120(7-8):390–396. **(LOE IV).**
39. Gautier E, Ziran BH, Egger B, Slongo T, Jakob RP. Growth disturbances after injuries of the proximal tibial epiphysis. *Arch Orthop Trauma Surg.* 1998;118(1-2):37–41. **(LOE IV).**

40. Kasser JR. Physeal bar resections after growth arrest about the knee. *Clin Orthop Relat Res.* 1990;(255):68–74. **(LOE V)**.

41. Pennig D, Baranowski D. Genu recurvatum due to partial growth arrest of the proximal tibial physis: correction by callus distraction. Case report. *Arch Orthop Trauma Surg.* 1989;108(2):119–121. **(LOE IV)**.

42. Skak SV, Jensen TT, Poulsen TD, Sturup J. Epidemiology of knee injuries in children. *Acta Orthop Scand.* 1987;58(1):78–81. **(LOE III)**.

43. Stanitski CL, Harvell JC, Fu F. Observations on acute knee hemarthrosis in children and adolescents. *J Pediatr Orthop.* 1993;13(4):506–510. **(LOE II)**.

44. Harris WR. The endocrine basis for slipping of the upper femoral epiphysis. An experimental study. *J Bone Joint Surg Br.* 1950;32-B:5–11. **(LOE III)**.

45. Tipton CM, Matthes RD, Martin RK. Influence of age and sex on the strength of bone-ligament junctions in knee joints of rats. *J Bone Joint Surg Am.* 1978;60(2):230–234. **(LOE N/A)**.

46. Tipton CM, Schild RJ, Flatt AE. Measurement of ligamentous strength in rat knees. *J Bone Joint Surg Am.* 1967;49(1):63–72. **(LOE N/A)**.

47. Cole PA, Ehrlich MG. Management of the completely stiff pediatric knee. *J Pediatr Orthop.* 1997;17(1):67–73. **(LOE IV)**.

48. Matelic TM, Aronsson DD, Boyd DW Jr, LaMont RL. Acute hemarthrosis of the knee in children. *Am J Sports Med.* 1995;23(6):668–671. **(LOE IV)**.

49. Smith AD, Tao SS. Knee injuries in young athletes. *Clin Sports Med.* 1995;14(3):629–650. **(LOE V)**.

50. Indelicato PA. Non-operative treatment of complete tears of the medial collateral ligament of the knee. *J Bone Joint Surg Am.* 1983;65(3):323–329. **(LOE IV)**.

51. King SJ, Carty HM, Brady O. Magnetic resonance imaging of knee injuries in children. *Pediatr Radiol.* 1996;26(4):287–290. **(LOE II)**.

52. King SJ. Magnetic resonance imaging of knee injuries in children. *Eur Radiol.* 1997;7(8):1245–1251. **(LOE III)**.

53. McDermott MJ, Bathgate B, Gillingham BL, Hennrikus WL. Correlation of MRI and arthroscopic diagnosis of knee pathology in children and adolescents. *J Pediatr Orthop.* 1998;18(5):675–678. **(LOE III)**.

54. Kocher MS, DiCanzio J, Zurakowski D, Micheli LJ. Diagnostic performance of clinical examination and selective magnetic resonance imaging in the evaluation of intraarticular knee disorders in children and adolescents. *Am J Sports Med.* 2001;29(3):292–296. **(LOE III)**.

55. Zobel MS, Borrello JA, Siegel MJ, Stewart NR. Pediatric knee MR imaging: pattern of injuries in the immature skeleton. *Radiology.* 1994;190(2):397–401. **(LOE IV)**.

56. Iobst CA, Stanitski CL. Acute knee injuries. *Clin Sports Med.* 2000;19(4):621–635. **(LOE III)**.

57. Williams JS Jr, Abate JA, Fadale PD, Tung GA. Meniscal and nonosseous ACL injuries in children and adolescents. *Am J Knee Surg.* 1996;9(1):22–26. **(LOE IV)**.

58. Zionts LE. Fractures around the knee in children. *J Am Acad Orthop Surg.* 2002;10(5):345–355. **(LOE V)**.

59. Abbasi D, May MM, Wall EJ, Chan G, Parikh SN. MRI findings in adolescent patients with acute traumatic knee hemarthrosis. *J Pediatr Orthop.* 2012;32(8):760–764. LOE: III.

60. Chen FS, Diaz VA, Loebenberg M, Rosen JE. Shoulder and elbow injuries in the skeletally immature athlete. *J Am Acad Orthop Surg.* 2005;13(3):172–185. **(LOE III)**.

61. Hoyt WA Jr. Etiology of shoulder injuries in athletes. *J Bone Joint Surg Am.* 1967;49(4):755–766. **(LOE V)**.

62. Cook C, Beaty S, Kissenberth MJ, Siffri P, Pill SG, Hawkins RJ. Diagnostic accuracy of five orthopedic clinical tests for diagnosis of superior labrum anterior posterior (SLAP) lesions. *J Shoulder Elbow Surg.* 2012;21(1):13–22. **(LOE IV)**.

63. Emery KH. Imaging of sports injuries of the upper extremity in children. *Clin Sports Med.* 2006;25(3):543–568, viii. **(LOE III)**.

64. Heyworth BE, Kocher MS. Shoulder instability in the young athlete. *Instr Course Lect.* 2013;62:435–444. **(LOE IV)**.

65. Rowe CR. Prognosis in dislocations of the shoulder. *J Bone Joint Surg Am.* 1956;38-A(5):957–977. **(LOE III)**.

66. Longo UG. Surgical vs nonoperative treatment in patients up to 18 years old with traumatic shoulder instability: a systematic review and quantitative synthesis of the literature. *Arthroscopy.* 2016;32(5):944–952. **(LOE III)**.

67. Mulroy MF, Larkin KL, Hodgson PS, et al. A comparison of the spinal, epidural, and general anesthesia for outpatient knee arthroscopy. *Anesth Analg.* 2000;91(4):860–864. **(LOE II)**.

68. Paxinos A, Walton J, Tzannes A, Callanan M, Hayes K, Murrell GA. Advances in the management of traumatic anterior and atraumatic multidirectional shoulder instability. *Sports Med.* 2001;31(11):819–828. **(LOE V)**.

69. Jones KJ, Wiesel B, Ganley TJ, Wells L. Functional outcomes of early arthroscopic Bankart repair in adolescents aged 11 to 18 years. *J Pediatr Orthop.* 2007;27(2):209–213. **(LOE III)**.

70. Owens BD, DeBerardino TM, Nelson BJ, et al. Long-term follow-up of acute arthroscopic Bankart repair for initial anterior shoulder dislocations in young athletes. *Am J Sports Med.* 2009;37(4):669–673. **(LOE IV)**.

71. Shymon SJ, et al. Traumatic anterior instability of the pediatric shoulder: a comparison of arthroscopic and open Bankart repairs. *J Pediatr Orthopc.* 2015;35(1):1–6. **(LOE III)**.

72. Baker Cl 3rd, Mascarenhas R, Kline AJ, Chhabra A, Pombo MW, Bradley JP. Arthroscopic treatment of multidirectional shoulder instability in athletes: a retrospective analysis of 2- to 5-year clinical outcomes. *Am J Sports Med.* 2009;37(9):1712–1720. **(LOE IV)**.

73. Bradley JP, et al. Arthroscopic capsulolabral reconstruction for posterior instability of the shoulder: a prospective study of 200 shoulders. *Am J Sports Med.* 2013;41(9):2005–2014. **(LOE II)**.

74. Echlin PS, Plomaritis ST, Peck DM, Skopelja EN. Subscapularis avulsion fractures in 2 pediatric ice hockey players. *Am J Orthop (Belle Mead NJ).* 2006;35(6):281–284. **(LOE IV)**.

75. Klasson SC, Vander Schilden JL, Park JP. Late effect of isolated avulsion fractures of the lesser tubercle of the humerus in children. Report of two cases. *J Bone Joint Surg Am.* 1993;75(11):1691–1694. **(LOE IV)**.

76. May MM, Bishop JY. Shoulder injuries in young athletes. *Pediatr Radiol.* 2013;43(suppl 1):S135–140. **(LOE V)**.

77. Eisner EA, Roocroft JH, Edmonds EW. Underestimation of labral pathology in adolescents with anterior shoulder instability. *J Pediatr Orthop.* 2012;32(1):42–47. **(LOE III)**.

78. Spiegl UJ, Warth RJ, Millet PJ. Symptomatic internal impingement of the shoulder in overhead athletes. *Sports Med Arthrosc Rev.* 2014;22(2):120–129. **(LOE III)**.

79. Edmonds EW, Eisner EA, Kruk PG, et al. Diagnostic shortcomings of magnetic resonance arthrography to evaluatve partial rotator cuff tears in adolescents. *J Pediatr Orthop.* 2015;35(4):407–411. **(LOE III)**.

80. Taylor DC, Krasinski KL. Adolescent shoulder injuries: consensus and controversies. *Instr Course Lect.* 2009;58:281–292. **(LOE V)**.

81. Veltri DM. Shoulder instability in the young athlete. *Conn Med.* 2010;74(8):465–468. **(LOE V)**.

82. Sommaire C, Penz C, Clavert P, Klouche S, Hardy P, Kempf JF. Recurrence after arthroscopic Bankart repair: is quantitative radiological analysis of bone loss of any predictive value? *Orthop Traumatol Surg Res.* 2012;98(5):514–519. **(LOE II)**.

83. Rowe CR. Acute and recurrent anterior dislocations of the shoulder. *Orthop Clin North Am.* 1980;11(2):253–270. **(LOE V)**.

84. Thomas SC, Matsen FA 3rd. An approach to the repair of avulsion of the glenohumeral ligaments in the management of traumatic anterior glenohumeral instability. *J Bone Joint Surg Am.* 1989;71(4):506–513. **(LOE IV)**.

85. Carreira DS, Mazzocca AD, Oryhon J, Brown FM, Hayden JK, Romeo AA. A prospective outcome evaluation of arthroscopic Bankart repairs: minimum 2-year follow-up. *Am J Sports Med.* 2006;34(5):771–777. **(LOE IV)**.

86. Kim SH, Ha KI, Kim SH. Bankart repair in traumatic anterior shoulder instability: open versus arthroscopic technique. *Arthroscopy.* 2002;18(7):755–763. **(LOE III)**.

87. Bottoni CR, Smith EL, Berkowitz MJ, Towle RB, Moore JH. Arthroscopic versus open shoulder stabilization for recurrent anterior instability: a prospective randomized clinical trial. *Am J Sports Med.* 2006;34(11):1730–1737. **(LOE I)**.

88. Lenters TR, Franta AK, Wolf FM, Leopold SS, Matsen FA 3rd. Arthroscopic compared with open repairs for recurrent anterior shoulder instability. A systematic review and meta-analysis of the literature. *J Bone Joint Surg Am.* 2007;89(2):244–254. **(LOE II)**.

89. Latarjet M. [Treatment of recurrent dislocation of the shoulder]. *Lyon Chir.* 1954;49(8):994–997. **(LOE V)**.

90. Haaker RG, Eickhoff U, Klammer HL. Intraarticular autogenous bone grafting in recurrent shoulder dislocations. *Mil Med.* 1993;158(3):164–169. **(LOE IV)**.

91. Warner JJ, Gill TJ, O'Hollerhan JD, Pathare N, Millett PJ. Anatomical glenoid reconstruction for recurrent anterior glenohumeral instability with glenoid deficiency using an autogenous tricortical iliac crest bone graft. *Am J Sports Med.* 2006;34(2):205–212. **(LOE IV)**.

92. Weng PW, Shen HC, Lee HH, Wu SS, Lee CH. Open reconstruction of large bony glenoid erosion with allogeneic bone graft for recurrent anterior shoulder dislocation. *Am J Sports Med.* 2009;37(9):1792–1797. **(LOE IV)**.

93. Lafosse L, Lejeune E, Bouchard A, Kakuda C, Gobezie R, Kochhar T. The arthroscopic Latarjet procedure for the treatment of anterior shoulder instability. *Arthroscopy.* 2007;23(11):1242.e1241–e1245. **(LOE V)**.

94. Provencher MT, Bhatia S, Ghodadra NS, et al. Recurrent shoulder instability: current concepts for evaluation and management of glenoid bone loss. *J Bone Joint Surg Am.* 2010;92(suppl 2):133–151. **(LOE V)**.

95. Shah AA, Butler RB, Romanowski J, Goel D, Karadagli D, Warner JJ. Short-term complications of the Latarjet procedure. *J Bone Joint Surg Am.* 2012;94(6):495–501. **(LOE IV)**.

96. Calandra JJ, Baker CL, Uribe J. The incidence of Hill-Sachs lesions in initial anterior shoulder dislocations. *Arthroscopy.* 1989;5(4):254–257. **(LOE III)**.

97. Hill HA, Sachs MD. The grooved defect of the humeral head. A frequently unrecognized complication of dislocations of the shoulder joint. *Radiology.* 1940;35:690–700. **(LOE IV)**.

98. Saito H, Itoi E, Minagawa H, Yamamoto N, Tuoheti Y, Seki N. Location of the Hill-Sachs lesion in shoulders with recurrent anterior dislocation. *Arch Orthop Trauma Surg.* 2009;129(10):1327–1334. **(LOE III)**.

99. Spatschil A, Landsiedl F, Anderl W, et al. Posttraumatic anterior-inferior instability of the shoulder: arthroscopic findings and clinical correlations. *Arch Orthop Trauma Surg.* 2006;126(4):217–222. **(LOE II)**.

100. Cho SH, Cho NS, Rhee YG. Preoperative analysis of the Hill-Sachs lesion in anterior shoulder instability: how to predict engagement of the lesion. *Am J Sports Med.* 2011;39(11):2389–2395. **(LOE II)**.

101. Kaar SG, Fening SD, Jones MH, Colbrunn RW, Miniaci A. Effect of humeral head defect size on glenohumeral stability: a cadaveric study of simulated Hill-Sachs defects. *Am J Sports Med.* 2010;38(3):594–599. **(LOE N/A)**.

102. Sekiya JK, Jolly J, Debski RE. The effect of a Hill-Sachs defect on glenohumeral translations, in situ capsular forces, and bony contact forces. *Am J Sports Med.* 2012;40(2):388–394. **(LOE N/A)**.

103. Skendzel JG, Sekiya JK. Diagnosis and management of humeral head bone loss in shoulder instability. *Am J Sports Med.* 2012;40(11):2633–2644. **(LOE IV)**.

104. Sekiya JK, Wickwire AC, Stehle JH, Debski RE. Hill-Sachs defects and repair using osteoarticular allograft transplantation: biomechanical analysis using a joint compression model. *Am J Sports Med.* 2009;37(12):2459–2466. **(LOE N/A)**.

105. Flury MP, Goldhahn J, Holzmann P, Simmen BR. Does Weber's rotation osteotomy induce degenerative joint disease at the shoulder in the long term? *J Shoulder Elbow Surg.* 2007;16(6):735–741. **(LOE III)**.

106. Boileau P, O'Shea K, Vargas P, Pinedo M, Old J, Zumstein M. Anatomical and functional results after arthroscopic Hill-Sachs remplissage. *J Bone Joint Surg Am.* 2012;94(7):618–626. **(LOE II)**.

107. Pagnani MJ. Open capsular repair without bone block for recurrent anterior shoulder instability in patients with and without bony defects of the glenoid and/or humeral head. *Am J Sports Med.* 2008;36(9):1805–1812. **(LOE IV)**.

108. Eisner EA, Roocroft JH, et al. Partial rotator cuff tears in adolescents: factors affecting outcomes. *J Pediatr Orthop.* 2013;33(1):2–7. **(LOE III)**.

109. Aglietti P, Insall JN, Cerulli G. Patellar pain and incongruence. I: measurements of incongruence. *Clin Orthop Relat Res.* 1983;(176):217–224. **(LOE IV)**.

110. Sabick MB, Kim YK, Torry MR, Keirns MA, Hawkins RJ. Biomechanics of the shoulder in youth baseball pitchers: implications for the development of proximal humeral epiphysiolysis and humeral retrotorsion. *Am J Sports Med.* 2005;33(11):1716–1722. **(LOE N/A)**.

111. Cahill BR, Tullos HS, Fain RH. Little League shoulder: lesions of the proximal humeral epiphyseal plate. *J Sports Med.* 1974;2(3):150–152. **(LOE IV)**.

112. Anton C, Podberesky DJ. Little League shoulder: a growth plate injury. *Pediatr Radiol.* 2010;40(suppl 1):S54. **(LOE V)**.

113. Brukner P. Stress fractures of the upper limb. *Sports Med.* 1998;26(6):415–424. **(LOE III)**.

114. Greyson ND. Humeral stress periostitis. The arm equivalent of "shin splints". *Clin Nucl Med.* 1995;20(3):286–287. **(LOE III)**.

115. Tibone JE. Shoulder problems of adolescents. How they differ from those of adults. *Clin Sports Med.* 1983;2(2):423–427. **(LOE V)**.

116. Osbahr DC, Kim HJ, Dugas JR. Little League shoulder. *Curr Opin Pediatr.* 2010;22(1):35–40. **(LOE IV)**.

117. Kocher MS, Waters PM, Micheli LJ. Upper extremity injuries in the paediatric athlete. *Sports Med.* 2000;30(2):117–135. **(LOE V)**.

118. Cain EL Jr, Dugas JR, Wolf RS, Andrews JR. Elbow injuries in throwing athletes: a current concepts review. *Am J Sports Med.* 2003;31(4):621–635. **(LOE IV)**.

119. Hurd WJ, Eby S, Kaufman KR, Murthy NS. Magnetic resonance imaging of the throwing elbow in the uninjured, high school-aged baseball pitcher. *Am J Sports Med.* 2011;39(4):722–728. **(LOE III)**.

120. Fleisig GS, Andrews JR, Dillman CJ, Escamilla RF. Kinetics of baseball pitching with implications about injury mechanisms. *Am J Sports Med.* 1995;23(2):233–239. **(LOE III)**.

121. Wilson FD, Andrews JR, Blackburn TA, McCluskey G. Valgus extension overload in the pitching elbow. *Am J Sports Med.* 1983;11(2):83–88. **(LOE IV)**.

122. Wilkins K. Fractures and dislocations of the elbow region. In: Wilkins KEK,RE, ed. *Fractures in Children.* Philadelphia: JB Lippincott, Co; 1991:509–828. **(LOE II)**.

123. Behr CT, Potter HG, Paletta GA Jr. The relationship of the femoral origin of the anterior cruciate ligament and the distal femoral physeal plate in the skeletally immature knee. An anatomic study. *Am J Sports Med.* 2001;29(6):781–787. **(LOE N/A)**.

124. Beck JJ, et al. What's new in pediatric medical epicondyle fractures? *J Pediatr Orthop.* 2016. **(LOE III)**.

125. Caine DJ, Nassar L. Gymnastics injuries. *Med Sport Sci.* 2005;48:18–58. **(LOE III)**.

126. Atanda AJ, et al. Factors related to increased ulnar collateral ligament thickness on stress sonography of the elbow in asymptomatic youth and adolescent baseball pitchers. *Am J Sports Med.* 2016;44(12):3179–3187. **(LOE III)**.

127. Cruz AIJ, et al. Medical epicondyle fractures in the pediatric overhead athlete. *J Pediatr Orthop.* 2016;36(1):S56–S62. **(LOE III)**.

128. Edmonds EW. How displaced are "nondisplaced" fractures of the medial humeral epicondyle in children? Results of a three-dimensional computed tomography analysis. *J Bone Joint Surg Am.* 2010;92(17):2785–2791. **(LOE III)**.

129. Souder CD, et al. The distal humerus axial view: assessment of displacement in medial epicondyle fractures. *J Pediatr Orthop.* 2015;35(5):449–454. **(LOE III)**.

130. Knapik DM, et al. Outcomes of nonoperative pediatric medial humeral epicondyle fractures with and without associated elbow dislocation. *J Pediatr Orthop.* 2017;37(4):e224–e228. **(LOE III)**.

131. Mubarak SJ, Carroll NC. Familial osteochondritis dissecans of the knee. *Clin Orthop Relat Res.* 1979;(140):131–136. **(LOE IV)**.

132. Cain EL Jr, Andrews JR, Dugas JR, et al. Outcome of ulnar collateral ligament reconstruction of the elbow in 1281 athletes: results in 743 athletes with minimum 2-year follow-up. *Am J Sports Med.* 2010;38(12):2426–2434. **(LOE IV)**.

133. Richard MJ, Aldridge JM 3rd, Wiesler ER, Ruch DS. Traumatic valgus instability of the elbow: pathoanatomy and results of direct repair. *J Bone Joint Surg Am.* 2008;90(11):2416–2422. **(LOE IV)**.

134. Savoie FH 3rd, Trenhaile SW, Roberts J, Field LD, Ramsey JR. Primary repair of ulnar collateral ligament injuries of the elbow in young athletes: a case series of injuries to the proximal and distal ends of the ligament. *Am J Sports Med.* 2008;36(6):1066–1072. **(LOE IV)**.

135. Makhni EC, et al. Arm pain in youth baseball players: a survey of healthy players. *Am J Sports Med.* 2015;43(1):41–46.

136. Klingele KE, Kocher MS. Little League elbow: valgus overload injury in the paediatric athlete. *Sports Med.* 2002;32(15):1005–1015. **(LOE V)**.

137. Ellman H. Anterior angulation deformity of the radial head. An unusual lesion occurring in juvenile baseball players. *J Bone Joint Surg Am.* 1975;57(6):776–778. **(LOE IV)**.

138. Rettig AC, Wurth TR, Mieling P. Nonunion of olecranon stress fractures in adolescent baseball pitchers: a case series of 5 athletes. *Am J Sports Med.* 2006;34(4):653–656. **(LOE IV)**.

139. Jans LB, et al. MR imaging findings and MR criteria for instability in osteochondritis dissecans of the elbow in children. *Eur J Radiol.* 2012;81(6):1306–1310. **(LOE IV)**.

140. Fujioka H, Tsunemi K, Takagi Y, Tanaka J. Treatment of stress fracture of the olecranon in throwing athletes with internal fixation through a small incision. *Sports Med Arthrosc Rehabil Ther Technol.* 2012;4(1):49. **(LOE IV)**.

141. Osbahr DC, Chalmers PN, Frank JS, Williams RJ 3rd, Widmann RF, Green DW. Acute, avulsion fractures of the medial epicondyle while throwing in youth baseball players: a variant of Little League elbow. *J Shoulder Elbow Surg.* 2010;19(7):951–957. **(LOE IV)**.

142. Kocher MS, Tucker R, Ganley TJ, Flynn JM. Management of osteochondritis dissecans of the knee: current concepts review. *Am J Sports Med.* 2006;34(7):1181–1191. **(LOE V)**.

143. Andrews JR, Jost PW, Cain EL. The ulnar collateral ligament procedure revisited: the procedure we use. *Sports Health.* 2012;4(5):438–441. **(LOE IV)**.

144. Petty DH, Andrews JR, Fleisig GS, Cain EL. Ulnar collateral ligament reconstruction in high school baseball players: clinical results and injury risk factors. *Am J Sports Med.* 2004;32(5):1158–1164. **(LOE III)**.

145. Eirickson BJ, et al. Exceeding pitch count recommendations in little league baseball increases the chance of requiring Tommy John surgery as a professional baseball pitcher. *Orthop J Sports Med.* 2017;5(3). **(LOE III)**.

146. Westermann RW, et al. Return to sport after operative management of osteochondritis dissecans of the capitellum: a systematic review and meta-analysis. *Orthop J Sports Med.* 2016;4(6). **(LOE IV)**.

147. Lyons ML, et al. Osteochondral autograft plug transfer for treatment of osteochondritis dissecans of the capitellum in adolescent athletes. *J Shoulder Elbow Surgery.* 2015;24(7):1098–1105. **(LOE III)**.

148. Maruyama M, et al. Outcomes of an open autologous osteochondral plug graft for capitellar osteochondritis dissecans: time to return to sports. *Am J Sports Med.* 2014;42(9):2122–2127. **(LOE IV)**.

149. DiFiori JP, Puffer JC, Aish B, Dorey F. Wrist pain, distal radial physeal injury, and ulnar variance in young gymnasts: does a relationship exist? *Am J Sports Med.* 2002;30(6):879–885. **(LOE III)**.

150. Lluch A, Garcia-Elias M. Etiology of Kienböck disease. *Tech Hand Up Extrem Surg.* 2011;15(1):33–37. **(LOE V)**.

151. Roy S, Caine D, Singer KM. Stress changes of the distal radial epiphysis in young gymnasts. A report of twenty-one cases and a review of the literature. *Am J Sports Med.* 1985;13(5):301–308. **(LOE IV)**.

152. Albanese SA, Palmer AK, Kerr DR, Carpenter CW, Lisi D, Levinsohn EM. Wrist pain and distal growth plate closure of the radius in gymnasts. *J Pediatr Orthop.* 1989;9(1):23–28. **(LOE IV)**.

153. Ellington MD, Edmonds EW. Pediatric elbow and wrist pathology related to sports participation. *Orthop Clin North Am.* 2016;47(4):743–748. **(LOE V)**.

154. Dwek JR, Cardoso F, Chung CB. MR imaging of overuse injuries in the skeletally immature gymnast: spectrum of soft-tissue and osseous lesions in the hand and wrist. *Pediatr Radiol.* 2009;39(12):1310–1316. **(LOE III)**.

155. Nakamoto JC, Saito M, Medina G, Schor B. Scaphoid stress fracture in high-level gymnast: a case report. *Case Rep Orthop.* 2011;2011:492407. **(LOE IV)**.

156. Mandelbaum BR, Bartolozzi AR, Davis CA, Teurlings L, Bragonier B. Wrist pain syndrome in the gymnast. Pathogenetic, diagnostic, and therapeutic considerations. *Am J Sports Med.* 1989;17(3):305–317. **(LOE IV)**.

157. Yamabe E, Nakamura T, Pham P, Yoshioka H. The athlete's wrist: ulnar-sided pain. *Semin Musculoskelet Radiol.* 2012;16(4):331–337. **(LOE V)**.

158. McAdams TR, Swan J, Yao J. Arthroscopic treatment of triangular fibrocartilage wrist injuries in the athlete. *Am J Sports Med.* 2009;37(2):291–297. **(LOE IV)**.

159. Auringer ST, Anthony EY. Common pediatric sports injuries. *Semin Musculoskelet Radiol.* 1999;3(3):247–256. **(LOE V)**.

160. Micheli LJ. *Pediatric and Adolescent Sports Medicine.* 1st ed. Boston: Little Brown; 1984. **(LOE N/A)**.

161. Vavken P, Wimmer MD, Camathias C, Quidde J, Valderrabano V, Pagenstert G. Treating patella instability in skeletally immature patients. *Arthroscopy.* 2013;29(8):1410–1422. **(LOE IV)**.

162. Harper DK, Craig JG, van Holsbeeck MT. Apophyseal injuries of the lesser tuberosity in adolescents: a series of five cases. *Emerg Radiol.* 2013;20(1):33–37. **(LOE IV)**.

163. Andrew JR, Baker CL, Curl WW, Gidumal R. *Surgical Repair of Acute and Chronic Lesions of the Lateral Capsuar Complex of the Knee. The Cruciate Ligaments: Diagnosis and Treatment of Ligamentous Injuries of the Knee.* New York: Livingstone; 1988. **(LOE N/A)**.

164. Rossi F, Dragoni S. Acute avulsion fractures of the pelvis in adolescent competitive athletes: prevalence, location and sports distribution of 203 cases collected. *Skeletal Radiol.* 2001;30(3):127–131. **(LOE III)**.

165. Balcarek P, Jung K, Frosch KH, Sturmer KM. Value of the tibial tuberosity-trochlear groove distance in patellar instability in the young athlete. *Am J Sports Med.* 2011;39(8):1756–1761. **(LOE III)**.

166. Combs J. Hip and pelvis avulsion fractures in adolescents: proper diagnosis improves compliance. *Physician and Sportsmedicine.* 1994;22(7):41–49. **(LOE III)**.

167. Dalzell D, Auringer ST. Problem children: common fractures commonly missed. *Postgraduate Radiology.* 1998;18:170–183. **(LOE IV)**.

168. McKinney BI, Nelson C, Carrion W. Apophyseal avulsion fractures of the hip and pelvis. *Orthopedics.* 2009;32(1):42. **(LOE V)**.

169. Irving MH. Exostosis formation after traumatic avulsion of the anterior inferior iliac spine. Report of two cases. *J Bone Joint Surg Br.* 1964;46:720–722. **(LOE IV)**.

170. Kong CG, In Y, Kim SJ, Sur YJ. Avulsion fracture of the iliac crest apophysis treated with open reduction and internal fixation. *J Orthop Trauma.* 2011;25(6):e56–e58. **(LOE IV)**.

171. Rajasekhar C, Kumar KS, Bhamra MS. Avulsion fractures of the anterior inferior iliac spine: the case for surgical intervention. *Int Orthop.* 2001;24(6):364–365. **(LOE IV)**.

172. Stanitski CL. Pediatric and adolescent sports injuries. *Clin Sports Med.* 1997;16(4):613–633. **(LOE V)**.

173. Bertin KC, Goble EM. Ligament injuries associated with physeal fractures about the knee. *Clin Orthop Relat Res.* 1983;(177):188–195. **(LOE III)**.

174. Rang M. *Children's Fractures.* Philadelphia: J.B. Lippincott; 1974. **(LOE N/A)**.

175. Delee JC. Ligamentous injury of the knee. In: Stanitski CL, Delee JC, Drez DJ Jr, eds. *Pediatric and Adolescent Sports Medicine.* Vol. 3. Philadelphia: W.B. Saunders; 1994:406–432. **(LOE N/A)**.

176. Buckley SL, Sturm PF, Tosi LL, Thomas MD, Robertson WW Jr. Ligamentous instability of the knee in children sustaining fractures of the femur: a prospective study with knee examination under anesthesia. *J Pediatr Orthop.* 1996;16(2):206–209. **(LOE II)**.

177. Goodrich A, Ballard A. Posterior cruciate ligament avulsion associated with ipsilateral femur fracture in a 10-year-old child. *J Trauma.* 1988;28(9):1393–1396. **(LOE IV)**.

178. Poulsen TD, Skak SV, Jensen TT. Epiphyseal fractures of the proximal tibia. *Injury.* 1989;20(2):111–113. **(LOE IV)**.

179. Sullivan JA, Anderson SJ. *Care of the Young Athlete.* [Rosemont, Ill.] [Elk Grove Village, Ill.]: American Academy of Orthopaedic Surgeons. American Academy of Pediatrics; 2000. **(LOE N/A)**.

180. Shea KG, Pfeiffer R, Wang JH, Curtin M, Apel PJ. Anterior cruciate ligament injury in pediatric and adolescent soccer players: an analysis of insurance data. *J Pediatr Orthop.* 2004;24(6):623–628. **(LOE V)**.

181. Swenson DM, Collins CL, Best TM, Flanigan DC, Fields SK, Comstock RD. Epidemiology of knee injuries among U.S. high school athletes, 2005/2006-2010/2011. *Med Sci Sports Exerc.* 2013;45(3):462–469. **(LOE IV)**.

182. Micheli LJ, Rask B, Gerberg L. Anterior cruciate ligament reconstruction in patients who are prepubescent. *Clin Orthop Relat Res.* 1999;(364):40–47. **(LOE IV)**.

183. Micheli LJ, Metzl JD, Di Canzio J, Zurakowski D. Anterior cruciate ligament reconstructive surgery in adolescent soccer and basketball players. *Clin J Sport Med.* 1999;9(3):138–141. **(LOE III)**.

184. Powell JW, Barber-Foss KD. Sex-related injury patterns among selected high school sports. *Am J Sports Med.* 2000;28(3):385–391. **(LOE IV)**.

185. Shea KG, Apel PJ, Pfeiffer RP, Showalter LD, Traughber PD. The tibial attachment of the anterior cruciate ligament in children and adolescents: analysis of magnetic resonance imaging. *Knee Surg Sports Traumatol Arthrosc.* 2002;10(2):102–108. **(LOE IV)**.

186. Shea KG, Apel PJ, Pfeiffer RP, Traughber PD. The anatomy of the proximal tibia in pediatric and adolescent patients: implications for ACL reconstruction and prevention of physeal arrest. *Knee Surg Sports Traumatol Arthrosc.* 2007;15(4):320–327. **(LOE IV)**.

187. Griffin LY, Agel J, Albohm MJ, et al. Noncontact anterior cruciate ligament injuries: risk factors and prevention strategies. *J Am Acad Orthop Surg.* 2000;8(3):141–150. **(LOE III)**.

188. Griffin LY, Albohm MJ, Arendt EA, et al. Understanding and preventing noncontact anterior cruciate ligament injuries: a review of the Hunt Valley II meeting, January 2005. *Am J Sports Med.* 2006;34(9):1512–1532. **(LOE III)**.

189. Aichroth PM, Patel DV, Zorrilla P. The natural history and treatment of rupture of the anterior cruciate ligament in children and adolescents. A prospective review. *J Bone Joint Surg Br.* 2002;84(1):38–41. **(LOE II)**.

190. Angel KR, Hall DJ. Anterior cruciate ligament injury in children and adolescents. *Arthroscopy.* 1989;5(3):197–200. **(LOE III)**.

191. Janarv PM, Nystrom A, Werner S, Hirsch G. Anterior cruciate ligament injuries in skeletally immature patients. *J Pediatr Orthop.* 1996;16(5):673–677. **(LOE II)**.

192. McCarroll JR, Rettig AC, Shelbourne KD. Anterior cruciate ligament injuries in the young athlete with open physes. *Am J Sports Med.* 1988;16(1):44–47. **(LOE IV)**.

193. Pressman AE, Letts RM, Jarvis JG. Anterior cruciate ligament tears in children: an analysis of operative versus nonoperative treatment. *J Pediatr Orthop.* 1997;17(4):505–511. **(LOE III)**.

194. Henry J, Chotel F, Chouteau J, Fessy MH, Berard J, Moyen B. Rupture of the anterior cruciate ligament in children: early reconstruction with open physes or delayed reconstruction to skeletal maturity? *Knee Surg Sports Traumatol Arthrosc.* 2009;17(7):748–755. **(LOE III)**.

195. Lawrence JT, Argawal N, Ganley TJ. Degeneration of the knee joint in skeletally immature patients with a diagnosis of an anterior cruciate ligament tear: is there harm in delay of treatment? *Am J Sports Med.* 2011;39(12):2582–2587. **(LOE III)**.

196. Millett PJ, Willis AA, Warren RF. Associated injuries in pediatric and adolescent anterior cruciate ligament tears: does a delay in treatment increase the risk of meniscal tear? *Arthroscopy.* 2002;18(9):955–959. **(LOE III)**.

197. Anderson AF. Transepiphyseal replacement of the anterior cruciate ligament in skeletally immature patients. A preliminary report. *J Bone Joint Surg Am.* 2003;85-A(7):1255–1263. **(LOE II)**.

198. Anderson AF. Transepiphyseal replacement of the anterior cruciate ligament using quadruple hamstring grafts in skeletally immature patients. *J Bone Joint Surg Am.* 2004;86-A (suppl 1) (Pt 2):201–209. **(LOE II)**.

199. Kocher MS, Garg S, Micheli LJ. Physeal sparing reconstruction of the anterior cruciate ligament in skeletally immature prepubescent children and adolescents. Surgical technique. *J Bone Joint Surg Am.* 2006;88 (suppl 1) Pt 2:283–293.**(LOE IV)**.

200. Cohen M, Ferretti M, Quarteiro M, et al. Transphyseal anterior cruciate ligament reconstruction in patients with open physes. *Arthroscopy.* 2009;25(8):831–838. **(LOE IV)**.

201. Kocher MS, Smith JT, Zoric BJ, Lee B, Micheli LJ. Transphyseal anterior cruciate ligament reconstruction in skeletally immature pubescent adolescents. *J Bone Joint Surg Am.* 2007;89(12):2632–2639. **(LOE IV)**.

202. Kumar S, Ahearne D, Hunt DM. Transphyseal anterior cruciate ligament reconstruction in the skeletally immature: follow-up to a minimum of sixteen years of age. *J Bone Joint Surg Am.* 2013;95(1):e1. **(LOE II)**.

203. Deitch J, Mehlman CT, Foad SL, Obbehat A, Mallory M. Traumatic anterior shoulder dislocation in adolescents. *Am J Sports Med.* 2003;31(5):758–763. **(LOE IV)**.

204. Matava MJ, Siegel MG. Arthroscopic reconstruction of the ACL with semitendinosus-gracilis autograft in skeletally immature adolescent patients. *Am J Knee Surg.* 1997;10(2):60–69. **(LOE IV)**.

205. McCarroll JR, Shelbourne KD, Porter DA, Rettig AC, Murray S. Patellar tendon graft reconstruction for midsubstance anterior cruciate ligament rupture in junior high school athletes. An algorithm for management. *Am J Sports Med.* 1994;22(4):478–484. **(LOE IV)**.

206. Barber FA. Anterior cruciate ligament reconstruction in the skeletally immature high-performance athlete: what to do and when to do it? *Arthroscopy.* 2000;16(4):391–392. **(LOE V)**.

207. Kocher MS, Sterett WI, Briggs KK, Zurakowski D, Steadman JR. Effect of functional bracing on subsequent knee injury in ACL-deficient professional skiers. *J Knee Surg.* 2003;16(2):87–92. **(LOE III)**.

208. Koman JD, Sanders JO. Valgus deformity after reconstruction of the anterior cruciate ligament in a skeletally immature patient. A case report. *J Bone Joint Surg Am.* 1999;81(5):711–715. **(LOE IV)**.

209. Fabricant PD, Jones KJ, Delos D, et al. Reconstruction of the anterior cruciate ligament in the skeletally immature athlete: a review of current concepts: AAOS exhibit selection. *J Bone Joint Surg Am.* 2013;95(5):e28. **(LOE III)**.

210. Frosch KH, Stengel D, Brodhun T, et al. Outcomes and risks of operative treatment of rupture of the anterior cruciate ligament in children and adolescents. *Arthroscopy.* 2010;26(11):1539–1550. **(LOE IV)**.

211. Shea KG, Jacobs JC Jr, Carey JL, Anderson AF, Oxford JT. Osteochondritis dissecans knee histology studies have variable findings and theories of etiology. *Clin Orthop Relat Res.* 2013;471(4):1127–1136. **(LOE V)**.

212. Anderson CN, Anderson AF. Tibial eminence fractures. *Clin Sports Med.* 2011;30(4):727–742. **(LOE V)**.

213. Cooper DE, Warren RF, Warner JJ. The posterior cruciate ligament and posterolateral structures of the knee: anatomy, function, and patterns of injury. *Instr Course Lect.* 1991;40:249–270. **(LOE II)**.

214. Shea KG, Grimm NL. Arthroscopic tibial spine or eminence repair - retraction tool for intermeniscal ligament to facilitate reduction of the tibial spine. *Tech Knee Surg.* 2010;9(4). **(LOE V)**.

215. Shea KG, Grimm NL, Laor T, Wall E. Bone bruises and meniscal tears on MRI in skeletally immature children with tibial eminence fractures. *J Pediatr Orthop.* 2011;31(2):150–152. **(LOE IV)**.

216. Chen SY, Cheng CY, Chang SS, et al. Arthroscopic suture fixation for avulsion fractures in the tibial attachment of the posterior cruciate ligament. *Arthroscopy.* 2012;28(10):1454–1463. **(LOE IV)**.

217. Sawyer GA, Anderson BC, Paller D, Schiller J, Eberson CP, Hulstyn M. Biomechanical analysis of suture bridge fixation for tibial eminence fractures. *Arthroscopy.* 2012;28(10):1533–1539. **(LOE N/A)**.

218. Schneppendahl J, Thelen S, Twehues S, et al. The use of biodegradable sutures for the fixation of tibial eminence fractures in children: a comparison using PDS II, Vicryl and FiberWire. *J Pediatr Orthop.* 2013;33(4):409–414. **(LOE N/A)**.

219. Hapa O, Barber FA, Suner G, et al. Biomechanical comparison of tibial eminence fracture fixation with high-strength suture, EndoButton, and suture anchor. *Arthroscopy.* 2012;28(5):681–687. **(LOE N/A)**.

220. Johnson DL, Durbin TC. Physeal-sparing tibial eminence fracture fixation with a headless compression screw. *Orthopedics.* 2012;35(7):604–608. **(LOE III)**.

221. Pan RY, Yang JJ, Chang JH, Shen HC, Lin LC, Lian YT. Clinical outcome of arthroscopic fixation of anterior tibial eminence avulsion fractures in skeletally mature patients: a comparison of suture and screw fixation technique. *J Trauma Acute Care Surg.* 2012;72(2):E88–E93. **(LOE III)**.

222. Anderson CN, Nyman JS, McCullough KA, et al. Biomechanical evaluation of physeal-sparing fixation methods in tibial eminence fractures. *Am J Sports Med.* 2013;41(7):1586–1594. **(LOE N/A)**.

223. Patel NM, Park MJ, Sampson NR, Ganley TJ. Tibial eminence fractures in children: earlier posttreatment mobilization results in improved outcomes. *J Pediatr Orthop.* 2012;32(2):139–144. **(LOE III)**.

224. Grood ES, Noyes FR, Butler DL, Suntay WJ. Ligamentous and capsular restraints preventing straight medial and lateral laxity in intact human cadaver knees. *J Bone Joint Surg Am.* 1981;63(8):1257–1269. **(LOE III)**.

225. Indelicato PA. Isolated medial collateral ligament injuries in the knee. *J Am Acad Orthop Surg.* 1995;3(1):9–14. **(LOE IV)**.

226. Warren LA, Marshall JL, Girgis F. The prime static stabilizer of the medial side of the knee. *J Bone Joint Surg Am.* 1974;56(4):665–674. **(LOE N/A)**.

227. Warren LF, Marshall JL. The supporting structures and layers on the medial side of the knee: an anatomical analysis. *J Bone Joint Surg Am.* 1979;61(1):56–62. **(LOE N/A)**.

228. Inoue M, McGurk-Burleson E, Hollis JM, Woo SL. Treatment of the medial collateral ligament injury. I: the importance of anterior cruciate ligament on the varus-valgus knee laxity. *Am J Sports Med.* 1987;15(1):15–21. **(LOE III)**.

229. Linton RC, Indelicato PA. Medial ligament injuries. In: Drez DJ Jr, ed. *Orthopaedic Sports Medicine.* Vol. 2. Philadelphia: W.B. Sanders; 1994:1261–1274. **(LOE N/A)**.

230. Muller W. *The Knee: Form, Function, and Ligament Reconstruction.* New York: Springer-Verlag; 1983. **(LOE N/A)**.

231. Kennedy JC, Fowler PJ. Medial and anterior instability of the knee. An anatomical and clinical study using stress machines. *J Bone Joint Surg Am.* 1971;53(7):1257–1270. **(LOE III)**.

232. Miller MD, Ritchie JR, Gomez BA, Royster RM, DeLee JC. Meniscal repair. An experimental study in the goat. *Am J Sports Med.* 1995;23(1):124–128. **(LOE N/A)**.

233. Bitar AC, Demange MK, D'Elia CO, Camanho GL. Traumatic patellar dislocation: nonoperative treatment compared with MPFL reconstruction using patellar tendon. *Am J Sports Med.* 2012;40(1):114–122. **(LOE I)**.

234. Bradley GW, Shives TC, Samuelson KM. Ligament injuries in the knees of children. *J Bone Joint Surg Am.* 1979;61(4):588–591. **(LOE IV)**.

235. Eiskjaer S, Larsen ST, Schmidt MB. The significance of hemarthrosis of the knee in children. *Arch Orthop Trauma Surg.* 1988;107(2):96–98. **(LOE III)**.

236. Kennedy JC. *The Injured Adolescent Knee.* Baltimore: Williams and Wilkins; 1979. **(LOE N/A)**.

237. Joseph KN, Fogrund H. Traumatic rupture of the medial ligament of the knee in a four-year-old boy. *J Bone Joint Surg Am.* 1978;60(3):402–403. **(LOE IV)**.

238. Hughston JC. Anterior cruciate deficient knee. *Am J Sports Med.* 1983;11(1):1–2. **(LOE IV)**.

239. O'Donoghue DH. An analysis of end results of surgical treatment of major injuries to the ligaments of the knee. *J Bone Joint Surg Am.* 1955;37-A(1):1–13; passim. **(LOE V)**.

240. Kannus P. Long-term results of conservatively treated medial collateral ligament injuries of the knee joint. *Clin Orthop Relat Res.* 1988;(226):103–112. **(LOE III)**.

241. Kannus P, Jarvinen M. Knee ligament injuries in adolescents. Eight year follow-up of conservative management. *J Bone Joint Surg Br.* 1988;70(5):772–776. **(LOE III)**.

242. Allen CR, Wong EK, Livesay GA, Sakane M, Fu FH, Woo SL. Importance of the medial meniscus in the anterior cruciate ligament-deficient knee. *J Orthop Res.* 2000;18(1):109–115. **(LOE N/A)**.

243. Woo SL, Jia F, Zou L, Gabriel MT. Functional tissue engineering for ligament healing: potential of antisense gene therapy. *Ann Biomed Eng.* 2004;32(3):342–351. **(LOE N/A)**.

244. Woo SL, Vogrin TM, Abramowitch SD. Healing and repair of ligament injuries in the knee. *J Am Acad Orthop Surg.* 2000;8(6):364–372. **(LOE V)**.

245. Hastings DE. The non-operative management of collateral ligament injuries of the knee joint. *Clin Orthop Relat Res.* 1980;147:22–28. **(LOE IV)**.

246. Indelicato PA. The importance of the posterior oblique ligament in repairs of acute tears of the medial ligaments in knees with and without an associated rupture of the anterior cruciate ligament. Results of long-term follow-up [letter; comment]. *J Bone Joint Surg Am.* 1995;77(6):969. **(LOE IV)**.

247. LaPrade RF. *The Medial Collateral Ligament Complex and Posterolateral Aspect of the Knee. Orthopaedic Knowledge Update.* Rosemont, IL: American Academy of Orthopaedic Surgeons; 1999:327–340. **(LOE N/A)**.

248. LaPrade RF, Resig S, Wentorf F, Lewis JL. The effects of grade III posterolateral knee complex injuries on anterior cruciate ligament graft force. A biomechanical analysis. *Am J Sports Med.* 1999;27(4):469–475. **(LOE N/A)**.

249. Derscheid GL, Garrick JG. Medial collateral ligament injuries in football. Nonoperative management of grade I and grade II sprains. *Am J Sports Med.* 1981;9(6):365–368. **(LOE III)**.

250. Sankar WN, Wells L, Sennett BJ, Wiesel BB, Ganley TJ. Combined anterior cruciate ligament and medial collateral ligament injuries in adolescents. *J Pediatr Orthop.* 2006;26(6):733–736. **(LOE III)**.

251. Krudwig WK, Witzel U, Ullrich K. Posterolateral aspect and stability of the knee joint. II. Posterolateral instability and effect of isolated and combined posterolateral reconstruction on knee stability: a biomechanical study. *Knee Surg Sports Traumatol Arthrosc.* 2002;10(2):91–95. **(LOE III)**.

252. Seebacher JR, Inglis AE, Marshall JL, Warren RF. The structure of the posterolateral aspect of the knee. *J Bone Joint Surg Am.* 1982;64(4):536–541. **(LOE IV)**.

253. Meister BR, Michael SP, Moyer RA, Kelly JD, Schneck CD. Anatomy and kinematics of the lateral collateral ligament of the knee. *Am J Sports Med.* 2000;28(6):869–878. **(LOE N/A)**.

254. Chen FS, Rokito AS, Pitman MI. Acute and chronic posterolateral rotatory instability of the knee. *J Am Acad Orthop Surg.* 2000;8(2):97–110. **(LOE III)**.

255. Pasque C, Noyes FR, Gibbons M, Levy M, Grood E. The role of the popliteofibular ligament and the tendon of popliteus in providing stability in the human knee. *J Bone Joint Surg Br.* 2003;85(2):292–298. **(LOE N/A)**.

256. Hagemeister N, Long R, Yahia L, et al. Quantitative comparison of three different types of anterior cruciate ligament reconstruction methods: laxity and 3-D kinematic measurements. *Biomed Mater Eng.* 2002;12(1):47–57. **(LOE N/A)**.

257. Ullrich K, Krudwig WK, Witzel U. Posterolateral aspect and stability of the knee joint. I. Anatomy and function of the popliteus muscle-tendon unit: an anatomical and biomechanical study. *Knee Surg Sports Traumatol Arthrosc.* 2002;10(2):86–90. **(LOE N/A)**.

258. Hughston JC. The importance of the posterior oblique ligament in repairs of acute tears of the medial ligaments in knees with and without an associated rupture of the anterior cruciate ligament. Results of long-term follow- up [see comments]. *J Bone Joint Surg Am.* 1994;76(9):1328–1344. **(LOE IV)**.

259. Hughston JC, Andrews JR, Cross MJ, Moschi A. Classification of knee ligament instabilities. Part I. The medial compartment and cruciate ligaments. *J Bone Joint Surg Am.* 1976;58(2):159–172. **(LOE IV)**.

260. LaPrade RF, Terry GC, Montgomery RD, Curd D, Simmons DJ. The effects of aggressive notchplasty on the normal knee in dogs. *Am J Sports Med.* 1998;26(2):193–200. **(LOE N/A)**.

261. Veltri DM, Deng XH, Torzilli PA, Warren RF, Maynard MJ. The role of the cruciate and posterolateral ligaments in stability of the knee. A biomechanical study. *Am J Sports Med.* 1995;23(4):436–443. **(LOE N/A)**.

262. Veltri DM, Warren RF. Posterolateral instability of the knee. *Instr Course Lect.* 1995;44:441–453. **(LOE V)**.

263. Veltri DM, Warren RF. Anatomy, biomechanics, and physical findings in posterolateral knee instability. *Clin Sports Med.* 1994;13(3):599–614. **(LOE V)**.

264. Veltri DM, Warren RF. Operative treatment of posterolateral instability of the knee. *Clin Sports Med.* 1994;13(3):615–627. **(LOE V)**.

265. Bergstrom R, Gillquist J, Lysholm J, Hamberg P. Arthroscopy of the knee in children. *J Pediatr Orthop.* 1984;4(5):542–545. **(LOE III)**.

266. Kendall NS, Hsu SY, Chan KM. Fracture of the tibial spine in adults and children. A review of 31 cases. *J Bone Joint Surg Br.* 1992;74(6):848–852. **(LOE IV)**.

267. Kovack TJ, Jacob PB, Tesner R, Papp G. Periosteal avulsion of the posterolateral corner of the knee in an adolescent: an unreported case. *Orthopedics.* 2011;34(10):791–794. **(LOE IV)**.

268. Cooper DE, Stewart D. Posterior cruciate ligament reconstruction using single-bundle patella tendon graft with tibial inlay fixation: 2- to 10-year follow-up. *Am J Sports Med.* 2004;32(2):346–360. **(LOE II)**.

269. Havranek P. Proximal fibular physeal injury. *J Pediatr Orthop B.* 1996;5(2):115–118. **(LOE IV)**.

270. Veltri DM, Warren RF. Isolated and combined posterior cruciate ligament injuries. *J Am Acad Orthop Surg.* 1993;1(2):67–75. **(LOE V)**.

271. LaPrade RF, Hamilton CD. The fibular collateral ligament-biceps femoris bursa. An anatomic study. *Am J Sports Med.* 1997;25(4):439–443. **(LOE N/A)**.

272. LaPrade RF, Terry GC. Injuries to the posterolateral aspect of the knee. Association of anatomic injury patterns with clinical instability. *Am J Sports Med.* 1997;25(4):433–438. **(LOE II)**.

273. Baker CL Jr, Norwood LA, Hughston JC. Acute combined posterior cruciate and posterolateral instability of the knee. *Am J Sports Med.* 1984;12(3):204–208. **(LOE III)**.

274. DeLee JC, Riley MB, Rockwood CA Jr. Acute posterolateral rotatory instability of the knee. *Am J Sports Med.* 1983;11(4):199–207. **(LOE IV)**.

275. Hughston JC, Bowden JA, Andrews JR, Norwood LA. Acute tears of the posterior cruciate ligament. Results of operative treatment. *J Bone Joint Surg Am.* 1980;62(3):438–450. **(LOE IV)**.

276. Hughston JC, Norwood LA Jr. The posterolateral drawer test and external rotational recurvatum test for posterolateral rotatory instability of the knee. *Clin Orthop Relat Res.* 1980;(147):82–87. **(LOE III)**.

277. Kannus P. Nonoperative treatment of grade II and III sprains of the lateral ligament compartment of the knee. *Am J Sports Med.* 1989;17(1):83–88. **(LOE II)**.

278. Chen CH, Chen WJ, Shih CH. Lateral collateral ligament reconstruction using quadriceps tendon-patellar bone autograft with bioscrew fixation. *Arthroscopy.* 2001;17(5):551–554. **(LOE IV)**.

279. Chen CH, Chen WJ, Shih CH. One-incision endoscopic technique for posterior cruciate ligament reconstruction with quadriceps tendon-patellar bone autograft. *Arthroscopy.* 2001;17(3):329–332. **(LOE IV)**.

280. Latimer HA, Tibone JE, ElAttrache NS, McMahon PJ. Reconstruction of the lateral collateral ligament of the knee with patellar tendon allograft. Report of a new technique in combined ligament injuries [see comments]. *Am J Sports Med.* 1998;26(5):656–662. **(LOE IV)**.

281. Noyes FR, Barber-Westin SD. The treatment of acute combined ruptures of the anterior cruciate and medial ligaments of the knee. *Am J Sports Med.* 1995;23(4):380–389. **(LOE II)**.

282. Lill H, Glasmacher S, Korner J, Rose T, Verheyden P, Josten C. Arthroscopic-assisted simultaneous reconstruction of the posterior cruciate ligament and the lateral collateral ligament using hamstrings and absorbable screws. *Arthroscopy.* 2001;17(8):892–897. **(LOE IV)**.

283. Shea KG, Apel PJ, Pfeiffer RP. Anterior cruciate ligament injury in paediatric and adolescent patients: a review of basic science and clinical research. *Sports Med.* 2003;33(6):455–471. **(LOE V)**.

284. Anderson AF, Anderson CN. Posterior cruciate and posterolateral ligament reconstruction in an adolescent with open physes. A case report. *J Bone Joint Surg Am.* 2007;89(7):1598–1604. **(LOE IV)**.

285. Harner CD, Hoher J. Evaluation and treatment of posterior cruciate ligament injuries. *Am J Sports Med.* 1998;26(3):471–482. **(LOE III)**.

286. Morgan CD, Kalman VR, Grawl DM. The anatomic origin of the posterior cruciate ligament: where is it? Reference landmarks for PCL reconstruction. *Arthroscopy.* 1997;13(3):325–331. **(LOE IV)**.

287. The knee: ligaments. In: Herring JA, ed. *Tachdjian's Pediatric Orthopaedics.* Vol. 3. Philadelphia: W.B. Saunders; 2002:2356. **(LOE N/A)**.

288. Harner CD, Livesay GA, Kashiwaguchi S, Fujie H, Choi NY, Woo SL. Comparative study of the size and shape of human anterior and posterior cruciate ligaments. *J Orthop Res.* 1995;13(3):429–434. **(LOE N/A)**.

289. Harner CD, Xerogeanes JW, Livesay GA, et al. The human posterior cruciate ligament complex: an interdisciplinary study. Ligament morphology and biomechanical evaluation. *Am J Sports Med.* 1995;23(6):736–745. **(LOE IV)**.

290. Greis PE, Georgescu HI, Fu FH, Evans CH. Particle-induced synthesis of collagenase by synovial fibroblasts: an immunocytochemical study. *J Orthop Res.* 1994;12(2):286–293. **(LOE III)**.

291. Frank C, Strother R. Isolated posterior cruciate ligament injury in a child: literature review and a case report. *Can J Surg.* 1989;32(5):373–374. **(LOE IV)**.

292. MacDonald PB, Black B, Old J, Dyck M, Davidson M. Posterior cruciate ligament injury and posterolateral instability in a 6-year-old child. A case report. *Am J Sports Med.* 2003;31(1):135–136. **(LOE IV)**.

293. Kim SJ, Jo SB, Kim SG, Park IS, Kim HP, Kim SH. Peel-off injury at the tibial attachment of the posterior cruciate ligament in children. *Am J Sports Med.* 2010;38(9):1900–1906. **(LOE IV)**.

294. Ross AC, Chesterman PJ. Isolated avulsion of the tibial attachment of the posterior cruciate ligament in childhood. *J Bone Joint Surg Br.* 1986;68(5):747. **(LOE V)**.

295. Torisu T. Avulsion fracture of the tibial attachment of the posterior cruciate ligament. Indications and results of delayed repair. *Clin Orthop Relat Res.* 1979;(143):107–114. **(LOE IV)**.

296. Itokazu M, Yamane T, Shoen S. Incomplete avulsion of the femoral attachment of the posterior cruciate ligament with an osteochondral fragment in a twelve-year-old boy. *Arch Orthop Trauma Surg.* 1990;110(1):55–57. **(LOE IV)**.

297. Lobenhoffer P, Wunsch L, Bosch U, Krettek C. Arthroscopic repair of the posterior cruciate ligament in a 3-year-old child. *Arthroscopy.* 1997;13(2):248–253. **(LOE IV)**.

298. Mayer PJ, Micheli LJ. Avulsion of the femoral attachment of the posterior cruciate ligament in an eleven-year-old boy. Case report. *J Bone Joint Surg Am.* 1979;61(3):431–432. **(LOE IV)**.

299. Suprock MD, Rogers VP. Posterior cruciate avulsion. *Orthopedics.* 1990;13(6):659–662. **(LOE V)**.

300. Fowler PJ, Messieh SS. Isolated posterior cruciate ligament injuries in athletes. *Am J Sports Med.* 1987;15(6):553–557. **(LOE III)**.

301. Parolie JM, Bergfeld JA. Long-term results of nonoperative treatment of isolated posterior cruciate ligament injuries in the athlete. *Am J Sports Med.* 1986;14(1):35–38. **(LOE IV)**.

302. Torg JS, Barton TM, Pavlov H, Stine R. Natural history of the posterior cruciate ligament-deficient knee. *Clin Orthop Relat Res.* 1989;(246):208–216. **(LOE III)**.

303. Boynton MD, Tietjens BR. Long-term followup of the untreated isolated posterior cruciate ligament-deficient knee. *Am J Sports Med.* 1996;24(3):306–310. **(LOE III)**.

304. Dandy DJ, Pusey RJ. The long-term results of unrepaired tears of the posterior cruciate ligament. *J Bone Joint Surg Br.* 1982;64(1):92–94. **(LOE IV)**.

305. Geissler WB, Whipple TL. Intraarticular abnormalities in association with posterior cruciate ligament injuries. *Am J Sports Med.* 1993;21(6):846–849. **(LOE IV)**.

306. Keller PM, Shelbourne KD, McCarroll JR, Rettig AC. Nonoperatively treated isolated posterior cruciate ligament injuries. *Am J Sports Med.* 1993;21(1):132–136. **(LOE III)**.

307. Shelbourne KD, Davis TJ, Patel DV. The natural history of acute, isolated, nonoperatively treated posterior cruciate ligament injuries. A prospective study. *Am J Sports Med.* 1999;27(3):276–283. **(LOE II)**.

308. Kocher MS, Shore B, Nasreddine AY, Heyworth BE. Treatment of posterior cruciate ligament injuries in pediatric and adolescent patients. *J Pediatr Orthop.* 2012;32(6):553–560. **(LOE IV)**.

309. Sanders WE, Wilkins KE, Neidre A. Acute insufficiency of the posterior cruciate ligament in children. Two case reports. *J Bone Joint Surg Am.* 1980;62(1):129–131. **(LOE IV)**.

310. Meyers MH. Isolated avulsion of the tibial attachment of the posterior cruciate ligament of the knee. *J Bone Joint Surg Am.* 1975;57(5):669–672. **(LOE IV)**.

311. Bovid KM, Salata MJ, Vander Have KL, Sekiya JK. Arthroscopic posterior cruciate ligament reconstruction in a skeletally immature patient: a new technique with case report. *Arthroscopy.* 2010;26(4):563–570. **(LOE IV)**.

312. Burns WC 2nd, Draganich LF, Pyevich M, Reider B. The effect of femoral tunnel position and graft tensioning technique on posterior laxity of the posterior cruciate ligament-reconstructed knee. *Am J Sports Med.* 1995;23(4):424–430. **(LOE IV)**.

313. Pearsall AT, Pyevich M, Draganich LF, Larkin JJ, Reider B. In vitro study of knee stability after posterior cruciate ligament reconstruction. *Clin Orthop.* 1996;(327):264–271. **(LOE N/A)**.

314. Covey DC, Sapega AA, Sherman GM. Testing for isometry during reconstruction of the posterior cruciate ligament. Anatomic and biomechanical considerations. *Am J Sports Med.* 1996;24(6):740–746. **(LOE IV)**.

315. Galloway MT, Grood ES, Mehalik JN, Levy M, Saddler SC, Noyes FR. Posterior cruciate ligament reconstruction. An in vitro study of femoral and tibial graft placement. *Am J Sports Med.* 1996;24(4):437–445. **(LOE IV)**.

316. Borden PS, Nyland JA, Caborn DN. Posterior cruciate ligament reconstruction (double bundle) using anterior tibialis tendon allograft. *Arthroscopy.* 2001;17(4):E14. **(LOE V)**.

317. Nyland J, Hester P, Caborn DN. Double-bundle posterior cruciate ligament reconstruction with allograft tissue: 2-year postoperative outcomes. *Knee Surg Sports Traumatol Arthrosc.* 2002;10(5):274–279. **(LOE IV)**.

318. Palilos LE. Bair BA. Transosseous reconstruction of the posterior cruciate ligament: single and double tunnel techniques. *Operative Techniques in Sports Medicine.* 2001;9(2):60–68. **(LOE V)**.

319. Stahelin AC, Sudkamp NP, Weiler A. Anatomic double-bundle posterior cruciate ligament reconstruction using hamstring tendons. *Arthroscopy.* 2001;17(1):88–97. **(LOE V)**.

320. Harner C, Giffin RB, Vogrin TM, Woo SL. Anatomy and biomechanics of the posterior cruciate ligament and posterolateral corner. *Operative Techniques in Sports Medicine.* 2001;9(2):39–46. **(LOE V)**.

321. Shea KG, Grimm NL, Belzer JS. Volumetric injury of the distal femoral physis during double-bundle ACL reconstruction in children: a three-dimensional study with use of magnetic resonance imaging. *J Bone Joint Surg Am.* 2011;93(11):1033–1038. **(LOE IV)**.

322. Accadbled F, Knorr J, Sales de Gauzy J. All inside transtibial arthroscopic posterior cruciate ligament reconstruction in skeletally immature: surgical technique and a case report. *Orthop Traumatol Surg Res.* 2013;99:361–365. **(LOE IV)**.

323. Warme WJ, Mickelson D. All-epiphyseal semitendinosus PCL reconstruction in a 10-year-old child. *J Pediatr Orthop.* 2010;30(5):465–468. **(LOE IV)**.

324. McManus F, Rang M, Heslin DJ. Acute dislocation of the patella in children. The natural history. *Clin Orthop Relat Res.* 1979;(139):88–91. **(LOE IV)**.

325. Buchner M. Acute traumatic primary patellar dislocation: long term result comparing conservative and surgical treatment. *Clin J Sport Med.* 2005;15(2):62–66. **(LOE III)**.

326. Harilainen A, Myllynen P, Antila H, Seitsalo S. The significance of arthroscopy and examination under anaesthesia in the diagnosis of fresh injury haemarthrosis of the knee joint. *Injury.* 1988;19(1):21–24. **(LOE II)**.

327. Nietosvaara Y, Aalto K, Kallio PE. Acute patellar dislocation in children: incidence and associated osteochondral fractures. *J Pediatr Orthop.* 1994;14(4):513–515. **(LOE III)**.

328. Atkin DM, Fithian DC, Marangi KS, Stone ML, Dobson BE, Mendelsohn C. Characteristics of patients with primary acute lateral patellar dislocation and their recovery within the first 6 months of injury. *Am J Sports Med.* 2000;28(4):472–479. **(LOE II)**.

329. Hinton RY, Sharma KM. Acute and recurrent patellar instability in the young athlete. *Orthop Clin North Am.* 2003;34(3):385–396. **(LOE V)**.

330. Fithian DC, Paxton EW, Cohen AB. Indications in the treatment of patellar instability. *J Knee Surg.* 2004;17(1):47–56. **(LOE III)**.

331. Fithian DC, Paxton EW, Post WR, Panni AS; International Patellofemoral Study Group. Lateral retinacular release: a survey of the International Patellofemoral Study Group. *Arthroscopy.* 2004;20(5):463–468. **(LOE IV)**.

332. Fithian DC, Paxton EW, Stone ML, et al. Epidemiology and natural history of acute patellar dislocation. *Am J Sports Med.* 2004;32(5):1114–1121. **(LOE II)**.

333. Cash JD, Hughston JC. Treatment of acute patellar dislocation. *Am J Sports Med.* 1988;16(3):244–249. **(LOE III)**.

334. Burks RT, Desio SM, Bachus KN, Tyson L, Springer K. Biomechanical evaluation of lateral patellar dislocations. *Am J Knee Surg.* 1998;11(1):24–31. **(LOE N/A)**.

335. Desio SM, Burks RT, Bachus KN. Soft tissue restraints to lateral patellar translation in the human knee. *Am J Sports Med.* 1998;26(1):59–65. **(LOE N/A)**.

336. Bassi RS, Kumar BA. Superior dislocation of the patella; a case report and review of the literature. *Emerg Med J.* 2003;20(1):97–98. **(LOE IV)**.

337. Beasley LS, Vidal AF. Traumatic patellar dislocation in children and adolescents: treatment update and literature review. *Curr Opin Pediatr.* 2004;16(1):29–36. **(LOE III)**.

338. Hughston JC, Deese M. Medial subluxation of the patella as a complication of lateral retinacular release. *Am J Sports Med.* 1988;16(4):383–388. **(LOE IV)**.

339. Joseph G, Devalia K, Kantam K, Shaath NM. Superior dislocation of the patella. Case report and review of literature. *Acta Orthop Belg.* 2005;71(3):369–371. **(LOE IV)**.

340. Choudhary RK, Tice JW. Intra-articular dislocation of the patella with incomplete rotation–two case reports and a review of the literature. *Knee.* 2004;11(2):125–127. **(LOE IV)**.

341. Dorizas JA, Stanitski CL. Anterior cruciate ligament injury in the skeletally immature. *Orthop Clin North Am.* 2003;34(3):355–363. **(LOE III)**.

342. Senavongse W, Farahmand F, Jones J, Andersen H, Bull AM, Amis AA. Quantitative measurement of patellofemoral joint stability: force-displacement behavior of the human patella in vitro. *J Orthop Res.* 2003;21(5):780–786. **(LOE N/A)**.

343. Arendt EA, Fithian DC, Cohen E. Current concepts of lateral patella dislocation. *Clin Sports Med.* 2002;21(3):499–519. **(LOE V)**.

344. Beals RK, Eckhardt AL. Hereditary onycho-osteodysplasia (Nail-Patella syndrome). A report of nine kindreds. *J Bone Joint Surg Am.* 1969;51(3):505–516. **(LOE IV)**.

345. Geary M, Schepsis A. Management of first-time patellar dislocations. *Orthopedics.* 2004;27(10):1058–1062. **(LOE V)**.

346. Schottle PB, Fucentese SF, Pfirrmann C, Bereiter H, Romero J. Trochleaplasty for patellar instability due to trochlear dysplasia: a minimum 2-year clinical and radiological follow-up of 19 knees. *Acta Orthop.* 2005;76(5):693–698. **(LOE IV)**.

347. Schottle PB, Fucentese SF, Romero J. Clinical and radiological outcome of medial patellofemoral ligament reconstruction with a semitendinosus autograft for patella instability. *Knee Surg Sports Traumatol Arthrosc.* 2005;13(7):516–521. **(LOE IV)**.

348. Lancourt JE, Cristini JA. Patella alta and patella infera. Their etiological role in patellar dislocation, chondromalacia, and apophysitis of the tibial tubercle. *J Bone Joint Surg Am.* 1975;57(8):1112–1115. **(LOE III)**.

349. Simmons E Jr, Cameron JC. Patella alta and recurrent dislocation of the patella. *Clin Orthop Relat Res.* 1992;(274):265–269. **(LOE IV)**.

350. Singerman R, Davy DT, Goldberg VM. Effects of patella alta and patella infera on patellofemoral contact forces. *J Biomech.* 1994;27(8):1059–1065. **(LOE N/A)**.

351. Airanow S, Zippel H. [Femoro-tibial torsion in patellar instability. A contribution to the pathogenesis of recurrent and habitual patellar dislocations]. *Beitr Orthop Traumatol.* 1990;37(6):311–316. **(LOE II)**.

352. Cameron JC, Saha S. External tibial torsion: an underrecognized cause of recurrent patellar dislocation. *Clin Orthop Relat Res.* 1996;328:177–184. **(LOE IV)**.

353. Elgafy H, El-Kawy S, Elsafy M, Ebraheim NA. Internal torsion of the distal femur as a cause of habitual dislocation of the patella: a case report and a review of causes of patellar dislocation. *Am J Orthop (Belle Mead NJ).* 2005;34(5):246–248. **(LOE IV)**.

354. Schoettle PB, Werner CM, Romero J. Reconstruction of the medial patellofemoral ligament for painful patellar subluxation in distal torsional malalignment: a case report. *Arch Orthop Trauma Surg.* 2005;125(9):644–648. **(LOE V)**.

355. Mizuno Y, Kumagai M, Mattessich SM, et al. Q-angle influences tibiofemoral and patellofemoral kinematics. *J Orthop Res.* 2001;19(5):834–840. **(LOE N/A)**.

356. Grelsamer RP, Bazos AN, Proctor CS. Radiographic analysis of patellar tilt. *J Bone Joint Surg Br.* 1993;75(5):822–824. **(LOE IV)**.

357. Pookarnjanamorakot C, Jaovisidha S, Apiyasawat P. The patellar tilt angle: correlation of MRI evaluation with anterior knee pain. *J Med Assoc Thai.* 1998;81(12):958–963. **(LOE III)**.

358. Maenpaa H, Lehto MU. Patellar dislocation has predisposing factors. A roentgenographic study on lateral and tangential views in patients and healthy controls. *Knee Surg Sports Traumatol Arthrosc.* 1996;4(4):212–216. **(LOE III)**.

359. Maenpaa H, Lehto MU. Patellar dislocation. The long-term results of nonoperative management in 100 patients. *Am J Sports Med.* 1997;25(2):213–217. **(LOE III)**.

360. Maenpaa H, Lehto MU. Patellofemoral osteoarthritis after patellar dislocation. *Clin Orthop Relat Res.* 1997;339:156–162. **(LOE II)**.

361. Balcarek P, Jung K, Ammon J, et al. Anatomy of lateral patellar instability: trochlear dysplasia and tibial tubercle-trochlear groove distance is more pronounced in women who dislocate the patella. *Am J Sports Med.* 2010;38(11):2320–2327. **(LOE III)**.

362. Stanitski CL. Articular hypermobility and chondral injury in patients with acute patellar dislocation. *Am J Sports Med.* 1995;23(2):146–150. **(LOE II)**.

363. Fucentese SF, Schottle PB, Pfirrmann CW, Romero J. CT changes after trochleoplasty for symptomatic trochlear dysplasia. *Knee Surg Sports Traumatol Arthrosc.* 2007;15(2):168–174. **(LOE IV)**.

364. Fucentese SF, von Roll A, Koch PP, Epari DR, Fuchs B, Schottle PB. The patella morphology in trochlear dysplasia–a comparative MRI study. *Knee.* 2006;13(2):145–150. **(LOE III)**.

365. Pfirrmann CW, Zanetti M, Romero J, Hodler J. Femoral trochlear dysplasia: MR findings. *Radiology.* 2000;216(3):858–864. **(LOE III)**.

366. Schottle PB, Scheffler SU, Schwarck A, Weiler A. Arthroscopic medial retinacular repair after patellar dislocation with and without underlying trochlear dysplasia: a preliminary report. *Arthroscopy.* 2006;22(11):1192–1198. **(LOE III)**.

367. Bharam S, Vrahas MS, Fu FH. Knee fractures in the athlete. *Orthop Clin North Am.* 2002;33(3):565–574. **(LOE V)**.

368. Smirk C, Morris H. The anatomy and reconstruction of the medial patellofemoral ligament. *Knee.* 2003;10(3):221–227. **(LOE N/A)**.

369. Sallay PI, Poggi J, Speer KP, Garrett WE. Acute dislocation of the patella. A correlative pathoanatomic study. *Am J Sports Med.* 1996;24(1):52–60. **(LOE IV)**.

370. Salter RB. *Textbook of Disorders and Injuries of the Musculoskeletal System.* Baltimore: Williams and Wilkins; 1970. **(LOE N/A)**.

371. Panagiotopoulos E, Strzelczyk P, Herrmann M, Scuderi G. Cadaveric study on static medial patellar stabilizers: the dynamizing role of the vastus medialis obliquus on medial patellofemoral ligament. *Knee Surg Sports Traumatol Arthrosc.* 2006;14(1):7–12. **(LOE N/A)**.

372. Putney SA, Smith CS, Neal KM. The location of medial patellofemoral ligament injury in adolescents and children. *J Pediatr Orthop.* 2012;32(3):241–244. **(LOE III)**.

373. Shea KG, Grimm NL, Belzer J, Burks RT, Pfeiffer R. The relation of the femoral physis and the medial patellofemoral ligament. *Arthroscopy.* 2010;26(9):1083–1087. **(LOE IV)**.

374. Schottle PB, Schmeling A, Rosenstiel N, Weiler A. Radiographic landmarks for femoral tunnel placement in medial patellofemoral ligament reconstruction. *Am J Sports Med.* 2007;35(5):801–804. **(LOE N/A)**.

375. Nelitz M, Dornacher D, Dreyhaupt J, Reichel H, Lippacher S. The relation of the distal femoral physis and the medial patellofemoral ligament. *Knee Surg Sports Traumatol Arthrosc.* 2011;19(12):2067–2071. **(LOE III)**.

376. Redfern J, Kamath G, Burks R. Anatomical confirmation of the use of radiographic landmarks in medial patellofemoral ligament reconstruction. *Am J Sports Med.* 2010;38(2):293–297. **(LOE N/A)**.

377. Kepler CK, Bogner EA, Hammoud S, Malcolmson G, Potter HG, Green DW. Zone of injury of the medial patellofemoral ligament after acute patellar dislocation in children and adolescents. *Am J Sports Med.* 2011;39(7):1444–1449. **(LOE II)**.

378. Seeley MA, Knesek M, Vanderhave KL. Osteochondral injury after acute patellar dislocation in children and adolescents. *J Pediatr Orthop.* 2013;33(5):511–518. **(LOE IV)**.

379. Mashoof AA, Scholl MD, Lahav A, Greis PE, Burks RT. Osteochondral injury to the mid-lateral weight-bearing portion of the lateral femoral condyle associated with patella dislocation. *Arthroscopy.* 2005;21(2):228–232. **(LOE IV)**.

380. Hawkins RJ, Bell RH, Anisette G. Acute patellar dislocations. The natural history. *Am J Sports Med.* 1986;14(2):117–120. **(LOE III)**.

381. Nikku R, Nietosvaara Y, Aalto K, Kallio PE. Operative treatment of primary patellar dislocation does not improve medium-term outcome: a 7-year follow-up report and risk analysis of 127 randomized patients. *Acta Orthop.* 2005;76(5):699–704. **(LOE IV)**.

382. Nikolai N. [Traumatic patellar dislocation and its sequelae]. *Monatsschr Unfallheilkd Versicherungsmed.* 1960;63:215–224. **(LOE V)**.

383. Bruce WD, Stevens PM. Surgical correction of miserable malalignment syndrome. *J Pediatr Orthop.* 2004;24(4):392–396. **(LOE III)**.

384. Dainer RD, Barrack RL, Buckley SL, Alexander AH. Arthroscopic treatment of acute patellar dislocations. *Arthroscopy.* 1988;4(4):267–271. **(LOE IV)**.

385. Murray TF, Dupont JY, Fulkerson JP. Axial and lateral radiographs in evaluating patellofemoral malalignment. *Am J Sports Med.* 1999;27(5):580–584. **(LOE II)**.

386. Inoue M, Shino K, Hirose H, Horibe S, Ono K. Subluxation of the patella. Computed tomography analysis of patellofemoral congruence. *J Bone Joint Surg Am.* 1988;70(9):1331–1337. **(LOE III)**.

387. Davies AP, Costa ML, Shepstone L, Glasgow MM, Donell S. The sulcus angle and malalignment of the extensor mechanism of the knee. *J Bone Joint Surg Br.* 2000;82(8):1162–1166. **(LOE III)**.

388. Martinez S, Korobkin M, Fondren FB, Hedlund LW, Goldner JL. Computed tomography of the normal patellofemoral joint. *Invest Radiol.* 1983;18(3):249–253. **(LOE III)**.

389. Martinez S, Korobkin M, Fondren FB, Hedlund LW, Goldner JL. Diagnosis of patellofemoral malalignment by computed tomography. *J Comput Assist Tomogr.* 1983;7(6):1050–1053. **(LOE IV)**.

390. McNally EG, Ostlere SJ, Pal C, Phillips A, Reid H, Dodd C. Assessment of patellar maltracking using combined static and dynamic MRI. *Eur Radiol.* 2000;10(7):1051–1055. **(LOE IV)**.

391. Koshino T, Sugimoto K. New measurement of patellar height in the knees of children using the epiphyseal line midpoint. *J Pediatr Orthop.* 1989;9(2):216–218. **(LOE III)**.

392. Pope TL Jr. MR imaging of patellar dislocation and relocation. *Semin Ultrasound CT MR.* 2001;22(4):371–382. **(LOE V)**.

393. Koskinen SK, Kujala UM. Patellofemoral relationships and distal insertion of the vastus medialis muscle: a magnetic resonance imaging study in nonsymptomatic subjects and in patients with patellar dislocation. *Arthroscopy.* 1992;8(4):465–468. **(LOE IV)**.

394. Koskinen SK, Taimela S, Nelimarkka O, Komu M, Kujala UM. Magnetic resonance imaging of patellofemoral relationships. *Skeletal Radiol.* 1993;22(6):403–410. **(LOE IV)**.

395. Kujala UM, Osterman K, Kormano M, Nelimarkka O, Hurme M, Taimela S. Patellofemoral relationships in recurrent patellar dislocation. *J Bone Joint Surg Br.* 1989;71(5):788–792. **(LOE III)**.

396. Lewallen LW, McIntosh AL, Dahm DL. Predictors of recurrent instability after acute patellofemoral dislocation in pediatric and adolescent patients. *Am J Sports Med.* 2013;41(3):575–581. **(LOE III)**.

397. Nikku R, Nietosvaara Y, Kallio PE, Aalto K, Michelsson JE. Operative versus closed treatment of primary dislocation of the patella. Similar 2-year results in 125 randomized patients. *Acta Orthop Scand.* 1997;68(5):419–423. **(LOE IV)**.

398. Vainionpaa S, Laasonen E, Patiala H, Rusanen M, Rokkannen P. Acute dislocation of the patella. Clinical, radiographic and operative findings in 64 consecutive cases. *Acta Orthop Scand.* 1986;57(4):331–333. **(LOE III)**.

399. Jarvinen M. Acute patellar dislocation–closed or operative treatment? *Acta Orthop Scand.* 1997;68(5):415–418. **(LOE V)**.

400. Palmu S, Kallio PE, Donell ST, Helenius I, Nietosvaara Y. Acute patellar dislocation in children and adolescents: a randomized clinical trial. *J Bone Joint Surg Am.* 2008;90(3):463–470. **(LOE II)**.

401. Ahmad CS, Stein BE, Matuz D, Henry JH. Immediate surgical repair of the medial patellar stabilizers for acute patellar dislocation. A review of eight cases. *Am J Sports Med.* 2000;28(6):804–810. **(LOE IV)**.

402. Brief LP. Lateral patellar instability: treatment with a combined open-arthroscopic approach. *Arthroscopy.* 1993;9(6):617–623. **(LOE IV)**.

403. Scuderi G, Cuomo F, Scott WN. Lateral release and proximal realignment for patellar subluxation and dislocation. A long-term follow-up. *J Bone Joint Surg Am.* 1988;70(6):856–861. **(LOE IV)**.

404. Fukushima K, Horaguchi T, Okano T, Yoshimatsu T, Saito A, Ryu J. Patellar dislocation: arthroscopic patellar stabilization with anchor sutures. *Arthroscopy.* 2004;20(7):761–764. **(LOE V)**.

405. Koskinen SK, Hurme M, Kujala UM. Restoration of patellofemoral congruity by combined lateral release and tibial tuberosity transposition as assessed by MRI analysis. *Int Orthop.* 1991;15(4):363–366. **(LOE IV)**.

406. Coons DA, Barber FA. Thermal medial retinaculum shrinkage and lateral release for the treatment of recurrent patellar instability. *Arthroscopy.* 2006;22(2):166–171. **(LOE IV)**.

407. Luscombe KL, Maffulli N. The three in one procedure: how I do it. *Surgeon.* 2004;2(1):32–36. **(LOE V)**.

408. Myers P, Williams A, Dodds R, Bulow J. The three-in-one proximal and distal soft tissue patellar realignment procedure. Results, and its place in the management of patellofemoral instability. *Am J Sports Med.* 1999;27(5):575–579. **(LOE IV)**.

409. Cossey AJ, Paterson R. A new technique for reconstructing the medial patellofemoral ligament. *Knee.* 2005;12(2):93–98. **(LOE IV)**.

410. Fernandez E, Sala D, Castejon M. Reconstruction of the medial patellofemoral ligament for patellar instability using a semitendinosus autograft. *Acta Orthop Belg.* 2005;71(3):303–308. **(LOE III)**.

411. Nelitz M, Dreyhaupt J, Reichel H, Woelfle J, Lippacher S. Anatomic reconstruction of the medial patellofemoral ligament in children and adolescents with open growth plates: surgical technique and clinical outcome. *Am J Sports Med.* 2013;41(1):58–63. **(LOE IV)**.

412. Aglietti P, Buzzi R, De Biase P, Giron F. Surgical treatment of recurrent dislocation of the patella. *Clin Orthop Relat Res.* 1994;(308):8–17. **(LOE IV)**.

413. Aglietti P, Pisaneschi A, De Biase P. Recurrent dislocation of patella: three kinds of surgical treatment. *Ital J Orthop Traumatol.* 1992;18(1):25–36. **(LOE V)**.

414. Dandy DJ, Desai SS. The results of arthroscopic lateral release of the extensor mechanism for recurrent dislocation of the patella after 8 years. *Arthroscopy.* 1994;10(5):540–545. **(LOE IV)**.

415. Harrison MH. The results of a realignment operation for recurrent dislocation of the patella. *J Bone Joint Surg Br.* 1955;37-B(4):559–567. **(LOE IV)**.

416. Macnab I. Recurrent dislocation of the patella. *J Bone Joint Surg Am.* 1952;34 A(4):957–967; passim. **(LOE IV)**.

417. Deie M, Ochi M, Sumen Y, Yasumoto M, Kobayashi K, Kimura H. Reconstruction of the medial patellofemoral ligament for the treatment of habitual or recurrent dislocation of the patella in children. *J Bone Joint Surg Br.* 2003;85(6):887–890. **(LOE IV)**.

418. Fondren FB, Goldner JL, Bassett FH 3rd. Recurrent dislocation of the patella treated by the modified Roux-Goldthwait procedure. A prospective study of forty-seven knees. *J Bone Joint Surg Am.* 1985;67(7):993–1005. **(LOE IV)**.

419. Vahasarja V, Kinnunen P, Lanning P, Serlo W. Operative realignment of patellar malalignment in children. *J Pediatr Orthop.* 1995;15(3):281–285. **(LOE III)**.

420. Oliva F, Ronga M, Longo UG, Testa V, Capasso G, Maffulli N. The 3-in-1 procedure for recurrent dislocation of the patella in skeletally immature children and adolescents. *Am J Sports Med.* 2009;37(9):1814–1820. **(LOE IV)**.

421. Jain NP, Khan N, Fithian DC. A treatment algorithm for primary patellar dislocations. *Sports Health.* 2011;3(2):170–174. **(LOE III)**.

422. Chotel F, Knorr G, Simian E, Dubrana F, Versier G, French Arthroscopy S. Knee osteochondral fractures in skeletally immature patients: French multicenter study. *Orthop Traumatol Surg Res.* 2011;97(suppl 8):S154–159. **(LOE III)**.

423. Kappis M. Weitese Beitrage zur Traumatisch-mechanischen Ent-stehung der "Spontanen" Knospelablosungen. *Dtsch Z Chir.* 1922;171:13–29. **(LOE I)**.

424. Dietrich TJ, Betz M, Pfirrmann CW, Koch PP, Fucentese SF. End-stage extension of the knee and its influence on tibial tuberosity-trochlear groove distance (TTTG) in asymptomatic volunteers. *Knee Surg Sports Traumatol Arthrosc.* 2014;22(1):214–218. **(LOE II)**.

425. Izadpanah K, Weitzel E, Vicari M, et al. Influence of knee flexion angle and weight bearing on the Tibial Tuberosity-Trochlear Groove (TTTG) distance for evaluation of patellofemoral alignment. *Knee Surg Sports Traumatol Arthrosc.* 2013. **(LOE IV)**.

426. Nelitz M, Theile M, Dornacher D, Wolfle J, Reichel H, Lippacher S. Analysis of failed surgery for patellar instability in children with open growth plates. *Knee Surg Sports Traumatol Arthrosc.* 2012;20(5):822–828. **(LOE IV)**.

427. Charles MD, Haloman S, Chen L, Ward SR, Fithian D, Afra R. Magnetic resonance imaging-based topographical differences between control and recurrent patellofemoral instability patients. *Am J Sports Med.* 2013;41(2):374–384. **(LOE III)**.

428. Deie M, Ochi M, Sumen Y, Adachi N, Kobayashi K, Yasumoto M. A long-term follow-up study after medial patellofemoral ligament reconstruction using the transferred semitendinosus tendon for patellar dislocation. *Knee Surg Sports Traumatol Arthrosc.* 2005;13(7):522–528. **(LOE IV)**.

429. Nonweiler DE, DeLee JC. The diagnosis and treatment of medial subluxation of the patella after lateral retinacular release. *Am J Sports Med.* 1994;22(5):680–686. **(LOE IV)**.

430. Sherman OH, Fox JM, Sperling H, et al. Patellar instability: treatment by arthroscopic electrosurgical lateral release. *Arthroscopy.* 1987;3(3):152–160. **(LOE IV)**.

431. Teitge RA, Torga Spak R. Lateral patellofemoral ligament reconstruction. *Arthroscopy.* 2004;20(9):998–1002. **(LOE V)**.

432. Panni AS, Tartarone M, Patricola A, Paxton EW, Fithian DC. Long-term results of lateral retinacular release. *Arthroscopy.* 2005;21(5):526–531. **(LOE III)**.

433. Letts RM, Davidson D, Beaule P. Semitendinosus tenodesis for repair of recurrent dislocation of the patella in children. *J Pediatr Orthop.* 1999;19(6):742–747. **(LOE III)**.

434. Marsh JS, Daigneault JP, Sethi P, Polzhofer GK. Treatment of recurrent patellar instability with a modification of the Roux-Goldthwait technique. *J Pediatr Orthop.* 2006;26(4):461–465. **(LOE IV)**.

435. Testa EA, Amsler F, Camathias C, Henle P, Freiderich N, Hirschmann MT. What is the evidence of trochleoplasty in treatment of patellofemoral instability? A systematic review and comparison with MPFL reconstruction outcomes. *Br J Sports Med.* 2013;47(10). **(LOE N/A)**.

436. Konig F. [Ueber freie Korper in den Glenken]. *Zeiteschr Chir.* 1888;27:90–109. **(LOE IV)**.

437. Paget J. On the production of some of the loose bodies in joints. *Saint Bartholomew's Hospital Reports.* 1870;6(1). **(LOE V)**.

438. Paré A, Malgaigne JF. *Œuvres Complètes d'Ambroise Paré.* Paris: J.-B. Baillière; etc.; 1840. **(LOE IV)**.

439. Edmonds EW, Shea KG. Osteochondritis dissecans: editorial comment. *Clin Orthop Relat Res.* 2013;471(4):1105–1106. **(LOE V)**.

440. Linden B. Osteochondritis dissecans of the femoral condyles: a long-term follow-up study. *J Bone Joint Surg Am.* 1977;59(6):769–776. **(LOE III)**.

441. Laor T, Zbojniewicz AM, Eismann EA, Wall EJ. Juvenile osteochondritis dissecans: is it a growth disturbance of the secondary physis of the epiphysis? *AJR Am J Roentgenol.* 2012;199(5):1121–1128. **(LOE III)**.

442. Stattin EL, Tegner Y, Domellof M, Dahl N. Familial osteochondritis dissecans associated with early osteoarthritis and disproportionate short stature. *Osteoarthritis Cartilage.* 2008;16(8):890–896. **(LOE IV)**.

443. Hefti F, Beguiristain J, Krauspe R, et al. Osteochondritis dissecans: a multicenter study of the European Pediatric Orthopedic Society. *J Pediatr Orthop B.* 1999;8(4):231–245. **(LOE II)**.

444. Kessler JI, Kikizad H, Shea KG, et al. The demographics and epidemiology of osteochondral dissecans of the knee in children and adolescents. *Am J Sports Med.* 2014;42(2):320–326. **(LOE III)**.

445. Linden B. The incidence of osteochondritis dissecans in the condyles of the femur. *Acta Orthop Scand.* 1976;47(6):664–667. **(LOE IV)**.

446. Jans LB, Ditchfield M, Anna G, Jaremko JL, Verstraete KL. MR imaging findings and MR criteria for instability in osteochondritis dissecans of the elbow in children. *Eur J Radiol.* 2012;81(6):1306–1310. **(LOE IV)**.

447. Jans LB, Jaremko JL, Ditchfield M, Huysse WC, Verstraete KL. MRI differentiates femoral condylar ossification evolution from osteochondritis dissecans. A new sign. *Eur Radiol.* 2011;21(6):1170–1179. **(LOE IV)**.

448. Hughston JC, Hergenroeder PT, Courtenay BG. Osteochondritis dissecans of the femoral condyles. *J Bone Joint Surg Am.* 1984;66(9):1340–1348. **(LOE IV)**.

449. Van Demark RE. Osteochondritis dissecans with spontaneous healing. *J Bone Joint Surg Am.* 1952;34:143–148. **(LOE IV)**.

450. Twyman RS, Desai K, Aichroth PM. Osteochondritis dissecans of the knee. A long-term study. *J Bone Joint Surg Br.* 1991;73(3):461–464. **(LOE II)**.

451. Chambers HG, Shea KG, Anderson AF, et al. American Academy of Orthopaedic Surgeons clinical practice guideline on: the diagnosis and treatment of osteochondritis dissecans. *J Bone Joint Surg Am.* 2012;94(14):1322–1324. **(LOE IV)**.

452. Chambers HG, Shea KG, Carey JL. AAOS Clinical Practice Guideline: diagnosis and treatment of osteochondritis dissecans. *J Am Acad Orthop Surg.* 2011;19(5):307–309. **(LOE IV)**.

453. Shea KG, Grimm NL, et al. Youth sports anterior cruciate ligament and knee injury epidemiology: who is getting injured? In what sports? When? *Clin Sports Med.* 2011;30(4):691–706. **(LOE V)**.

454. Shea KG, Grimm NL, Ewing CK, Aoki SK. Youth sports anterior cruciate ligament and knee injury epidemiology: who is getting injured? In what sports? When? *Clin Sports Med.* 2011;30(4):691–706. **(LOE V)**.

455. Su AW, Larson AN. Pediatric ankle fractures: concepts and treatment principles. *Foot Ankle Clin.* 2015;20(4):705–719. **(LOE V)**.

456. Wuerz TH, Gurd DP. Pediatric physeal ankle fracture. *J Am Acad Orthop Surg.* 2013;21(4):234–244. **(LOE V)**.

457. van den Bekerom MP, Raven EE. The distal fascicle of the anterior inferior tibiofibular ligament as a cause of tibiotalar impingement syndrome: a current concepts review. *Knee Surg Sports Traumatol Arthrosc.* 2007;15(4):465–471. **(LOE V)**.

458. Schlesinger I, Wedge JH. Percutaneous reduction and fixation of displaced juvenile Tillaux fractures: a new surgical technique. *J Pediatr Orthop.* 1993;13(3):389–391. **(LOE V)**.

459. Kaya A, Altay T, Ozturk H, Karapinar L. Open reduction and internal fixation in displaced juvenile Tillaux fractures. *Injury.* 2007;38(2):201–205. **(LOE V)**.

460. Stefanich RJ, Lozman J. The juvenile fracture of Tillaux. *Clin Orthop Relat Res.* 1986;210:219–227. **(LOE IV)**.

461. Jennings MM, Lagaay P, Schuberth JM. Arthroscopic assisted fixation of juvenile intra-articular epiphyseal ankle fractures. *J Foot Ankle Surg.* 2007;46(5):376–386. **(LOE IV)**.

462. Leetun DT, Ireland ML. Arthroscopically assisted reduction and fixation of a juvenile tillaux fracture. *Arthroscopy.* 2002;18(4):427–429. **(LOE IV)**.

463. Thaunat M, Billot N, Bauer T, Hardy P. Arthroscopic treatment of a juvenile Tillaux fracture. *Knee Surg Sports Traumatol Arthrosc.* 2007;15(3):286–288. **(LOE IV)**.

464. Ertl JP, Barrack RL, Alexander AH, VanBuecken K. Triplane fracture of the distal tibial epiphysis. Long-term follow-up. *J Bone Joint Surg Am.* 1988;70(7):967–976. **(LOE III)**.

465. Birch JG. *Tachdjian's Pediatric Orthopaedics.* 4th ed. Philadelphia: Saunders; 2008. **(LOE N/A)**.

466. Eismann EA, Stephan ZA, Mehlman CT, et al. Pediatric triplane ankle fractures: impact of radiographs and computed tomography on fracture classification and treatment planning. *J Bone Joint Surg Am.* 2015;97(12):995–1002. **(LOE III)**.

467. Biswas D, Bible JE, Bohan M, Simpson AK, Whang PG, Grauer JN. Radiation exposure from musculoskeletal computerized tomographic scans. *J Bone Joint Surg Am.* 2009;91(8):1882–1889. **(LOE III)**.

468. Konig F. Uber freie Körper in den Gelenken. (Translated by Drs. Richard A. Brand and Christian-Dominik Peterlein. Clin Orthop Rel Res. 2013;471:1107-15.). *Dtsch Z Klin Chir.* 1887;27:90–109. **(LOE IV)**.

469. Wolff AA. Osteochondritis dissecanstalo-cruralleddet. *Hospitalstidende.* 1926;78:36. **(LOE N/A)**.

470. Talusan PG, Milewski MD, Toy JO, Wall EJ. Osteochondritis dissecans of the talus: diagnosis and treatment in athletes. *Clin Sports Med.* 2014;33(2):267–284. **(LOE V)**.

471. Higuera J, Laguna R, Peral M, Aranda E, Soleto J. Osteochondritis dissecans of the talus during childhood and adolescence. *J Pediatr Orthop.* 1998;18(3):328–332. **(LOE V)**.

472. Letts M, Davidson D, Ahmer A. Osteochondritis dissecans of the talus in children. *J Pediatr Orthop.* 2003;23(5):617–625.

473. Berndt AL, Harty M. Transchondral fractures (osteochondritis dissecans) of the talus. *J Bone Joint Surg Am.* 1959;41-A:988–1020.

474. Perumal V, Wall E, Babekir N. Juvenile osteochondritis dissecans of the talus. *J Pediatr Orthop.* 2007;27(7):821–825. **(LOE III)**.

475. Bruns J, Rosenbach B. Osteochondrosis dissecans of the talus. Comparison of results of surgical treatment in adolescents and adults. *Arch Orthop Trauma Surg.* 1992;112(1):23–27. **(LOE III)**.

476. Amendola A, Panarella L. Osteochondral lesions: medial versus lateral, persistent pain, cartilage restoration options and indications. *Foot Ankle Clin.* 2009;14(2):215–227. **(LOE V)**.

477. Anders S, Lechler P, Rackl W, Grifka J, Schaumburger J. Fluoroscopy-guided retrograde core drilling and cancellous bone grafting in osteochondral defects of the talus. *Int Orthop.* 2012;36(8):1635–1640. **(LOE II)**.

478. Taranow WS, Bisignani GA, Towers JD, Conti SF. Retrograde drilling of osteochondral lesions of the medial talar dome. *Foot Ankle Int.* 1999;20(8):474–480. **(LOE II)**.

479. Kumai T, Takakura Y, Kitada C, Tanaka Y, Hayashi K. Fixation of osteochondral lesions of the talus using cortical bone pegs. *J Bone Joint Surg Br.* 2002;84(3):369–374. **(LOE II)**.

480. Zengerink M, Struijs PA, Tol JL, van Dijk CN. Treatment of osteochondral lesions of the talus: a systematic review. *Knee Surg Sports Traumatol Arthrosc.* 2010;18(2):238–246. **(LOE IV)**.

20 Nonaccidental Trauma: Inflicted Skeletal Injuries or Child Physical Abuse

Jeffrey Shilt | Christopher Greeley

INTRODUCTION

Inflicted physical abuse to children is a grotesque act that no one likes to diagnose. This phenomenon accounts for nearly 20% of all child maltreatment cases, which encompass a spectrum of offenses including neglect, sexual and physical abuse, and psychological maltreatment.[1] Many terms have been used to describe the orthopedic manifestations of physical abuse and include battered child syndrome, nonaccidental trauma, and the current convention of child physical abuse (CPA).[2,3]

Unlike many chapters in this book in which technologic advances have changed the care of children's fractures, such advances are unlikely to help treat child abuse. Instead, this chapter will provide the basis for greater education, training, and awareness that will enable physicians to better recognize child abuse, reduce missed diagnoses, and aid in the reporting of CPA. The topic remains in the forefront of the American Academy of Orthopaedic Surgeons (AAOS), Pediatric Orthopaedic Society of North America, and pediatric orthopedic thought leaders who continue to update diagnostic workup indications for femur fractures. These changes have been included in the most recent clinical practice guidelines by the AAOS in an effort of continued education in identifying at-risk patients.[4]

LEGAL ASPECTS

In 1961, the Children's Bureau of the US Department of Health, Education, and Welfare published a model law that required mandatory reporting by physicians and other medical professionals. Although the exact reading of the law in various communities may differ, all statutes require prompt identification of any suspected case of abuse. Typically, physicians are granted immunity from civil and criminal liability if a report is made in good faith.

Maliciously reporting abuse when it is not the cause of injury, however, may expose an individual to the risk of litigation. Unfortunately, the litigious environment in which we live has given concomitant rise to the number of lawsuits from parents who feel they have been falsely accused. This risk of litigation leads to healthcare providers' reluctance to become involved in child protective matters, which is a trend that must be avoided.[5] Conversely, civil suits have been filed against physicians for failure to report acts of child abuse, and most laws impose a criminal penalty for failure to report suspected child abuse. Fortunately, the trend in most parts of the world is that of increasing recognition of the

phenomenon and improved healthcare education about it.[6,7] Heightened awareness should improve legal protection for reporting healthcare providers.

HISTORICAL PERSPECTIVE

Although the radiographic findings of child abuse have been known for more than a century, it was not until 1946 that Caffey[8] studied six children with chronic subdural hematomas and fractures of long bones with no history of injury. He stated that they did not have a systemic disease that could explain the radiographic findings and believed that injury to the children was responsible for the findings. He further suggested that children with unexplained long bone fractures should be investigated for chronic subdural hematomas and vice versa.

In 1953, Silverman[9] described periosteal new bone formation associated with irregular fragmentation of the metaphyses in children and believed that this injury was part of the syndrome that Caffey originally described. In 1960, Altman and Smith[10] reported cases of unrecognized trauma in children, and in 1972, Kempe and Helfer[11] coined the term *battered child syndrome*.

Reporting continues to increase, demonstrating a nearly 15% rise from 2012 to 2016. Unfortunately, fatalities have continued to rise despite an overall decrease in physical abuse previously reported.[1,12]

FORMS OF ABUSE AND NEGLECT

This chapter will focus on the orthopedist's role in the care of children who are victims of CPA and their assistance with injury evaluation and management in physical abuse. However, the treating surgeon must be familiar with other forms of child maltreatment. Recognition of the signs of neglect, sexual abuse, or emotional maltreatment may lead the treating physician to consider child abuse as a possibility.

Child neglect has been defined as "an omission in care by caregivers that results in significant harm or the risk of significant harm."[13] Neglect, accounting for 75% of all child maltreatment, is the most common form of child maltreatment and includes categories such as physical, medical, supervisional, educational, and emotional.[1] Neglect can be acute or chronic and may be quantified by the severity, frequency, and chronicity of the caregiver's omissions. Physical signs of neglect include malnutrition, pica, constant fatigue and listlessness, poor hygiene, and inadequate clothing for the circumstances. Behavioral signs of physical neglect include lack of appropriate adult supervision and even "role reversal," in which the child becomes the parental caretaker. Other signs include drug or alcohol abuse, poor school attendance, and exploitation by the parents, such as being forced to beg or steal. Importantly, although the rates of physical and sexual abuse have been decreasing over the past 3 decades, child neglect remains stubbornly unchanged.[14]

Unfortunately, when one form of child maltreatment has been identified (e.g., neglect), it is not uncommon for additional types to be present (e.g., physical abuse). The presence of multiple types may have a negative synergistic effect on the child's physical and mental well-being, as the worst outcomes associated with child maltreatment include the comorbidities of physical neglect, emotional neglect, verbal abuse, and physical abuse.[15]

Child sexual abuse has been defined as ". . . the involvement of dependent, developmentally immature children and adolescents in sexual activities that they do not fully comprehend, to which they are unable to give informed consent, or that violate the social taboos of family roles."[16] Child sexual abuse encompasses both contact abuse (e.g., genital, oral, anal, or fondling) and noncontact sexual exploitation of a minor (e.g., child pornography).[17] Most orthopedists are poorly trained in the evaluation of sexual abuse. Fortunately, the American Academy of Pediatrics and its Committee on Child Abuse and Neglect summarize the epidemiology of child sexual abuse, appropriate care of child victims, and the physical and emotional consequences. They have developed specific protocols for the evaluation of sexual abuse, for which there is now specialty certification.[17,18]

Sexual exploitation is usually perpetrated by someone known to the child and may continue over a prolonged period. A description of the physical signs of sexual abuse is beyond the scope of this text; however, the behavioral signs should be recognized because their presence may alert the physician that the child is a victim of sexual abuse. A child who is a victim of sexual abuse may demonstrate internalizing behaviors (i.e., withdrawn, depressed) or externalizing behaviors (anxiety, emotional outbursts, aggressiveness), engage in sexually reactive behaviors, develop eating disorders, and/or develop substance abuse problems.[19] These children may also become sexually promiscuous and may sexually abuse a sibling.

PHYSICAL ABUSE

Although soft tissue injuries are the most common finding in child abuse,[20] 10% to 70% of physically abused children manifest some form of skeletal trauma. It is estimated that 30% to 50% of physically abused children are seen by orthopedists for fractures or other orthopedic problems.[21,22] An orthopedist caring for injured children must be familiar with abuse-related injuries and the clinical manifestations of such injuries to appropriately diagnose and intervene in suspicious cases.

Recognition of physical abuse is extremely important in protecting the involved child, in addition to other children living in the home. Approximately 9% to 12% of child household contacts or siblings of the abuse victims will have a history or injuries consistent with abuse.[23,24] Of children

returned to an abusive home without intervention, 35% to 50% will be abused again, and the second incident may be fatal in 5% to 10%.[25,26] Early identification and intervention in cases of child abuse cannot be overemphasized, and the results are encouraging for reducing rates of future CPA among abusive parents. The effectiveness of programs varies depending on the type of intervention, with parent-child interaction therapy seemingly most promising.[27,28]

AGE DEMOGRAPHICS

The younger the child, the more vulnerable he or she is to maltreatment. In 2016, an astounding 29% of all cases of CPA occurred in children younger than 3 years of age.[1] Furthermore, 50% of fractures in children younger than 1 year of age are attributable to abuse.[29,30,31] These figures alone are just cause for thorough workup in young children, particularly infants, who are seen with fractures. Multiple reports further substantiate these findings. Victims of CPA seen in the emergency department have similar age demographics. In fact, 10% of the total trauma population younger than 3 years is nonaccidental, as are 30% of head and limb injuries in this age group.[32,33] Highest rates of child maltreatment fatalities occur in the youngest age group: nearly 80% of the deaths occur in children younger than 3 years and more than 40% in children younger than 1 year.[1] Even though only 58% of the children in the study by Herndon[34] were younger than 3 years, they accounted for 94% of the fractures. A pattern of decreasing incidence of *nonaccidental* fractures with increasing age corresponds to the increasing incidence of *accidental* fractures with increasing age up to 12 years. In fact, children older than 5 years account for less than 10% of the fractures related to abuse.[35]

HISTORY OF INJURY

Historical clues remain one of the most important tools in diagnosing child abuse. Additionally, tools have been created to help investigate CPA. One such tool is the injury plausibility method, which helps tabulate historical data into the likelihood of injury from falling from stairs, a common occurrence yet also a common false explanation excuse for child abuse.[36] Differentiating CPA from unintentional injuries has also been described in a Likert-like fashion, with the use of criteria to determine the likelihood of abuse within a spectrum of "definitely not inflicted injury" to "definite inflicted injury."[37] This highlights the fact that diagnosing CPA often requires clinical judgement. Although many of the skeletal findings associated with CPA are highly specific, there is no single injury that, in and of itself, is diagnostic.

Various societies and professional organizations have developed practice guidelines for interviewing in cases of alleged child abuse.[17,38,39] These guidelines detail the purpose of the *forensic* investigative interview, background and procedures of the interviewers, the context and content of the interview, and special issues for law enforcement investigators. Orthopedists should be aware of guidelines so that the information obtained will be useful to those who must later make difficult decisions regarding the placement of children back in the home of the involved patients.

Orthopedists must be cognizant that numerous disciplines have trained specialists who are competent in performing specialized interviews, including law enforcement personnel, child protection services personnel, members of the district attorney's office (e.g., assistant district attorneys), and child forensic interviewers (e.g., social workers, psychologists, or physicians), and who are members of specialized child assessment teams. If available, children should be referred to specialty clinics (i.e., child advocacy centers) for evaluation. It is vital that people with appropriate training in this interview method be allowed to conduct a proper interview in a timely manner.

Recommendations intended to improve the quality of the information obtained include these:

- Children should undergo an interview as soon as possible after the initial disclosure of the abuse.
- The child should be separated from the parent, if possible, for the interview, to prevent undue influence (intentional or unintentional).
- If not previously established, the interviewer should develop a rapport with the child by initially asking about nonthreatening issues.
- The interviewer should not ask leading or suggestive questions. The interviewer should begin with open-ended questions to encourage a narrative response and then transition into more direct questions, if necessary.
- Questions should be asked with the use of developmentally appropriate language. A description of the abuse should be recorded word for word, with the use of quotation marks.
- The interviewer should not urge or coerce the child to talk about the abuse, should be supportive and show respect toward the patient, and should avoid appearing shocked or upset if/when the patient describes the abuse.

The orthopedist's role is to treat the child's injuries while carefully documenting the child's and caregiver's provided history in a nurturing manner. The facts gathered and documented are important in helping investigative agencies that will eventually compare stories and corroborate facts. The parent or caregiver's account of the injury can be vague and incomplete; he or she may be evasive or contradictory or fail to volunteer details regarding the incident. The degree of physical injury may be inconsistent with the history given, and often the reported time of injury does not correlate with the obvious age of the injury. A delay in seeking treatment is suspicious. A history of repeated trauma in which the child has been treated at several different facilities should arouse suspicion.

The parents' response to the situation may be inappropriate. They may be critical of or angry with the child for being injured, or they may ignore the child completely. Other parents may become overly involved.

The social history will provide additional information in identifying children at risk. Children with birth defects and families with disabled children are at higher risk of child abuse in the home.[40] Socially isolated families with no external support system tend to be more abusive. Abuse is also more common in families in which the parents are involved in a violent interpersonal relationship. Adults who were childhood victims of abuse are more likely to become abusive parents, as are those with unrealistic expectations for their children (i.e., expectations inconsistent with the child's developmental or intellectual abilities). Families with increased stress are vulnerable. Drug or alcohol abuse

increases the likelihood of abuse.[1] Mental illness of caregivers is also a significant risk factor for child maltreatment.

Any condition that interferes with normal parent-child bonding and results in lack of normal parental contact increases the risk of child abuse. Irritable or hyperactive children or children with physical or developmental disabilities are more likely to suffer abuse from their parents or caretakers. Premature or low-birth-weight infants, who may require more care and attention, are abused three times as often as full-term infants.[40,41] In a report reviewing infant homicide, a mother younger than 17 years of age, a second or subsequent birth in a mother 19 years or younger, no prenatal care, and a low level of education were cited as the strongest risk factors. Because infanticide occurs most often in the first few months of life, intervention during pregnancy and the postpartum period is recommended.[42]

PHYSICAL EXAMINATION

An orthopedist caring for children's fractures will probably be confronted with children who have sustained musculoskeletal injuries as a result of abuse. The possibility of CPA must always be considered, and a complete and systematic examination of the child must be performed.

Important general considerations for physical examination findings that should raise concern for CPA include:[2]

- *any* injury to a young, preambulatory infant, including bruises, mouth injuries, fractures, and intracranial or abdominal injury;
- injuries to multiple organ systems;
- multiple injuries in different stages of healing;
- patterned injuries; for example, blunt instrument marks or burns, circumferential immersion burns, human hand or bite marks;
- injuries to nonbony or other unusual locations, such as over the torso, ears, face, neck, or upper arms;
- significant injuries that are unexplained; and
- additional evidence of child neglect.

Careful documentation of skin and soft tissue injuries is required, including the size, shape, location, and estimated stage of healing of any lesions. The entire axial and appendicular skeleton is then examined. The injured area is examined last to lessen the child's anxiety. Whereas tenderness, crepitus, or instability may be present in acute fractures, palpable callus without associated tenderness may be noted in healing fractures. Any of the aforementioned findings warrant radiographic examination.

Soft tissue injuries may include bruises or welts over any part of the body. Areas particularly subject to trauma are the face, head, and neck, including the lips, mouth, ears, and eyes.[20] Bruises about the trunk, back, buttocks, and thighs are also common. Bruises may form regular patterns resembling the shape of the object that was used to inflict the injury, such as a hand, fist, belt or belt buckle, or electric cord. A common mnemonic for suspicious bruises is "TEN-4"[43]: which stands for:

T: torso;
E: ear;

N: neck;

4: in children less than 4 years of age and any bruise in an infant under 4 months of age.

Multiple body surface involvement or multiple injuries in various stages of resolution suggest abuse and warrant further investigation.

Burns are also commonly seen and may be noted in conjunction with other injuries. Cigarette burns may be present, especially on the palms, soles, back, or buttocks. Immersion burns form a regular pattern. If the child is pushed into a tub or sink of very hot water, the burns will occur around the buttocks and genitalia. However, if one of the extremities is dipped in hot water, a stocking-glove distribution of the burn may be seen. Pattern burns may result if the child is burned with an instrument such as an iron, grill, or some other hot object with a recognizable shape.

Lacerations may occur anywhere on the body, including rope burns on the wrists, ankles, neck, or torso. Lacerations about the head and face are frequently noted and may even be seen inside the mouth or ears. One must also look for injuries to the genitalia and other body surfaces.

Injuries to the abdomen and to the components of the abdominal cavity may result from child abuse. Bruises of the abdominal wall and bleeding within the wall of the small intestine may be seen. Rupture of an abdominal viscus has been reported, including the intestine, spleen, liver, pancreas, and blood vessels. The kidneys, adrenal glands, and bladder may also be injured.

Trauma to the central nervous system is common and may be severe. Subdural hematomas in an abused infant may result from blunt trauma, violent shaking, or a combination of both. Hematoma is a frequent finding in abusive head trauma (historically known as shaken baby syndrome).[44] Ophthalmologic examination will demonstrate the presence of retinal hemorrhage.[45] The presentation of nonaccidental head injury is different from that seen in motor vehicle crashes. When seen, patients with inflicted head injuries are more often lucid and have higher Glasgow Coma Scale scores than those involved in motor vehicle accidents.[46]

An abused child is likely to have behavioral characteristics that may be the result of physical or emotional abuse. Abused children may be less compliant and more negative and unhappy than the average child. Abused children may be hypervigilant and wary of any contact with adults. They tend to be angry, feel isolated, and show destructive behavior. They may be abusive toward others and have difficulty developing normal relationships.[47] Parental separation is frequently difficult, but occasionally an abused child will be indifferent to separation from the parents. These children may constantly seek attention and may also show developmental delays.

RADIOGRAPHIC EVALUATION

In cases of suspected physical abuse, conventional skeletal radiography by way of a skeletal survey is the primary screening examination.[3] This survey should consist of anteroposterior (AP) views of arms, forearms, thighs, and legs; posteroanterior views of hands and feet; frontal and lateral views of the thoracolumbar spine with adequate penetration for visualization of the ribs; AP views of the abdomen/lumbosacral spine/bony pelvis; lateral views of the lumbar spine; AP and lateral views of the cervical spine; and frontal and lateral views of the skull. The American College of Radiology (ACR) and the Section on Radiology of the American Academy of Pediatrics recommend that a high-quality radiographic skeletal survey (1) involve the use of a high-detail imaging system, with technical factors designed to optimize image contrast and spatial resolution; and (2) include the addition of Townes and right and left lateral views of the skull, at least two views of all areas suggestive of skeletal injuries during the initial survey that require orthopedic treatment, and additional oblique views of the thorax for rib fractures. Skull films may be foregone if the child is receiving a head computed tomography (CT) scan with three-dimensional reconstruction, as that modality is superior to plain films of the skull for identifying fractures.[48,49] The "babygram" with the entire child on one radiograph has long been considered unacceptable and is likely to miss fractures.[50]

The methods in which the plain films are obtained have rapidly changed over the past decade. Conventional film-screen imaging has historically been the method in which radiographs were obtained. However, computed radiography is rapidly becoming the standard. It was estimated by 2004 that nearly 80% of pediatric healthcare imaging facilities in the United States had migrated to digital technology, and this is likely higher currently. The advantages of this process are many; those that are applicable to diagnosis in CPA lie in the postprocessing abilities that are available. When used optimally, postprocessing improves the visualization of pathology while improving local contrast.[51]

Recent discussion about radiation safety in the pediatric population indicates that clinicians need to be aware of the risks versus benefits of medical imaging studies. In suspected child abuse cases, the consequences of unrecognized inflicted trauma can be devastating. Jenny and Crawford-Jakubiak[17] published a study describing 173 cases of abusive head trauma. Of the cases, 54 (31%) were misdiagnosed on initial presentation, and 19 of the 54 misdiagnosed children sustained additional injuries after the missed diagnosis, including 4 fatalities. Although the risks of radiation exposure are not necessarily negligible, they are relatively small compared with the expected benefit of timely recognition of physical abuse and protection from additional inflicted or fatal injuries.

Although CPA in children can present with nearly any injury pattern, some injuries observed in battered children are more characteristic of this population and are more likely to be the result of inflicted injury. These are skeletal injuries, including fractures of the ribs, metaphyses, and skull. The appropriate selection of radiographic imaging can facilitate detection of these injuries. In particular, detection of a metaphyseal fracture depends on high-quality, small field-of-view radiographs. Postimage processing allowed by computed radiography is helpful in improving the quality of films for this type of injury investigation. The injury appears as a radiographically lucent area within the subphyseal metaphysis, extending completely or partially across the metaphysis, roughly perpendicular to the long axis of the bone. Acute rib fractures in children younger than 2 years are highly suggestive of CPA. These fractures appear as linear lucent areas but are very difficult to visualize, and some suggest the

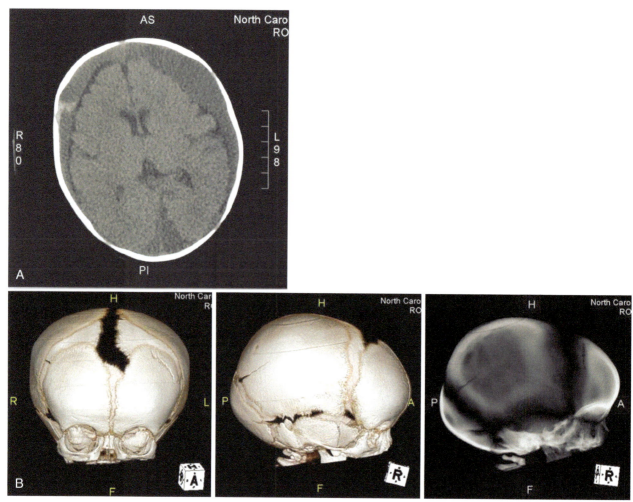

Fig. 20.1 (A) Axial computed tomographic (CT) scan of the skull. (B) Reformatted images. The findings and anatomic relationships are not adequately characterized with the use of the axial images alone. In this case, supplemental three-dimensional/multiplanar reformatted images were generated, clearly identifying the left frontal and right parietal skull fractures existing with the mixed-density subdural hematomas, bulging fontanelle, and widened sutures noted on the axial CT.

sensitivity of plain films to be less than 50%. Thus, follow-up radiography increases detection of these fractures, and chest films on follow-up are warranted. For skull injuries, plain radiography is historically the gold standard. However, there is evidence that CT is superior for detecting fractures.[48,49] Adopting this modality as standard protocol is controversial. However, in cases in which a high suspicion exists, CT should be used. CT and magnetic resonance imaging (MRI) best depict intracranial injury[52] (Fig. 20.1).

Follow-up skeletal surveys (approximately 2 weeks after the initial evaluation) have been shown to be helpful in identifying and dating skeletal injuries in cases of suspected child abuse.[53,54,55,56] In one study reviewing 796 cases, additional information regarding skeletal injury was obtained in 21% of those cases.[57] The use of bone scintigraphy is considered complementary, but not an alternative, to skeletal survey. It is sensitive for pelvis, rib, spine, acromion, and subtle diaphyseal trauma, but is considered inferior in the classic metaphyseal lesions.[58] Unfortunately, an abnormal bone scan is not specific for trauma and may be seen in a variety of other conditions. In addition, interpretation of bone scans in children is often difficult, and even minor errors in positioning may simulate focal abnormality.[59] The

ACR considers this modality a "problem solving rather than a first-line study" in its ACR Appropriateness Criteria on suspected physical child abuse.[60]

Historically, ultrasound and arthrography were considered for cartilage or joint injuries, and this continues to be the case for distal humeral epiphyseal separation in young children.[61] For these injuries and an increasing number of other clinical indications, MRI is being used. However, MRI has a low sensitivity for classic metaphyseal lesions and rib fractures. It does have utility in identifying soft tissue abnormalities or in the differential diagnosis to rule out other causes of periosteal reaction, for example, osteomyelitis.[62]

As indicated previously, CT scan of the head is the examination of choice for intracranial injury in child abuse. CT of the ribs can also be helpful.[63,64,65] These areas are often difficult to assess for fractures with the use of plain film radiography. In difficult cases, platforms exist to assist with manipulation of digital images and volume renderings that can make the diagnosis clearer (Fig. 20.2).

RADIOGRAPHIC DATING OF INJURIES

A basic knowledge of the stages of fracture healing that can be detected radiographically is imperative for orthopedists

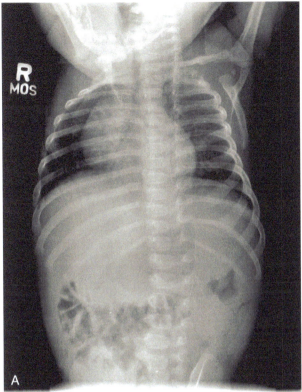

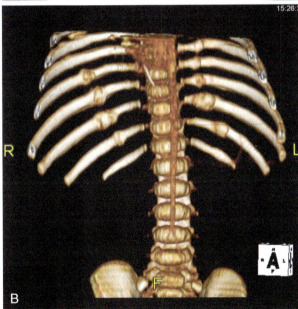

Fig. 20.2 (A) Plain radiograph of ribs, in which fractures are difficult to diagnose. (B) Computed tomographic scan after volume rendering with a TeraRecon Aquarius workstation (San Mateo, CA). This represents a sophisticated platform using a combination of task-specific hardware and software specifically designed to rapidly manipulate large digital imaging and communications in medicine data sets and provide surface-shaded and multiplanar renderings in real time.

caring for injured children.[66] A fracture in a radiographic stage of healing that does not correspond to the stated date of injury should arouse suspicion. Table 20.1 gives a general timetable for the various stages of fracture healing, and a brief outline is presented here. Very young infants may

exhibit an accelerated rate of response, so the timetable should be considered only an estimate.[67]

1. Resolution of Soft Tissues

   Obliteration of the normal fat planes and muscle boundaries occurs as a result of hemorrhage and inflammation. These changes are the first and sometimes the only evidence of a fracture immediately after injury. Depending on the magnitude of injury, these changes may persist for several days.[62,68]

2. Periosteal New Bone

   Radiographically, periosteal new bone formation is not evident until it calcifies, usually between 7 and 14 days in an infant; however, it may occur in as few as 4 days. Continued subperiosteal hemorrhaging caused by repetitive trauma to a fracture that is not immobilized may result in extensive, or "exuberant," fracture callus.[62,68]

3. Loss of Fracture Line Definition

   As necrotic bone is resorbed, the sharply defined margins of fresh fractures become blurred. The fracture gap appears to widen and becomes indistinct. It reaches a peak between 2 and 3 weeks but is not generally apparent before 1 week. Bucket-handle metaphyseal fractures or corner fractures can frequently be dated only by this method because periosteal new bone formation does not occur.[62,68]

4. Hard Callus Order

   Approximately 1 week after soft callus is visible, the fracture site is bridged by lamellar bone. This phase of healing is complete between 3 and 6 weeks.[62,68]

5. Remodeling Order

   Patient age, the degree of displacement, and the amount of callus formation are all variables involved in bone remodeling. A young child with a nondisplaced fracture may complete remodeling in a few months; however, an older child with a displaced or angulated fracture may continue remodeling for more than a year.[62,68]

FRACTURE PATTERNS

Almost any bone can be fractured; the extremities, skull, and rib cage are the most common sites of injury. However, in one series, fractures of the long bones accounted for 68% of all fractures in patients who were the victims of child abuse.[69] Although no fracture pattern is absolutely pathognomonic of physical abuse, certain fracture patterns have been found to be more characteristic of abuse than others. These patterns include metaphyseal or epiphyseal fractures (e.g., corner fractures, bucket-handle fractures, and chip fractures), posterior rib fractures, multiple or wide complex skull fractures, scapular and sternal fractures, multiple fractures, and unreported fractures.[70] Single fractures, linear narrow parietal skull fractures, long bone shaft fractures, and clavicular fractures are all associated with child abuse but have low specificity.[35,71,72,73] Whereas spiral fractures were the most common long bone fracture pattern reported by earlier authors,[74,75] more recent data suggest that single, transverse long bone fractures are the

Table 20.1   Timetable of radiographic changes on children's fractures

Category	Early	Peak	Late
Resolution of soft tissues	2–5 days	4–10 days	10–21 days
Periosteal new bone	4–10 days	10–14 days	14–21 days
Loss of fracture line definition	10–14 days	14–21 days	—
Soft callus	10–14 days	14–21 days	—
Hard callus	14–21 days	21–42 days	42–90 days
Remodeling	3 months	1 year	2 years to epiphyseal closure

(Modified from O'Connor JF, Cohen J. Dating fractures. In: Kleinman P, ed. *Diagnostic Imaging of Child Abuse*. Baltimore: Williams Wilkins;1987:103-113.)

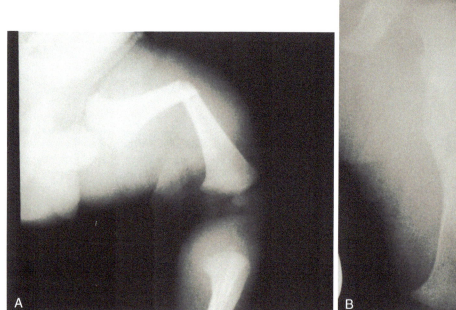
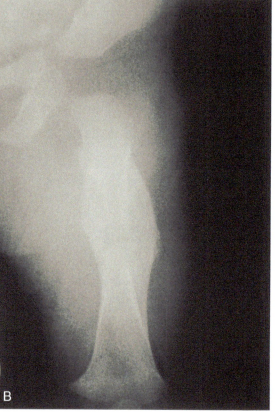

Fig. 20.3 Fracture of the midshaft of the femur in an infant that was caused by child physical abuse. (A) A radiograph of the femur demonstrates a midshaft fracture of the femur with marked angulation. Fractured femurs in infants that result from child abuse may be spiral fractures but may also be simple transverse diaphyseal fractures such as seen here. This fracture was undoubtedly the result of significant force. (B) Healing of the fracture is demonstrated after the fracture had been reduced and the limb immobilized in a hip spica cast.

most common fractures in child abuse.[72,76] Because these fractures are also seen in accidental trauma, they are not specific for abuse.[73]

DIAPHYSEAL FRACTURES

It cannot be overemphasized that one of the most difficult problems in the diagnosis of abuse is the child seen with an isolated long bone fracture with unlikely history but no other stigmata of abuse.[77] These fractures can be ubiquitous

and are seen in every pattern: spiral, oblique, and transverse fractures. Equally difficult is that long bone shaft fractures may result from accidental or CPA (Figs. 20.3 and 20.4). Transverse fractures are the result of direct injury, whereas spiral fractures result from rotational or torsional forces (Fig. 20.5). An abusive parent may use either mechanism, so both fracture patterns may be seen in abuse. An isolated diaphyseal fracture is the most common fracture pattern identified in child abuse,[72,76] and diaphyseal fractures occur four times as often as "classic" metaphyseal fractures.[78] The

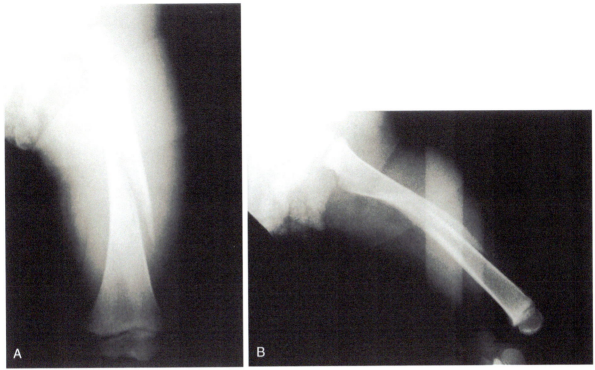

Fig. 20.4 Fracture of the femur in a toddler that occurred as a result of accidental trauma. (A) Anteroposterior radiograph of the femur of a 2-year-old child who tripped while running. This fracture pattern is quite typical of fractures in the toddler age group. Investigation of the family showed no evidence for suspicion, and the child had no other injuries or warning signs of abuse. (B) Lateral radiograph demonstrating the long spiral fracture of the femur.

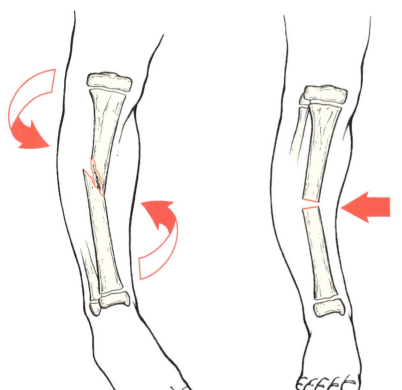

Fig. 20.5 The mechanism of injury that produces either a spiral fracture, which is the result of a twisting injury (A) or a transverse fracture, which is the result of a direct blow to a long bone (B).

humerus, femur, and tibia are the most frequently injured long bones in cases of child abuse. Fracture of the diaphysis of a long bone in a nonambulatory child without a history consistent with the injury is highly suggestive of inflicted trauma. Abuse should be suspected if either an unreasonable history of the cause of the fracture is described, such as a fracture occurring during a diaper change, or no true history of trauma is reported. Abuse should also be suspected if the delay in seeking medical care is inappropriate or if physical evidence of other trauma is observed. The diagnosis of abuse should be made if the child has, in addition to a diaphyseal fracture, radiologic evidence of fractures in varying stages of healing or multiple acute fractures without evidence of accidental trauma or bone disease.

Femoral shaft fractures are seen in both accidental trauma and CPA; however, in children younger than 12 months, abuse accounts for 60% to 80% of these fractures.[79–81] Abuse should be considered when a child younger than 2 years is seen with a femoral fracture.[82] Fractures associated with CPA tend to occur in the distal femur or in combination with the distal femur more commonly.[83] As many as 30% of femoral shaft fractures in children younger than 4 years may be the result of child abuse, and the most common cause of a femur fracture in the nonambulatory infant is CPA.[84–86] Long spiral fractures of the femur are common in toddlers as a result of accidental trauma and should not be considered solely the result of abuse; several authors have recently shown that femoral shaft fracture patterns are unreliable in differentiating accidental from nonaccidental injury.[87,88,89]

Humeral shaft fractures in young children have historically had a high association with child abuse and have not generally been reported as a result of accidental trauma.[79,90] Worlock and colleagues[35] found no cases of accidental humeral shaft fracture in children younger than 5 years; all the cases documented were the result of abuse. In contrast, all the supracondylar and condylar fractures of the distal end of the humerus in their series were the result of accidental trauma. However, more recent reports dispute these findings. In evaluating humeral fractures in children younger than 3 years, Strait and colleagues[31] documented abuse in only 58% of humeral shaft fractures but found that 20% of the supracondylar fractures evaluated were associated with abuse. Abuse-related injuries in this study were significantly associated with an age younger than 15 months. Given these data, abuse should be considered in the differential diagnosis of all humeral fractures (including supracondylar fractures) in children younger than 15 months.[31] Fractures of the radius and ulna, commonly seen in accidental trauma, are the least fractured long bones in child abuse.[72,74,75]

One must be careful when assessing the cause of tibial shaft fractures in children of walking age.[79] A nondisplaced spiral tibial shaft fracture ("toddler's fracture") is very common and is a result of accidental trauma. A toddler's fracture typically occurs in the second or third years of life, and frequently the history of trauma is not always clear on initial examination. The parents may be unaware of the trauma because it occurred out of their sight. These facts all make differentiation from CPA very difficult. A metaanalysis, however, strongly recommends close evaluation of these injuries because of the high risk of inflicted trauma.[29,91,92]

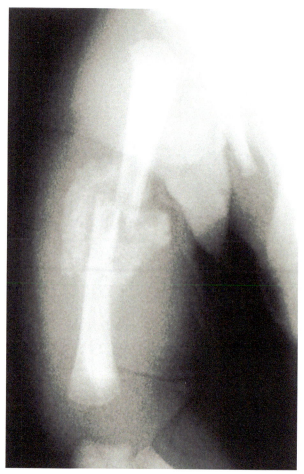

Fig. 20.6 Fracture of the humerus in an infant. An anteroposterior radiograph of the humerus demonstrates a transverse, mid-diaphyseal fracture of the humerus that was the result of child physical abuse. When the child was seen, the fracture was already healing, as demonstrated by the radiograph. The child was found to have other skeletal and soft tissue injuries.

TREATMENT

Diaphyseal fractures of the long bones are optimally treated with immobilization. Fractures of the shaft of the femur are best treated with a Pavlik harness in the young infant. If this is deemed insufficiently stable, application of an immediate spica cast is indicated. Some fractures of the shaft of the femur may be very unstable if the trauma has been significant enough to disrupt the periosteum. Therefore close observation with repeated radiographs is necessary until union of the fracture is complete, usually within 6 weeks. Hospitalization is necessary for completion of a social services investigation of the family and the circumstances of the injury.

Humeral shaft fractures should also be treated with immobilization, which is best accomplished with the application of a Velpeau bandage. Such fractures heal very quickly in an infant (Fig. 20.6).

EPIPHYSEAL-METAPHYSEAL FRACTURES

Although epiphyseal-metaphyseal fractures are much less common than diaphyseal fractures, they are much more specific for child abuse. The forces necessary to produce such

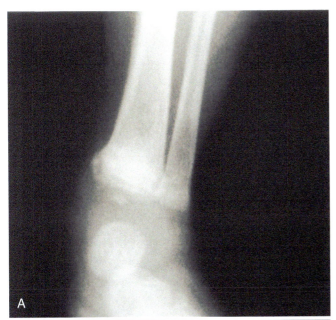

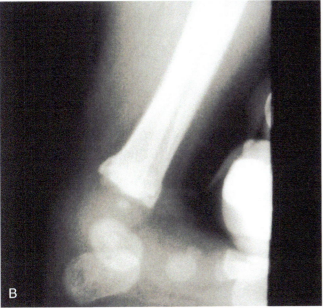

Fig. 20.7 Corner fractures of the distal end of the tibia in an infant who was abused. (A) Anteroposterior radiographs showing the corner fractures of both sides of the metaphysis at the level of the physis. Evidence of new bone formation is present and indicates that the fracture is more than a week old. (B) A lateral radiograph of the same ankle also shows the corner fractures.

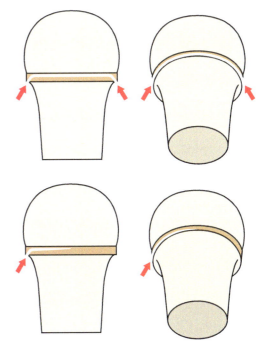

Fig. 20.8 Corner fractures and bucket-handle fractures have been shown to be the same lesion viewed from different projections.

fractures (traction and torsion) are unlikely to be generated from falls or other accidents[69] (Figs. 20.5 and 20.6). It was once believed that these fractures represented focal avulsion of the metaphysis, but recent pathologic radiographic studies have shown that corner fractures and bucket-handle fractures are probably the same lesion viewed in different projections[93,94] (Figs. 20.7 and 20.8). The shearing forces associated with rapid acceleration-deceleration in violent shaking cause fracture through the primary spongiosa, and a disk of bone and calcified cartilage is left attached to the epiphysis. Subsequent subperiosteal new bone formation does not occur because the periosteum in this area is tightly adherent and is not disrupted.[70] If present at all, periosteal

reaction is often subtle. Massive periosteal reaction occurs only with displacement of the metaphyseal fragment or shearing of the periosteum itself[50,70] (Fig. 20.9). The fracture margins become indistinct with further healing.[50] These fractures may be easily overlooked early on, and high-quality radiographs are necessary to make the diagnosis.[95] In addition, the absence of periosteal elevation in the healing phase makes detection of these fractures difficult. As a result, the true incidence of these fractures may be underestimated.[50]

The presence of radiolucent epiphyseal extensions of hypertrophied cartilage into the metaphysis has also been documented during the healing phase. The depth of penetration into the metaphysis is related to the age of the injury, and the configuration of the extensions is related to the degree of injury. These radiolucent epiphyseal extensions are single and focal in minor injuries and multiple and broad in extensive ones.[96]

True physeal fractures with separation of the epiphysis frequently result from violent traction or rotation rather than shaking and may be complicated by growth disturbance and deformity.[75] These fractures are uncommon in an abused child except in the distal end of the humerus and proximal ends of the humerus and femur (Fig. 20.10).

SPECIFIC FRACTURES

TYPE I DISTAL HUMERAL FRACTURES

At one time, this injury was thought to be rare, but it is now acknowledged to be underdiagnosed.[61,97] Two clear associations are seen with this fracture: birth trauma and abuse. Child abuse is the probable cause after the neonatal period. One must therefore strongly suspect the possibility of child abuse when one sees this fracture in a young child.[98]

These children are seen with marked swelling about the elbow, and the physical appearance of the elbow resembles a dislocation. On an AP radiograph, the radius and ulna

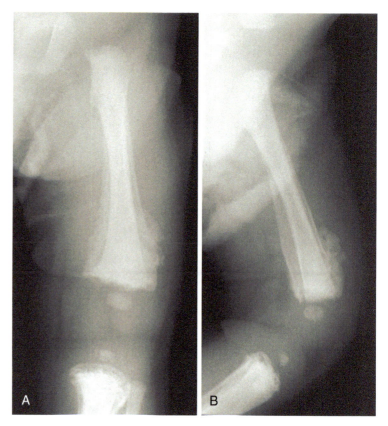

Fig. 20.9 Infant with multiple injuries sustained as a result of child abuse. (A) An anteroposterior radiograph of the leg in this child shows significant periosteal reaction about the distal end of the femur and proximal portion of the tibia. The child sustained both distal femoral and proximal tibial physeal fractures. The proximal tibial fracture was a so-called corner fracture. (B) Lateral radiograph of the same extremity again showing the remarkable periosteal reaction in the femur. The periosteum was significantly stripped well beyond the midpoint of the femur, which indicates the enormous amount of trauma that the infant sustained.

are displaced in relation to the humerus. However, the radius and ulna are in their normal relationship to each other (Fig. 20.11). This injury must be distinguished radiographically from an elbow dislocation, displaced lateral condylar fracture, and supracondylar humeral fracture.

Cubitus varus is the most common complication, likely the result of malunion, osteonecrosis of the medial condyle, or growth arrest.[98] Holda and colleagues[99] found cubitus varus deformity in five of their seven patients.

Surgical management with closed reduction and pinning using the aid of arthrogram is recommended for timely diagnosed fractures.[98] DeLee and associates[100] recommended closed reduction if the fracture was fresh, but if the fracture was old, they recommended splinting the arm until the fracture was solid, without any attempt at reduction. The results presented by Holda and colleagues[99] tend to corroborate such management because their results with more aggressive treatment were poor. Mizuno and colleagues[101] obtained good results with open reduction through a posterior approach, although this is seldom necessary.

The authors' preference is to investigate the possibility of child abuse first. The child may be admitted to the hospital to facilitate this investigation, if necessary. Admission may also be warranted for observation of circulatory changes. If reduction is required, gentle traction on the forearm first corrects coronal plane deformity followed by flexion of the elbow to correct sagittal plane deformity. The elbow flexion is commonly performed with the forearm pronated to prevent medial displacement, which can occur with the forearm in supination. If pins are placed, external rotation of the upper arm will maintain rotational instability, if present. The fracture is percutaneously pinned so that splinting in less flexion is allowed.

TYPE I PROXIMAL FEMORAL FRACTURES

Type I fractures of the proximal end of the femur are rare and are usually the result of significant trauma, such as a motor vehicle accident or a fall from a great height. Displaced type I fractures may be associated with dislocation of the femoral head. The prognosis, particularly in the case of dislocation, is generally poor because of the extremely high incidence of avascular necrosis.

If a type I fracture of the proximal part of the femur is seen and the history of the injury does not include violent trauma, the orthopedic surgeon should be suspicious of child abuse, especially in a child younger than 5 years. A 60% prevalence of child abuse has been documented in type I fractures of the proximal end of the femur in young children.[102]

Although the prognosis for a markedly displaced type I fracture is poor, minimally displaced fractures of the proximal femoral physis do well in the authors' experience. Forlin and colleagues[102] showed that avascular necrosis of the femoral head is not as common as once feared if the femoral head is not dislocated. Treatment of these fractures in a spica cast until union is complete is recommended. Remodeling of the fracture is usually extensive because of the wide range of motion of the hip (Fig. 20.12).

Other Salter-Harris injuries of the physis are commonly seen in children as a result of accidental trauma but are only rarely seen in victims of child abuse.

RIB FRACTURES

After fractures of the skull and long bones, the ribs are the third most common site of skeletal injury in children who are abused,[103,104,105] and 90% of abuse-related rib fractures

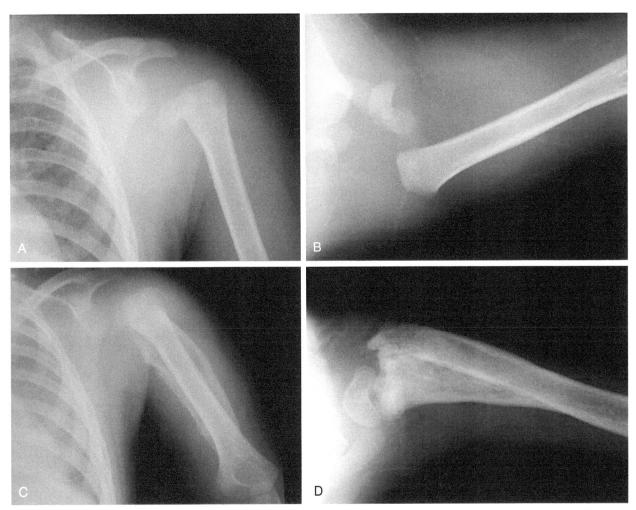

Fig. 20.10 A 20-month-old child who sustained a violent injury to her shoulder. When seen, she had an enormously swollen shoulder and would not move her arm. The family gave no history of trauma, but it was subsequently proved that the child had been abused. (A) This anteroposterior (AP) radiograph demonstrates a totally displaced fracture of the proximal humeral physis. The epiphysis sits inferior to the metaphysis and the inferior portion of the glenoid. (B) A lateral radiograph of the same shoulder and proximal part of the humerus again demonstrates the remarkable displacement of the fracture that occurred through the proximal humeral physis. (C) This AP radiograph taken 1 month postinjury demonstrates the enormous amount of periosteal new bone formation that is occupying the entire shaft of the humerus. This finding demonstrates that this fracture was the result of violent trauma with a significant amount of periosteal stripping all the way to the distal humeral metaphysis. (D) A lateral radiograph of the humerus 5 months after injury demonstrates that the fracture is healed with all the early remodeling. One can expect complete subsequent remodeling. At this juncture, the child had complete full range of motion of the shoulder with no pain and normal use of the arm.

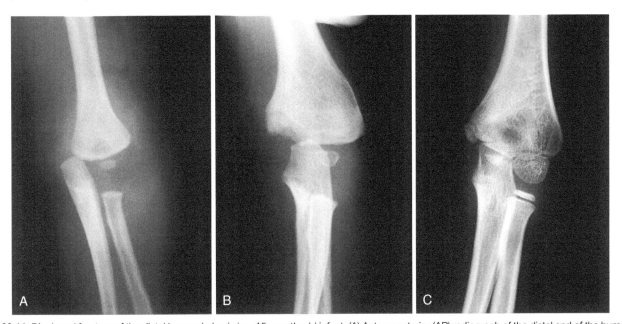

Fig. 20.11 Displaced fracture of the distal humeral physis in a 15-month-old infant. (A) Anteroposterior (AP) radiograph of the distal end of the humerus at the time of injury demonstrating medial displacement of the capitellum. Note that the longitudinal axis of the radius intersects the capitellum, which is displaced laterally. (B) AP radiograph of the elbow 3 months after injury. The displacement was not corrected at the time of immobilization. (C) Follow-up radiograph 5 years postinjury demonstrating remodeling of the distal portion of the humerus. Clinically, the patient had full mobility in the elbow.

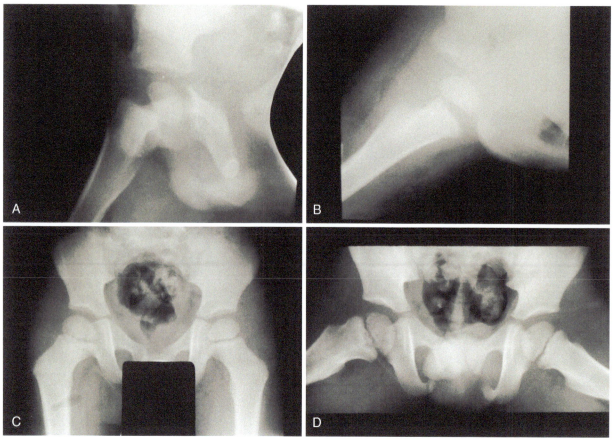

Fig. 20.12 A 3-year-old child sustained a type I physeal injury of the proximal end of the femur as a result of child abuse. (A) An anteroposterior (AP) radiograph demonstrates the angulation of the fracture but without complete displacement. (B) A lateral radiograph of the hip and proximal end of the femur also shows the displacement of the fracture. (C) An AP radiograph of both hips shows nearly complete remodeling of the fracture 1.5 years after the injury. The fracture was not reduced, but the child was placed in a hip spica cast for 6 weeks. No evidence of avascular necrosis of the femoral head can be found. (D) A lateral radiograph of both hips demonstrates nearly complete remodeling of the fracture.

are seen in children younger than 2 years.[104] The relatively pliant rib cage of infants and toddlers affords protection against fracture of the ribs from falls, and accidental fracture is rare.[103] Multiple studies have shown that rib fractures from cardiopulmonary resuscitation are extremely rare in children.[106,107,108] In the series by Worlock and colleagues,[35] none of the rib fractures in the infants and toddlers were the result of accidental trauma. Moreover, all the children and infants with rib fractures had an additional skeletal injury. Most of the rib fractures were identified incidentally on skeletal surveys.

Although often clinically unsuspected, abusive rib fractures are frequently multiple and most occur posteriorly.[109] These posterior fractures result from maximal mechanical stress at the costovertebral junction as the child is grasped and shaken. Lateral rib fractures are much less commonly seen in child abuse and are thought to be caused by anterior compression of the chest (Fig. 20.13). Anterior rib fractures involving the costochondral junctions have also been reported in association with major abdominal visceral injuries.[110] Rib fractures in abused children may be very difficult to diagnose radiographically in the acute care setting. In a postmortem study of infants who died with inflicted injuries, only 36% of the rib fractures identified were detected by the skeletal survey.[105] These fractures are best visualized radiographically after fracture callus is evident (Fig. 20.14). In the

postmortem setting, a detailed anthropologic dissection can improve the identification of rib fractures at autopsy.[109,111] Repeated chest films or CT scan on follow-up are highly indicated for detection of fractures not seen earlier.[63,64,65]

FRACTURES OF THE SHOULDER GIRDLE

Most accidental and abuse-related clavicular fractures were believed to involve the midshaft of the clavicle.[71] However, avulsion fractures of either end of the clavicle or an acromion process fracture can result from traction or the violent acceleration-deceleration in shaking.[50] Additionally, distal clavicular fractures in an infant are particularly suggestive and may be associated with proximal humeral fractures.[71,112]

SPINAL FRACTURES

Vertebral fractures remain unusual in child abuse,[71,113] but more recent reports describe several spinal lesions attributed to CPA. Hangman fractures and flexion-extension thoracolumbar injuries, in particular, appear to be recognized more commonly. Hangman fractures are cited with increasing frequency in the literature, and some authors suggest that the increased reporting should prompt the inclusion of a lateral view of the cervical spine in the routine skeletal survey done for suspected child abuse.[114–116]

Thoracolumbar injuries commonly occur through the neurocentral synchondrosis, the junction between the vertebral

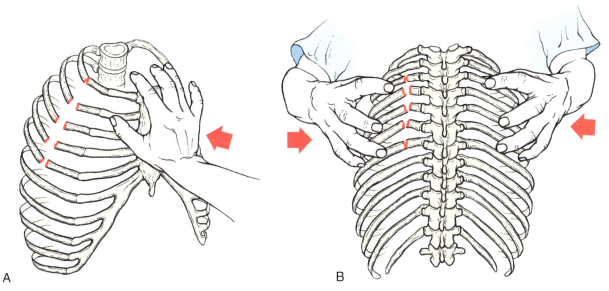

Fig. 20.13 Mechanism of injury that produces rib fractures. Anteroposterior compression of the chest most commonly results in fractures of the ribs laterally (A). Compression of the ribs from the side, however, produces posterior rib fractures (B). This mechanism of injury is most commonly seen in children who have been abused from side-to-side compression of the infant by an adult's hands.

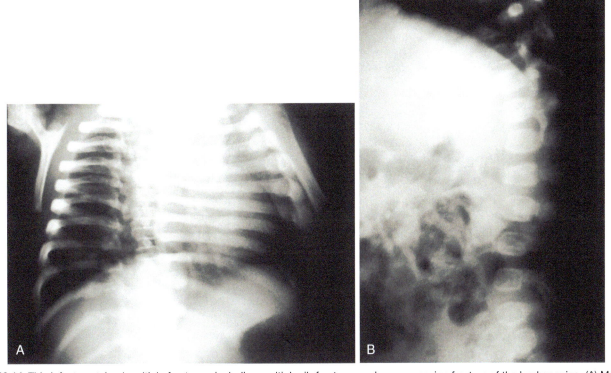

Fig. 20.14 This infant sustained multiple fractures, including multiple rib fractures and a compression fracture of the lumbar spine. (A) Multiple posterior fractures of the ribs on both sides of the chest in this infant were seen on a radiograph of the ribs taken on the day of admission to the hospital. These fractures were all healed, evidence that these injuries had occurred before admission. (B) A lateral radiograph of the spine demonstrates a compression fracture of the second lumbar vertebra. Both these injuries were thought to be the result of intentional trauma.

body and posterior elements. Because of this area's fragility during growth, traumatic injuries can occur until it fuses, usually by 5 or 6 years but as late as adolescence. In these fractures, the vertebral body and the vertebral arches with their articular processes remain intact, and vertebral body displacement can be anterior or posterior.[117,118]

There is increasing evidence that cervical spine injury can be identified in infant victims of abuse. With the improvement in imaging technology and software, the more modern CT and MRI images have identified spinous process and ligamentous injury in victims of abusive head trauma.[119–123]

However, differentiation from congenital defects is necessary. This can be accomplished with additional imaging by CT or MRI. If needed in fatal cases, postmortem analysis may be performed.[118,124,125]

> **Box 20.1   Differential Diagnosis of Inflicted Fractures in Children**
>
> Normal variants
> Birth trauma
> Osteogenesis imperfecta
> Osteopenia of prematurity
> Osteomyelitis
> Rickets
> Copper deficiency
> Congenital syphilis
> Leukemia
> Scurvy
> Drug-induced bone changes

Finally, injury to the spinal cord itself is rare but may be seen in association with particularly violent trauma.[113,125]

SKULL FRACTURES

Skull fractures are common in children who have been physically abused. These fractures are second in frequency only to fractures of the long bones. A child under the age of 6 with a skull fracture has a 1 in 3 chance of having been abused. Most abuse-related skull fractures are linear fractures in the parietal bone, similar to those seen in accidental trauma[79]; the more specific, depressed, wide, and complex lesions are found less frequently.[126] Although planar radiology has been the standard imaging modality, there is increasing data that three-dimensional reconstructed CT images are a preferable modality when available.[48,49] Cerebral damage associated with the skull injury is of greatest concern. One most commonly associates cerebral injury with trauma to the skull, but brain injury can occur without external signs of head trauma.[127]

In 1974, Caffey[8] coined the term *whiplash shaken infant syndrome*, also known as the *shaken baby syndrome*, or more appropriately, abusive head trauma.[128] A crying infant with an overwhelmed, frustrated caregiver is a scenario that not uncommonly results in severe and violent shaking of the baby. Injuries associated with abusive head trauma often include subdural, subarachnoid, and retinal hemorrhages. Axonal injury, cerebral edema, skull fractures (when shaking is associated with head impact injury), rib fractures, and long bone fractures may also be present.[129]

DIFFERENTIAL DIAGNOSIS

A suggestive history may lead one to investigate CPA. Differentiating the nonaccidental infliction of fractures from physiologic causes is anxiety provoking for both the physician and caregiver. The well-being of the child is paramount yet preserving a working relationship with the caregivers can be done with care and time. Understanding the demographics and different disease processes responsible for CPA can assist in narrowing the differential diagnosis (Box 20.1). Although a thorough history and physical examination usually provide the diagnosis, additional tests may occasionally be necessary for confirmation.

NORMAL VARIANTS

Healthy infants may exhibit periosteal new bone formation along the shafts of the long bones during the first few months of life. Spurring and cupping of the metaphysis are also frequently observed. These findings are initially seen between 2 and 3 months and resolve by 8 months.[130,131] The periosteal new bone formation is identical to that seen in trauma, and the clinical findings must be taken into account.

BIRTH TRAUMA

Birth trauma should be considered a possible cause when a child with a fracture is seen during the first few weeks of life. Clavicular fractures are the most common fractures related to birth trauma. Fractures missed in the delivery room or nursery are frequently found incidentally on chest radiographs or when palpable callus is noted by the parents. The humerus is the most commonly fractured long bone in birth trauma, and these fractures usually involve the midshaft. Long bone fractures of the lower extremities occurring during birth are often seen in association with neuromuscular disease or bone abnormality, whereas epiphyseal fractures are most commonly associated with breech delivery. Rib fractures from birth trauma are rare,[132–135] and rib fractures found incidentally, without a history of severe trauma, are usually as a result of abuse.[103] Callus develops in birth fractures within 2 weeks, and lack of callus formation after this time interval strongly suggests that the injury did not occur during delivery.[130]

OSTEOGENESIS IMPERFECTA

Osteogenesis imperfecta (OI) is the entity most often raised in the differential of cases of CPA. It has been historically divided into four main types based on clinical features described by Sillence since 1979.[136,137] The understanding of inheritance patterns in OI is evolving, and the many mutations responsible for the subsequent phenotypical expression have been expanded.[138] For simplicity's sake, the disease is discussed here based on the more obvious clinical features. Type I is most common and accounts for 80% of all cases. The sclerae are blue, and the skeletal manifestations are mild and associated with fewer fractures and less bone deformity than seen in the other types. Type II is a very severe form of the disease that leads to intrauterine or early infant death. Type III is similar to type II but milder; however, both types are characterized by extreme bone fragility, fractures at birth, and obvious bony deformity. Typically the severity of these two types makes them less likely to be mistaken for child abuse. Type IV is associated with less bone fragility than types II and III, the sclerae are normal or gray, and there is no dental involvement. Types I and IV are most likely to be mistaken for child abuse.

Radiographic features help differentiate OI from CPA. The severe forms of OI have ultrasound findings present before birth during the second trimester and are rarely confused with CPA. The less severe forms may have a degree of osteopenia and deformity, in addition to fractures, that may be helpful in distinguishing the diagnosis. Deformities, such as occipital prominence "Darth Vader appearance," cranial vault flattening "Tam O'Shanter skull," mosaic or "paving" wormian appearance in bone, pelvic coxa vara, or diaphyseal cortical thinning have been reported.[139] Occasionally, both osteopenia and deformity are radiographically absent, thereby making the diagnosis difficult. Although fractures in OI usually involve the shafts of the long bones,[140] Gahagan and Rimsza[141] have also reported metaphyseal corner-type fractures. In one study of children with OI,[140] metaphyseal fractures were seen in 15% of patients. If, in addition, the child is a member of an at-risk family, one may be quick to diagnose child abuse.

A review of a cohort of 68 children with OI revealed that OI can be readily identified on a clinical basis.[142] Rib fractures can rarely be seen in children with OI, but do not appear in infancy. Rib fractures can occur with delivery and in childhood, but would be unexpected during the first year of life. Importantly, children with OI, although they fracture easily, outside of the neonatal period, they typically present with two or fewer fractures at the time of diagnosis.[142] An infant or child with three or more fractures is more likely to have been a victim of CPA than OI.

A history that is incompatible with the injury is one of the hallmarks of child abuse; however, such is also the case in patients with OI. Fractures in these children may be sustained with minimal, even trivial, trauma. A careful family history is important. Because of the occurrence of new mutations, a negative history does not exclude the diagnosis of OI. Although the majority of children with OI can be comfortably diagnosed clinically,[142] genetic or fibroblast testing may be of value.[143,144] Currently, no single biochemical or genetic test is completely sensitive in identifying children with OI.[145] Biochemical analysis of skin fibroblast collagen to identify the abnormalities of type I collagen seen in children with OI is available, but 10% to 15% of individuals with nonlethal forms of OI are not identified with the correct screening test.[146] The determination of OI or abuse can usually be made by careful clinical evaluation by physicians familiar with the variability of OI. However, when the clinical examination and history are insufficient to make the diagnosis, laboratory testing for OI is a valuable adjunct.

OSTEOPENIA OF PREMATURITY

Osteopenia (or metabolic bone disease) of prematurity is a complication in low-birth-weight infants. The condition can be compounded by prolonged parenteral nutrition. Osteopenia of prematurity is multifactorial, with factors including inadequate calcium and phosphorus stores, inadequate mineral intake to support rapid growth, effects of medications used to treat complications of preterm birth, and limited patient mobility. It is radiographically defined by diffuse osteopenia or rickets, but these patients are prone to fractures as a result of the osteopenia that can present in similar fashion to CPA. This condition usually resolves by 6 to 12 weeks postnatally.[147]

TEMPORARY BRITTLE BONE DISEASE

Temporary brittle bone disease (TBBD) was initially hypothesized by Paterson and colleagues[148] to be a temporary deficiency of an enzyme involved in the posttranslational processing of collagen. They reported 39 patients who sustained fractures only in the first year of life and had findings similar to those seen in infantile copper deficiency; however, in addition, several features of so-called TBBD (fractures in the first year of life, preponderance of rib and metaphyseal fractures, and lack of an external mechanism of trauma) are factors associated with child abuse, creating doubt in the validity of this diagnosis. TBBD was subsequently proposed by Miller and Hangartner (1999) as a transient defect in copper metabolism,[149] but this perspective equally lacks meaningful empiric supporting data. This theory has been refuted by others as lacking any scientific data and is not widely accepted.[150–152] Neither of these theories is supported by any clinical or laboratory studies. The very nature of bone maturation and development makes it unlikely that bones would quickly change from fragile to normal. TBBD is neither clinically validated nor generally accepted by expert professionals and should not be invoked to explain multiple fractures in an infant.[153,154]

OSTEOMYELITIS

Multifocal metaphyseal lesions with periosteal reaction may be seen in osteomyelitis in young infants. The classic systemic signs and symptoms of infection may not be present in a neonate, thus making the diagnosis difficult. However, true corner fractures are not present, and the metaphyseal radiolucencies are less well-defined in osteomyelitis. Over time, the bone destruction seen in osteomyelitis is easily differentiated from the bone formation seen in healing fractures.[62]

RICKETS

Although metaphyseal abnormalities, fractures, and periosteal reaction may be seen in both rickets and child abuse, the additional radiographic characteristics seen in rickets allow proper diagnosis; however some controversy remains.[155] Fraying of the metaphysis, widening of the physis, and Looser zones (sharply defined, symmetric, transverse stress fractures in the shafts of long bones) are all seen in rickets but not in child abuse.[93,156] Multiple long bone and rib fractures are more prominent in premature infants in whom rickets develops in association with total parenteral nutrition. Laboratory tests confirm the diagnosis.[157]

COPPER DEFICIENCY

Kinky hair disease, or Menkes syndrome, is associated with inadequate copper absorption. Although often presented as a mimic of CPA, Menkes syndrome is exceedingly rare and is clinically easy to distinguish. The metaphyseal fractures and periosteal reaction observed in this disorder are similar to those seen with abuse. Long bone metaphyseal spurring and wormian bones in the skull help differentiate this condition from CPA. Serum levels of copper and ceruloplasmin are reduced and confirm the diagnosis.[158]

CONGENITAL SYPHILIS

The prevalence of congenital syphilis is increasing in the United States and, if unrecognized, may lead to a delay in treatment, progression of the disease, or a misdiagnosis of child abuse.[159,160] Congenital syphilis may be mistaken for

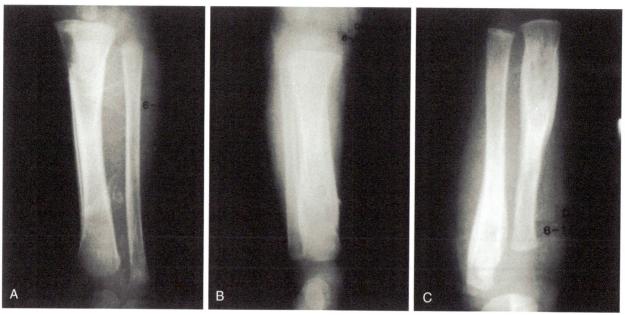

Fig. 20.15 Radiographs of multiple bones of an infant with congenital syphilis. (A and B) The radiographs show periosteal new bone in both tibias. (C) Periosteal new bone formation in the radius and ulna.

child abuse because of the periosteal new bone formation and the corner metaphyseal erosions that may be mistaken for corner fractures. Wimberger sign is a classic finding in congenital syphilis and refers to a medial tibial metaphyseal defect. Congenital syphilis is frequently diffuse and can involve not only the long bones but also the skull and the small bones of the hands and feet. The epiphyses and spine are spared. The bone lesions of congenital syphilis are usually symmetric, and serologic testing confirms the diagnosis (Fig. 20.15).

CONGENITAL INSENSITIVITY TO PAIN

Inherited as an autosomal recessive trait, this rare syndrome is difficult to differentiate from abuse. Afflicted children are normal in every aspect except for indifference to painful stimuli and occasionally temperature. Multiple fractures and epiphyseal separations may be seen in various stages of healing. A detailed clinical history, careful neurologic sensory examination, and genetic analysis for mutation in the *SCN9A* gene are helpful in making the diagnosis.[161]

CAFFEY DISEASE

Infantile cortical hyperostosis is a painful periosteal reaction that results in cortical thickening. It occurs in infants younger than 6 months, and its cause is unknown. Although any bone may be involved, the mandible, clavicle, and ulna are the most common sites. The mandible is involved in 95% of cases. Metaphyseal lesions and fractures are not seen in Caffey disease, and it is more commonly confused with osteomyelitis because of the laboratory results and clinical picture associated with inflammation (elevated erythrocyte sedimentation rate, alkaline phosphatase, total leukocyte count, immunoglobulin levels, C-reactive protein, and platelet count; and decreased hemoglobin) (Fig. 20.16).[162]

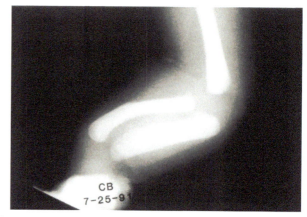

Fig. 20.16 Caffey disease is a rare cause of periosteal new bone formation. A radiograph of the forearm in this infant shows periosteal new bone formation in both the radius and, especially, the ulna. Frequently, such children may have fever and evidence of local inflammation, which makes the differential diagnosis of osteomyelitis more common than child abuse.

VITAMIN A INTOXICATION

Fractures are rare with hypervitaminosis A. However, widening of the cranial sutures and a thick, undulating periosteal reaction of the tubular bones is frequently seen, particularly in the ulna and metatarsals. Early on, the epiphyseal and metaphyseal areas are radiographically normal, but late deformities secondary to premature epiphyseal fusion have been reported. This is more commonly mistaken for infantile cortical hyperostosis. The diagnosis is confirmed by the history and vitamin A levels.[163]

LEUKEMIA

Diffuse demineralization and periosteal reaction are both features of leukemia. Multiple localized osteolytic lesions are characteristic of leukemia, whereas sclerotic lesions are unusual. Narrow, radiolucent metaphyseal bands, or *leukemic lines*, may be seen, but the associated osteopenia and lack of bony fragments easily distinguish them from the metaphyseal lesions in child abuse.

SCURVY

Scurvy is much less common than rickets and is unusual before the age of 6 months. It is caused by inadequate vitamin C intake. Some of the radiographic changes seen in scurvy, such as subperiosteal hemorrhage and metaphyseal fractures, may also be seen in child abuse. However, bone mineralization in scurvy is impaired, and thin cortices and osteopenia allow differentiation from child abuse.[70]

SPONTANEOUS FRACTURES SECONDARY TO OSTEOPENIA

The term *spontaneous fractures secondary to osteopenia* is used to define fractures that occur without any known external cause and is a diagnosis of exclusion. It is more commonly found in children with neuromuscular syndromes, such as cerebral palsy with spasticity or myelodysplasia.[164]

DRUG-INDUCED BONE CHANGES

Periosteal reaction of the ribs and long bones may be seen in association with the use of prostaglandin E_1. The diagnosis is determined by the history because the radiologic findings are identical to those of traumatic periostitis.[70] Previously, fractures and osteopenia were reported in children treated with methotrexate, but current treatment protocols using lower doses of the drug make such fractures rare today.

A careful history and physical examination combined with thoughtful interpretation of the radiographs and confirmatory laboratory testing generally allow for a correct diagnosis, even if the condition results from obscure causes.

MANAGEMENT

Evaluation of suspected child abuse is best handled by a multidisciplinary team of healthcare professionals. It is crucial that those involved have appropriate training and continuing medical education in evaluation and treatment of CPA because diagnostic accuracy improves with such experience.[165] This child protection team may include a board-certified child abuse pediatrician, a social worker, a nurse, and a pediatric orthopedic surgeon. Consultants may include a pediatric radiologist, a pediatric neurosurgeon, a pediatric neurologist, and a pediatric ophthalmologist. One individual, such as the social worker, should be designated as the contact person for the child abuse team. Such an arrangement facilitates reporting of suspected abuse in that all contacts are made through the same person or office.

The physician should remain nonjudgmental and, if possible, attempt to establish a normal relationship with the family. If a child is seen with a suspicious fracture, the physician should explain to the family that the injury is one that may be seen in abused children. One should never accuse the family but explain in a nonjudgmental manner that the injuries raise concern for the child's safety and

that physicians are required by law to contact appropriate investigative agencies. So that the patient's continued safety can be ensured, the abused child may be hospitalized even if admission is not indicated based on injury severity. This will allow time for child protective agencies and law enforcement to ensure the safety of the home environment and conduct their investigation. If necessary, the child may be placed in emergency foster care. Abuse of siblings must also be considered, and care must be provided for them. In one study, approximately 12% of siblings of abused children were noted to have at least one abusive fracture.[24] Although orthopedic surgeons do not usually assume the primary responsibility for complete evaluation and reporting of suspected child abuse, they should be aware of the process so that appropriate steps are taken to ensure the future safety of the child.

The vast majority of orthopedic injuries associated with child abuse occur in very young children. Healing is therefore rapid, and treatment primarily consists of simple immobilization of the injured area until the fracture has healed. Frequently, many of these children are seen some time after the original injury, and some degree of healing may already be present. Rarely do the orthopedic injuries associated with child abuse require urgent operative treatment. Particularly in this young age group, significant remodeling is advantageous and most often results in complete correction of the deformity over time. Because these lesions pose the highest risk of permanent deformity, it is fortunate that injuries to the physis itself are rare.

CONCLUSION

Ultimately, good judgment and experience continue to be the best guide in the diagnosis of CPA. The nature of the injuries likely precludes a technologic advancement that guarantees diagnosis, although standardized workups that include laboratory testing in addition to standard radiographic imaging are becoming more prominent.[166,167] However, it is critical that physicians educate themselves on historical cues and injury characteristics that lead to this diagnosis. Furthermore, physicians must be aware of the role they play in identifying suspicious childhood injuries and reporting them to child protective services.

REFERENCES

The level of evidence (LOE) is determined according to the criteria provided in the Preface.

1. U.S. Department of Health & Human Services, A. f. C. a. F. *Administration on Children, Youth and Families.* Children's Bureau. U.S. Department of Health & Human Services, Administration for Children and Families, Administration on Children, Youth and Families, Children's Bureau; 2018. Child Maltreatment 2016. 2016. Available from: https://www.acf.hhs.gov/cb/research-data-technology/statistics-research/child-maltreatment. **(LOE V)**.
2. Christian CW, et al. The evaluation of suspected child physical abuse. *Pediatrics.* 2015;135(5):e1337–1354. **(LOE V)**.
3. Flaherty EG, et al. Evaluating children with fractures for child physical abuse. *Pediatrics.* 2014;133(2):e477–489. **(LOE V)**.
4. Jevsevar DS, et al. AAOS clinical practice guideline on the treatment of pediatric diaphyseal femur fractures. *J Am Acad Orthop Surg.* 2015;23(12):e101. **(LOE V)**.

5. Williams C. United Kingdom General Medical Council fails child protection. *Pediatrics.* 2007;119(4):800–802. **(LOE III)**.

6. Kocher MS, Kasser JR. Orthopaedic aspects of child abuse. *J Am Acad Orthop Surg.* 2000;8(1):10–20. **(LOE III)**.

7. Lee PY, et al. Nurse reporting of known and suspected child abuse and neglect cases in Taiwan. *Kaohsiung J Med Sci.* 2007;23(3):128–137. **(LOE IV)**.

8. Caffey J. Multiple fractures in the long bones of infants suffering from chronic subdural hematoma. *Am J Roentgenol Radium Ther.* 1946;56(2):163–173. **(LOE III)**.

9. Silverman FN. The roentgen manifestations of unrecognized skeletal trauma in infants. *Am J Roentgenol Radium Ther Nucl Med.* 1953;69(3):413–427. **(LOE IV)**.

10. Altman DH, Smith RL. Unrecognized trauma in infants and children. *J Bone Joint Surg Am.* 1960;42-a:407–413. **(LOE III)**.

11. Kempe CH, Helfer RE. *Helping the Battered Child and His Family.* Philadelphia: Lippincott; 1972. **(LOE V)**.

12. Sedlak AJ, Mettenburg J, Basena M, et al. *Fourth National Incidence Study of Child Abuse and Neglect (NIS–4): Report to Congress.* Washington, DC: U.S. Department of Health and Human Services; 2010. **(LOE V)**.

13. Dubowitz H. Preventing child neglect and physical abuse: a role for pediatricians. *Pediatr Rev.* 2002;23(6):191–196. **(LOE V)**.

14. Finkelhor D, Saito K, Jones L. *Updated Trends in Child Maltreatment, 2014.* Durham, NH: Crimes against Children Research Center; 2016. **(LOE IV)**.

15. Ney PG, et al. The worst combinations of child abuse and neglect. *Child Abuse Negl.* 1994;18(9):705–714. **(LOE III)**.

16. Kempe CH. Sexual abuse, another hidden pediatric problem: the 1977 C. Anderson Aldrich lecture. *Pediatrics.* 1978;62(3):382–389. **(LOE V)**.

17. Jenny C, Crawford-Jakubiak JE. The evaluation of children in the primary care setting when sexual abuse is suspected. *Pediatrics.* 2013;132(2):e558–567. **(LOE III)**.

18. Kellogg N. The evaluation of sexual abuse in children. *Pediatrics.* 2005;116(2):506–512. **(LOE III)**.

19. McPherson P, et al. Barriers to successful treatment completion in child sexual abuse survivors. *J Interpers Violence.* 2012;27(1):23–39. **(LOE III)**.

20. McMahon P, et al. Soft-tissue injury as an indication of child abuse. *J Bone Joint Surg Am.* 1995;77(8):1179–1183. **(LOE IV)**.

21. Council on Scientific Affairs. AMA diagnostic and treatment guidelines concerning child abuse and neglect. Council on Scientific Affairs. *JAMA.* 1985;254(6):796–800. **(LOE V)**.

22. Akbarnia BA, Akbarnia NO. The role of orthopedist in child abuse and neglect. *Orthop Clin North Am.* 1976;7(3):733–742. **(LOE V)**.

23. Lindberg DM, et al. Predictors of screening and injury in contacts of physically abused children. *J Pediatr.* 2013;163(3):730–735. e731-733. **(LOE III)**.

24. Lindberg DM, et al. Prevalence of abusive injuries in siblings and household contacts of physically abused children. *Pediatrics.* 2012;130(2):193–201. **(LOE IV)**.

25. Galleno H, Oppenheim WL. The battered child syndrome revisited. *Clin Orthop Relat Res.* 1982;162:11–19. **(LOE III)**.

26. Schmitt M, et al. Battered child syndrome. *Pediatric trauma. R. Touloukin.* St. Louis, Mosby-Year Book: 1990;161. **(LOE V)**.

27. Chaffin M, et al. Parent-child interaction therapy with physically abusive parents: efficacy for reducing future abuse reports. *J Consult Clin Psychol.* 2004;72(3):500–510. **(LOE I)**.

28. Macmillan HL, et al. Interventions to prevent child maltreatment and associated impairment. *Lancet.* 2009;373(9659):250–266. **(LOE II)**.

29. Carty H, Pierce A. Non-accidental injury: a retrospective analysis of a large cohort. *Eur Radiol.* 2002;12(12):2919–2925. **(LOE III)**.

30. Skellern CY, et al. Non-accidental fractures in infants: risk of further abuse. *J Paediatr Child Health.* 2000;36(6):590–592. **(LOE IV)**.

31. Strait RT, et al. Humeral fractures without obvious etiologies in children less than 3 years of age: when is it abuse? *Pediatrics.* 1995;96(4 Pt 1):667–671. **(LOE IV)**.

32. Holter JC, Friedman SB. Child abuse: early case finding in the emergency department. *Pediatrics.* 1968;42(1):128–138. **(LOE IV)**.

33. Parry N, Goldsworthy L, Melsom S, Fryer J, Haythornthwaite G. Non-accidental injury: an important cause of pediatric major trauma. *Emerg Med J.* 2016;33:937–938. **(LOE III)**.

34. Herndon WA. Child abuse in a military population. *J Pediatr Orthop.* 1983;3(1):73–76. **(LOE IV)**.

35. Worlock P, et al. Patterns of fractures in accidental and non-accidental injury in children: a comparative study. *Br Med J.* 1986;293 (6539):100–102. **(LOE II)**.

36. Pierce MC, et al. Femur fractures resulting from stair falls among children: an injury plausibility model. *Pediatrics.* 2005;115(6):1712–1722. **(LOE IV)**.

37. Lindberg DM, et al. Variability in expert assessments of child physical abuse likelihood. *Pediatrics.* 2008;121(4):e945–953. **(LOE IV)**.

38. Lamb ME, et al. A structured forensic interview protocol improves the quality and informativeness of investigative interviews with children: a review of research using the NICHD Investigative Interview Protocol. *Child Abuse Negl.* 2007;31(11–12):1201–1231. **(LOE II)**.

39. Pence D, et al. *Investigative Interviewing in Cases of Alleged Child Abuse: Practical Guidelines.* Proceedings from APSAC Task Force on Investigative Interviews in Cases of Alleged Child Abuse: Chicago. **(LOE V)**.

40. Van Horne BS, et al. Maltreatment of children under age 2 with specific birth defects: a population-based study. *Pediatrics.* 2015;136(6):e1504–1512. **(LOE III)**.

41. Wu SS, et al. Risk factors for infant maltreatment: a population-based study. *Child Abuse Negl.* 2004;28(12):1253–1264. **(LOE IV)**.

42. Overpeck MD, et al. Risk factors for infant homicide in the United States. *N Engl J Med.* 1998;339(17):1211–1216. **(LOE IV)**.

43. Pierce MC, et al. Bruising characteristics discriminating physical child abuse from accidental trauma. *Pediatrics.* 2010;125(1):67–74. **(LOE III)**.

44. Greeley CS. Abusive head trauma: a review of the evidence base. *AJR Am J Roentgenol.* 2015;204(5):967–973. **(LOE III)**.

45. Wilkinson WS, et al. Retinal hemorrhage predicts neurologic injury in the shaken baby syndrome. *Arch Ophthalmol.* 1989;107(10): 1472–1474. **(LOE IV)**.

46. Arbogast KB, et al. Initial neurologic presentation in young children sustaining inflicted and unintentional fatal head injuries. *Pediatrics.* 2005;116(1):180–184. **(LOE III)**.

47. Salzinger S, et al. The effects of physical abuse on children's social relationships. *Child Dev.* 1993;64(1):169–187. **(LOE II)**.

48. Culotta PA, et al. Performance of computed tomography of the head to evaluate for skull fractures in infants with suspected non-accidental trauma. *Pediatr Radiol.* 2017;47(1):74–81. **(LOE III)**.

49. Dundamadappa SK, et al. Skull fractures in pediatric patients on computerized tomogram: comparison between routing bone window images and 3D volume-rendered images. *Emerg Radiol.* 2015;22(4):367–372. **(LOE III)**.

50. Merten DF, Carpenter BL. Radiologic imaging of inflicted injury in the child abuse syndrome. *Pediatr Clin North Am.* 1990;37(4):815–837. **(LOE V)**.

51. Offiah AC, et al. Diagnostic accuracy of fracture detection in suspected non-accidental injury: the effect of edge enhancement and digital display on observer performance. *Clin Radiol.* 2006;61(2):163–173. **(LOE IV)**.

52. Lonergan GJ, et al. From the archives of the AFIP. Child abuse: radiologic-pathologic correlation. *Radiographics.* 2003;23(4):811–845. **(LOE III)**.

53. Bennett BL, et al. Retrospective review to determine the utility of follow-up skeletal surveys in child abuse evaluations when the initial skeletal survey is normal. *BMC Res Notes.* 2011;4:354. **(LOE III)**.

54. Harlan SR, et al. Follow-up skeletal surveys for nonaccidental trauma: can a more limited survey be performed? *Pediatr Radiol.* 2009;39(9):962–968. **(LOE II)**.

55. Powell-Doherty RD, et al. Examining the role of follow-up skeletal surveys in non-accidental trauma. *Am J Surg.* 2017;213(4):606–610. **(LOE IV)**.

56. Sonik A, et al. Follow-up skeletal surveys for suspected non-accidental trauma: can a more limited survey be performed without compromising diagnostic information? *Child Abuse Negl.* 2010;34(10):804–806. **(LOE IV)**.

57. Harper NS, et al. The utility of follow-up skeletal surveys in child abuse. *Pediatrics.* 2013;131(3):e672–678. **(LOE II)**.

58. Mandelstam SA, et al. Complementary use of radiological skeletal survey and bone scintigraphy in detection of bony injuries in suspected child abuse. *Arch Dis Child.* 2003;88(5):387–390; discussion 387-390. **(LOE IV)**.

59. Sty JR, Starshak RJ. The role of bone scintigraphy in the evaluation of the suspected abused child. *Radiology.* 1983;146(2):369–375. **(LOE II)**.

60. Meyer JS, et al. ACR Appropriateness Criteria® on suspected physical abuse-child. *J Am Coll Radiol.* 2011;8(2):87–94. **(LOE V)**.

61. Supakul N, et al. Distal humeral epiphyseal separation in young children: an often-missed fracture-radiographic signs and ultrasound confirmatory diagnosis. *AJR Am J Roentgenol.* 2015; 204(2):W192–W198. **(LOE IV)**.

62. van Rijn RR, Sieswerda-Hoogendoorn T. Educational paper: imaging child abuse: the bare bones. *Eur J Pediatr.* 2012;171(2): 215–224. **(LOE III)**.

63. Dankerl P, et al. Evaluation of rib fractures on a single-in-plane image reformation of the rib cage in CT examinations. *Acad Radiol.* 2017;24(2):153–159. **(LOE III)**.

64. Kleinman PK, et al. Detection of rib fractures in an abused infant using digital radiography: a laboratory study. *Pediatr Radiol.* 2002;32(12):896–901. **(LOE V)**.

65. Wootton-Gorges SL, et al. Comparison of computed tomography and chest radiography in the detection of rib fractures in abused infants. *Child Abuse Negl.* 2008;32(6):659–663. **(LOE IV)**.

66. Pickett TA. The challenges of accurately estimating time of long bone injury in children. *J Forensic Leg Med.* 2015;33:105–110. **(LOE III)**.

67. Drury A, Cunningham C. Determining when a fracture occurred: does the method matter? Analysis of the similarity of three different methods for estimating time since fracture of juvenile long bones. *J Forensic Leg Med.* 2018;53:97–105. **(LOE V)**.

68. O'Connor J, Cohen J. Dating fractures. *Diagnostic Imaging of Child Abuse.* 2nd ed. St. Louis: Mosby; 1998:168–177. **(LOE V)**.

69. Al Ayed IH, et al. The spectrum of child abuse presenting to a university hospital in Riyadh. *Ann Saudi Med.* 1998;18(2):125–131. **(LOE III)**.

70. Kleinman PK, ed. *Diagnostic Imaging of Child Abuse.* 3rd ed. Cambridge: Cambridge University Press; 2015. **(LOE I)**.

71. Kogutt MS, et al. Patterns of injury and significance of uncommon fractures in the battered child syndrome. *Am J Roentgenol Radium Ther Nucl Med.* 1974;121(1):143–149. **(LOE III)**.

72. Loder RT, Bookout C. Fracture patterns in battered children. *J Orthop Trauma.* 1991;5(4):428–433. **(LOE IV)**.

73. Thomas SA, et al. Long-bone fractures in young children: distinguishing accidental injuries from child abuse. *Pediatrics.* 1991;88(3):471–476. **(LOE IV)**.

74. Helfer RE, et al. Injuries resulting when small children fall out of bed. *Pediatrics.* 1977;60(4):533–535. **(LOE V)**.

75. O'Neill JA Jr, et al. Patterns of injury in the battered child syndrome. *J Trauma.* 1973;13(4):332–339. **(LOE III)**.

76. King J, et al. Analysis of 429 fractures in 189 battered children. *J Pediatr Orthop.* 1988;8(5):585–589. **(LOE III)**.

77. Blakemore LC, et al. Role of intentional abuse in children 1 to 5 years old with isolated femoral shaft fractures. *J Pediatr Orthop.* 1996;16(5):585–588. **(LOE II)**.

78. Merten DF, et al. The abused child: a radiological reappraisal. *Radiology.* 1983;146(2):377–381. **(LOE IV)**.

79. Kemp AM, et al. Patterns of skeletal fractures in child abuse: systematic review. *BMJ.* 2008;337:a1518. **(LOE II)**.

80. McClelland CQ, Heiple KG. Fractures in the first year of life. A diagnostic dilemma. *Am J Dis Child.* 1982;136(1):26–29. **(LOE III)**.

81. Son-Hing JP, Deniz Olgun Z. The frequency of nonaccidental trauma in children under the age of 3 years with femur fractures: is there a better cutoff point for universal workups? *J Pediatr Orthop B.* 2018;27(4):366–368. **(LOE IV)**.

82. Baldwin K, et al. Femur fractures in the pediatric population: abuse or accidental trauma? *Clin Orthop Relat Res.* 2011;469(3):798–804. **(LOE III)**.

83. Rewers A, et al. Childhood femur fractures, associated injuries, and sociodemographic risk factors: a population-based study. *Pediatrics.* 2005;115(5):e543–e552. **(LOE III)**.

84. Capra L, et al. Characteristics of femur fractures in ambulatory young children. *Emerg Med J.* 2013;30(9):749–753. **(LOE III)**.

85. Hui C, et al. Femoral fractures in children younger than three years: the role of nonaccidental injury. *J Pediatr Orthop.* 2008;28(3):297–302. **(LOE IV)**.

86. Schwend RM, et al. Femur shaft fractures in toddlers and young children: rarely from child abuse. *J Pediatr Orthop.* 2000;20(4):475–481. **(LOE III)**.

87. Murphy R, et al. Transverse fractures of the femoral shaft are a better predictor of nonaccidental trauma in young children than spiral fractures are. *J Bone Joint Surg Am.* 2015;97(2):106–111. **(LOE IV)**.

88. Rex C, Kay PR. Features of femoral fractures in nonaccidental injury. *J Pediatr Orthop.* 2000;20(3):411–413. **(LOE IV)**.

89. Thompson NB, et al. Intraobserver and interobserver reliability and the role of fracture morphology in classifying femoral shaft fractures in young children. *J Pediatr Orthop.* 2014;34(3):352–358. **(LOE III)**.

90. Pandya NK, et al. Humerus fractures in the pediatric population: an algorithm to identify abuse. *J Pediatr Orthop B.* 2010;19(6): 535–541. **(LOE III)**.

91. Coffey C, et al. The risk of child abuse in infants and toddlers with lower extremity injuries. *J Pediatr Surg.* 2005;40(1):120–123. **(LOE III)**.

92. Pandya NK, et al. Child abuse and orthopaedic injury patterns: analysis at a level I pediatric trauma center. *J Pediatr Orthop.* 2009;29(6):618–625. **(LOE III)**.

93. Kleinman PK, et al. The metaphyseal lesion in abused infants: a radiologic-histopathologic study. *AJR Am J Roentgenol.* 1986;146(5):895–905. **(LOE III)**.

94. Kleinman PK, Marks SC Jr. Relationship of the subperiosteal bone collar to metaphyseal lesions in abused infants. *J Bone Joint Surg Am.* 1995;77(10):1471–1476. **(LOE III)**.

95. Kleinman PK, Marks SC Jr. A regional approach to the classic metaphyseal lesion in abused infants: the proximal tibia. *AJR Am J Roentgenol.* 1996;166(2):421–426. **(LOE IV)**.

96. Osier LK, et al. Metaphyseal extensions of hypertrophied chondrocytes in abused infants indicate healing fractures. *J Pediatr Orthop.* 1993;13(2):249–254. **(LOE IV)**.

97. Gilbert SR, Conklin MJ. Presentation of distal humerus physeal separation. *Pediatr Emerg Care.* 2007;23(11):816–819. **(LOE III)**.

98. Abzug JM, et al. Transphyseal fracture of the distal humerus. *J Am Acad Orthop Surg.* 2016;24(2):e39–44. **(LOE V)**.

99. Holda ME, et al. Epiphyseal separation of the distal end of the humerus with medial displacement. *J Bone Joint Surg Am.* 1980;62(1):52–57. **(LOE IV)**.

100. DeLee JC, et al. Fracture-separation of the distal humeral epiphysis. *J Bone Joint Surg Am.* 1980;62(1):46–51. **(LOE IV)**.

101. Mizuno K, et al. Fracture-separation of the distal humeral epiphysis in young children. *J Bone Joint Surg Am.* 1979;61(4):570–573. **(LOE III)**.

102. Forlin E, et al. Transepiphyseal fractures of the neck of the femur in very young children. *J Pediatr Orthop.* 1992;12(2):164–168. **(LOE III)**.

103. Bulloch B, et al. Cause and clinical characteristics of rib fractures in infants. *Pediatrics.* 2000;105(4):E48. **(LOE III)**.

104. Garcia VF, et al. Rib fractures in children: a marker of severe trauma. *J Trauma.* 1990;30(6):695–700. **(LOE III)**.

105. Kleinman PK, et al. Rib fractures in 31 abused infants: postmortem radiologic-histopathologic study. *Radiology.* 1996;200(3):807–810. **(LOE IV)**.

106. Betz P, Liebhardt E. Liebhardt Rib fractures in children–resuscitation or child abuse? *Int J Legal Med.* 1994;106(4):215–218. **(LOE III)**.

107. Feldman KW, Brewer DK. Child abuse, cardiopulmonary resuscitation, and rib fractures. *Pediatrics.* 1984;73(3):339–342. **(LOE II)**.

108. Hoke RS, Chamberlain D. Skeletal chest injuries secondary to cardiopulmonary resuscitation. *Resuscitation.* 2004;63(3):327–338. **(LOE III)**.

109. Love JC, et al. Novel classification system of rib fractures observed in infants. *J Forensic Sci.* 2013;58(2):330–335. **(LOE III)**.

110. Ng CS, Hall CM. Costochondral junction fractures and intra-abdominal trauma in non-accidental injury (child abuse). *Pediatr Radiol.* 1998;28(9):671–676. **(LOE V)**.

111. Love JC, Sanchez LA. Recognition of skeletal fractures in infants: an autopsy technique. *J Forensic Sci.* 2009;54(6):1443–1446. **(LOE V)**.

112. Carty HM. Fractures caused by child abuse. *J Bone Joint Surg Br.* 1993;75(6):849–857. **(LOE V)**.

113. Swischuk LE. Spine and spinal cord trauma in the battered child syndrome. *Radiology.* 1969;92(4):733–738. (LOE: V).

114. Kleinman PK. Hangman's fracture caused by suspected child abuse. *J Pediatr Orthop B.* 2004;13(5):348. author reply 348. **(LOE IV)**.

115. Oral R, et al. Intentional avulsion fracture of the second cervical vertebra in a hypotonic child. *Pediatr Emerg Care.* 2006;22(5):352–354. **(LOE V)**.

116. Ranjith RK, et al. Hangman's fracture caused by suspected child abuse. A case report. *J Pediatr Orthop B.* 2002;11(4):329–332. **(LOE V)**.

117. Levin TL, et al. Thoracolumbar fracture with listhesis—an uncommon manifestation of child abuse. *Pediatr Radiol.* 2003;33(5):305–310. **(LOE IV)**.

118. Vialle R, et al. Spinal fracture through the neurocentral synchondrosis in battered children: a report of three cases. *Spine.* 2006;31(11):E345–E349. **(LOE V)**.

119. Choudhary AK, et al. Imaging of spinal injury in abusive head trauma: a retrospective study. *Pediatr Radiol.* 2014;44(9):1130–1140. **(LOE III)**.

120. Governale LS, et al. A retrospective study of cervical spine MRI findings in children with abusive head trauma. *Pediatr Neurosurg.* 2018;53(1):36–42. **(LOE IV)**.

121. Gruber TJ, Rozzelle CJ. Thoracolumbar spine subdural hematoma as a result of nonaccidental trauma in a 4-month-old infant. *J Neurosurg Pediatr.* 2008;2(2):139–142. **(LOE V)**.

122. Kadom N, et al. Usefulness of MRI detection of cervical spine and brain injuries in the evaluation of abusive head trauma. *Pediatr Radiol.* 2014;44(7):839–848. **(LOE IV)**.

123. Kemp AM, et al. What are the clinical and radiological characteristics of spinal injuries from physical abuse: a systematic review. *Arch Dis Child.* 2010;95(5):355–360. **(LOE II)**.

124. Aronica-Pollak PA, et al. Coronal cleft vertebra initially suspected as an abusive fracture in an infant. *J Forensic Sci.* 2003;48(4):836–838. **(LOE IV)**.

125. Brennan LK, et al. Neck injuries in young pediatric homicide victims. *J Neurosurg Pediatr.* 2009;3(3):232–239. **(LOE III)**.

126. Merten DF, et al. Craniocerebral trauma in the child abuse syndrome: radiological observations. *Pediatr Radiol.* 1984;14(5):272–277. **(LOE III)**.

127. Morris MW, et al. Evaluation of infants with subdural hematoma who lack external evidence of abuse. *Pediatrics.* 2000;105(3 Pt 1):549–553. **(LOE IV)**.

128. Christian CW, Block R. Abusive head trauma in infants and children. *Pediatrics.* 2009;123(5):1409–1411. **(LOE V)**.

129. Hymel KP, Deye KP. *Abusive Head Trauma. Child Abuse and Neglect.* Elsevier; 2010:349–358. **(LOE V)**.

130. Brill PW, et al. *Differential Diagnosis 1: Diseases Simulating Abuse. PK Kleinman Diagnostic Imaging of Child Abuse.* St. Louis: Mosby, Inc.; 1998:178–196. **(LOE V)**.

131. Glaser K. Double contour, cupping and spurring in roentgenograms of long bones in infants. *Am J Roentgenol Radium Ther.* 1949;61(4):482–492. **(LOE V)**.

132. Barry PW, Hocking MD. Infant rib fracture–birth trauma or non-accidental injury. *Arch Dis Child.* 1993;68(2):250. **(LOE IV)**.

133. Hartmann RW Jr. Radiological case of the month. Rib fractures produced by birth trauma. *Arch Pediatr Adolesc Med.* 1997;151(9):947–948. **(LOE V)**.

134. Rizzolo PJ, Coleman PR. Neonatal rib fracture: birth trauma or child abuse? *J Fam Pract.* 1989;29(5):561–563. **(LOE V)**.

135. Thomas PS. Rib fractures in infancy. *Ann Radiol.* 1977;20(1):115–122. **(LOE V)**.

136. Ben Amor IM, et al. Genotype-phenotype correlations in autosomal dominant osteogenesis imperfecta. *J Osteoporos.* 2011:540178. **(LOE III)**.

137. Kocher MS, Shapiro F. Osteogenesis imperfecta. *J Am Acad Orthop Surg.* 1998;6(4):225–236. **(LOE III)**.

138. Ben Amor M, et al. Osteogenesis imperfecta. *Pediatr Endocrinol Rev.* 2013;2(suppl 10):397–405. **(LOE III)**.

139. Renaud A, et al. Radiographic features of osteogenesis imperfecta. *Insights Imaging.* 2013;4(4):417–429. **(LOE V)**.

140. Dent JA, Paterson CR. Fractures in early childhood: osteogenesis imperfecta or child abuse? *J Pediatr Orthop.* 1991;11(2):184–186. **(LOE III)**.

141. Gahagan S, Rimsza ME. Child abuse or osteogenesis imperfecta: how can we tell? *Pediatrics.* 1991;88(5):987–992. **(LOE V)**.

142. Greeley CS, et al. Fractures at diagnosis in infants and children with osteogenesis imperfecta. *J Pediatr Orthop.* 2013;33(1):32–36. **(LOE IV)**.

143. Byers PH, et al. Genetic evaluation of suspected osteogenesis imperfecta (OI). *Genet Med.* 2006;8(6):383–388. **(LOE V)**.

144. Pereira EM. Clinical perspectives on osteogenesis imperfecta versus non-accidental injury. *Am J Med Genet C Semin Med Genet.* 2015;169(4):302–306. **(LOE III)**.

145. Steiner RD, et al. Studies of collagen synthesis and structure in the differentiation of child abuse from osteogenesis imperfecta. *J Pediatr.* 1996;128(4):542–547. **(LOE IV)**.

146. Wenstrup RJ, et al. Distinct biochemical phenotypes predict clinical severity in nonlethal variants of osteogenesis imperfecta. *Am J Hum Genet.* 1990;46(5):975–982. **(LOE IV)**.

147. Rustico SE, et al. Metabolic bone disease of prematurity. *J Clin Transl Endocrinol.* 2014;1(3):85–91. **(LOE III)**.

148. Paterson CR, et al. Osteogenesis imperfecta: the distinction from child abuse and the recognition of a variant form. *Am J Med Genet.* 1993;45(2):187–192. **(LOE III)**.

149. Miller ME, Hangartner TN. Temporary brittle bone disease: association with decreased fetal movement and osteopenia. *Calcif Tissue Int.* 1999;64(2):137–143. **(LOE III)**.

150. Jenny C. Evaluating infants and young children with multiple fractures. *Pediatrics.* 2006;118(3):1299–1303. **(LOE III)**.

151. Mendelson KL. Critical review of 'temporary brittle bone disease'. *Pediatr Radiol.* 2005;35(10):1036–1040. **(LOE III)**.

152. Sprigg A. Temporary brittle bone disease versus suspected non-accidental skeletal injury. *Arch Dis Child.* 2011;96(5):411–413. **(LOE V)**.

153. Greeley CS. The evolution of the child maltreatment literature. *Pediatrics.* 2012;130(2):347–348. **(LOE V)**.

154. Lang C. Letter to the editor: unexplained fractures: child abuse or bone disease: a systematic review. *Clin Orthop Relat Res.* 2011;469(11):3253–3254. **(LOE V)**.

155. Kleinman PK. Classic metaphyseal lesions. *AJR Am J Roentgenol.* 2014;202(6):W603. **(LOE V)**.

156. Wood BP. Commentary on a critical review of the classic metaphyseal lesion: traumatic or metabolic? *AJR Am J Roentgenol.* 2014;202(1):197–198. **(LOE V)**.

157. Kaushal S, et al. Spiral fracture in young infant causing a diagnostic dilemma: nutritional rickets versus child abuse. *Case Rep Pediatr.* 2017:7213629. **(LOE V)**.

158. Bacopoulou F, et al. Menkes disease mimicking non-accidental injury. *Arch Dis Child.* 2006;91(11):919. **(LOE IV)**.

159. Connors JM, et al. Syphilis or abuse: making the diagnosis and understanding the implications. *Pediatr Emerg Care.* 1998;14(2):139–142. **(LOE V)**.

160. Lim HK, et al. Congenital syphilis mimicking child abuse. *Pediatr Radiol.* 1995;25(7):560–561. **(LOE V)**.

161. Golshani AE, et al. Congenital indifference to pain: an illustrated case report and literature review. *J Radiol Case Rep.* 2014;8(8):16–23. **(LOE V)**.

162. Mishra P, et al. Infantile cortical hyperostosis: two cases with varied presentations. *J Clin Diagn Res.* 2014;8(10):PJ01–PJ02. **(LOE V)**.

163. Canadian Paediatric Society. The use and abuse of vitamin A. *Can Med Assoc J.* 1971;104(6):521–522. **(LOE V)**.

164. Torwalt CR, et al. Spontaneous fractures in the differential diagnosis of fractures in children. *J Forensic Sci.* 2002;47(6):1340–1344. **(LOE V)**.

165. Lane WG, Dubowitz H. What factors affect the identification and reporting of child abuse-related fractures? *Clin Orthop Relat Res.* 2007;461:219–225. **(LOE III)**.

166. Trout AT, et al. Abdominal and pelvic CT in cases of suspected abuse: can clinical and laboratory findings guide its use? *Pediatr Radiol.* 2011;41(1):92–98. **(LOE III)**.

167. Center TC.s.H.E.B.O. Suspected Child Physical Abuse Guidelines. 2018 [accessed 3/9/2019]; Available from: http://connect2search.texaschildrens.org/Pages/Results.aspx?k=e-boc%20guidelines%20child%20abuse&s=All%20Sites. **(LOE IV)**.

Anesthesia and Analgesia for the Ambulatory Management of Children's Fractures

21

Sheila M. Jones | Andrea C. Bracikowski

INTRODUCTION

The goal of anesthesia in the management of fractures in children is to provide analgesia and relieve anxiety so that successful closed treatment of the skeletal injury is facilitated. Optimal pain management in the emergency department or other ambulatory setting is delivered by the combined efforts of the orthopedic surgeon and anesthesiologist or emergency medicine specialist. Numerous techniques are available to control pain associated with fractures in children, including blocks (i.e., local, regional, and intravenous [IV]), sedation (i.e., moderate or deep), and general anesthesia. Important factors in choosing a particular technique include safety, efficacy, and ease of administration. Additional considerations include patient and parent acceptance and cost.

Local and regional techniques such as hematoma, brachial plexus, and IV regional blocks are particularly effective for upper extremity fractures. Sedation with inhalational agents such as nitrous oxide, parenteral narcotic and benzodiazepine combinations, ketamine, and propofol are not region specific and are suitable for patients over a wide range of ages. With all of these techniques, protocol-based monitoring and adherence to hospital sedation safety guidelines are essential.

Fractures in children are common. The majority (approximately 65%) involve the upper extremity. Most are closed and best treated by closed reduction. Time, logistics, and cost favor treatment in the emergency department or other ambulatory setting, as opposed to the operating room, when possible. In a study of axillary block anesthesia for the treatment of pediatric forearm fractures in the emergency department, Cramer and colleagues[1] estimated a cost reduction of almost 70% compared with similar treatment in the operating room.

Performance of satisfactory closed treatment of displaced musculoskeletal injuries in an ambulatory setting requires effective and safe levels of sedation and analgesia so that pain is minimized and the apprehensions of the child are allayed.[2,3] A variety of anesthetic techniques are available to the orthopedic surgeon faced with the challenge of treating a child with a closed fracture. The purpose of this chapter is to describe current methods of sedation and analgesia for fracture management in children.

PRINCIPLES OF PAIN MANAGEMENT IN CHILDREN

Children with fractures typically have significant pain and apprehension. Psychologically, their perceptions of the emergency department and the impending treatment of their injury often exacerbate their level of discomfort and anxiety.[4] Children with painful injuries about to undergo an additionally painful procedure are entitled to adequate analgesia and sedation. Despite the rationale of this concept, the problem of undertreatment of pain in children in the emergency department has been documented but occurs less frequently due to more recent extensive residency training of emergency physicians and fellowship training of pediatric emergency physicians.[5–13] Ignorance of the problem of pain in children, lack of familiarity with the methods of anesthesia and sedation for children, and concern for complications such as respiratory depression and hypotension are reasons for the often inadequate management of pain in the pediatric population.[4,6–11,13–16] Additionally, children with developmental disabilities, specifically autism spectrum disorders, require a more cautious approach in selection of procedural sedation and analgesia (PSA). Specifically, the need for additional time, specialized personnel, and personalized nonpharmacologic behavioral management strategies will optimize the efficiency and satisfaction for the orthopedic surgeon and for patients and their families.

In recognition of the increase in the number of minor procedures performed on children in a variety of ambulatory settings, the American Academy of Pediatrics (AAP) and the American Society of Anesthesiologists (ASA) have both developed goals for sedation and analgesia in children. Their purpose is to ensure the child's safety and welfare while minimizing the physical discomfort and negative psychological repercussions frequently associated with treatment of painful injuries, as well as returning the child to a state in which safe discharge is possible.[17] From a practical perspective, the method of analgesia-sedation must also allow for the satisfactory treatment of the primary problem. Thus, efficacy, safety, ease of administration, patient-parent acceptance, and cost are all important factors to be considered in selecting a technique.[3]

From an orthopedic perspective, the ultimate goal of anesthesia for the child with a closed fracture requiring manipulation is to facilitate the satisfactory reduction of the injury and obviate the need for a trip to the operating room. The ideal method should include management of preprocedure pain and anxiety, efficaciously and safely eliminate procedural pain, promote patient compliance, and produce amnesia of the procedure. It should be easy to administer, predictable in its action, and reliable for a wide range of ages. It should have a rapid onset and short duration of action, result in little or no complications or side effects, and be reversible. Finally, it should be relatively inexpensive to administer and completely satisfactory to the child and his or her parents.[1,3,4,14,15,18–31]

ANESTHETIC TECHNIQUES

A variety of techniques short of general anesthesia have been used to achieve analgesia and sedation in children with closed fractures requiring treatment in the ambulatory setting. The techniques can be grouped into two broad categories: blocks (i.e., local, regional, and IV) and moderate (formerly referred to as *conscious*) or deep sedation (i.e., anxiolytics, narcotic analgesics, or dissociative agents alone or in combination). Each technique incorporates various aspects of the "ideal" method described earlier. It is incumbent on the orthopedic surgeon treating children's fractures to be aware of the various techniques and the potential benefits, side effects, and complications of each to be able to make an educated decision about which to use in a particular situation.[32,33]

TECHNIQUES TO BE AVOIDED

Vocal, or "O.K.," anesthesia is a technique that provides only the verbal assurance to the child that the manipulation of the fracture will be briefly painful. The concept that children are somehow more resilient to pain has been disproved as knowledge of the developmental and psychological makeup of children and their perception of pain has become better understood.[6,7,34] The notion that it is acceptable for children to endure pain during the performance of therapeutic or diagnostic procedures has become dated with the evolution of techniques in pediatric pain management.[10,15,30] Given the availability of many safe and effective options for pain management during the reduction of children's fractures, the technique of "verbal reassurance" should be avoided if possible.

Chloral hydrate and the so-called lytic cocktail, a combination of meperidine (Demerol), promethazine (Phenergan), and chlorpromazine (Thorazine) (DPT), two techniques of sedation used frequently in the past, have fallen out of favor.[34,35] Chloral hydrate was introduced in 1832 and was used commonly for children undergoing painless diagnostic procedures.[34] Although it has been demonstrated to be effective for the sedation of young children (<6 years of age) undergoing therapeutic procedures, it has several disadvantages for the management of fractures in children.[15] The onset of sedation is slow (40–60 minutes), and recovery can be prolonged, taking up to several hours, with residual effects lasting as long as 24 hours. Moreover, chloral hydrate has no analgesic properties, and children can become disinhibited and agitated in response to painful stimuli. For these reasons, chloral hydrate is not a preferred technique for sedation in the management of fractures in children.[4,11,14,15,30,36,37]

DPT has been the second most commonly used method of sedation for children undergoing painless diagnostic tests and the one most widely used in children undergoing therapeutic procedures since 1989.[35] DPT is typically administered in a single intramuscular (IM) injection and provides sedation with some analgesia.

Despite widespread usage, the drugs in the lytic cocktail have many undesirable characteristics. The combination is poorly titrated and has a delayed onset of action (20–30 minutes). The duration of sedation can last 20 hours, but the duration of analgesia is only 1 to 3 hours. The mixture does not have any anxiolytic or amnestic properties. Recently, it was demonstrated that the DPT cocktail is a largely empiric mixture of three drugs, not based on sound pharmacologic data, with a relatively frequent occurrence of therapeutic failure (29%) and a relatively high rate (approximately 4%) of serious adverse effects such as seizures, respiratory depression, and death.[15,31,35,38] For these reasons, the use of DPT is discouraged by both the US Agency for Health Care Policy and Research and the AAP.[35,38]

LOCAL AND REGIONAL ANESTHESIA

Local anesthetics work by blocking the conduction of nerve impulses. At the cellular level, they depress sodium ion flux across the nerve cell membrane and, in this way, inhibit the initiation and propagation of action potentials.[39] After injection, local anesthetics diffuse toward their intended site of action and also toward nearby vasculature, where uptake is determined by the number of capillaries, the local blood flow, and the affinity of the drug for the tissues. Elimination occurs after vascular uptake by metabolism in the plasma or liver. Vasoconstrictors such as epinephrine are mixed with local anesthetics to decrease the vascular uptake and prolong the anesthetic effect.

Local anesthetics are classified chemically as either amines or esters (Table 21.1). After absorption in the blood, esters are broken down by plasma cholinesterase, but amides are bound by plasma proteins and are then metabolized in the liver. Local adverse effects include erythema, swelling, and, rarely, ischemia when injected into tissues supplied by terminal arteries. Adverse systemic effects are caused by high blood levels of local anesthetics and include tinnitus, drowsiness, visual disturbances, muscle twitching, seizures, respiratory depression, and cardiac arrest. Bupivacaine is a long-acting amide that is particularly dangerous because it binds with high affinity to myocardial contractile proteins and can cause cardiac arrest. Ropivacaine, which is closely related to bupivacaine structurally, is a newer long-acting amide that, at clinically relevant doses, provides a greater sensorimotor differential block, has an increased cardiovascular safety profile, and has a shorter elimination half-life with lower potential for accumulation than bupivacaine. The lower systemic toxicity and cardiotoxicity is desirable when the potential exists for high plasma concentrations of local anesthetics, such as in peripheral nerve blocks or after inadvertent intravascular injections.[40]

A number of local and regional techniques, including hematoma, IV regional, and regional nerve blocks, have been reported to be variably effective in providing anesthesia for fracture treatment in children. These methods require the surgeon to be familiar with regional anatomy, have working knowledge of the pharmacokinetics and dosing of local anesthetic drugs, and be proficient in the techniques of administering them. Compared with the performance of these techniques in adults, the performance of these techniques in children is often technically easier because anatomic landmarks are more readily identifiable.[41] Physiologically,

Table 21.1 Local Anesthetics

Generic Name	Brand Name	Onset	Duration	Maximum Dose
Amines				
Lidocaine	Xylocaine	Fast	1.0–2.0 hours	5 mg/kg, 7 mg/kg (epinephrine)
Mepivacaine	Carbocaine	Fast (infiltration)	1.5–3.0 hours	5 mg/kg
Ropivacaine	Naropin	Slow (block) Fast (infiltration)	2.0–8.0 hours	3 mg/kg
Bupivacaine	Marcaine	Slow	4.0–12.0 hours	3 mg/kg
Esters				
Chloroprocaine	Nesacaine	Fast	30–60 min	15 mg/kg
Procaine	Novocain	Slow (block) Fast (infiltration)	30–60 min	7 mg/kg
Tetracaine	Pontocaine	Slow (topical)	30–60 min	2 mg/kg

the relatively smaller calibers of the peripheral nerves in children are more susceptible to the pharmacologic actions of anesthetic agents.[42]

HEMATOMA BLOCK

The hematoma block has been a popular method of anesthesia for the reduction of fractures, particularly in the distal radius but also about the ankle.[43–47] In this technique, a local anesthetic agent is injected directly into the hematoma surrounding the fracture. The anesthetic inhibits the generation and conduction of painful impulses primarily in small nonmyelinated nerve fibers in the periosteum and local tissues.[30] This block is quick and relatively simple to administer. The skin is prepared with a bactericidal agent and draped at the site of infiltration. The fracture hematoma is aspirated with a 20- or 22-gauge needle and then injected with plain lidocaine. The typical dose of lidocaine is 3 to 5 mg/kg, which should be concentrated so as to limit the total amount of fluid injected to less than 10 mL; limiting the fluid will avoid elevating soft tissue compartment pressures and minimize the risk of creating a compartment syndrome or other neurovascular problem.[48] Although direct injection of the hematoma theoretically converts a closed fracture into an open one, no infections have been reported with this technique.[45]

Recent studies of hematoma blocks administered to children have shown its safety and efficacy. Studies have shown parental satisfaction and shorter length of stays in the emergency department. In three separate studies authored by Dinley and Michelinakis,[46] Case,[45] and Johnson and Noffsinger[47] with a combined total of 491 adult and pediatric patients, hematoma block was shown to be effective for the reduction of a variety of fractures of the distal upper extremity in patients of all ages. Despite the generally favorable experience with hematoma block anesthesia, other methods of regional anesthesia have been shown to be more effective for the management of upper extremity fractures.[48] A study by Abbaszadegan and Johnson[22] found that analgesia during fracture reduction was superior with

IV regional (Bier block) anesthesia compared with hematoma block and that fracture alignment after reduction was also better. The authors concluded that the more favorable outcomes achieved with the Bier block were related to better analgesia and muscle relaxation.

INTRAVENOUS REGIONAL ANESTHESIA

IV regional anesthesia was originally described in 1908 by August Bier, who used IV cocaine to obtain analgesia.[19,29] Subsequently, a number of studies have described the effective use of this technique of anesthesia for the treatment of upper extremity fractures in children in an ambulatory setting.[18,19,21,29,49–58] The block has also been described for use in lower extremity fractures but is less common.[56]

The technique for administering the Bier block in the upper extremity involves placement of a deflated pneumatic cuff above the elbow of the injured extremity. Holmes[55] introduced the concept of two cuffs in an effort to minimize tourniquet discomfort with prolonged inflation, but the practice has not proven to be necessary for the limited amount of time it takes for fracture reduction in a child.[18,19,21] The tourniquet should be secured with tape to prevent Velcro failure.[57] IV access is established in a vein on the dorsum of the hand of the injured extremity with a 22- or 23-gauge butterfly needle. The arm is exsanguinated by elevating it for 1 to 2 minutes. Although exsanguination with a circumferential elastic bandage is described classically, this method can be more painful and difficult to perform in an injured extremity and is no more efficacious than the gravity method.[19,21,26,29] The blood pressure cuff is then rapidly inflated to either 100 mm Hg above systolic blood pressure or between 200 and 250 mm Hg.[18,19,21,26,29,57] The arm is lowered after cuff inflation. Lidocaine is administered, the IV catheter is removed, and reduction of the fracture is performed. In the traditional technique, the lidocaine dose is 3 to 5 mg/kg[18,29,57] and in the "mini-dose" technique, the dose is 1 to 1.5 mg/kg.[19,29,41,52] The tourniquet is kept inflated until the fracture is immobilized and radiographs are obtained in case repeated manipulation is necessary. In any event, the tourniquet should remain inflated for at least 20 minutes so that the lidocaine can diffuse and become adequately fixed to the tissues, thus minimizing the risk of systemic toxicity.[57,59] The blood pressure cuff may be deflated in either a single stage or graduated fashion, although single-stage release has proven to be clinically safe and easier technically.[18,29,57]

During the entire procedure, basic monitoring is required, and cardiac monitoring is suggested in case toxic effects occur. Routine IV access in the noninjured extremity may be beneficial but is not required.[18,26] Patients should be observed for at least 30 minutes after cuff deflation for any adverse systemic reactions. Motor and sensory function typically returns during this period, allowing assessment of neurovascular status of the injured extremity before discharge.[59]

The literature within the past decade certainly speaks to the effectiveness of the traditional Bier block, using a lidocaine dose of 3 to 5 mg/kg, in managing forearm fractures in children. Four large series with a total of 895 patients undergoing this technique[18,21,57,58] demonstrated satisfactory anesthesia and successful fracture reduction in more than 90% of cases (Table 21.2). The most common adverse effect of the procedure in these studies was tourniquet pain in about 6% of patients.[21,58] One patient experienced transient dizziness and circumoral paresthesia.[58] One patient

developed persistent myoclonic twitching after tourniquet deflation and was admitted for observation.[57]

Despite the efficacy and relatively low number of complications with the "traditional" Bier block (lidocaine, 3–5 mg/kg), concerns and anecdotal reports of systemic lidocaine toxicity (i.e., seizures, hypotension, tachycardia, and arrhythmias) have prompted development of a mini-dose (lidocaine, 1–1.5 mg/kg) technique of IV regional anesthesia.[19,28,52] Reports by Farrell and colleagues[52] and Bolte and associates[19] using a lidocaine dose of 1.5 mg/kg and by Juliano and colleagues[29] using a dose of 1.0 mg/kg in a total of 218 patients have shown the mini-dose Bier block to be effective in achieving adequate anesthesia in 94% of children studied (Table 21.3).

The primary site of action of the IV regional block is thought to be the small peripheral nerve branches. At this anatomic level, blockade is better achieved with a larger volume of anesthetic that can be distributed more completely to the peripheral nerve receptors. It appears to be the quantity (i.e., volume) and not the dose of anesthetic that predicates success of the block. For any given dose of lidocaine, diluting the concentration permits the administration of a larger volume of fluid (Table 21.4). This mechanism explains the success of the mini-dose technique. In the series by Juliano and colleagues,[29] forearm fracture reduction was

---

Table 21.2   Results With Traditional[a] Intravenous Regional Anesthesia (Bier Block) for Forearm Fracture Reduction in Children

Author	Lidocaine Dose	Good/Excellent Anesthesia	Successful Fracture Reduction (%)	Adverse Effects
Turner et al (1986)	0.5%, 3 mg/kg	177/205 (72%)	98	Tourniquet pain (12), dizziness (1), circumoral paresthesias (1)
Olney et al (1988)	0.5%, 3 mg/kg	361/401 (90%)	98	Myoclonus (1)
Barnes et al (1991)	0.5%, 3–5 mg/kg	100/100 (100%)	100	None
Colizza and Said (1993)	0.5%, 3 mg/kg	139/139 (100%)	96	Tourniquet pain (10)

[a]Traditional technique uses 3 to 5 mg/kg of 0.5% lidocaine.
IV, Intravenous.
(Modified from McCarty EC, Mencio GA, Green NE. Anesthesia and analgesia for the ambulatory management of fractures in children. *J Am Acad Orthop Surg.* 1999;7:84. With permission.)

Table 21.3   Results With Minidose[a] Bier Block for Forearm Fracture Reduction in Children

Author	Lidocaine Dose	Good/Excellent Anesthesia	Successful Fracture Reduction	Adverse Effects
Farrell et al (1985)	0.5%, 1.5 mg/kg	29/29 (100%)	100%	None
Juliano et al (1992)	0.125%, 1.0 mg/kg	43/44 (98%)	100%	Tourniquet pain (1)
Bolte et al (1994)	0.5%, 1.5 mg/kg	61/66 (92%)	100%	Tourniquet pain (2), local reaction (3)

[a]Mini-dose technique uses 1.0 to 1.5 mg/kg lidocaine.
(Modified from McCarty EC, Mencio GA, Green NE. Anesthesia and analgesia for the ambulatory management of fractures in children. *J Am Acad Orthop Surg.* 1999;7:84. With permission.)

Table 21.4   Effect of Lidocaine Dose and Concentration on Infusion Volume

Lidocaine dose (mg/mL) = lidocaine concentration (mg%) × 10
Examples: 1.0% lidocaine = 10 mg/mL 0.125% lidocaine = 1.25 mg/mL
Calculations of infusion volumes for a 20-kg child with traditional[a] and mini-dose technique[b]
Dose (mg/kg) × Body weight (kg) ÷ lidocaine concentration (mg/mL) = IV infusion volume (mL)
3 mg/kg[a] × 20 kg ÷ 5 mg/mL (0.5% lidocaine) = 12 mL of 0.5% lidocaine
1 mg/kg[b] × 20 kg ÷ 1.25 mg/mL (0.125% lidocaine) = 16 mL of 0.125% lidocaine
Decreasing the concentration of lidocaine with the mini-dose technique permits the infusion of a large volume (mL) of anesthetic with lower risk of systemic toxicity because the total amount (mg) of lidocaine is much lower than with the traditional technique.

IV, Intravenous.

pain free in 43 of 44 patients (98%) after IV regional block achieved with a very dilute lidocaine solution (0.125%) and a relatively small total dose (1 mg/kg).

IV regional anesthesia, with the use of either the traditional or mini-dose technique, has several advantages. The technique is fairly easy to administer. The onset of action of the block is relatively fast (<10 minutes) but also of relatively short duration, which allows for assessment of neurovascular function in the extremity after fracture reduction and immobilization. An empty stomach is not required. Tourniquet discomfort is the most common adverse side effect. Inadvertent cuff deflation with loss of analgesia or systemic toxicity is a potentially significant problem. Compartment syndrome has also been reported. Technically, placing the tourniquet and obtaining IV access in the injured extremity can be a challenge in the uncooperative child, and application of the splint or cast can be cumbersome with the tourniquet in place.

In a retrospective study comparing Bier block (600 patients) to procedural sedation (645 patients) for treatment of displaced forearm fractures in children over a 2-year period, Aarons et al found shorter average time from initiation of treatment to discharge (47 min vs. 1 hour 45 min) and lower average cost ($4956 vs. $6313) in the Bier block group, with similar outcomes (complications requiring admission, compartment syndrome, cast complications) otherwise in regard to fracture treatment.[60]

AXILLARY BLOCK

The brachial plexus supplies all of the motor function to the upper extremity and sensation to the lower two-thirds of the limb. It is formed from the fifth through eighth cervical and first thoracic nerve roots with occasional contributions from the fourth cervical and second thoracic nerves. A continuous fascial sheath that extends from the cervical transverse processes to the axilla encases it. Regional blockade of the brachial plexus within this sheath may be performed at the interscalene, supraclavicular, infraclavicular, or axillary level (Fig. 21.1).

Axillary block provides excellent anesthesia for the forearm and hand. Initial use of the technique is attributed to Halsted and Hall, who first used axillary block for outpatient procedures in 1884. The technique has since proven

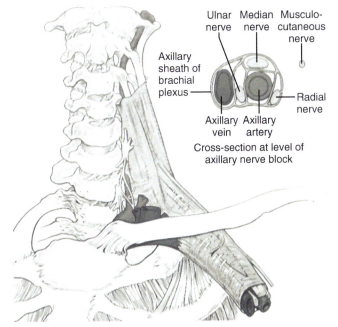

Fig. 21.1 Brachial plexus sheath. A continuous fascial sheath, extending from the cervical transverse processes to just beyond the axillary region, completely surrounds the brachial plexus. Common sites for blockade of the brachial plexus within this sheath include the interscalene, infraclavicular, and axillary regions. (Modified from Bridenbaugh LD. The upper extremity: somatic blockade. In: Cousins MJ, Bridenbaugh PO, eds. *Neural Blockade in Clinical Anesthesia and Management of Pain.* 2nd ed. Philadelphia: J.B. Lippincott; 1988:392. With permission.)

to be a safe and reliable method of anesthesia for a variety of outpatient surgical procedures in the upper extremity in both adults and children.[42] It is an excellent choice of anesthesia for treatment of fractures below the elbow because it provides muscle relaxation in addition to analgesia. Cramer and colleagues[1] reported on the successful use of axillary anesthesia by orthopedic surgeons in the emergency department for the reduction of forearm fractures in children. In this study, effective anesthesia was achieved in 105 of 111 children (95%) with no complications.

One administers axillary block anesthesia by placing the child in a supine position with the injured arm abducted and externally rotated 90 degrees. IV access is usually established in the uninjured extremity. Mild sedation may be helpful before the procedure. The axilla is prepared with a bactericidal solution and draped with sterile towels. The block is performed with the use of a 1.0% lidocaine solution at a dose of 5 mg/kg. As with the Bier block, a larger volume of local anesthetic is preferable and can be achieved by use of a more dilute concentration of drug. The target for delivery of the anesthetic agent is the axillary sheath, which contains the axillary artery and vein surrounded by the radial nerve (behind), median nerve (above), and ulnar nerve (below). The musculocutaneous nerve courses outside this sheath through the coracobrachialis muscle and, for this reason, may escape blockade, which explains the unreliability of this technique for anesthesia above the elbow.

Several techniques have been described, including blind injection into the neurovascular sheath, patient-reported paresthesias, use of a nerve stimulator, and transarterial puncture, that ensure accurate delivery of the anesthetic into the axillary sheath. Elicitation of paresthesias provides reliable evidence of position within the neurovascular sheath but may be uncomfortable and requires a conscious and cooperative patient. For these reasons, it cannot be used in most children. The use of a nerve stimulator and insulated needle to elicit a motor response is another effective method for determination of accurate location within the sheath. However, this technique requires special equipment (nerve stimulator and insulated needles), which may not be readily available in an ambulatory setting; threshold stimulation of the nerves may also be distressful to the conscious patient.

The transarterial method is the most popular technique of axillary block and, as described in the study by Cramer and colleagues,[1] has been shown to be an effective way to administer this block in children (Fig. 21.2). With this method, the axillary artery is palpated, and a 23-gauge butterfly needle, connected via extension tubing to a syringe containing lidocaine, is inserted perpendicular to the artery. The needle is advanced while being continuously aspirated until a flash of arterial blood is seen and is then advanced through the artery. Approximately two-thirds of the lidocaine is injected into the sheath deep to the artery; a check should be performed by aspiration after every 5 mL so that extravascular positioning is ensured. The needle is withdrawn to the superficial side of the artery, and the remaining lidocaine is injected. Pressure is held over the puncture site for 5 minutes, and fracture manipulation can usually begin shortly thereafter.

In most children, the axillary sheath is superficial because of the dearth of subcutaneous fat, which makes for a technically easier procedure in a child than in an adult. Of course, this advantage can be offset if the child is obese or uncooperative. From a pharmacokinetic standpoint, the local anesthetic diffuses more rapidly and with enhanced blockade of the nerves, which are smaller in diameter in children than in adults.[42] The duration of the block is usually prolonged enough to allow repeated manipulation of the fracture in the event of an unsatisfactory reduction.

Potential complications of axillary block anesthesia include systemic lidocaine toxicity, hematoma formation, and persistent neurologic symptoms. Horner syndrome has also been reported. In actuality, complications of axillary block anesthesia are rare.[42] None were encountered in the series reported by Cramer and colleagues[1] of 111 children with displaced forearm fractures treated in an emergency department setting. Contraindications to axillary block anesthesia are the presence of a coagulopathy of any type, a preexisting neurologic or vascular abnormality of the extremity, axillary lymphadenitis, or an uncooperative or combative patient.

WRIST AND DIGITAL BLOCKS

Whereas brachial plexus anesthesia may be efficacious for any fracture of the upper extremity below the elbow, more distal upper extremity blocks at the wrist or of the digital nerves in the hand may be useful for treatment of fractures or minor surgical procedures of the hand. Anesthesia to the

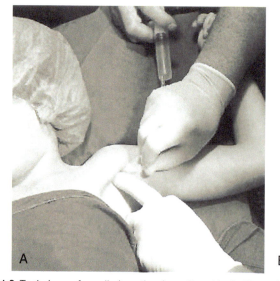
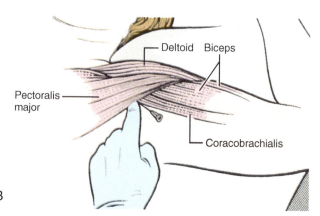

Fig. 21.2 Technique of needle insertion for axillary block. The axillary artery is palpated (A), and the needle is inserted at the lateral edge of pectoralis major parallel to the coracobrachialis (B). (A, Courtesy of Gregory A. Mencio, MD, Professor, Department of Orthopaedics, Vanderbilt University Medical Center, Nashville, TN; B, Modified with permission from Bridenbaugh LD. The upper extremity: somatic blockade. In: Cousins MJ, Bridenbaugh PO, eds. *Neural Blockade in Clinical Anesthesia and Management of Pain*. 2nd ed. Philadelphia: J.B. Lippincott; 1988:401.)

digits can be achieved by block of the common digital nerves near the point of bifurcation at the level of the metacarpal heads or by block of the radial and ulnar digital nerves at the base of each finger. This technique is most useful for treatment of phalangeal fracture(s) of a single digit. For injuries involving multiple digits or the metacarpals, anesthesia of the hand can be achieved with blockade of the three major nerves of the upper extremity at the wrist (wrist block). The median nerve is located on the radial side of the palmaris longus tendon approximately 2 cm proximal to the wrist crease and can be blocked with 3 to 5 mL of local anesthetic (Fig. 21.3A,B). The ulnar nerve is blocked on the radial side of the flexor carpi radialis, about 2 cm proximal to the volar wrist crease with 3 to 5 mL of local anesthetic, and the dorsal and volar cutaneous branches of the nerve are blocked by subcutaneous injection of an additional 2 to 3 mL of anesthetic (see Fig. 21.3A,B). Alternatively, the ulnar nerve may be approached from the ulnar side of the wrist, just dorsal to the flexor carpi ulnaris tendon (Fig. 21.3C). The terminal branches of the radial nerve are blocked by injection of 1 to 2 mL of anesthetic along the extensor pollicis longus tendon as it crosses the base of the first metacarpal and across the snuff box to the radial side of the extensor pollicis brevis tendon (Fig. 21.3D).

FEMORAL NERVE BLOCK

Femoral nerve blockade is another type of regional anesthesia that is often used in the treatment of femoral fractures.[61-64] Although the majority of children with femoral fractures are not treated on an outpatient basis, femoral nerve blockade can provide excellent anesthesia and analgesia for the initial management of this injury, including manipulation of the fracture, application of an immediate spica cast, or placement of a traction pin. It is a good option for children unable to undergo general anesthesia or for those who cannot be sedated for any reason. This technique is most effective for fractures of the middle third of the femur and less so for fractures of the proximal and distal thirds of the bone because these areas also receive sensory innervation from branches of the obturator and sciatic nerves, respectively.

Blockade of the femoral nerve involves preparation and draping of the inguinal area and palpation of the femoral artery (Fig. 21.4). A 22- or 23-gauge needle on a syringe containing a local anesthetic agent (typically 0.5% bupivacaine, dosed at 1–1.5 mg/kg) is inserted one fingerbreadth lateral to the artery and 1 to 2 cm below the inguinal ligament. The needle is advanced at a 30 to 45 degree angle

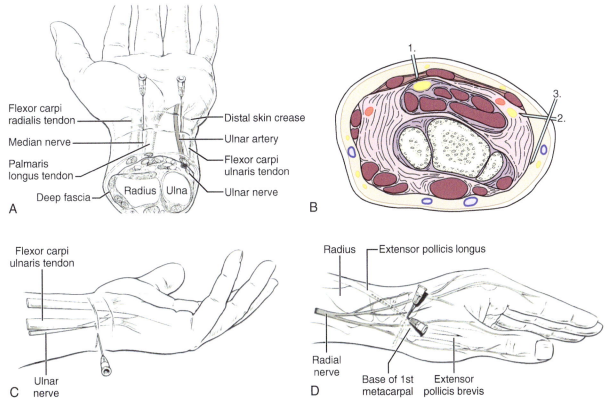

Fig. 21.3 (A and B) Technique for median and ulnar nerve blockade at the wrist. The median nerve is approached from the palmar side of the wrist between the palmaris longus and flexor carpi radialis (*needle 1* in B). The ulnar nerve can be approached between the flexor carpi ulnaris tendon and the ulnar artery. (C) Alternative method for ulnar nerve blockade. The ulnar can also be approached from the ulnar side of the wrist just dorsal to the flexor carpi ulnaris tendon (*needles 2 and 3* in B). (D) Technique for radial nerve block at the wrist. The needle is inserted where the extensor pollicis longus tendon crosses the base of the first metacarpal, and approximately 2 to 3 mL of local anesthetic is injected as the needle is advanced along the tendon to the radial tubercle. The needle is then redirected at a right angle across the anatomic snuff-box, and an additional 1 to 2 mL is injected into the radial border of the extensor pollicis longus tendon. (A, Courtesy of Stephen Hays, MD, FAAP, Assistant Professor, Departments of Anesthesiology and Pediatrics, Vanderbilt University Medical Center, Nashville, TN; B, Modified with permission from Bridenbaugh LD. The upper extremity: somatic blockade. In: Cousins MJ, Bridenbaugh PO, eds. *Neural Blockade in Clinical Anesthesia and Management of Pain*. 2nd ed. Philadelphia: J.B. Lippincott; 1988:410-411.)

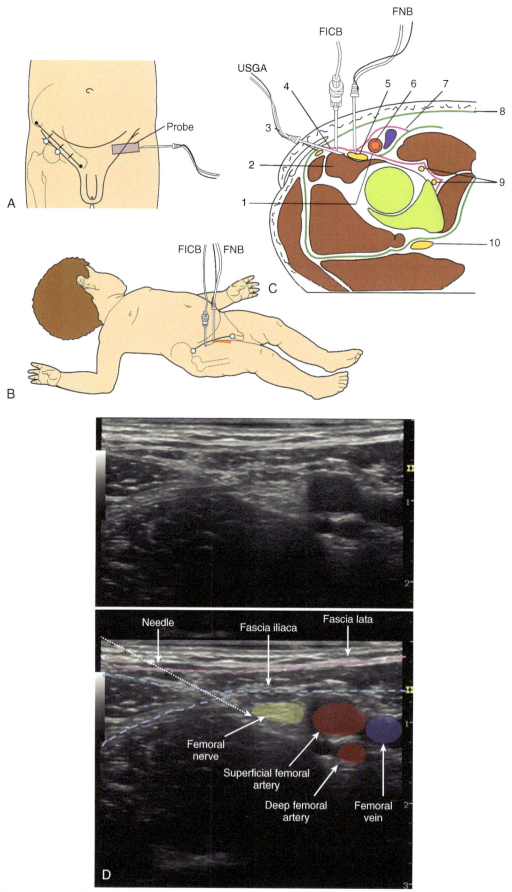

Fig. 21.4 (A–C) Blockade of the femoral nerve. (D) Ultrasound view of femoral nerve blockade. (1) Fascia iliaca (floor of femoral sheath) (2) Iliacus muscle (3) Lateral femoral cutaneous nerve (4) Fascia iliaca (5) Femoral nerve (6) Superficial femoral artery (7) Fascia iliaca (floor of femoral sheath) (8) Obturator nerve branches (9) Sciatic nerve (10) sciatic nerve *FICB* = Fascia Iliac Compartment Block *FNB* = Femoral Nerve Block USGA: ultrasound-guided approach. (From Miller RD, et al. *Miller's Anesthesia.* 8th ed. Philadelphia: Elsevier; 2015.)

to the skin, and the syringe is aspirated as the needle passes through the deep fascia into the femoral triangle. If no blood is aspirated, the anesthetic agent is injected around the femoral nerve. Alternatively, the nerve can be blocked more proximally within the fascia iliaca compartment if the needle enters just above the inguinal ligament, which gives the advantage of accessing all branches of the nerve before it starts to arborize. As with axillary block, the volume of the anesthetic is the key to achieving anesthesia with this technique. The onset of analgesia occurs within 10 minutes and, with the use of long-acting agents such as bupivacaine, may last up to 8 hours.[62] In one randomized controlled study,[65] regional blockade of the femoral nerve was shown to provide clinically superior pain relief compared with IV morphine sulfate throughout the initial 6 hours of management in children age 16 months to 15 years with isolated femoral shaft fractures.

In the reports of this technique, there have been few inadvertent arterial punctures and no long-term sequelae or neurologic complications.[62-64] Other potential complications include systemic toxicity from intravascular injection, infections, and injury to the nerve. As with the axillary block, this method may be difficult in obese children and in young or uncooperative children. Contraindications include any preexisting neurologic abnormality of the injured lower extremity and the inability to manage systemic toxicity.

SEDATION

Sedation is a continuum of various states of consciousness. For purposes of classification, two levels are recognized: *moderate* (previously termed *conscious*) and *deep*. All levels of sedation short of deep are characterized by a state of depressed consciousness in which a patent airway and protective reflexes are maintained and from which the individual can be aroused by physical stimulation or verbal command. *Deep sedation* is a more profound state of depressed consciousness during which patients cannot be easily aroused but respond purposefully after repeated or painful stimulation. In deep sedation, the ability to independently maintain ventilatory function may be impaired and may require assistance in maintaining a patent airway.[66] Sedation can be achieved with the use of inhalational agents, such as nitrous oxide, or parenteral techniques including opioids, benzodiazepines, dissociative agents (e.g., ketamine), and hypnotic agents (e.g., propofol and etomidate), alone or in combination. The AAP and ASA have established guidelines for equipment and monitoring for all levels and methods of sedation in an attempt to protect patient welfare during sedation and emergence and to allow safe discharge home afterward[17,33] (Table 21.5). The safe and efficacious use of PSA specifically by nonanesthesiologists in a pediatric emergency department has been demonstrated. In a study performed at Children's Hospital of Pittsburgh,[67] PSA was successfully provided in 1177 (98.6%) of 1194 sedation events, which is a little more than half of whom were admitted for fracture reduction (643 patients, or 52.9%), with the use of parenteral (IM or IV) ketamine hydrochloride, fentanyl citrate, or midazolam in various combinations. Complications occurred in approximately 18% of patients and most commonly consisted of hypoxia that was easily treated.

Table 21.5   American Academy of Pediatrics Guidelines for Conscious Sedation

Monitoring
Preprocedure vital signs Continuous monitoring of O_2 saturation/heart rate
Intermittent monitoring of respiratory rate and blood pressure every 5 minutes Personnel responsible *only* for administering drugs and monitoring patients; individual skilled in airway management

Equipment
Pulse oximeter Positive-pressure oxygen delivery system and suctioning equipment *in room* Emergency cart with appropriate medications, ECG monitor with defibrillator, equipment for airway management *immediately available*

Recommended Discharge Criteria
Cardiovascular function and airway patency are satisfactory and stable.
The patient is easily arousable, and protective reflexes are intact.
The patient can talk (if age appropriate).
The patient can sit up unaided (if age appropriate). For a very young or handicapped child, incapable of the usually expected responses, the presedation level of responsiveness or a level as close as possible to the normal level has been achieved.
The state of hydration is adequate.

ECG, Electrocardiograph.
(Modified from American Academy of Pediatrics Committee on Drugs. Guidelines for monitoring and management of pediatric patients during and after sedation for diagnostic and therapeutic procedures. *Pediatrics* 1992;89(6):1110-1115. With permission.)

NITROUS OXIDE

Dentists have used nitrous oxide extensively since the 1950s to provide anesthesia for patients undergoing office dental procedures. Its use in the ambulatory setting for fracture management is more recent.[23,27,28,68] Nitrous oxide is a relatively weak inhalational anesthetic with low solubility. It acts quickly on the central nervous system and has a fairly short duration of action, which makes it a good anesthetic option for fracture treatment. Other desirable effects of nitrous oxide include a variable degree of analgesia, sedation, anxiolysis, and amnesia.[4,23,28]

Nitrous oxide has been shown to be most effective when it is administered as a 50% mixture of nitrous oxide and oxygen.[15,68] This mixture of gases is most commonly delivered through a machine that controls the rate of flow of the gases, regulates the mix, and scavenges stray nitrous oxide from the surrounding environment. The gas is self-administered through inspiratory effort, and the child holds the face mask. Once adequate sedation occurs, the child relaxes and drops the mask. When the mask seal is broken, the flow of nitrous oxide is stopped. As a safeguard against overdosing, it is important that the mask not be held by anyone but the patient. Fracture reduction can begin within a few minutes of administration of the nitrous oxide.[4] After the fracture has been immobilized, 100% oxygen is administered to the child for approximately 5 minutes to wash out the nitrous oxide and prevent diffusion hypoxia.[4,23,28,68] Monitoring guidelines for sedation must be followed.

This technique of sedation is relatively easy to administer, works quickly, and does appear to be safe. Nitrous oxide is quickly eliminated and does not appear to suppress laryngeal reflexes. IV access is not required.[28,68] This method is obviously not region specific and can be used for fractures in all extremities. On the negative side, administration of nitrous oxide can be a problem in the child who is uncooperative or anxious with the face mask and in the child who has difficulty obtaining a tight seal with the mask.[27,68] Other potential problems are nausea, vomiting, diffusion hypoxia, and respiratory depression. Contraindications for the use of nitrous oxide include the presence of significant cardiac or pulmonary disease, prior administration of narcotics or sedatives, presence of a pneumothorax or abdominal distention, middle ear infection, or altered mental status.

Studies suggest that nitrous oxide does provide effective sedation for the management of fractures but that its analgesic effects vary.[23,26,28,68] Evans and colleagues[23] found nitrous oxide to provide similar analgesia but also to have a faster onset of action, a shorter recovery time, and better patient satisfaction than IM meperidine. Gregory and Sullivan[26] compared nitrous oxide with IV regional anesthesia (Bier block) in a prospective study of 28 children with upper extremity fractures and found that fracture reduction was completed in less time with nitrous oxide, although the pain response, as measured by a visual analog scale, was worse. In two separate studies by Hennrikus and associates[28] and Wattenmaker and colleagues[68] with a combined total of 76 children, in whom nitrous oxide was used as the sole anesthetic agent, fracture reduction was successful in 95%, and no complications were encountered. However, "moderate" or "significant" pain was observed in 41% of the patients during fracture reduction,

and in the Wattenmaker study, analgesia was completely ineffective in 9%.

NITROUS OXIDE AND HEMATOMA BLOCK COMBINATION

Because of the unpredictable nature of analgesia with nitrous oxide alone, some have suggested it be combined with a regional technique. Hennrikus and associates[27] reported on the use of nitrous oxide and hematoma block in 100 children from age 4 to 17 years with various closed fractures treated in the emergency department. In the combined technique, preliminary administration of nitrous oxide provided sedation and anxiolysis that facilitated placement of the block as well as an amnestic response to fracture reduction. The hematoma block provided additional analgesia both during and after the reduction. The study found a significant decrease in behavior, suggestive of pain with this technique compared with an earlier study in which only nitrous oxide was used.[28,68]

PARENTERAL SEDATION

A variety of medications are used for sedation of pediatric patients (Table 21.6). For many years, narcotics and benzodiazepines have been safely administered to children with painful injuries to provide analgesia or to supplement other methods of anesthesia in the emergency department setting.[3,4,15,30,32,33,69–76] Narcotics produce analgesia by reversibly binding to opioid receptors. In higher doses, they also have some sedative properties. Benzodiazepines are primarily sedatives. They produce hypnosis, anxiolysis, muscle relaxation, and some antegrade amnesia but have no analgesic properties. When these two different classes of drugs are given in combination, they act synergistically to induce a moderate to deep level of sedation and analgesia.[30] The IV route of administration is preferred over others (e.g., IM, nasal, oral, or rectal) because it is the most reliable and manageable.[4] The effect after IV administration is rapid in onset, can be readily titrated, and is reversible, if necessary. One should obtain IV access in a noninjured extremity and adhere to the guidelines for deep sedation.[66] The benzodiazepine is ideally administered before the narcotic so that a sedative effect is provided. Low doses of medications should be given initially and titrated for effect within recommended dosage levels[66] (see Table 21.6). Supplemental oxygen should be administered if oxygen saturation falls below 90%, and capnography should be used unless unavailable. Reversal agents such as naloxone (Narcan) for the narcotic and flumazenil (Romazicon) for the benzodiazepine should be readily available. Fracture reduction typically can begin when the patient becomes drowsy.[3]

The more common benzodiazepines used for IV sedation are midazolam (Versed) and diazepam (Valium). Midazolam is a rapid-acting benzodiazepine that has three to four times the potency of diazepam. Its onset of action is usually within 2 to 3 minutes.[30] It is also eliminated rapidly and thus has the shortest duration of action of any of the benzodiazepines. Because of these characteristics, it has supplanted diazepam as the benzodiazepine of choice for sedation for noxious procedures in most emergency departments.[77] Diazepam has a slightly longer onset and a more protracted

Table 21.6   Common Medications Used for Sedation in the Reduction of Children's Fractures

Medications	Dosages	Comments
Midazolam (Versed)	0.05–0.2 mg/kg IV	Rapid onset; brief duration of action
Diazepam (Valium)	0.04–0.3 mg/kg IV	Good muscle relaxant
Morphine	0.1–0.2 mg/kg IV	Long duration of action
Meperidine (Demerol)	1–2 mg/kg IV	Long duration of action
Fentanyl (Sublimaze)	1.0–5.0 mcg/kg IV	Potent, rapid onset of action; titrate slowly
Ketamine	1–2 mg/kg IV 3–4 mg/kg IM	Manage emergence reactions with small doses of midazolam
Propofol (Diprivan)	1–2 mg/kg IV	Initial dose titrate to effect; rapid onset, short acting
Naloxone (Narcan)	1.0–2.0 mcg/kg IV	Narcotic reversal agent
Flumazenil (Mazicon, Romazicon)	0.003–0.006 mg/kg IV	Benzodiazepine reversal agent
Atropine	0.04 mg/kg IV or IM; minimum, 0.1mg; maximum, 1.0 mg	Antisialogogue
Glycopyrrolate (Robinul)	0.05 mg/kg IV or IM; maximum, 0.25 mg	Antisialogogue

IM, Intramuscular; *IV,* intravenous.
Dexmedetomidine, 2–3 mcg/kg IV over 10 min, infusion 1–2 mcg/kg. Modest analgesic effect, 2 mcg/kg IV for short procedures, 2–3 mcg/kg intranasal, buccal.
(Modified from McCarty EC, Mencio GA, Green NE. Anesthesia and analgesia for the ambulatory management of fractures in children. *J Am Acad Orthop Surg.* 1999;7:84. With permission.)

duration of action, making it less desirable than midazolam from a pharmacokinetic standpoint. However, it is an excellent muscle relaxant and continues to be a good choice for fracture and joint reduction.[4,15]

Morphine sulfate and fentanyl citrate (Sublimaze) are the most common narcotics used for IV management of acute pain and painful procedures in the emergency department.[15] Morphine is the standard by which other narcotics are judged. However, it tends to be more effective for continuous dull pain than the sharp pain typically associated with fractures.[30] It is the least lipid soluble of the narcotics listed and, as a consequence, has a slower onset and longer duration of action (3 to 4 hours). As a result, it is difficult to titrate.[30] Meperidine was a commonly used narcotic in the emergency department, although it has some characteristics that make it less desirable than other narcotics. It is one-tenth as potent as morphine but has better euphoric properties. It has a slightly faster onset and shorter duration of action (2–3 hours) than morphine. Like morphine, meperidine is also difficult to titrate. When used for initial pain management, both drugs, but meperidine in particular, have been shown to cause a significant increase in sedation recovery times.[78] Fentanyl is a narcotic analgesic that is 100 times more potent than morphine. It is highly lipid soluble, and its onset of action (peak analgesia in 2–3 minutes) is rapid.[30] Its duration of action is shorter than either meperidine or morphine (20–30 minutes) and it can be titrated more easily. Infants younger than 6 months metabolize fentanyl more slowly than older children and should be dosed more conservatively (one-third normal).[4] Fentanyl can also be administered intranasally for a rapid-onset analgesic effect. Intranasal fentanyl, in the dose of 2 mcg/kg given with a nasal atomizer, is an effective alternative to nitrous oxide when used in combination with a hematoma block.[79]

When IV sedation is administered with both a narcotic and a benzodiazepine, dosing should begin low and be titrated slowly, and the synergistic effect of these drugs should be kept in mind. If respiratory depression occurs, immediate airway support should be given, and reversal agents may need to be administered. Typically, the narcotic is reversed first with naloxone. If respiratory depression persists after 1 to 2 minutes, the benzodiazepine should be reversed with flumazenil.[68] Both reversal agents have a shorter half-life than the drugs they are reversing; therefore, monitoring must continue until all respiratory effects have dissipated. IV sedation should never be used in children with a history of apnea or airway disease, altered mental status, or hemodynamic instability, or in infants younger than 2 months.

PROPOFOL

Propofol (Diprivan) is a nonopioid, nonbarbiturate, short-acting, potent sedative/hypnotic agent that must be administered intravenously. Although originally used almost exclusively in operating rooms and intensive care units, it has become increasingly popular in the ambulatory care setting for procedural sedation because it has the advantage of rapid induction and short recovery time. Propofol has comparable amnestic properties to midazolam with the advantages of more rapid onset of sedation (about 40 seconds), faster recovery, smoother emergence, and antiemetic properties.[80–82] Disadvantages of propofol include high incidences of hypotension and apnea compared with both midazolam and ketamine (discussed in the following section) and a lack of analgesic properties. For painful fracture reductions, propofol should be used concurrently with opioid analgesics such as fentanyl or morphine, but this may further increase the risk of respiratory depression and hypotension. There is no reversal agent for propofol, so adverse events must be treated supportively until the drug is metabolized; competent airway management skills must be available from the sedation provider.

KETAMINE

Ketamine is a pharmacologic analog of phencyclidine that causes dissociation between the thalamoneocortical and limbic areas of the brain and induces a cataleptic, trance-like state. Ketamine interferes with perception of visual, auditory, and noxious stimuli.[25,30] Children under ketamine sedation appear to be awake, with eyes open and with nystagmus, yet are unresponsive to stimuli. Ketamine provides a combination of sedation, analgesia, and amnesia without cardiovascular depression. With ketamine sedation, normal function of the orotracheal airway, including protective reflexes, is preserved.[25] Respiratory depression is rare and is dose related. The onset of sedation with ketamine is rapid, the effect is short-lived, and recovery is rapid.[4,24,30] It can be used for injuries in all extremities.

Ketamine can be administered either by IV or IM routes.[24,25] The IV route is attractive because dosing can be titrated, and a smaller cumulative dose can be given to achieve the desired effect. The onset of action is also quicker, and recovery is more rapid.[24] The IV dose of ketamine is 1 to 2 mg/kg and should be administered slowly so that respiratory depression is avoided. The IM route can be used when IV access is unobtainable. The IM dose is 4 mg/kg. Pain reduction has actually been shown to be better after IM administration; however, recovery times are significantly longer, and nausea and vomiting are more common, which makes the IV route preferable.[83] Typically, fracture manipulation may begin within 1 to 2 minutes after IV administration and 5 minutes after IM administration. A repeated IM dose can be given after 10 to 15 minutes if the initial effect is inadequate.[24,25] AAP and ASA guidelines for equipment and monitoring of patients undergoing deep sedation must be followed. Empiric preprocedural fasting guidelines for anesthesia and sedation are followed in most centers, although several studies have reported no significant association between the preprocedural fasting state and adverse events. In a study of 2085 patients undergoing procedural sedation in a pediatric emergency department, adverse events occurred in 344 patients, including desaturations and vomiting. No difference in events was noted between those who met fasting criteria and those who did not.[3]

Ketamine increases upper airway secretions, and an anti-sialogogue such as atropine or glycopyrrolate can be effective in minimizing this effect.[4,25,30] Ketamine may cause hallucinations during emergence from sedation, although this problem rarely occurs in children younger than 10 years.[24,25] In older children, prophylactic administration of a low-dose benzodiazepine (midazolam, 0.05 mg/kg) can effectively prevent this side effect from occurring.[4,30] However, the benzodiazepine may prolong recovery by delaying the metabolism of ketamine.[24] Other potential problems associated with ketamine include nausea, emesis, rash, elevated intracranial pressure, tachycardia and hypertension, rigidity or hypertonicity, and random movements. Ketamine is contraindicated in patients with hypertension who have demonstrated hypersensitivity to the drug. Relative contraindications for the use of ketamine are pulmonary disease or upper respiratory infections, the presence of an intracranial mass, a closed head injury, psychiatric history, children younger than 10 years (because of emergence phenomena), heart disease, porphyria, glaucoma, a penetrating eye injury, and hyperthyroidism.[24,25]

Ketamine has been in clinical use since the 1960s. During that time, the safety and efficacy of ketamine sedation for children undergoing painful procedures in an emergency department setting have been established.[4,15,24,25,30] In 1990, Green and Johnson[24] performed a metaanalysis of 97 studies of ketamine sedation that included administration to 11,589 children. Only two children (0.017%) required intubation for laryngospasm. The incidence of emesis was 8.5%, but no cases of aspiration occurred. Because of its unique properties and safe track record, ketamine is, in many ways, an ideal drug for PSA in children in the emergency department.[25]

Until the end of the last millennium, there had been limited experience with ketamine for sedation of children during fracture treatment or management of other musculoskeletal problems. Of the studies reviewed by Green and Johnson[24] in their extensive analysis of the literature on ketamine use in the emergency department, only one[84] mentioned fracture treatment as one of the indications for sedation by this method. A subsequent investigation by Green and associates[25] on the use of IM ketamine sedation in the emergency department reported successful use in seven (of 108) children with fractures. Physician satisfaction with the sedation was excellent. Most of the patients (82.9%) were able to undergo fracture reduction within 5 minutes of ketamine injection. Several minor complications, including hypersalivation, hypertonicity, rash, and vomiting, did occur, but no major problems were reported. Overall parental satisfaction was high in this study.

In the early 1970s, several reports were published in the European literature regarding the use of ketamine in children with fractures.[85–87] McCarty and colleagues[88] reported excellent results with ketamine sedation for the treatment of fractures in 114 children in the emergency department. The time from administration of the ketamine to manipulation of the fracture averaged less than 2 minutes after IV dosing and less than 5 minutes after IM administration. Pain scale scores reflected minimal or no pain during fracture reduction. Parental satisfaction was high, and 99% of parents responded that they would allow it to be used again in a similar situation. Airway patency and independent respiration were maintained. Minor adverse effects, including nausea (13 patients) and vomiting (8 patients), occurred but only well into the emergence phase of the sedation. No major problems were encountered.

ETOMIDATE

Etomidate is an ultrashort-acting nonbarbiturate hypnotic that has several uses in the emergency department. In lower doses (0.15 mg/kg), it is an excellent sedation medication, and in larger doses (0.3 mg/kg), it is an excellent sedation medication for intubation.[89] Its onset of action is within 1 minute and it has a duration of action ranging from 4 to 15 minutes. Etomidate has minimal hemodynamic effects and does not have analgesic properties, so it can be used in conjunction with an opioid for painful procedures. Myoclonus, however, has been reported in up to 22% of pediatric patients who received etomidate, which makes its utility in some orthopedic reductions less than ideal.[90] Some studies have also shown that cortisol production may be blocked by one dose of etomidate.[91]

DEXMEDETOMIDINE

Dexmedetomidine is an alpha-2 adrenergic agonist that provides modest analgesia and sedation that parallels natural sleep. It is useful for prolonged motionless sedation and may be used in combination with ketamine, midazolam, or opioids. An advantage of dexmedetomidine is it maintains ventilation and airway patency in the presence of deep sedation. If used for painful procedures, the addition of other analgesics may increase the risk for airway intervention. For prolonged procedures, induction dose of 2 to 3 mcg/kg is administered over 10 min followed by a maintenance infusion of 1 to 2 mcg/kg/hour. For short procedures, a single dose of 2 mcg/kg has shown to be effective. Intranasal and buccal dosing is 2 to 3 mcg/kg.

COMPARATIVE STUDIES

Over the past 20 years, several studies have compared drug combinations for procedural sedation in the pediatric emergency department setting. Kennedy and colleagues[70] compared the safety and efficacy of ketamine- versus fentanyl-based protocols in the emergency management of pediatric fractures. In this study, patients 5 to 15 years of age needing emergency fracture or joint reduction were randomly assigned to receive IV midazolam plus either fentanyl (F/M) or ketamine (K/M). During fracture reduction, K/M subjects ($n = 130$) had lower distress scores and parental ratings of pain and anxiety than did F/M subjects ($n = 130$). Although both regimens equally facilitated fracture treatment, deep sedation, and procedural amnesia, orthopedists favored the ketamine-based technique. Recovery was 14 minutes longer for K/M, but fewer K/M subjects had hypoxia (6% vs. 25%), needed breathing cues (1% vs. 12%), or required oxygen (10% vs. 20%) than did F/M subjects. Two K/M subjects did require assisted ventilation briefly, and more K/M subjects vomited. Adverse emergence reactions were rare but equivalent between regimens. The authors concluded that K/M is more effective for pediatric fracture reduction than F/M for pain and anxiety relief and was associated with fewer respiratory complications, although vomiting was slightly more frequent and recovery was more prolonged (mean, 15 minutes) with K/M.

Roback and colleagues[92] compared the frequency and severity of adverse events associated with four major parenteral drug combinations used for procedural sedation in the emergency department in 2500 children (mean age, 6.7 years): ketamine alone ($n = 1492$; 59.7%), ketamine/midazolam ($n = 299$; 12.0%), midazolam/fentanyl ($n = 336$; 13.4%), and midazolam alone ($n = 260$; 10.4%). They identified a total of 458 adverse events (respiratory or nausea/vomiting) in 426 patients (17%) and found that patients receiving ketamine with or without midazolam experienced fewer respiratory adverse events than those sedated with the combination of midazolam and fentanyl. Patients who received ketamine did experience more vomiting, although none aspirated. In a systematic review of the literature to assess safety and efficacy of various forms of analgesia and sedation for fracture reduction in the emergency department, Migita and associates[71] identified eight randomized, controlled trials with a total of 1086 patients that showed, among parenteral drug combinations, K/M to be associated with less distress during fracture manipulation than F/M or propofol and fentanyl (P/F) and that patients receiving K/M required significantly fewer airway interventions than those in whom either F/M or P/F was used. In another comparative study of K/M versus P/F, Godambe and colleagues[93] found that P/F was comparable to K/M in reducing procedural distress associated with painful orthopedic procedures in children in an emergency department setting and that P/F was associated with a shorter recovery time than ketamine. However, propofol had a greater potential for respiratory depression and airway obstruction than ketamine.

Administering ketamine and propofol simultaneously, a combination referred to as "ketofol," has been shown to be very effective for procedural sedation.[94] This combination of drugs takes advantage of the benefits of both drugs while counteracting the other agent's unwanted effects. The rapid onset and short duration of propofol is added to the analgesic properties of ketamine. With the addition of propofol, the dosage of ketamine is reduced; therefore, it effects a more rapid recovery. Ketamine causes hypertension and tachycardia and aids in counteracting the bradycardia and hypotension seen with propofol. This mixture requires strict adherence to deep sedation monitoring because the potential need for airway intervention is increased.[95]

SUMMARY

Numerous techniques for analgesia and sedation exist for the outpatient management of fractures in children. The method chosen should be safe, reliable, and efficacious so that the child is kept free from pain and anxiety is minimized, parents are satisfied, and, ultimately, satisfactory treatment of the fracture is permitted, obviating a trip to the operating room.

DPT and chloral hydrate are outmoded methods and should *not* be used. Local and regional techniques such as the hematoma block, axillary block, and IV regional anesthesia (Bier block) can be effective for upper extremity fractures. Sedation with nitrous oxide or a parenterally administered narcotic-benzodiazepine combination are not region specific and are suitable for a wide range of ages. Ketamine, propofol, and etomidate are excellent choices for procedural sedation for treatment of fractures or other orthopedic procedures. With any method of sedation, state and institutional guidelines for appropriate physiologic monitoring should be followed, and equipment and expertise for rescue of a patient from deeper levels of sedation than intended (including advanced airway management) should be available.

ACKNOWLEDGMENT

The authors would like to acknowledge and thank Dr. Eric C. McCarty and Dr. Gregory A. Mencio for their contributions to the previous versions of this chapter.

REFERENCES

The level of evidence (LOE) is determined according to the criteria provided in the Preface.

1. Cramer K, Glasson S, Mencio GA, et al. Reduction of forearm fractures in children using axillary block anesthesia. *J Orthop Trauma.* 1995;9:407–410. **(LOE III)**.
2. Ogden J. *Skeletal Injury in the Child.* 2nd ed. Philadelphia; WB Saunders.
3. Roback MG, Bajaj L, Wathen J, Bothner J. Preprocedural fasting and adverse events in procedural sedation and analgesia in a pediatric emergency department: are they related? *Ann Emerg Med.* 2004;44(5):454–459. **(LOE III)**.
4. Sacchetti A, Schafermeyer R, Gerardi M, et al. Pediatric analgesia and sedation. *Ann Emerg Med.* 1994;23:237–250. **(LOE V)**.
5. Beales J, Kean J, Lennox-Holt P, Mellor V. Children with juvenile chronic arthritis: their beliefs about their illness. *J Rheumatol.* 1983;10:61–65. **(LOE IV)**.
6. Haslam D. Age and the perception of pain. *Psychonomic Sci.* 1969;15:86. **(LOE IV)**.
7. Jay S, Ozolins M, Elliott C, et al. Assessment of children's distress during painful medical procedures. *Health Psych.* 1983;2:133–147. **(LOE IV)**.
8. Paris P. Pain management in children. *Emerg Med Clin North Am.* 1987;5:699–707. **(LOE V)**.
9. Schechter N. Pain and pain control in children. *Curr Probl Pediatr.* 1985;15:1–67. **(LOE V)**.
10. Schechter N. The undertreatment of pain in children: an overview. *Pediatr Clin North Am.* 1989;36:781–794. **(LOE V)**.
11. Selbst S. Managing pain in the pediatric emergency department. *Pediatr Emerg Care.* 1989;5:56–63. **(LOE V)**.
12. Selbst S, Henretig F. The treatment of pain in the emergency department. *Pediatr Clin North Am.* 1989;36:965–977. **(LOE V)**.
13. Zeltzer L, Jay S, Fisher D. The management of pain associated with pediatric procedures. *Pediatr Clin North Am.* 1989;36:941–963. **(LOE V)**.
14. Proudfoot J, Roberts M. Providing safe and effective sedation and analgesia for pediatric patients. *Emerg Med Rep.* 1993;14:207–217. **(LOE V)**.
15. Sacchetti A, Gerardi M. Pediatric sedation and analgesia. *Acad Emerg Med.* 1995;2:240–241. **(LOE V)**.
16. Stehling L. Anesthesia update #11: unique considerations in pediatric orthopaedics. *Orthop Rev.* 1981;10:95–99. **(LOE V)**.
17. American Academy of Pediatrics, Committee on Drugs. Guidelines for monitoring and management of pediatric patients during and after sedation for diagnostic and therapeutic procedures. *Pediatrics.* 1992;6:1110–1115. **(LOE V)**.
18. Barnes C, Blasier R, Dodge B. Intravenous regional anesthesia: a safe and cost-effective outpatient anaesthetic for upper extremity fracture treatment in children. *J Pediatr Orthop.* 1991;11:717–720. **(LOE IV)**.
19. Bolte R, Stevens P, Scott S, et al. Mini-dose Bier block intravenous regional anesthesia in the emergency department treatment of pediatric upper-extremity injuries. *J Pediatr Orthop.* 1994;14:534–537. **(LOE II)**.
20. Chudnofsky C, Wright S, Pronen S. The safety of fentanyl use in the emergency department. *Ann Emerg Med.* 1989;18:635–639. **(LOE III)**.
21. Colizza W, Said E. Intravenous regional anesthesia in the treatment of forearm and wrist fractures and dislocations in children. *Can J Surg.* 1993;36:225–228. **(LOE II)**.
22. Cook B, Bass J, Nomizu S, et al. Sedation of children for technical procedures. *Clin Pediatr.* 1992;31:137–142. **(LOE V)**.
23. Evans J, Buckley S, Alexander A, et al. Analgesia for the reduction of fractures in children: a comparison of nitrous oxide with intramuscular sedation. *J Pediatr Orthop.* 1995;15:73–77. **(LOE II)**.
24. Green S, Johnson N. Ketamine sedation for pediatric procedures: part 2, review and implications. *Ann Emerg Med.* 1990;19:1033–1046. **(LOE V)**.
25. Green S, Nakamura R, Johnson N. Ketamine sedation for pediatric procedures: part 1, a prospective series. *Ann Emerg Med.* 1990;19:1024–1032. **(LOE II)**.
26. Gregory P, Sullivan J. Nitrous oxide compared with intravenous regional anesthesia in pediatric forearm fracture management. *J Pediatr Orthop.* 1996;16:187–191. **(LOE II)**.
27. Hennrikus W, Shin A, Klingelberger C. Self-administered nitrous oxide and a hematoma block for analgesia in the outpatient reduction of fractures in children. *J Bone Joint Surg Am.* 1995;77:335–339. **(LOE IV)**.
28. Hennrikus W, Simpson R, Klingelberger C, et al. Self-administered nitrous oxide analgesia for pediatric reductions. *J Pediatr Orthop.* 1994;14:538–542. **(LOE IV)**.
29. Juliano P, Mazur J, Cummings R, et al. Low-dose lidocaine intravenous regional anesthesia for forearm fractures in children. *J Pediatr Orthop.* 1992;12:633–635. **(LOE IV)**.
30. Proudfoot J. Analgesia, anesthesia, and conscious sedation. *Emerg Med Clin North Am.* 1995;13:357–378. **(LOE V)**.
31. Snodgrass W, Dodge W. Lytic/"DPT" cocktail: time for rational and safe alternatives. *Pediatr Clin North Am.* 1989;36:1285–1291. **(LOE V)**.
32. Kennedy RM, Luhmann JD, Luhmann SJ. Emergency department management of pain and anxiety related to orthopedic fracture care: a guide to analgesic techniques and procedural sedation in children. *Paediatr Drugs.* 2004;6:11–31. **(LOE V)**.
33. McCarty EC, Mencio GA, Green NE. Anesthesia and analgesia for the ambulatory management of fractures in children. *J Am Acad Orthop Surg.* 1999;7:81–91. **(LOE V)**.
34. McGrath P, Craig K. Developmental and psychological factors in children's pain. *Pediatr Clin North Am.* 1989;36:823–836. **(LOE V)**.
35. American Academy of Pediatrics, Committee on Drugs. Reappraisal of lytic cocktail/Demerol, Phenergan, and Thorazine (DPT) for the sedation of children. *Pediatrics.* 1995;95:598–602. **(LOE V)**.
36. Binder L, Leake L. Chloral hydrate for emergent pediatric procedural sedation: a new look at an old drug. *Am J Emerg Med.* 1991;9:530–534. **(LOE V)**.
37. Lowe S, Hershey S. Sedation for imaging and invasive procedures. In: Deshpande J, Tobias J, eds. *The Pediatric Pain Handbook.* St. Louis: Mosby;263–317.
38. U.S. Department of Health and Human Services PHS, Agency for Health Care Policy and Research, Acute Pain Management Guideline Panel. *Clinical Practice Guideline. Acute Pain Management: Operative or Medical Procedures and Trauma.* Washington, DC: U.S. Department of Health and Human Services.
39. Winnie A. Regional anesthesia. *Surg Clin North Am.* 1975;54:861–892. **(LOE V)**.
40. Wang RD, Dangler LA, Greengrass RA. Update on ropivacaine. *Expert Opin Pharmacother.* 2001;2(12):2051–2063. **(LOE V)**.
41. Grey W. Regional blocks and their difficulties. *Aust Fam Physician.* 1977;6:900–906. **(LOE V)**.
42. Wedel D, Krohn J, Hall J. Brachial plexus anesthesia in pediatric patients. *Mayo Clin Proc.* 1991;66:583–588. **(LOE IV)**.
43. Abbaszadegan H, Jonsson H. Regional anesthesia preferable for Colles' fracture: controlled comparison with local anesthesia. *Acta Orthop Scand.* 1990;61:348–349. **(LOE II)**.
44. Alioto R, Furia J, Marquardt J. Hematoma block for ankle fractures: a safe and efficacious technique for manipulations. *J Orthop Trauma.* 1995;9:113–116. **(LOE III)**.
45. Case R. Haematoma block—A safe method of reducing Colles' fractures. *Injury.* 1985;16:469–470. **(LOE III)**.
46. Dinley R, Michelinakis E. Local anesthesia in the reduction of Colles' fractures. *Injury.* 1973;4:345–346. **(LOE IV)**.

47. Johnson P, Noffsinger M. Hematoma block of distal forearm fractures: is it safe? *Orthop Rev.* 1991;20:977–979. **(LOE III)**.

48. Bear DM, Friel NA, Lupo CL, Pitetti R, Ward WT. Hematoma block versus sedation for the reduction of distal radius fractures in children. *J Hand Surg Am.* 2015;40(1):57–61. **(LOE II)**.

49. Bell H, Slater E, Harris W. Regional anesthesia with intravenous lidocaine. *JAMA.* 1963;186:544–549. **(LOE V)**.

50. Carrel E, Eyring E. Intravenous regional anesthesia for childhood fractures. *J Trauma.* 1971;11:301–305. **(LOE IV)**.

51. Colbern E. The Bier block for intravenous regional anesthesia: technic and literature review. *Anesth Analg.* 1970:935–940. **(LOE V)**.

52. Farrell R, Swanson S, Walter J. Safe and effective IV regional anesthesia for use in the emergency department. *Ann Emerg Med.* 1985;14:239–241. **(LOE III)**.

53. Fitzgerald B. Intravenous regional anaesthesia in children. *Br J Anaesth.* 1976;48:485–486. **(LOE IV)**.

54. Gingrich T. Intravenous regional anaesthesia of the upper extremity in children. *JAMA.* 1967;200:235. **(LOE V)**.

55. Holmes C. Intravenous regional analgesia: a useful method of producing analgesia of the limbs. *Lancet.* 1963;1:245–247. **(LOE V)**.

56. Lehman W, Jones W. Intravenous lidocaine for anesthesia in the lower extremity. A prospective study. *J Bone J Surg Am.* 1984;66:1056–1060. **(LOE II)**.

57. Olney B, Lugg P, Turner P, et al. Outpatient treatment of upper extremity injuries in childhood using intravenous regional anaesthesia. *J Pediatr Orthop.* 1988;8:576–579. **(LOE IV)**.

58. Turner P, Batten J, Hjorth D, et al. Intravenous regional anaesthesia for the treatment of upper limb injuries in childhood. *Aust NZ J Surg.* 1986;56:153–155. **(LOE IV)**.

59. Urban B, McKain C. Onset and progression of intravenous regional anesthesia with dilute lidocaine. *Anesth Analg.* 1982;61:834–838. **(LOE IV)**.

60. Aarons CE, Fernandez MD, Willsey M, Peterson B, Key C, Fabregas J. Bier block regional anesthesia and casting for forearm fractures: safety in the pediatric emergency department setting. *J Pediatr Orthop.* 2014;34(1):45–49. **(LOE IV)**.

61. Chu RS, Browner GJ, Cheng NG, et al. Femoral nerve block for femoral shaft fractures in a paediatric emergency department: can it be done better? *Eur J Emerg Med.* 2003;10:258–263. **(LOE IV)**.

62. Denton J, Manning M. Femoral nerve block for femoral shaft fractures in children: brief report. *J Bone Joint Surg Br.* 1988;70:84. **(LOE V)**.

63. Grossbard G, Love B. Femoral nerve block: a simple and safe method of instant analgesia for femoral shaft fractures in children. *Aust NZ J Surg.* 1979;49:592–594. **(LOE V)**.

64. Ronchi L, Rosenbaum D, Athouel A, et al. Femoral nerve blockade in children using bupivacaine. *Anesthesiology.* 1989;70:622–624. **(LOE IV)**.

65. Wathen JE, Gao D, Merritt G, et al. A randomized controlled trial comparing a fascia iliaca compartment nerve block to a traditional systemic analgesic for femur fractures in a pediatric emergency department. *Ann Emerg Med.* 2007;50:162–171. **(LOE II)**.

66. American Society of Anesthesiologists Task Force on Sedation and Analgesia by Non-Anesthesiologists. Practice guidelines for sedation and analgesia by non-anesthesiologists. *Anesthesiology.* 2002;96(4):1004–1017. **(LOE V)**.

67. Pitetti RD, Singh S, Pierce MC. Safe and efficacious use of procedural sedation and analgesia by nonanesthesiologists in a pediatric emergency department. *Arch Pediatr Adolesc Med.* 2003;157:1090–1096. **(LOE IV)**.

68. Wattenmaker I, Kasser J, McGravey A. Self-administered nitrous oxide for fracture reduction in children in an emergency room setting. *J Orthop Trauma.* 1990;4:35–38. **(LOE IV)**.

69. Friedland L, Kulick R. Emergency department analgesic use in pediatric trauma victims with fractures. *Ann Emerg Med.* 1994;23:203–207. **(LOE IV)**.

70. Kennedy RM, Porter FL, Miller JP, et al. Comparison of fentanyl/midazolam with ketamine/midazolam for pediatric orthopedic emergencies. *Pediatrics.* 1999;104(5 Pt 1):1167–1168. **(LOE III)**.

71. Migita RT, Klein EJ, Garrison MM. Sedation and analgesia for pediatric fracture reduction in the emergency department: a systematic review. *Arch Pediatr Adolesc Med.* 2006;160:46–51. **(LOE I)**.

72. Pruitt J, Goldwasser M, Sabol S, et al. Intramuscular ketamine, midazolam, and glycopyrrolate for pediatric sedation in the emergency department. *J Oral Maxillofac Surg.* 1995;53:13–17. **(LOE IV)**.

73. Luhmann JD, Schootman M, Luhmann SJ, Kennedy RM. A randomized comparison of nitrous oxide plus hematoma block versus ketamine plus midazolam for emergency department forearm fracture reduction in children. Pediatrics. *Pediatrics.* 2006;118(4):e1078–1086. **(LOE II)**.

74. Patel M, Grunwell J, Bryan L, et al. A survey of procedural sedation in children with autism spectrum disorders. *Crit Care Med.* 2018;46(1):222. **(LOE V)**.

75. Roback MG, Carlson DW, Babl FE, Kennedy RM. Update on pharmacological management of procedural sedation for children. *Curr Opin Anaesthesiol.* 2016;29(suppl 1):S21–S35. **(LOE V)**.

76. Younge D. Haematoma block for fractures of the wrist: a cause of compartment syndrome. *J Hand Surg Br.* 1989;14(2):194–195. **(LOE V)**.

77. Krauss B, Zurakowski D. Sedation patterns in pediatric and general community hospital emergency departments. *Pediatr Emerg Care.* 1998;14:99–103. **(LOE V)**.

78. Losek JD, Reid S. Effects of initial pain treatment on sedation recovery time in pediatric emergency care. *Pediatr Emerg Care.* 2006;22:100–103. **(LOE III)**.

79. Saunders M, Adelgais K, Nelson D. Use of intranasal fentanyl for the relief of pediatric orthopaedic trauma pain. *Acad Emerg Med.* 2010;17(11):1155–1161. **(LOE IV)**.

80. Havel CJ, Strait RT, Hennes H. A clinical trial of propofol vs midazolam for procedural sedation in a pediatric emergency department. *Acad Emerg Med.* 1999;6:989–997. **(LOE I)**.

81. Skokan EG, Pribble C, Bassett F, et al. Use of propofol sedation in a pediatric emergency department: a prospective study. *Clin Pediatr.* 2001;40:663–671. **(LOE IV)**.

82. Vardi A, Salem Y, Padeh S, et al. Is propofol safe for procedural sedation in children? A prospective evaluation of propofol vs ketamine in pediatric critical care. *Crit Care Med.* 2002;30:1231–1236. **(LOE III)**.

83. Roback MG, Wathen JE, Bajaj L. A randomized, controlled trial of IV versus IM ketamine for sedation of pediatric patients receiving emergency department orthopaedic procedures. *Ann Emerg Med.* 2006;48:605–612. **(LOE I)**.

84. Caro D. Trial of ketamine in an accident and emergency department. *Anaesthesia.* 1974;29:227–229. **(LOE IV)**.

85. Caroli G, Lari S, Serra G. La ketamina in ortopedia e traumatologia: indicazioni e limiti. *Chir Organi Mov.* 1972;61:99–104. **(LOE V)**.

86. Muncibi S, Santoni R. Utilizzazione della ketamina in ortopedia e traumatologia. *Minerva Anestesiol.* 1973;39:370–376. **(LOE V)**.

87. Pagnani I, Ramaioli F, Mapelli A. Prospettive sull'impiego clinico della ketamina cloridrato in ortopedia e traumatologia pediatrica. *Minerva Anestesiol.* 1974;40:159–162. **(LOE II)**.

88. McCarty EC, Mencio GA, Walker LA, et al. Ketamine sedation for the reduction of children's fractures in the emergency department. *J Bone Joint Surg Am.* 2000;82:912–918. **(LOE III)**.

89. Wolters Kluwer Health, Inc. Etomidate. Drug facts and comparisons, Efacts. http://www.wolterskluwerhealth.com/Search/Pages/Results.aspx?k=etomidate. **(LOE V)**

90. Di Liddo L, D'Angelo A, Nguyen B, et al. Etomidate versus midazolam for procedural sedation in pediatric outpatients: a randomized controlled trial. *Ann Emerg Med.* 2006;48:433–440. **(LOE I)**.

91. Donmez A, Kaya H, Haberal A, et al. The effect of etomidate induction on plasma cortisol levels in children undergoing cardiac surgery. *J Cardiothorac Vasc Anesth.* 1998;12:182–185. **(LOE II)**.

92. Roback MG, Wathen JE, Bajaj L, et al. Adverse events associated with procedural sedation and analgesia in a pediatric emergency department: a comparison of common parenteral drugs. *Acad Emerg Med.* 2005;12:508–513. **(LOE III)**.

93. Godambe S, Elliot V, Matheny D, Pershad J. Comparison of propofol/fentanyl versus ketamine/midazolam for brief orthopedic procedural sedation in a pediatric emergency department. *Pediatrics.* 2003;112(1 Pt 1):116–123. **(LOE II)**.

94. Willman EV, Andolfatto G. A prospective evaluation of "ketofol" (ketamine/propofol combination) for procedural sedation and analgesia in the emergency department. *Ann Emerg Med.* 2007;49:23–30. **(LOE IV)**.

95. Andolfatto G, Willman E. A prospective case series of pediatric procedural sedation and analgesia in the emergency department using single-syringe ketamine-propofol combination (Ketofol). *Acad Emerg Med.* 2010;17(2):194–201. **(LOE IV)**.

22

Rehabilitation of the Child with Multiple Injuries

Eric D. Shirley | Louise Z. Spierre

INTRODUCTION

Trauma is the most common cause of death and disability for children in the United States, with up to half of injuries resulting in long-term sequelae.[1–4] Children with multiple injuries present particular challenges to both their families and the medical teams that care for them. The rehabilitation goal for children with multiple injuries is to maximize function and return them to their home and community as soon as possible.[5] The purpose of this chapter is to review the important aspects of rehabilitation treatment in this setting.

> ### Key Points
> - Multidisciplinary care and early rehabilitation are essential to optimize outcomes of children with polytrauma, spinal cord injury, or traumatic brain injury.
> - Criteria for inpatient rehabilitation include the need for moderate/maximum assistance, the ability to participate in 3 hours of therapy per day, the ability to follow at least simple commands, and the need for at least two different therapies.
> - Spasticity should be classified as localized or generalized and graded by severity.
> - Psychologic rehabilitation of an injured child is as important as the physical rehabilitation.

INPATIENT REHABILITATION

Inpatient rehabilitation plays an integral role in the recovery of patients following a severe trauma or a disabling illness. Admission to an inpatient rehabilitation facility is indicated for patients requiring moderate to maximum assistance due to deficits in mobility, function, cognition, and/or speech. The majority of patients meeting criteria have sustained severe head injuries. Admission is also considered for patient with multiple fractures but no central nervous system involvement to become facile with orthoses and adaptive equipment. Patients must be able to participate in 3 hours per day of therapy and follow at least simple commands, although patients with lower levels of function may be admitted to specialized disorders of consciousness programs.[6] Patients must also be medically stable before transfer from the hospital.

Candidates for inpatient rehabilitation need at least two different therapies, such as physical therapy, occupational therapy, speech therapy, or cognitive therapy, for insurance companies to provide approval. Insurance authorization typically takes 3 days for commercial insurance and 7 days for public insurance.[7] Thus, patients with private insurance are more likely to receive inpatient rehabilitation and have a shorter hospital stay before admission.[7] Although children are often transferred a long distance to trauma centers for acute care, efforts should be made to find a rehabilitation facility close to the family's home. However, some trauma centers also have inpatient rehabilitation services, and the continuity between patients and their initial care team is likely beneficial.

The rehabilitation team consists of members from physiatry, physical therapy, occupational therapy, speech therapy, orthotics, nutrition, psychology, psychiatry, social work, and case management. The team is usually led by a physiatrist. Communication between the rehabilitation team and the orthopedist is critical, particularly at the beginning of therapy, to define weight-bearing or range and motion restrictions. Fractures do not have to be completely healed before admission, but achieving the benefits of therapy is facilitated by greater fracture stability. If a child is non-weight-bearing on more than two limbs, it is often better to delay rehabilitation until this restriction is lifted.

The goals of inpatient rehabilitation are to increase the child's level of function to transition to outpatient rehabilitation. Programs also teach families how to care for their injured child and facilitate integration back into the community.[5] Length of stay is influenced by the underlying condition, functional status, insurance, and psychosocial factors.[8] The median length of stay in rehabilitation is 32 days for spinal cord injury (SCI), 26 days for traumatic brain injury (TBI), and 13 days for orthopedic conditions.[8] A lack of available stepdown (subacute or chronic) rehabilitation facilities may contribute to longer lengths of stay.[8]

Although inpatient rehabilitation leads to improvements in quality of life and function for the majority of patients,[9–13] residual disability requiring further care (particularly in patients with SCI or TBI) is often present at discharge.[13] The transition from inpatient rehabilitation to outpatient management is stressful, and families may be overwhelmed by the complexity of care for their previously healthy child.[14,15] Families may even feel abandoned by the healthcare system.[15] Therefore, proper discharge from inpatient rehabilitation is essential. Phone calls after discharge from a rehabilitation nurse can facilitate difficulties with appointments, medications, and equipment.[14]

Successful rehabilitation not only results in returning the child to their home but also into their school and community. In adolescents who are of driving age, a driver's capacity evaluation should be done to assess the patient's safety and ability to drive. Children who require prolonged rehabilitation will have their schooling interrupted, in many cases for an extended period. This interruption in schooling may put them significantly behind the level of their peers, which adds to their problems when they are ready to return. It is important to initiate schooling and tutoring as soon as the patient's condition allows while recognizing that the duration of tutoring may be lengthy. Potential barriers for attending school are identified and addressed by the rehabilitation team in advance, and communication with the school regarding the child's needs is essential.

REHABILITATION OF FRACTURES

THERAPEUTIC EXERCISE

Fractures are typically immobilized during the protection phase of rehabilitation to allow adequate healing.[16] However, it is important to consider fracture and fixation stability to avoid excessive immobilization that delays rehabilitation. Therapy then progresses to controlled range of motion (ROM). Although isolated fractures in children often return to full ROM on their own,[17,18] ROM and physical therapy are critical for patients with head injuries, spine injuries, or multiple fractures to avoid joint contractures. Communication between the orthopedist and therapist facilitates rehabilitation at the proper pace.

Active ROM exercises (movement generated by the patient) are performed if possible. These are facilitated by active-assistive ROM exercises that consist of having the child actively move through as much of the range as possible and then passively completing as much movement as possible through the normal range. The use of body weight often increases the effectiveness of ROM exercises. For example, the best stretch of the gastrocnemius muscles is obtained when the patient is standing. Children are encouraged to participate in their ROM exercise program, and young children may be able to perform simple stretches if properly supervised. Passive ROM is performed if the child is too young, weak, or unable to cooperate. Standards for full and functional ROM have been established (Table 22.1).[19,20]

After additional fracture healing is well established, therapy then transitions to strengthening exercises. These exercises usually involve extremely simple equipment such as a ball, putty, or exercise band. Strengthening programs may also include isometric exercises, which maintain muscle length with increasing tension during contraction, or isotonic exercises with muscle shortening and steady tension. Isotonic exercises include open kinetic chain exercises, such as with free weights, and closed kinetic chain exercises, such as with pulley systems. Closed kinetic chain exercises are often favored in the early postinjury period because they provide a more predictable path of movement. During this phase, progress is also made with balance and proprioception exercises.[16] Sports-specific and functional training are also helpful before return to activities.[16] Return to play is not allowed until pain relief, full strength, and full ROM have been restored.[21]

Table 22.1 Normal and Functional Joint Range of Motion

Joint	Degrees of Normal (and Functional) Range of Motion
Shoulder	
Abduction	180 (120)
Adduction	45 (30)
Flexion	180 (120)
Extension	60 (40)
Internal rotation (arm in abduction)	80 (45)
External rotation (arm in abduction)	90 (45)
Elbow	
Flexion	140–160 (130)
Extension	0–5 (–30)
Supination	80–90 (50)
Pronation	70–80 (50)
Wrist	
Flexion	75 (15)
Extension	70 (30)
Radial deviation	20 (10)
Ulnar deviation	35 (15)
Hip	
Flexion	125–128 (90–110)
Extension	0–20 (0–5)
Abduction	45–48 (0–20)
Adduction	40–45 (0–20)
Internal rotation	40–45 (0–20)
External rotation	45 (0–15)
Knee	
Flexion	130–140 (110)
Extension	0 (0)
Ankle	
Plantar flexion	45 (20)
Dorsiflexion	20 (10)
Inversion	35 (10)
Eversion	25 (10)

(Modified from Hoppenfield S, Murthy VI. *Treatment and Rehabilitation of Fractures*. Philadelphia: Lippincott Williams & Wilkins; 2000.)

ORTHOSES AND ADAPTIVE EQUIPMENT

Casts and braces for fracture healing are discontinued as soon as possible to facilitate recovery. Lower extremity orthoses are often prescribed for abnormal gait dynamics in patients with associated spinal cord or TBI. These orthoses are named according to the region of the body that they help control, such as ankle-foot orthoses and knee-ankle-foot orthoses. Generally, the more joints controlled by the orthosis, the bulkier it becomes and the greater the potential to interfere with balance, gait, and function.

Adaptive devices can be helpful in extending reach, providing grasp, reducing force, and improving safety.[22] Examples include reachers, sock aids, a long-handled sponge or shoe horn, grooming aids, built-up feeding utensils, a rocker knife, a raised toilet seat, tub chair, and built-up door handles (Fig. 22.1).[22] Velcro or elastic shoe closures also may be helpful. Such devices can provide increased independence in activities of daily living including feeding, dressing, bathing, grooming, and toileting. Evaluation by an occupational therapist is valuable for problem-solving to increase independence and quality of life during recovery.

Gait aids are prescribed taking into account the child's function and any cognitive or balance limitations. These aids may be useful for a child with weight-bearing restrictions on the lower extremity. Initial crutch training is needed to prevent axillary irritation and injury from falls. A child who requires additional support because of instability or reduced lower extremity strength may require a walker. For patients with concurrent wrist or hand injuries, the walker or crutches can be modified with an upper extremity platform support to distribute the weight through the forearm and elbow. Wheelchairs are used if both lower extremities are involved or the patient cannot comply with weight-bearing restrictions. A sliding board may be helpful in increasing a child's independence in transfers for children who can weight bear on more than two limbs. Otherwise, a lift is prescribed, and caregivers are taught how to perform transfers.[23]

PAIN CONTROL

Adequate pain control in children after sustaining multiple fractures is required for successful rehabilitation. Providing a description of their pain is difficult for preschool-age children who do not possess the language ability or the understanding to correctly identify the location and characteristics of the pain.[24] Pain management is facilitated by using age-specific objective measurement scales based on expressive capability to quantify pain levels.[25] The Children's Hospital of Eastern Ontario Pain Scale and the Objective Pain Scale are used in infants and very young children.[26] For children 3 to 6 years of age, visual progression of happy to sad faces such as the McGrath Facial Affective Scale and Beyer Oucher Scale are frequently used. Older children have improved abstract and numeric reasoning and may be able to use more adult measures, such as the visual analog scale.[26] Inadequate pain control should be included in the differential diagnosis of unexplained agitation or vital sign changes such as tachycardia or hypertension in patients who are uncommunicative because of age or neurologic insult.

Pain relief should not be achieved with the indiscriminate use of narcotics. It has been shown that nonopioid analgesics such as acetaminophen and ibuprofen are as effective as opioids for acute fracture pain management.[27–30] In addition, ibuprofen is also as effective as morphine for postoperative management following minor orthopedic procedures.[30] However, for a multiply injured child, pain may be an ongoing

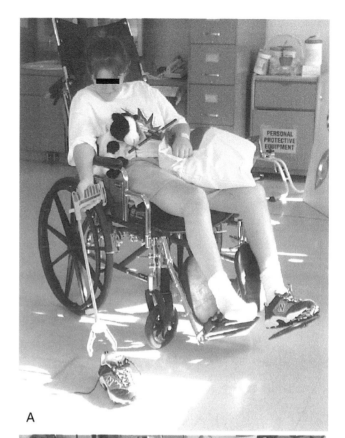

A

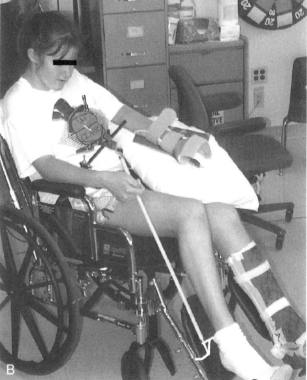

B

Fig. 22.1 This 17-year-old driver sustained multiple injuries in a motor vehicle crash, including pelvic and sacral fractures and traumatic brain injury resulting in left hemiparesis. She remained non-weight-bearing in bilateral lower extremities until the time of discharge from early rehabilitation and had significant motor impairment in her left upper extremity because of the neurologic injury. Provision of adaptive equipment, including a reacher (A) and sock aid (B), reduced caregiver assistance required in self-care.

problem such that narcotics are required. In this setting, efforts are made to slowly wean the child from the opioids while managing their side effects. Weaning is often started by switching to longer-acting medications.

PREVENTION OF REINJURY

The effort to prevent reinjury is an integral part of the rehabilitation process. This effort includes a discussion of safety equipment such as car seats, seat belts, helmets, and proper sports equipment. Children with fractures may have higher rates of conduct disorder, psychosomatic complaints, and impulsive/hyperactive behavior.[32] Thus, injury prevention methods include behavioral interventions in an attempt to decrease or at least better manage the impulsive behavior that may have contributed to the child's injury. Prevention can be a sensitive subject, particularly if the injury was potentially avoidable with improved parental supervision or appropriate use of safety devices. However, if this discussion is avoided, the child and family may incur worse trauma if recurrent injuries are sustained.

SPINAL CORD INJURY

SCI is an uncommon complication of pediatric skeletal trauma and occurs in only 2% of pediatric trauma cases.[33] However, the mental, physical, and economic consequences can be devastating. Multidisciplinary care and early rehabilitation are essential to optimize outcomes.[34]

COMPLICATIONS OF SPINAL CORD INJURY

The limitations in function and mobility secondary to the SCI are associated with numerous complications. The risk of venous thromboembolism (VTE) is increased in individuals with SCIs. However, the incidence of VTE is lower in patients younger than 14 years of age (1.1%) than adolescents (14–19 years of age, 4.8%), and adults (5.4%).[35] Thus the indications for mechanical or pharmacologic VTE prophylaxis are more controversial in younger patients than children who are showing signs of pubertal development or who are 14 years or older.[35,36] In addition to making careful decisions regarding prophylaxis, regular physical examinations should be performed to detect clinical signs of VTE, and a low threshold is recommended for ordering diagnostic tests when VTE is suspected.

Patients with SCIs are at risk for autonomic dysreflexia, which is characterized by a sudden increase in blood pressure in response to a stimulus below the level of injury. Compensatory bradycardia may occur in effort to decrease blood pressure. Symptoms include headache, sweating, and flushing.[34] The most common cause of autonomic dysreflexia is bladder irritation secondary to distention, renal stones, or infection.[34] Other causes include bowel distension from stool impaction, pressure ulcers, ingrown toenails, deep venous thrombosis, fractures, surgery, and hyperthermia.[34] Patients with lesions above T5–6 are particularly at risk due to low baseline sympathetic tone. As healthcare providers may be unfamiliar with this condition, it is important to educate families and provide them with a treatment card that they can bring to treatment facilities in the event of emergency

(Table 22.2). Treatment consists of immediately alleviating noxious stimuli such as an overdistended bladder or other painful areas and providing antihypertensive medications to prevent stroke.

Hypercalcemia occurs in 10% to 23% of patients with SCI, usually in the first 3 months after injury as bones demineralize from immobility.[34,37] Symptoms include abdominal pain, nausea, vomiting, lethargy, polyuria, polydipsia, and dehydration. Hypercalcemia may also result in behavioral changes or acute psychosis. Treatment with intravenous hydration and furosemide is required to prevent the development of renal stones or failure.[38,39]

Fractures in children with SCIs may occur immediately as a result of the initial trauma or later as chronic immobility leads to osteoporosis.[40] The increase in osteoclast activity after SCI results in bone density levels 60% of normal when homeostasis is reached.[41] Therefore, patients are at risk for low-energy fractures, particularly of the distal femur.[42] As pain may be absent, fractures may only present with swelling or general malaise.[34] Casts or splints used in treatment of non- or minimally displaced fractures must be well padded and removable to inspect the insensate skin.[43,44] There are mixed results of methods to decrease the loss of bone mineral density including exercise, supported standing, and functional electric stimulation.[45,46]

Heterotopic ossification may also occur after SCI. The most common location is the hip, followed by the knee and shoulder.[47,48] Heterotopic ossification typically occurs later in children (mean, 14 months) than adults (mean, 1–4 months).[34] The risk is lower in pediatric patients, and pharmacologic prophylaxis is not usually required.[34] Early ROM is still encouraged, as the risk of heterotopic ossification is higher when ROM is delayed more than 1 week after injury.[48,49]

Pressure sores and decubitus ulcers have the potential for significant morbidity and mortality in patients with SCIs. Common areas include the skin overlying the occiput, heels, and sacrum. These sores are the result of prolonged compression on insensate skin with subsequent hypoxia, necrosis, and possibly ulceration.[50] Prophylactic measures to prevent pressure sores are mandatory. These measures include ensuring proper nutrition, frequent weight shifts, Multi Podus boots, and fitting of braces and wheelchairs to minimize friction on the skin.[34] Patients are turned every 2 hours while in bed if they are insensate or have decreased bed mobility. Specialized mattresses can help decrease pressure but do not replace turning frequently and good nursing care. Patients are also instructed to avoid hot plates, curling irons, heated car seats, and other hot items on insensate areas to prevent unrecognized burns. Skin should be checked twice daily, and as soon as the first stage of a decubitus ulcer (nonblanching erythema) is identified, ways to relieve pressure from that area should be sought immediately.[51]

Neuropathic pain is common after SCI. Gabapentin can be prescribed to alleviate this pain, using a lower dose than for seizures. In a child 3 to 12 years of age, a starting dose of 10 to 15 mg/kg/day, divided three times a day and increased every 3 days to a maximum of 50 mg/kg/day, is recommended. In a patient older than 12 years, the maximum dose is 3600 mg/day. Adverse effects include sedation and the potential for abuse. When gabapentin is no longer needed, it should be tapered over 7 days because of the risk of seizures.

Table 22.2   Autonomic Dysreflexia Guidelines for Patients and Physicians

Definition

A sudden increase in blood pressure, 20–40 mm Hg systolic higher than usual, resulting from painful stimuli applied below neurologic levels in persons with spinal cord injuries. Without emergent treatment, it can lead to stroke, seizures, and death.

Common Signs and Symptoms

Above Level of Injury	Below Level of Injury
Hypertension	Nausea
Bradycardia or tachycardia	Chills without fever
Pounding headache	Cool
Apprehension/anxiety/uneasy feeling	Pale
Changes in vision	
Nasal congestion	
Sweating	
Flushed skin	
Goosebumps	
Tingling sensation	

Common Causes

Distended bladder
Constipated bowel
Pressure ulcers
Fractured bones
Skin burns
Urinary tract infections
Ingrown toenails
Any condition or procedure that may cause pain or discomfort but that is located below the neurologic injury level

What to Do

Sit up.
Take off or loosen any restrictive clothing.
Check blood pressure every 5 minutes until at baseline.
Check bladder; empty/catheterize. If indwelling catheter, check for kinks and blockages.
Check bowel; disimpact, if needed, using anesthetic jelly.
Check skin.
Assess for any other sources of painful stimuli or irritant.
If systolic blood pressure is more than 150 mm Hg, give antihypertensive agent with rapid onset and short duration while cause is being determined.
Monitor symptoms and blood pressure at least 2 hours after the resolution of an autonomic dysreflexia episode.

(From the Christopher and Dana Reeve Foundation website, http://www.christopherreeve.org. Accessed March 2018.)

Muscular spasticity develops in approximately half of patients with SCIs and is most common in incomplete lesions.[52] The spasticity may result in loss of joint motion, pressure ulcers, and difficulty for caregivers.[34] Treatment is indicated when spasticity results in functional consequences, and management options are discussed below.

REHABILITATION PRINCIPLES FOR SPINAL CORD INJURY

The goal of SCI rehabilitation is to maximize the child's functional mobility to perform activities of daily living. ROM exercises started in the acute setting are continued to prevent contractures. Strengthening exercises are performed for muscles involved in functional activities such as the shoulder and core stabilizers.[34] Activities of daily living often need to be relearned.

The level and completeness of SCIs, which are determined using the International Standards for Neurological Classification of Spinal Cord Injury grading scale,[53] are prognostic for neurologic recovery and functional independence.[54] Wheeled and upright mobility recommendations are also based on level of injury (Table 22.3). Proper wheelchair seating is essential for pressure sore prevention.[55] The reciprocal gait orthosis can be used for upper thoracic lesions that preserve hip flexion.[34] Community ambulation is feasible for lesions at L3 and below. Gait aids include walkers, crutches, and canes. Reverse walkers may be preferred in children as they facilitate an erect posture.[34] Lofstrand crutches have the functional advantage of permitting grasping of objects but do have less trunk support than axillary crutches.[34]

Recently, the efficacy of locomotor training has been evaluated in adolescent patients. The goal of locomotor training is to retrain walking after SCI by using preinjury movement patterns to activate the neuromuscular system below the level of injury. Behrman et al[56] evaluated locomotor training using repetitive stepping in three adolescents; age 15 T5

Table 22.3   Wheeled and Upright Mobility Recommendations

Neurological level (AIS A & B)	Wheelchair Type	Standing	Ambulation
C1–C4	Power WC base	Tilt table or standing frame	Not indicated
C5–C6	Power WC base or adjustable manual WC frame with power assist wheels	Tilt table or standing frame	Not indicated
C7–C8	Adjustable manual WC frame +/- power assist wheels	Tilt table or standing frame	Not indicated
T1–T9	Adjustable manual WC frame	Standing frame	RGOs or HKAFOs and assist device
T10–L1	Adjustable manual WC frame	Standing frame	RGOs, HKAFOs, or KAFOs and assist device
L2–S5	Adjustable manual WC frame	Standing frame	KAFOs or AFOs and often assist device

AFOs, Ankle-foot orthoses; *AIS,* American Spinal Injury Association Impairment Scale; *HKAFOs,* hip-knee-ankle-foot orthoses; *KAFOs,* knee-ankle-foot orthoses; *RGOs,* reciprocating gait orthoses; *WC,* wheelchair.
(Modified from Calhoun CL, Schottler J, Vogel LC. Recommendations for mobility in children with spinal cord injury. *Top Spinal Cord Inj Rehabil.* 2013;19(2):142-151.)

AIS D (primary wheelchair user), age 14 T5 AIS C (primary wheelchair user), and age 14 C2, AIS D (primary ambulatory). Locomotor training was performed four to five times weekly for 75, 293, and 40 total sessions. Two patients progressed from using a wheelchair for community mobility to walking 90% of the time. The primary ambulator improved their locomotor skills, kinematics, and endurance. The authors concluded that locomotor therapy can be effectively used in adolescents.

Although working to improve mobility and prevent contractures, rehabilitation also seeks to optimize function of the respiratory, urinary, and gastrointestinal systems. Thus, in addition to the traditional rehabilitation team, patients with SCIs often require members from respiratory therapy, SCI specialty nursing, pediatric medicine, and urology.[34] Measures are instituted to prevent deep venous thrombosis and skin breakdown as described above. Children with lesions at the thoracic and cervical levels need aggressive pulmonary management ranging from assisted ventilation (invasive and noninvasive) to instruction in quad cough techniques.

Urinary continence is desirable for both independence and quality of life. A clean, intermittent catheterization program is initiated to achieve this and also helps to prevent urinary infections, renal stones, and autonomic dysfunction.[57,58] The catheterization program also helps to keep volumes at or below the maximal bladder volume for age. Anticholinergics may be prescribed to prevent elevated bladder pressure, frequent urination, and hydronephrosis, whereas alpha-blocker medications can be prescribed for bladder-sphincter dyssynergy.[59]

Age-appropriate bowel continence without stool impaction is also desirable for independence and quality of life.[60] Bowel programs often include timing, digital stimulation, dietary recommendations, and medications. Timed programs can be initiated as early as age 3.[61] Medications to facilitate emptying and prevent impaction include stool softeners, laxatives, and suppositories.

TRAUMATIC BRAIN INJURY

TBI is the result of an external force such as direct blow, penetration, or rapid acceleration or deceleration.[62] TBI is classified into three types based on the Glasgow Coma Scale (GCS) score after resuscitation: mild (13–15), moderate (9–12), and severe (≤8).[63,64] The pathophysiology of TBI includes two lesions. The irreversible primary injury occurs at impact and is due to tearing of axons, hematoma, edema, and ischemia.[65] Secondary insults are due to the release of neurotransmitters and free radicals with subsequent ischemia and inflammation.[65,66] Initial management includes standard trauma assessment with neuroimaging to identify the primary insult.[67,68] The head of the bed is elevated 30 degrees, and a cervical collar is worn to allow venous drainage and prevent increases in intracranial pressure.[64] Additional methods to control intracranial pressure include adequate sedation, hyperventilation, osmotic agents, drainage of cerebrospinal fluid, and placement of an external ventricular drain.[64] Anticonvulsants are provided due to the high rate of posttraumatic seizures.[69] Nutrition is optimized, and a tracheostomy may be required in the setting of severe TBI.[70]

Due to the high rate of clinically silent fractures, patients with TBIs have screening radiographs of the cervical, thoracic, and lumbar spine, as well as the pelvis and possibly the knees.[71] Fracture treatment should assume that the patient will regain full mobility. The early mobilization afforded by internal fixation is preferred when possible.[71] If delayed internal fixation of long bone fractures is planned, traction should be considered to avoid excess shortening. If closed treatment is chosen, it is important to allow monitoring of the skin, as the patient may not be able to communicate or feel pain from excessive skin pressure. A high index of suspicion is maintained for peripheral nerve injuries as well. Electrodiagnostic studies may be helpful when the clinical recovery of motor function is not typical of the associated central nervous system injury.[71]

COMPLICATIONS OF TRAUMATIC BRAIN INJURY

TBI is a major cause of acquired disability in children.[72] Complications include problems with cognition, behavior, balance, sleep, headaches, hearing, vision, speech, and swallowing.[73,74] Patients are also at risk for seizures, hydrocephalus, and sensory disturbances. Outside the neurologic system, complications include pulmonary symptoms, autonomic instability, feeding intolerance, and endocrine disorders.[75–77] Endocrine disturbances such as growth hormone deficiency may also impact cognition.[78]

Many complications from TBI are similar to SCI including VTE, heterotopic ossification, pressure sores, and hypercalcemia.[72,75] Children with lower GCS scores (usually <8) are associated with an increased risk of VTE (Table 22.4).[79,80] Mechanical prophylaxis and ambulation are encouraged. Pharmacologic prophylaxis for patients with TBI is typically not required except in patients 14 to 21 years of age with impaired mobility and other risk factors for VTE, although formal guidelines have not been developed.[75,81] Heterotopic ossification occurs in approximately 11% of patients with TBIs and is most commonly found in the hips and knees.[47,82] Evidence to support the benefit of prophylactic antiinflammatory agents or radiation therapy in children is lacking.[83] Prevention of pressure sores in TBI is similar to patients with SCI.[84]

Children who have sustained moderate or severe TBI are at high risk for motor disturbances.[76] Motor system damage can have both negative and positive effects. Negative effects include weakness, loss of sensation, and the loss of muscle tone and reflexes often seen immediately after an upper motor neuron injury. As recovery proceeds, positive effects often become more prominent with hyperreflexia, increased resting muscle tone, abnormal patterns of muscle tone (dystonia), or a velocity-dependent increase in tone with passive stretching (spasticity).[85] Spasticity is seen in 17% to 50% of patients with TBI and is discussed at the end of this chapter.[86,87]

PRINCIPLES OF REHABILITATION FOR TRAUMATIC BRAIN INJURY

Evaluations from physical, occupational, and speech therapy are necessary during the acute hospitalization to determine rehabilitation needs and facilitate planning.[88] The goals of inpatient rehabilitation for TBI are to improve motor skills, learn how to perform activities of daily living, maximize recovery of the brain, and facilitate integration into the community.[75] Therapy plans include measures to address posttraumatic seizures, tone or movement disorders, and altered sleep patterns. Pain management is essential to address the nociceptive and neuropathic pain that occur in TBI. Nociceptive pain is due to stimulation of peripheral nociceptors and is treated with medications such as acetaminophen, nonsteroidal antiinflammatory agents, or opioids.[75] Neurogenic pain is due to somatosensory system damage and is treated with medications such as gabapentin, similar to patients with SCI.[75] Inpatient rehabilitation after TBI leads to improvements in cognitive function, functional independence, and long-term outcomes.[13,89–91] Thus, outcomes can be hindered by the failure to recognize the need for further care in the acute setting or the lack of available rehabilitation centers.[92]

The neurocognitive and neurobehavioral sequelae of TBI can be disabling and require extensive therapy beyond discharge from inpatient rehabilitation.[90] These disturbances are more extensive in patients with severe and moderate TBI. Problems with memory and executive function can impact school and social performance.[75,93,94] In addition, 40% of children with severe TBI and 20% with moderate TBI will develop behavior problems.[95] Approximately 60% of children will develop psychiatric disorders such as attention-deficit hyperactivity disorder (ADHD) and oppositional defiant disorder.[96,97] Methylphenidate can be prescribed for ADHD, whereas cognitive rehabilitation therapy is more helpful for problems with memory and attention.[98] Technology-assisted interventions such as applications and online problem-solving therapy may facilitate improvements in behavior, executive, and family function.[94]

Table 22.4 Risk factors for Venous Thromboembolism

Acute Conditions	Chronic Medical Conditions	Historical Factors
Major lower extremity orthopedic surgery	Obesity	Previous history of VTE
Spinal cord injury	Weight >80 kg in age 14–16 years	Family history of VTE in first-degree relative younger than 40 years
Major trauma to the lower extremities	Weight >85 kg in those older than 16 years	
Lower extremity central venous catheter	Estrogen-containing medications	
Acute infection	Inflammatory bowel disease	
Burns	Nephrotic syndrome	
Pregnancy	Known acquired or inherited thrombophilia	

VTE, Venous thromboembolism.

(From Raffini L, Trimarchi T, Beliveau J, Davis D. Thromboprophylaxis in a pediatric hospital: a patient-safety and quality-improvement initiative. *Pediatrics* 2011;127(5):e1326-e1332, Fig. 22.2.)

SPASTICITY MANAGEMENT

Management of spasticity is rapidly evolving. However, most studies on spasticity management in children involve individuals with cerebral palsy, and it is not clear how directly this translates to the management of spasticity due to TBI or SCI. No guidelines exist on when to proceed with different interventions, and conflicting opinions are common. However, some basic principles can help make treatment decisions.

The first step is to establish the pattern of spasticity via serial clinical evaluations, as spasticity may be difficult to differentiate from dystonia, volitional guarding, and contractures. Mixed patterns may be present as well.[75] Ideally, a relaxed patient should be evaluated in a variety of different positions and different situations. Spasticity should be classified as localized or generalized, and the severity should be graded using scales such as the Modified Ashworth Scale (Table 22.5).[99]

The next step is to understand the possible functional implications of spasticity for a patient. Spasticity is not always harmful. Mild spasticity may help preserve muscle bulk, and extensor tone in the legs may assist with weight-bearing, standing, or transfers. However, severe or dysfunctional tone leads to problems such as joint contractures, pain, difficulty tolerating casting, and skin breakdown. It can also interfere with individual care and functional use of affected limbs.[100] Severe spasticity may also complicate fracture healing (Fig. 22.2).

Spasticity management requires a multidisciplinary approach involving the patient, family or other caregivers, therapists, and medical specialists. Family and patient input is particularly important for both establishing functional goals and managing expectations. It is important to convey that whereas the spasticity may be decreased through treatment, often the loss of strength and sensation in an affected limb is too severe to allow substantial functional improvement. The patient may only achieve more modest goals of improved ROM or ease of care by family members. Treatment options for spasticity are physical interventions, oral medications, injections, and surgery.

PHYSICAL INTERVENTIONS FOR SPASTICITY

Physical interventions for spasticity include ROM exercises, splinting, and casting. Maintaining muscle ROM not only decreases contractures but may also decrease the severity of spasticity because a longer muscle tendon unit and increased static stretch response are maintained.[85] A ROM program requires initial supervision and instruction from a therapist to ensure that the targeted muscle is receiving an effective stretch. Static splints are commonly used, particularly at night, to maintain ROM. Daytime use is limited because the splints may interfere with function. Dynamic splints may allow more functional use of the limb.[85]

Serial casting can be used to maintain or increase the length of a muscle. These casts are typically changed every 5 to 7 days until no further effect occurs or the desired ROM is achieved. Serial casting has the advantages of good patient compliance and a sustained stretch. The risk of serial casting includes atrophy of muscles, skin breakdown, edema, circulatory impairment, and injury from falls while the cast is worn. The impact of injecting botulinum toxin before initiating serial casting is unclear.

ORAL MEDICATIONS FOR SPASTICITY

There are multiple medication options for spasticity, although many of these have not been specifically studied in children (Table 22.6). Medication selection should consider potential side effects and the patient's general medical condition. For patients with SCI, oral baclofen is often the first-line agent.[34] Recommendations regarding oral baclofen for TBI are controversial.[76] Alternatives for TBI include diazepam, tizanidine, dantrolene, and clonidine.[75] Dosages are increased as needed while monitoring for side effects that often limit the effectiveness of these medications.

Table 22.5 Modified Ashworth Scale

0: No increase in muscle tone

1: Slight increase in muscle tone, manifested by catch and release or by minimal resistance at the end of the range of motion in which the affected part is moved in flexion or extension

2: Slight increase in muscle tone, manifested by a catch, followed by minimal resistance throughout the remainder (less than half) of range of motion

3: More marked increase in muscle tone through most of the range of motion, but affected parts are easily moved

4: Considerable increase in muscle tone; passive movement is difficult

5: Affected parts are rigid in flexion or extension

Fig. 22.2 (A) Postoperative anteroposterior (AP) radiograph illustrating elastic stable intramedullary nail fixation of a femur shaft fracture of 9-year-old boy struck by a truck while on a scooter. (B) AP pelvis radiograph illustrating pelvic and sacroiliac fixation. (C) Lateral radiograph of the femur illustrating fracture angulation secondary to spasticity/head injury.

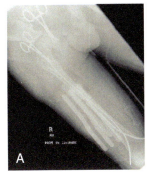
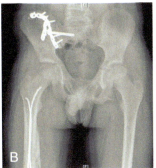
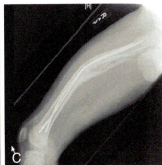

Table 22.6 Oral Medications for Treating Spasticity

Medication	Pediatric dose	Mechanism	US FDA Approval	Adverse Effects	Comments
Baclofen	Age 2–7 years, start 2.5–5 mg by mouth tid. Increase 5–15 mg/day as needed every 3 days to a maximum of 40 mg/day divided tid–qid. Age 8–11 years, maximum of 60 mg/day divided tid–qid. Age 12 years to adult, start 5 mg by mouth tid. Increase by 15 mg/day as needed every 3 days to a maximum of 80 mg/day divided tid–qid.	Centrally acting muscle relaxant. Thought to be a GABA agonist. Exact mechanism of action unknown.	Older than 12 years only.	Sedation, respiratory depression, seizures, withdrawal symptoms (particularly with abrupt withdrawal), muscle weakness, constipation, variety of central nervous system side effects. Other rare but serious side effects.	Caution against abrupt withdrawal. Increase dose slowly to ensure use of lowest effective dose and allow time for adjustment to sedation. Monitor creatinine level at baseline and EEG if epilepsy.
Tizanidine	Pediatric dosing not well established. In adults, start 4 mg by mouth once a day. Increase by 2–3 mg/day to a maximum of 12 mg tid and a daily maximum of 36 mg.	Centrally acting muscle relaxant. Thought to be a GABA agonist. Exact mechanism of action unknown.	No	Hepatotoxicity, bradycardia, hypotension, sedation, variety of central nervous system and cardiovascular side effects. Other rare but serious side effects.	Begin low dose and increase slowly. Taper slowly if discontinuing. Watch for drug interactions. Monitor liver function test, blood pressure, and creatinine level.
Dantrolene	Age 5 years and older, begin 0.5 mg/kg/day by mouth once a day. Increase by up to 1 mg/kg/day every 7 days as needed to a maximum of the lesser of 12 mg/kg/day divided 2–3 times a day or 400 mg a day.	Direct muscle relaxant. Inhibits calcium release at the sarcoplasmic reticulum. Affects all skeletal muscle. However, because spastic muscles fire more frequently, may have greater effect on spastic muscles.	Older than 5 years only.	Hepatotoxicity; GI side effects, including diarrhea. Other rare but serious side effects.	Hepatotoxicity may not be reversible. Check liver function tests at baseline and periodically thereafter. Typically, liver function tests are monitored every 3–6 months. May have a synergistic effect with baclofen.
Diazepam	Age 6 months to 12 years, 0.12–0.8 mg/kg/day divided every 6–8 hr. Maximum, lesser of 0.6 mg/kg/per 8 hour or 10 mg/day.	Centrally acting. Binds to benzodiazepine receptors and enhances GABA effects.	Older than 6 months.	Respiratory distress, cardiovascular depression, sedation. Other rare but serious side effects.	Monitor complete blood count and liver function tests if prolonged treatment. Although benzodiazepines have a long history of use in children, cognitive side effects generally limit use. Wean slowly to decrease risk of withdrawal symptoms. Long half-life so sedating effects may persist for days after discontinuation.

bid, Twice a day; *EEG*, electroencephalogram; *FDA*, US Food and Drug Administration; *GABA*, gamma-aminobutyric acid; *GI*, gastrointestinal; *qid*, four times a day; *tid*, three times a day.

Please read package inserts for complete list of adverse effects.

INJECTIONS FOR SPASTICITY

In a patient with localized spasticity, it is often more helpful to use localized interventions such as injections to avoid these systemic side effects.[101,102] Injections can be precisely localized to spastic muscles and have effects that are at least partially reversible. Two different strategies exist for localized injections for spasticity. One is to target a peripheral nerve or its distal branches with near-nerve injections (using phenol) to weaken and decrease spasticity in all of the distally innervated muscles. The other approach is to block the neuromuscular junction in the target muscle with the use of botulinum toxin injections.

The use of phenol blocks has decreased since the introduction of botulinum toxin. Phenol blocks involve the injection of phenol at concentrations between 1% and 6% as close as possible to a peripheral nerve. A nerve stimulator is used for localization. Injections are painful, and children require some form of sedation to remain still and to tolerate the injections. Either the main trunk of the nerve or its terminal branches can be targeted. Commonly targeted nerves include the obturator, tibial, musculocutaneous, and median nerves.[102] More proximal targeting of the nerve has the advantage of greater efficacy but the disadvantage of causing undesired damage to associated sensory portions of the nerve, which may lead to persistent paresthesias. Great care should be taken to inject only small amounts as close as possible to the targeted nerve to avoid injury to adjacent muscles or nontargeted nerves. In addition, phenol should never be injected in the vicinity of the spinal cord because spinal cord infarction could occur. Phenol blocks last from 1 to 12 months, depending on the amount of phenol used and the concentration. Repeated injections or higher concentrations may lead to more permanent damage to the nerve.[103,104] Possible side effects include nerve pain and paresthetic pain, infection at the injection site, and deep venous thrombosis. Overdose or inadvertent direct vascular injection may lead to convulsions, central nervous system depression, and cardiovascular collapse.

Botulinum toxin is a naturally occurring toxin produced by *Clostridium botulinum* bacteria. It temporarily blocks the presynaptic release of acetylcholine at the neuromuscular junction. Of the many types of botulinum toxins, only botulinum toxin types A and B are used medically. Botulinum toxin type A is available in the United States from different manufacturers as onabotulinum toxin, abobotulinum toxin, or incobotulinum toxin, and botulinum toxin type B as rimabotulinum toxin.[105] Onabotulinum toxin A injection (Botox; Allergan Inc., Irvine, CA) has been approved by the US Food and Drug Administration (FDA) for upper limb spasticity in adults, although it is commonly also used in children.[106] Abobotulinum toxin (Dysport, Ipsen Biopharmaceuticals, Basking Ridge, NJ) has been FDA approved for lower limb spasticity in children 2 years and older.[107]

Botulinum toxin can only be delivered via direct injection into the targeted muscle. It should be mixed according to the manufacturer's directions. Generally, the lowest effective dose should be used so that the risk of side effects and decreasing patient responsiveness over time are minimized. However, using larger doses may allow more muscle groups to be targeted for better disruption of pathologic tone patterns.[108] Topical analgesia such as cooling spray or topical lidocaine may be helpful in decreasing the pain of the needle entering the skin. This usually provides adequate analgesia for adults or cooperative older children. However, the injection of medication is still painful. Children are often afraid of injections and may become more fearful after serial injections. Children also have difficulty sitting still for adequate localization. Therefore, oral or intravenous sedation is often essential for proper localization and relief of anxiety. Sedation does expose children to additional risks; thus, children should be carefully monitored according to sedation protocols.[105]

Techniques for injecting botulinum toxin vary. They include anatomic location alone, electromyography (EMG) guidance with or without patient activation of muscles, electric stimulation, ultrasonography, and radiologic (computed tomography or fluoroscopic) guidance.[109] The forearm pronator and flexor muscles are more difficult to localize, particularly in a contracted arm, so EMG localization, particularly with patient activation of muscles or ultrasound, is useful.[110] In the forearm, ulnar wrist flexor and pronator groups are in close proximity, so diffusion of botulinum may help with targeting motor groups. EMG localization is limited by the fact that children with brain injuries and SCIs are often too scared or neurologically impaired to volitionally activate a muscle. Passively stretching the muscle may activate a spastic response and help with EMG localization. Electric stimulation or ultrasound may help with localization, and neither require the active participation of the child. Deep muscles such as the psoas can be difficult and dangerous to inject without direct visualization via computed tomography, ultrasound, or fluoroscopy.[110]

Tone patterns vary, so planning of botulinum toxin injection should be individualized. However, some common patterns are followed in treating spasticity in children. In the upper extremity, flexion and adduction of the shoulder, flexion of the elbow, pronation of the forearm, and flexion of the wrist and hand predominate. Frequently injected muscles in the shoulder include the pectoralis major, latissimus dorsi, teres major, and subscapularis. For the elbow, injecting the biceps, brachioradialis, and brachialis may be helpful. Flexor and pronator muscles most frequently targeted in the forearm include the pronator quadratus, pronator teres, flexor carpi radialis, flexor carpi ulnaris, flexor pollicis longus and brevis, adductor pollicis, and flexor digitorum superficialis and profundus.[111] In the lower extremity, frequently targeted flexor muscles of the hip and knee include the iliacus, psoas, rectus femoris, and the medial or lateral hamstrings. For knee extensor tone, the quadriceps group, particularly the rectus femoris, is targeted. The triceps surae are involved in toe walking and excessive plantar flexor tone at the ankle. For varus tone, the tibialis posterior is targeted, whereas for a valgus foot, injection of the peroneus longus and brevis may be helpful.[111]

Botulinum takes effect in 2 to 3 days and generally lasts 3 months, although in some individuals, it may last up to 6 months. Botulinum toxin injections may be a one-time event to help achieve a specific goal or given every 3 months or longer for spasticity management. Serial use of botulinum toxin can lead to resistance caused by the formation of antibotulinum antibodies or muscle atrophy.[112] Using lower doses and less frequent administration can lower the risk of resistance. However, botulinum toxin resistance may be misdiagnosed. Lack of responsiveness can often be better explained by underdosing a muscle, poor localization, or increasing spasticity. Repeating trials of botulinum toxin with larger doses and more precise localization is often a helpful first step in the face of diminished responsiveness.[111]

Botulinum toxin is generally well tolerated in children.[113] However, of particular concern is the risk of systemic reaction to botulinum toxin, including respiratory compromise and even death. Children treated for limb spasticity appear to be particularly at risk. The FDA recommends that patients and families be alerted to the risk of systemic side effects, including respiratory and swallowing problems, after botulinum toxin injection. Any suspected systemic reaction should receive prompt medical attention.[106] The FDA website and package inserts should be consulted for further details of side effects and monitoring.[106,107]

SURGERY FOR SPASTICITY

If spasticity fails to resolve or improve after an acute central nervous system injury, surgery may be required to restore ROM or improve muscle imbalance. Muscle and tendon lengthening is an option but may further weaken a muscle already weak from neurologic injury. Implantation of a baclofen pump is an option for diffuse and severe spasticity that fails to respond to oral medications and is not expected to resolve otherwise.[34,76,114]

The baclofen pump delivers baclofen medication intrathecally. This method allows delivery of a much higher effective dose of baclofen to the spinal cord with fewer sedating side effects than oral baclofen. A trial of intrathecal baclofen should be performed before definitive pump placement. A positive result occurs when the Modified Ashworth Score decreases by 2 or more.[34] Pump placement is not advised if a positive response has not been achieved with three trials.[34] Catheter dysfunction may occur after baclofen pump insertion, resulting in symptoms of withdrawal such as increased spasticity, agitation, itching, and seizures.[34] Baclofen withdrawal can also cause end organ damage and therefore be life-threatening if not managed emergently.[34] Deep implant infection may also occur.

Pearls and Pitfalls

- The more joints controlled by orthosis, the greater chance it will interfere with function.
- Providers should be vigilant for autonomic dysreflexia in patients with spinal cord injuries.
- Gabapentin for neuropathic pain should be tapered to decrease the risk of seizures.
- Injections may be more helpful for localized spasticity to avoid the risk of systemic side effects from medications.

Outcomes

- The rehabilitation goal for children with polytrauma is to maximize function and return them to their home and community as soon as possible.
- Inpatient rehabilitation leads to improvements in quality of life and function for the majority of patients.
- Inpatient rehabilitation after TBI leads to improvements in cognitive function and functional independence.

PSYCHOSOCIAL FACTORS

Psychologic rehabilitation of an injured child is as important as the physical rehabilitation.[40,115] After the initial traumatic event, the patient is faced with continued pain from the injury or necessary treatments, disfigurement and loss of body image, and prolonged separation from family and friends. Up to 60% of children with severe multiple-system traumatic injuries have personality changes 1 year after hospital discharge, and up to 50% have social, affective, and learning disabilities.[116] Twenty-five percent of children will demonstrate signs of posttraumatic stress disorder after a road accident.[117]

This psychologic trauma is not limited to the child but also affects the family, who may feel responsible for the injury. Two-thirds of uninjured siblings show psychologic disturbances, and parents may have marital problems traceable to the event. Family stress is worse in families with difficulties functioning before the injury.[40] For these reasons, social work and psychology should play an active role in providing family guidance and reassurance. Finally, the economic stress on the family can be significant, and all patients with SCIs, TBIs, or long-term limitations should begin the process of assessment for long-term disability shortly after injury.

REFERENCES

The level of evidence (LOE) is determined according to the criteria provided in the Preface.

1. Centers for Disease Control and Prevention. Injury prevention and control. Data and statistics (WISQARS). Available at http://www.cdc.gov/injury/wisqars/leadingcauses.html. Accessed April, 2018 **(LOE IV)**.
2. Letts M, Davidson D, Lapner P. Multiple trauma in children: predicting outcome and long-term results. *Can J Surg.* 2002;45:126–131 **(LOE IV)**.
3. Myers SR, Branas CC, French B, et al. A national analysis of pediatric trauma care utilization and outcomes in the United States. *Pediatr Emerg Care.* 2016. https://doi.org/10.1097/PEC.0000000000000902 **(LOE IV)**.
4. Valadka S, Poenaru D, Dueck A. Long-term disability after trauma in children. *J Pediatr Surg.* 2000;35:684–687 **(LOE IV)**.
5. Jaffe KM. Pediatric trauma rehabilitation: a value-added safety net. *J Trauma.* 2008;64:819–823 **(LOE V)**.
6. McKesson Health Solutions LLC. Rehabilitation adult and pediatric. *InterQual Level of Care Criteria.* 2010:71–84 **(LOE V)**.
7. Nguyen HT, Newton C, Pirrotta EA, et al. Variations in utilization of inpatient rehabilitation services among pediatric trauma patients. *J Pediatr.* 2017;182:342–348 **(LOE IV)**.
8. Kim CT, Greenberg J, Kim H. Pediatric rehabilitation: trends in length of stay. *J Pediatr Rehabil Med.* 2013;6:11–17 **(LOE IV)**.
9. Dumas HM, Haley SM, Ludlow LH, Rabin JP. Functional recovery in pediatric traumatic brain injury during inpatient rehabilitation. *Am J Phys Med Rehabil.* 2002;81:661–669 **(LOE IV)**.
10. Kramer ME, Suskauer SJ, Christensen JR, et al. Examining acute rehabilitation outcomes for children with total functional dependence after traumatic brain injury: a pilot study. *J Head Trauma Rehabil.* 2013;28:361–370 **(LOE IV)**.
11. Rice SA, Blackman JA, Braun S, et al. Rehabilitation of children with traumatic brain injury: descriptive analysis of a nationwide sample using the WeeFIM. *Arch Phys Med Rehabil.* 2005;86:834–836 **(LOE IV)**.
12. Allen DD, Mulcahey MJ, Haley SM, et al. Motor scores on the functional independence measure after pediatric spinal cord injury. *Spinal Cord.* 2009;47:213–217 **(LOE IV)**.
13. Zonfrillo MR, Durbin DR, Winston FK, et al. Physical disability after injury-related inpatient rehabilitation in children. *Pediatrics.* 2013;131:e206–e213 **(LOE IV)**.

14. Biffl SE, Biffl WL. Improving transitions of care for complex pediatric trauma patients from inpatient rehabilitation to home: an observational pilot study. *Patient Saf Surg.* 2015;9:33 (**LOE III**).

15. Kirk S, Fallon D, Fraser C, et al. Supporting parents following childhood traumatic brain injury: a qualitative study to examine information and emotional support needs across key care transitions. *Child Care Health Dev.* 2015;41:303–313 (**LOE III**).

16. Paterno MV. Unique issues in the rehabilitation of the pediatric and adolescent athlete after musculoskeletal injury. *Sports Med Arthrosc Rev.* 2016;24:178–183 (**LOE V**).

17. Keppler P, Salem K, Schwarting B, Kinzl L. The effectiveness of physiotherapy after operative treatment of supracondylar humeral fractures in children. *J Pediatr Orthop.* 2005;25:314–316 (**LOE I**).

18. Schmale GA, Mazor S, Mercer LD, Bompadre V. Lack of benefit of physical therapy on function following supracondylar humeral fracture: a randomized controlled trial. *J Bone Joint Surg Am.* 2014;96:944–950 (**LOE I**).

19. American Academy of Orthopaedic Surgeons. Committee for the Study of Joint Motion: method of measuring and recording joint motion. American Academy of Orthopaedic Surgeons: Chicago. (**LOE V**).

20. Hoppenfeld S, Murthy VL, ed. *Treatment And Rehabilitation of Fractures.* Philadelphia: Lippincott, Williams & Wilkins. (**LOE V**).

21. Thomas MA. Treatment and rehabilitation of fractures: assistive devices and adaptive equipment for activities of daily living (ADL). Philadelphia: Lippincott, Williams & Wilkins. (**LOE V**).

22. Thomas MA. Assistive devices and adaptive equipment for activities of daily living. In: Hoppenfeld S, Murthy VI, eds. *Treatment and Rehabilitation of Fractures.* Philadelphia: Lippincott, Williams & Wilkins. (**LOE V**).

23. Leach J. Physical therapy in children. Philadelphia: W.B. Saunders. (**LOE V**).

24. Joseph MH, Brill J, Zeltzer LK. Pediatric pain relief in trauma. *Pediatr Rev.* 1999;20:75–84 (**LOE V**).

25. Poonai N, Kilgar J, Mehrotra S. Analgesia for fracture pain in children: methodological issues surrounding clinical trials and effectiveness of therapy. *Pain Manag.* 2015;5:435–445 (**LOE V**).

26. Steward S, O'Connor J. Pediatric pain, trauma, and memory. *Curr Opin Pediatr.* 1994;6:411–417 (**LOE IV**).

27. Clark E, Plint AC, Correll R, et al. A randomized, controlled trial of acetaminophen, ibuprofen, and codeine for acute pain relief in children with musculoskeletal trauma. *Pediatrics.* 2007;119:460–467 (**LOE I**).

28. Friday JH, Kanegaye JT, McCaslin I, et al. Ibuprofen provides analgesia equivalent to acetaminophen–codeine in the treatment of acute pain in children with extremity injuries: a randomized clinical trial. *Acad Emerg Med.* 2009;16:711–716 (**LOE I**).

29. Koller DM, Myers AB, Lorenz D, Godambe SA. Effectiveness of oxycodone, ibuprofen, or the combination in the initial management of orthopedic injury-related pain in children. *Pediatr Emerg Care.* 2007;23:627–633 (**LOE I**).

30. Le May S, Gouin S, Fortin C, et al. Efficacy of an ibuprofen/codeine combination for pain management in children presenting to the emergency department with a limb injury: a pilot study. *J Emerg Med.* 2013;44:536–542 (**LOE I**).

31. Poonai N, Datoo N, Ali S, et al. Oral morphine versus ibuprofen administered at home for postoperative orthopedic pain in children: a randomized controlled trial. *CMAJ.* 2017;189:e1252–1258 (**LOE I**).

32. Loder RT, Warschausky S, Schwartz EM, et al. The psychosocial characteristics of children with fractures. *J Pediatr Orthop.* 1995;13:41–46 (**LOE IV**).

33. American Pediatric Surgical Association. *National Pediatric Trauma Registry.* Boston: Department of Rehabilitative Medicine, Tufts New England Medical Center; 2001 (**LOE IV**).

34. Greenberg JS, Ruutiainen AT, Kim H. Rehabilitation of pediatric spinal cord injury: From acute medical care to rehabilitation and beyond. *J Pediatr Rehabil Med.* 2009;2:13–27 (**LOE V**).

35. Jones T, Ugalde V, Franks P, et al. Venous thromboembolism after spinal cord injury: incidence, time course, and associated risk factors in 16,240 adults and children. *Arch Phys Med Rehabil.* 2005;86:2240–2247 (**LOE IV**).

36. Price V, Chan A. Venous thrombosis in children. *Expert Rev Cardiovasc Ther.* 2008;6:411–418 (**LOE IV**).

37. Maynard FM. Immobilization hypercalcemia following spinal cord injury. *Arch Phys Med Rehabil.* 1986;67:41–44 (**LOE V**).

38. Lteif AN, Zimmerman D. Bisphosphonates for treatment of childhood hypercalcemia. *Pediatrics.* 1998;102:990–993 (**LOE IV**).

39. Vogel LC. The child with a spinal cord injury. *Spasticity: Diagnostic Workup and Medical Management.* Rosemont, IL: American Academy of Orthopaedic Surgeons; 1996 (**LOE V**).

40. Stancin T, Taylor HG, Thompson GH, et al. Acute psychosocial impact of pediatric orthopedic trauma with and without accompanying brain injuries. *J Trauma.* 1998;45:1031–1038 (**LOE III**).

41. Garland DE, Stewart CA, Adkins RH, et al. Osteoporosis after spinal cord injury. *J Orthop Res.* 1992;10:371–378 (**LOE IV**).

42. Sabo D, Blaich S, Wenz W, et al. Osteoporosis in patients with paralysis after spinal cord injury: a cross sectional study in 46 male patients with dual-energy X-ray absorptiometry. *Arch Orthop Trauma Surg.* 2001;121:75–78 (**LOE IV**).

43. Cochran TP, Bayley JC, Smith M. Lower extremity fractures in paraplegics: pattern, treatment and functional results. *J Spinal Disord.* 1988;1:219–223 (**LOE IV**).

44. Ragnarsson KT, Sell GH. Lower extremity fractures after spinal cord injury: a retrospective study. *Arch Phys Med Rehabil.* 1981;62:418–423 (**LOE IV**).

45. de Bruin ED, Frey-Rindova P, Herzog RE. Changes of tibia bone properties after spinal cord injury: effects of early intervention. *Arch Phys Med Rehabil.* 1999;80:214–220 (**LOE IV**).

46. Stein RB. Functional electrical stimulation after spinal cord injury. *J Neurotrauma.* 1999;16:713–717 (**LOE IV**).

47. Citta-Pietrolungo TJ, Alexander MA, Steg NL. Early detection of heterotopic ossification in young patients with traumatic brain injury. *Arch Phys Med Rehabil.* 1992;73:258–262 (**LOE IV**).

48. Hurvitz EA, Mandac BR, Davidoff G, et al. Risk factors for heterotopic ossification in children and adolescents with severe traumatic brain injury. *Arch Phys Med Rehabil.* 1992;73:450–461 (**LOE IV**).

49. Daud O, Sett P, Burr RG. The relationship of heterotopic ossification to passive movements in paraplegic patients. *Disabil Rehabil.* 1993;15:114–118 (**LOE IV**).

50. Kosiak M. Prevention and rehabilitation of pressure ulcers. *Decubitus.* 1991;4:60–62 (**LOE IV**).

51. Levine SM, Sinno S, Levine JP, Saadeh PB. Current thoughts for the prevention and treatment of pressure ulcers: using the evidence to determine fact or fiction. *Ann Surg.* 2013;257:603–608 (**LOE V**).

52. Vogel LC, Betz RR, Mulcahey MJ. Spinal cord injuries in children and adolescents. *Handb Clin Neurol.* 2012;109:131–148 (**LOE V**).

53. Kirshblum SC, Burns SP, Biering-Sorensen F, et al. International standards for neurological classification of spinal cord injury. *J Spinal Cord Med.* 2011;34:535–546 (**LOE V**).

54. Mange KC, Ditunno JF, Herbison GJ, Jaweed MM. Recovery of strength in the zone of injury in motor complete and motor incomplete cervical spinal cord injured patients. *Arch Phys Med Rehab.* 1990;71:562–565 (**LOE IV**).

55. Burns SP, Betz KL. Seating pressures with conventional and dynamic wheelchair cushions in tetraplegia. *Arch Phys Med Rehabil.* 1999;80:566–571 (**LOE IV**).

56. Behrman AL, Watson E, Fried G. Restorative rehabilitation entails a paradigm shift in pediatric incomplete spinal cord injury in adolescence: an illustrative case series. *J Pediatr Rehabil Med.* 2012;5:245–259 (**LOE V**).

57. Generao SE, Dall'era JP, Stone AR, Kurzrock EA. Spinal cord injury in children: long term urodynamic and urologic outcome. *J Urol.* 2004;172:1092–1094 (**LOE IV**).

58. Francis K. Physiology and management of bladder and bowel continence following spinal cord injury. *Ostomy Wound Manage.* 2007;53:18–27 (**LOE V**).

59. Pandya NK, Upasani VV, Kulkarni VA. The pediatric polytrauma patient: current concepts. *J Am Acad Orthop Surg.* 2013;21:170–179 (**LOE V**).

60. Mitrofanoff P. Trans-appendicular continent cystostomy in the management of the neurogenic bladder. *Chir Pediatr.* 1980;21:297–305 (**LOE IV**).

61. Gleeson RM. Bowel continence for the child with a neurogenic bowel. *Rehabil Nurs.* 1990;15:319–321 (**LOE V**).

62. Menon DK, Schwab K, Wright DW, et al. Position statement: definition of traumatic brain injury. *Arch Phys Med Rehabil.* 2010;91:1637–1640 (**LOE V**).

63. Jaffe KM, Polissar NL, Fay GC, et al. Recovery trends over three years following pediatric traumatic brain injury. *Arch Phys Med Rehabil.* 1995;76:17–26 (**LOE IV**).

64. Mtaweh H, Bell MJ. Management of pediatric traumatic brain injury. *Curr Treat Options Neurol.* 2015;17:348 (**LOE V**).

65. Maas AI, Stocchetti N, Bullock R. Moderate and severe traumatic brain injury in adults. *Lancet Neurol.* 2008;7:728–741 **(LOE V)**.

66. Nestler EJ, Hyman SE, Malenka RC, eds. *Molecular Neuropharmacology: A Foundation for Clinical Neuroscience.* New York: McGraw-Hill; 2000 **(LOE V)**.

67. Adelson PD, Bratton SL, Carney NA, et al. Guidelines for the acute medical management of severe traumatic brain injury in infants, children, and adolescents. *Pediatr Crit Care Med.* 2012;13:252 **(LOE V)**.

68. Kochanek PM, Carney N, Adelson PD, et al. Guidelines for the acute medical management of severe traumatic brain injury in infants, children, and adolescents: second edition. *Pediatr Crit Care Med.* 2012;13:S1–S82 **(LOE V)**.

69. Arndt DH, Lerner JT, Matsumoto JH, et al. Subclinical early posttraumatic seizures detected by continuous EEG monitoring in a consecutive pediatric cohort. *Epilepsia.* 2013;54:1780–1788 **(LOE III)**.

70. Valadka A. Surgery of cerebral trauma and associated critical care. *Neurosurgery.* 2007;64:203–221 **(LOE V)**.

71. Kushwaha VP, Garland DG. Extremity fractures in the patient with a traumatic brain injury. *J Am Acad Orthop Surg.* 1998;6:298–307 **(LOE V)**.

72. McLean DE, Kaitz ES, Keenan CJ, et al. Medical and surgical complications of pediatric brain injury. *J Head Trauma Rehabil.* 1995;10:1–12 **(LOE V)**.

73. Frattalone AR, Ling GS. Moderate and severe traumatic brain injury: pathophysiology and management. *Neurosurg Clin N Am.* 2013;24:309–319 **(LOE V)**.

74. Webb TS, Whitehead CR, Wells TS, et al. Neurologically-related sequelae associated with mild traumatic brain injury. *Brain Inj.* 2015;29:430–437 **(LOE IV)**.

75. Cantore L, Norwood K, Patrick P. Medical aspects of pediatric rehabilitation after moderate to severe traumatic brain injury. *Neuro Rehabilitation.* 2012;30:225–234 **(LOE V)**.

76. Pérez-Arredondo A, Cázares-Ramírez E, Carrillo-Mora P, et al. Baclofen in the therapeutic scale of traumatic brain injury: Spasticity. *Clin Neuropharmacol.* 2016;39:311–319 **(LOE V)**.

77. Munjal SK. Audiological deficits after closed head injury. *J Trauma.* 2010;1:13–18 **(LOE IV)**.

78. Norwood K. Traumatic brain injury in children and adolescents: surveillance for pituitary dysfunction. *Clini Pediatr.* 2010;10:1044–1049 **(LOE IV)**.

79. Azu MC, McCormack JE, Scriven RJ, et al. Venous thromboembolic events in pediatric trauma patients: is prophylaxis necessary? *J Trauma.* 2005;59:1345–1349 **(LOE IV)**.

80. Cyr C, Michon B, Pettersen G, et al. Venous thromboembolism after severe injury in children. *Acta Haematol.* 2006;115:198–200 **(LOE IV)**.

81. Raffini L, Trimarchi T, Beliveau J, Davis D. Thromboprophylaxis in a pediatric hospital: a patient-safety and quality-improvement initiative. *Pediatrics.* 2011;127:e1326–1332 **(LOE III)**.

82. Cipriano CA. Heterotopic ossification following traumatic brain injury and spinal cord injury. *J Am Acad Orthop Surg.* 2009;17:689–697 **(LOE V)**.

83. Mavrogenis AF, Soucacos PN, Papagelopoulos PJ. Heterotopic ossification revisited. *Orthopedics.* 2011;34:177 **(LOE V)**.

84. Suddaby EC. Skin breakdown in acute care pediatrics. *Dermatol Nurs.* 2008;18:155–161 **(LOE V)**.

85. Meythaler JM, Kraft GH, eds. *Physical Medicine and Rehabilitation Clinics of North America: Spastic Hypertonia.* Philadelphia; W.B. Saunders. **(LOE V)**.

86. Aras MD, Kaya A, Cakc A, et al. Functional outcome following traumatic brain injury: the Turkish experience. *Int J Rehabil Res.* 2004;27:257–260 **(LOE IV)**.

87. Williams G, Banky M, Olver J. Distribution of lower limb spasticity does not influence mobility outcome following traumatic brain injury: an observational study. *J Head Trauma Rehabil.* 2015;30:e49–57 **(LOE III)**.

88. Bennett TD, Niedzwecki CM, Korgenski EK, Bratton SL. Initiation of physical, occupational, and speech therapy in children with traumatic brain injury. *Arch Phys Med Rehabil.* 2013;94:1268–1276 **(LOE IV)**.

89. Jimenez N, Osorio M, Ramos JL, et al. Functional independence after inpatient rehabilitation for traumatic brain injury among minority children and adolescents. *Arch Phys Med Rehabil.* 2015;96:1255–1261 **(LOE IV)**.

90. Zonfrillo MR, Durbin DR, Winston FK, et al. Residual cognitive disability after completion of inpatient rehabilitation among injured children. *J Pediatr.* 2014;64:130–135 **(LOE IV)**.

91. Tepas JJ, Leaphart CL, Pieper P, et al. The effect of delay in rehabilitation on outcome of severe traumatic brain injury. *J Pediatr Surg.* 2009;44:368–372 **(LOE IV)**.

92. Greene NH, Kernic MA, Vavilala MS, et al. Variation in pediatric traumatic brain injury outcomes in the United States. *Arch Phys Med Rehabil.* 2014;95:1148–1155 **(LOE IV)**.

93. Babikian T, Asarnow R. Neurocognitive outcomes and recovery after pediatric TBI: meta-analytic review of the literature. *Neuropsychology.* 2009;23:283–296 **(LOE IV)**.

94. Wade SL, Narad ME, Shultz EL, et al. Technology-assisted rehabilitation interventions following pediatric brain injury. *J Neurosurg Sci.* 2018;62:187–202 **(LOE V)**.

95. Schwartz L, Taylor HG, Drotar D, et al. Long-term behavior problems following pediatric traumatic brain injury: incidence, predictors, and correlates. *J Pediatr Psychol.* 2003;28:251–263 **(LOE IV)**.

96. Bloom DR, Levin H, Ewing-Cobbs L, et al. Lifetime and novel psychiatric disorders after pediatric brain injury. *J Am Acad Child Adolesc Psychiatry.* 2001;40:572–579 **(LOE IV)**.

97. Max JE, Robin DA, Lindgren SD, et al. Traumatic brain injury in children and adolescents: psychiatric disorders at two years. *J Am Acad Child Adolesc Psychiatry.* 1997;36:1278–1285 **(LOE IV)**.

98. Backeljauw B, Kurowski BG. Interventions for attention problems after pediatric traumatic brain injury: what is the evidence? *PMR.* 2014;6:814–824 **(LOE V)**.

99. Bohannon RW, Smith MB. Interrater reliability of a modified Ashworth scale of muscle spasticity. *Phys Ther.* 1987;67:206–2067 **(LOE IV)**.

100. Sheehan G. The pathophysiology of spasticity. *Eur J Neurol.* 2002;9:3–9 **(LOE V)**.

101. Danan-Oliel N, Kasaai B, Montpetit K, Hamdy R. Effectiveness and safety of botulinum toxin type A in children with musculoskeletal conditions: what is the current state of evidence? *Int J Pediatr.* 2012:898–924 **(LOE V)**.

102. Gracies JM, Elovic E, McGuire J. Traditional pharmacological treatments for spasticity part II: general and regional treatments. *Muscle Nerve Suppl.* 1997;6:S92–120 **(LOE V)**.

103. Bodine-Fowler SC. The course of muscle atrophy and recovery following a phenol-induced nerve block. *Muscle Nerv.* 1996;19:497–504 **(LOE IV)**.

104. Westerlund T. The endoneurial response to neurolytic agents is highly dependent on the mode of application. *Reg Anesth Pain Med.* 1999;24:294–302 **(LOE II)**.

105. Bell KR, William E. Use of botulinum toxin type A and type B for spasticity in upper and lower limbs. *Phys Med Rehabil Clin N Am.* 2003;14:821–835 **(LOE V)**.

106. Food and Drug Administration. Highlights of prescribing information. Botox. Available at https://www.accessdata.fda.gov/drugsatfda_docs/label/2017/103000s5302lbl.pdf. Accessed April, 2018 **(LOE V)**.

107. Food and Drug Administration. Highlights of prescribing information. Dysport. Available at https://www.accessdata.fda.gov/drugsatfda_docs/label/2016/125274s107lbl.pdf.Accessed April, 2018 **(LOE V)**.

108. Kinnett D. Botulinum toxin type A injections in children: technique and dosing issues. *Am J Phys Med Rehabi.* 2004;83:S54–S64 **(LOE III)**.

109. Schroeder AS, Berweck S, Lee SH, et al. Botulinum toxin treatment of children with cerebral palsy – a short review of different injection techniques. *Neurotox Res.* 2006;9:189–196 **(LOE V)**.

110. Chin TY, Nattras GR. Accuracy of intramuscular injection of botulinum toxin A in juvenile cerebral palsy: a comparison between manual needle placement and placement guided by electrical stimulation. *J Pediatr Orthop.* 2005;25:286–289 **(LOE I)**.

111. Koman LA, Smith BP, Goodman A, ed. *Botulinum Toxin Type A in The Management of Cerebral Palsy.* Winston-Salem, NC: Wake Forest University Press. **(LOE V)**.

112. Mathevon L, Michel F, Decavel P, et al. Muscle structure and stiffness assessment after botulinum toxin type A injection: a systematic review. *Ann Phys Rehabil Med.* 2015;58:343–350 **(LOE III)**.

113. Danan-Oliel N, Kasaai B, Montpetit K, Hamdy R. Effectiveness and safety of botulinum toxin type A in children with musculoskeletal conditions: what is the current state of evidence? *Int J Pediatr.* 2012:898924 **(LOE III)**.

114. Loubser PG, Akman NM. Effects of intrathecal baclofen on chronic spinal cord injury pain. *J Pain Symptom Manage.* 1996;12:241–247 **(LOE IV)**.

115. Stancin T, Kaugars AS, Thompson GH, et al. Child and family functioning 6 and 12 months after a serious pediatric fracture. *J Trauma.* 2001;51:69–76 **(LOE I)**.

116. American College of Surgeons Committee on Trauma. *Advanced Trauma Life Support for Doctors. Student Course Manual.* Chicago: Pediatric Trauma American College of Surgeons; 2008: Chapter 10 **(LOE IV)**.

117. Miele V, Di Giampietro I, Ianniello S, et al. Diagnostic imaging in pediatric polytrauma management. *Radiol Med.* 2015;120:33–49. **(LOE V)**.

Index

Note: Page numbers followed by "f" indicate figures, "t" indicate tables and "b" indicate boxes.